HANDBUCH DER MEDIZINISCHEN RADIOLOGIE

ENCYCLOPEDIA OF MEDICAL RADIOLOGY

HERAUSGEGEBEN VON · EDITED BY

L. DIETHELM F. HEUCK

O. OLSSON F. STRNAD H. VIETEN

A. ZUPPINGER

BAND/VOLUME XIV
TEIL/PART 1 A

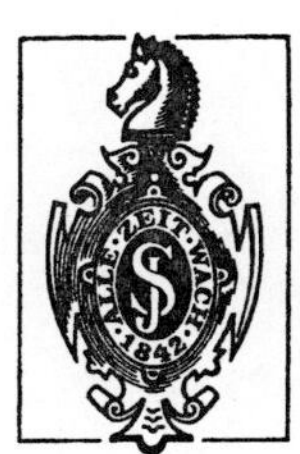

SPRINGER-VERLAG BERLIN · HEIDELBERG · NEW YORK 1981

RÖNTGENDIAGNOSTIK DES ZENTRALNERVENSYSTEMS

TEIL 1 A

ROENTGEN DIAGNOSIS OF THE CENTRAL NERVOUS SYSTEM

PART 1 A

VON · BY

E. BETZ · P. HUBER · H. H. JACOBSEN
M. NADJMI · M. RATZKA · K. J. ZÜLCH

REDIGIERT VON · EDITED BY

L. DIETHELM · S. WENDE

MAINZ

MIT 410 ABBILDUNGEN (795 EINZELDARSTELLUNGEN)
WITH 410 FIGURES (795 SEPARATE ILLUSTRATIONS)

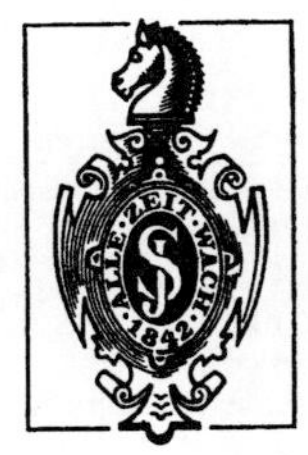

SPRINGER-VERLAG BERLIN · HEIDELBERG · NEW YORK 1981

Professor Dr. L. DIETHELM
Institut für Klinische Strahlenkunde der Universität, Langenbeckstraße 1
D-6500 Mainz

Professor Dr. S. WENDE
Abteilung für Neuroradiologie an der Neurochirurgischen Universitätsklinik,
Langenbeckstraße 1, D-6500 Mainz

CIP-Kurztitelaufnahme der Deutschen Bibliothek
Handbuch der medizinischen Radiologie – Encyclopedia of medical radiology / hrsg. von L. Diethelm ...
Berlin ; Heidelberg ; New York : Springer.
NE: Diethelm, Lothar [Hrsg.]; PT
Bd. 14. → Röntgendiagnostik des Zentralnervensystems

Röntgendiagnostik des Zentralnervensystems – Roentgen diagnosis of the central nervous system. – Berlin ; Heidelberg ; New York : Springer.
NE: PT
Teil 1. / von J. Ambrose ... Redigiert von L. Diethelm u. S. Wende Teil 1, A. – 1979
(Handbuch der medizinischen Radiologie ; Bd. 14)

ISBN-13:978-3-642-95334-7 e-ISBN-13:978-3-642-95333-0
DOI: 10.1007/978-3-642-95333-0

NE: Diethelm, Lothar [Hrsg.]; Ambrose, J. [Mitverf.]

Softcover reprint of the hardcover 1st edition 1981

Gesamtherstellung: Universitätsdruckerei H. Stürtz AG, Würzburg
2122/3020-543210

Vorwort

Die Röntgendiagnostik cerebraler und spinaler Erkrankungen – die Neuroradiologie – hat in den letzten Jahren so große Fortschritte gezeigt, daß ihr 3 Bände dieses Handbuches zur Verfügung gestellt wurden.

Die einzelnen Kapitel umfassen die spezielle Diagnostik der Hirntumoren, der cerebralen Gefäßerkrankungen, des Schädel-Hirn-Traumas, die Diagnostik der Orbita und die Diagnostik des Spinalkanals.

Besonderer Wert wurde auf die neueste Untersuchungsmethode, auf die cerebrale Computer-Tomographie, gelegt, die in ihrer Aussagekraft eine führende Stelle in der Neuroradiologie einnimmt. Eine ausführliche Darstellung der angiographischen und luftencephalographischen Technik und der Untersuchungsbefunde bei raumfordernden intracraniellen Prozessen mit diesen Methoden war jedoch auch erforderlich, da die Neuroradiologie nicht nur aus der Computer-Tomographie besteht, die als alleinige Untersuchungsmethode nicht immer ausreicht.

Ferner ist es auch heute noch nicht möglich, daß überall in der Welt ein CT-Gerät zur Verfügung steht.

Den Indikationen zu jeder Untersuchung ist in allen Kapiteln ein großer Raum gewidmet; die Normalbefunde, die Physiologie, Pathophysiologie und die Neuropathologie werden in speziellen Kapiteln abgehandelt.

Das Gebiet „Neuroradiologie“ ist damit von Spezialisten in allen Abschnitten umfassend dargestellt.

S. Wende

Preface

So much progress has been made in the past years in neuroradiology – X-ray investigation of neurological disorders in the cranial and spinal regions – that three volumes of this Handbook are now devoted to it.

Computer tomography of the cranial region receives particular emphasis because it is such a powerful new tool and can provide vital and otherwise inaccessible information. Yet computer tomography alone is sometimes inadequate, and not every hospital in all parts of the world has such an expensive piece of equipment. Thus angiography and gas encephalography are described in detail, as are the results obtained by these methods in cases of space-occupying intracranial lesions.

There are separate chapters dealing with the specialized diagnostic techniques for brain tumors, head injuries, cranial vascular disorders, the orbits, and the spinal canal. In each chapter the indications for each type of investigation are discussed thoroughly. Separate chapters are devoted to normal findings, physiology, pathophysiology, and neuropathology respectively. In this way all sections of neuroradiology have been comprehensively reviewed by specialists in their own fields.

S. Wende

Inhaltsverzeichnis – Contents

Cerebrovascular Pathology and Pathogenesis as a Basis of Neuroradiological Diagnosis

By K.J. ZÜLCH

Physiologie und Pathophysiologie der Gehirndurchblutung. Von E. BETZ

Mitarbeiter von Band XIV/1A – Contributors to Volume XIV/1A

Professor Dr. E. BETZ, Universität Tübingen, Physiologisches Institut, Lehrstuhl I, Gmelinstraße 5, D-7400 Tübingen

Professor Dr. P. HUBER, Inselspital Bern, Institut für Diagnostische Radiologie der Universität Bern, CH-3010 Bern

Dr. H.H. JACOBSEN, Rigshospitalet Neuroradiologisk, Afdeling XN 3023, Blegdamsvej 9, DK-2100 Kopenhagen

Professor Dr. M. NADJMI, Universität Würzburg, Abteilung für Neuroradiologie in der Kopfklinik, Josef-Schneider-Straße 11, D-8700 Würzburg

Dr. M. RATZKA, Universität Würzburg, Abteilung für Neuroradiologie in der Kopfklinik, Josef-Schneider-Straße 11, D-8700 Würzburg

Professor Dr. K.J. ZÜLCH, Max-Planck-Institut für Hirnforschung, Neurologische Klinik, Abteilung für Allgemeine Neurologie, Ostmerheimer Straße 200, D-5000 Köln 91

Cerebrovascular Pathology and Pathogenesis as a Basis of Neuroradiological Diagnosis*

by

K.J. ZÜLCH

With 183 Figures

Carl Christlieb Bethke: Über Schlagflüsse und Lähmungen, Leipzig 1797:
Man findet so mancherlei Meinungen über die Natur und Heilung der Schlagflüsse und Lähmungen, daß es ein wichtiger Gegenstand ist, sich mit der Untersuchung derselben zu beschäftigen.
One meets many concepts of the nature and cure of stroke and palsies, therefore it seems important to occupy himself with their investigation.

A. Foreword

The following chapter has been prepared as an introduction to the morphological and pathomorphological background information required to understand and interpret neuroradiological methods in patients with cerebrovascular disease. To try to fulfill this demand completely one would have to provide such a wealth of data that a separate handbook would be required solely for this topic. The material included must therefore be selected carefully. The selection naturally has been a personal one dictated by the fact that for more than two decades the author has been interested in the pathomorphology, clinical aspects and angiography of cerebrovascular disease and may suffice to explain any omissions from the description.**

I. Introductory Remarks

Cerebral angiography attempts to show as much of the morphological characteristics of the normal or diseased brain and its circulation as are available by radiographic methods. It attempts to visualize vessels by injecting contrast material into the circulation, and to deduce the "circulation time" by seriography. Vascular patterns including congenital "variants" and acquired pathological changes in the vessel wall, as well as the normal and pathological anastomoses and collateral pathways, "hyperemia" consequent to dilatation of normal or pathological vessels and finally their sequelae in the brain, such as hemorrhages and infarcts will be described and illustrated.

Profound knowledge of the normal anatomy and pathological alterations of the intracranial vessels and their sequelae, mainly infarctions and mass hemorrhages, permits one more easily to diagnose cerebrovascular disease in all its angiographic aspects. For example, a reasonable analysis of a computed tomogram is possible only with a clear understanding of the underlying pathology.

---

* Dedicated to Dr. Derek DENNY-BROWN who initiated so much in cerebrovascular pathophysiology.

** I greatly appreciate the help given to me by Frau Margot GÖLDNER and Herr Hans GÖLDNER in the preparation of this chapter, the assistance of Dr. Helen COOPER and Dr. W.S. FIELDS in the translation and the financial support provided by Frau Andrea MÖLLER, Hamburg.

A general terminology and classification of cerebrovascular disease has been described by the World Health Organization (1971: Annexe 2 (classification) and 3 (glossary) of "Série de Rapports Techniques" and of "Atherosclerotic Lesions" (1958) and Atherosclerosis of the Aorta (KAGAN and UEMURA, 1976) as "Focus on Atherosclerosis" (KAGAN, 1977).

B. Morphology and Primary Pathomorphology of the Arterial and Venous Vasculature

I. Embryology

When "reading" an angiogram, one of the most difficult problems is to distinguish congenital "variants" from pathological vessel patterns. This difficulty can be overcome only by acquiring adequate knowledge of embryology because the embryonal development of the extra- and intracranial brain vessels into their ultimate pattern may influence many vascular disorders, e.g., arteriovenous malformations, saccular aneurysms, aplasia or hypoplasia and other abnormalities. The most decisive factor is the original anlage of the vascular system as a network (see BERGSTRAND et al., 1936; GOUAZE et al., 1973) of "sinusoidal" vessels of more or less equal caliber and formed around the neural tube. Some elements of this vasculature may finally develop into arteries, capillaries and veins, thereby leading to the foundation of the ultimate structure of the cerebral vasculature.

It is important to understand that in the first phase of development a differentiation does not yet exist between the vessel walls of either an artery or a vein. The same undifferentiated type of wall also occurs in most arteriovenous malformations, which only in some parts of the supplying vessels of the original *rete* show the formation of an "arterial" wall. The meningeal network of the vessels in the Sturge-Weber angioma which corresponds to the anterior vascular plexus of the brain and eye appears similarly undifferentiated.

In this process of "maturation" of arteries, capillaries and veins some pathways are favored and further developed while some may even become atretic and still others remain in the original state until the final pattern is reached.

The following steps may be observed: (1) During early development the "neural tube" is mainly supplied by circumferential arteries. (2) Later these vessels anastomose to form longitudinal chains, i.e., the internal carotid system with its main distributing arteries. This directly supplies the supratentorial space of the brain, whereas the infratentorial parts obtain their supply from the caudal branch of the carotid, the trigeminal artery. (3) The carotid during further development becomes connected to a system of ascending longitudinal arteries including the two vertebral and the anterior spinal arteries. (4) Eventually the rostral segments of the two vertebral arteries fuse to form the basilar artery. The "button-hole" and window formations in the basilar artery may be explained by this process of fusion of the two parallel parts. They are usually of no clinical importance (see however Fig. 2). When this vertebro-basilar system of longitudinal arteries is continuous and is connected to the posterior part of the carotid system later by the two communicating arteries, the trigeminal artery becomes hypoplastic and disappears. Only rarely is it preserved as a post-natal variant (carotico-basilar anastomosis). Similarly, during fetal development two more such interconnecting arteries are first formed and later regress: the primitive hypoglossal and the – smaller – primitive otic artery. These also may persist but as even rarer variants.

The vertebral artery actually originates from six longitudinal anastomoses of intersegmental transverse arteries. The longitudinal anastomoses by which the caudal – vertebrobasilar – system finds access to the oral-carotid system through the posterior communicating arteries has been mentioned.

The origin of these arteries is the system of six branchial arteries of which some parts are still evolving at a time when others are already regressing. It is important to note that most *cerebral arteries have no accompanying veins,* with the exception of the "perforating" paramedian and median vessels of the primary tube (such as the median and lateral striate arteries, the peduncular, pontine and bulbar arteries).

The general pattern of the vascular supply in the brain changes: the median and paramedian arteries pierce into the brain substance in order to supply mainly the basal ganglia, the mass of the cerebral substance, namely cortex and white matter are supplied by a network penetrating from the surface into the depth (see however, SCHEINKER'S textbook 1948, Fig. 13 and TÖNDURY, 1959, Fig. 256).

The normal site and course of the cerebral vessels has been thoroughly studied and equally well described in textbooks (excellent descriptions in STEPHENS and STILWELL, 1969; SALAMON, 1971, 1973; GÄNSHIRT, 1972; SALAMON and HUANG, 1976; and others), although some undescribed anomalies can be found.

Angioarchitecture has been described first by R.A. PFEIFER (1930) from injected specimens, and more recently by X-ray microscopy and histochemistry (SAUNDERS and BELL, 1971).

II. Variants

Common variations in the vascular pattern. In the complex process of embryogenesis of the cerebral vessels, many variants may develop which are of importance in explaining cerebrovascular insufficiency. Before describing them however, we should be acquainted with some other rules in the formation of vascular networks (ROUX, 1978).

If a smaller vessel branches from a larger one, the latter deviates from its original direction toward the side opposite from the branching vessels. Yet small vessels as they leave (approximately at the same point to both sides) do not influence the direction of the main trunk. If, however, the main vessel divides into equal branches, both diverge at equal angles to the original direction (as the branching of the posterior cerebral arteries from the basilar artery). If the branching vessel is small, the change of direction in the main trunk is also only small.

Many of these arterial channels are formed only transiently. The principal members of the final system consist of the external and internal carotid arteries, the subclavian arteries and the aortic arch. Anomalies may give rise to varied patterns of flow but seldom lead to clinical disturbances. In the system defined above, the normal pattern may be reached only during this process of regression with certain variations (or malformations); in only 70% of the general population there is a "normal" textbook pattern of the four main arteries, e.g., the brachiocephalic, the left carotid and the vertebral arteries originate separately from the aortic arch.

In about 30% of the population the left carotid originates more to the right and directly from the brachiocephalic artery. In about 15% there is one trunk only for the carotid and vertebral arteries of the left side; in some 8% the right vertebral artery originates from the brachiocephalic trunk; in 5% the left carotid, vertebral and subclavian arteries branch singly from the aortic arch, in 1% the right carotid and subclavian arteries originate separately and in 2% bifurcation of the common carotid artery is observed to occur lower in the neck than at the usual level opposite the body of the fourth cervical vertebra (for details see TOOLE and PATEL, 1974).

The vertebral artery itself may have certain variants:

a) There may be an atresia of one of the arteries (5% MITTERWALLNER, 1955; KRAYENBÜHL and YASARGIL, 1957).

b) The vertebral artery may end in the posterior inferior cerebellar artery and thereby not gain access to the basilar system.

c) The caliber of the vertebral arteries may be quite different, the right one – according to own observations – being more commonly hypoplastic (Fig. 1) (see also ATKINSON, 1949), in which case the partner will usually be more voluminous.

However, the data concerning differences in lumen size are somewhat variable. In the series of C.M. FISHER et al. (1965a) the right vertebral artery was larger in 35% of cases, the left in 47% and they were equal in 15%; whereas according to MITTERWALLNER (1955) the left vertebral artery is larger in 30%–50% and in up to 72% of the cases in the series of LOEB and MEYER (1965).

d) The left vertebral artery in 5% of the population does not originate from the left subclavian artery but from the aortic arch directly.

e) Very rarely the left vertebral artery is supplied by the common or the external carotid artery.

The caliber of the various parts of the vertebro-basilar system depends upon the pattern of the carotid system and is smaller when the carotid artery supplies one or two posterior cerebral arteries ("embryonal" pattern).

Coiling of the vertebral arteries (see p. 56) near the atlanto-occipital joints is "physiological" and necessary for the maintenance of the circulation in the case of extreme rotation of the head. In rare cases such extreme rotation can occlude one of the vertebral arteries even under physiological conditions (KRAYENBÜHL and YASARGIL, 1957, Fig. 149a, b). A double basilar artery in which there has been no unification between the "two vertebrals" is an extreme rarity. Formation of windows and buttonholes, however, (Fig. 2) is not so rare. Whether this process

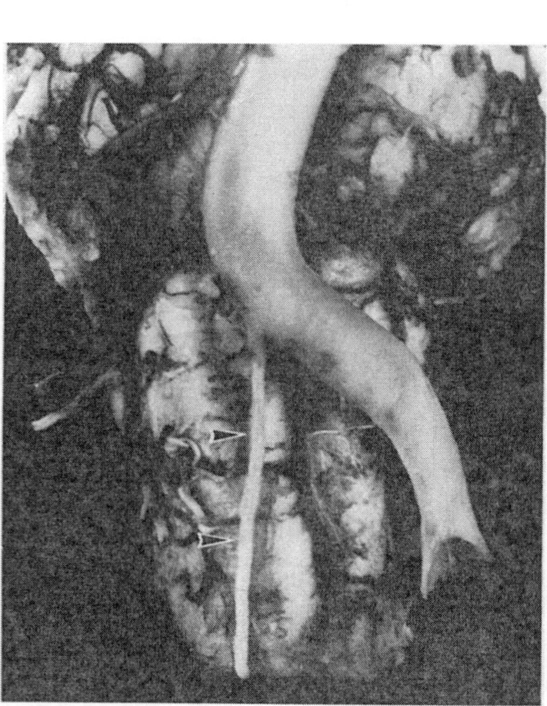

Fig. 1

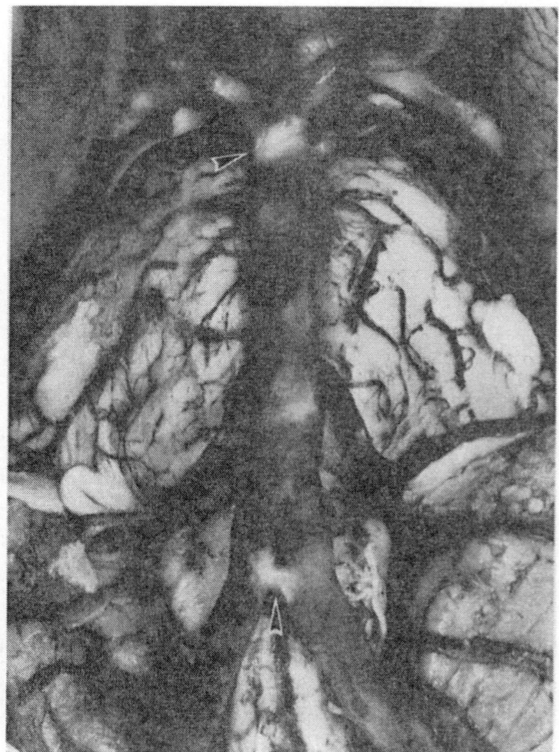

Fig. 2

Fig. 1. Marked difference in width of the vertebral arteries (right almost atretic; *arrows*)

Fig. 2. Atherosclerotic plaques occur mainly in segments with curves, branchings or divisions (turbulence!) in this case especially *(arrows)* at junction of vertebral arteries ("button-hole anomaly") and at division of basilar artery (origin of posterior cerebral and superior cerebellar arteries; see also Fig. 44, 45)

of fusion produces weak points in the vessel wall and gives rise to the formation of the not infrequent large fusiform aneurysms (Fig. 44) has not yet been sufficiently investigated.

There are many branches leaving the vertebral arteries on their way through the foramina in the transverse processes of the cervical vertebrae which run over the unco-vertebral joints to the neighboring muscles.

Hypoplasia of the carotid artery – in contrast to the vertebral – is thought to be very rare and does not usually cause cerebral ischemia (SMITH et al., 1968; LHERMITTE et al., 1968). Agenesis of the internal carotid artery is usually compensated by anastomotic supply to the brain through the contralateral carotid and the vertebro-basilar systems (BURMESTER and STENDER, 1961; TURNBULL, 1962; STEIMLE et al., 1969; TEAL et al., 1973) and has even been observed bilaterally (FISHER, 1913; HILLS and SAMENT, 1968 review; LIE, 1968, 1972). The case of a long narrow caliber in the angiogram leaves "hypoplasia", atherosclerotic stenosis, fibromuscular hyperplasia or angiospasm as possible diagnoses (it is necessary here to assess the width of the carotid canal or foramen!). Anomalous loops and coils have been noted to exist even in healthy children (FIELDS et al., 1965) (see also p. 56).

According to PADGET (1944, 1948) the primitive internal carotid artery has two main divisions: the "anterior", giving rise to the anterior and middle cerebral and the anterior chorioidal arteries, and the "posterior" which persists as the posterior communicating artery from which the posterior chorioidal and the posterior cerebral arteries may originate ("embryonal" type).

In 20% of cases the posterior cerebral artery originates from the carotid system (Fig. 3), whereas in another 10% the distribution of the supply from the carotid and vertebro-basilar systems is equal (see KAMEYAMA and OKINAKA, 1963) and the posterior communicating artery correspondingly wide.

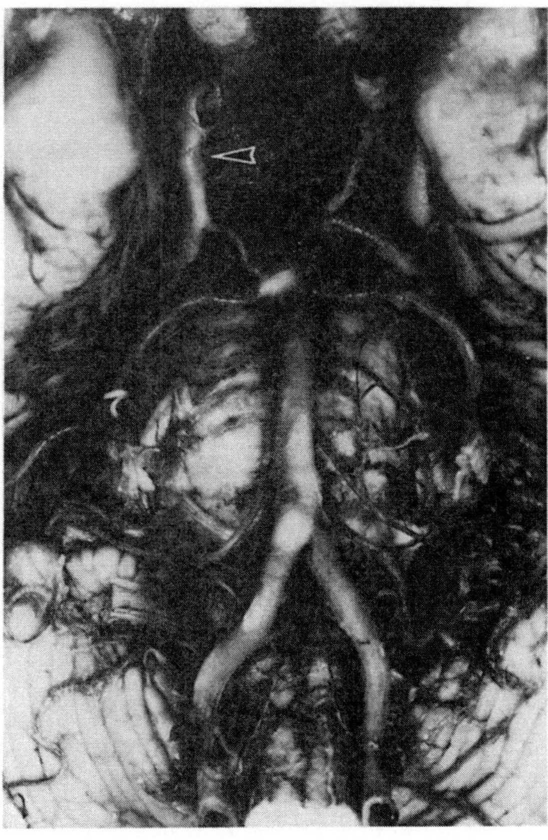

Fig. 3. Typical course of an "embryonal" posterior cerebral artery originating from the carotid. Atherosclerotic plaques at origin and branching of basilar artery *(arrow)*

We have already mentioned the three possible variants of intercommunications between the carotid and basilar artery systems of which the "primitive" trigeminal artery has the largest caliber, the otic the smallest, and the hypoglossal artery lies between.

Other "primitive" arteries are the communications between the ophthalmic artery and the tentorial artery of Bernasconi or the middle meningeal artery. Originally there is another anastomotic channel between the stapedial artery and the ophthalmic but this usually undergoes involution. It sometimes persists, however, as a branch of the carotid artery to the tympanum. There is also a temporary olfactory artery which may persist with collaterals to the anterior cerebral artery thereby supplying the anterior perforated substance as well as parts of the territory of Heubner's middle striate artery.

Such "fetal" primitive arteries can be of importance in the case of vascular occlusions by serving as a base for a collateral circulation ("rete" patterns).

An additional "median" anterior cerebral artery occurs in 8% of cases (LAZORTHES et al., 1956). The bihemispheric distribution of one normal anterior cerebral artery over the corpus callosum has been illustrated by ZÜLCH et al., (1964, Fig. 4; 1979; see also BAPTISTA, 1963).

RIGGS and RUPP (1963) found in 8% of 1647 autopsies hypoplasia of the horizontal part of the anterior cerebral artery together with an "embryonal" origin of the posterior cerebral artery. (The anomalies of the circle of Willis will be described in the Chap. B. III.)

Origination of the ascending pharyngeal or the occipital artery from the internal carotid artery is extremely rare. The distal trunk of the internal carotid artery has, however, two other very constant communications with the external: the branches to the trigeminal ganglion and to the hypophysis (Fig. 6). These are important for *retrograde* filling of the carotid siphon by the ophthalmic artery down to the origin of these two branches (ZÜLCH, 1963a) in the presence of occlusion of the internal carotid artery.

These persistent anastomoses are usually of no clinical importance and are merely detected by angiography. Only in the presence of stenosis or occlusion may they be of great value by serving as collateral pathways.

The complex formation of the carotid siphon was thought to be a protection of the brain against sudden rise of blood pressure and forceful pulsation. However, this explanation is not readily substantiated. The four main cerebral arteries, after perforating the dura, remain for longer distances within the cisternae and are therefore easily movable. This is particularly apparent in the ectatic type of atherosclerosis, where coils of the anterior cerebral artery or the vertebrobasilar system (Fig. 44) pass freely over the midline to the other side or those of the posterior inferior cerebellar artery pass downwards (KAUTZKY, ZÜLCH et al., 1976), even through the foramen magnum into the spinal canal. (For literature see LAZORTHES et al., 1950 and 1956 and the excellent chapter in the text-book of TOOLE and PATEL, 1974, pp. 9, 31, 46.)

The variations of the middle cerebral artery are now well-known as a result of numerous angiographic observations (see RING and WADDINGTON, 1967 and DELONG, 1973).

III. Anastomoses and Collateral Pathways (Physiological and Pathological)

1. Morphology

In the analysis of infarction, the naturally present anastomoses play a decisive role, provided that the hemodynamic conditions allow a perfusion pressure sufficient to make these operative.

The morphological development of such an auxiliary circulation and the resulting patterns in cases of stenosis or occlusion of supply arteries must be therefore extensively described. Only then is it possible for the neuroradiologist to interpret an angiogram intelligently for the clinician (EINSIEDEL-LECHTAPE and KLEIHUES, 1977).

Embryonic development is well-known from texbooks and has been discussed above (for details see FIELDS et al., 1965). Embryological anomalies have to be distinguished from "secondary" channels, widened after the initiation of an unphysiological change in direction of the blood stream after stenosis or occlusion of a "primary" vessel.

As an example it should be re-emphasized that if one vertebral artery is very small or absent, the larger caliber of the other may be the result of a discrepancy in the anlage – resulting in one of small, the other large caliber (Fig. 1) – or partly the result of increasing demand as in the case of a stenosing process. In such cases vessels may be come widened if they are not already atherosclerotic.

Since the most common anomalies have been mentioned above without indicating their value in providing collateral circulation in case of emergency, the most frequent patterns of such an actual collateral circulation will be described based upon neuroradiological experience.

2. Terminology

When we describe the more important anastomoses of the four main arteries to the brain we encounter semantic difficulties with terminology. In clinical parlance as in neuoradiology, we are accustomed to use the terms "collateral circulation" and "anastomoses" synonymously, whereas in fact, they originally had different meanings.

"Anastomoses" are network-like intercommunications of one or many supply systems, where the direction of the pathway and the caliber are not defined. "Anastomosis" may be even used as a technical term. "Collaterals", on the other hand, are morphological pathways which run parallel and can substitute for each other (in the case of inadequacy of one!); in other words, they are parallel supply systems to one organ (Fig. 4).

This is particularly true for the arterial channels around the joints – such as the elbow joint – where in the case of impedance of the medial channels by flexion the lateral pathways take over.

If we were to apply such a strict definition of "collaterals" to our subject, only the two vertebrals could fit this definition, both running parallel to the same organ and being able to substitute for each other when of normal caliber (Fig. 4). In teleological terms, this is a sound arrangement since the possibility of mechanical strangulation is very great, both at the entrance into the foramen costotransversarium and later in the vertebral column itself, as for example at the level of the atlanto-occipital joint or while piercing the dura (see KRAYENBÜHL

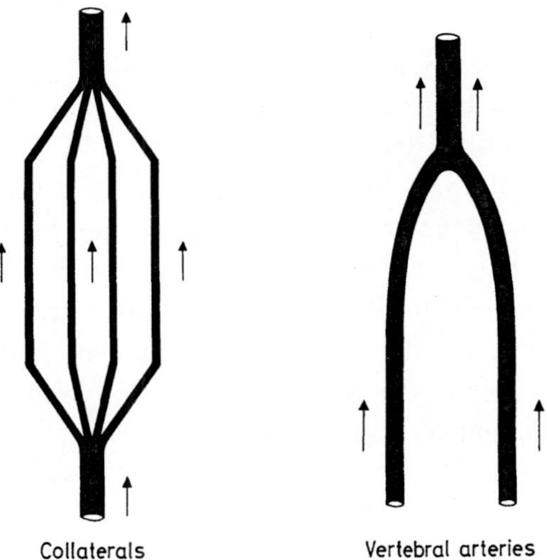

Fig. 4. The only example of true "collaterals" is in the field of cerebral circulation: the two vertebral arteries

and YASARGIL, 1957, Fig. 149a, b). This is particularly true when hyperostoses due to cervical osteochondrosis are formed near the foramina costotransversaria (see ZÜLCH, 1970, Fig. 19).

To summarize. Collaterals are – by their original definition – double, triple or multiple parallel supply systems substituting for one another in case of inadequacy; anastomoses, on the other hand, are network-like intercommunications within one or between two or more functionally separate systems, allowing the possibility of draining blood from them. An auxiliary supply may occur, usually after widening of the channel, and flow in either direction may result.

In spite of these logical distinctions in the use of the above two terms, they have been introduced into clinical parlance as though they were synonyms. In the following discussion however, we will adhere as far as possible, to their original definitions.

Several systems of anastomoses seem particularly worthy of more detailed description. As a logical subdivision we would distinguish three types: (1) The various *"extracranial"* systems, (2) the proximal *(basal) intracranial* system of anastomoses, i.e. the circle of Willis, and (3) the *"distal" intracranial* anastomosing communications, i.e., mainly the "meningeal" anastomoses of Heubner.

True arteriovenous anastomoses have never been shown physiologically in cerebral vessels (for the pathological "widening" of the arterio- (capillary)-venous pathways; see p. 17ff.).

3. Extracranial Anastomoses

a) Transverse Anastomoses Between the Two External Carotid Arteries

These become operative in cases of a thrombotic occlusion (or surgical ligation) of one common carotid artery with the intention of supplying the internal carotid artery of the involved side. The two external carotid systems in the neck are interconnected by a particularly dense network of anastomoses in their terminal supply areas (ZÜLCH and HERBERG, 1949) (Fig. 5).

If only the common carotid artery is blocked (see also LABAUGE et al., 1967), the external remains open. There will be immediate intercommunication between the external carotids with a retrograde flow into the internal carotid, the blood passing through the transverse anastomoses (Fig. 5). Between the two superior thyroid arteries, the lingual, ascending pharyngeal, internal maxillary, mental, coronal, labial, inferior angular arteries etc. (see FIELDS et al., 1965, Figs. 2–10, especially Fig. 9, as well as tables plate 230/232). The collateral circulation between the two vertebral arteries in the case of occlusion of a subclavian artery ("subclavian steal") is too well known to be described here in detail (see Fig. 9).

b) Ophthalmic Anastomoses

The role of the ophthalmic artery as a potent source of supply in the case of occlusion of the internal carotid artery has been discussed in recent years (DILENGE et al., 1961; ZÜLCH, 1963a, Figs. 2, 3, 4; WIENER et al., 1964; GUNNING et al., 1964; CASTAIGNE et al., 1970; RING, 1971). However, the pattern of bypassing a blocked internal carotid artery via the ophthalmic anastomoses of the external to the internal carotid artery is fairly complex.

The ophthalmic artery and its branches are normally supplied through the internal carotid artery with anastomoses available from the system of the external carotid artery by (1) the frontal artery via the superficial temporal, (2) the ethmoidal via the internal maxillary, and (3) the dorsal nasal artery via the external maxillary artery. Even the middle meningeal artery may participate in these communications (Fig. 6).

In the angiogram retrograde flow through the ophthalmic artery can be observed to provide satisfactory supply to the internal carotid and its distal branches through retrograde filling of the siphon of the carotid artery down to its entrance into the cranial cavity at the base of the skull.

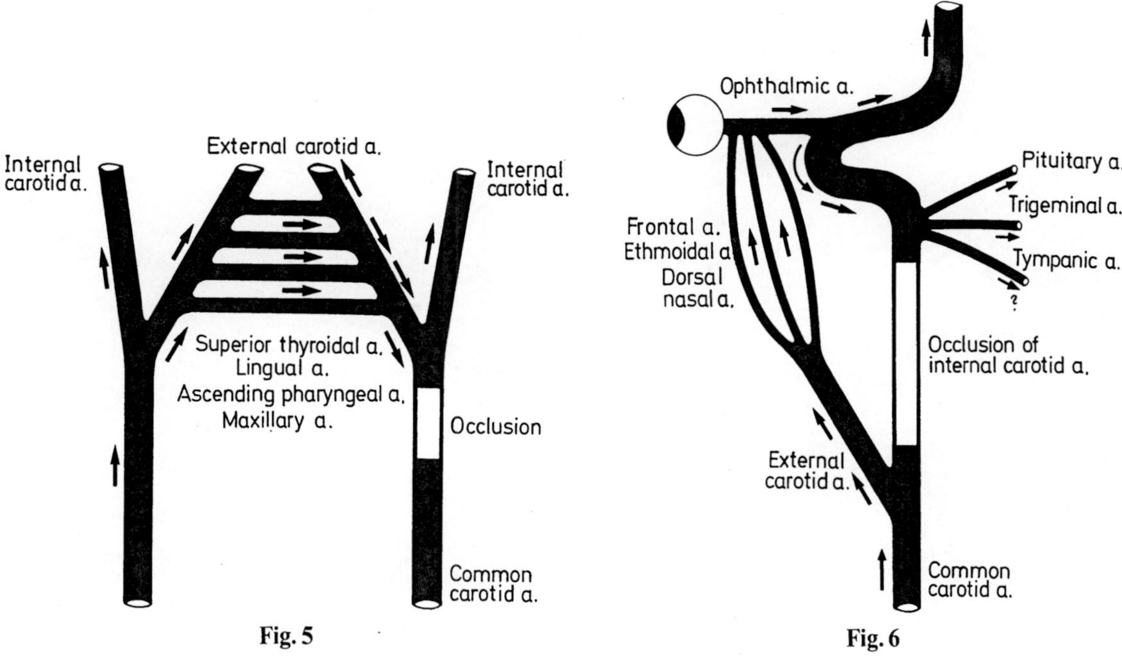

Fig. 5. The two parallel systems of the external carotid arteries are interconnected by numerous transverse anastomoses

Fig. 6. In case of occlusion of the internal carotid artery, anastomoses between the external and distal internal carotid artery form a detour around the occlusion via the ophthalmic artery

According to FIELDS et al. (1965) this is due to the presence of the caroticotympanic artery, which fills the carotid stump from the external carotid system (see their Fig. 37a). In our cases, we have never been able to see such an artery even with subtraction (ZÜLCH, 1963a, Figs. 2 and 3). In my opinion, the explanation is a different one, namely, that the carotid is filled in a retrograde manner through the ophthalmic artery down to the point where the branches to the pituitary gland and trigeminal ganglion (see PERNKOPF, 1957, Fig. 66b) originate.

In two of MARX's (1949) cases, the ophthalmic artery was supplied by a branch of the middle meningeal, in a case of SACHS' series (1954) by the internal maxillary and in VAERNET's report (1954) by the facial; in Case 5 of the paper of ELVIDGE and WERNER (1951), Fig. 8 shows very clearly the retrograde influx from the internal maxillary into the ophthalmic artery.

Occasionally the dilated pulsating superficial temporal artery of this ophthalmic collateral pathway from the external carotid artery may be seen with the naked eye and the increased pulsation may be apparent to the patient (ZÜLCH, 1963a, Fig. 4).

c) The Transverse Anastomoses Between the Carotid and Vertebral Systems

The external carotid → occipital → vertebral anastomoses. Other transverse anastomoses exist extracranially between the carotid and the vertebrobasilar system. Here the unimpaired systems are – as always – substituted for those which are deficient. However, circulatory intercommunication is possible in either direction (Fig. 7). In this case, it is achieved by an arterial anastomosis between the occipital and vertebral arteries, which is very commonly present and is well described by many anatomists (SOBOTTA, 1948; RAUBER-KOPSCH, 1948; CORNING, 1949; TÖNDURY, 1959; HAFERL, 1953; SCHULZE and SAUERBREY, 1956). It was shown by SCHÜRMANN (1954) in angiography of the external carotid artery when the vertebral artery was occluded. We have similar pictures in a case of occlusion of the vertebral artery (Fig. 7) on one side, where the external carotid system is the source of supply.

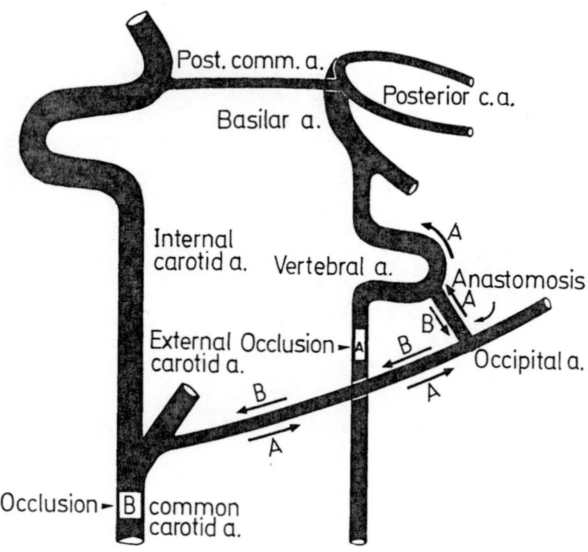

Fig. 7. The vertebral and the carotid systems are anastomosed by the greater occipital arterial channel, which can work either way in occlusion (*A* or *B*)

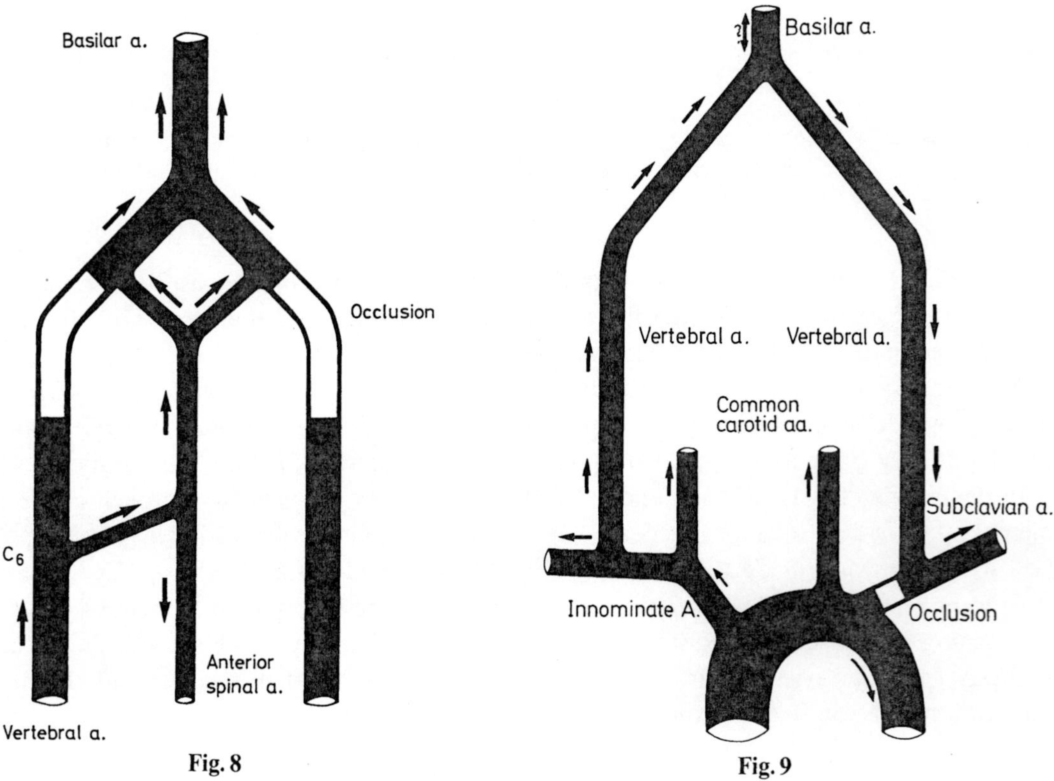

Fig. 8. In an occlusion of both vertebrals, the anterior spinal artery is used as a detour around the blockage

Fig. 9. The confluence of the two vertebrals may provide a very long anastomotic source of supply in case of occlusion of one subclavian artery. This may even be temporarily detrimental to the basilar artery circulation (so-called "subclavian steal")

The reverse flow pattern also exists in occlusion of the common carotid where we find a draining of the vertebral artery via the occipital anastomosis into the external carotid artery and from there the internal carotid can be filled proximal to the siphon.

Apart from this direct arterial intercommunication between the external carotid and the vertebral arteries, terminal muscular branches of the external carotid (KRAYENBÜHL and RICHTER, 1952,

Fig. 100) also exist, and the parallel thyrocervical plexus may anastomose with the vertebral artery. It may serve to supply the vertebro-basilar system as shown by a recent personal observation where the vertebral artery was occluded at the tuberculum anterious but refilled distal to this point through the aforementioned anastomoses.

d) The Vertebral → Anterior Spinal → Vertebral Anastomoses

The same ground pattern of a temporary "parallel" detour which again finds access to the original supply system is seen when both vertebral arteries are blocked distally near the entrance into the cranial cavity. Then, the segmental branches from the vertebral artery (Fig. 8) on one or both sides supply the anterior spinal artery which communicates with both vertebrals intracranially (SCHECHTER and ZINGESSER, 1965, 1966; FIELDS et al., 1965, Fig. 35). All of these arteries then dilate very markedly and a convergence of flow is only seen in the upper part of the anterior spinal artery, where, however, the direction of flow normally changes according to whether the position of the body is upright or lying – the so-called Teilströmchentheorie of Adamkiewicz (ZÜLCH, 1976).

The extra-intracranial anastomosis of the "subclavian steal" syndrome (Fig. 9) is very well-known and therefore need not be described here in detail (see p. 11).

4. Intracranial Anastomoses

In the intracranial arterial circulation the main anastomotic system is the circle of Willis. It is actually a polygonal transverse anastomosis (a) between two equal supply systems, namely, the two internal carotid arteries and coincidentally (b) between two different systems, namely, the carotid supply and the vertebrobasilar supply. This ring system seems predisposed towards a purposeful "redistribution" (Fig. 10) between three systems in the case there is temporary or permanent deficiency of any one of them; each of these three probably carries about one-third of the total blood supply. How often and to what extent this anastomotic ring is needed under physiological conditions (extreme turning or bending of the neck and head with strangulation of one carotid or one vertebral artery) has not yet been definitely clarified.

In some of our angiograms different parts of this polygonal system may be visualized without our full understanding of the hemodynamic conditions which may be responsible. Early neurosurgical investigations postulated that the pressure in the circle of Willis up to the source arteries may not be increased by the injection pressure during carotid or vertebral angiography. However, these data are questioned today.

For instance, many neuroradiological observations prove that a small bolus may be injected from the vertebrobasilar system temporarily into the carotid via the posterior communicating artery (TÖNNIS and SCHIEFER, 1959; ZÜLCH, 1970, Figs. 15, 16) or from one carotid system to the contralateral (through the anterior communicating artery and then into the opposite middle cerebral). This may be explained by low pressure during diastole where the pressure gradient is overcome by the injection pressure. Of great importance is the problem of maintainance of the injection pressure and also the limit, where "pulsatile" flow passes into "steady" flow (see p. 41).

Collateral circulation through the circle of Willis depends upon its patency and the adequacy of the perfusion pressure. Unfortunately the circle of Willis is normal only in 20%–30% of the general population (see STEHBENS, 1972, Tables 1–7; and also WINDLE, 1887; FAWCETT and BLACKFORD, 1906; BLACKBURN, 1907; FETTERMAN and MORAN, 1941; KLEISS, 1942; MOREL and WILDI, 1953; SYMONDS, 1955; MITTERWALLNER, 1955; ALPERS et al., 1959; MCCULLOUGH, 1962; ALPERS and BERRY, 1963; RIGGS and RUPP, 1963; C.M. FISHER, 1965c; FAZIO et al., 1966; BATTACHARJI et al., 1967), whereas in 25% it may be "open" and its function as a distributing

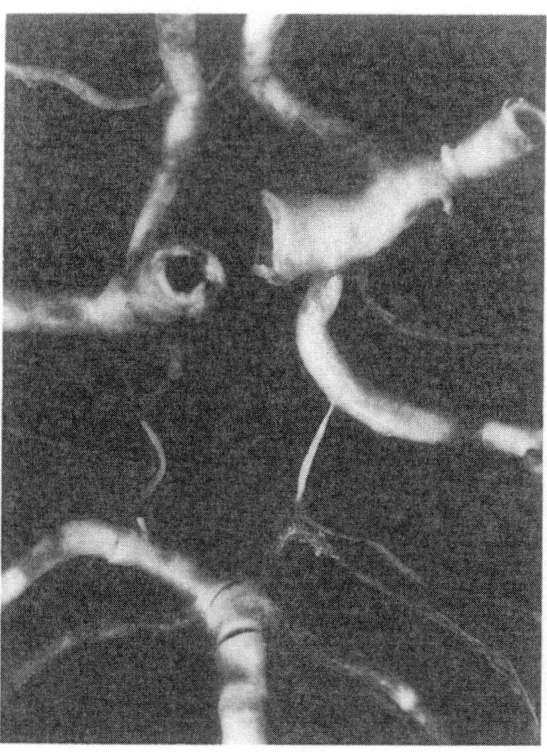

Fig. 10. Circle of Willis, in which the anterior and the posterior communicating arteries are noted to be only thin threads. The usual anastomosing function of this markedly arteriosclerotic specimen must have been lacking. At the right of the picture the "embryonal" type of posterior cerebral artery is seen

system deficient; in the remaining cases, blocking of one of the three great supply systems may have unexpected and dramatic consequences due to hypoplasia of parts of the circle of Willis (see Fig. 51 in KRAYENBÜHL and YASARGIL, 1957, after PADGET, 1944; or Fig. 1 in GILLILAN, 1959; FAZIO et al., 1966; Fig. 29ff in FIELDS et al., 1965; Table 1 in BATTACHARJI et al., 1967).

A recent study of BATTACHARJI et al. (1967) described the circle of Willis in 137 autopsies of which 49 with cerebral infarction were compared with the 88 controls. The most common abnormalities were a small posterior communicating artery and an anomalous origin of the posterior cerebral artery from the carotid. The incidence of all varieties of anomalous vessels was higher in the infarct cases than in the control series. GILLILAN (1959) emphasized the significance of the "entire ventral complex of arteries" and also the superficial anastomoses between the posterior cerebral artery and branches of the basilar artery (300 morphological cases).

Although there are angiographic tests for the functioning of the circle (KRAYENBÜHL and YASARGIL, 1957, p. 47; DECKER, 1960, 1966) and also methods in electroencephalography such as compression of one carotid artery (GASTAUT and BEHREND, 1961), a reliable study of the function of this ring system is not yet available. This is regrettable since atherosclerosis of the posterior communicating arteries is not infrequent (Fig. 10). The fact, however, that its supplementary function may also be "ideal" is proven by clinical observations (ZÜLCH und HERBERG, 1949, Fig. 1) or autopsy (HULTQVIST, 1942). On the other hand, a "paradoxical" functioning of the circle can occur in which the supply to the normal hemisphere also supplies the compromised side to such an extent by "interhemispheric" anastomoses that it suffers from ischemia (ZÜLCH and ESCHBACH, 1972). The actual hemodynamic relations in the ring system in these "steal" conditions ("redistribution") is not yet elucidated (FAZIO et al., 1971; see also p. 111ff., 122) nor is the interesting phenomenon of general flow reduction in infarcts (LAVY et al., 1975).

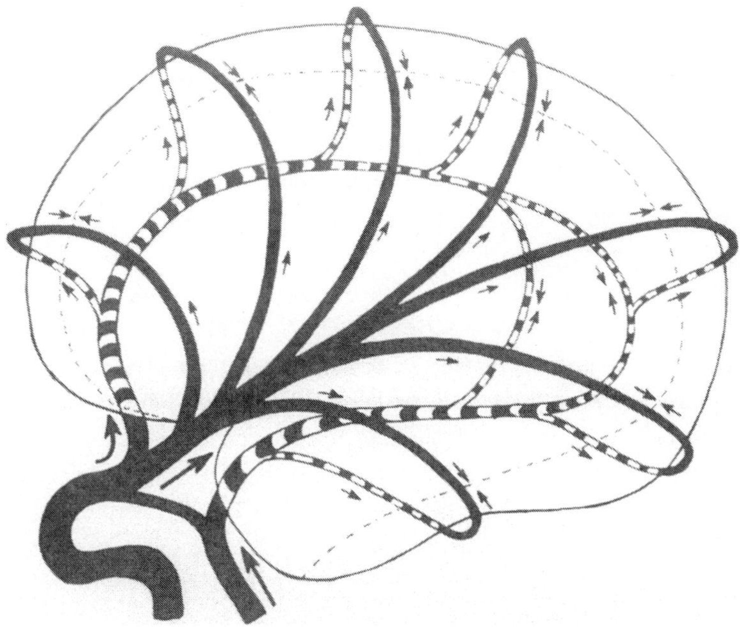

Fig. 11. A network-like arterial anastomotic system is provided by the "meningeal anastomoses" of Heubner between the three great cerebral source arteries

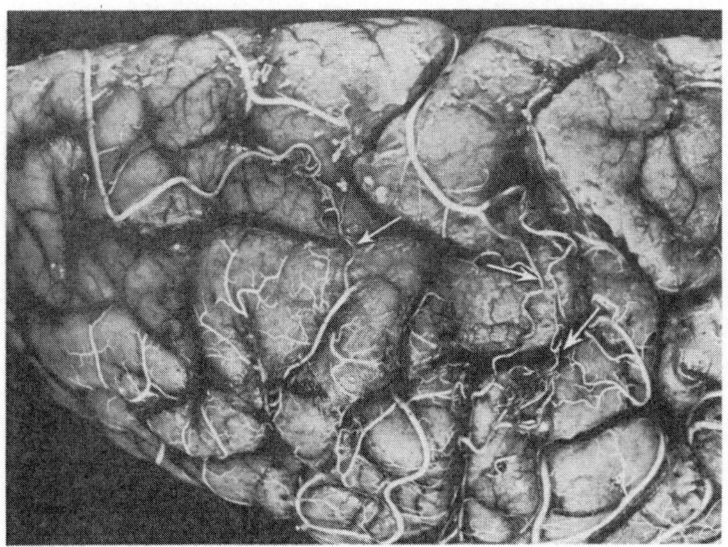

Fig. 12. Meningeal anastomoses (*arrows*) after contrast injection into the arteries; *above*: the median fissure with branches of anterior cerebral artery; *below*: the middle cerebral artery (Sylvian vessels)

a) Meningeal Anastomoses

Transverse intercommunications also exist between the large intracranial source arteries, Heubner's "meningeal anastomoses" which are of the greatest importance in occlusions of the carotid and the middle cerebral arteries. We are indebted to the elder HEUBNER (1872, 1874) and maybe even to RUYSCH (1699) for the observation that practically all of the large cerebral and cerebellar arteries form a network (Fig. 11) on the surface of the brain, the anastomotic channels of which consist of smaller arteries (caliber 500–1000 μ) sufficient in size to supply blood to the deficient regions in case of emergency (Fig. 12).

COHNHEIM's theory that the brain arteries are "end arteries" must be rejected. This concept – with the exceptions discussed on p. 112 – is valid only for the arteries of the basal ganglia and the brainstem (Heubner's anterior circumflex artery, the lenticulo-striate and lenticular-optic and the anterior chorioidal arteries; also the tegmental, pontine and oblongata branches, the median, paramedian, short and long circumflex arteries). Only the anterior chorioidal may have a more definitive anastomosis with its posterior partner (i.e., posterior chorioidal artery) which may, however, vary in size and function (see COOPER, 1956).

HEUBNER'S (1872, 1874) concept of a reticular arterial network on the surface (for pictures in the fetus see Fig. 2 in GOUAZE et al., 1973) of the brain was, however, long rejected (CHARCOT, 1878) although confirmed by anatomists (BEEVOR, 1907; TESTUT and LATARJET, 1929). However, French clinicians at the beginning of this century reconfirmed Heubner's findings and showed the decrease of the size of an infarct due to the action of Heubner's "meningeal anastomoses" (LECENE and J. LHERMITTE, 1920). Temple FAY (1925) proved the existence of these arterial intercommunications, but it was not until 1951 that they were rediscovered by VAN DER EECKEN and ADAMS (1953) and VAN DER EECKEN (1959; see also WEIDNER et al., 1965).

The first angiographic proof of such anastomotic channels was seen in FISCHER-BRÜGGE'S angiogram of 1944, published in 1949 (his Figs. 1, 2), and honored in the meantime by his name as the "corpus callosum anastomosis" of FISCHER-BRÜGGE (see p. 14). Further observations have been made by MOUNT and TAVERAS (1953), ROSEGAY and WELCH (1954), GREITZ (1956, 1967) and many others.

Experimentally the operative effect of these meningeal anastomoses has been shown in the classical experiments of D. DENNY-BROWN and J.S. MEYER (1957), and also by THOMPSON and RHODE (1950), HARVEY and RASMUSSEN (1951), METTLER et al. (1954), RALSTON et al. (1955).

The various types of potential intercommunication by the "meningeal anastomoses" were rediscovered and masterfully described by VAN DER EECKEN and ADAMS (1953) and by VAN DER EECKEN (1959). If we try to analyze the basic pattern operative in most of these cases of either middle cerebral or anterior cerebral occlusion, it can be defined as the draining (stealing) by a parallel but separate neighborhood system through "transverse anastomoses" resulting in reversal of flow in the occluded artery (Fig. 13). For instance, in an occlusion of the middle cerebral artery (Fig. 13) the blood may be drained from the anterior and the posterior cerebral arteries via Heubner's meningeal anastomoses (see GILLILAN, 1959). In the case of an occlusion of one of the anterior cerebral arteries apart from transverse supracallosal anastomoses (Fig. 14)

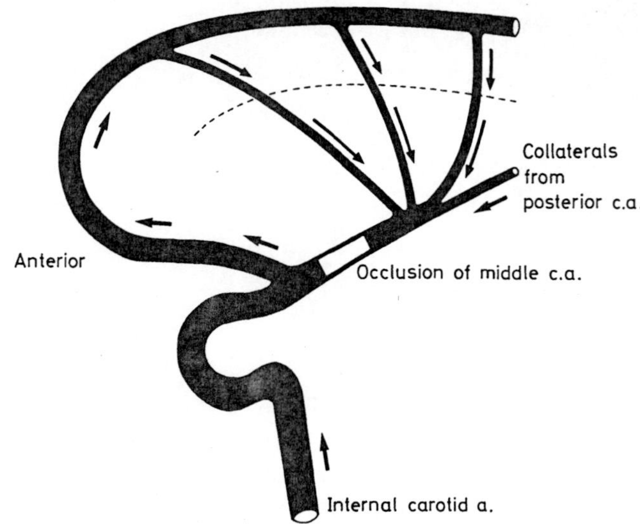

Fig. 13. In occlusion of the middle cerebral artery the parallel systems of the anterior and posterior cerebral arteries are drained by "Heubner's meningeal anastomoses"

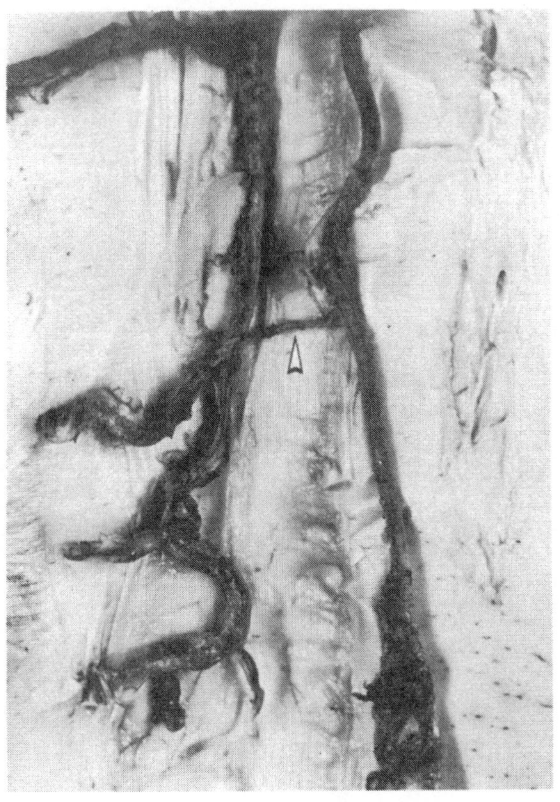

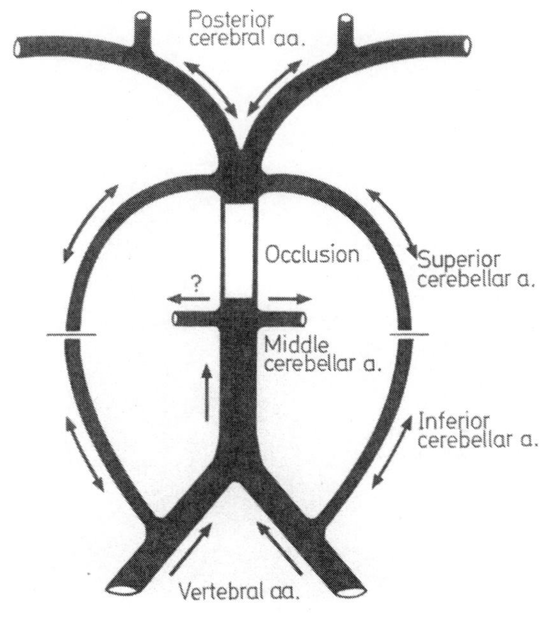

Fig. 14 **Fig. 15**

Fig. 14. Transverse ("supracallosal") anastomoses between two anterior cerebral arteries overlying the corpus callosum *(arrow)*

Fig. 15. In an occlusion of the basilar artery anastomoses between the superior and posterior inferior cerebellar arteries may become operative

the posterior system is particularly used for drainage through the "corpus callosum anastomosis" of Fischer-Brügge (1949) which works in either direction between the vertebrobasilar and the carotid systems (Kautzky, Zülch et al., 1976, Fig. 125).

Another example of functional meningeal anastomoses is the series of "transverse" anastomoses between the two independent but parallel systems of the two anterior cerebral arteries which may be situated on the superior aspect of the corpus callosum (Zülch et al., 1964, Fig. 4).

A final example of "meningeal anastomosis" is the pathway over the cerebellum from the posterior inferior cerebellar to the superior cerebellar artery. This anastomotic system may be called into play in the case of an occlusion of the middle segment of the basilar artery (Fig. 15). This may even be sufficient to prevent the syndrome of "basilar thrombosis" accompanied by the catastrophe of tetraplegia provided that the block does not occlude the main perforating pontine arteries at the same time.

b) Micronetwork of Meningeal Ring Anastomoses (Arachnoidal Arterial Ring Systems)

These small arterial rings on the surface of the brain were well studied by Schmidt (1955a). They do not appear to provide any considerable supply service in the case of an "acute" *emergency* and do not fit into any of the auxiliary patterns thus far described. However, in *chronic* obliteration of the lumina of smaller surface arteries (250 to 1000 μ lumen), as in the case of thromboangiitis obliterans v. Winiwarter-Buerger, they form an anastomotic network (Fig. 16) which macroscopically resembles "hyperemia" of the meninges but is, however, of "arterial" origin and different

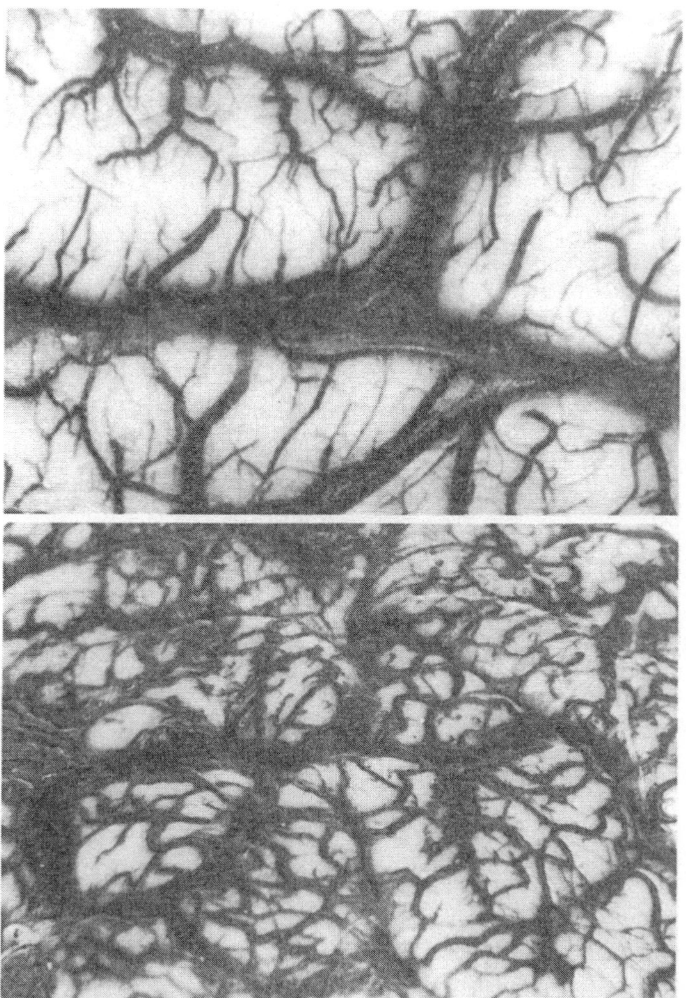

Fig. 16. Marked hyperemia of the small cortical superficial arteries in thromboangiitis obliterans. They form ring-like collateral anastomotic systems *(below)*. For comparison a venous hyperemia is shown in the upper part

from the usual venous "hyperemia" (Fig. 16; see also ZÜLCH et al., 1964, Fig. 3; ZÜLCH, 1969a, Fig. 4).

Cerebral thromboangiitis obliterans (or v. Winiwarter-Buerger's disease) is until now ill-defined and diagnosed clinically far too commonly. Morphologically, we have had two cases in about 800 brains with obvious vascular disease. The morphological findings consisted of thromboses, fresh and organized, in the arteries of $^1/_4$ to $^3/_4$ mm diameter which are pseudosystematically distributed over the cerebrum and cerebellum (see also p. 61ff.).

I have taken the risk (in 1966 at the International Academy of Angiology in Madrid; ZÜLCH, 1969a, Fig. 4) of drawing a hypothetical angiogram of the cerebral form of v. Winiwarter-Buerger's disease. We have, however, never seen angiographically such a case as first demonstrated by HACKER (1968). His angiogram showed the breaking up of the small terminal arteries in the middle cerebral artery territory on one side and the anterior cerebral on the other. In the borderline zone a "blush" is visualized, demonstrating the hyperemia of the arachnoidal rings. By this demonstration one may come to the conclusion this was the characteristic angiogram of v. Winiwarter-Buerger's disease (see ZÜLCH, 1969a).

c) *"Capillary Anastomoses"*

These transverse intracerebral microchannels so well studied by R.A. PFEIFFER (1931; "Pfeiffer's capillary anastomoses") do not have any significant function in the supply of blood to a deficient

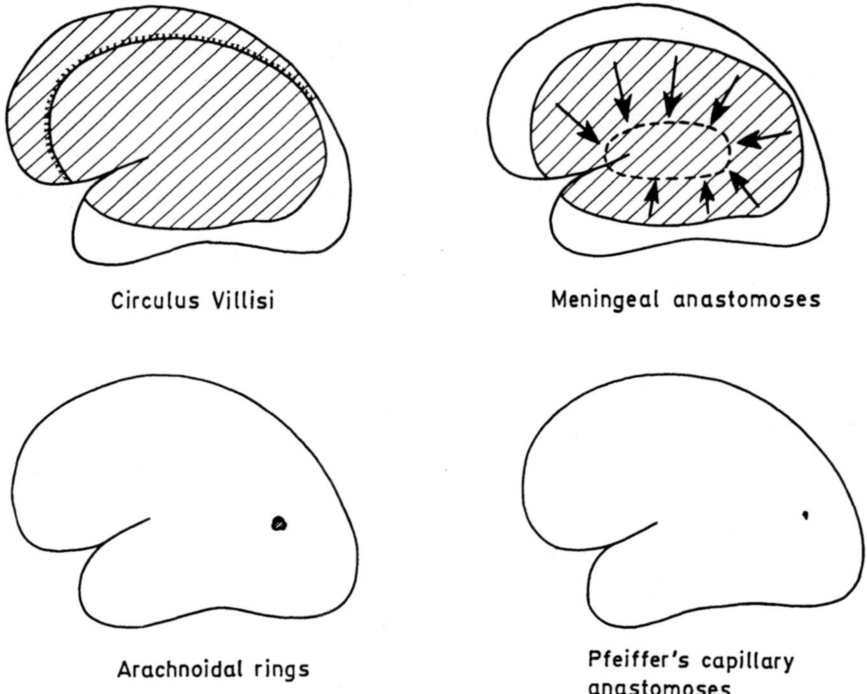

Fig. 17. Different size of brain territories, when the collateral circulation of the various systems become operative in emergencies

area in case of an acute emergency. This is particularly detrimental for the "brainstem" where the arteries seem to have no major intercommunications apart from the capillaries. Consequently, in case of an occlusion of a lenticulostriate or a paramedian pontine artery at its origin, a total infarct of the supply area was supposed to result (see above). Unfortunately satisfactory explanation has not yet been provided as to why the morphological findings fail to confirm such a concept. It may be true, however, that in chronic stenoses the capillary anastomoses begin to work and thereby decrease the size of an infarct, though not to any considerable extent.

There seems to be one exception as in the case of very slow development of a compromise of the small arteries of the basal ganglia, as is found in the "Moya-Moya syndrome" (see p. 18ff.).

In summary, it seems reasonable to assume that with respect to the efficiency of the various intracranial anastomotic systems that the circle of Willis and the meningeal anastomoses may be very important, but the two other systems are probably only of very limited value (see Fig. 17) for redistribution of the blood supply.

IV. The Moya-Moya Type of Collateral Arteries – Do "Transcerebral Anastomoses" Exist?

An unusual arterial vascular formation was first described by TAKEUCHI (1961) in Japan and was confirmed two years later by SUZUKI et al. (1963) in six cases. In the following year NISHIMOTO and SUGIU (1964) reported details of two similar cases. This pattern has been named Moya-Moya (puff of tobacco smoke) by SUZUKI, and also described as "Nishimoto's disease" or juvenile occlusion of the circle of Willis (KUDO, 1965), cerebral arterial rete (HANDA et al., 1967; HANDA and HANDA, 1972), cerebral juxta-basal teleangiectasia (SANO, 1965), cerebral basal rete mirabile (NISHIMOTO and TAKEUCHI, 1967) etc.

By 1966 KUDO had collected 146 cases in Japan and in 1968 NISHIMOTO and TAKEUCHI gave a clinical survey of 96 cases based on information from the Japanese neurosurgical hospitals. However, cases have also been observed outside Japan (e.g. a Japanese woman living in the USA, by WEIDNER et al., 1965; two Japanese children by LEEDS and ABBOTT, 1965). The first case of a white American male is said to have been observed by MERRITT in 1968.

In the literature (SUZUKI and KODAMA, 1971; DUMAS et al., 1972; see also PICARD et al., 1974) it has been mentioned that DECKER (1960), TAVERAS and WOOD (1964), KRAYENBÜHL and YASARGIL (1965) and GERLACH et al. (1967) have described similar cases. We have seen a really convincing description and picture only in the book by KRAYENBÜHL and YASARGIL (1965, Fig. 307a, b: described as "bilateral capillary diffuse cerebral angioectasia"). Furthermore, DUMAS et al. (1972) observed five cases among Senegalese patients, GALLIGIONI et al. (1971) four patients of Mediterranean origin and ANDRIOLI et al. (1971) one patient from Padua. The case described by BALBO et al. (1972) is difficult to identify from his pictures. HANDA and HANDA (1972) have also made an extensive report on this desease.

The pathogenesis of this curious syndrome has been unexplained from the outset. NISHIMOTO and SUGIU (1964) suspected a malformation whereas SUZUKI et al. (1963) considered it to be an acquired disease parallel to Takayasu's disease.

In these Moya-Moya cases there is always a stenosis or a proximal occlusion in the carotid siphon, with or without a middle cerebral occlusion and often an occlusion of the anterior cerebral artery as well. A bundle of spiral, thickly twisted arterial channels extends "from the siphon" towards the basal ganglia, i.e. along the general course of the medial and lateral striate vessels, as well as along other perforating arteries supplying the basal ganglia. In some cases (observation by ZÜLCH et al., 1974a) a connection has been noted with cortical arteries *perforating deep into and through the centrum semiovale.*

These new collateral systems appear to originate in the following areas: medial and lateral lenticulostriate vessels, Heubner's artery, the perforating branches of the communicating arteries, as well as those posterior arteries supplying the thalamus and originating from the posterior cerebral artery. Apparently the group of the vessel involved differs from case to case and depends on the location and degree of the stenosis or occlusion as for example in the distinction between the "orbital" and "ethmoidal" types of Moya-Moya, formed from the external carotid artery.

Furthermore, SUZUKI et al. (1963) were able to distinguish several phases in the gradual development of the Moya-Moya system as noted for instance in (1) initial stenosis of the siphon, and (2) stenosis turning into an occlusion.

Some authors believe that Moya-Moya disease is a special form of cerebral arterial collateral system. As proof they point to the fact that occasionally these systems disappear when the stenosis becomes an occlusion. Then extracranial communications by way of the ophthalmic and vertebral arteries are formed.

The authors assume that the abnormality is an "acquired" formation which develops in an attempt to compensate for an endangered arterial circulation resulting from stenosis or occlusion, as may also be observed in cases of tuberculous or syphilitic arteritis.

To the contrary, NISHIMOTO's opinion was that Moya-Moya disease must be a vascular malformation parallel to the "rete mirabile" which are present in some mammals such as cats, pigs, goats, sheep and oxen. This opinion is shared by DUMAS et al. (1972) and also by GALLIGIONI et al. (1971). The lack of progress seemed to support their interpretation. However, this is in contrast to the cases of MAKI and NAKATA (1965) as well as KUDO (1965, 1966), who have observed the progress of the disease in a boy by means of repeated angiographies. Such morphological variants as the rete formations, however, have been seen also in adult males and show a certain parallel to the Moya-Moya picture.

We made a very important observation in a man of 27 with an occlusion of one carotid artery. The contralateral signs and symptoms eventually disappeared. Seven years later he was readmitted to the clinic with a hemilateral syndrome, contralateral to the original, and apparently due to a fresh occlusion of the second carotid artery. Later, various rete systems, not seen on the first angiography, were demonstrated angiographically. These were also confirmed morphologically at autopsy.

Moreover, we have described angiographically (ZÜLCH et al., 1974a) the case of a 52 year old white female in whom the first carotid angiogram showed a stenosis of the carotid siphon and an occlusion of the left middle cerebral artery distal to the lenticulostriate arteries. These were patent as was the anterior cerebral artery. Twenty-three months later the angiogram of

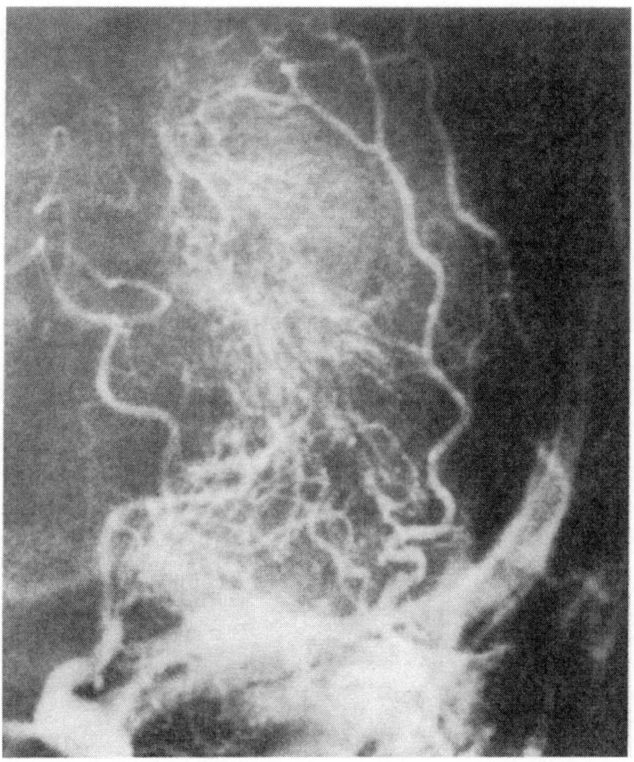

Fig. 18. Moya-Moya pattern of angioma-like vessels, probably an attempt to form a transcerebral anastomosis after middle cerebral artery occlusion

the major arteries was similar with the exception of a nonfilling of the anterior cerebral artery. *Moreover the lenticulostriate arteries were replaced by bundles of larger corkscrew-like (Moya-Moya) (Fig. 18) arteries that ran from the base into the centrum semiovale, where they connected with the parieto-occipital cortical supply.* This case suggests the possibility of an *acquired* formation of such systems typical of Moya-Moya disease and must be discussed in detail, because of the fundamental significance of such an unusual observation.

Are we then entitled to adopt the concept that *intracerebral arteries of the basal ganglia may rarely form a collateral supply system?* Although probably an exception to the rule, this case would prove that they can be formed as an angioma-like system originating from medial and lateral striate arteries. However, whether this is of any actual value for a better supply of the tissue is still an open question. The very fact that the lumina of the lenticulostriate vessels are so much enlarged and many smaller ones – hardly visible on the ordinary angiogram – are markedly dilated, and that the circulation time of this system is relatively short, proves that this new supply system is functioning. It must be emphasized that this system apparently is formed as a result of great demand for blood to the otherwise deprived area.

It is by no means the arterial pressure which provokes this dilatation as is true in the case of the vascular systems of a carotid-cavernous fistula. It definitely did not preexist in this form, but the objection that it could have been a certain *microscopical* congenital "anlage" which was already present cannot be rejected.

We have to learn therefore that not only extra- and intracranial collateral pathways of many varieties (WEIBEL and FIELDS, 1969; ZÜLCH, 1971d) can be formed in cases of high grade stenosis or occlusion, but also *on a macroscopical level within the cerebrum.*

Other cases were kindly demonstrated to me by TAKEUCHI in 1979 (personal communication). Here the similarity to the end stage of thromboangiitis obliterans was surprisingly great. At another hospital in Japan the microscopic picture was more similar to atherosclerosis. The basic vascular process may be therefore different, and the vascular patterns a "phenomenon" (TAKEUCHI) of a stereotyped pattern. I would suggest then to introduce the term of a "Moya-Moya syndrome" of different causation.

I had the privilege of seeing a microscopic slide of a typical Moya-Moya artery in a Peking hospital during a 1978 visit to China. Proximally it showed a high-grade collagenous stenosing process of the arterial lumen almost deprived of cells. This seemed to be the final stage of an earlier mainly cellular proliferation as seen in a smaller more distal branch artery. No hint as to the pathogenesis of this process could be deduced from this slide.

Therefore our thesis developed above, that within the cerebrum there were only small marginal anastomoses between the capillaries without any significant function, must be enlarged. Occasionally specific cases will be encountered where such anastomoses are formed at the level of the small arteries. In this circumstance not only dilatation, *but a transcerebral collateral system of arteries may* be *formed*, probably 2–3 mm thick, arising from the base and extending to the perforating vessels within the parieto-occipital cortex. Through these vessels there is rapid circulation into the venous system.

Finally the question arises why these Moya-Moya systems have been observed particularly in Japan and China (see also LEE and CHEUNG, 1973), and even in the Japanese ethnic population outside their home country. In our opinion, SUZUKI's hint regarding the frequency of Takayasu's disease (FUKUSHIMA et al., 1975) may give a clue as to the cause, which probably has an allergic/hyperergic origin, e.g. a slowly proliferating endovascular lesion at the cellular level. Other varieties of neuroallergic disease also occur in Japan with greater frequency than seen in the western world (neuromyelitis optica which is encountered more commonly than in the western world). My recent visit to Chinese (1978) hospitals confirmed a similar incidence of Moya-Moya within the Chinese population.

We will be able to gain more exact knowledge of the unexplained formation of collateral arterial anastomoses only after obtaining a more exact morphological description of the arteries in Moya-Moya. The possibility of an "acquired" origin on the basis of an otherosclerotic occlusion, at least in European patients, is demonstrated by our case (ZÜLCH et al., 1974a).

The factors responsible for making collateral channels or anastomoses operative. The consequences of the inadequacy of arterial channels depend on the presence or absence of anastomoses able to form a collateral pathway. The general rule is that the more proximal the lesion the higher the probability of the formation of a collateral supply system able to prevent neurological deficit. Moreover the speed of the developing impairment is of utmost importance: very sudden lesions such as thromboembolic processes usually have a lesser chance of being compensated by anastomoses than do more slowly developing occlusive processes. Proximal lesions such as atherosclerotic stenosis or occlusion of the internal carotid artery in the neck are often never detected during life (HULTQVIST, 1942). The well-known case of WÜLLENWEBER (1928: with occlusion of both carotid arteries) or the recent description of VITEK et al. (1972: with occlusion of four vessels) and also DONIGER (1963) and many other cases in the literature indicate the potential for very good functioning collaterals in such cases.

Which are then the factors which make an efficient collateral system operative? The causes are (1) a temporary or (2) a permanent impairment of an arterial channel. We have mentioned already that some of these "temporary" impairments (pp. 4, 7) responsible for the opening of collateral pathways through existing large anastomoses may be "physiological".

This may be the case in strangulations of one carotid in extreme rotation or extension of the neck, where the circle of Willis will compensate, or by extreme positions at the atlanto-occipital joint where one vertebral artery may support or substitute for the supply of the other (pp. 4, 7).

In "pathologic" conditions the resulting collateral systems will be more rapidly and more satisfactorily developed if the stenoses or occlusions progress *slowly*, and they will depend on the hemodynamic situation within the systemic circulation, e.g. the perfusion pressure. Therefore, time and the perfusion pressure through the four main source arteries are decisive factors.

V. Venous Drainage System

After examining a large number of phlebograms (Krayenbühl and Yasargil, 1965; Zülch, 1964) as well as anatomical descriptions (K.-A. Hossmann, 1966; see Padget, 1956, 1957; also the excellent atlas of Stephens and Stilwell, 1969 and Salamon and Huang, 1976) the morphologic variability of the large cerebral veins and sinuses becomes evident. The outer venous system drains toward the sagittal sinus (predominantly the Rolandic vein, vein of Trolard and the anastomotic veins) whereas the Sylvian veins and vein of Labbé drain toward the basal sinuses (transverse sinus, sigmoidal sinus, superficial petrosal sinus) (for morphological details see Tournade et al., 1972). The veins of the posterior fossa as seen in angiograms have been excellently described by Huang and Wolf (1963, 1964b, 1965, 1966, 1967) and Huang et al. (1968).

The sphenoparietal sinus forms a connection between the sagittal and the basal sinuses but there may be extreme variations in this pattern. In contrast the system of the inner cerebral veins (septum pellucidum or internal cerebral veins, basal vein of Rosenthal, chorioidal vein, great vein of Galen) seems to be built more uniformly (Hacker, 1968; Huang and Wolf, 1964a, 1964b, 1965; Huang et al., 1968). Also very variable is the circulation through the torcular Herophili. There is a definite tendency for the sagittal sinus to drain more often into the right transverse sinus and the sinus rectus into the left one (Zülch, 1964, K.-A. Hossmann, 1966). Both may drain simultaneously though, with a smaller branch, towards the other side. However, a complete mixture of blood with symmetrical drainage is found in only 10% of cases. This finding is important with respect to the need for operative ligature or during mechanical occlusion of a sinus.

The development of the venous system has been described by Padget (1956, 1957).

VI. Malformations

(Capillary, Arteriovenous, Cavernomatous Malformations, Berry – Saccular – Aneurysms)

1. Angiomas and Arteriovenous Malformations

Angiomas are frequently not space-occupying lesions. They may, however, produce a mass effect either through rupture and hemorrhage or through reactive changes. A modern classification (Bergstrand et al., 1936; Paterson and McKissock, 1956; Pool and Potts, 1965; Lange-Cossack, 1966; McCormick, 1966; Stehbens, 1972 – excellent review of literature –; Zülch, 1956a, 1965, 1975a) must include:

cavernous angiomas
capillary angiomas
venous angiomas
capillary and venous angiomas in combination (Sturge-Weber's disease)
arteriovenous malformations or angiomas.

Cavernous angiomas occur within the skull and vertebral column as well as in the brain and spinal cord. They are bluish-red tumor-like masses of vessels which do not possess a capsule and over which the vessels of the leptomeninges cross unchanged. The surrounding tissue may form scars and often contains calcification. By definition one wall harbors two cavities without much interstitial tissue. They are not like the common angiomas which occur elsewhere in the brain or near the sella (Kautzky et al., 1976).

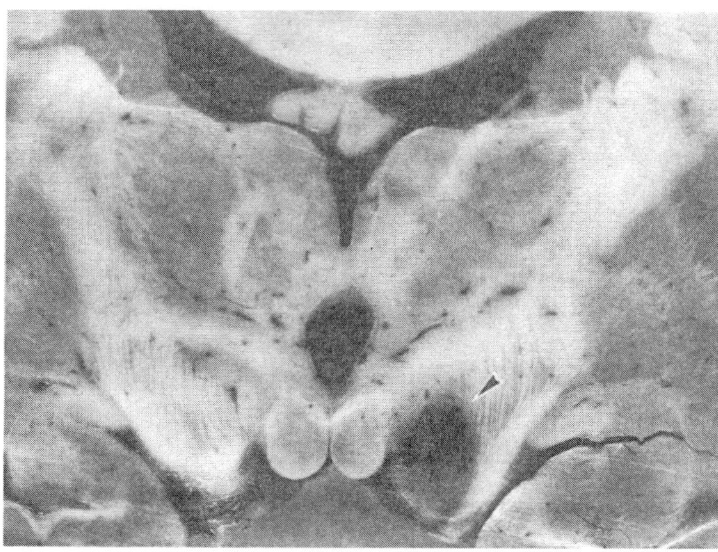

Fig. 19. Pea-sized capillary angioma in the cerebral peduncle (incidental finding; *arrow*)

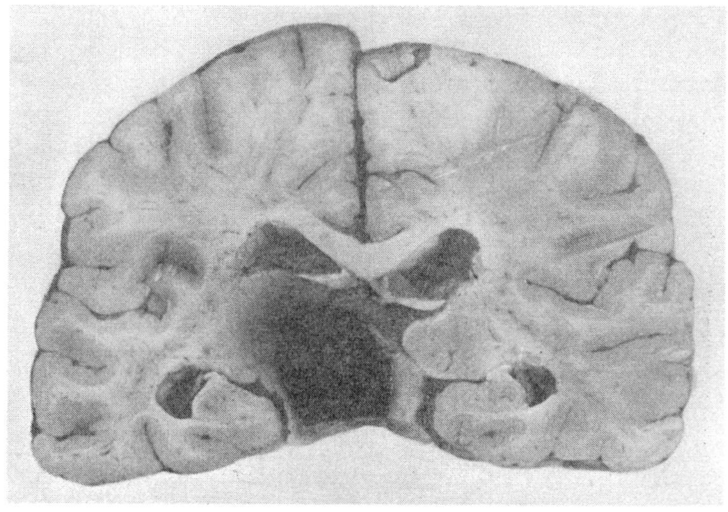

Fig. 20. Cherry-sized, fatal mass-hemorrhage from a capillary angioma of the left peduncle (c.f. Fig. 19)

More frequently observed are the *capillary angiomas* (teleangiectasias) of the central nervous system which are usually pea-sized and are sometimes discovered only incidentally. They may, however, be a source of hemorrhage ("microangiomas"; Fig. 19). They form a tangled knot of capillaries and lie in the brainstem (Fig. 20) or over the hemispheres. The overlying leptomeningeal vessels are unchanged.

The *venous* angiomas are, as yet, not well defined. They are supposed to be varicocele-like accumulations of veins (more often seen in the Sylvian fissure or over the spinal cord).

The combined *capillary and venous angiomas* of Sturge-Weber's disease form a vascular network within the leptomeninges and consist of venous and capillary channels, usually not thicker than a matchstick, overlying the cortex. The adjacent brain parenchyma becomes atrophic, scarred and grossly calcified. The typical pattern of calcification seen radiographically is deposited in parallel "linear, serpentine or convoluted configurations". This is probably a secondary conse-

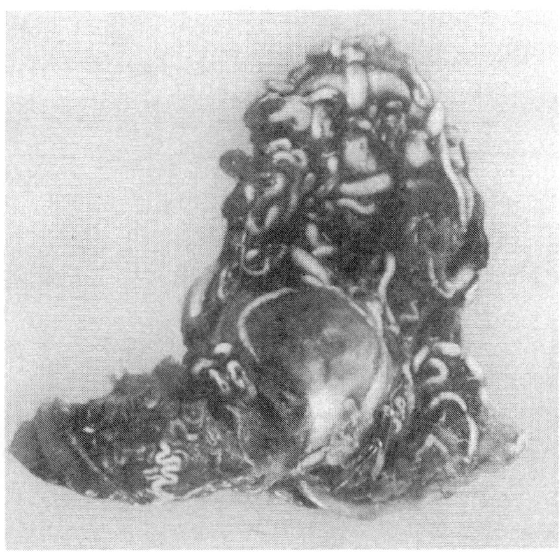

Fig. 21. Large arteriovenous malformation (AVM) surgically removed from the parieto-occipital region. The angioma was injected with contrast medium postoperatively

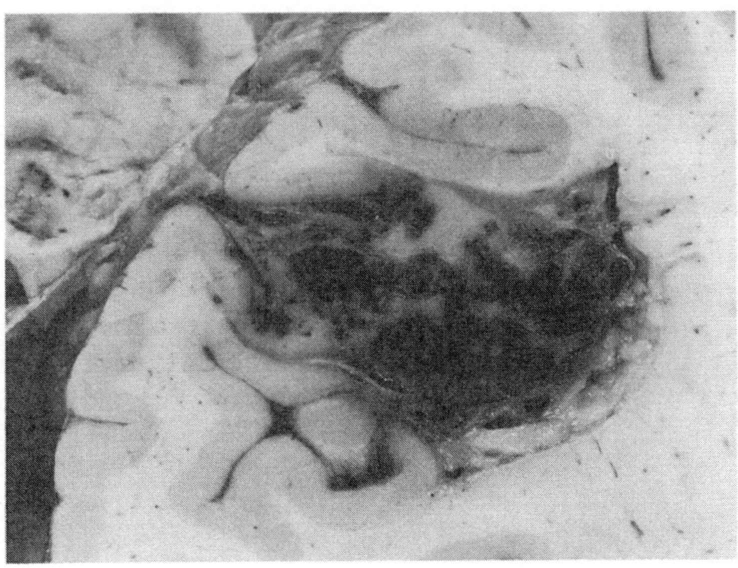

Fig. 22. A large arteriovenous malformation (AVM) in the medial portion of the occipital lobe

quence of the disturbed circulation. These intracranial are frequently coincident with facial angiomas (Kautzky, 1949; Fazio et al., 1966 – meningeal angioma).

The most important angiomas are the *arteriovenous malformations* (or arteriovenous angiomas or aneurysms). By means of angiography it has been possible to fully analyse them. These angiomas consist of a circumscribed network of arteries and veins, some of which may be as thick as half a centimeter. They are connected in part by large fistulous vessels of intermediate wall structure, and in part by a capillary network. They vary in size (from 2–6 cm or more in diameter; Fig. 21), predominantly involve the cerebral cortex, but may extend down to the ventricle and even reach the ependymal zone. A plexus of tangled vessels may be seen on the surface of the cortex but these vessels may also be buried within the brain substance (Fig. 22). The vascular channels themselves vary in size, may loop around one another and may become thrombosed.

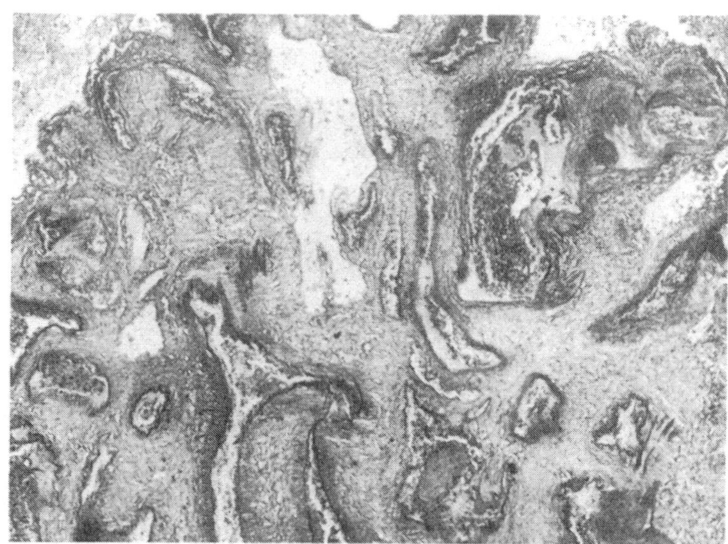

Fig. 23. Small (pea-sized) arteriovenous malformation which gave rise to a fatal hemorrhage (microangioma)

Small arteriovenous malformations which have been termed "cryptic" (CRAWFORD and D. RUSSELL, 1956; MCCORMICK and NOFZINGER, 1966) fall into our group of "microangiomas" (up to the size of 1 cm^3; GERLACH and JENSEN, 1961, 1965, JENSEN, 1979; HENSCH, 1979). The most susceptible age range for these to be observed is between 18 and 30 years, and overall, males outnumber females by two to one (Fig. 23).

Probably the majority of cases of "varicosis spinalis" really belong to this group of arteriovenous malformations, as has been shown by selected angiography (M. DJINDJIAN, 1976; R. DJINDJIAN et al., 1976).

2. Dissecting Aneurysms of Cerebral Arteries

A special form of subacute posttraumatic "apoplexy" with infarction relates to a dissecting aneurysm usually involving the middle cerebral artery. It may occur following the sudden impact of the arterial wall against a bony surface such as the lesser wing of the sphenoid bone (NEDWICH et al., 1963).

We have observed such an occurrence in a patient who suffered, as a consequence, total infarction of the Sylvian territory resulting in death (Fig. 24). Preexisting atherosclerotic changes seem to be the prerequisite for this splitting of the arterial wall and should be considered in any medico-legal evaluation of such a case (WOLMAN, 1959; DUMAN and STEPHENS, 1963; ZÜLCH, 1969c).

Dissecting aneurysms also occur at the level of the carotid artery (FRANTZEN et al., 1961; OJEMANN et al., 1972) and may be of infectious origin (see FINKEMEYER, 1950).

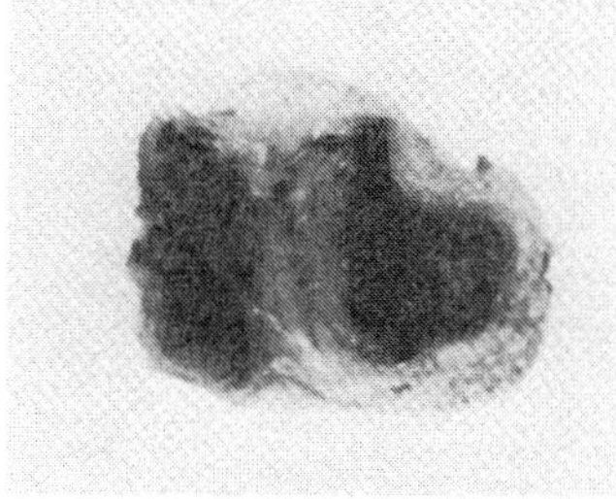

Fig. 24. Dissecting aneurysm of middle cerebral artery in a 70 year old woman after fall on edge of bed. Death occurred three days later due to huge infarct of anterior and middle cerebral artery (c.f. Fig. 154)

3. Aneurysms and Varices

Aneurysms are most frequently secondary to congenital defects in the arterial wall. Therefore they have sites of predilection which are well-known both clinically and morphologically from large series of reported cases (see Figs. of McDonald and Korb, 1939). Hassler (1961) has shown microscopically that these congenital defects arise in the vessel walls usually at points of branching. Probably secondary factors such as hypertension tend to promote the clinical manifestation of these wall defects in the form of saccular (berry) aneurysms, after disintegration of the elastic lamellae has occurred. Atherosclerosis also is considered to play a role in their formation (discussion of the so-called Charcot-Bouchard aneurysms see p. 94).

In the analysis of 363 cases made by Pakarinen (1967) the following locations of aneurysms were observed during angiography:

Anterior cerebral artery	89, of these at the
Communicating artery	40
A. pericallosa	5
Proximal anterior artery	1
Internal carotid artery	71, of these at the
Posterior communicating artery	26
Bifurcation	4
Ophthalmic artery	3
Anterior chorioidal artery	1
Middle cerebral artery	135
Vertebral system	14
Multiple	50
Site not specified	4

The total series comprised 144 cases proven by angiography and 219 by autopsy.

About 90% of saccular aneurysms will be found in the anterior half of the circle of Willis and only 10% in the vertebrobasilar system.

Aneurysms are small *berry*-like outpouchings from an arterial wall of any size (see Fig. 25). They may be partly or totally obliterated by organized thrombus. Adherence to the neighboring tissue is common if the aneurysm has bled and the adjacent brain maybe yellowish because of earlier deposition of blood pigment.

Extensive aneurysms of the *fusiform* type are most common in the basilar artery (Fig. 26). They may have their origin in the embryological fusion of the two vertebral arteries (p. 4). An ectatic atherosclerotic wall lesion may also be important. The definition "fusiform aneurysm" is based upon a 50% increase in the size of the lumen. Probably 50% of arteries which first appear as microaneurysmatic and ballooning, later appear as "true" saccular aneurysms at the time of rupture. In the series of McDonald and Korb (1939) only about 25% had not ruptured.

Aneurysms may be multiple in 10%–20% of cases. Their incidence is said to be between 10 and 16 per 100.000 of a normal population and in Finland half of that.

The figures reported from the large United States cooperative study (Locksley, 1966) based on 3321 cases contained 320 cases (9.6%) which had not bled and were discovered only by angiography. The ratio of males to females in this study was 2:3. Only below the age of 20 years was there a predominance of males. There was an age-dependent pattern, the group of 50–54 years being that most represented (407 cases), the group of 55–59 being the second (398) and the group of 45–49 the third (369 cases).

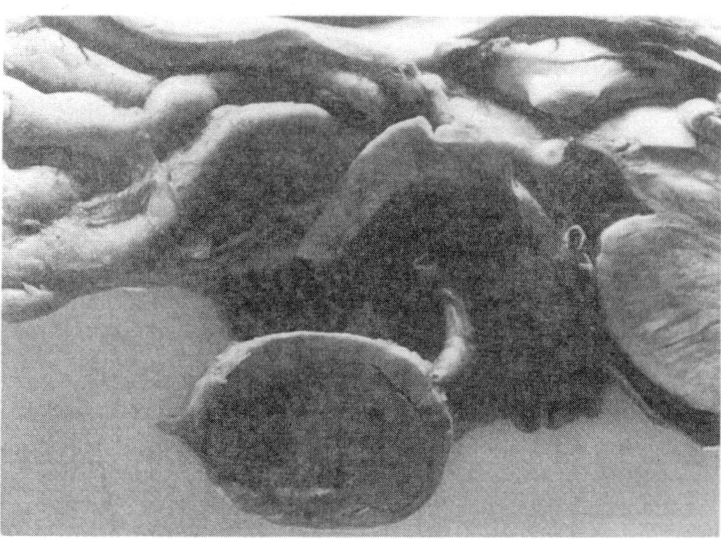

Fig. 25. Chestnut-sized, completely thombosed, supraclinoid aneurysm of the internal carotid artery

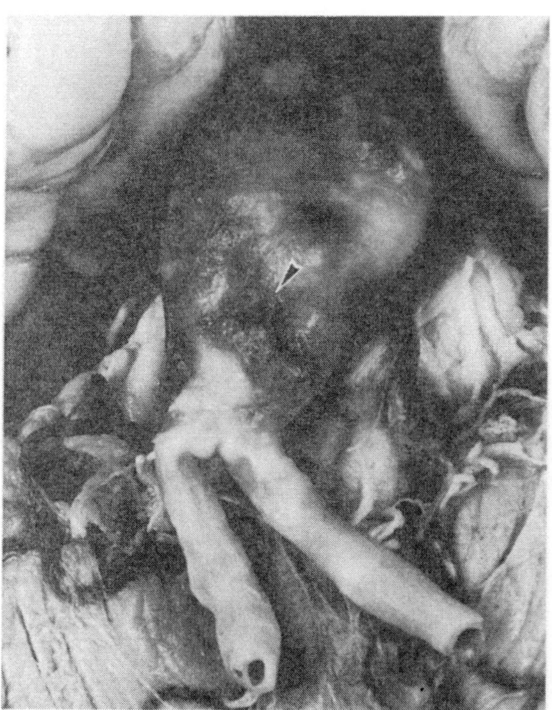

Fig. 26. Enormous, ruptured fusiform aneurysm of the basilar artery *(arrow)*

The relationship to a particular activity (see also KRAYENBÜHL and YASARGIL, 1958), during which the hemorrhage started is also interesting:

sleeping	820	coughing	49
unspecified circumstances	734	trauma	63
lifting or bending of the body	273	urination	45
emotional strain	100	surgery	10
defaecation	99	parturition	8
coitus	87		

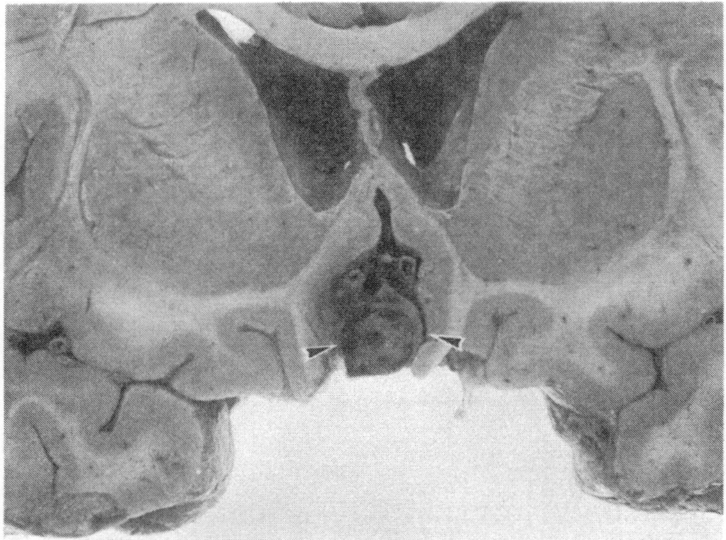

Fig.27. Cherry-sized saccular aneurysm of the anterior communicating artery *(arrows)*

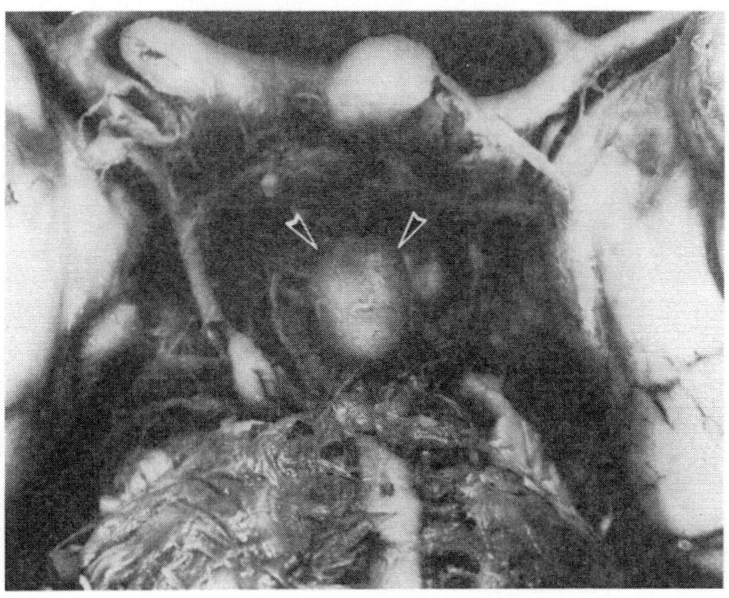

Fig. 28. Bean-sized aneurysm at the bifurcation of the basilar artery into the posterior cerebral arteries *(arrows)*

It is important to note that more than two-thirds bled during sleep or unspecified circumstances (1554 of 2288 cases).

The sex distribution in a larger combined series by nine authors comprised 904 males and 1974 females with an age peak in the fifth and sixth decades. In still another report by 21 authors there were 3076 males (43.9%) and 3934 females (56.1%).

Of subarachnoidal hemorrhages 50%–70% are related to berry aneurysms and 15% to arteriovenous or other malformations. KRAYENBÜHL and YASARGIL (1958) could not find the source of the subarachnoid hemorrhage in 155 of 431 of their cases, nor could MCKISSOCK et al. (1958)

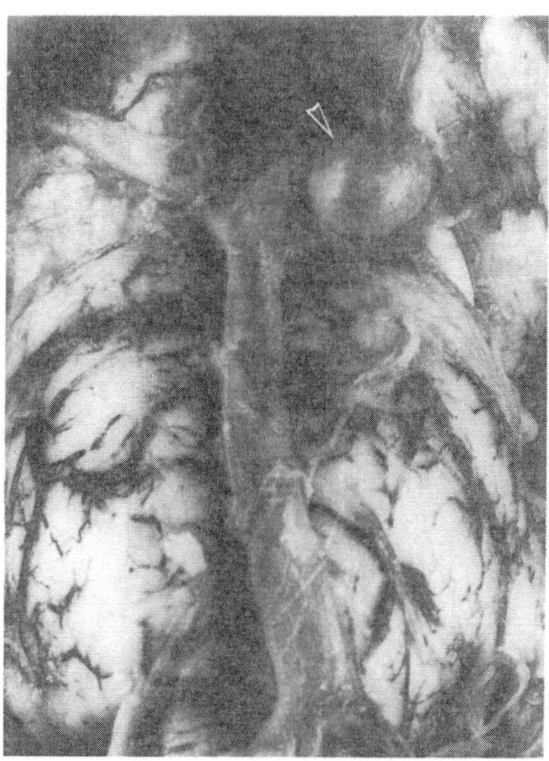

Fig. 29. Bean-sized aneurysm of the posterior cerebral artery *(arrow)*

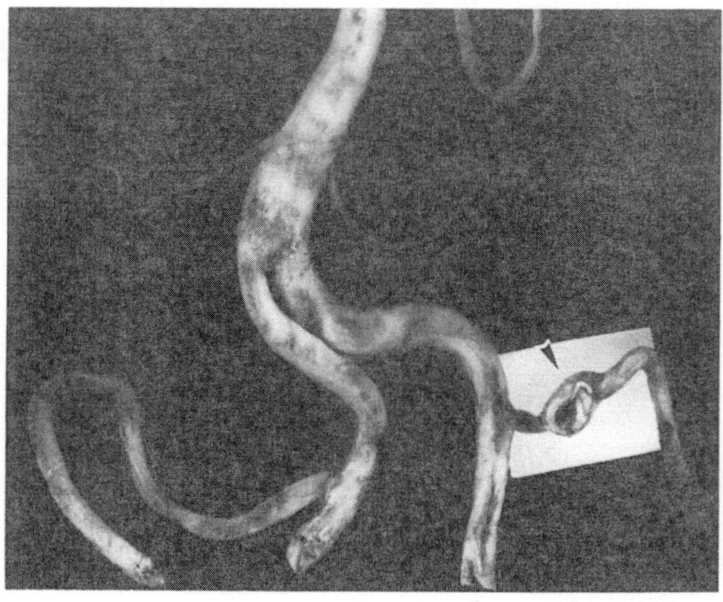

Fig. 30. Small ruptured aneurysm of the left posterior inferior cerebellar artery *(arrow)*

in 140 of 455 in their series. In autopsy cases where a precise dissection is undertaken (RICHARDSON and HYLAND, 1941) positive observations are more frequent. This has been confirmed by our own large experience. However, it is not always easy to detect the aneurysm within a hard formalin-fixed blood clot.

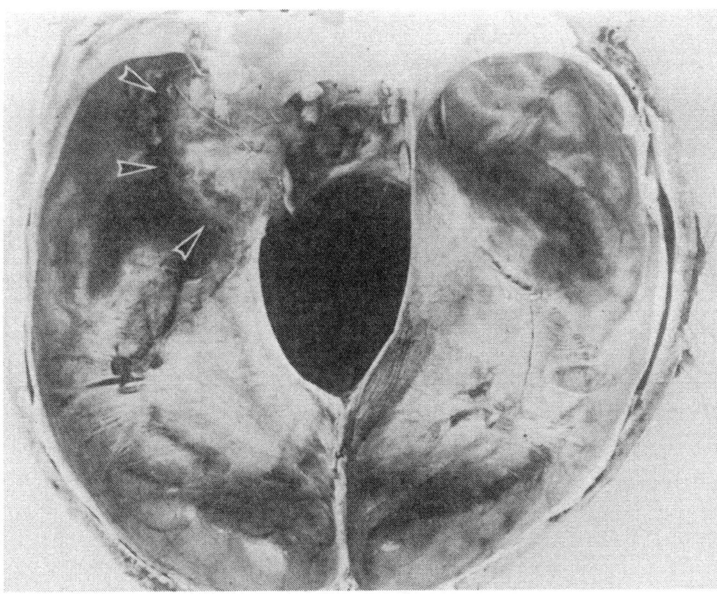

Fig. 31. Huge infraclinoid aneurysm of the left carotid artery (*arrows;* c.f. Fig. 32)

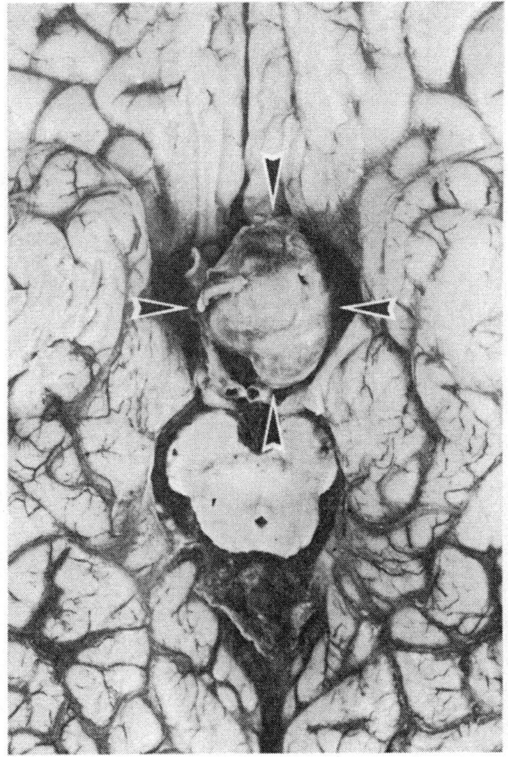

Fig. 32. Large supraclinoid aneurysm of the left carotid artery. Aneurysms of this size may have a mass effect similar to that of a chiasmatic tumors *(arrows)*

Within the anterior intracranial circulation berry aneurysms are found most commonly on the anterior and posterior communicating arteries (Figs. 27, 28) and in the vertebrobasilar circulation at the distal end of the basilar artery (Figs. 29, 30). Distinction is made between the infra- (Fig. 31) and supraclinoid (Figs. 25, 32) carotid aneurysms, the latter location being the more common. The site and extension of a hemorrhage from a ruptured aneurysm is very typical and usually diagnostic (see p. 82 and Figs. 81–83). Today, it can easily be ascertained by computed tomography which may lead also to the detection of the site in angiographically negative cases. In any case the computed tomography will determine the plan for angiography.

"Venous varicosis" is occasionally seen as an accumulation of varicose, enlarged veins in a network. True "varices", e.g. phlebectasias, occur most commonly near the sinuses, for example near the superior sagittal sinus, in the form of an enlarged Pacchionian granulation and also near the great vein of Galen in a spherical form (see Fig. 197 in KAUTZKY et al., 1976; references see also chapter "subarachnoid hemorrhage", p. 81).

C. Pathomorphology and Pathophysiology of the Vasculature (Secondary)

I. Atherosclerosis – Classification – Macroscopical Description – Grading

1. Atherosclerosis – Arteriosclerosis

"Atherosclerosis – the principal killer of western man" (ROSS et al., 1979) and the main cause of most disturbances of cerebral circulation.

Atherosclerosis has had a significant role in world politics as demonstrated by three old men, namely WILSON, v. HINDENBURG and LENIN (FRIEDLANDER, 1972).

Atherosclerosis (atheros = pap, scleros = hardened) is the term more commonly used in the English speaking world than arteriosclerosis. In a semantic discussion one would define arteriosclerosis as a broader term combining atherosclerosis and arteriolar sclerosis or angiosclerosis as a lesion of arteries, capillaries and veins such as is observed in hypertensive encephalopathy. Cerebral atherosclerosis is only a regional manifestation of a general disease, but with some interesting differences:

a) The gross calcification (particularly as Mönckeberg's form), an essential feature in such changes in the rest of the body, is almost never observed after passage of the "brain vessels" through the dura. We have only scarce observations on complete calcification of a vertebral and basilar artery (KLEIHUES et al., 1964; ZÜLCH, 1962a, 1964; see also Fig. 33).

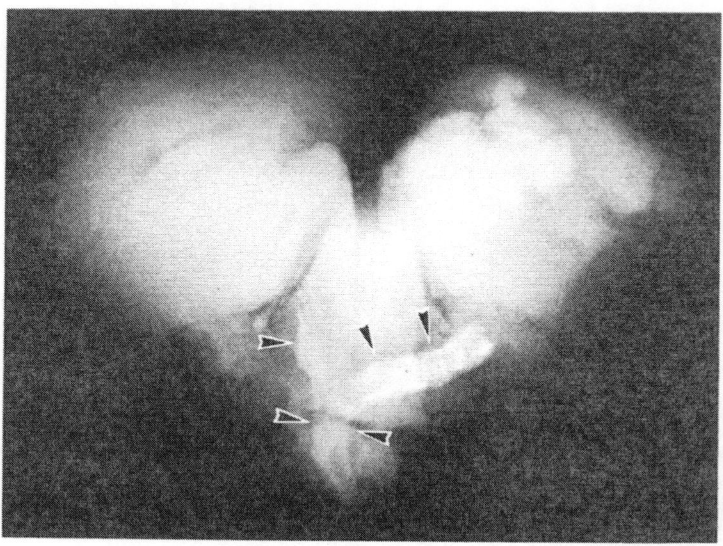

Fig. 33. Unexplained total calcification in the vertebro-basilar system (x-ray; *arrows*)

b) The manifestation of *cerebral* atherosclerosis is usually of a lower grade than in other organs (p. 52ff.; see also NUUTILA, 1973).

c) The causal relationship with hypertension is less marked in cerebral atherosclerosis (see pp. 50ff., 119ff.) than in other regions of the body.

The highest grade of atherosclerosis is usually reached in the abdominal aorta and the hypogastric arteries, then in the thoracic aorta and the coronaries, and in the intracranial arteries only as the third or lowest grade. A similar discrepancy is seen with reference to the time of clinical manifestation. Severe grades of atherosclerosis of the coronary arteries are usually observed 1–2 decades before that of the cerebral arteries, the earliest coronary lesions having been found in "healthy" people of 20–25 years (World Wars I and II, also in the Korean War).

a) Classification of Atherosclerosis

It is possible to differentiate three main types of atherosclerosis: (1) the *stenosing* type *generalized* (Figs. 41 and 42), (2) the stenosing type *localized* (Figs. 34–36, 38) and (3) the *dilating*-ectatic-fibrotic alteration of the vessel (Fig. 37). The stenosing type of atherosclerosis can affect the vessel concentrically (Fig. 38) or eccentrically and can occur (Fig. 34) either diffusely or localized appearing as narrow bands or rings (see p. 34ff. and Figs. 36, 39).

In the classification of the World Health Organization, three types of atherosclerosis are distinguished the "lipid-rich", the "fibrous", and the "complex" type, the latter being the most disastrous for the coronary arteries.

There may also be marked differences in the type of atherosclerosis at various sites in the body:

1) Very marked fibrous plaques
2) Fibrous plaques plus lipid infiltration
3) Fibro-lipid plaques with ulceration
4) As 3 plus thrombosis
5) As 2 plus calcification.

These types may be differently represented in the extra- and intracranial arteries and in arteries with different sized lumina.

The classification of the World Health Organization Technical Report Series (1958) employs the terminology (fatty streak, fibrous plaque, atheroma, etc.).

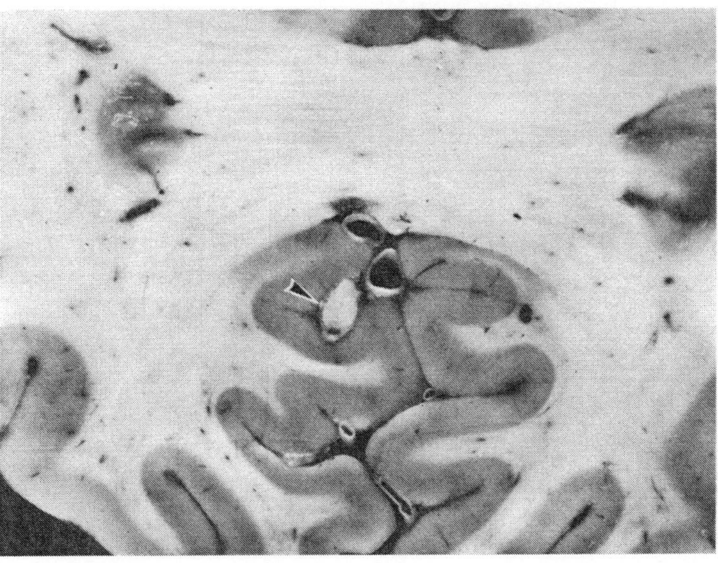

Fig. 34. Almost complete atherosclerotic occlusion of the left anterior cerebral artery *(arrow)*, whereas the contralateral is almost uncompromised

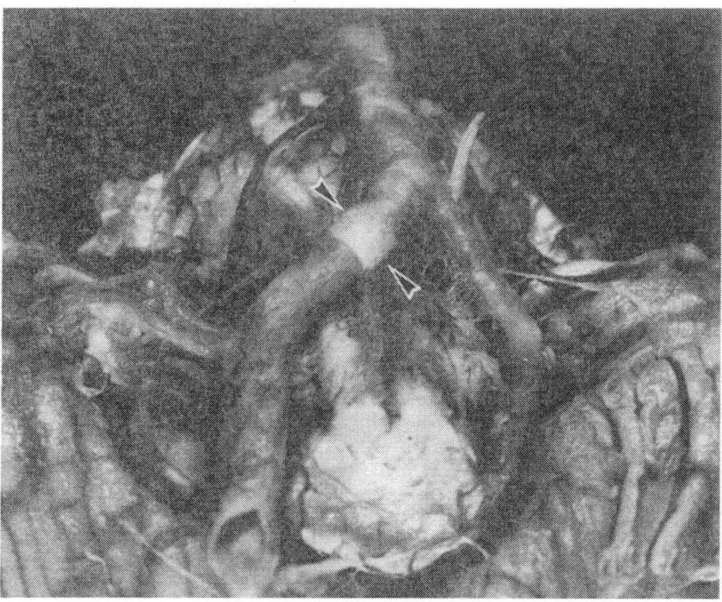

Fig. 35. Band-like atherosclerotic plaque in the right vertebral artery *(arrows)*. Another smaller plaque is visible in the middle segment of the basilar artery

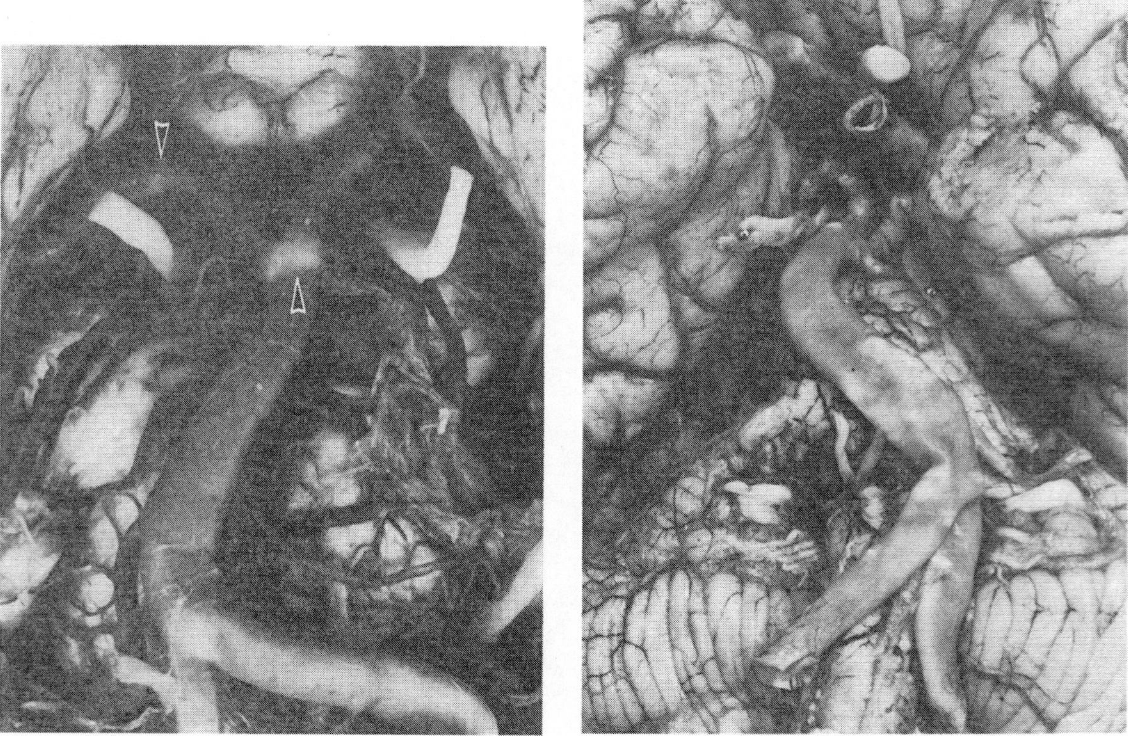

Fig. 36 **Fig. 37**

Fig. 36. The predilection site for the first (earliest) atherosclerotic intracranial plaque is usually the branching point of the basilar artery *(arrows)*

Fig. 37. "Ectatic" type of atherosclerosis with lengthening and widening of the artery. Only single, non-stenosing atherosclerotic plaques are visible. Such pictures can be seen in the "megadolicho"-basilar artery

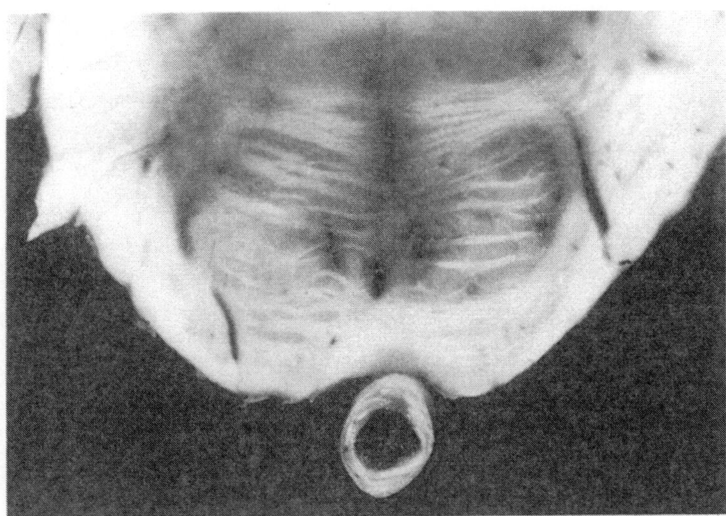

Fig. 38. Concentric atherosclerosis of the basilar artery narrowing the lumen by about 50%

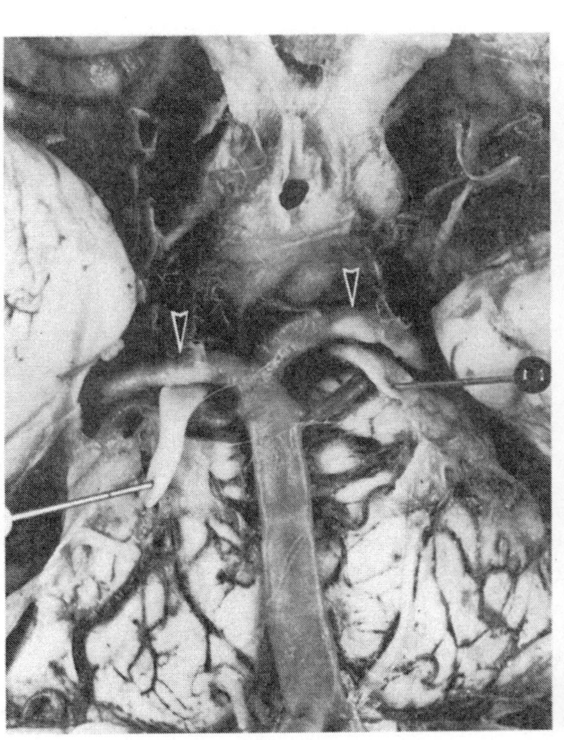

Fig. 39

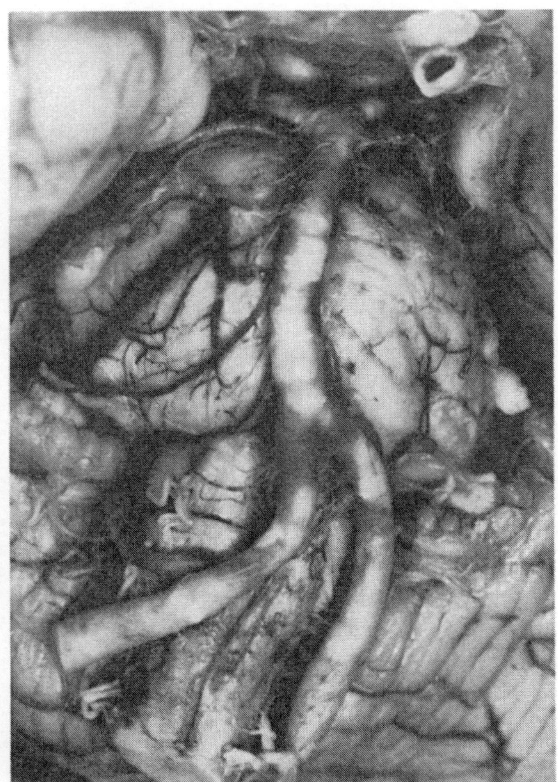

Fig. 40

Fig. 39. The basilar artery is not yet compromised by atherosclerosis. However, both posterior cerebral arteries show the first plaques above the course of the oculomotor nerve *(arrows)*

Fig. 40. Patchy atherosclerosis in the vertebral and basilar arteries (first stage of the "goose-gurgle" type of atherosclerosis)

b) General Macroscopic Appearance

A characteristic feature of stenotic atherosclerosis is narrowing of the lumen. This results from thickening of the wall associated with formation of small flecks or plaques (Fig. 36) of fatty acid ("athero" = fatty) and cholesterol material as well as a productive cellular proliferation,

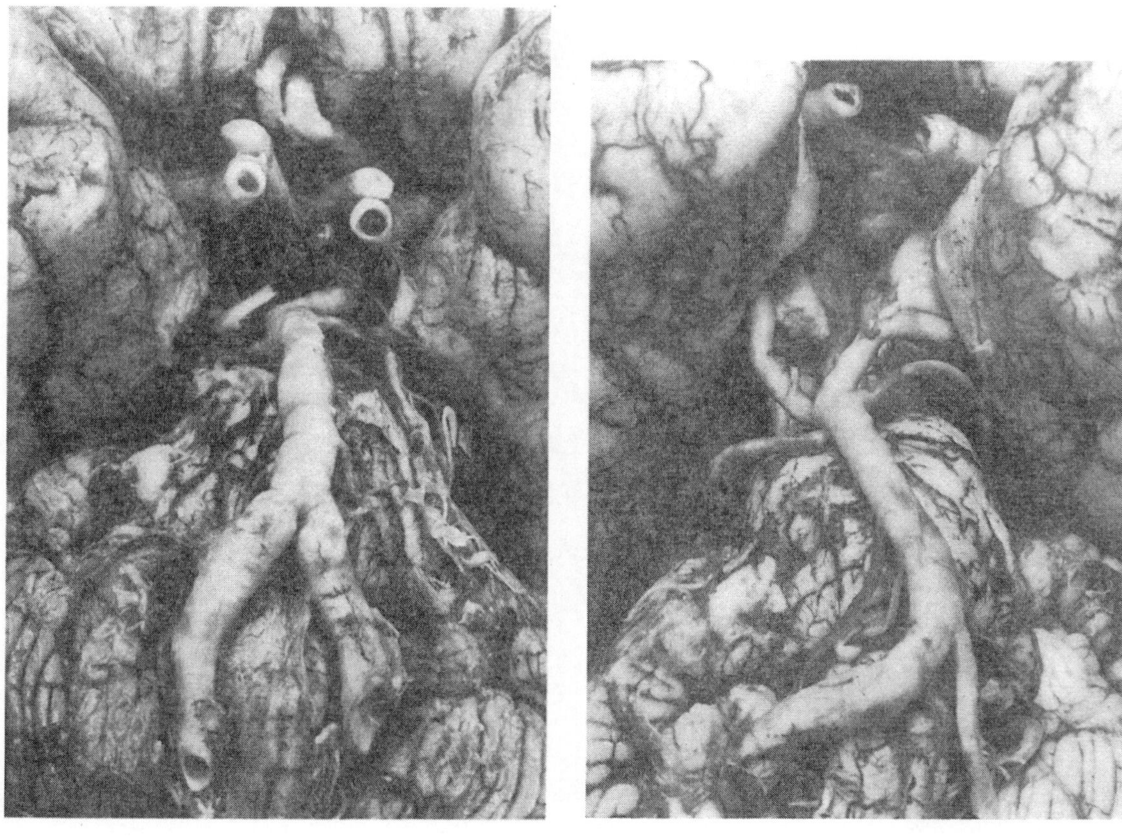

Fig. 41 **Fig. 42**

Fig. 41. "Birch-bark" type of atherosclerosis (see Fig. 40) in the vertebrobasilar system and right carotid artery

Fig. 42. "Maccaroni" type of atherosclerosis of the vertebral and basilar arteries and their branches

mainly of the intima (see p. 54). These nodules or plaques arise usually at sites of turbulence (Fig. 36, see also p. 40ff.) in contrast with less affected segments in the remainder of the vessel. In the course of time, atherosclerotic arteries may become more rigid and their caliber either stenotic or enlarged while their surface becomes uneven and knobbed (Fig. 40) and stains yellowish with a siderotic pigmentation. These vessels become firm and brittle but it is extremely rare for them to calcify (Fig. 33). Small plaques are rarely visible in the x ray and are more commonly seen microscopically in the intracranial segment of the carotid siphon (ZÜLCH 1961a, Fig. 4).

Gradually the plaques increase and the entire arterial wall is transformed into atherosclerotic material. The surface is irregular, nodular, and sometimes like bark ("birch-bark type", Fig. 41, which according to BOTTON (1955a, b) is supposed to occur in malignant hypertension). Alternatively, atherosclerosis starts with ring- or band-like (Figs. 35, 38) greyish-yellowish changes and lesions of the "goose-gurgle" (Fig. 40) type may ensue. Small elevations like warts may arise on the surface, looking sometimes like saccular aneurysms. Another type results in a smoother change in the entire wall and may develop into what is called a "macaroni" or "pipe-stem" vessel (Fig. 42). These changes may involve the wall either in a more concentric or in an eccentric way (Fig. 43), and correspondingly narrow the lumen (Figs. 37, 38).

Ectatic cerebral atherosclerosis is characterized by an elongation (Fig. 44) of the vessel, enlargement of its lumen and associated with fibrosis and sclerosis of the wall (Fig. 34).

Excellent descriptions of the pathology of atherosclerosis are given in the books of STEHBENS (1972), of TOOLE and PATEL (1974) and in the chapter of EINSIEDEL-LECHTAPE and KLEIHUES (1977).

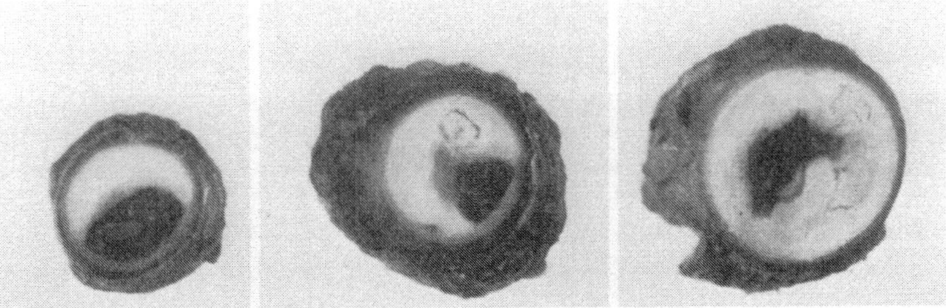

Fig. 43. Three levels of stenosing atherosclerosis in the basilar artery narrowing the lumen by 85%

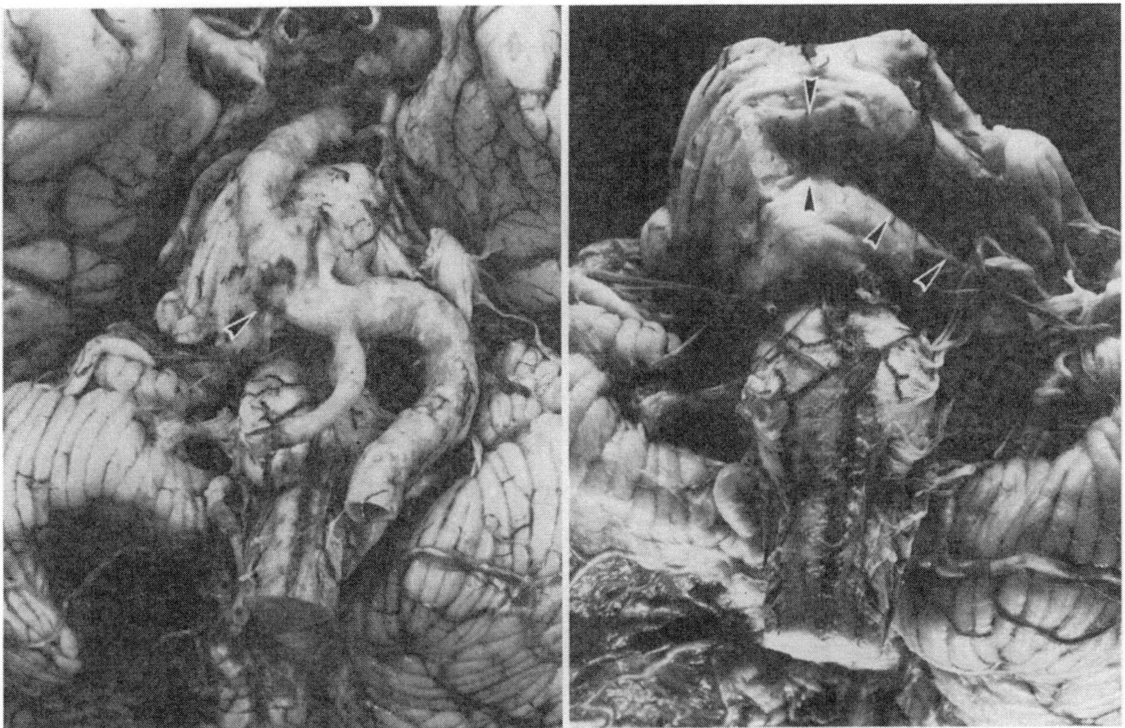

Fig. 44. Prominent tortuosity of the vertebro-basilar system associated with fusiform – ruptured – atherosclerotic aneurysm impressing itself into the adjacent pons *(arrows)* (clinically: syndrome of intermittent basilar insufficiency)

c) Grading of Atherosclerosis

Our own investigations of atherosclerosis in the "brain vessels" were based on the excellent "grading" recommendations of BAKER et al. (1967, 1973) and RESCH et al. (1969, 1970), who followed the coding guide of the World Federation of Neurology (WFN) and the National Institutes of Health, Bethesda (1959).

The grades in the WFN classification are defined as:

I. eccentric, very thin plaque without lumen narrowing

II. thin plaque involving over half of the circumference with minimal narrowing

III. concentric, thick plaque with mild lumen narrowing (25%–50%)

IV. concentric, very thick plaque with moderate or marked (pipe-stem) narrowing (over 50%).

We have measured the lumina of the main intracranial arteries as RESCH et al. (1969, 1970) have done systematically with the basal arteries of the brain. Based on these measurements

(ZÜLCH, 1971 c) we felt entitled to define, for comparison, the following sized lumina as "normal" for:

A. cerebri anterior	1.3–2.0 mm	A. cerebri interna	2.1–3.8 mm
A. cerebri media	1.6–2.9 mm	A. basilaris	2.2–3.8 mm
A. cerebri posterior	1.6–2.4 mm	A. vertebralis	1.4–3.2 mm

The lumina of cerebral arteries in another series of 30 cases (MD. thesis of ALBUS, 1970) were reported on the basis of age in decades 30–75 years (ibidem Figs. 11–14).

DEI POLI and ZUCHA (1940) have made their own system of "grading" of the atherosclerotic changes in the carotid and vertebral arteries. These are important for comparison:

Carotid channel-segment	I=4.5	Siphon segment	I=13
Carotid channel-segment	II=5.6	Siphon segment	II=12

Extracranial bifurcation of carotid artery in the neck=24. This trend is confirmed by DÖRFLER (1935). According to LINDENBERG (1957), the carotid arteries are said to remain almost free of changes in the upper neck region, but tend to show calcification at branching points and in the siphon segment.

2. General Definition – Frequency – Formal Pathogenesis

a) Statistics: Frequency of Stenosing Atherosclerosis and Ensuing Infarcts

Atherosclerosis is a universal disease, occurring in almost every human but to a variable extent. There are authors who have alleged that one third of patients in the sixth decade exhibit no atherosclerosis and that even in the ninth decade some 5% may remain uninvolved. One may differentiate the different lesions of cerebral atherosclerosis as:

1) cellular proliferation and lipid infiltration
2) localized plaque formation
   a) stenosis or b) stenosis plus appositional thrombus leading to occlusion
3) plaque formation plus ulceration and thrombus formation leading to microembolization
4) generalized stenosing forms
5) generalized stenosing forms plus formation of aneurysms
6) ectatic forms.

Autopsy statistics. In order to define the general representation of brain infarcts in autopsy cases the following figures will be interesting: FOIX et al. (1927) found – after exclusion of embolism – in 63 cases of infarcts that 25% had occlusion or severe stenosis and more than 50% a partial narrowing. An excellent review article of the most important papers of the laboratory and neurological wards of FOIX has been given by MISCH (1929). MOOSSY (1966a, b) in 2650 brain dissections found that 527 (19.8%) contained areas of encephalomalacia out of which there were 58 (2.2%) with recent, 84 (3.1%) with recent and old, and 385 (14.5) with old softening. In 55% of 142 cases suitable for that study a thrombus was demonstrated in an anatomically appropriate artery while, in the other cases, no thrombus was observed. No attempt was made in these cases to assess the pathogenesis. C.M. FISHER et al. (1965a) observed in 178 unselected autopsy cases, 16 with one or more total vascular occlusions in the neck, 16 intracranially, and of the remainder about 40% showed some degree of vascular stenosis. Further general frequency data are obtained from the papers of R. ADAMS and VAN DER EECKEN (1953): from

740 brains 17.4% had infarcts; YATES and HUTCHINSON (1961): 35%; HICKS and WARREN (1951): 33% with cerebral infarcts.

PRIBRAM (1963) found on *angiographic* examination of 170 patients with suspected cerebrovascular lesions, 84 instances of extracranial arterial stenosis and 64 instances of intracranial stenosis. Postmortem angiographic studies (STEIN et al., 1962) reveal that 28% of the cases had stenosis of more than 50% of the intracranial arteries; nine patients with neurological symptoms had stenosis of 100%. In ZÜLCH's morphological series of 329 infarcts, KLEIHUES et al. (1964) found 137 cases with occlusions.

However, the most striking results in this respect were published by BRUETSCH (1955); BRUETSCH and WILLIAMS (1959) who found among 20 atherosclerotic brains no instance of thrombosis as cause of the softenings and pointed out that apparently sometimes adherent coagulated blood, which histologically is no true thrombus, is often mistaken as such (see also CRONQVIST, 1969; CRONQVIST et al., 1965; PRIBRAM, 1961). CASTAIGNE et al. (1970) in assessing the cause for a stroke in 50 cases encountered 60% thromboses and 21% emboli.

b) Formal Pathogenesis of the Atherosclerotic Process

Atherosclerosis is an arterial disease which is thought to be influenced by many factors: nutritional and trophic, hemodynamic, genetic, immunologic, dysmetabolic, endocrinologic and enzymatic and even psychological factors have been suggested. The morphological and clinical risk factors will be discussed in detail below (see pp. 50 and 110).

Such ideas first started in the 1880's with the classical theory of ROKITANSKI (1852, 1856) that blood elements infiltrate the vessel wall; the accumulation of fibrin components and platelets was described by BIZZOZERO (1882) before the beginning of this century. His antagonist VIRCHOW (1856) had emphasized that lipids probably infiltrated the arterial wall and compromised the endothelium; the fibrin was located beneath the vessel endothelium and therefore probably had a local origin. According to him the process started during a cellular exudative inflammation, BIZZOZERO (1882), however, although clearly depicting the apposition of platelets, never had his interpretation generally accepted in general pathology. For long time the whole discussion on the genesis of atherosclerosis was in the hands of the German school of pathologists (MARCHAND, 1902; MÖNCKEBERG, 1914; THOMA, 1914; HUECK, 1920; BÜCHNER, 1960, 1964; BREDT, 1961; DOERR, 1964 etc.).

The various and somewhat contradictory concepts of different schools concerning the pathogenesis of atherosclerosis will not be discussed here. Relatively complete information may easily be obtained from the books of RATSCHOW (1959), SCHETTLER (1961), JONES (1970), STEHBENS (1972), HEBERER et al. (1974). The general concept of the German school of pathologists is best described by BREDT (1961).

In any current discussion of the pathogenesis of atherosclerosis the following factors should be mentioned:

a) the role of metabolic factors
b) increase of lipoproteins in the blood
c) aggregation of platelets
d) increased intrusion of plasma proteins into the arterial wall, caused by hypertension, anoxia, toxins or an increase of amines stemming from platelets
e) decrease of metabolism of cells within the media
f) proliferation of media cells
g) accumulation of lipoproteins and ensuing necrosis of media cells (GOFMAN et al., 1956; WISSLER, 1974, 1977).

Russell ROSS, one of the leading researchers in experimental atherosclerosis has examined the three main components (ROSS and GLOMSET, 1973; ROSS et al., 1979), (1) proliferation of intima cells, (2) increase of connective tissue, (3) deposition of fat. Step one – according to his concept – is injury of endothelium at particular sites with attraction of platelets. Substances "released" from these platelets are able to stimulate the underlying smooth muscle cells, particularly if the "injury" is chronic. The proliferation of smooth muscle cells in culture is not stimulated by cell-free blood serum, a mitogenic protein derived from platelets being necessary for this purpose. It was proved subsequently that this platelet-derived growth factor was also necessary in subhuman primates whose arteries were "injured" experimentally by a mechanical lesion and placed on a high cholesterol diet. Inhibition of platelet function was one means of preventing the formation of atherosclerotic lesions. Prevention of endothelial lesions, inhibition of platelet function and the invention of an inhibition to the mitogenic action of the platelet-derived protein presumably would help to protect humans as well from atherosclerosis.

MOOSSY's (1971) concept of pathogenesis considered the following steps: fatty infiltration → fibrous plaque → thrombosis. His belief was that the lipids were formed intrinsically in the wall – as VIRCHOW (1856) suggested – and did not come from the blood stream.

Those who have followed the concepts of the pathogenetic significance of nutrition in atherosclerosis will recall that these have changed considerably during the last three decades. This also becomes quite apparent in assessment of the Framingham study, the recommendations of which have also changed considerably.

Over a period of time, cholesterol, saturated fatty acids, carbohydrates and particularly a high caloric diet were accused of promoting atherosclerosis. These concepts were recently discussed critically by H. KAUNITZ (Columbia University, 1977). The author came to the drastic conclusion that "longterm studies in man for testing the serum cholesterol-lowering action of the "unsaturated" vegetable oils include serious errors of method and permit no confirmed conclusions."

Modern research tries to clarify certain features of this concept. Two patients (METTINGER et al., 1977) admitted for carotid surgery were given 100–150 μCi of ^{125}I-fibrogen preoperatively. Various parts of removed plaque material were submitted to scintillation counting. The activity in ulcerated regions was twice as high as in non-ulcerated regions. In a pilot study of five cases it was concluded that ^{125}I is not suitable for external detection by scintigraphy. Further studies using ^{125}I-labeled fibrinogen showed external detection by gamma camera to be possible, at least in some cases. Additional studies using isotope-labeled platelets are now in progress.

The modern concept of atherosclerosis was first put forward by DUGUID (1948, 1952), who postulated an appositional thrombus of platelets at the beginning of the process, as first discussed and illustrated by BIZZOZERO as early as 1882. One can describe the process in detail as follows:

Atherosclerosis begins with a lesion of the endothelial cells and thereby the subendothelial connective tissue consisting mainly of collagenous fibers is exposed to invasion by "low density" lipids. This endothelial lesion can, however, be transient and reversible, but when certain "risk factors" (see p. 50) or other causes come into play, the lesion may be more protracted. Next, it appears that blood platelets settle on this lesion to form an appositional platelet thrombus. During the dissolution of the platelets amines will be liberated. If plasma proteins invade under the intima, muscle cells of the media will begin to proliferate and enter the zone of the proteins, and then a mixed plaque consisting of lipids, proteins and cells will be formed. This is the first step in the development of atherosclerosis. R. ROSS et al. (1979) speak of amines stemming from the platelets and bringing the smooth muscle cells into proliferation.

However, the physical chemist BÖTTCHER/Leiden (1965) and BÖTTCHER et al. (1959) are of the opinion that there is no infiltration of lipids, but rather synthesis in situ (see VIRCHOW, 1856). They have developed the very important concept that there are probably several types of atherosclerosis, which differ in the qualitative and quantitative composition of the spectrum of lipids, phosphatides and acid mucopolysaccharides and, moreover, that these chemical differences determine the type and site of the atherosclerosis as it may develop in the aorta or the coronary arteries in one individual and in the cerebral arteries in another (see p. 52ff.).

α) *Mechanical Factors in the Origin of Atherosclerosis*

Local predilection. As in all other organs, the brain has predilection sites for atherosclerosis. However, according to ROBERTS (1977), this is only slightly demonstrable in the heart although there may be a local tendency for a major stenosis, for instance in the left coronary artery 2 cm after dividing into the two major branches. But we also find that there are marked discre-

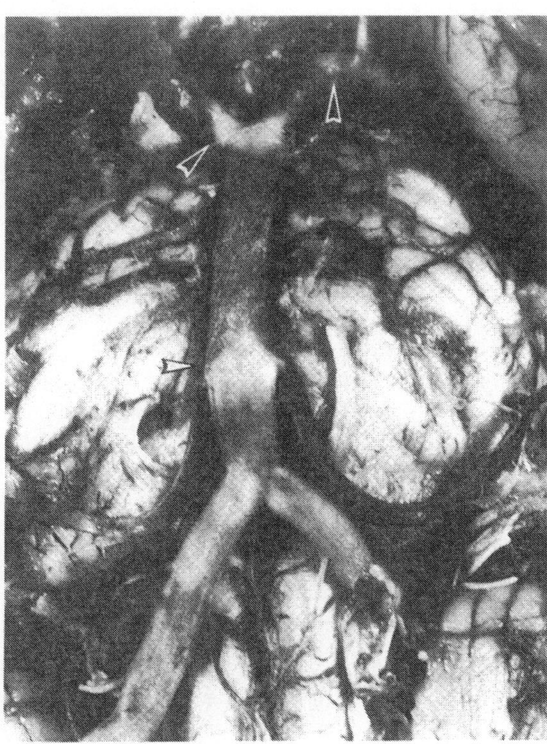

Fig. 45. Vertebro-basilar system showing atherosclerosis at the predilection sites; branching into the posterior inferior and superior cerebellar artery, middle segment of basilar at origin of anterior inferior cerebellar artery, atherosclerotic plaques also at the origin of posterior communicating artery *(arrows)*

pancies. In the intracranial arterial circulation for instance, there can be a stenosing atherosclerosis down to the level of the "meningeal anastomoses", but virtually rarely any further (see, however, Binswanger's disease; p. 67). This statement can be partly explained by the correlation of atherosclerosis with the size of the lumen.

However, it may be noted occasionally that there is a predominant involvement of the arteries at the base of the brain with exclusion of the carotids, or marked atherosclerosis of one or both intracranial carotid arteries, without involvement of the vertebrobasilar system. Patchy atherosclerosis (Figs. 2, 45) may be encountered or the process may have a fairly even distribution (Fig. 10).

The *first manifestations* of atherosclerosis visible to the naked eye are in the large cervical arteries, where they appear as "fatty streaks" (see Moossy, 1971, Fig. 105-12), they are particularly marked by a "staircase" pattern. This is due probably to specific mechanical factors (turbulence?) between the vertebrae, which tend to promote atherosclerotic plaques. The first plaque in the intracranial arteries is seen at the bifurcation (Figs. 36, 45) of the basilar artery (see Zülch, 1962a, Figs. 5 and 6), and may be mainly fibrotic, but shortly thereafter (as in the fatty streaks) lipoproteins also will infiltrate (see the histochemical study of H.H. Hoff, 1972).

"Mechanical factors" (Krafka, 1937) mentioned in the literature include: A "shearing effect" (Allbutt, 1915), a "loosening of connective tissue" (Virchow, 1856; Aschoff, 1925, 1939), "mechanical strain", "pulsatile stress" (Azuma and Fukushima, 1979), "suction-like action", "converging boundaries", "branching", bifurcations", "abrupt curvatures", "fixation of arteries" etc. (Thoma, 1914, 1920, 1923; and recently Blumenthal et al., 1954), "fixation of arteries" (Lauda, 1921; Doerfler, 1935; Dei Poli and Zucha, 1940), "missing movements (gymnastics)" (Oberndorfer, 1911), "physical factors" (in 5031 cases Resch et al., 1970).

Stehbens (1959) studied in serial sections the turbulence of flow in glass models as well as (1965) the arterial bifurcations in sheep and steers. In the latter investigation he found intimal proliferation at specific sites. In steers only traces of lipids could be demonstrated whereas in sheep, spontaneous lipid deposition occurred in the intimal thickenings. In comparing these findings with human pathology it would suggest that intimal thickenings and sites of predilection like the "face" and the "dorsum" of arteries are universal in mammals having blood vessels of comparable size. The plaques in the apex (carina) are probably extensions of the facial and dorsal thickenings.

This is consistent with the findings of TEXON (1960, 1963; TEXON et al., 1960) in a published study of 100 brains at autopsy where the predilection of atherosclerotic lesions corresponded to the exact sites determined by the laws of fluid mechanics. These were:

1) tapering vessels with decrease of lateral pressure (suction)
2) areas of curvature with decrease along the inner curvature
3) branchings and bifurcations with a relative decrease in lateral pressure at the medial walls
4) areas of external attachment with predilection for the "dorsal wall". These areas of predilection, in correspondence with theoretical hydrodynamics, corroborate the concept that hemodynamics play the primary role in the etiology and pathogenesis of local atherosclerosis (see also FRIEDE, 1962).

β) Hemodynamics and Turbulence

Intracranial atherosclerosis develops primarily in the arteries within the confines of the basal cisterns, in which the large pulsating arteries lie free. There they are surrounded by the spinal fluid but are not protected by the neighboring brain tissue; indeed, WILLIS (1954) considers this to be one of the important factors for the manifestation of atherosclerosis. However, this seems erroneous since the internal carotid artery will be most markedly involved by atherosclerosis within the bony canal, a fact which is denied by WILLIS (1954) contrary to DEI POLI and ZUCHA (1940). According to the latter authors, atherosclerosis in this segment is of grade 5.6 on their scale of 24, but according to angiographic findings this is probably too low a grade (see Figs. 100–104 in KAUTZKY et al., 1976).

Unfortunately local predilection of atherosclerosis in the cerebral arteries thus far has been studied insufficiently and has been described only globally (BAKER et al., 1967; BOTTON, 1955a, b; D.R. DOW, 1925; EROS, 1951; LANZA, 1938; LIEBEGOTT, 1959; MOOSSY, 1971; STEHBENS, 1965; WILLIS, 1954; ZÜLCH, 1961a, 1971b, c).

In this concept of the pathogenesis of atherosclerosis the primary endothelial lesion plays the important role. But which were the compromising factors? The fact that cerebral atherosclerosis shows a remarkable tendency for predilection sites (see p. 41ff.) and that these locations correspond to certain features in flow – namely to turbulence? – has led to an interest in the particular local hemodynamics within the arteries.

We should investigate therefore those regional factors which promote the formation of atherosclerotic lesions in the "four brain vessels". Atherosclerosis develops especially in places which are hemodynamically unstable. This development is probably provoked by turbulence in the blood stream, which produces the endothelial lesions and the accumulation of platelets on the vessel wall.

Hemodynamic considerations suggest that pressure is exerted by the pulsatile blood stream on the convex wall of a curvature. On the concave side of the curve however, the pressure is low and in addition there is probably a certain degree of "turbulence". This deviation from laminar blood flow is supposed to be responsible for the manifestation of atherosclerosis on the concave side of a curve (TEXON, 1960, 1963, TEXON et al., 1960; DROPMAN, 1963; KIKUCHI et al., 1973, Fig. 3). Correspondingly, at a bifurcation, atherosclerosis will be seen on the inner wall of the curves or directly at the carina i.e. the dividing point of the two branches. The atherosclerotic process which occurs near orifices of branches has been explained by the fact that the waves of dilation and contraction of the free wall are dampened at the relatively fixed orifices (LEARY, 1936). Whether atheromas really form on the inner surface of a curving vessel (TEXON, 1960, 1963, TEXON et al., 1960; O. HASSLER, 1961) was doubted by C.M. FISHER et al. (1965a), but SAKO (1962) and WESOLOWSKI et al. (1965) subscribed to this theory of turbulence.

There seems to be a direct linear relation between the radius of an artery and the degree of atherosclerosis (BLUMENTHAL et al., 1954).

AZUMA and FUKUSHIMA (1979) were able to show patterns of turbulence in tubes with axisymmetric or eccentric constriction, both in steady and pulsatile flow. There was a definite relation of the formation of vortices at a certain distance from the obstacle. These were then broken down into turbulence. Intensity of turbulence was far greater in pulsatile than in steady flow (pulsatile flow is probably still present in the arteries within the basal-cisterns). His excellent film proves this concept. The effects of turbulence and hypertension were studied by SAKO (1962) and found to be additive factors in the production of experimental atherosclerosis.

The laws of circulation within the brain arteries are fairly complex and cannot be derived only from the theoretical laws of fluid mechanics since the stream in the cerebral arteries is still pulsatile proximally. On the other hand the circulation is physiologically steady, since there is only very little increase of local circulation with an increase in function (LASSEN et al., 1978: 20%; LENIGER-FOLLERT and K.-A. HOSSMANN, 1979: more than 60%). This is in contrast to the muscle arteries (five times) or the coronary arteries, where we encounter a 20 fold increase in circulation at the time of highest functional demand. Moreover, there is a decisive difference in the smaller coronary arteries and arterioles which are "squeesed" in systole, so that flow within them almost ceases.

γ) Special Site of Involvement of Various Arteries

MOOSSY (1959) found the earliest involvement by atherosclerosis in the carotid and vertebral arteries, followed by the basilar and middle cerebral vessels. The anterior cerebral and cerebellar arteries showed less frequent and less extensive involvement. The posterior inferior cerebellar (Wallenberg's) artery was the earliest of the cerebellar vessels affected and it was usually more severely involved than the others.

MOOSSY (1959) observed that aortic lesions were first evident with fatty streaks in the first decade, that coronary lesions became evident in the second decade and cerebral artery involvement in the third.

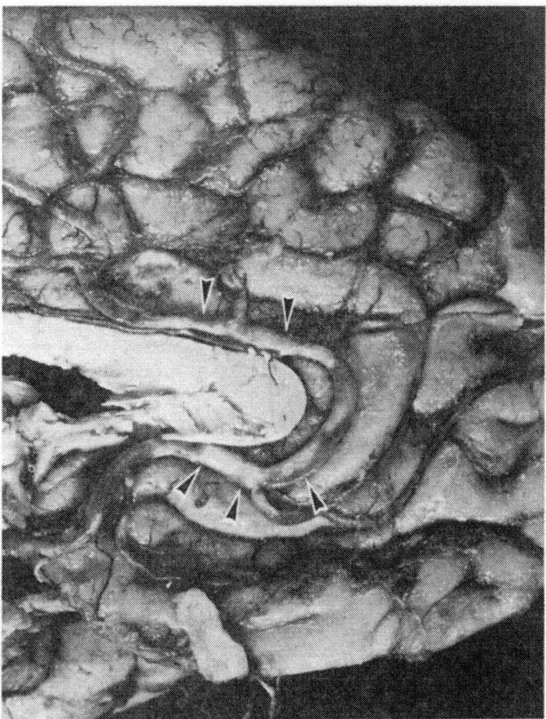

Fig. 46. The predilection sites for atherosclerosis in the anterior cerebral artery are visible. The most prominent changes have occurred below and above the rostrum corporis callosi (*arrows*)

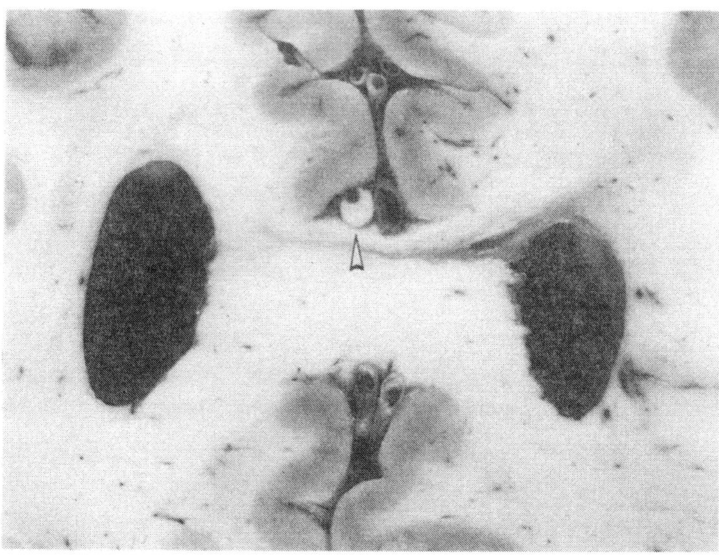

Fig. 47. Eccentric atherosclerosis with high grade narrowing of the lumen of the left pericallosal artery just distal to its point of division. View from in front of a slice of brain

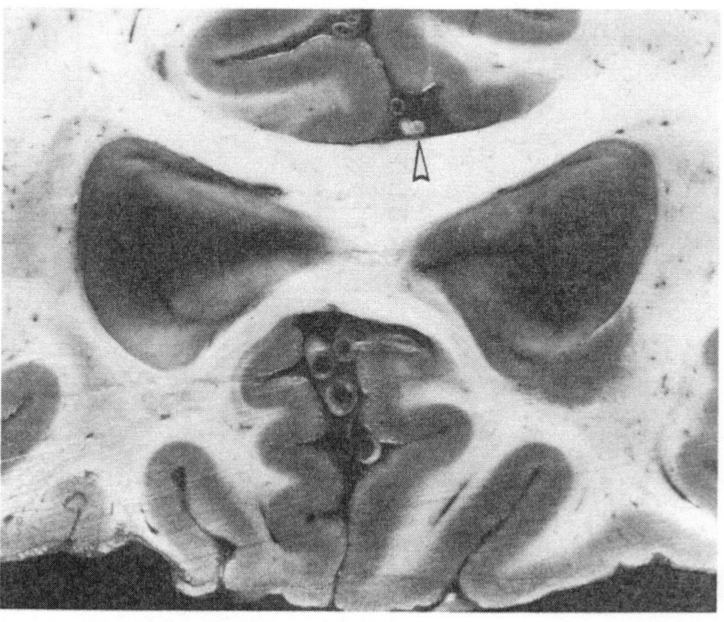

Fig. 48. Only mild stenosing atherosclerosis in the dividing branches of the anterior cerebral artery. An epicallosal artery above the rostrum shows an old thrombosis in process of organization

The carotid stumps, the junctions between the vertebral arteries and the proximal and middle section of the basilar artery (Figs. 35, 40) are typical sites of primary arterial involvement. Although these sites may be involved early in the course of the disease, they do not necessarily severely stenose throughout its course. Most often, severe stenosis occurs in the anterior and posterior cerebral arteries as they curve around the genus corporis callosi or the cerebral peduncles respectively and in the middle cerebral artery during its course along the lesser sphenoid wing.

In the *anterior* cerebral artery the main plaque is located more frequently at the lower part of the curve around the rostrum than in the upper part (Figs. 46–49). Occasionally both locations are involved (Fig. 46). The frequently observed eccentric plaque (Fig. 47) favors the inward sections

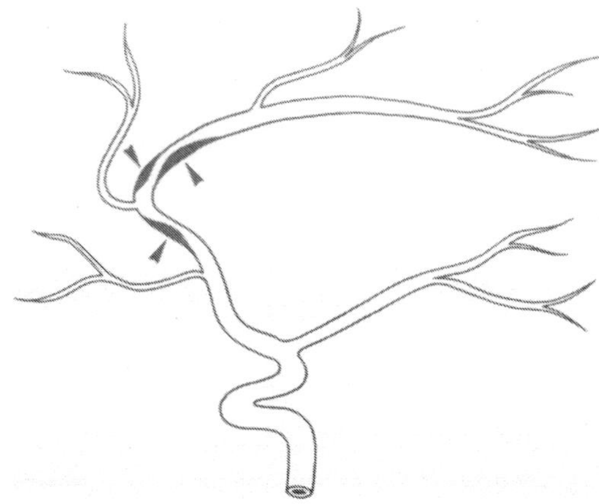

Fig. 49. The most frequent types of stenosis of the anterior cerebral artery at the rostrum

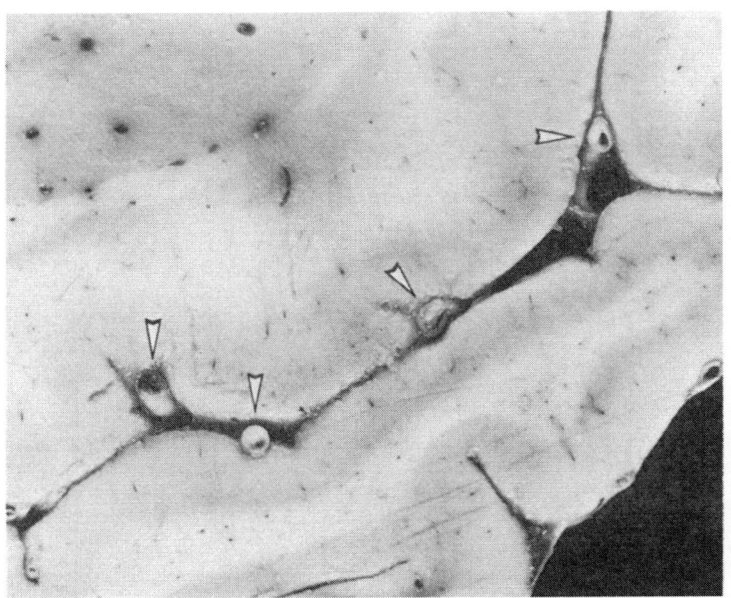

Fig. 50. Marked atherosclerosis in smaller arteries of the Sylvian fissure *(arrows)*

of the curve (ZÜLCH, 1961 a, Fig. 31; 1971 c, Fig. 22). Multiple plaques resembling a string of pearls are rarely encountered, but demonstrated at magnification angiography (KAUTZKY, ZÜLCH et al., 1976, Fig. 124).

In the atherosclerotic process the middle cerebral arteries may be involved at four sites (Figs. 50–52):

1) 5–15 mm beyond their origin from the internal carotid artery, but still proximal to origin of the striate arteries (Figs. 51 a, 53)
2) the plaque may extend to the point of origin of the striate arteries whereby either only the medial (Fig. 51 b) or
3) both groups of the striate arteries are occluded (Fig. 51 c)
4) the plaque lies at the branching into the candelabra arteries (Fig. 51 d).

The first and the last localization provide the best opportunity for preservation of the brain tissue supplied by the middle cerebral artery subject to the adequacy of the anastomotic retrograde supply.

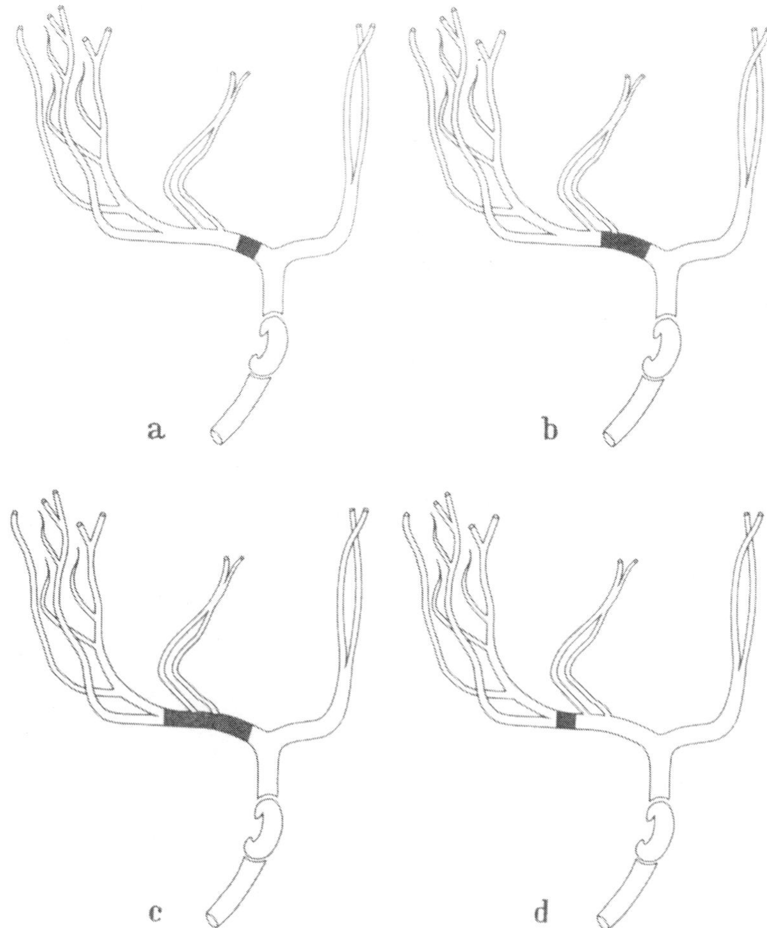

Fig. 51. The four predilection sites of stenosis or occlusion of the middle cerebral artery

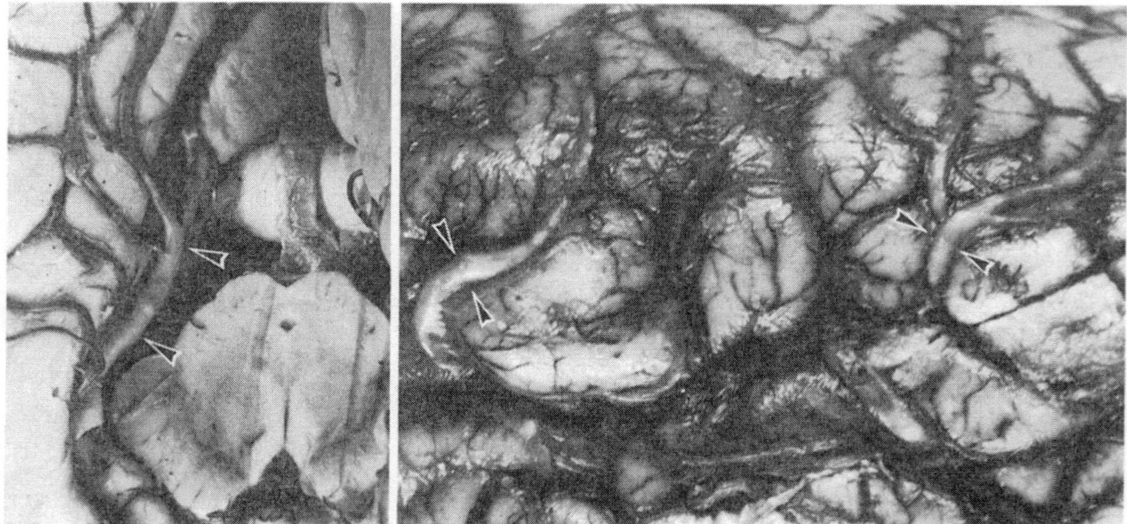

Fig. 52. *Right:* Pronounced distal type of atherosclerosis: one recognizes the arteries of the first distribution extending out of the Sylvian fissure onto the convexity. They are severely altered by stenosing atherosclerosis *(arrows)*. *Left:* Mainly proximal type of atherosclerosis in which the changes cease when the posterior cerebral artery leaves the cisterns *(arrows)*

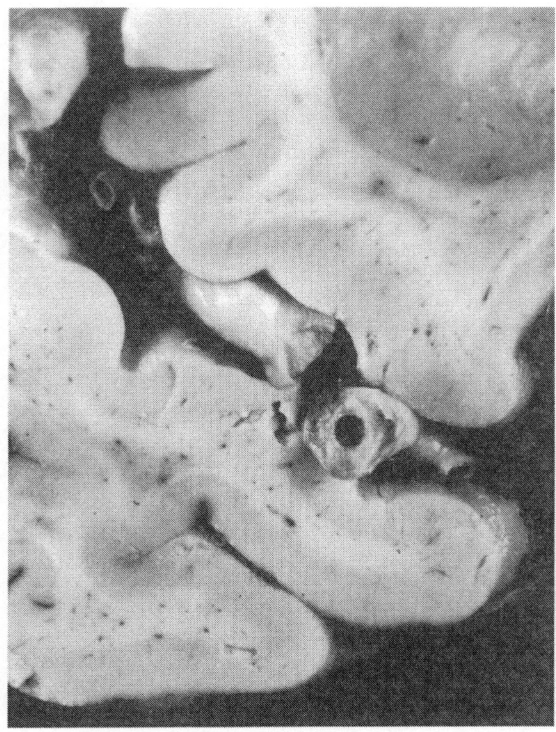

Fig. 53

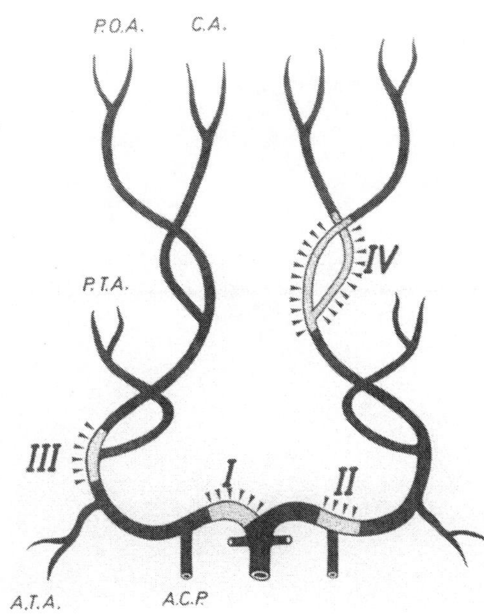

Fig. 54

Fig. 53. A predilection site for atherosclerosis in the middle cerebral artery is situated 1–2 cm beyond its origin (here: a concentric plaque of $1^1/_2$ cm length narrowing its lumen by 70%)

Fig. 54. The four main types of stenosis and occlusion of the posterior cerebral arteries: I proximal, II intermediate, III peduncular, IV distal type

In the *posterior* cerebral artery also four different locations of the stenosing plaque are recognized (LECHTAPE-GRÜTER, 1978) (Figs. 52, 54):

1) directly at or shortly after the origin, whereby the posterior communicating artery is not compromized (Fig. 54 I), or
2) more distantly directly at the origin of the posterior communicating artery, e.g. 1 to 2 cm from its origin (Fig. 54 II), or
3) a distal plaque is encountered at the end of the curve around the cerebral peduncle (Fig. 54 III). More commonly the plaque lies eccentrically (ZÜLCH, 1971c, Figs. 19, 22)
4) The last involvement lies at the points of branching as in the middle cerebral artery (Fig. 54 IV).

The vertebral artery. A stenosing plaque is seen very frequently at the point of perforation of the dura where a poststenotic dilation is very marked and the lumen sometimes aneurysmatic (Fig. 55). The differences in caliber of these arteries have been described above (p. 4, Fig. 1). A stenosing plaque or even an occlusion is not infrequently seen beyond the origin of the posterior inferior cerebellar artery. RESCH et al. (1970) on the other hand, reported that the basilar artery is more frequently involved.

The basilar artery shows two sites of predilection for stenosing atherosclerosis. The first is at the branching into the or superior cerebellar and posterior cerebral arteries (Figs. 2, 3, 55) but this is more frequently fibrotic and less stenosing. Stenosis characterizes plaque formation in the middle segment of the basilar artery (Figs. 35, 40, 55). Any malformation (see p. 4, Fig. 2) is liable

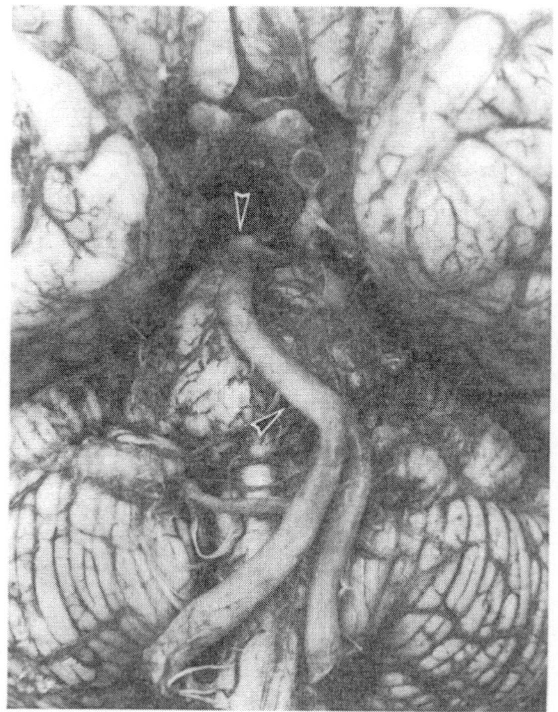

Fig. 55

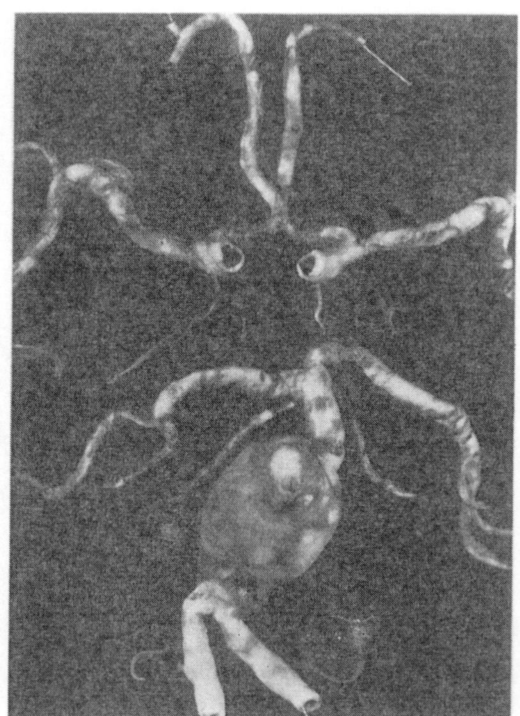

Fig. 56

Fig. 55. Atherosclerosis is only seen at the branching point of the basilar artery and above its origin from the vertebrals where the anterior inferior cerebellar artery originates. There is, however, ectasia, lengthening and marked tortuosity *(arrows)*

Fig. 56. Panatherosclerosis of the circle of Willis and the six great cerebral arteries. The posterior communicating arteries are very narrow. They were also compromised so that an anastomotic function in vivo was very unlikely. Large aneurysm of the basilar artery

to give rise to plaques (Fig. 2). With a severe degree of atherosclerosis the artery (Fig. 56) can produce an impression into the pons (Fig. 44). It is in this middle segment that aneurysms occur. The *ectatic* type of atherosclerosis is, from our experience, more marked in the vertebrobasilar system than in carotid arteries. The distal vertebral and the basilar artery may become dilated and elongated up to the formation of a *megadolicho-basilar artery* (GREITZ and LÖFSTEDT, 1954; BOERI and PASSERINI, 1964; SACKS and LINDENBERG, 1969). The elongated segment of the vertebral artery usually swings over to the side of the more hypoplastic partner (Fig. 44), sometimes by as much as several centimeters (ESCHBACH and ZÜLCH, 1969; METZINGER, 1971; KAUTZKY, ZÜLCH et al., 1976). It may extend up to the height of the foramen of Monroe.

In *the carotid artery*, although the same ectatic and lengthening process occurs as in the vertebrobasilar system, only rarely is a megadolicho-carotid artery formed which may extend similarly up to the height of the foramen of Monroe. The range of the stenosing process has been described by DEI POLI and ZUCHA (1940), HUTCHINSON and YATES (1956), MARTIN et al. (1960), WHISNANT et al. (1961) and STEIN et al. (1962).

The carotid *siphon* shows atherosclerosis in its supra- or infraclinoidal segments with three predilection sites, namely (Fig. 57):

a) proximal to the origin of the ophthalmic artery
b) when piercing the dura and
c) most frequently and markedly in the distal (cisternal) segment (see KAUTZKY, ZÜLCH et al., 1976, Figs. 100–104).

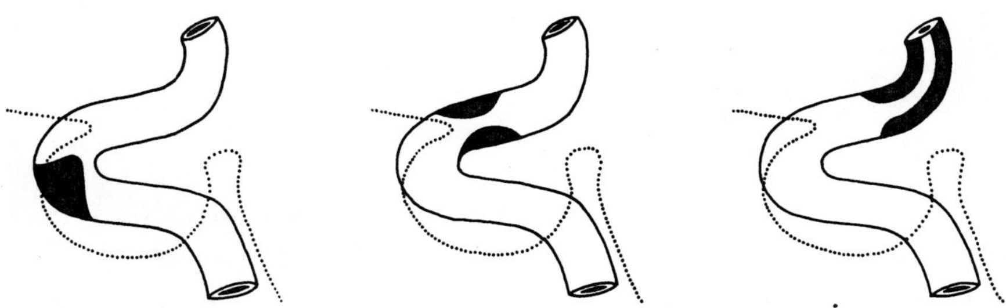

Fig. 57. Predilection site for stenosis in the carotid siphon segments

Atherosclerosis of the *circle of Willis* has been studied by BAKER and IANONE (1959a) and NUUTILA (1973) and is dependant upon the general type of lesions at the base. Together with the proximal segments of the large cerebral arteries it has formed the basis of grading. Stenosis is not infrequent at the origin of the posterior communicating arteries.

δ) Summary of General Rules for the Local Development of Atherosclerosis

If we apply the laws of hemodynamics to the cerebral arterial tree the following morphological locations may be considered in that regard:

1) The *origin* of arteries, the most prominent example being the stenosing atherosclerosis at the origin of the vertebral artery from the subclavian.
2) The formation of *curves* and *bends*:
   a) at the anterior cerebral artery as it swings around the rostrum of the corpus callosum (Figs. 47/49),
   b) at the middle cerebral artery around the lesser wing of the sphenoid bone (Fig. 53),
   c) at the posterior cerebral artery around the cerebral peduncle (Figs. 52 below, 54).
3) The *mechanical fixation* of an artery to surrounding structures:
   a) of the vertebral artery at the entrance to the vertebral column (C 6), and in the foramina costotransversaria.
   In the intravertebral course of the vertebral artery fatty streaks are formed at each cervical bony segment ("ladder-effect") by strangulation (see also MOOSSY, 1971, Fig. 105-12),
   b) of the vertebral artery at the perforation of the dura in the posterior fossa,
   c) the strangulation of the posterior cerebral artery by the oculomotor nerve (Fig. 39),
   d) the siphon of the carotid in its bony bed.
4) The *branchings* or *bifurcations* which impede the circulation in the new branch during the pulse beat, e.g. at bifurcation of large arteries such asthe basilar artery where it branches into the posterior cerebral arteries or superior cerebellar arteries the first intracranial atherosclerotic plaque is formed (see p. 4ff., Figs. 2, 3 and Fig. 36), the common carotid artery at its bifurcation in the neck or more rarely, at its origin from the aorta.

Concentric atherosclerosis is seen as a product of a "converging boundary" lesion, whereas "branch" and "curvature" lesions tend to become *eccentric*. In bifurcation, "Y" or "crotch" lesions the medial walls are preferred in the production of atherosclerosis. "Attachment" lesions have a predilection for the "dorsal wall". These general laws have been deduced from cardiac pathology (TEXON, 1957) but correspond fairly well to what we have observed in the brain vessels.

Usually atherosclerosis stops when the arteries are leaving cisterns (Fig. 52 left; proximal type). Rarely atherosclerosis is extended beyond the cisterns to the convexity (Fig. 52) right of the brain.

II. Epidemiology and Geographic Pathology – Risk Factors of Atherosclerosis

1. Epidemiology – Geographic Pathology

Intensive studies on the incidence and frequency of cerebral atherosclerosis in various geographic (McGill, 1968) and ethnic populations are being undertaken in order to isolate the important pathogenetic factors which would explain the gross differences in atherosclerotic involvement in various regions and populations (Baker et al., 1967). We know now that probably geographic location, climate, economic and social status, but also racial and ethnic factors may exert a marked influence on the atherosclerotic process. Clinical studies may even more definitely point to pronounced differences in population groups and ethnic communities since outer – social – variables may play a pronounced role in the *clinical outcome*. The radiologist, however, may be more interested in the morphological studies of the vasculature in autopsy material, for instance Hutchinson and Yates (1956) and C.M. Fisher (1965c). Here the greater weight must be given to those series based on a large number of cases (Resch and Baker, 1964: 3839 cases; Baker et al., 1967: 5035 cases, in contrast to Hannah, 1958, who investigated – understandably – only 42 cases in the Bantu tribe.

The methods of assessment of atherosclerosis are also of importance (Gore and Tejada, 1957; Daoud et al., 1962; Wanscher et al., 1951). The most reliable and most frequently-used grading and recording system is that of the World Federation of Neurology (Baker et al., 1967, page 687) which we have also used (Grade I–IV, "A"-concentric and "B"-eccentric situation of the stenosing lesion, see pp. 31, 35).

A blind study and screening by several investigators was adopted for control. Since most studies suggest that atherosclerosis is extremely infrequent in Orientals, Baker, Resch and many co-workers compared a large Minnesota population with a Japanese population where at the circle of Willis, at least, atherosclerotic lesions in the American white population were as severe as in the Asiatic. Yet, morphological and angiographic studies showed a greater involvement of the smaller vessels by atherosclerosis (hyalinosis?) in a Japanese autopsy group of 375 cases as compared with the Minnesota population (Resch et al., 1969). Even more so (Resch, 1972) this seemed to be true of an endogenous Israeli population (see also Kameyama and Okinaka, 1963; Kurland, 1958a, b, 1966, 1971; Kurtzke, 1969; Yates, 1966; Yates and Hutchinson, 1961; see also for atherosclerosis in the Japanese Nakamura et al., 1976a, b; Kikuchi et al., 1973).

Most studies suggest, that atherosclerosis is extremely rare among Orientals (Oppenheim's study (1925) of Shanghai Chinese). Foster (1927) reported a low incidence of atherosclerosis among 4000 Chinese with no cases of angina pectoris. More recent figures are not available due to the smaller number of autopsies performed nowadays (at the most 10%–15%). Furthermore, on my recent visit to Chinese hospitals (1978, 1979) an exact figure of atherosclerosis could not be assessed.

The following statement is very important. Of the three major causes of death in Japan "stroke" ranks first, followed by cancer and heart disease, a correlation which is the reverse of that seen in the western world (Kimura, 1977). Apparently hypertension among other factors relates closely to development of stroke and ischemic heart disease in Japan. The data from China appear to be similar.

Gross differences are encountered between the African population in Nigeria (Williams and Wilson, 1962; Williams et al., 1963; Williams et al., 1975), where the prevalence and severity of atherosclerosis is said to be surprisingly low, and the Blacks of America who are ethnologically related to West Africans. The American Blacks, however, had a degree of involvement similar to that of the Minnesota whites. In the more primitive parts of Africa atherosclerosis in the aorta and coronary arteries seems to be conspicuously lower than in the West, and similarly in the Central American and Caribbean States. South American peoples on the other hand appear to be subject to a more severe involvement. According to the observations of BAKER's group (BAKER et al., 1973) the atherosclerotic process within Norway, Denmark, Germany, Czechoslovakia and Poland (MOSSAKOWSKI et al., 1964) was without any marked differences, however, it was higher in German and Finnish populations. Russia apparently has a lower atherosclerosis index. Italians are said to have a higher involvement in the aorta and coronary arteries than in the cerebral vessels. The frequency of coronary atherosclerosis in the USA is similar to that reported in Italy but higher than that of other European countries (References see BAKER et al., 1967; STEHBENS, 1972). With regard to the "small vessels" the Japanese cases present more severe involvement than the Minnesota cases (RESCH et al., 1969) probably due to the high frequency of hypertension.

In the International Atherosclerosis Project the conclusion was that environmental factors were of more importance than was racial or ethnic origin. Differences were found in the aortic lesions seen in autopsy studies in New Orleans, Guatemala and Costa Rica or in the African Bantu and non-Bantu populations (MOOSSY, 1966c). However, no statements were given concerning risk factors. Therefore the results of such controlled studies – as the Framingham study – seem to weigh more in this regard although autopsy control is still scare and the full importance is in the problem of morbidity and not morphology.

KURTZKE (1969) in his provocative comment and conclusions in his comprehensive book emphasizes the following items:

1) That exclusive of subarachnoidal hemorrhage (SAH) cerebral hemorrhage constitutes about $^1/_3$ of cerebrovascular disease cases; and that nearly $^9/_{10}$ of the remainder are "cerebral thrombosis".

2) Cerebral hemorrhage and thrombosis are not related to geographically determined environmental factors, but rather occur quite uniformly within and among countries, where we have good data.

3) Cerebrovascular disease as a whole shows essentially equal occurrence in males and in females regardless of age or location. Cerebral hemorrhage too appears of equal frequency. However, for some inexplicable reason TIAs (transient ischemic attacks) are reported twice as often in males.

4) There is no racial predilection for cerebrovascular disease in American Blacks or in Japan.

NAKAYAMA (1977) came even to the conclusion, that a significant correlation existed in Japan between cigarette smoking and ischemic heart disease and that the inverse relationship between smoking and stroke was not explainable. It might even inhibit the development of stroke in hypertensive men.

Japan is an interesting model for such studies with its different life styles: "farmland type" (rice), "fishing village type" (fish) and "urban type" (similar food to the western world as for instance studied by KATSUKI and HIROTA, 1966). Strokes were seven times more common in a farming village and three times in a fishing village. It is interesting to follow the development of the incidence of strokes in Japan. According to KIMURA (1977) cerebral infarction has lead to death in 3.9/100000 persons a year in 1950 and 37.1/100000 in 1970. This is a tenfold increase in the last 20 years. (The fact "intake" showed a threefold increase in that period.) Any general conclusion cannot yet be warranted but it seems as if low levels of serum albumin and cholesterol caused by malnutrition of protein and fat constitute a low risk factor for strokes in the Japanese.

In a study of 543 autopsied cases SOLBERG (1977) found the following relations: a strong independent relationship between cerebral infarction and intracranial atherosclerosis and some weaker relationship between cerebral infarction and vertebral and coronary atherosclerosis. The relationship to other factors including hypertension was weak. There was a strong independent relationship between cerebral hemorrhage and hypertension and some weaker relationship between cerebral hemorrhage and atherosclerosis.

However, after long discussions about risk factors in atherosclerosis the divergences are expressed by the phrase of the Symposium "Atherosclerosis IV" (J.P. STRONG, 1977, pp. 671–674):

"The major questions remaining are:

a) What fraction of the variability in the extent of atherosclerosis in humans can be explained

by knowledge of known risk factors such as age, sex, race, serum lipid levels, blood pressure levels, cigarette smoking habits, and measure of obesity, glucose tolerance, and physical activity?
b) What is the cause or what are the causes of the remaining variability?
c) Are there other risk factors, as yet unknown, for atherosclerosis?" (End of STRONG's citation).

5) Hypertension, coronary artery disease, and thromboembolic cerebrovascular disease are three essentially unrelated entities.

6) Hemorrhage and thrombosis are "endogenous" rather than "exogenous" disease. There is nothing apparent in the macroclimate that can be manipulated to alter their frequency. Even in the microclimate the author could not find good evidence that the control of hypertension and diabetes alters the occurrence of non-hemorrhagic stroke (KURTZKE, 1969).

The most dramatic factor in cerebrovascular disease is its relationship to age, which is one of a logarithmic increase (for the latter see also RESCH and BAKER, 1964, Figs. 2 and 3).

It is evident that epidemiological studies are devoted less commonly to the morphological phenomenon of atherosclerosis than to the clinical pathogenesis and risk factors of stroke. The available data therefore depend on whether they come from general population samples, hospitalized cases or autopsy material (KANNEL, 1971). Even the epidemiological studies are hampered by the undefined non-uniform criteria for "stroke" and the inability to distinguish between the major stroke entities [DAWBER, 1975; DAWBER et al., 1977; ADLER, 1969; STEHBENS, 1972; World Health statistics, 1947–1950, 1958; the Framingham Study (see DAWBER, KANNEL etc.), and the Thule Symposium/Sweden, 1967].

For example in his summary, ADLER (1969) includes the following facts for stroke in Israel:
1) Embolism is far more frequent among Oriental Jews.
2) Thrombosis is diagnosed more often and hemorrhages less often than they actually occur.
3) The overall death rate seems to be lower than in the rest of the world except for the first year after the cerebral event when it is as high as it is elsewhere.
4) Females above 61 and even more particularly above 71 years show a higher mortality rate than males.

In ADLER'S (1969) series of 5486 patients hospitalized because of cerebrovascular disease 52% were males; 84% of the men and 85% of the women were over 50 years and there were slightly more males than females in each age group except over 71 years. In Israel cerebrovascular disease is the third main killer of people above 45 years. The same sex-ratio was present in the fatal cases as in the total series.

In Norway and Sweden deaths from "apoplexy" have always been slightly higher than in Denmark. In Norway an increase began in about 1945 and seemed in 1960 to be still in progress (RIISHEDE, 1967).

2. Risk Factors for Atherosclerosis

MOOSSY (1966c) emphasizes that all investigations on the epidemiology and the risk factors for atherosclerosis are difficult to compare (owing to differences in terms, concepts and methods). *One has to distinguish risk factors promoting atherosclerosis and those inducing stroke.* Hypertension allegedly (BAKER et al., 1969) may promote atherosclerosis in the cerebral vessels but this occurs probably more often in combination with other risk factors, such as diabetes. According to our own observations hypertension definitely triggers the origin of *arteriolo*sclerosis or hyalinosis, which is the main cause of mass hemorrhages and lacunae in the brain (see p. 98). Hypertension is, however, also a prominent risk factor for "stroke", since it promotes cardiovascular insufficiency and may undergo a dramatic fall of blood pressure (hypotensive crises in the hypertensive patient! see p. 119).

Mortality rates for coronary heart disease have been falling significantly in USA, Canada, Australia. The wide differences in the incidence of *coronary heart disease* in a variety of populations (FEINLEIB, 1979) are probably partly due to personal characteristics ("risk factors") such as life styles, particularly diet, physical activity and urban stress. The most important of these "risk factors" are sex, age, high blood cholesterol levels, hypertension, cigarette smoking, glucose intolerance and obesity according to this author.

Diabetes as a risk factor for intracranial atherosclerosis was studied by ARONSON (1973) in a sub-sample of 5479 consecutive complete autopsies upon individuals 25 years of age or older. Diabetes mellitus appeared to increase the frequency of encephalomalacia, particularly in the older age groups, and did so conspicuously against a background of sustained hypertension. This observation had to be reconciled with the clinically based statement of other authors that cerebrovascular atherosclerosis as a cause of death was not more frequent in the diabetic than the non-diabetic population. ARONSON (1973) observed a vastly increased number of cerebral infarctions in the diabetic group in the form of small multiple lacunar lesions typically situated in the paramedian perforating arteries (see p. 147). The crude frequency of cerebral hemorrhage was significantly lower in the diabetic sample. Again the desire to differentiate between the risk factors for the promotion of morphological atherosclerosis or arteriolosclerosis and their sequela such as stroke is not followed.

Nutrition. Nutrition, global and specific, and consequent overweight has been put forward (KLASSEN et al., 1974; NAKAMURA et al., 1976a, b) as being a risk factor for atherosclerosis, however, this was not confirmed by BAKER et al., 1961b).

In BETZ's model (BETZ and SCHLOTE, 1979) of experimental atherosclerosis caused by transluminal electrical square wawe stimulations and cholesterol diet, the lesions showed regression, when after the end of stimulation normal diet was given (the atheromatous plaques included necrosis and calcification). On the significance of various fats in human nutrition, see H. KAUNITZ (1977) who calls them "outdated".

BÖTTCHER (1965; BÖTTCHER et al., 1959) investigated biochemically the various plaques of atherosclerosis on a broad scientific front. He claims that a "nutritional factor" has a role in the production of atherosclerosis, but that this factor is different from the factors usually incriminated (see below), and probably is due to a fault in the *individual's* metabolism of lipid and fatty acids. He has shown that in atherosclerotic plaques (whether in the aorta or the coronary of cerebral arteries) it is always possible to demonstrate an abnormal but *locally specific* individual spectrum of lipids and fatty acids. In this way, he explained how in one patient there may be a local predilection for disease of the coronary arteries, and in another, for the cerebral arteries. Thus, one can understand "familial" constitutions with predilections for stenosing atherosclerosis in different vascular territories. We know families in whom all men at the age of about fifty years die from coronary infarction or progressive cerebral atherosclerosis.

In particular, BÖTTCHER et al. (1959) found that the triglyceride content was particularly high in the coronary arteries whereas in the aorta and cerebral arteries (circle of Willis) it remained roughly the same. The amount of lipids extracted from coronary or brain arteries was extremely small. An unusual feature in the aorta was the comparatively high amount of cholesterol esters coupled with the extremely low level of free cholesterol.

In general, BÖTTCHER's concept seems plausible. It may be stated here – and will be seen later – that the topical predilection for the atherosclerotic plaques and the (later) occlusions of arteries are widely identical.

However, data of "atherothrombotic brain infarction" (ABI) may be informative though the circulatory component is included. The definite blood pressure-ABI correlations are only partly important (DAWBER et al., 1977) and the cholesterol level is much less predictable for ABI than previously believed, but a significant increase is observed in the incidence rate in the diabetic population. Obesity also is an important risk factor for ABI, whereas cigarette smoking *may* have an effect; however, all these data count for the *clinical* manifestation of ABI, not strictly for its atherosclerotic origin; *they are, as we have seen, surprisingly contradictory.*

3. Familial Incidence of Atherosclerosis

Most data on familial incidence of atherosclerosis are based on coronary patients (SCHETTLER, 1961). Familial aggregation of cerebral atherosclerosis or stroke is less well demonstrated than that of coronary atherosclerosis (BLOOR, 1972; see also the study of THOMAS and COHEN, 1955). However, although clinically single cases frequently seem to prove such influences as inheritance a statistical study seems to show genetic (familial) factors act only when the atherosclerosis occurs before the 50th year of age; in the later decades a separation of environmental and genetic factors does not seem possible (EPSTEIN and ECKHOFF, 1967; EPSTEIN, 1974).

A short investigation of the families of psychiatric patients has certainly shown that a familial predilection for cerebral atherosclerosis did not exist (CONSTANTINIDIS, 1965). Perhaps the number of probands was too small and perhaps there was a negative selection. With a positive selection (if one of the familial probands has severe cerebral atherosclerosis) the result may develop differently. A detailed study on 160 parents and 384 sibs has been made by ALTER and KLUZNIK (1972) and no great genetic risk discovered.

4. Age and Sex Distribution

Development of *cerebral* intracranial atherosclerosis starts after the 40th year of age (see RESCH and BAKER, 1964, Fig. 3), a decade later than in the coronary vessels, although we have detected the first changes in autopsies of patients aged 25. The extracranial and the intracranial parts of the vertebral artery show the same general pattern. The extracranial internal carotid and the common carotid artery have a pattern of development of atherosclerotic lesions similar to the coronary artery. The youngest patient with atherosclerotic lesions in MOOSSY's observations (1959) was a 26 year old Black female. These early lesions appeared to be sudanophilic "fatty streaks" (MOSSY, 1971). The earliest sites were the extracranial carotid and vertebral arteries (see p. 41).

Generally atherosclerosis (HOLMAN et al., 1958) may already start in childhood with aortic fatty streaks (STRONG and MCGILL jr., 1969). Basilar atherosclerosis can even be detected in the second decade of life. Women up to menopause have a marked retardation of atherosclerotic involvement but after the sixth decade of life women are said to have reached the age standard of males (RESCH and BAKER, 1964).

In autopsy populations males are affected with extracranial carotid disease more frequently, and more extensively than females between the ages of 50 and 60 (see also FLORA et al., 1968a, b: in 5033 cases). After that, atherosclerosis in females increases considerably due to the lack of protective sexual hormones following the menopause. Also structural differences in the arterial wall of males and females account for this difference in atherosclerosis proliferation. By the 9th decade, females have more atherosclerosis than males (unadjusted data). Since diabetes is strongly atherogenic beyond the fourth decade, a diabetic female will have more and more severe atherosclerosis than the diabetic male of the same age.

The Japanese autopsy group of RESCH et al. (1969) showed an earlier onset of detectable atherosclerosis than the Minnesota cases and the females a higher frequency of the disease. According to MCGILL (1968) based on 1547 sets of cerebral arteries, men have more fibrous plaques than women. General remarks on studies of age-sex distributions were made by MCMAHAN (1962).

It must be concluded that data on risk factors, age and sex predilections are still very fragmentary and often contradictory.

III. Comparison with Atherosclerosis of Other Systems – Histology of Atherosclerosis

1. Comparison of Atherosclerosis in Various Parts of the Body

Atherosclerosis of the cerebral vessels is the third most common site of manifestation in all body organs following the aorta and coronary arteries. According to some authors (BOTTON, 1955a, b) intracranial atherosclerosis is altogether rare, representing only 10%. However, more detailed data are given by HULTQVIST (1942), DEI POLI and ZUCHA (1940), DÖRFLER (1935), HUTCHINSON and YATES (1956) and BAKER et al. (1967). In the Institute of Rutishauser and Wildi, BOTTON (1955a, b) found 87 cases with involvement of the internal carotid arteries in 50% and the anterior cerebral arteries only in 19% of the instances represented. They emphasized that the highest involvement is seen in the circle of Willis with 100% in the 8th decade, however, to a lesser degree than in the coronary arteries. There is no exact correlation visible between extracranial and intracranial atherosclerosis of the brain arteries (see also the detailed study of NUUTILA, 1973).

The autopsy studies (347 cases) in atherosclerosis of ROBERTS et al. (1959a, b) show the different participation of the cerebral vessels as compared to the aorta, coronary, iliac, mesenteric and renal arteries (see their Figs. 1–7 with excellent analyses of the atherosclerosis of various vessels in the different age groups). This work support the general view that atherosclerosis increases with age and involves primarily the large arteries. The picture of the cerebral arteries was extremely variable. Most important: 30% of the patients over 70 showed no gross atherosclerotic lesions in the 12 cerebral vessels examined. At all ages, there were few lesions of the anterior cerebral artery and the anterior communicating artery but the posterior cerebral artery and vertebral artery showed somewhat more and the middle cerebral artery the most atherosclerosis. However, vertebral atherosclerosis was less severe than that in visceral arteries of the same size.

ROBERTS et al. (1979) have examined recently segments of the coronary arteries in fatal coronary disease in order to determine the site and degree of narrowing. Surprisingly the constriction was less than 25% only in one fourth to one third of the cases and this with slight differences in the various clinical types. About one third, however, was more than 75% narrowed. Isolated plaques with topographic predilection as has been considered typical for cerebrovascular ischemia were apparently rare, the majority corresponding to the generalized birch-bark or pipe-stem type (see also ROBERTS et al., 1959a, b, ROBERTS, 1977).

Very curious, and not consistent with the more modern observations, were the results of a study of 500 cases by WARTMAN (1933). He found that the most frequently involved large vessels were the cerebral arteries, followed by the heart and renal vessels. In the small vessels the spleen was most frequently involved followed in descending order by the brain, kidneys, heart and liver. On the other hand HSIEH (1967) in 204 autopsy cases adopting the standard coding system of the World Federation of Neurology observed striking dissimilarities in the degenerative changes of the brain, heart, liver and kidney arteries. Atherosclerotic changes were most frequent and severe in the kidneys, followed by brain and heart and there was a positive correlation between heart weight over 450 g (hypertension!) and changes in the cerebral and renal arteries.

It is generally believed that atherosclerosis of the cerebral arteries is strictly correlated though not by "grade" but by occurrence with that of other organs. This does not correspond, however, to our own observations. There are rare cases which have considerable cerebral atherosclerosis, while the alterations in the coronaries and aorta are not pronounced. More common are cases in which aorta, heart, and extremities have extensive, partly thrombotic atherosclerosis. We know of only one example of an all over atherosclerotic arteriopathy, with equal involvement of periphery, and that is the extreme case of diabetes mellitus. In this case, the entire intracranial vascular system of the base was transformed into a net of "macaroni" arteries, or finally the birch-bark or pipe-stem type.

Why cerebral atherosclerosis develops so differently from that in other territories is not yet clarified. There are certainly differences in the morphological pattern of the arterial wall. The general morphological particularities are: less elastic layers and material, spiral pattern of the media (!) (GÄNSHIRT, 1957), no existence of vasa vasorum. In particular the internal elastic layer in the cerebral arteries is especially well developed, the media is lacking any elastic fibers and the adventitia has only a few such fibers. Atherosclerosis is formed under the endothelium and the underlying elastic layer (see p. 54).

The relation of intima and media in the coronary arteries changes up until the twentieth year, when they become *physiologically* (ROBERTS, 1977) equal in thickness following intimal proliferation. This, however, cannot be said for the cerebral arteries.

Our own investigations (PABELICK, 1967) show that the wall of the cerebral vessels is in relation to the lumen thinner than in other organ arteries. ROBERTS (1977) emphasizes that atherosclerosis in the heart is not a "focal" process, but that in autopsies no segment of the extramural arteries will be found free from atherosclerosis. Again this is different in the intracranial arteries. Interesting is the degree of constriction or even the fact of occlusion of the three major coronary arteries. So, the 75% stenosis of one of the three may not induce insufficiency (in the field of coronary circulation we have apparently one "bonus" artery!). The three fourths stenosis seems then to be the decisive grade, in the cerebral it is the 80%–90% (BRICE et al., 1964). An extensive survey about the epidemiology of coronary atherosclerosis was presented by EPSTEIN (1977).

Atherosclerosis of the visceral arteries is described in textbooks, a recent contribution was made by HSIEH (1967). An extensive publication on atherosclerosis of the aorta may be found in the WHO Bulletin 1976.

2. Experimental Atherosclerosis – Spontaneous Atherosclerosis in Animals

The subject of experimental atherosclerosis will not be discussed here, although in recent years much weight – perhaps too much – has been put on the results of this type of research. Suffice it to mention here, as a comparison, the occurrence of spontaneous atherosclerosis in animals. Data about spontaneous atherosclerosis in most animals are still scarce (see FANKHAUSER and LUGINBÜHL, 1968; FANKHAUSER et al., 1965) because most species are only rarely investigated in the older age groups. However, atherosclerosis has been observed in aged monkeys and even more frequently in horses and pigs.

LUGINBÜHL (1966) reported on his studies in Philadelphia with a litter of old lean sows aged eight to twelve years. These animals lived without stress and, quite surprisingly, had gross stenosing atherosclerosis of the internal carotid at necropsy. It is not surprising, therefore, to find that two-thirds of the cases showed deep border zone infarcts in the forebrain such as have been described in man (see p. 131 ff.). This atherosclerosis, however, remains entirely intracranial; one never finds a trace of it in the cervical bifurcation (can this be a result of the upright posture of man and the severe rotation to which his neck is subjected?). Furthermore thrombus is never formed nor is there coating of the walls by platelets. The age of the sows at the time of natural death corresponds to from sixty to eighty years for humans. The cholesterol level lies between 60–80 and never exceeds 100 mg%. The sows have never had any overweight and had no contact with tobacco, and other chemical factors do not seem to play a role. This is in striking contrast to all the factors we consider in the genesis of atherosclerosis in man!

3. Histology of Cerebral Atherosclerosis

The microscopic appearance will be described here only in its major characteristics. It starts with the local formation (see Fig. 58) of cellular and fibrotic tissue or of a diffuse thickening of the intima associated with loss of elastic tissue in the internal elastic layer. This process may increase with the formation of multiple plaques which become infiltrated with lipids and cholesterol material. There is extensive destruction of elastica and a thinning of media. The form of these plaques may be concentric (Fig. 38) or eccentric (Fig. 34). Gradually the cellular content of the intimal proliferation disappears and in advanced atherosclerosis, most of the wall may consist of foam cells filled with lipids and cholesterol crystals, the elastic laminae are degenerated, the vessel walls are acellular and even partly hyalinotic, and even hemorrhages – which are rare in cerebral arteries – may occur within the plaque. Usually the atherosclerotic process *alone* does not lead to an occlusion, but the rest of the severely narrowed lumen is occluded by appositional thrombosis (see p. 69) or embolism (see p. 72). *Ulceration* may occur in atherosclerotic plaques (see pp. 56, 122) in 10% of cases (GOMENSORO et al., 1973).

MOOSSY (1959) found calcification within intimal plaques in 17 out of 122 cases invariably limited to the internal carotid and extracranial vertebral arteries. The calcium content is supposed to be very low in the walls of intracranial arteries, a fact which is consistent with the phenomenon

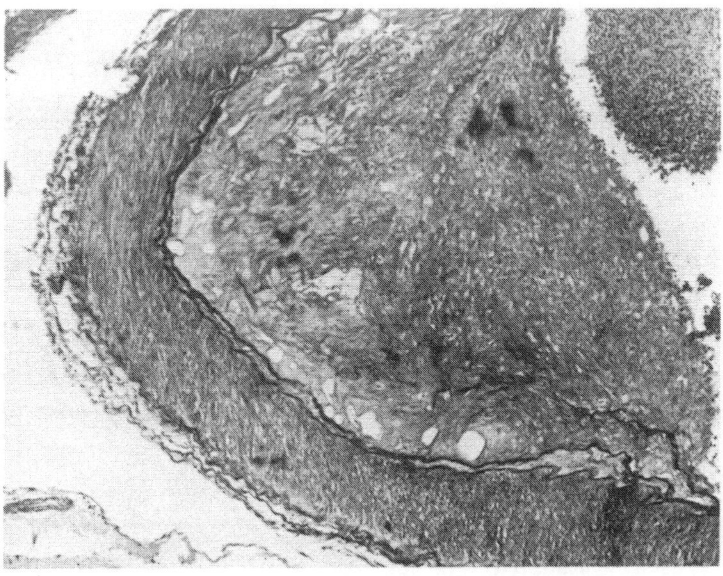

Fig. 58. Typical atherosclerosis in a Sylvian artery. Pronounced cell proliferation with plaque formation on the intima. The elastic layer is sometimes split, yet readily visible. v. Gieson stain ×50

of the non-calcification of these vessels after piercing the dura (see the small deposit in Fig. 4, ZÜLCH 1961a). Calcification is almost never seen in computed tomography, which is very sensitive for visualization of calcium deposits. We have seen calcium deposits inside the dura only in the carotid and verebrobasilar arteries as an exception from the rule (see Fig. 33).

In electron microscopical studies smooth muscle cells and blood monocytes were observed to be filled with lipid droplets, cell debris and plasma lipoproteins. Apparently the picture is similar in cerebral vessels and in arteries of other organs so that the differing prevalence of atherosclerosis of specific sites has not bearing on structure or content. For information regarding the histochemistry of atherosclerosis see FRIEDE (1962).

IV. Ectatic Type of Atherosclerosis – Coiling, Kinking and Megadolicho-Type of Atherosclerosis

Two main types of cerebral "atherosclerosis": the atheromatous or stenosing and the fibrous-ectatic type may be distinguished (ZÜLCH, 1971b). Calcification is seen after perforation of the dura only in very rare cases (Fig. 33) or as small microscopical plaques in the very proximal segments (ZÜLCH, 1961a, Fig. 4). Intimal thickening with the formation of plaques consisting of collagenous fibers and the infiltrated lipids make up the characteristic picture of atherosclerosis (see p. 54). On the other hand widening and extension of the lumen with a certain fibrous hardening even up to a local bulging is typical for the ectatic form. The stenosing type may involve any arteries down to 500 μ (Fig. 52). The ectatic form of atherosclerosis is found mainly in the extracranial arteries as well as in the intradural section of the vertebral and carotid artery and in the basilar artery. This lesion may simulate locally a fusiform aneurysm, which in one of our cases (Fig. 44) impressed itself into the adjacent brain (pons and medulla oblongata) and mimicked the intermittent basilar insufficiency syndrome (Fig. 44). BREIG et al. (1967) have even observed hydrocephalus secondary to obstruction of the cerebrospinal fluid pathway.

Combined forms – stenosing and ectatic – of atherosclerosis are infrequent. FIELDS (personal communication) found ectatic atherosclerosis far more common in the angiograms of Uruguayan patients in the Hospital de Clinicas (Montevideo), which was the only non-USA unit taking part in the "Joint Study" (HASS et al., 1968; FIELDS et al., 1968, 1970). This, however, would tend to point to the co-effect of an "outer" environmental factor. Kinks and coils can lead to neurological symptoms (DESAI and TOOLE, 1975).

Coiling and kinking at a later state may be the consequence of this ectatic lengthening of the artery and occurs more commonly in the carotid than in the vertebral artery. Such extension are somewhat difficult to detect at autopsy, whereas they are strikingly well demonstrated in the angiogram. This is particularly true in a special form of extension seen in the "megadolicho" types of basilar or carotid artery although the latter is far more rarely involved (see p. 46).

1. Ulceration

In larger extracranial arterial plaques there may be an ulceration as at the bifurcation of the common carotid artery in the neck (WEIBEL and FIELDS, 1965; GOMENSORO et al., 1973; METTINGER et al., 1977). Its ulcerative destruction may introduce the formation of little grooves or craters which can be partly covered by thrombotic material. This can be seen, though not so frequently as is usually assumed. For instance there were *13 cases with ulceration* in 160 cases of TOOLE et al. (1975) while the surface was *smooth* in 110 of his cases with more than 50% constriction. Ulceration and apposition of thrombotic material gives rise to fairly specific arteriographic appearances. Ulceration practically never occurs in arteries after they have perforated the dura.

One of the hypotheses for the pathogenesis of Transient Ischemic Attacks (TIAs) is based on the morphological observation of thrombotic material on ulcerated atherosclerotic plaques at the common carotid bifurcation. These ulcerated plaques are interpreted as the source of microembolization (MARSHALL, 1971; R. RUSSELL, 1971). The opposite – mainly hemodynamic – hypothesis has been emphasized since 1966 by the author and has been developed in the III International Symposium on TIA, Valencia (see 1977, p. 177ff.).

2. Hemorrhages

Sometimes hemorrhages into an atherosclerotic plaque are seen which may increase its volume and its stenosing effect. More frequently, however, hemorrhages are only of microscopic size. Hemorrhages almost never occur in the atherosclerotic wall of intracranial vessels, apart from those seen with dissecting aneurysms (see p. 24).

3. Tortuosity, Kinking and Coiling

In a one sixth of elderly subjects the cervical segment of the carotid arteries may show tortuosity, sometimes bilaterally (CAIRNEY, 1924). These variations in the normal course of the arteries are observed in angiograms but are often difficult to assess at autopsy. The ectatic form of atherosclerosis in particular may lead to lengthening of these arteries and thereby to tortuosity, to coiling, which may assume circular patterns, and kinking. Especially involved are the internal carotid, the basilar and the vertebral arteries (ZIMMERMAN and FARELL, 1970). Kinking may be seen in a case of particularly marked lengthening where circular formation is prevented by the surrounding structures. METZ et al. (1961) saw kinking of the internal carotid in 60 (!) out of 100 carotid angiograms.

The formation of coils is sometimes seen in infants even in the first year after birth, so it must be congenital and have no great hemodynamic consequences. However, it can according to some authors, produce some signs or symptoms (GURDJIAN et al., 1964a, b; SARKARI et al., 1970; DESAI and TOOLE, 1975).

Coiling and kinking is, as mentioned above, more common in ectatic atherosclerosis and is mainly to be observed in the upper one third of the vertebral and carotid arteries; TOOLE and PATEL (1974) found in 17% of all their cases a hemodynamic barrier. WEIBEL and FIELDS (1965) investigated such arterial deformations and divided them into three groups namely:

a) Tortuosity: any "S" or "C" shaped forms.

They found in a total of 328 bilateral carotid angiograms (1965): bilateral tortuosity occurred in 223 cases and no stenosis or aneurysmal dilatation in 65 of these. Unilateral tortuosity occurred in the remaining bilateral angiographies of which 39 showed no stenosis or aneurysmal dilatation. If the number of patients having occlusive disease with or without associated aneurysmal dilatation and those having aneurysmal dilatation only are combined, the incidence of concomitant arterial degenerative disease was 71% in patients with bilateral tortuosity and 63% in those with unilateral tortuosity of the internal carotid artery.

b) Coiling: exaggerated "S" or circular formations.

c) Kinking: angulation associated with subsequent stenosis.

4. Widening of arteries

The question was considered at the Thule Symposium (1967) as to whether arterial vascular channels will dilate in case of "need", this is answered partly by the results of the study by GURDJIAN et al. (1960, 1961 a, b) on possible "arterial training" of the cerebral collateral circulation. The answer is further elucidated through the establishment by GREITZ (1967) at the Symposium that markedly dilated vessels can, in the course of time, functionally return to normal size, for example, after an operation for a large arteriovenous malformation. The large "meningeal anastomoses" from the anterior cerebral artery seen coursing towards the stump of an occluded middle cerebral artery, as shown in Fig. 13, are indicative of such a functional dilatation. This is also true of arteries with smaller lumen (cross-sectional diameter 1–2 mm) provided that they are not yet affected by atherosclerosis.

In children with normal "soft" arteries a functional dilatation may develop very rapidly but it is much less likely to occur in older persons with more rigid arteries. (For the discussion of vasoconstriction or angiospasm respectively see p. 75ff.)

V. Hyalinosis, Arteriolosclerosis, Small Vessel Disease

The smaller intracerebral vessels have a distinct pathology, the degree of which is age related (BAKER and IANONE, 1959b; ELLINGTON, 1970). The most characteristic but different form is hyalinosis (SCHOLZ and NIETO, 1938), also called "small vessel disease", arteriolosclerosis or fibrinoid degeneration (W.F. ROBERTSON, 1900; HUECK, 1920; ASCHOFF, 1925, 1939) of the cerebral arterioles which is located mainly in the small vessels of the basal ganglia and lower brainstem and less frequently in cortical arteries. It affects deep perforating arteries with a lumen of around 200 μ (Fig. 59). Its etiologic relation to hypertension is well known. SPATZ (1939), ANDERS and EICKE (1939), ZÜLCH (1961 a, 1971 a), and ROTHEMUND and FRISCHE (1973) observed it in cases of longstanding high blood pressure. It comprises a separate and distinct entity among the degenerative arterial diseases (YATES, 1976).

Epidemiologically in Japan the small vessels show the same incidence of plaques as the larger caliber vessels (RESCH et al., 1969). This type of pathological process bears no relation to common atherosclerosis nor are there any changes provoked by the direction of flow such as turbulence (as seen in atherosclerosis, see p. 40). Instead it has a close quantitative relation to the pathogenesis of hypertensive hemorrhage (see p. 94, also for a particular morphology and the ensuing micro-infarcts – "lacunar infarcts").

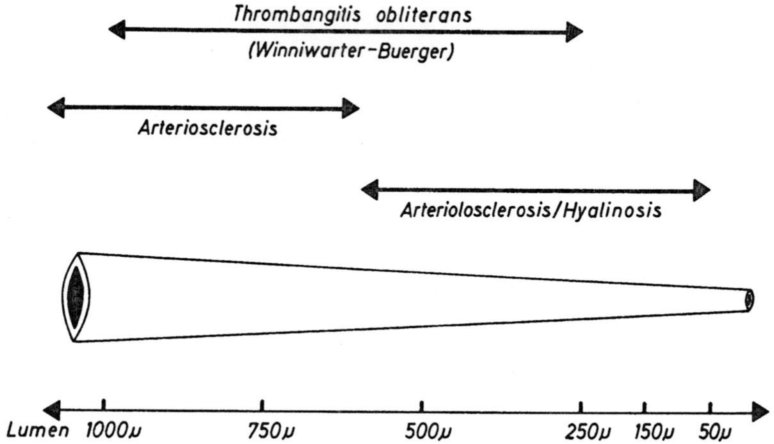

Fig. 59. Predilection of the three vascular diseases: atherosclerosis, thromboangiitis obliterans (Winiwarter-Buerger), arteriolosclerosis-hyalinosis for the various segments of an artery

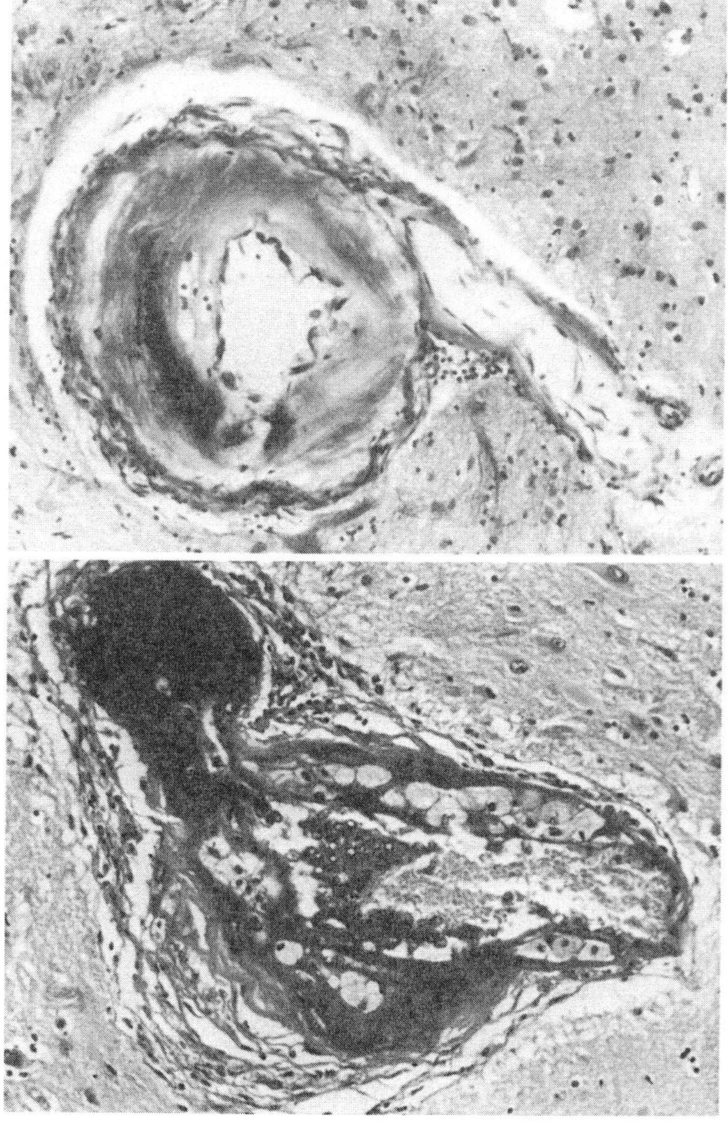

Fig. 60. Concentric hyalinotic transformation of the wall of a striate artery. The media is particularly involved, enlarged and homogenous *(above)*. Prominent hyalinotic process in a striatal artery. Foam cells are visible in the hyalinotic mass *(below)*. This pattern has also been called arterionecrosis

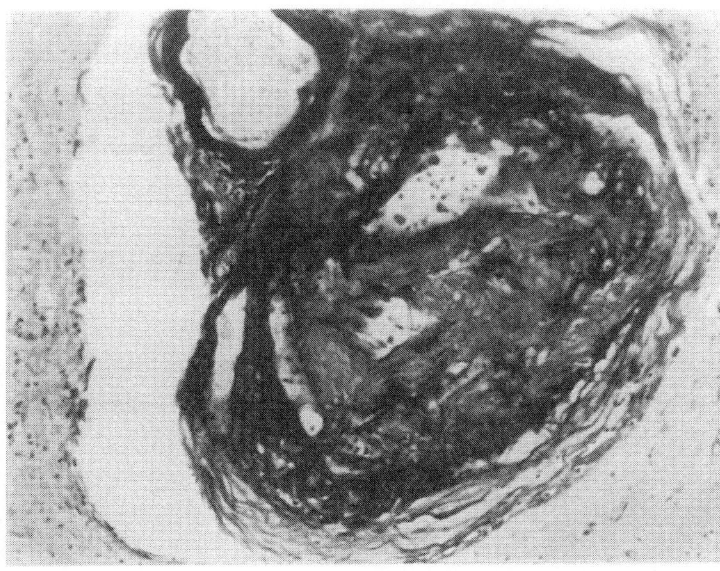

Fig. 61. Hyaline outpouching near the ramification of a striate artery. Attempts at recanalization of the hyalinotic mass

Morphologically (ZÜLCH, 1961a, page 56, Fig. 3a, b), it starts with changes – broadening – in the intima (BAKER and IANONE, 1959b) which begins to swell, probably by the infiltration of "plasmatic substances" from the blood and degeneration of the elastic lamina (Fig. 60 below). The normal structure of the inner vessel wall is blurred and the lumen severely stenosed (Fig. 60 above). The invading plasma substances have special staining properties. Hyalinosis usually has a concentric localization but it may also accumulate eccentrically as a periarteriolar bulging (Fig. 61), thereby mimicking a microaneurysm (for details see p. 101 ff.).

Experimentally MUIRHEAD et al. (1951) have produced hyalinosis in "Goldblatt" dogs with hypertensive levels of 150–200 mmHg. After 10 days there is an acute necrosis of the media, after 20 days a transformation of the media into hyaline, and by the 30th day true hyalinosis has been observed (see also MONTGOMERY and MUIRHEAD, 1954; R. ROSS et al., 1979; STEHBENS, 1979; and p. 103). This process has been termed "plasmatic atheronecrosis" or arterionecrosis (OONEDA et al., 1976; see p. 100 ff.).

An extensive examination in our laboratory (see PABELICK, 1967, and p. 58) has shown that it is only in arteries with a lumen of 200 μ or less that hyalinosis is observed. It occurs scarcely at all proximally and hence gives rise to the term art*eriolo*sclerosis. Although in the proximal parts of the arteries slight atherosclerotic changes may develop (see p. 95) much changes cease abruptly beyond a lumen size of 200 μ where they change into "small artery disease", i.e. hyalinosis (see Fig. 59).

Our investigations were carried out on arteries of the basal ganglia on the uninvolved side and not on the side affected by the cerebral hemorrhage. Hyalinosis began to be observed in the lenticulostriate arteries in a histological investigation of blocks taken from above a horizontal plane through the anterior commissure. We can readily establish, as have all our predecessors, the occurrence of "hyaline balls" in such cases (about "microaneurysms", see p. 101, and also ZÜLCH, 1971a, Fig. 13).

However, in general the statement of MOSCHCOWITZ (1929) may be accepted that as a rule when "atherosclerosis" affects the arteries in one circulatory system (either the larger or the smaller vessels), it will be absent in the other.

With respect to the clinical consequences of hyalinosis, of which the most overwhelming entity is mass hemorrhage, the following observations are important (see p. 101).

The origin of microinfarctions runs parallel to the promotion of hyalinosis in the terminal zones of the paramedian arteries of the brainstem. The so-called "lacunae" as seen in the striatum, thalamus, mesencephalon and pons (see p. 84ff.) also have been shown very convincingly as a consequence of hyalinotic occlusion by C.M. FISHER (1965b) in serial sections. FISHER correctly correlates some of "little strokes" (ALVAREZ, 1955) with these sudden vascular events ("lacunar strokes", C.M. FISHER, 1967). When mechanical stress on the vascular wall is considered the pulsatile impact of hypertension comes into discussion. However, in order to define its action properly, we should probably first determine whether or not hypertension may provoke three major effects on the arterial wall:

a) atherosclerosis in medium sized and larger vessels but this is rare in the brain
b) arteriolosclerosis or hyalinosis in small arteries, and
c) in the general circulation
   1. when acutely provoking: "hypertensive" crises in normotensives
   2. when acting chronically: left cardiac insufficiency by small vessel disease.

We therefore distinguish between the *acute* and the *chronic effects* of hypertension on the vascular wall and its *clinical significance* in the actual production of catastrophic stroke, which we will discuss later (p. 119).

The existence of hypertension was determined according to the "highest systolic and diastolic readings found in the patients chart". The authors admit the adherent weakness in the use of these data and we have constantly stressed this point (ZÜLCH, 1961a; 1962b; ZÜLCH and V. HOSSMANN, 1967; see p. 118).

Hypertension in addition to other factors is considered by many authors to promote atherosclerosis of the *large cerebral vessels*, but this concept should probably be somewhat limited. The statement may be valid for the special form of "renal hypertension", particularly in the younger age groups (LIEBEGOTT, 1959) although BAKER, RESCH and their group (see BAKER et al., 1969) found a strong general association between the grade of cerebral atherosclerosis and hypertension.

However, the significance of chronic hypertension is still open in respect to the general problem of cerebral atherosclerosis. From *our experience*, long lasting hypertension does not necessarily result in general atherosclerosis of the intracranial cerebral arteries, as ANDERS and EICKE (1939), SPATZ (1939), EICKE (1952) and finally LINDENBERG (1957) were inclined to believe. LINDENBERG (1957) for instance, when writing about atherosclerosis of the "birch bark" type in the basilar artery states that "according to our experience this finding is almost always an indication of a malignant fast-developing hypertension".

C.M. FISHER (1965b) expressed the opinion that hypertension aggravates cerebral atherosclerosis in general, and basilar atherosclerosis and stenosis in particular.

Our observations also are contrary to the above-mentioned concept of LIEBEGOTT (1959). This may be due to the fact that his material was highly selected including predominantly young patients with hypertension of renal origin.

From our large series from a Municipal General Hospital of "average" cases (see also Doctor-thesis of PABELICK, 1967) with long-lasting ("benign"?) hypertension and mass hemorrhage, in one third there was *no intracranial vessel atherosclerosis*; in another third a mild degree while only the last third showed atherosclerosis to a severe degree. FREITAG (1968) counted the arterial atheromas in her cases of cerebral hemorrhage: only one third showed grade III to IV plaques. This supports very well our observations in cerebral hemorrhage. For the statistical correlation between these two conditions see p. 95, Fig. 101.

In the two groups which were studied by PRINEAS and MARSHALL (1966), the difference lay in the levels of diastolic blood pressure (below and above 110 mmHg). The former group presented large cortical and subcortical lesions while the latter was associated with a high incidence of stenotic and occlusive lesions. The latter (high pressure) group presented a picture of small deeply situated lesions, as reported by C.M. FISHER (1965b). It appears therefore that SAKO (1962) emphasized correctly that turbulence and increased blood flow and intraluminal pressure following hypertension are abetting factors in experimental atherosclerosis.

However, atherosclerosis and the associated clinical pictures as seen in men, are the end result of *multiple contributing factors, partly morphological, partly functional in nature.*

In the "small vessels" of the coronary circulation (100–1000 μ) subintimal hyaline-like deposits and perivascular fibrosis have been observed in hypertension. Moreover, in diabetes, thrombus formation and diabetic angiopathies with atherosclerotic and nonatherosclerotic vascular lesions have been noted. That participation of "smaller vessels" in the ischemic lesions of the brain does not necessarily mean "hyalinosis" is convincingly shown by ELLINGTON (1970).

Diabetic angiolopathy (W.W. MEYER, 1974a, b) consists of hyalinotic thickening of arteries in which cellular intimal proliferations may be seen in the "small arteries" of retina and brain. The veins and even capillaries may be involved.

VI. Regression of Atherosclerosis

The concept of a regression of atherosclerosis (GRESHAM, 1976) was discussed shortly after the first world war (ASCHOFF, 1925; BEITZKE, 1928): such regression was noted during the final years of the war and immediately thereafter, when in general only very low fat diets could be given to the population. However, it is difficult to follow morphologically an atherosclerotic lesion other than by angiography (BLANKENHORN, 1977); clinical "regression" alone is not always convincing (SCHLIERF, 1976). In recent animal experiments many pertinent and interesting facts have been reported, although they are based only on regression of so-called advanced atherosclerotic lesions in animals, which may have very limited parallels to genuine atherosclerosis in man. ARMSTRONG et al. (1970) showed that in monkeys, fairly advanced atheromatous lesions could regress with either a *low* cholesterol diet or with combined polyunsaturated fat and low cholesterol rations. In addition to cholesterol even collagen decreased in the plaques. This has been shown similarly in pigs (DAOUD et al., 1975; WISSLER, 1977). These endothelial lesions probably are repaired permanently if the provoking factors are removed or if additional risk factors are avoided. There are some indications from experimental morphology and clinical observations that even gross changes may be partly reversible (BETZ and SCHLOTE, 1979; STEHBENS, 1979). Two of the components, the lipid and calcareous deposits definitely disappear after prolonged protein deficiency (see WISSLER, 1977). It has been observed for a long time that in fasting disease, insufficient protein intake or starvation, lipids (BAKER et al., 1961b) and even calcification in the atherosclerotic vessels may disappear.

In dystrophic prisoners of World War II luminar stenosis of the coronary arteries was apparently fairly small (ROBERTS, 1977). This has been observed also with cachexia accompanying maligant tumors.

The same has been in "dystrophic" members of various sorts of camps both during and after the war. Observations at autopsy (RANDERATH) have proved that following prolonged starvation atherosclerosis is markedly reduced (lipids, calcification). On the other hand these lipid and calcareous deposits "fill up" very rapidly in the arterial lesions during the "feeding-up" period.

As mentioned above, atherosclerosis produced experimentally is not identical to atherosclerosis in man. This has been emphasized by BLUMENTHAL et al. (1954). Even spontaneous atherosclerosis in animals gives no clue to the pathogenesis (see LUGINBÜHL, 1966) of atherosclerosis in man (see p. 54).

Since, in man, modifications in diet leading to reduction of weight, modifications in smoking habits, and normalization of blood pressure etc. seem at least to reduce the risks of progression of atherosclerosis, it may become possible in the future to achieve regression of atherosclerotic lesions with specific treatment.

VII. Thromboangiitis Obliterans (von Winiwarter-Buerger's disease)

We once chose the provocative title of "The Cerebral Form of von Winiwarter Buerger's Disease: Does it exist?" for a paper because scientists of such international standing as

VON ALBERTINI (1946), C.M. FISHER (1957) and R. ADAMS (1958) denied the existence of such a vascular disease entity. Definitions of the pathology, etiology, pathogenetic factors and the clinical diagnosis would lead us to endless and fatiguing enumeration of details (see v. WINIWARTER, 1879; BUERGER, 1924, 1939; v. HASSELBACH, 1939; LLAVERO, 1948; J.E. MEYER, 1948, 1958; EICKE, 1957; SPATZ, 1935, 1939, 1942; LINDENBERG and SPATZ, 1940; ZÜLCH, 1969a).

The *cerebral* form of thromboangiitis may be most suitable for discussion because, in contrast to the limbs, the brain is best protected from influences of external pathogenetic factors such as cold and superimposed infection and gangrene unrelated to the primary disease (see original cases of v. WINIWARTER, 1879). This disease occurs predominantly in men (HORTON and BROWN, 1932; HORTON and DORSEY, 1932; WESSLER et al., 1960) and is always thought to be an affliction of the younger age group although it may occur also in elderly people.

In many thousands of brain autopsies of which more than 800 were vascular cases, *we only saw two instances* of this condition.

Thromboangiitis of the brain, therefore, is judged to be a very rare disease.

1. Size of the Arterial Caliber Involved

Both thromboangiitis and atherosclerosis have predilections for a certain caliber of cortical arteries. Thromboangiitis as a rule affects vessels below 1 mm diameter (Fig. 59) whereas atherosclerosis, on the other hand, affects vessels having a lumen above $^1/_2$ mm. It is not necessary to add that hyalinosis (or arteriolosclerosis), the third major form of arterial disease and the usual cause of mass hemorrhage in the brain, is mainly localized in the arteries of the basal ganglia, especially those below 500 μ, i.e. distal to the size affected by thromboangiitis (see pp. 16, 55 and Fig. 59).

2. Morphology

On the surface the terminal arteries of the cortex appear "whitish, bloodless, solid, shrunken" (Figs. 62, 66). These findings, being systemically observed over all the cerebral and cerebellar convexity (Fig. 63), seem to be the principal macroscopical characteristic of this disease, particularly near the zone of granular atrophy (Fig. 64). However, *single* vessels of this type found

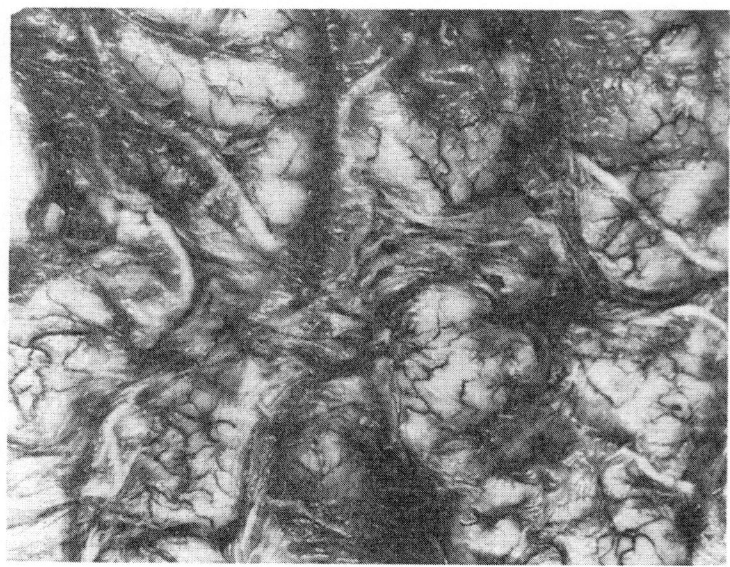

Fig. 62. In the leptomeninges the arteries are seen as whitish, bloodless, solid strings

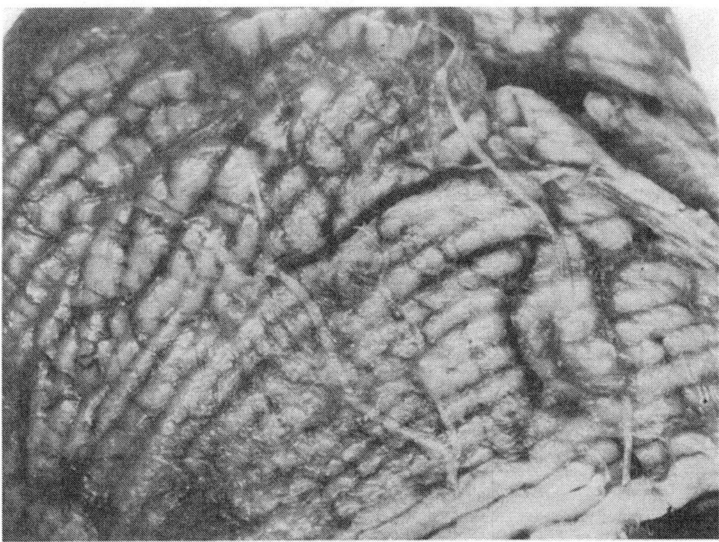

Fig. 63. One sees these white solid arteries also over the surface of the cerebellum

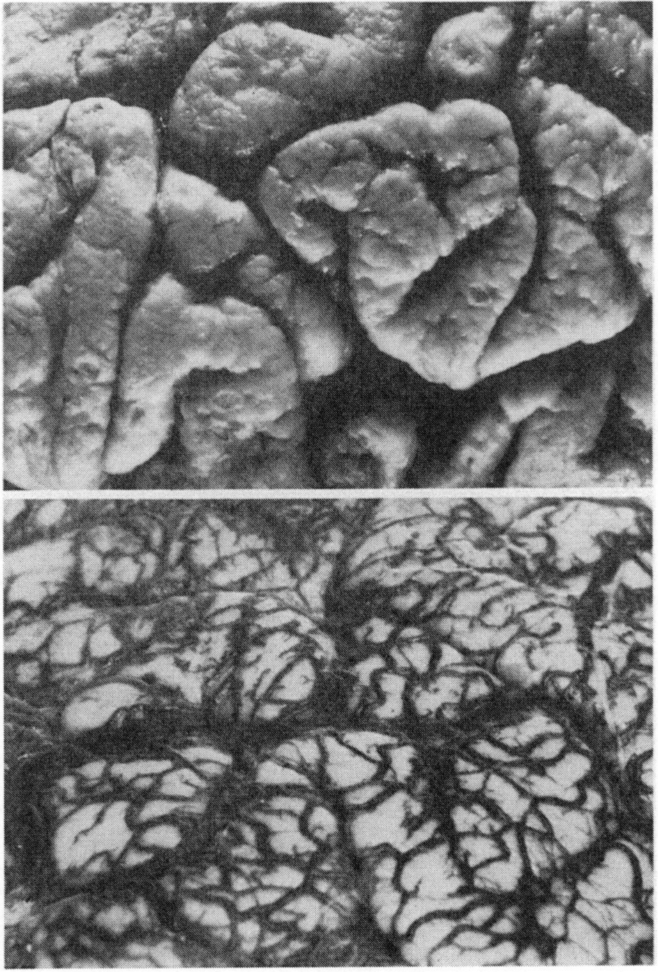

Fig. 64. *Above:* "Granular atrophy" of the cerebral convolutions. Small scars are seen, resembling the granular surface of similar kidney disease. *Below:* Marked hyperemia of the small cortical superficial arteries. They form annular collateral anastomotic rings

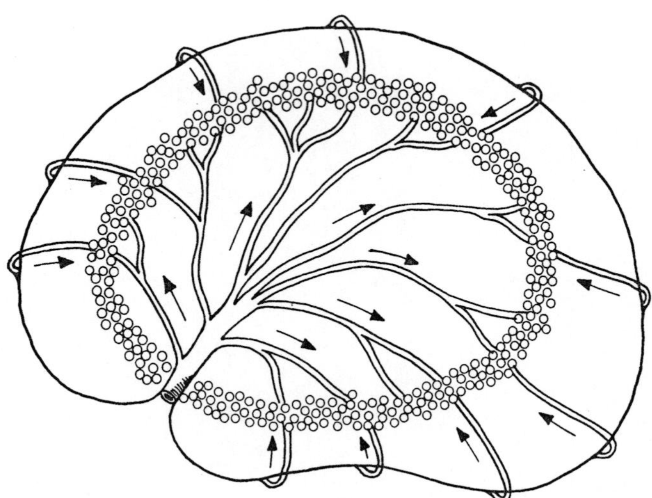

Fig. 65. Schematic ("synthetic") drawing of the probable pattern of an angiogram (lateral view) in thromboangiitis obliterans

distal to a major vessel thrombosis are by no means a rare occurrence, as C.M. Fisher (1957) has correctly pointed out.

Another characteristic observation in such cases is the above-mentioned "granular atrophy" of the cortex (Fig. 64), developing from the accumulation of small cortical scars. It is best seen after removal of the meninges, and has its common predilection (Pentschew, 1934; Lindenberg and Spatz, 1940; Lippmann, 1952) in a *ring shaped zone between the areas supplied by the anterior, middle and posterior cerebral arteries* (Romanul and Abramovicz, 1964; see Fig. 65). However, this granular atrophy is not specific for thromboangiitis. On the contrary, it also occurs in atherosclerosis or infantile circulatory disturbances of the cerebrum (see J.E. Meyer, 1948, 1958).

The third remarkable finding in this disease is hyperemia due to vigorously filled meningeal arterial rings (Fig. 64) which are by no means similar to simple venous congestions (see p. 115ff.). This collateral system of arteriolar anastomoses indicates a completely different condition. It seems to be the only disease where the annular rings of Schmidt (1955a, b; see p. 15) fulfill partly a function as an anastomosing system. Finally as described by J.E. Meyer (1948, 1958) the cerebellar arteries are involved in the alterations (Fig. 63).

Histologically, the occluded small arteries are filled with a loose connective tissue (Fig. 66) as has been described earlier by Pentschew, 1934, R. Lindenberg and H. Spatz (1940). In the center of the vessel one or two newly formed vascular lumina (Fig. 66) may be seen. In case illustrated here, it should be emphasized that the patient was 31 years of age. No major changes are seen in the arterial media and interna (Fig. 66), the otherwise normal elastic layer remaining free from any splitting or other degenerative change. If the patient had been older, minor atherosclerotic alterations might have been observed in the larger arteries. However, these are never the predominant features of the cerebral form of thromboangiitis. The most characteristic sign then is the occlusion of many otherwise healthy small arteries of the convexities by a loose connective tissue, commonly occurring together with the formation of one or two new smaller lumina (Fig. 66) apart from older or fresh thromboses.

The cerebral form of thromboangiitis is considered to occur in a 1:50 ratio among patients with the generalized form of von Winiwarter-Buerger's disease. Since the cerebrum is well protected against external influences, we must assume that an almost ("pseudo") "systemic" thrombotic process affects superficial arteries of a special size, i.e. below 1 mm. In contrast to C.M. Fisher (1957) we do not believe that thrombosis of only one single artery has much to do with this pseudosystemic effect on the small arteries even if there is histologic similarity. Lindenberg

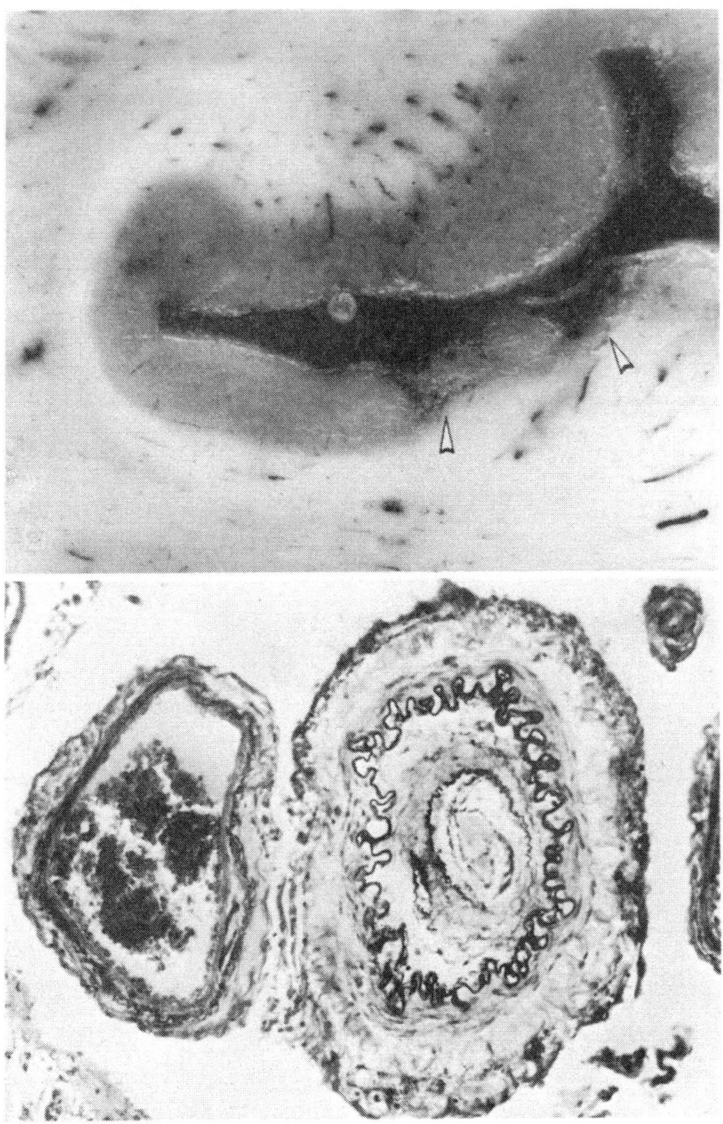

Fig. 66. *Above:* Magnification of an artery in the Sylvian fissure. The lumen is closed by gelatinous connective tissue. One can easily recognize two small scars in the upper part of the convolution *(arrows)*. *Below:* Free new lumina with a new elastica interna in a small artery occluded by loose connective tissue. Elastica-van Gieson stain × 50

and SPATZ (1940) distinguished a *second type* of thromboangiitis obliterans in the major arteries. We think that this second type of thromboangiitis obliterans, i.e. thrombosis of the carotid etc. should be better defined. If it belongs at all to the entity it occurs even more rarely and we have observed it only once clinically in a man aged 34 years (see also SORGO, 1939).

The cause of this apparently primarily thrombotic (Fig. 67) process in small arteries is still unknown and there are no clinical observations which would shed full light on the genesis of the disease. Our first patient was completely healthy until the day of his sudden death from *traumatic* hemorrhage; prior to that, he was mentally normal and very active in his professional and social life, although he had already developed the severe granular atrophy of the cerebrum previously described.

None of the theories so far propounded in the literature is very satisfying. In our cases there were no thrombi of the carotid arteries or the heart which would support the idea of a "morbus

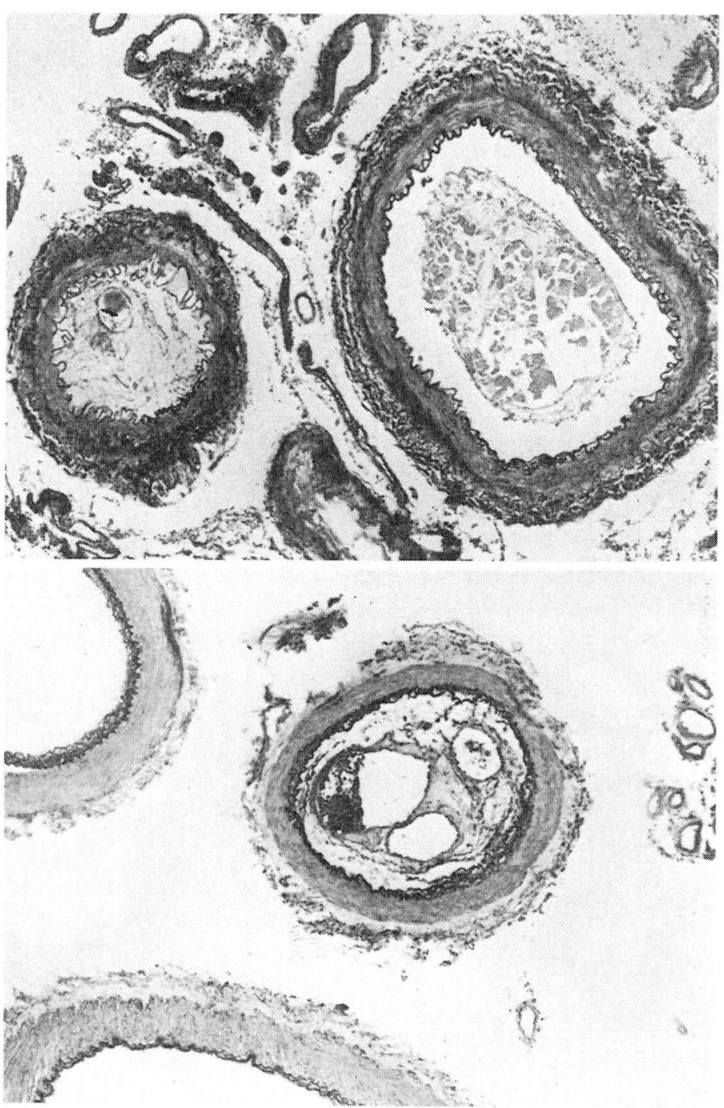

Fig. 67. *Above:* Apart from a total occlusion of the smaller artery one sees a recent thrombus in the larger vessel, of which the internal elastic layer is hardly changed. *Below:* Recanalization of a vascular thrombus

embolicus" (v. ALBERTINI, 1946) a multilocular macroembolism; also from our observations with experimental microembolization of the brain this seems very unlikely since quite different lesions occur (see ZÜLCH and TZONOS, 1965). Furthermore, the cerebellum (see J.E. MEYER, 1948, 1953) could never be affected by carotid emboli.

We do not know the etiology or the details of pathogenesis of this morphologically fairly well-defined cerebral arterial disease of young or middle-aged men. From the beginning I have doubted the "angiitic" origin of this lesion, a concept which does not find any support from the histology of our cases. It may have been suggested from the inflammatory lesions which can be seen along the peripheral vessels (artery, vein, lymph vessel and encasing connective tissue) in cases where gangrene for instance in the foot has been the primary involvement.

The concept of a chronic intermittent insufficiency in the arterial border zones (see ROTTER, 1949; ROMANUL and ABRAMOWICZ, 1964; QUANDT and SOMMER, 1969) also seems very unsatisfactory.

This fact of an obscure pathogenesis and even inadequate definition (if only made angiographically) leads us to the assumption that von Winiwarter-Buerger's disease apparently has been diagnosed far too often both peripherally and in the brain. The differential diagnosis from early atherosclerotic lesions has not always been sufficiently clear. Clinical diagnosis alone does not seem to be sufficient in view of the increasingly early atherosclerotic lesions, at least not for the cerebral form in which clinical symptoms may be entirely lacking as in both of our cases. Furthermore, diagnosis has been based too often on cerebral angiography although the pathologic descriptions of the angiograms do not correspond exactly to the morphologic picture of occlusion of the terminal segments of the cortical arteries (see below).

I once risked predicting the angiogram (Fig. 65) of "real" cases of cerebral thromboangiitis obliterans on the base of the morphological findings (VIIIth Annual Meeting International College of Angiology, see ZÜLCH, 1969a, Fig. 9). The cutting-off of all the middle-sized arteries ("terminal branches"), linked instead by the arachnoidal arterial rings (seen as a "blush") must be regarded as the characteristic pattern. This synthetic angiogram was later confirmed by HACKER's first three cases (1968). Therefore, in the future, some hope for an early angiographic diagnosis seems to exist.

For instance the early angiographic description given by KRAYENBÜHL and WEBER (1944), and KRAYENBÜHL (1945) did not correspond to this morphological definition of thromboangiitis obliterans; in their cases, the large carotid artery and medium-sized anterior and middle cerebral arteries were involved, also BROBEIL's (1950) interpretation of an angiogram in thromboangiitis obliterans ("wirres Gefäßknäuel") has turned out to be erroneous.

VIII. Binswanger's Disease

Subcortical atherosclerotic encephalopathy or Binswanger's disease – clinically leading to dementia – seems to be caused by stenosing lesions in *intra*cerebral vessels. Although not yet sufficiently defined a subcortical demyelination seems to be the most prominent feature. According to our own observations and figures in the literature the beginning of the process seems to be perivenous. I have discussed its origin amongst the perivenous syndromes (ZÜLCH, 1973a). For more extensive discussions see also FRIEDE (1962), BLACKWOOD (1963), BURGER et al. (1976).

IX. Mechanical Obstructions of the Arterial Lumen

1. Pathogenesis

Occlusion of cerebral vessels can be formed slowly by atherosclerosis, acutely by embolism, or subacutely by thrombosis (see also H.J. PETERS and CHANDLER, 1971). Mechanical obstructions may be acute or chronic.

Thrombotic lesions in the main arteries can act as a source for *macro-* (above 1000 μ) (Fig. 68) or *microembolization* (pp. 72ff., 122). In addition, the valves, the valleculae, and the cardiac endothelium itself overlying a myocardial infarct or aneurysm or in rare cases vallecular tumors (fibromyxoma, see STEINMETZ et al., 1973) may serve as sources for macroembolization. Moreover the arterial wall in the aorta or carotid artery can act as a source.

One has to distinguish therefore between two sources of emboli:

1) cardiac, 2) arterial intraluminal.

Thrombosis (primary) is supposed to result from a lesion or interruption of the endothelium of an artery, at a point overlying an arterial plaque, by traumatic rupture or even on a relatively uncompromised surface (ADAMS and GRAHAM, 1967) by an unknown process (tearing, desquama-

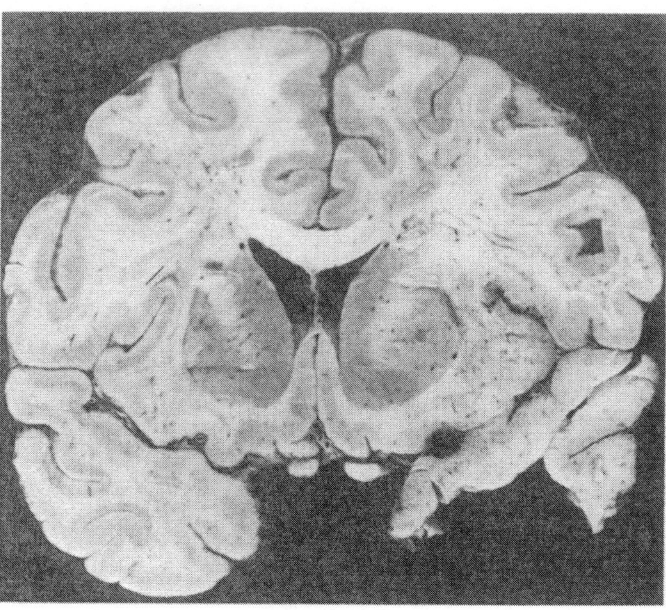

Fig. 68. Thrombosis of the middle cerebral artery. The vessels of the Sylvian group are not yet compromised by atherosclerosis

tion, sloughing of the intima). When an atheroma is compromised, material like collagen, which induces adherence of blood platelets, and the release of platelet factors which activate aggregation, come into action. One theory emphasizes, that the beginning of atherosclerosis is the formation of a flat thrombus (p. 37).

2. Frequency

In larger series, the incidence of embolism as a cause of cerebro-vascular accidents is given as around 11%. The origin was from coronary infarcts 22%, acute endocarditis 8%, and atherosclerotic heart lesions (patients in a medical department) 18%; in 6% the carotid artery was implicated, and in 5% they were of unknown origin. In the series of WRIGHT et al. (1954) 4.9% of the 442 patients with coronary infarcts had cerebral emboli. In BERNSMEIER'S (1963) series (13.1% of all cases) the source of cerebral embolism in 88% was the left heart. In our clinical retrospective series of 1000 patients we observed 23.6% (probable!) arterial thromboses and 6.1% embolism, i.e. the former was four times more frequent (ZÜLCH and v. EINSIEDEL-LECHTAPE, 1977).

3. Distribution of Thromboses

STAEMMLER (1958) reports an incidence of thrombosis of cerebral arteries in 93 cases (46 male, 47 female) from 3600 autopsies. This corresponds to 2% arising in men (average age 64) and 3.6% in women (average age 68). STAEMMLER found thrombi in the internal carotid artery in 30 cases, in the middle cerebral in 45 and in the anterior cerebral artery in 6 cases (total 81) in contrast to 25 cases within the vertebral-basilar arterial system (vertebral artery 6, basilar artery 8, posterior cerebral artery 11). METZINGER and ZÜLCH (1971) gave a detailed report on 45 cases of vertebral or vertebrobasilar thromboses, including the description of 96 infarcts in the dependent supply territories (p. 146) however, without any mention of incidence. In MOOSSY'S (1966a) 2650 completely dissected cases there were 19.8%, e.g. 527 cases of old and new infarction, out of which 5.4% (142 cases) were fresh and 55% had thrombosis.

Other statistics report that the middle cerebral artery is most commonly thrombosed (for instance SCHEID, 1963: 69% thrombosis of middle cerebral artery, 19% of posterior cerebral artery, 12% of anterior cerebral artery, i.e. a similar distribution). KLEIHUES et al. (1964) found in ZÜLCH's material (137 cases) the following localization of the thromboses: A. cerebri ant. 20=14.6%, A. cerebri med. 50=36.5% (Fig. 68), A. cerebri post. 15=11.0%.

4. Sex

Thrombosis definitely occurs more frequently in women. In our series of 1000 patients with cerebrovascular disease the male/female ratio was 1.8 for thrombosis, and 0.9 for embolism (ZÜLCH and EINSIEDEL-LECHTAPE, 1977). Thrombo-embolism associated with oral contraceptive medication is not the cause of this, because it is a rare occurrence.

5. Arterial Thrombosis

Thrombosis or stenosis of the common carotid artery in the neck region plays a special role in the infarct theory of the brain (Fig. 69). We found a detailed review of the literature in the monograph by HULTQVIST (1942) and angiographic evaluation has been described already by MONIZ, 1934, 1940; SORGO, 1939; RIECHERT, 1943; KRAYENBÜHL and WEBER, 1944 and JOHNSON and A.E. WALKER, 1951.

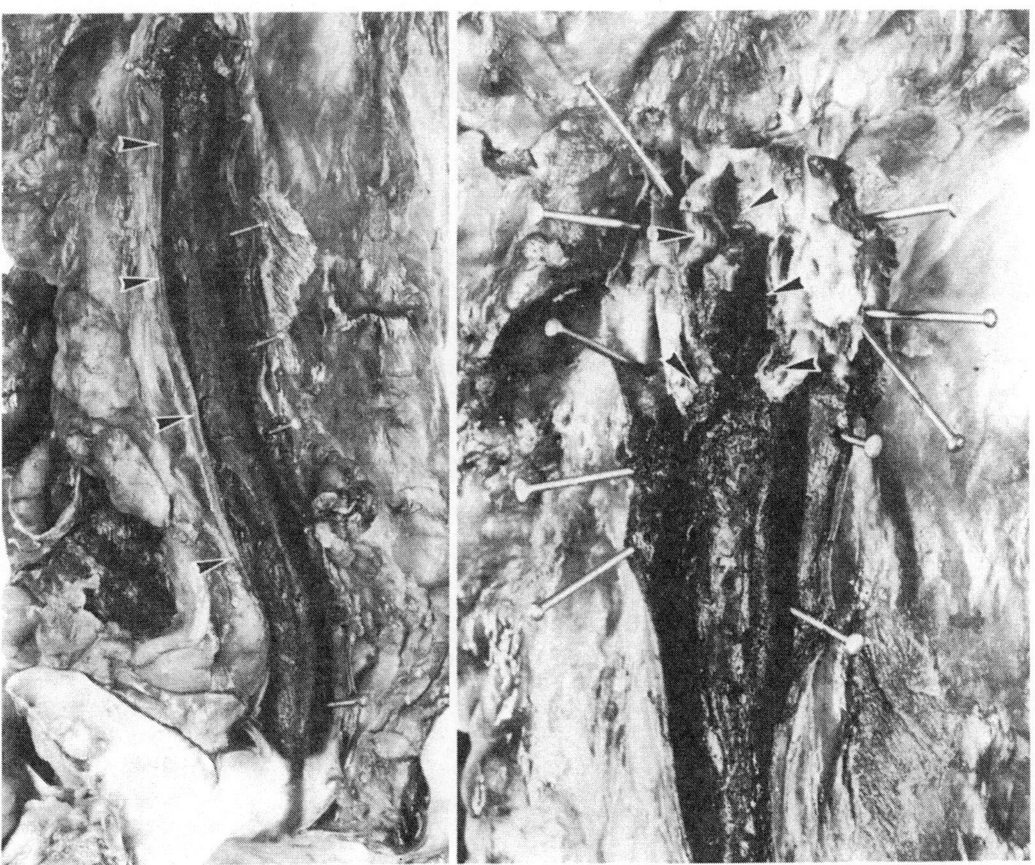

Fig. 69. *Left:* 12 cm long thrombus proximal to the carotid bifurcation in the neck. *Right:* closer view of the upper part; the stenosis of the internal carotid artery ("calcified") is recognizable *(arrows)*

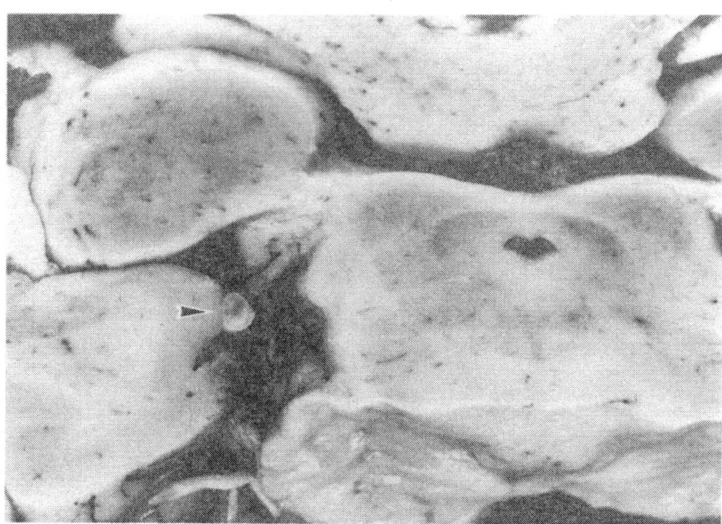

Fig. 70. Occlusion of the posterior cerebral artery by an old "organized" thrombosis *(arrow)*

The importance of the carotid artery for the cerebral circulation was well known in antiquity as is shown by the choice of name (ho karos – deep sleep, unconsciousness). BEHREND and GASTAUT (1962) recently called attention to the trick of ancient wrestlers who tried to compress the carotid artery of the opponent to induce unconsciousness. The consequences of thrombosis have been described by ELVIDGE and WERNER (1951). We know, however, since HULTQVIST'S paper (1942) that thrombosis of the common carotid artery occurs in an average autopsy material in 2%–4% of cases without clinical evidence. Therefore, it appears possible that there is very frequently a sufficient collateral circulation to meet with the emergency situation if pathogenesis is slow. This has been mentioned in a previous chapter on anastomoses (p. 11). Thrombosis of the middle cerebral arteries and the posterior (Fig. 70) and vertebral arteries are the next most common types. There are also rare cases of multiple progressive occlusions (MASTRI et al., 1973). For acute occlusions of the carotid artery see ZÜLCH and HERBERG (1949).

6. Venous Thrombosis and Its Sequelae

Up to now, little is known about the occurrence and sequelae of cerebral venous thromboses (ZÜLCH, 1964) but what is known is mentioned in detail in textbooks and therefore our description will be short (Fig. 71). These are hemorrhagic infarcts with "flea-bite" hemorrhages located in the white matter (Fig. 72) in contrast with arterial hemorrhagic infarcts (ESCOLA, 1962; NOETZEL and JERUSALEM, 1965; KALBAG and WOOLF, 1967), in which the cortex is involved (see also page 128 and Figs. 125, 126). The occurrence of venous thromboses has been shown to be more common since serial angiograms have made possible the demonstration of the venous system and since retrograde opacification of the veins has been successfully carried out (sinus demonstration by GEJROT and LAUREN, 1964; see ZÜLCH, 1964).

In sinus thrombosis, the supplying "bridging veins" are usually congested and the thrombosis advances into them (Fig. 71). If the venous flow is obstructed (vein, sinus) a transudative cerebral edema develops, the severity of which depends on the possibility of venous drainage via anastomoses. Furthermore, congestion occurs in the deep cerebral veins of the white matter with perivenous hemorrhages and less often in the cortex with smaller perivenous hemorrhages. These hemorrhages are located mainly in the cerebrum on one or both sides of the sagittal sinus. Thrombosis of the "deep" veins, for instance of the great vein of Galen, leads to "red infarcts" of their drainage areas (NOETZEL, 1965). These have been observed also in birth trauma particularly involving the basal ganglia which occasionally become calcified (KAUTZKY, 1948).

Sinus obstructions occur in: 1. marasmus, 2. blood diseases (i.e. in sickle-cell anemia), 3. neighborhood infections, particularly suppurative diseases of the peri-nasal sinuses and of the

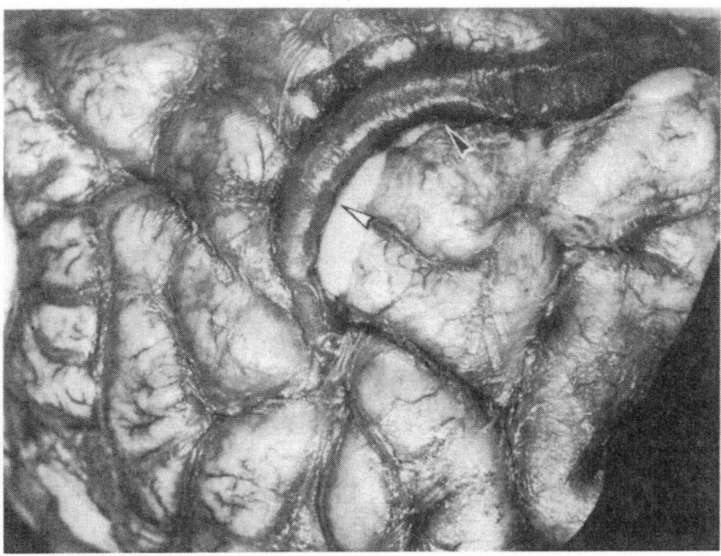

Fig. 71. Thrombosis of the superior sagittal sinus with propagation of clot to the bridging veins *(arrows)*

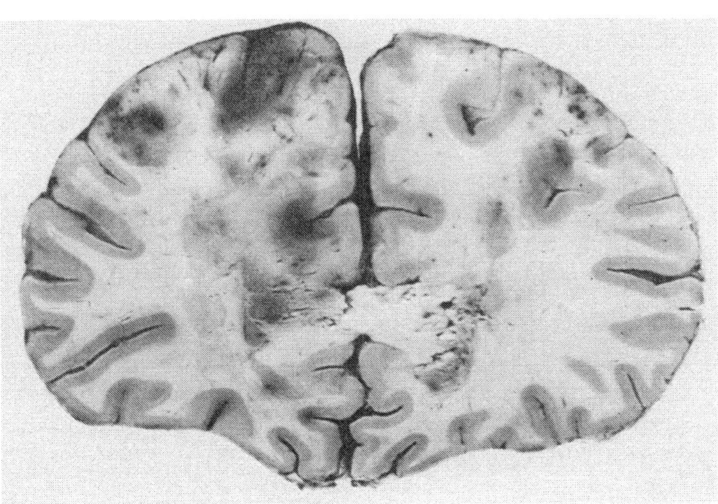

Fig. 72. Occlusion of the superior sagittal sinus. The sections show a hemorrhagic infarction in the appropriate distribution, which is similar to that of the anterior cerebral artery. Note, however, that the white matter is relatively more involved and the veins and venules more engorged than in the infarct of the anterior cerebral artery

ear. However, in cases of tumor growth into the sinus there is only slight obstruction of blood flow because the venous collateral system has enough time to become functional due to the slowness of the growth. In thrombosis of the transverse sinus congestion with massive edema is well known. For a long time this clinical condition was called "otogenic hydrocephalus" (SYMONDS, 1937; ZÜLCH, 1964).

The best description of venous and sinus thrombosis as a complication or rhinotologic disease is found in the textbooks (NOETZEL and JERUSALEM, 1965; KALBAG and WOOLF, 1967; O.T. BAILEY, 1971) and in the monograph and the papers by COURVILLE (1937, 1944, 1955). The monograph by GARCIN and PESTEL (1949) gives a survey of the clinical importance of cortical thrombophlebitis. Angiographic data about the obstruction of veins and sinuses is found also in the otologic literature (ASKENASY et al., 1962; MONTRIEUL and JANNY, 1962; ZÜLCH, 1964; HELMS, 1978).

7. Embolism

Traditionally, three large groups of emboli may be distinguished, namely:

1. thrombotic emboli,
2. fat emboli,
3. air emboli.

The distinction of macroemboli – above 1 mm size – and microemboli – below – is arbitrary, yet seems necessary.

8. Macroembolism

In the past thrombotic embolism seemed to be of greatest importance (FOWLER, 1950). However, the number of such cases seems to decrease continually, especially so since thrombotic embolism formerly was postulated most often from the alleged sequelae, i.e., the development of a softening, without demonstration of thrombus in the vessels.

This is, for instance, true of embolism which was described repeatedly by Ph. SCHWARTZ (1930, 1961) and SCHWARTZ and GOLDSTEIN (1925) in the striolenticular artery and the alleged subsequent hemorrhagic infarcts in the caudate nucleus and putamen. It is certainly extremely difficult to differentiate at autopsy from gross inspection between thrombosis and embolism. The microscopic examination may then be decisive.

Heart diseases, especially disease of the mitral valve, as well as thrombi in the left heart originating from other causes (rheumatic diseases) and the increasing number of artificial heart valves are still the foremost cause of thrombotic emboli.

In the statistics of STAEMMLER (1927, 1936, 1955, 1958), there were 19 cases with recurrent endocarditis and with mural thrombi (in contrast to 93 atherosclerotic softenings). HILLER (1935, 1936, 1951, 1952, 1953) found 15 embolic softenings in contrast to 16 atherosclerotic infarcts. In POPPER'S material (1949), there were 45 stenoses of cardiac valves (32 mitral) and 12 mural thrombi in 88 fatal cases while in another 12 cases, there were "peripheral" thrombi. SCHEID (1963), however, believes that mural thrombi are more common. Emboli from left atrial myxoma are not so rare (STEINMETZ et al., 1973; ZÜLCH et al., 1976).

The frequency data are still discrepant. We have mentioned above the "probable" representation of embolism as 6.1% in our series of 1000 patients. Other authors cite figures of 5%–20% of emboli causing brain infarcts (ARING and MERRITT, 1935; GLYNN, 1956; MURRAY, 1957). In other series this went up to 50% (ADAMS and VAN DER EECKEN, 1953), a figure which may be influenced by their interpretation of the hemorrhagic type of brain infarct (see p. 128ff.); KURTZKE'S (1969) figure of 10% seems to me to be more representative of the real occurrence in general practice or general hospitals.

It has not been proven whether secondary macroemboli occur from primary thrombi of the carotid artery. They are most frequent *after heart diseases proper*. The emboli from *infectious* diseases are second in importance, although these have decreased steadily (scarlet fever, influenza, smallpox, typhoid fever, diphtheria, endocarditis lenta; see also for septic embolism MOLINARI, 1972) since the advent of antibiotic therapy.

Embolization by "atheromatous mush" from atherosclerotic vessels – mainly the aortic arch – postulated again and again (in classic pathology observed by LÖWENFELD, 1886), was demonstrated beyond doubt by DAVID et al. (1963), and also after surgical manipulation of the carotid artery (FIELDS et al., 1958; FLORY, 1945; W.W. MEYER, 1947; SAYRE and CAMPBELL, 1959).

9. Age

The average age of patients with brain embolism (clinically observed) is *high* due to the fact that heart diseases are the main source of emboli; according to HILLER (1936) the average age is sixty-three and according to W. SCHEID (1963) sixty-four.

The preference of emboli which was reported earlier, for the left side of the brain in all forms of embolism (SAWELIEW, 1894) could not be statistically proven (HILLER, 1936).

Among 15 cases, HILLER (1936) found the right side involved 10 times. W. SCHEID (1963) found among 19 fatal cases of embolism, 10 involving the right middle cerebral artery, 3 involving the left, 3 situated in the right carotid artery, and 1 in the left. According to BÖHNE (1927, 1931a, b), the first large surface branch of the middle cerebral artery is supposed to be most often involved. Allegedly, the embolic infarct is frequently hemorrhagic (POPPER, 1949: 40%). However, this statement and also the general statistics of brain embolism need further checking. The concept developed at the Massachusetts General Hospital (R. ADAMS and C.M. FISHER, 1961) assumed that the emboli would progress and split up and thus give rise to the hemorrhagic form of infarct (p. 128ff.). For these authors the statistical correlation between hemorrhagic infarction and embolism is high.

10. Circulatory Sequelae After Embolism

If an artery is occluded by an embolus, the collaterals (PENRY and NETSKY, 1960) go into action as they do in thrombosis (see above). However, this process is often not sufficiently rapid for sufficient restoration of circulation to occur within 4–6 min. J.S. MEYER et al. (1954), by clamping the middle cerebral artery in the rhesus monkey, demonstrated that the meningeal anastomoses are indeed immediately called into play. Reversal of the blood stream could be observed after 10–30 s. The effectiveness of collaterals following an embolic occlusion of the middle cerebral artery has been demonstrated arteriographically. It has been proven also angiographically that cerebral emboli may split up (CRONQVIST, 1969) and "disappear" (see p. 72). They may also be "recanalized" (DALAL et al., 1965).

11. Microembolism

The entrance of fat droplets into the bloodstream occurs most frequently after fracture of the long bones or pelvis and less frequently after contusions of large fat cushions. Depending upon its size, the fat embolus is retained in the lung or passes through the lung capillaries (or through an open foramen ovale) eventually to cause life-endangering disturbances in the cerebral circulation. Macroscopically the picture is characterized by "flea-bite" hemorrhages in the white matter, especially in the corpus callosum and centrum semiovale; first reported by RIBBERT in 1894, 1900). Again depending on size, the emboli are usually retained in the capillaries where they block the flow of blood. Only rarely is an arteriole occluded but occlusion of an arteriole leads to microinfarction. Occlusion of the capillaries apparently causes morphological tissue damage only if the capillaries of several, closely adjoining cylinders of Krogh are involved. This leads to damage of the capillary endothelium and to tiny pericapillary hemorrhages. It is always astonishing to see how few nerve cells are damaged in an area in which the capillaries are extensively occluded by fat emboli. However, edematous and metabolic changes have been experimentally reproduced in our laboratory and have been shown to lead to massive intra- and extracellular edema and raised intracranial pressure (ZÜLCH and TZONOS, 1964, 1965; VISE et al., 1977; SCHUIER et al., 1978; TAMURA and ZÜLCH 1979).

The main damage in fat embolism is not in the cortex, which indeed also exhibits minor circulatory damage, but in the subjacent white matter (ZÜLCH et al., 1976). Perivascular edema occurs very early (in animal experiments after 4 h), from the large veins resulting in demyelination in the immediate vicinity and small perivenous necroses containing a large amount of fibrin also occur. On the second or third day diapedetic hemorrhages may develop around them in man, but are only rarely observed in animal experiments. The pathogenetic mechanism of this "distant" lesion in microembolism is not yet clarified.

SWANK and HAIN (1952), J.S. MEYER et al. (1962) and particularly ZÜLCH and TZONOS (1964, 1965) described the effect of experimental microemboli. We succeeded in revealing the mechanism of the damage in experiments employing plastic emboli of 30–37 μ diameter. Obviously, an obstruction of blood flow occurs either in the arterioles (in animal experiments) or in the capillaries (in human experiments) or in experiments with 15 μ emboli (TAMURA and ZÜLCH, 1979), causing delay of flow and sludging in the deep veins of the white matter. The ensuing endothelial alteration permits a transudation of serum which causes demyelination. It has not been explained why diapedesis of erythrocytes occurs in the human while it is absent in the animal. The postedematous perivenous demyelination is the main cause of permanent damage or a fatal outcome in humans. The pathological entity *microembolism of thrombotic* and/or atheromatous material from ulcerated atherosclerotic intraarterial plaques plays an important role in the discussion of transient ischemic attacks (TIAs). For details see p. 122.

12. Air Embolism

The pathogenesis in air embolism is much more complex. The damage may vary depending on whether the embolism was caused by entrance of air from the inside (Caisson disease), from the outside (criminal abortion or during pneumothorax) or by nonabsorbable administrations into the bloodstream. ROER (1949) also discussed the possibility of entrance of air from the nasal cavities into the dural sinuses as a result of basal skull fracture. The tissue alterations consist of tiny foci of nerve cell loss, selective parenchymal necroses, etc. The experimental observations of NAQUET were of great importance for electro-encephalography (NAQUET, 1965; NAQUET and VIGOUROUX, 1966; NAQUET et al., 1966; GASTAUT et al., 1971).

Air embolism leads to endothelial lesions, transudation of plasma and erythrocytes and to ischemic foci predominantly in the cortex as described in the ischemic cell disease of SPIELMEYER (1922) etc. These lesions are less severe than those of fat embolism but show a similar pattern and a topographical predilection for the "Dreiländereck" (EEG-Colloque de Marseille à Cologne, 1964; GASTAUT et al., 1971; see also p. 139).

Unique observations are those of CHASON et al. (1963) and others, and of SILBERMAN et al., (1960) describing cotton fiber embolism in angiography.

X. Vascular Lesions of Nonatherosclerotic Origin

Vessels may be involved by other types of lesions, particularly those of an *inflammatory* nature. Tuberculous meningitis with arteritis and periphlebitis of the basal vessels is still encountered but syphilitic lesions (infarcts) are rare. The still somewhat obscure condition of thromboangiitis obliterans is discussed on p. 61 ff.

In rare cases a parasite – cysticercus – may cause *granulomatous* restriction and stenosis of the carotid artery (Figs. 1 and 2 in BEHREND et al., 1966). Allergic conditions are presumed to be involved in temporal arteritis, Takayashu's ("pulse less") disease, periarteritis nodosa and lupus erythematosis ("collagen disease"). The arterial wall proliferation in Moya-Moya disease (see p. 17) may also have an allergic component. (For references see textbooks of BLACKWOOD et al., 1949, PETERS, 1970, and STEHBENS, 1972.)

Hypertensive encephalopathy (see p. 119) will not be discussed here (see ZIEGLER et al., 1965).

Fibromuscular dysplasia (RINALDI et al., 1976) is a condition which until now has been poorly defined and which is usually angiographically diagnosed (CONNET and LAUSCHE, 1965; HOUSER et al., 1971). It is said to present itself in 1% of angiograms (LIE, 1968). It may also occur in the smaller arteries (HUBER and FUCHS, 1967). Histologically, ring-like hyperplasia of fibrous or muscular tissue is considered to be causative.

1. Functional Arterial Changes: Vasospasm

The consequence of vasospasm is said to be twofold: a cause of arteriolosclerosis and provoking cerebrovascular insufficiency.

Older theories considered primary vasospasm as the main factor leading to arteriolosclerosis and even more so to atherosclerosis (SPATZ, 1939; ANDERS and EICKE, 1939). There is data today, which proves the old theory of BAYLISS (1902) of vasospasm in the smaller arteries following sudden hypertension (e.g. a "hypertensive crisis"). This was the basis for the concept of the "angiospastic insult" of the German school (v. BERGMANN, 1932; Fr. KAUFFMANN, 1925). However, this theory was opposed by the "hemodynamic" concept of DENNY-BROWN (1951) and for a long time cerebral angiospasm was denied. Meanwhile, new observations on cerebral vasospasm have been made (Review article: SIMEONE, 1979) in the field of neuroradiology particularly following puncture of arteries, and also very commonly in cases of subarachnoid hemorrhage. Its pros and cons have been discussed extensively by ZÜLCH (1962b, 1967, 1971a) and LECHTAPE-GRÜTER and ZÜLCH (1971).

Recent experimental investigations confirm the possibility of local "vasospasm" following a hypertensive crisis alternating with "dilatation" (HÄGGENDAL and JOHANSSON, 1971/72; EKSTRÖM-JODAL et al., 1975). It is, however, associated with a "break-through" of the blood-brain barrier. Either may cause the ensuing neurological symptoms (see MCHEDLISHVILI et al., 1970/71; WHITE et al., 1975; WHITE, 1979).

2. Arterial Innervation

Innervation of the cerebral arteries has been morphologically proven since the classical observations of FORBES and WOLFF (1928), CHOROBSKI and PENFIELD (1932), FORBES and COBB (1938), etc. (for references see NELSON and RENNELS, 1970; BLAUMANIS, 1979; OWMAN, 1979; R. WHITE, 1979; ZERVAS, 1979). It is, however, difficult to analyse its functional significance. NELSON and RENNELS (1970) are of the opinion that the majority of vascular smooth muscle cells must be without direct innervation, though transmitters may stimulate them at some distance by diffusion. The authors could not explain the significance of intracranial arterial innervation, and although much experimental data is available today it is often dissenting (EDVINSSON and OWMAN, 1979).

Vasospasm following subarachnoid hemorrhage (SAH) is common knowledge now. It can definitely be the cause of diminished flow through the spastically stenosed vessels.

XI. Sequelae of Vascular Changes: Hematomas and Infarction

1. Intracranial Hemorrhages (for short review see ZÜLCH, 1968a)

a) Epidural Hemorrhage

In the majority of cases epidural hemorrhage follows a traumatic rupture of the middle meningeal artery, but occasionally venous oozing during decreased intracranial pressure may be responsible. The site and extension of epidural bleeding may be explained by anatomical fixation of the dura to the skull (Fig. 73). The localization may therefore be different from that of a typical subdural hematoma for which the site of predilection in the free subdural fronto-temporo-parietal space is well known (ZEHNDER, 1937). The epidural hemorrhage on the other hand may be more frontal, temporal or occipital-parietal according to the site of the fracture affecting a branch of the middle meningeal artery. The second, postoperative form

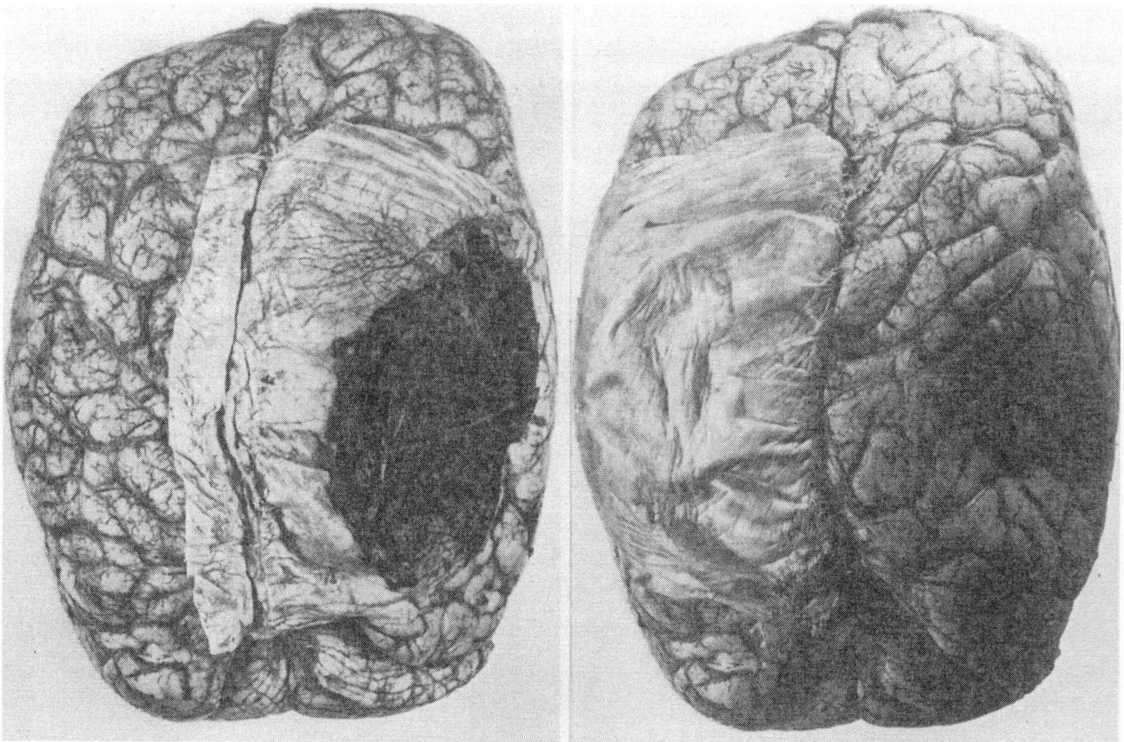

Fig. 73. Fresh epidural parietal hematoma; note the impression on the hemisphere

arising from venous oozing into the epidural space is naturally related to the site of the surgical flap since the dura is fixed to the bone. Therefore there is no predilection site for epidural hematomas. This is different than for subdural hematoma.

b) Subdural Hemorrhages – Acute– Chronic (Encapsulated)

Subdural (acute and chronic) hemorrhages including chronic subdural encapsulated hemorrhages can spread more easily than the epidural ones because of the open subdural space. Its predilection site is in the centre of the three great lobes, that is over the fronto-temporo-parietal region (Fig. 74). This may be explained by the site and direction of movement of the brain substance giving way to the blood clot (ZEHNDER, 1937; BRUETMAN et al., 1963). These lateral shifts are determined by the mobility of the brain underneath the falx and its fixation at the base, and by its internal structure (great fasciculi of the white matter). Its mobility is therefore dependent upon the local resistance of the brain tissue to compression or deformation by the hematoma. This, in turn, may be influenced by the cerebrospinal fluid pressure, by the intra-arterial pressure, and by fixation of the brain itself (pituitary stalk, vessels, nerves) within the cranial cavity (see ZÜLCH, 1959; ZÜLCH et al., 1974b).

These facts regarding a site of predilection seem to be of importance in echoencephalography, conventional radiography and computed tomography for the differential diagnosis between an epidural and an acute or a chronic encapsulated subdural hematoma (ZÜLCH, 1968b).

One point should be added in order to explain some figures from DANDY's "Surgery of the Brain" (1932): in rare cases an encapsulated subdural hematoma may be accompanied by a congenital arachnoidal cyst, a phenomenon which DANDY in his textbook on brain surgery calls (1932) a "subdural hygroma" (his Figs. 171, 172).

We have also had such a patient, aged 48, who died in spite of evacuation of the subdural hematoma because of a space-occupying arachnoidal cyst in the Sylvian fissure underneath the hematoma. The cyst

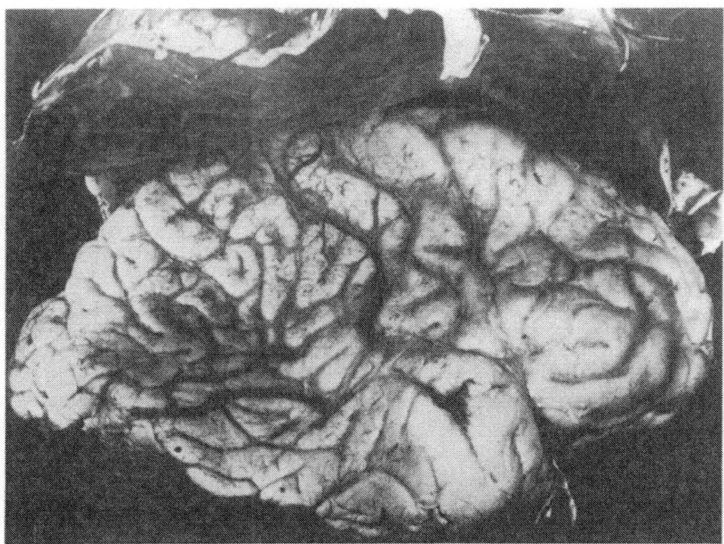

Fig. 74. Marked impression on the convexity of a brain with consequent displacement by an old subdural capsulated hematoma (upper margin)

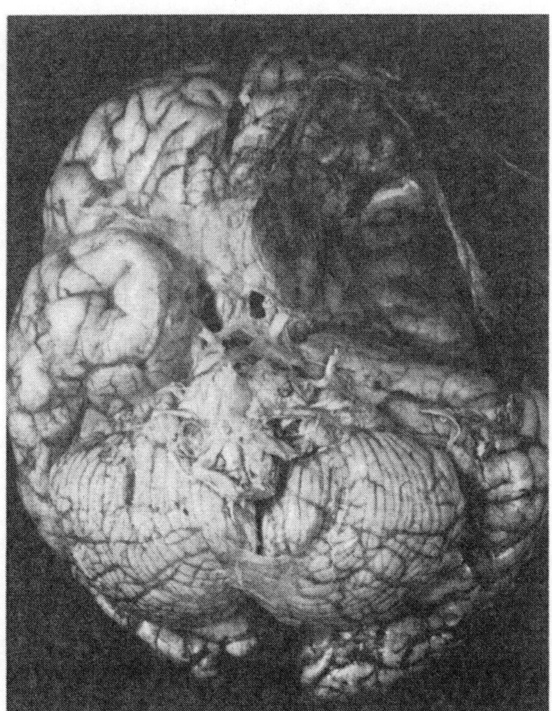

Fig. 75. Old "congenital" temporal arachnoidal cyst with overlying subacute subdural capsulated hematoma. Death from traffic accident

was not recognized through the burr holes at surgery and was only revealed at autopsy (ZÜLCH, 1954a, Fig. 8). Usually in the plain skull films a protrusion of the bone will indicate the presence of such a congenital cyst (Fig. 75).

An *acute traumatic subdural hematoma* (KRAULAND, 1950; LOEW and WÜSTNER, 1960) stems from a laceration of a major arterial vessel (Fig. 76) usually on the surface of the brain, as in our own case of a man aged 56. If diagnosed promptly and correctly, surgery ought to be easy. The predilection site of an *acute* subdural hematoma corresponds to that of the subacute or *chronic* type.

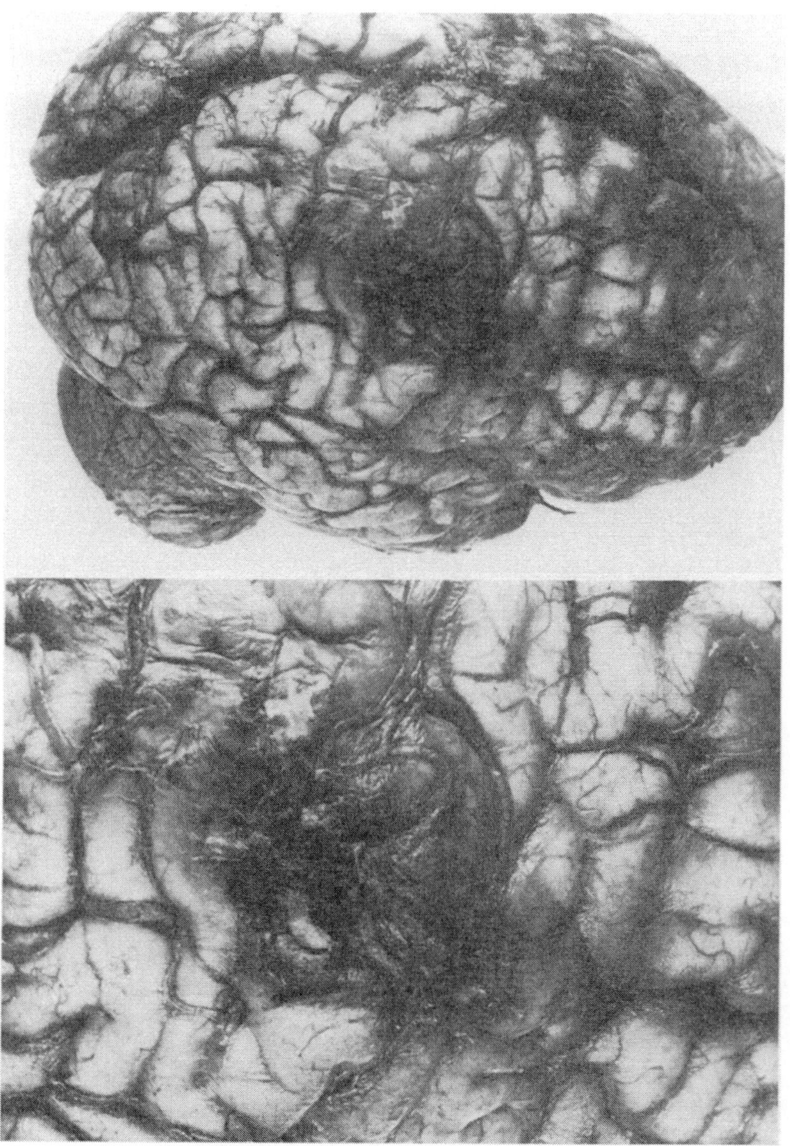

Fig. 76. Traumatic laceration of cortical arteries giving rise to acute subdural, space-occupying hematoma

Posttraumatic chronic encapsulated subdural hematoma. It is still controversial as to whether a chronic subdural hematoma (LINK, 1945, 1950; JACOB, 1950; PETERS, 1950, 1951; OKONEK, 1950) always is traumatic in origin or is dependent upon a disease *sui generis* of the dura mater. The time required for its formation after trauma (which is often minor and may be called "bagatelle trauma") is usually up to 3 months. The supposed traumatic origin stems from the observations and theories of TROTTER (1914), PUTNAM and CUSHING (1925), GARDNER (1932, 1935) and recent microscopical findings. The bleeding is of venous origin, coming usually from torn "bridging" veins. Yet, in general medicine and forensic pathology, very often the older theory of VIRCHOW (1856), of a "pachymeningitis hemorrhagica" as a "genuine" disease of the dura is favored, that is, the hemorrhage follows a granulating (intra-) dural process. This has been discussed thoroughly in neurosurgical meetings and extensively published (for history see also LINK, 1945, 1950; LOEW and WÜSTNER, 1960).

The fact of a predilection site for subdural encapsulated hematomas is now better understood (ZÜLCH, 1956b, 1968a) since we have a clearer insight into pathogenesis, where we distinguish be-

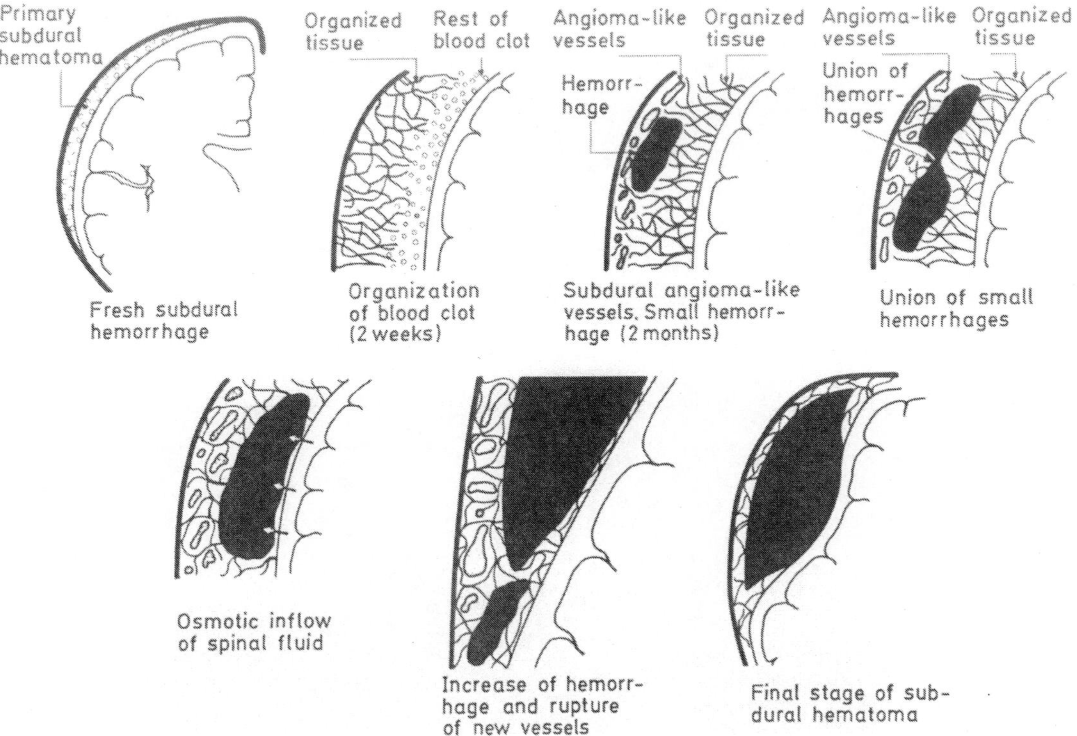

Fig. 77. Various stages in the pathogenesis of the chronic subdural encapsulated hematoma

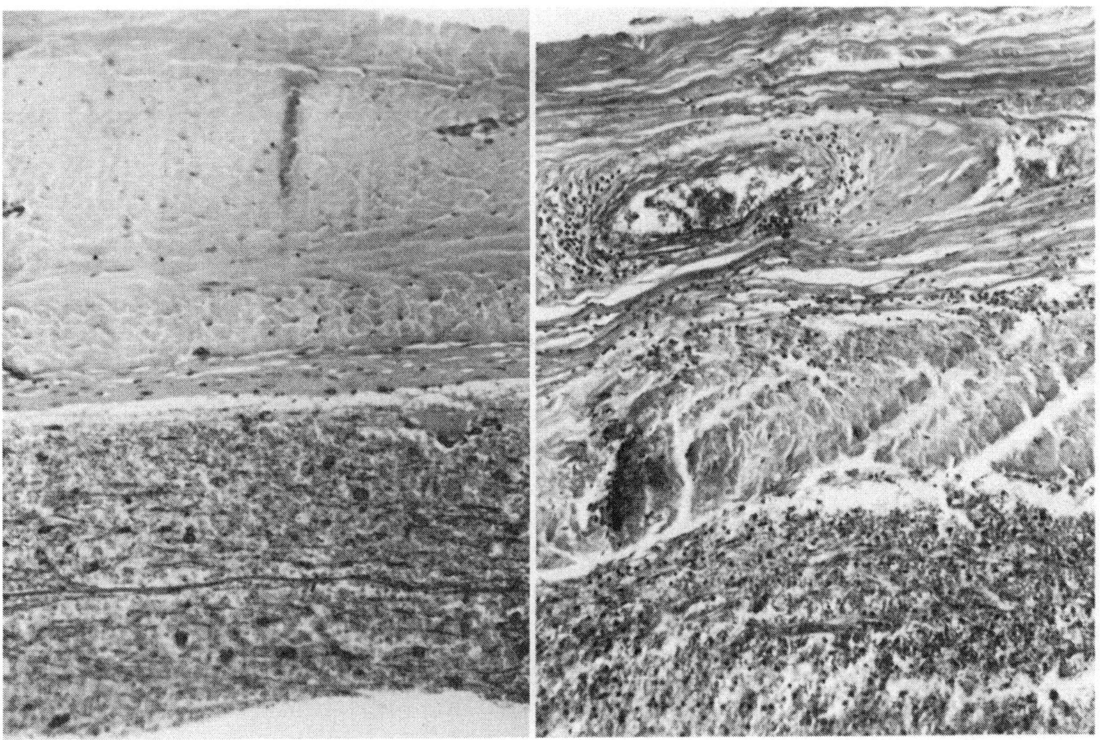

Fig. 78. Organization of the fresh blood film by fibroblastic invasion from the dura "endothelium". *Left:* from a healthy dura, HE, ×125; *Right:* from a dura with lymphoid infiltration and degenerative changes of the layers of the dura, HE, ×125

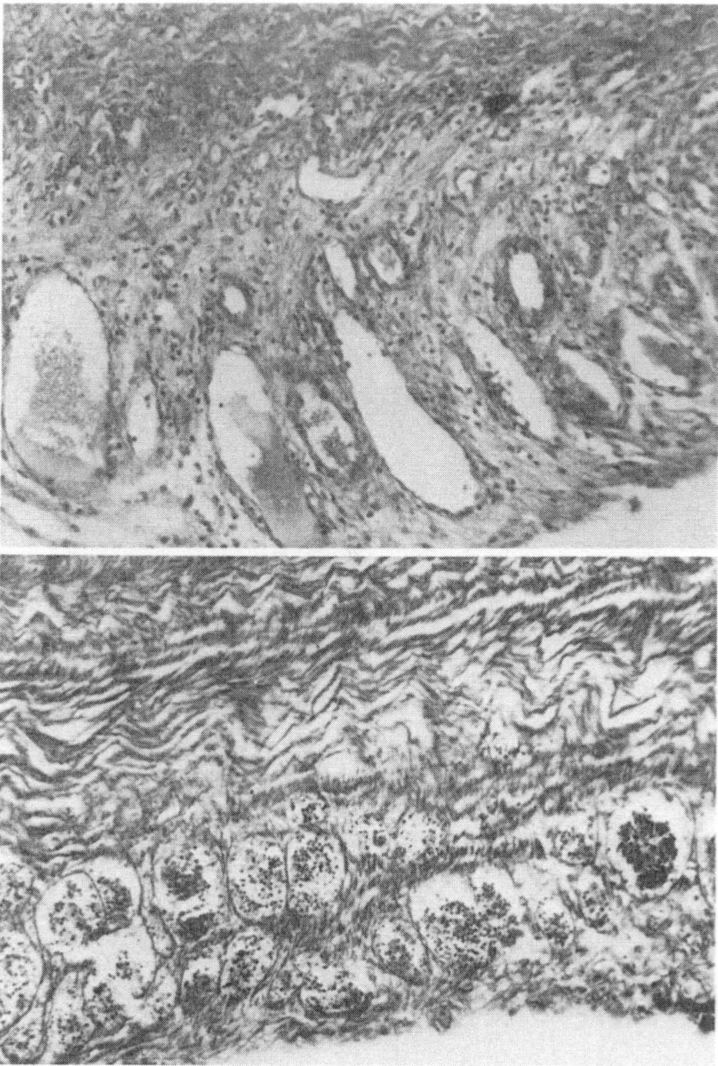

Fig. 79. Formation of new vessels in an organized blood clot near the dura in an angioma-like condensation; *above:* HE, ×125; *below:* Wilders impregnation, ×125

tween two forms: (1) a primary degenerative process of the dura, in the old-age group, called the true "pachymeningitis" or "pachymeningosis" of Virchow and (2) the post-traumatic subdural hematoma which is later encapsulated and is more common in younger people (ZÜLCH, 1956b). Macroscopically they both seem to be very similar, but there are histological differences in the dura. In pachymeningosis we find primary degenerative changes and/or lymphoid infiltration, whereas in the traumatic form the dura is unchanged or only secondarily affected. The various steps in the development of the encapsulated hematoma commence with a small blood film underneath (Figs. 77, 78, published in LOEW and WÜSTNER, 1960, as Fig. 16) the dura which becomes organized and forms capillaries and a cavernoma-like accumulation of vessels (Figs. 77, 78, 79, 80) which may break and form small blood clots (Figs. 77, 80). These blood clots attract cerebro-spinal fluid by osmosis according to the postulates of GARDNER (1932, 1935) who defined the inner membrane of the hematoma as an osmotic membrane. Thus, small hematomas grow in size by taking up cerebrospinal fluid. They then tear other vessels in the granulation tissue, and new blood is added, the internal osmotic tension is reinforced and cerebrospinal fluid is absorbed by increase in osmotic pressure. Finally these small hematomas unite, form a larger blood clot, and once again new blood is added.

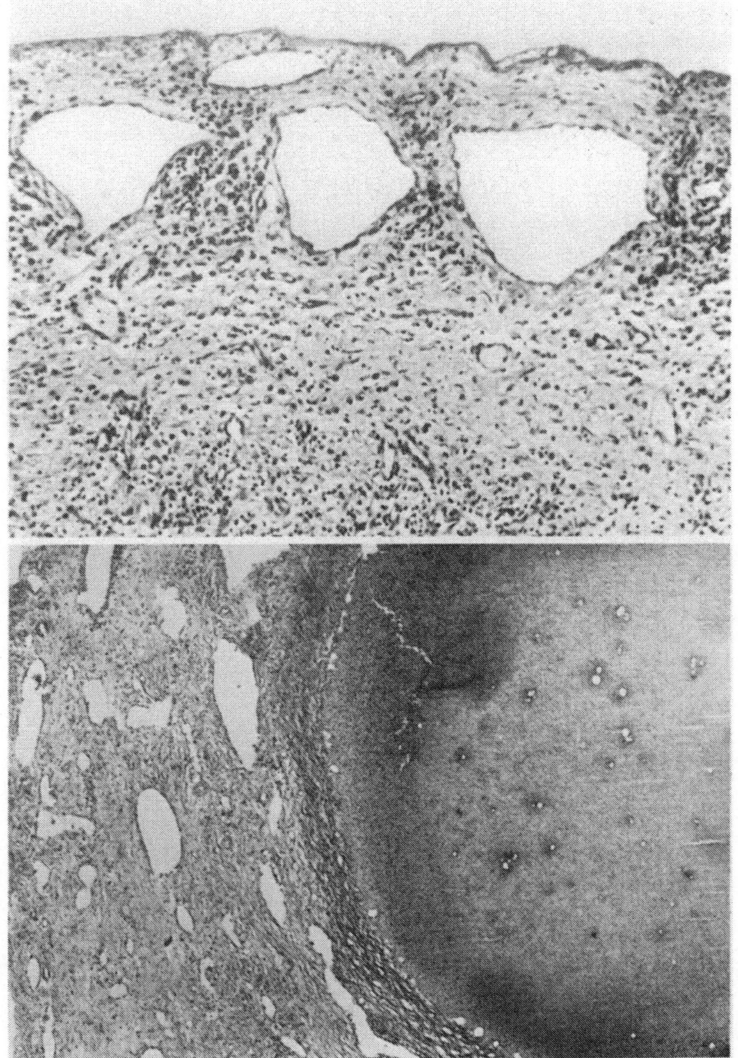

Fig. 80. *Above:* Great angioma-like vessels in an organized blood clot near the dura; HE, ×125; *Below:* Rupture of these vessels and formation of fresh hemorrhage; HE, ×50

Eventually it becomes too large for the available space in the internal and external "reserve" channels of the cerebrospinal fluid, even though these spaces may already be larger as a result of atrophy of the aged brain. Finally the point of decompensation is reached, intracranial pressure begins to rise, and neurological symptoms appear (Fig. 77).

In summary, for *legal cases* in the younger age group trauma may be regarded as the main cause whereas in older patients pachymeningosis, i.e., a primary degenerative process in the dura may be the primary lesion, while the formation of a hematoma by a trauma is only secondary (see Jacob, 1950; Okonek, 1950; Peters, 1950, 1951; Zülch, 1950).

c) *Subarachnoid Hemorrhage* (see also p. 25ff.)

Subarachnoid hemorrhage (Locksley, 1966: 6368 cases) may be local, e.g., near the bleeding vessel, or generalized. It has however, a predilection and is most marked in the cisterns neighboring the bleeding vessel. It may invade the ventricles through the foramina of the 4th ventricle but does not usually extend beyond the 4th ventricle. Traumatic subarachnoid hemorrhage is usually associated with simultaneous subdural hemorrhage (see p. 76ff.) whereas subarachnoid

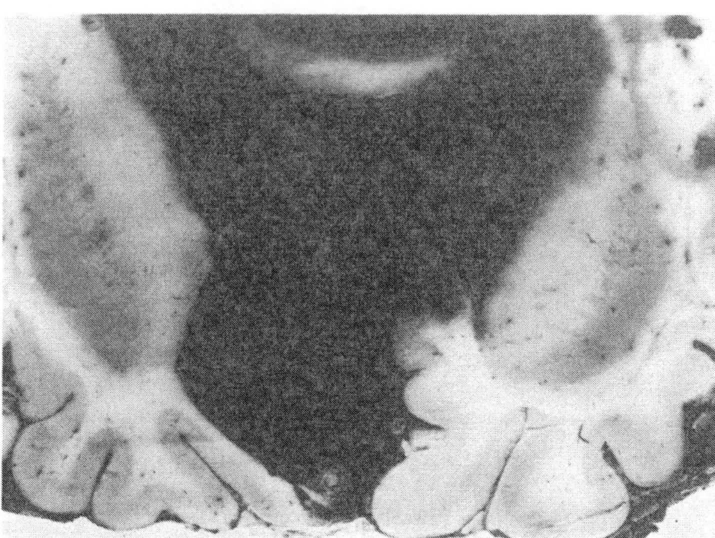

Fig. 81. Large blood clot around ruptured saccular aneurysm of the anterior cerebral artery

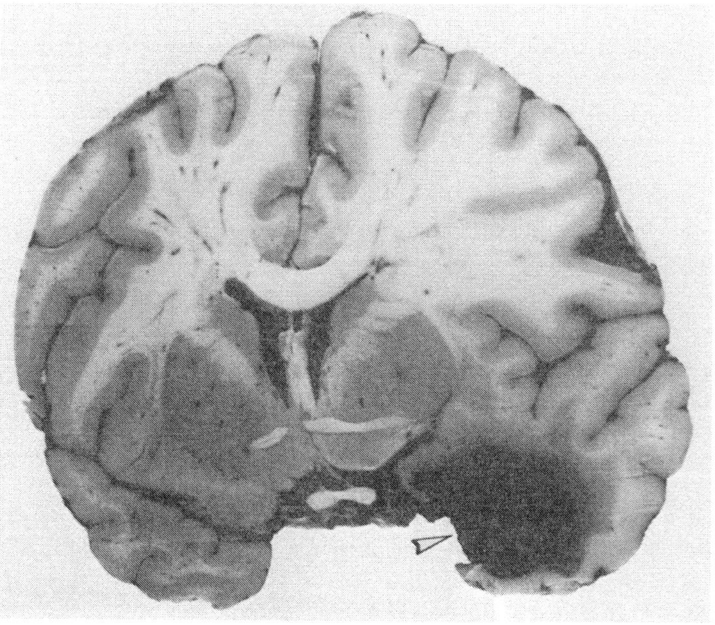

Fig. 82. Hemorrhage near a ruptured saccular aneurysm of the posterior communicating artery. Typical localization

hemorrhage from ruptured saccular aneurysms or arteriovenous malformations and angiomas tends to destroy and invade the surrounding brain tissue in a region typical for the site of the aneurysm (see Figs. 81–83). It is interesting to know that bleeding aneurysm, therefore, have predilection sites. They give a very typical picture for each of the three main groups of aneurysms of the basal arterial system. Thus we see a double-sided penetration of blood into the base of the medial frontal (Fig. 81) lobes from ruptured aneurysms of the anterior communicating artery. From the posterior communicating artery we see a rupture (Fig. 82) into the temporal horn while finally we may find a hemorrhage in the Sylvian fissure breaking into the adjacent frontal and/or temporal lobe tissue from aneurysms of the middle cerebral artery (Fig. 83). These bleedings are at present easily shown by computed tomography and will be the requirements for angiography.

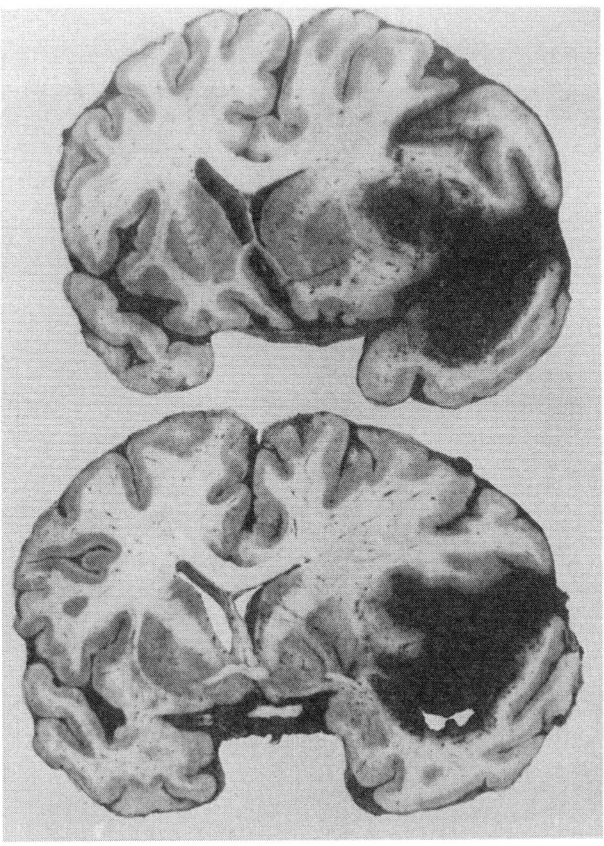

Fig. 83. Typical localization of hemorrhage in a case of ruptured saccular aneurysm of middle cerebral artery

Hemorrhage from ruptured angiomas may penetrate into the brain substance, into the subarachnoid space (Sturge-Weber: ANDERSON and DUNCAN, 1974) or into the ventricles. Many cerebral mass hemorrhages, particularly in younger poeple, are seen in an atypical site which is easily distinguished from that of hypertensive hemorrhages into the basal ganglia (see p. 103) or the other predilection sites. These other forms are caused very often by the rupture of a "microangioma" (Fig. 23), a term customary in clinical jargon. Morphologically it may correspond to the "telangiectatic" or "capillary angioma" or more rarely to the cavernoma or even a small arteriovenous angioma. We have seen these particularly in the mesencephalothalamic region (Fig. 20).

Subarachnoid hemorrhage may also follow the rupture of a hypertensive mass hemorrhage through the cortex (see p. 88 and Fig. 84), or a hemorrhage into a tumor (preferably oligodendroglioma, glioblastoma, clear cell carcinoma of kidney, malignant melanoma, chorioepithelioma). The source of the bleeding is detected infrequently either angiographically or at autopsy because this may be difficult in a formalin-hardened blood clot (however, 10–20% have been reported in some autopsy-series, see HYLAND, 1950; WOLFE, 1953; MCKISSOCK and PAINE, 1959).

The "spontaneous" subarachnoid hemorrhage of the Internist in any case is, if real at all, a rarity. Inflammatory conditions, venous thromboses, systemic vascular disease, or hematologic conditions may be other very rare causes. Yet there will be some help in ascertaining the source of a subarachnoid hemorrhage by referring to a table listing (see GILROY and MEYER, 1969) the possible (rarer) causes. (For references see OLIVECRONA and LADENHEIM, 1957; TÖNNIS et al., 1957; MCKISSOCK and PAINE, 1959; POOL and POTTS, 1965; LANGE-COSACK, 1966; LOCKSLEY, 1966; PAKARINEN, 1967; HEIDRICH, 1970, 1972; LIE, 1972; MORELLO and BORGHI, 1973).

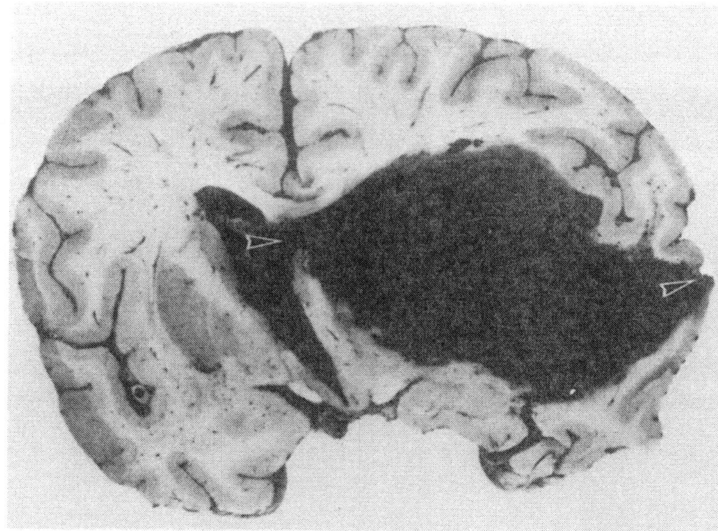

Fig. 84. Enormous, typical massive hemorrhage with pronounced shift to the contralateral side associated with rupture both into adjacent ventricle and through the cortex *(arrows)*

d) Associated Ischemic Lesions

Meanwhile it is well known that aneurysmal bleedings may be complicated by ischemic lesions. The causes may be:

a) arterial spasm, which is probably the most frequent event (for further references see E.G. ROBERTSON, 1949; CROMPTON, 1964; LANDAU and RANSOHOFF, 1968; HANAU and REDONDO, 1973). In the observations of SYMON (1967), MCHEDLISHVILI (1972), HANAU and REDONDO (1973) and WHITE et al. (1975) ischemic lesions were encountered in 80% of cases (136 out of 169), some of them even contralateral (see also angiospasm, p. 75).
b) an impairment of vessels by the hemorrhage invading the cerebral tissue (for instance thrombosis).

2. Cerebral Hemorrhages

a) Typical Mass Hemorrhages, Surgical Treatment, Angiographic Classification

For the radiologist dealing with cases of cerebral hemorrhage it is still important to be acquainted with their morphology and pathogenesis although there has been a drastic reduction in their frequency and a relative increase in cerebral infarction (KRUEGER et al., 1967, for Memphis/USA; KATSUKI et al., 1971). In spite of this decrease among adequately treated hypertensives, hemorrhage still remains persistently high in the older age group (MOSER and GOLDMAN, 1967). Moreover, some authors still recommend surgical treatment (MIZUKAMI et al., 1976). Furthermore, differential diagnosis by computed tomography has become exceedingly important (H.R. MÜLLER et al., 1975).

α) Morphological Fact

"Striatal hemorrhage". It occurs predominantly in association with hypertension. It produces acorn to fist-sized areas of destruction (Fig. 85) of brain tissue which are filled with blood and cellular debris and disrupt the integrity of the surrounding grey and white substance. As seen at the time of operation or autopsy, these hemorrhagic cavities contain fresh or older blood which is either fluid or coagulated and mixed with remnants of nervous tissue and isolated blood vessels. In the border zone, punctiform, petechial hemorrhages designated "flea-bite" hemorrhages, occur in the course of the first 2–3 days (Fig. 86) (STAEMMLER's "marginal hemor-

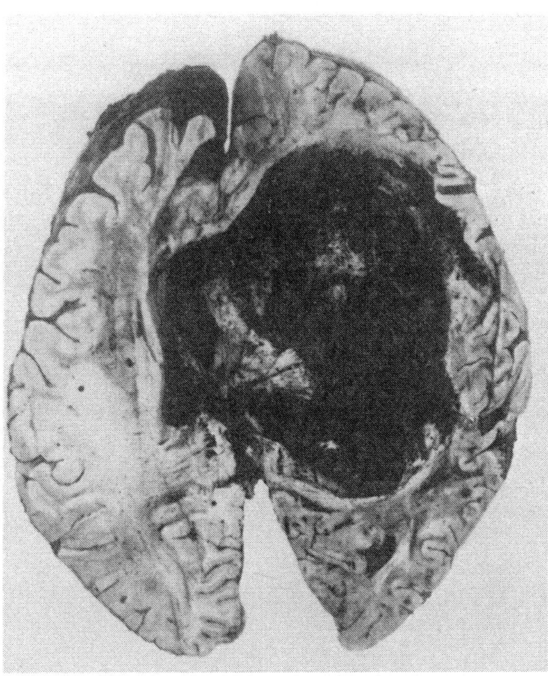

Fig. 85. Fist-sized hypertensive hemorrhage arising from the striatal arteries and pushing to the contralateral side

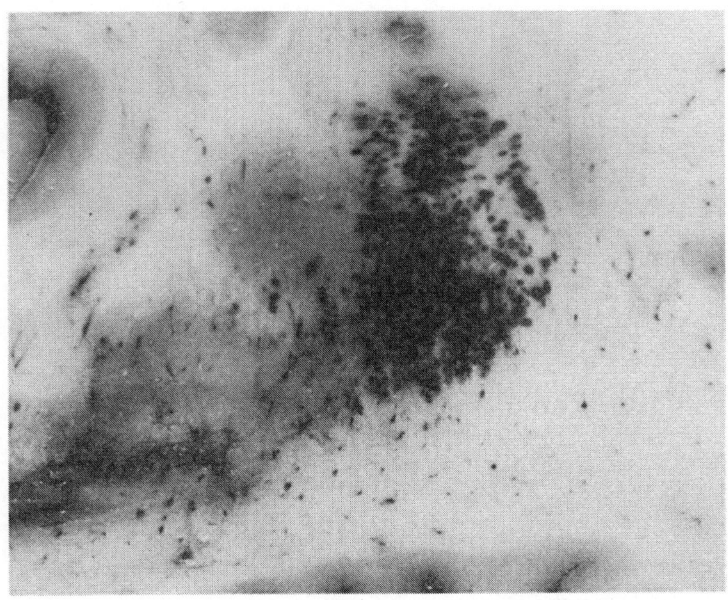

Fig. 86. Pericapillary bleeding adjacent to a cerebral mass hemorrhage (so-called STAEMMLER's hemorrhages)

rhages", 1936). After several hours there is formation of a penetrating extracellular brain edema which first develops perivascularly and then diffusely invades the tissue spaces (Fig. 87).

Macroscopically massive hemorrhage in the striatum must be distinguished from hemorrhagic infarction in the same territory (lenticulo-striate artery) (Figs. 96, 97, 142) since this occasionally has been misinterpreted in the literature (ROSENBLATH, 1918, 1927; Ph. SCHWARTZ, 1930).

The massive hemorrhage usually takes on rather large dimensions rapidly (Fig. 88) – possibly within at most a few hours – and becomes an important space-occupying lesion. This leads

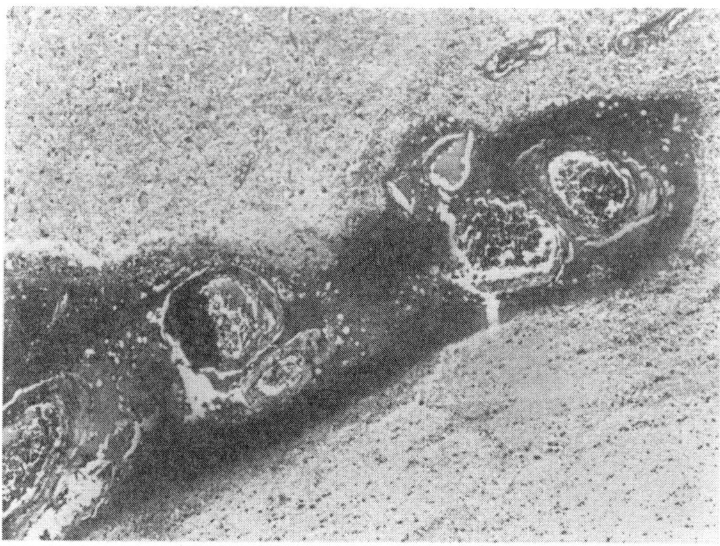

Fig. 87. Perivascular edema, rich in albumin, in the vicinity of a "striatal" mass hemorrhage. HE, ×50

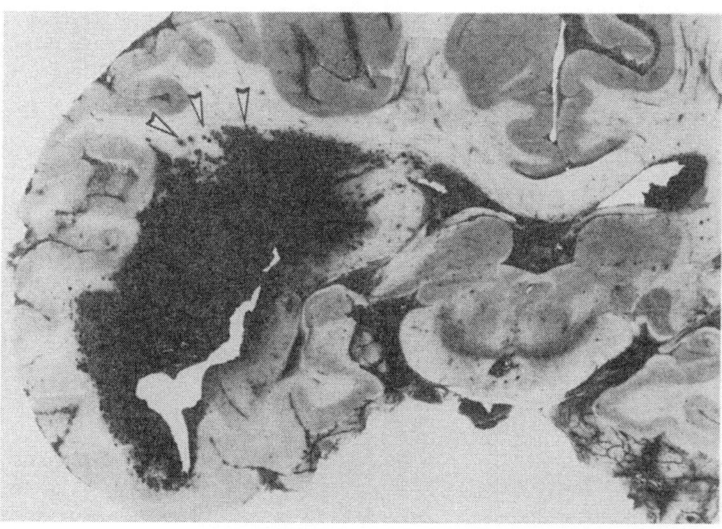

Fig. 88. Typical massive hemorrhage with extension into the temporal lobe. In the marginal zone pericapillary bleedings (petechiae, STAEMMLER's hemorrhages) *(arrows)*

to the displacement of tissue and to its known consequences: a *lateral* shift 1) to the opposite side including the susceptible parts of the brain stem: hypothalamus and especially the midbrain (Fig. 84), 2) of the basal temporal lobe in a lateral and also the brainstem and the medulla oblongata in an *"axial"* direction towards the posterior fossa with the formation of a temporal and/or cerebellar pressure cone.

This axial shift may cause stretching of the vessels of the lower brainstem and lead to secondary hemorrhages in the midbrain (Fig. 89) and pons by rupture or congestion of the paramedian and circumferential arteries and veins (HUTCHINSON and YATES, 1956; FRIEDE and ROESSMANN, 1966; LINDENBERG, 1957). Similar hemorrhages occur with other space-occupying lesions (see ZÜLCH et al., 1974b, and pp. 89, 162ff.; 54% of FREITAG's cases, 1968; 47% in MARKS' series, 1960, when the patient died within 3 days) and in acute trauma (see ZÜLCH, 1959, Fig. 71). The perifocal brain edema progressing in the first two days adds an additional space-occupying factor, which is thought to have a volume of at least 50 cc (COHEN and ARONSON, 1968).

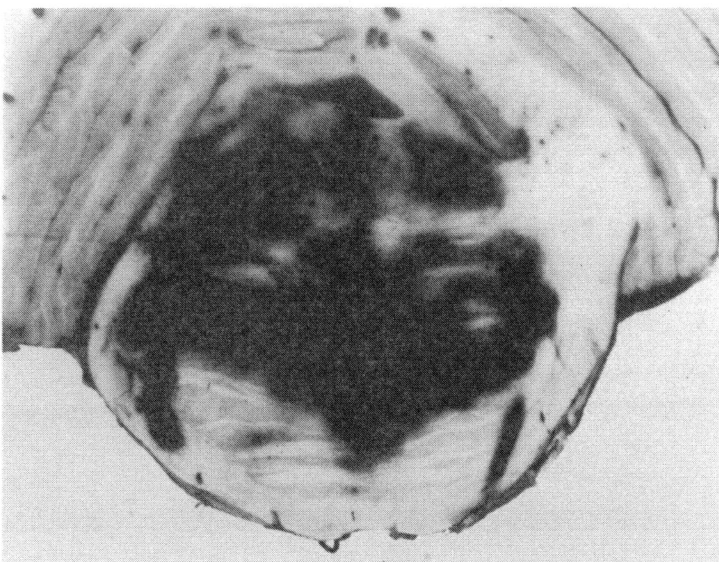

Fig. 89. Typical secondary hemorrhages around pontine veins and arteries in a case of marked "axial shift" produced by supratentorial tumor surrounded by gross brain edema

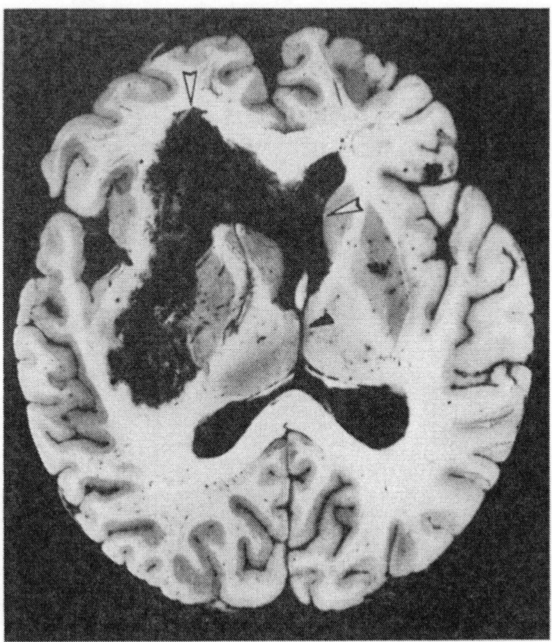

Fig. 90. Massive left cerebral hemorrhage arising in typical location in putamen. Invasion of the left frontal and parietal white matter. Rupture into anterior horn of the left lateral ventricle *(arrows)*. Internal hematocephalus. Contralateral displacement

The hematoma may also rupture into the ventricular system, usually into the frontal horn (in 42 of our 70 cases, PABELICK, 1967; 75% in FREITAG'S cases, 1968; see Figs. 84 and 91), and less frequently into the region of the cella media and the trigone or the occipital horn of the lateral ventricle. The bursting into the lateral ventricles follows characteristic tears with a predilection for the corners of the ventricles (Figs. 90, 91; see also HARRIS et al., 1968; FREITAG, 1968).

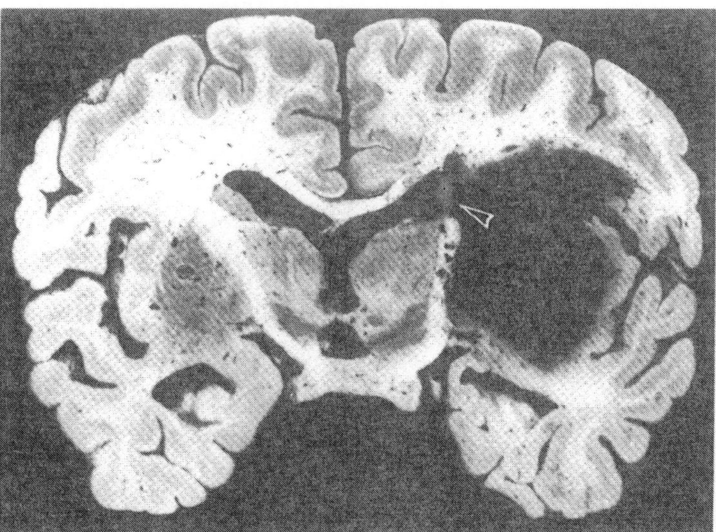

Fig. 91. Typical hypertensive hemorrhage arising from the striatal arteries and rupturing into the adjacent frontal horn *(arrow)*. A lacuna is seen in the contralateral putamen

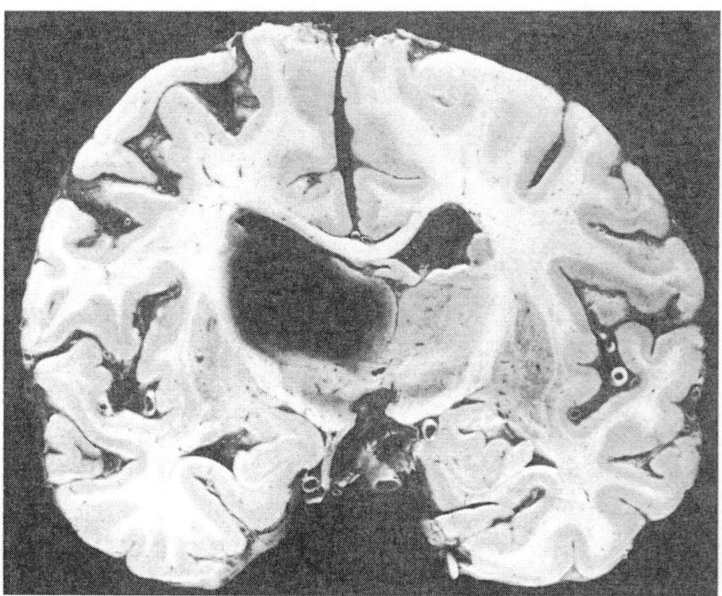

Fig. 92. Typical thalamic hemorrhage with rupture into lateral ventricle. Severe stenosing atherosclerosis especially in vessels of the Sylvian fissure. General convolutional atrophy with widening of sulci

Further complications may arise by extension – "rupture" – of this "striatal" hemorrhage into the neighboring white matter of the frontal (Fig. 90), temporal (Fig. 84) or parieto-occipital lobe. The cortex (Fig. 84) may also be torn and blood may escape into the subarachnoid space (ZÜLCH, 1961a; FREITAG, 1968: 15% of her cases) or even into the subdural space (FREITAG, 1968: 6% of her cases).

Thalamic hemorrhage. Hemorrhage within the more caudal areas of the thalamus, excluding the lenticular nucleus, is a rare form associated with hypertension (3.1% in our series; ZÜLCH, 1971a, see also Figs. 92 and 93). It may also rupture into the more posterior parts of the lateral ventricle (Fig. 93) or the third ventricle. In thalamic hemorrhage it is presumably the thalamo-perforating or geniculate arteries that rupture.

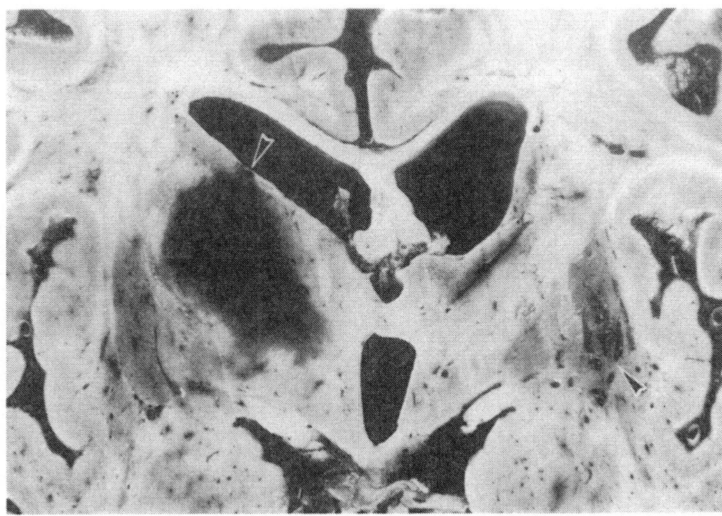

Fig. 93. Typical thalamic hemorrhage with rupture into lateral ventricle *(arrow)*. Severe "criblures" in contralateral putamen *(arrow)*. Arteries are hardly compromised by atherosclerosis

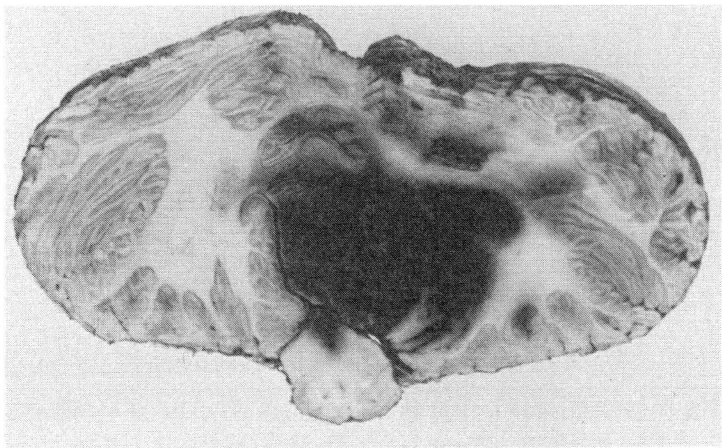

Fig. 94. Typical *(small)* cerebellar hemorrhage near the dentatum

Cerebellar hemorrhage. Hemorrhages into the cerebellum are rare (about 5.4% of our cases; ZÜLCH, 1971a). They most often occur in the region of the dentate nucleus and extend either to the cortex or to the fourth ventricle (Fig. 94; see also REY-BELLET, 1960; C.M. FISHER et al., 1965b; LICHTENSTEIN, 1968). They arise from the superior cerebellar artery (A. nucl. dentati; see A. THOMAS, 1925; POOR, 1967).

Pontine hemorrhage. Primary pontine hemorrhages are not so rare. They amounted to 11.0% (ZÜLCH, 1971a) in our series (Fig. 95; cf. 7.5% SILVERSTEIN, 1967), while according to other authors they are more frequent and particularly prone to occur in severe hypertension. However, it appears to depend on how *critically they are interpreted and classified* as primary or secondary hemorrhages (see Fig. 89, 95) as mentioned previously (GOWERS, 1892; v. MONAKOW, 1897; OPPENHEIM, 1908; BÖHNE, 1927, 1931a, b, etc.). Hypertension was present in 90% of our cases (see PABELICK, 1967, p. 55).

Degeneration and organization. If the hemorrhage – rarely! – stops and the patient survives, organization of the blood clot occurs and the perifocal tissues become softened. Also, as a result of edema (Fig. 87), the diffusely damaged areas of the brain begin to liquefy. Many

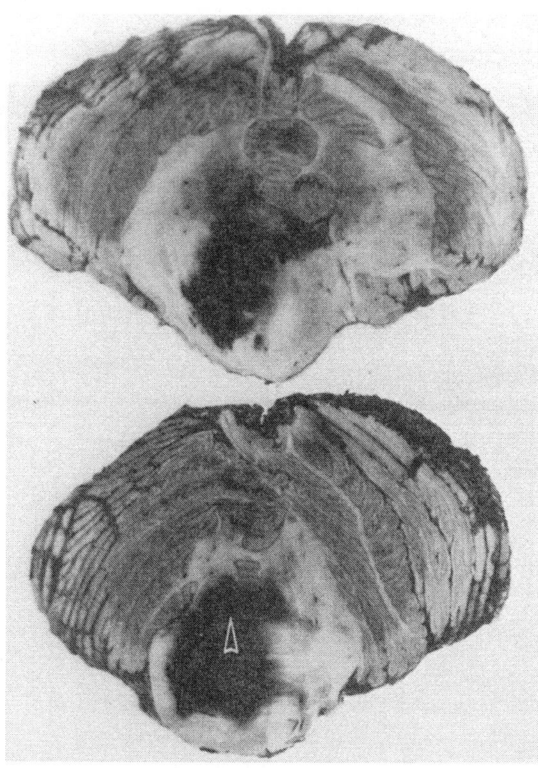

Fig. 95. Primary pontine hemorrhage with rupture into fourth ventricle (*arrow*, c.f. Fig. 155)

scavenger cells, some laden with blood pigment, are seen especially around veins. They may remain for a long time. Glial and mesodermal scars may surround the focus.

β) Localizations – Relative Frequency

The putamen-claustrum-striatum location is the predominant site of hemorrhage in hypertensive patients and was the locus in 72,3% of our cases (ZÜLCH, 1971a).

Some authors believe that 70% of cerebral hemorrhages occur in the area of the internal capsule, 10% in other regions of the cerebral hemispheres and 20% in subtentorial structures. According to FASANO and BROGGI (1956) the direction in which the hematoma will extend (precapsular, capsular, postcapsular segment) depends on the particular segment of the ruptured artery. The frequency of the hemorrhage in other locations varies. Our own cases (141 cases) showed a preferential site: 72,3% striatum, 9,9% pons, 2,8% thalamus, 5% cerebellum and 9.9% white matter (atypical). The ordered preference of sites in FREITAG'S (1968) cases was: 42% striatum, 16% pons, 15% thalamus, 12% cerebellum, 10% white matter; in Dorothy RUSSELL'S series (1954): 66% basal ganglia, 14% pons and midbrain, 8% cerebellum, 9% cerebral white matter.

"Atypical hemorrhages" (see p. 105)

γ) Relative Frequency of Cerebral Mass Hemorrhage and Infarcts

Although it is the rule that only one or the other of these lesions occurs, they may be seen simultaneously, though of different age (Figs. 96, 97). The data about the relative frequency of cerebral hemorrhage therefore may be somewhat inadequate even in autopsy studies because of the greater lethal effect of cerebral hemorrhage. Clinical observations provide figures (DELACHAUX, 1959) of a ratio of 1 hemorrhage to 10 infarcts.

The frequency of cerebral hemorrhages in series of autopsies from most general hospitals is around 3% (ROSE, 1948: 3.2%; FISHER and ADAMS, 1951: 3.8%; FANG and FOLEY, 1954: 2.86%; ZIMMERMAN, 1949: 2.3%).

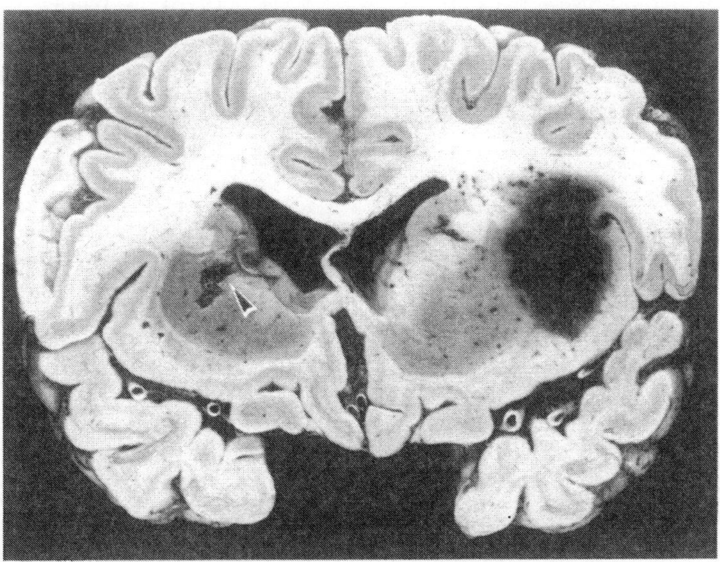

Fig. 96. Very small, fresh striatal hemorrhage associated with old "frontier zone" *(watershed)* infarct on the contralateral side *(arrow)*. Marked atherosclerosis

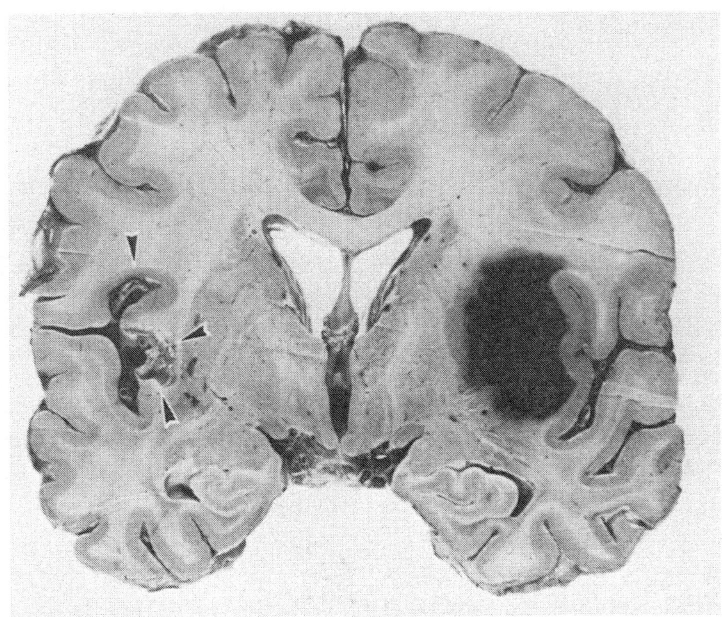

Fig. 97. Small, typical striatal hemorrhage associated with small old infarct in the insular cortex *(arrows)*

In earlier statistics the ratio between cerebral hemorrhages and infarctions was around 3:1 (LOCKSLEY, 1966), 10:7 (ZIMMERMAN, 1949), 3:2 (JOHANSSON and MELIN, 1960), 13:11 (POPPER, 1949), 7:6 (CARTER, 1964), 19:14 (LYAGER, 1955), 3:4 (FAHR, 1937), 11:12 (BELL, 1940), 11:13 (ARING and MERRITT, 1935), 4:7 (REISNER, 1954), 1:4 (FOIX and LEY, 1927), 2:5 (FISHER and ADAMS, 1951), 4:19 (SCHEID, 1963), 1:9 (BÖHNE, 1931b) (see also ZÜLCH, 1971b, p. 1500).

However, the data of KURLAND et al. (1958a, b, 1966) on the US mortality shows a 3:1 (!) ratio (62% intracerebral hemorrhage versus 21% infarction). It may be interesting to note the low incidence in the Framingham study (KANNEL et al., 1965) where the ratio between hemorrhage and infarcts was about 1:10. This corresponds to our own observations in the last decade. In our stroke ward the ratio of hemorrhage to infarction was 1:10.

Many data about epidemiology are given by P. YATES (1976). A recent Stockholm statistical analysis revealed the occurrence of intracerebral hemorrhage in 1000 stroke patients with 88 (8.8%: 40 males, 48 females) supra- and 0.9% infratentorial; the average age was 60 and 62.8 respectively (SJÖSTRÖM et al., 1977).

δ) Age and Sex – Familial Incidence

Prevalence data at autopsy (YATES, 1976) oscillate between 2 and 5/100 on autopsies. Even in Japan, where the frequency was supposed to be very high, KATSUKI'S very thorough study showed a figure of 2.2/100, as compared to 2/100 for cerebral infarction (KATSUKI and HIROTA, 1966), at the Salpêtrière it was 5.4/100 (see YATES, 1976). The figures depend on the "genius loci", the hospital and the indication for hospitalisation. In the USA fatal cerebral hemorrhage below the age of 45 is proved to be much more common than infarcts, but above 65 years of age it occurs to the same extent as infarction (KANE and ARONSON, 1969).

The peak of the *age curve* of the patients suffering mass hemorrhage was in the sixth decade according to ZIMMERMAN (1949) and FREITAG (1968); the average age was 58.4 years in the series of JOHANSSON and MELIN (1960). In our series it was 68 years. This will be more fully discussed again in the section on "Race". However, a different aspect of the curves will be more interesting namely, the correlation of age and sex (see Fig. 98).

The distribution of the *sexes* in the various decades in cases of mass hemorrhage is shown (Fig. 98), which emphasizes 1) the higher frequency in males (see also FREITAG, 1968, twice as frequent in men than in women in the sixth decade; KANE and ARONSON, 1969, Fig. 1), 2) the later manifestation in women. This is in contrast to the figures for cerebral infarction, where there was no predominance of either sex in the Framingham Study (KANNEL et al., 1965; see, however, own Fig. 99).

There are two points of interest which may explain this. 1) Atherosclerosis commences later in women, since there is some apparent protection prior to the menopause. Females lagged about 15 years behind men in middle age but in the ninth decade they had even slightly more atherosclerosis than males (GIERTSEN, 1966). The sex difference was significant only in the fifth decade. 2) The same difference in age of manifestation is seen with regard to hypertension.

The only exception to this general rule of predominance of hemorrhage in males and the lack of such a predominance in cerebral infarcts is with carotid occlusion, which was three times more common in men (ZÜLCH, 1973a; HENSCH, 1979; see also: predilections in the manifestation of atherosclerosis and infarct, Fig. 100). J. MARSHALL (1973) found no significant excess of death by cerebral hemorrhage in one family (brothers and sisters) among 180 patients.

ε) Race

The interesting data reported in the American literature regarding the preferential incidence of cerebral hemorrhage in Blacks (KANE and ARONSON, 1969), again more so in males, are well documented by FREITAG (1968). The percentage of such cases in Blacks was also high as compared with the occurrence in the general population. Blacks were on the average 12 years younger at the time of the cerebrovascular accident and pontine hemorrhage was by far more frequent (39 versus 24 cases in Whites). After the age of 59 years the average participation by Blacks was – in contrast – only one third that of the White patients.

Myocardial infarction was twice as frequent in White males and females as in their Black counterparts. The predominance of lethal cerebral hemorrhage was reversed in Blacks, in whom it was twice the figure observed in Whites. It is interesting also that this relationship reversed with age; below 60, Blacks were more frequently represented than Whites and over 60, Whites more than Blacks.

It is noteworthy that lethal cerebral hemorrhage in Blacks and Whites with *normal heart weight* occurs with essentially similar frequency.

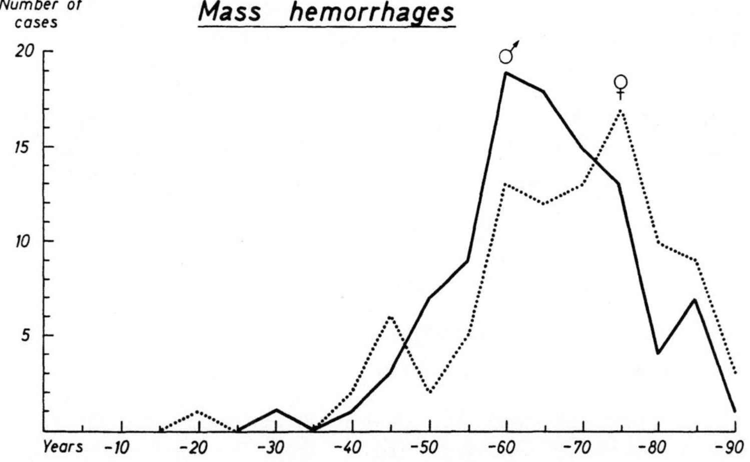

Fig. 98. Age and sex distribution of fatal cases of mass hemorrhage

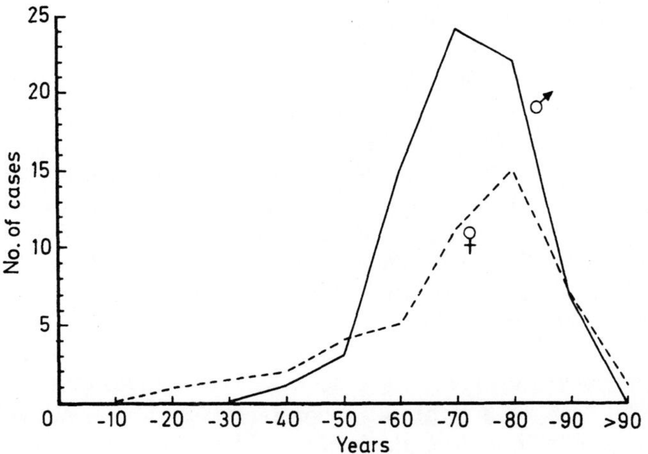

Fig. 99. Age curve and sex distribution of fatal brain infarcts (118 cases)

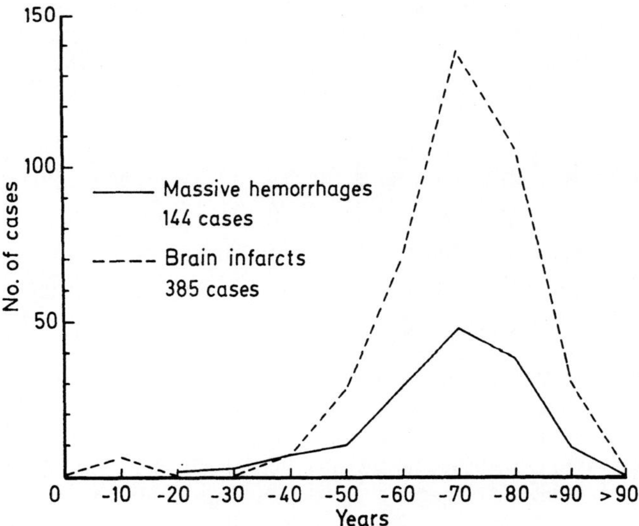

Fig. 100. Age curve of fatal cerebral hemorrhages and infarcts combined

The recent figures obtained in Japan are also interesting. KATSUKI et al. (1971) reported on observations in Kyushu where there were 113 males and 34 females with cerebral infarction. The cases of cerebral hemorrhage consisted of 24 males and 10 females, the ratio being 2.4:1. This is in marked contrast to the figures previously published for Japan and similar to the figures in the Western World apart from the low figures for infarcts in women. The general low incidence of hospitalization may, however, have social and cultural implications, particularly between the sexes and thus explain the discrepancies.

ζ) *Pathogenesis*

The discussion of pathogenesis must begin with an explanation of the site of predilection of the hemorrhages; the site may be due to peculiarities in the ruptured vessel.

History: The problem is best approached from the historical viewpoint since all present day theories have been discussed by classical scientists. Systematic exploration of the pathogenesis did not start before the nineteenth century when it was debated whether massive hemorrhage of the brain was due to arterial rupture or due to diapedesis from small vessels. CRUVEILHIER (1829a) distinctly differentiated between these two types. In the first type he saw an accumulation or sedimentation of blood among the destroyed cerebral tissues, in the second an infiltration of the capillaries of the softened brain tissue with blood. The same distinction was made by R. VIRCHOW (1856). Even in MORGAGNI's (1769) time an arterial tear was thought to be the cause of cerebral hemorrhages as already suggested by WEPFER (1658) in his excellent book in Latin.

However, ROKITANSKI (1856) and later CHARCOT and BOUCHARD (1868) made this clear when they showed the so-called miliary cerebral aneurysms. Other authors including HASSE (1855) and PAGET (1850) demonstrated alterations of the small arteries, KÖLLIKER (1849) and PESTALOZZI (1849) first showed intramural hemorrhages and mentioned false aneurysms. KOELLIKER (1849) and HASSE (1846) spoke of "aneurysmata spuria" and finally VIRCHOW (1856) described the (dissecting) "ampullary" ectasia which corresponded morphologically to the "miliary aneurysms". EPPINGER (1887, 1888) and ROBERTSON (1900) were also of this view. ELLIS (1909) and PICK (1910) were the first to succeed in identifying these morphologic entities as "supermiliary aneurysms", however, dissenting about the true nature, as did ZENKER (1872) and EPPINGER (1888), who had previously disagreed with this explanation.

Even before CHARCOT a different interpretation of the development of massive hemorrhage was offered by ROUCHOUX (1833, "ramollissement hémorrhagique"), followed by DURAND-FARDEL (1854) and later by PARISOT and CORNIL (1927). They believed that the hemorrhage takes place in brain substance which is already disorganized. For several decades the leader of this interpretation was ROSENBLATH (1918, 1927) who postulated an unknown damaging factor with extremely potent chemical properties (probably originating from the kidneys) which supposedly could destroy a circumscribed area of the brain to such a degree that hemorrhages from capillaries and veins resulted. It was believed that these hemorrhages due to diapedesis coalesced into massive hematomas. WESTPHAL (1926a, b) – partly in collaboration with BAER (WESTPHAL and BAER, 1926) – thought that the initial disintegration of tissue was caused by vascular spasm leading to necrosis of brain substance and vessel walls from which bleeding then occurred. In other words, the hemorrhage was supposed to result from necrosis. But they could be understood only on the basis of v. BERGMANN's (1932) theory of the "Functional Pathology of the Internal Diseases". In regard to diseases of the heart, peripheral circulation, gallbladder, intestines and other organs, v. BERGMANN (1932) assumed "spasm of the smooth musculature" to be the forerunner of morphologic alterations.

What this theory describes in the brain is, in fact, a *hemorrhagic infarct*. This must be distinguished from mass hemorrhage since both may arise at the same site and may have superficial resemblances. With hemorrhagic softening, it is a question of pericapillary bleeding into a tissue with the tissue maintaining its integrity; in the case of mass hemorrhage, it is clear that from the beginning the tissue is broken up and separated.

The reaction of pathologists to this interpretation of massive hemorrhage was very violent. FAHR (1937) and especially RÜHL (1927) named atherosclerosis and increased blood pressure (see also LÖWENFELD, 1886) as the two responsible factors for massive hemorrhage – while STAEMMLER (1927, 1936, 1958), WOLFF (1932, 1937) and HILLER (1936, 1951) favored the old interpretation of vascular "rupture". STAEMMLER (1927, 1936, 1958) could prove that marginal hemorrhages develop from diapedesis but could not "give an indication of the pathogenesis of large hematomas". They are present also in many other processes. Thus, the main point of discussion was the alteration of the vascular wall in the vicinity of the hemorrhages, so-called angionecrosis which, however, could be shown to be of "secondary" nature (STAEMMLER, 1927, 1936, 1958; HILLER, 1936, 1951; see below).

Finally, the pendulum swung back to the interpretation of massive hemorrhage as being caused by a vascular tear when ANDERS and EICKE (1939, 1940) and also SPATZ (1939) could prove by careful investigations that "hyalinosis" was the predisposing factor (ROBERTSON, 1900: "fibroid" disease).

They saw in the "micro"-ball hemorrhage ("Kugelblutung") a model for the development of the large massive hematoma. SPATZ (1939) interpreted the angiospasm at the periphery as a chronic pathoplastic factor, initiated by high blood pressure, which caused "hyalinosis" of the smaller vessels. This condition had been described in greater detail and named by SCHOLZ and NIETO (1938). Hyalinosis was thought to cause loss of elasticity and rupture of the vessel under the influence of blood pressure. The causes for massive hemorrhage were recently studied anew by MCCORMICK and ROSENFIELD (1973).

We proceed then into a discussion of the pathogenesis of massive hemorrhage and ask:

1) which vessels rupture?
2) at which site is there rupture and
3) why?

With reference to this problem it can be shown that the relevant arteries when observed in cadavers of hypertensive patients can be ruptured only by applying high pressure (1520 mmHG, LAMPERT and MÜLLER, 1926) and this only in two cases.

What changes do we see in the arteries of hypertensives who have previously suffered mass hemorrhages?

Again, a historical survey provides the best clues to the actual problems, where we meet a very close statistical correlation to hypertension. We find a detailed description of the disturbances of the cerebral circulation and their sequelae in the excellent book by WEPFER in Latin (1658) and by CARL CHRISTLIEB BETHKE in Germany a century later (1797), by BAILLIE (1761–1823) in London and by CRUVEILHIER (1829b). However, the anatomists of the middle ages already knew the relationship between cerebral hemorrhage and organic heart disease, especially hypertrophy of the left ventricle (VALSALVA, MORGAGNI, LIEUTAUD). The detailed historical introduction in the excellent monograph by ROBERTSON (1900) should be consulted and also the works of GLOBUS and EPSTEIN (1953).

Risk factors. The general risk of hypertension in provoking cerebral mass hemorrhage has been well studied. In the series by SOKOLOW and PERLOFF (1961) the risk was 18% for a male hypertensive and 28% for a female. In Dorothy RUSSELL's (1954) series of a total of 461 cases 232 were hypertensive. One of the important figures came from the report by JOHANSSON and MELIN (1960), where the cerebral hemorrhages were statistically 4 times more common in hypertensives when located in the basal ganglia: little difference was noted when the hemorrhage was anywhere in the brain (atypical hemorrhage see p.105). The high incidence of cerebral hemorrhage in hypertensives is emphasized both by older and newer statistics (PAULLIN et al., 1926/1927: 7.2% cerebral hemorrhage in a series of 500 patients; SMITH et al., 1950: 56 patients out of 376). The risk factors initiating hypertension are fully discussed in the Framingham study (KANNEL et al., 1965; see also DAWBER, 1977). MCCORMICK and ROSENFIELD (1973) found hypertension as a cause only in about one fourth of their patients (144 cases with cerebral hemorrhage).

In our own investigations we tried to analyse these changes in the arteries of the basal ganglia. For this purpose we investigated, histologically, the striatum on the side *opposite* the hemorrhage in a large number of cases i.e. using the same procedure as NEUBUERGER (1930). The following were our presuppositions: That the hemorrhage occurred with *equal frequency* on both sides, that at the time of hemorrhage, the vascular changes on both sides would be of equal *magnitude* and that probably the arterial changes are the same *type* on both sides.

The following *vascular changes* were found in brains with hypertensive mass hemorrhage: a) *Atherosclerosis*: We found atherosclerosis to a marked degree in about one third of the basal arteries, moderate in one third and in the last third practically absent (see also SCHOOP, 1967). *There was no statistical correlation between atherosclerosis of the basal arteries and the appearance of mass bleeding.* In contrast: the degrees of atherosclerosis observed in the patients (see Fig. 101) with mass hemorrhage corresponded almost to the frequency of this disease observed

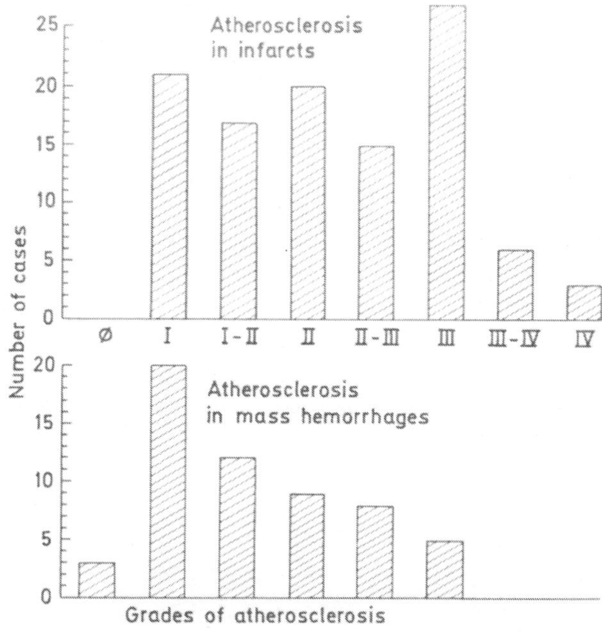

Fig. 101. The fundamental difference between high grade atherosclerosis in mass hemorrhage and in infarction is shown. In the former only the mean incidence of a normal population is observed

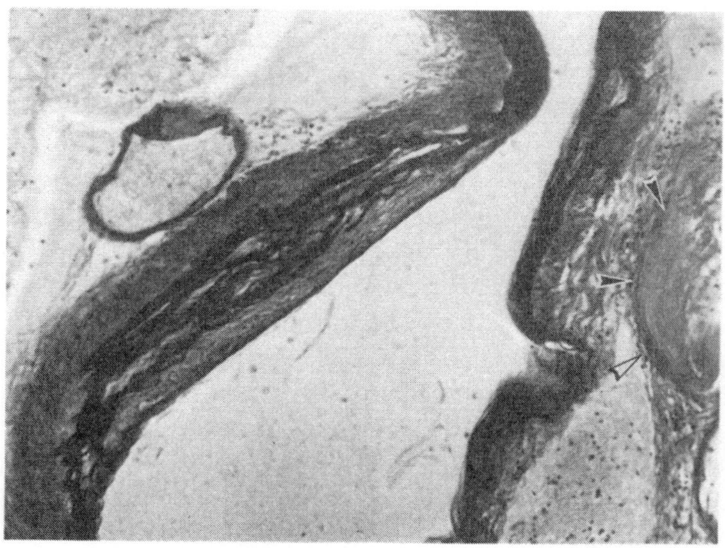

Fig. 102. Atherosclerosis at its intracerebral proximal segment: splitting of the internal elastic layer, cellular and fibroblastic proliferation. A smaller branch of this *(arrows)* artery is entirely hyalinotic (to the right)

normally in a cross-section of the population of the same age. In her detailed morphological study of cases of mass hemorrhage, FREITAG (1968) noted atherosclerosis of degree I in 25%, II in 17%, III in 22%, IV in 11%. In summary, in 75% of all cases atherosclerosis of various degrees was seen and in the remaining 25% there was no atherosclerosis whatsoever; these are figures similar to those we have observed.

In the *intracerebral* arteries of the basal ganglia atherosclerotic changes occurred with an almost similar frequency. This atherosclerosis (Figs. 101, 102) attacked predominantly the *proximal segment* (Fig. 103) of the arteries of the basal ganglia, while the *distal segments*, in contrast, were affected primarily with "hyalinosis" (arter*iolo*sclerosis). This will be described later. The

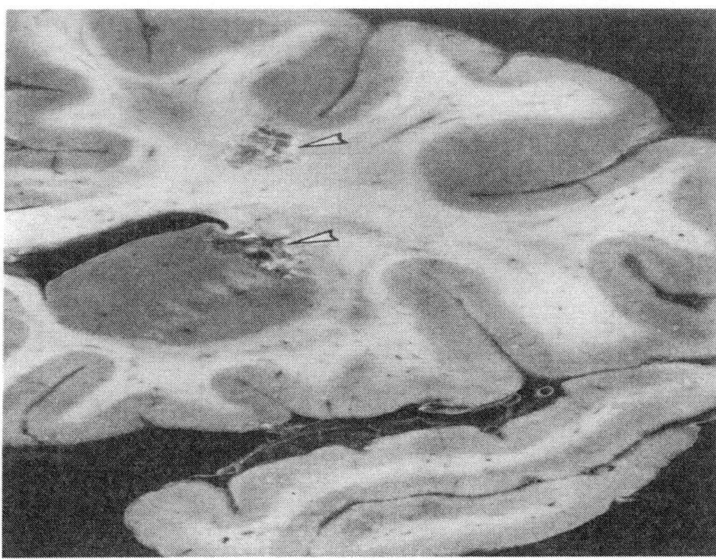

Fig. 103. Transverse section through a lenticulo-striate artery (proximal segment), typical atherosclerotic changes

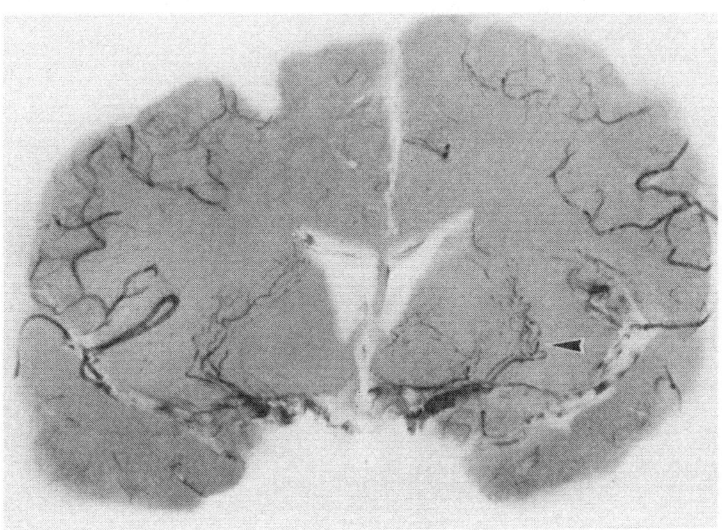

Fig. 104. Injection specimen of arteries of the basal ganglia. Arrow points to the probable site of rupture in case of hypertensive mass hemorrhage

lenticulo-striate arteries make – as is demonstrated by injection of dye and by angiography – a gentle arc against the putamen at the beginning and continue (Fig. 104) to and through the putamen. At a later age, this arc at the base adopts a rather acute angle (less than 90°) and the vessel shows coiling. The atherosclerotic changes are situated on both the inner and outer side of the bend of the basal ganglia arteries, which is interesting from the point of turbulence as a predisposing factor (see O. HASSLER, 1961).

The distribution of the atherosclerotic changes within the brain is quite interesting. They occur predominantly below a *horizontal plane* passing through the anterior commissure. Dorsal to this plane, the arteries begin to branch and it is here where the well-known hyalinotic process (arteriolosclerosis) starts.

The changes of atherosclerosis consist of splitting of the elastica into many lamellae, deposition of collagen and, now and then, also hyaline fibers and, in addition, cellular proliferation of the endothelium in the form of plaques, lipid deposits, foam cells etc.

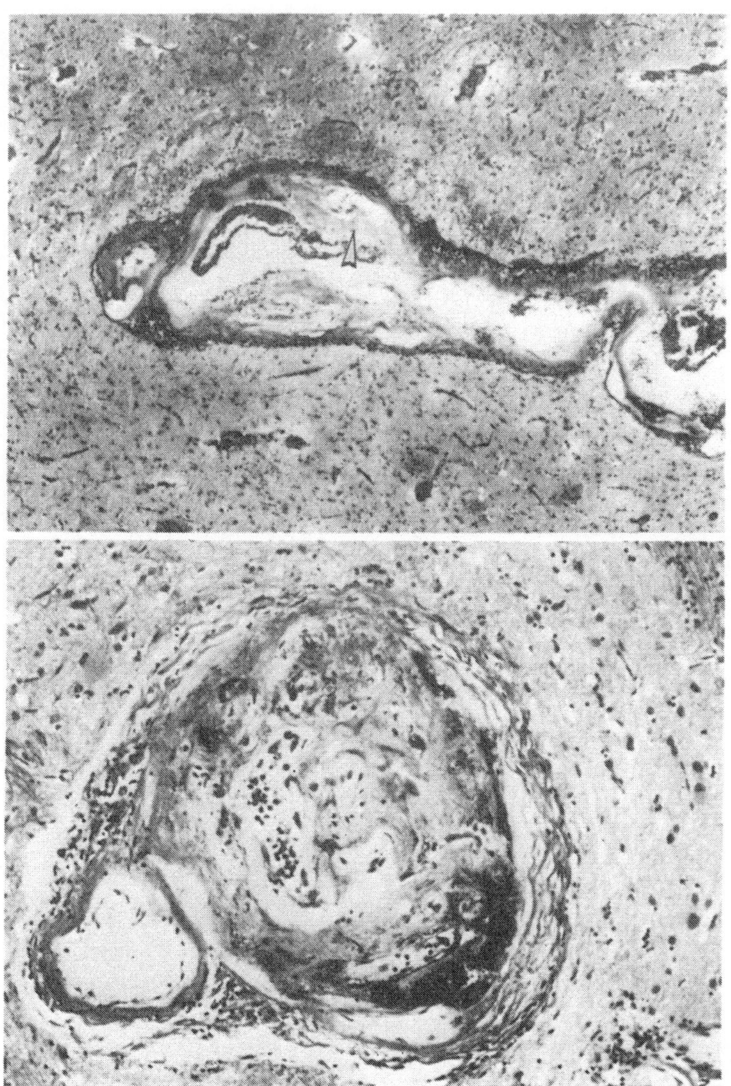

Fig. 105. *Above:* The hyaline substance stems partly from the blood and is *(arrow)* pressed beneath the endothelium and between the mesodermal lamellae. Masson's stain, ×50. *Below:* Complete occlusion of an artery by hyaline masses, which stain either red *(dark)* or blue *(light)* by Masson's stain, ×125

Hyaline change. Even in the older literature, this "hyalinosis" is mentioned (fibroid changes, ROBERTSON, 1900). To clarify the importance of hyalinosis for cerebral mass hemorrhage we have to answer the following questions:

1) What is the pathogenesis of the hyaline changes and where does the hyaline change takes place?

2) Is it reversible?

3) What are the consequences on the circulation?

4) What are the relations with a) atherosclerosis, b) arterionecrosis

However, at present it is impossible to answer all these questions satisfactorily in detail.

Hyalinosis can lead to a uniform transformation of the entire media and intima into a hyaline mass (Figs. 60, 61, 105, 106).

According to LETTERER (1959) this is the first form of hyaline and it arises from collagen. The second form of hyaline is different: it is a deposit of an unorganized hyaline mass under the intima arising from the blood, and it is precipitated either concentrically, or, more frequently eccentrically within the vessel wall.

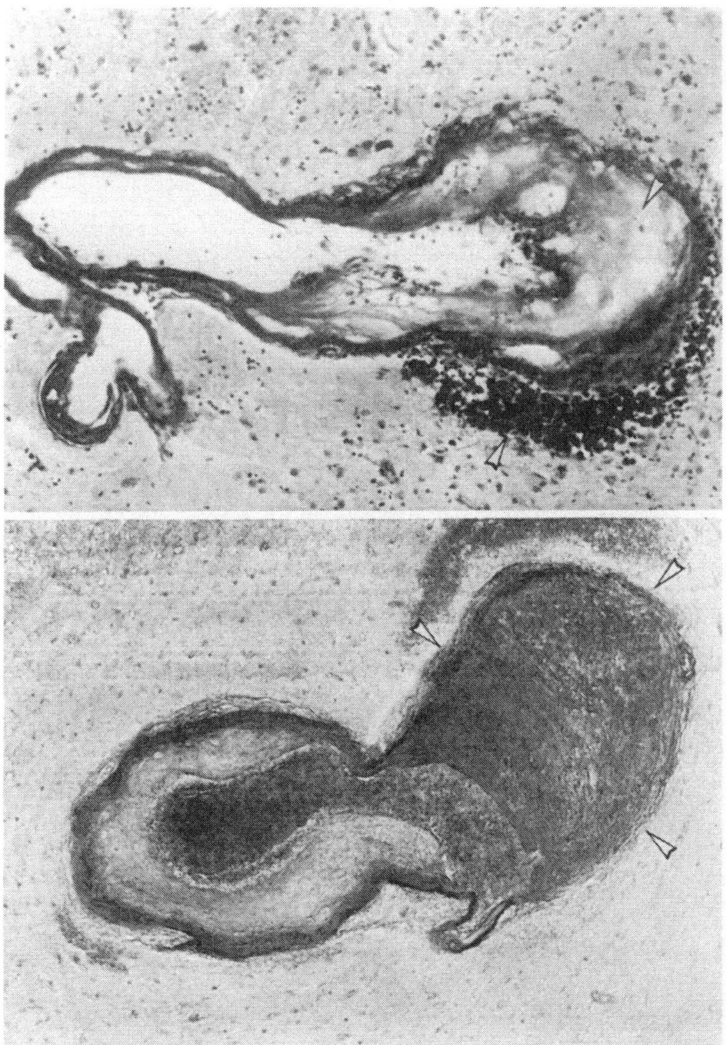

Fig. 106. *Above:* The lenticulo-striate artery is very thin-walled. Part of its wall has undergone hyaline changes *(arrow)*. An accumulation of macrophages laden with blood pigment speaks for a former bleeding *(arrow)*. Elastica-van Gieson stain, ×125. *Below:* Tearing of an arterial wall and formation of a small hemorrhage with halfmoon shaped fibrin mantle. Also, subendothelial bleeding is seen *(arrows)*. Elastica-van Gieson stain, ×50

These hyaline masses may form spherical outpouchings of the arteries. Such deposits of hyaline, besides occurring occasionally in the proximal basal ganglia arteries, are particularly evident in their small branches. Occasionally even a capillary is also involved. How such hyaline transformations and depositions develop as a result of hypertension has not been adequately clarified. We have observed that hyalinosis is usually patchy and one has to examine often 20–30 serial sections (!) to meet it.

EICKE (1952) held the view that hyalinosis of the cerebral arteries in man could follow already half a year of hypertension. Similar to the changes in the cerebral arteries, the factors producing cardiomegaly exert an increasing influence with age on the frequency of coronary arterial disease and subsequently on myocardial infarct. The theory of German pathologists (BREDT, 1961; STOCHDORPH and MEESSEN, 1957) is that deposits of proteins are compressed in the intima as a result of small tears or spaces in the subintimal space and that these then consolidate and precipitate there. DUGUID and ANDERSON (1952), however, thought that the hyaline thrombus-material was deposited upon the endothelium and was later covered by it (details see p. 38). PH. SCHWARTZ (1930, 1961) observed that "hyalinosis of the cerebral arteries is affected by adventitial amyloidosis which is a newly discovered disease".

More substantial evidence supporting the true explanation of the pathogenesis of these hyaline transformations of the arteries comes from the experiments of MUIRHEAD et al. (1951) and MONTGOMERY and MUIRHEAD (1954). They showed by means of the Goldblatt-model that arteries undergo acute necrosis following prolonged hypertension of 150–200 mmHg (STERN, 1938; ROSENBERG, 1940; GLOBUS and EPSTEIN, 1953; BYROM, 1954 etc.). After 10 days an acute necrosis of the media was found, after 20 days beginning of a transformation into hyaline and after 70 days a classical and true hyalinosis of the arterial wall was present. Similarities were also seen in the "hypertensive rat" experiments of YAMORI et al. (1976).

Hyalinotic processes change the structure of the arterial wall so fundamentally that this is regarded as *irreversible* while some atherosclerotic changes may disappear for a time (lipoid and calcareous deposits! see p. 61) as has been shown for periods of severe prolonged starvation (so-called dystrophy). The hyaline changes lead to stenosis or occlusion of the smaller arterial branches to the basal ganglia (Fig. 105). The result is generally a microinfarct, described in the classical literature as a "lacuna", located most commonly (Figs. 107, 108) in the lateral putamen: then a small softened infarct formed in a characteristic fashion may become transformed into a cyst. These lacunae will be mentioned later. C.M. FISHER (1965b, 1969, 1971) has convincingly shown, by means of serial sections, the formation of such softenings – i.e. the lacunae – distal to the hyalinized vascular obstruction. They have nothing to do directly with the formation of hemorrhages.

Arterionecrosis. In the older literature (see WESTPHAL and BAER, 1926) and also in the more recent articles (STAEMMLER, 1927, 1936, 1958; K. WOLFF, 1932; STOCHDORPH and MEESSEN, 1957) changes are designated as "arterionecrosis", a term which has no uniform definition. ARENDT

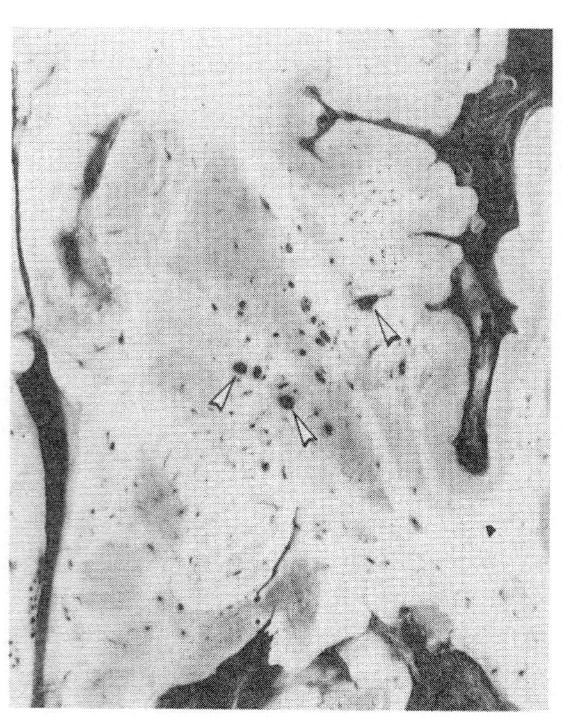

Fig. 107

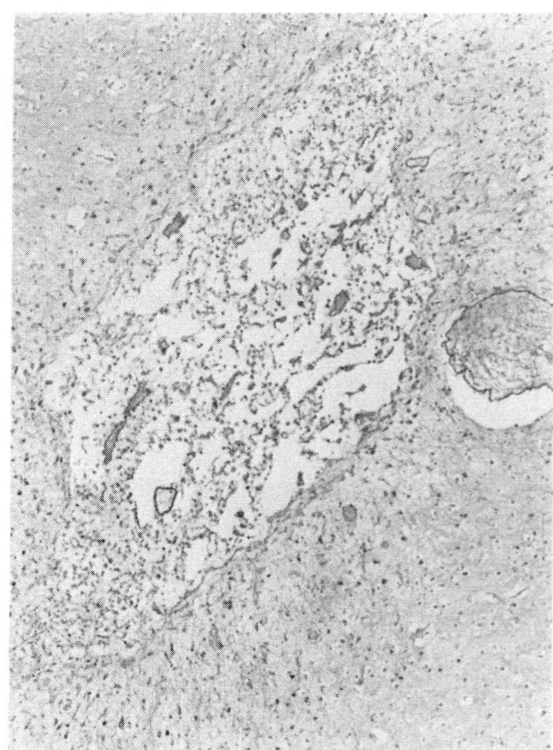

Fig. 108

Fig. 107. The little holes dispersed equally over the basal ganglia are usually "lacunae", e.g. cystic tissue defects after microinfarcts. These occur after hyalinotic occlusion of the striate arteries (see Fig. 105); so-called "status lacunaris" *(arrows)*

Fig. 108. Histologic picture of a "lacuna", i.e. small softened cyst. Network of capillaries and glial trabeculae; meshes filled with compound granular corpuscles (see Fig. 107); HE, ×50

and BACHMANN (1966) have tried in a very precise microscopical study to distinguish arterionecrosis and hyalinosis by their staining properties and the location of the changes (see OONEDA et al., 1976).

Arterionecrosis was regarded by WESTPHAL and BAER (1926) as a sequel to primary angiospasm, PICKERING (1948) found arteriolar necrosis in malignant hypertension and BYROM (1954) spoke of spasms with anoxic changes.

Many think of arterionecrosis as a degeneration of the vessel wall (Fig. 60) resulting from hyaline deposition and, simultaneously, infiltration by lymphoid cells within the layers of the vessel wall (STAEMMLER, 1958, Fig. 115–117). Others understand it to be splitting of the vessel wall (WESTPHAL and BAER, 1926; POLLAK and REZEK, 1928) especially involving the elastica as is always seen after periarterial hemorrhages (FRIEDE, 1952; GREENFIELD and TINDALL, 1965). The most severe (Fig. 106) arterionecrosis is always found when a small perivascular bleeding has existed for a sufficient time or if a vessel lies in a clotted hemorrhage (see BEITZKE'S Fig. in HILLER'S chapter, 1936, Fig. 88). Almost complete digestion of the vessel wall occurs and such a vessel can only be recognized by using special stains (see also HERXHEIMER, 1924; LINDEMANN, 1924; RÜHL, 1927; SCHULTZ, 1930; BÖHNE, 1931a, b; WIRTZ, 1936 etc.). MATSUOKA (1952) emphasized that angionecrosis is directly related to cerebral apoplexy. Later descriptions by OONEDA et al. (1976) discuss plasmatic arterionecrosis, which was also studied electron-microscopically by SHINKAI et al. (1976).

What relationships exist between hyalinosis and arterionecrosis? It is my belief that hyaline changes in these arteries should not be designated as "arterionecrosis" since "necrosis" represents a relatively acute process. Hyalinosis, itself, is a change which takes months or years to occur in *man* except perhaps in certain extreme cases of renal hypertension. Only the acutely developing forms of splitting or destruction of the vessel wall should be called arterionecrosis (Fig. 106). These are not too frequently encountered.

To come back to the various forms of arterial disease. The distinction between hyalinosis and atherosclerosis is morphologically fundamental. Moreover the caliber of the vessels changed by these transformations differs markedly.

Arterial diseases have a special predilection for vessels with a specific size lumen. Atherosclerosis attacks especially these vessels with a lumen of $^1/_2$ to 1 mm, and more, hyalinosis primarily involves arteries in the diameter range of 60 to 250 μ, while thromboangiitis obliterans (Fig. 59) affects vessels of an intermediate size of 150 to 750 μ (ZÜLCH, 1971a, Fig. 11). Hyalinosis is almost always present in the arteries of the basal ganglia of hypertensives (PABELICK, 1967 in our own series: in 58 out of 70 cases).

On the basis of our serial sections it must be emphasized that: Not only do the lesions of atherosclerosis of the large arteries but even more so, those of hyalinosis have a spotty distribution. Thirty to fifty serial sections of the basal ganglia are often cut in order to find one hyalinotic area. A negative finding in 1 or 2 blocks means little.

Lacunae and status cribrosus. We mentioned above the development of micro-infarcts of the "lacunar" type (ALZHEIMER, 1895; Pierre MARIE, 1901; C. and O. VOGT, 1919: état lacunaire; ZÜLCH, 1961a, Figs. 5–7). Lacunae are little holes in the tissue filled with a loose network of connective tissue. C.M. FISHER (1965b) observed that lacunae occur 65% in the lenticular nucleus, 39% in the pons and 32% in the thalamus.

A second form of multi-loculated hole is found in brain tissue at the site of the acute bending of the arteries of the basal ganglia and behaves as a so-called "status cribrosus" (Figs. 109, 110) (C. and O. VOGT, 1919: état criblé; see also CATOLA, 1904; ZÜLCH, 1961a, Fig. 6), which usually contains an artery and its accompanying vein. The tissue around such arteries is almost absent, and replaced by a very loose reticulated connective tissue containing a few macrophages. To my belief *it comes about as a result of the pressure effects on the surrounding tissues during hypertension. The artery is stretched at the site of the angle formation at each pulse beat and, as with an aortic aneurysm pounding the ribs and sternum, this leads to loosening of the nervous tissue surrounding the striate arteries and to enlarging of periarterial spaces.*

"Aneurysms" of the striate arteries. The "aneurysm" has been repeatedly mentioned above and been studied in the old literature (PESTALOZZI, 1849; KÖLLIKER, 1896, "spurious aneurysms;

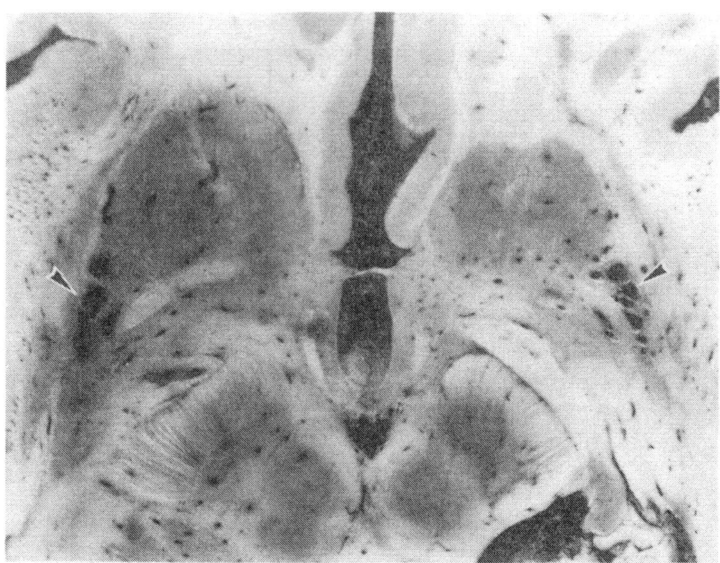

Fig. 109. The holes in the lateral part of the lenticular nucleus are usually "criblures", e.g. periarterial tissue defects beaten out by the pulsating vessel in hypertensive patients (see Fig. 110, so-called "status cribrosus")

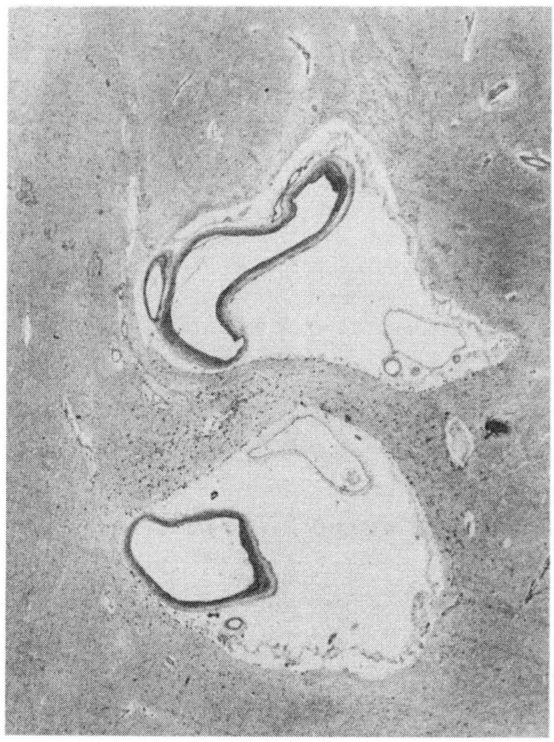

Fig. 110. Histologic picture of two foci in status cribrosus: relatively small artery with accompanying vein at the base of a large, apparently empty space (see Fig. 109). HE, ×15

VIRCHOW, 1851, "dissecting ectasia"; CHARCOT and BOUCHARD, 1868, in 77 cases) they were well described by ELLIS (1909) and PICK (1910). What is their significance? I believe that with this macroscopically fairly uniform condition we are dealing with several different forms a) the previously mentioned and described hyaline spheres which primarily involve the smaller vessels, b) another by our findings (see ZÜLCH, 1979) represents the outpouching of proximal vessels; c) a third form shows a vessel undergoing arterionecrosis or having periarterial hemorrhage. Moreover, since the basal ganglia arteries possess a high degree of bending and coiling, simulated aneurysms (outpouchings!) are often present. Serial sections are necessary to confirm accurately their nature (Figs. 60, 61, 103, 105 above).

In rereading more thoroughly the literature and the illustrations provided, one finds interesting facts; the size of the aneurysms described by COLE and YATES (1967) and YATES (1976) was below 250 μ, and their site was in the basal ganglia, the dentate nucleus, pons and the subcortical white matter.

In the investigation of COLE and YATES (1967) 53 of 200 brains showed that "some 15–25 aneurysms were found in each brain... not one was found on the main striate vessel, e.g., Charcot's artery of cerebral hemorrhage" (see Lancet, 1967).

Ross RUSSEL's (1963) aneurysms in contrast exceeded 300 μ and went up to 900. They occurred particularly at points of branching and were often multiple.

MATUOKA (1939) examined 146 brains in serial sections and found aneurysms of a size of 200–700 μ, which were strictly correlated with hypertension. The arteries had a lumen of 70–200 μ and there was no correlation with atherosclerosis. Hemorrhages were by no means always a consequence of such aneurysms.

STEHBENS (1972) has reproduced larger aneurysms which were similar in size to those which I have observed and which correspond to the original macroscopic pictures by CHARCOT and BOUCHARD (1868) and ELLIS (1909) and PICK (1910). Many of these authors see a close causal relation between the formation of these aneurysms and the occurrence of cerebral mass hemorrhage. However, C.M. FISHER (1969, 1971) holds that aneurysm formation at the site of rupture was not evident in his cases examined by serial section. MOOSSY (1966a) pointed to the fact that there were a great many more aneurysms than hemorrhages and that curiously enough they also occurred in normotensives. To the contrary the fact that the formation of these "microaneurysms" was in causal relation to hypertension was proved by R. RUSSELL (1963). He demonstrated multiple microaneurysms by angiography in 9 out of 10 patients with hypertension. We shall mention our own interpretation below. (For details see ZÜLCH, 1979).

η) The Rupture

Why and where do the arterial walls tear? Previously, I have discussed (1961a) several points, of which four appear to me to remain important after our recent investigations:

1) The walls of the lenticulostriate artery and the lenticulooptic artery are relatively thin (15–100 μ) for the size of their lumen 150–600 μ as compared with other arteries (BAKER and IANNONE, 1959c).

COOK and YATES (1972) measured the lumina of the vessels and reported that the small cerebral arteries were half as thick as the renal ones and that hypertension caused an appropriate "hypertrophy" in all sizes. Our own measurements have confirmed that.

2) The statistical correlation between hemorrhage and hypertension has been known since preclassical times.
3) One seldom encounters final massive bleeding without the signs of cerebral hypertensive arterial disease before, "little strokes" usually caused by a hypertensive crisis, corresponding to little forme fruste hemorrhages around the arteries inducing arterionecrosis.
4) Clinically we know that hemorrhages usually follow an *acute* hypertensive crisis, either during emotional stress or physical exertion with pressure similar to the type produced by Valsalva-experiments. Both lead to acutely increased blood pressure (hypertensive crisis).

Where does the artery tear? There may be found in addition to the large hemorrhage, "formes frustes" hemorrhages (see above) detectable in the lenticulostriate and lenticulooptic arteries on the opposite – "healthy" – side approximately at, or above, the level of a horizontal plane

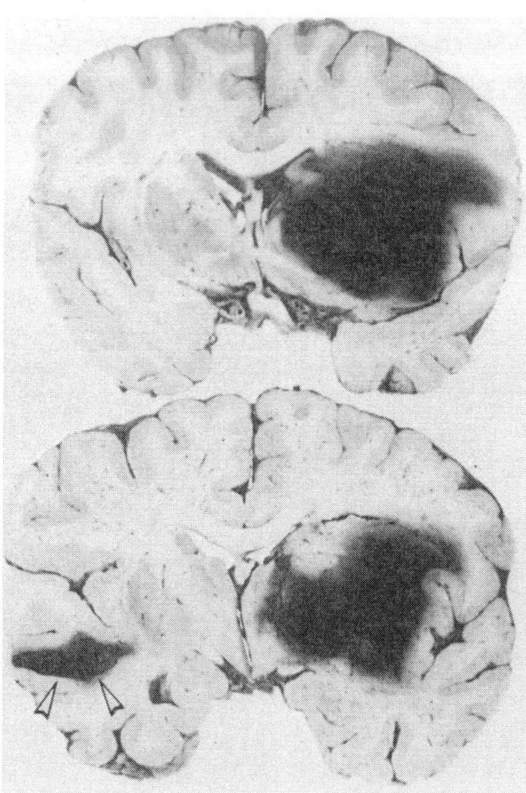

Fig. 111. In addition to typical right-sided striatal hemorrhage, smaller left-sided hemorrhage in the second temporal convolution (*arrows*)

passing through the anterior commissure. I should here mention a picture by HILLER (1936, Fig. 90) and similar illustrations from our own material. At this level there is a ramification of the arteries of the basal ganglia into their branches and it is here that the arterial segments are prone to arterionecrosis and hyalinosis. Signs of earlier tissue damage, namely periarterial bleedings, are also frequently found (Fig. 106) and these are probably remnants of earlier hypertensive events. Some vessels may be necrobiotic due to such previous hemorrhages as shown by macrophages filled with hemosiderin. *The old thesis of previous acute damage to a vessel wall – which leads to arterionecrosis – certainly has its basis. Possibly these findings on the "healthy" side show the real etiology and pathogenesis of the opposite massive bleeding which cannot be studied properly in a direct manner because of destruction produced by the hemorrhage.*

How then does the massive bleeding occur? There is an age predilection in the 6th to 7th decade as we have seen. In some statistics the age in men may be lower than in women. The patients have usually had hypertensive disease for many years. Minor neurological events (small perivascular bleedings?) may become noticeable many months or years earlier and are significant as indicators of later massive bleeding. Morphologically, we described the small, periarterial hemorrhages in hypertensive crises which may lead to arterionecrosis and vascular occlusion due to hyalinosis, which produces a micro-infarct by *closing* the lumina of a substantial number of end arteries. This then may raise the intra-arterial pressure in their proximal parts! Aneurysmic outpouchings of the vessel walls may arise at sites of arterionecrosis. The arterial changes are progressive if hypertension persists. *Finally, rupture occurs if the arterial pressure at some stage of development during an acute hypertensive crisis is greater than the necrotic vessel wall can endure.* Once bleeding starts, other vessels in this zone will be ruptured and "additional bleeders" will be initiated in an avalanche fashion (C.M. FISHER, 1971). Within a few minutes this may disrupt the surrounding tissues; the inner capsule tears and then there is a break through into the surrounding white matter or even the ventricular system.

The arterial wall must be weakened first because SATINSKY and BRASLOW reported in 1969 that large rises in blood pressure alone did not rupture vessels.

It seems evident by now that the number of cerebral hemorrhages associated with hypertension is *decreasing everywhere* when current methods of treatment of hypertension are adopted. MOSER and GOLDMAN reported in 1967 about the disappearance of cerebral hemorrhage when hypertensive patients were sufficiently controlled and treated while under 55 years of age. AURELL and HOOD (1964) were able to state the same for patients under 65 years.

In summary, the pathogenesis of hypertensive mass hemorrhage is still not entirely explained although we know that hyalinosis (arteriolosclerosis) of the lenticulo striate and lenticulo-optic arteries is the predisposing factor for the hemorrhages of the "basal ganglia". Hyalinosis follows long-standing hypertension. Forme fruste of periarterial hemorrhage may induce arterionecrosis some time before the actual hemorrhage, which is usually provoked by an additional acute rise of blood pressure ("hypertensive crisis").

We repeat a statement by LUGINBÜHL (1966) that "this unique type of hemorrhage is not known to occur in animal species and could not be reproduced experimentally" (see GLOBUS and EPSTEIN, 1955; RASCHER, 1979). In other words cerebral hemorrhage of the hypertensive is an extraordinary human event.

b) Atypical Hemorrhages

Particularly important to the neurosurgeon are the "atypical" hemorrhages – atypical in location and in a younger age (9.9% in our series) – which lack any relationship to the putamen, thalamus, dentate nucleus or pons. They will be discussed separately because they are generally not the result of hypertensive conditions but rather of a rupture of a micro-angioma (Figs. 112–115; see also ZÜLCH, 1961a, Fig. 18; GERLACH and JENSEN, 1961, 1965; THIENEMANN, 1975, Figs. 1–2e; JENSEN, 1979). Their pathogenesis, however, may not be always clear (LAZORTHES, 1956).

c) Other Forms of Hemorrhages

Traumatic hematomas. The pathology of trauma will not be here described but only those conditions in which in small contusions produce vascular rupture. These bleedings will be discussed here for purposes of differential diagnosis.

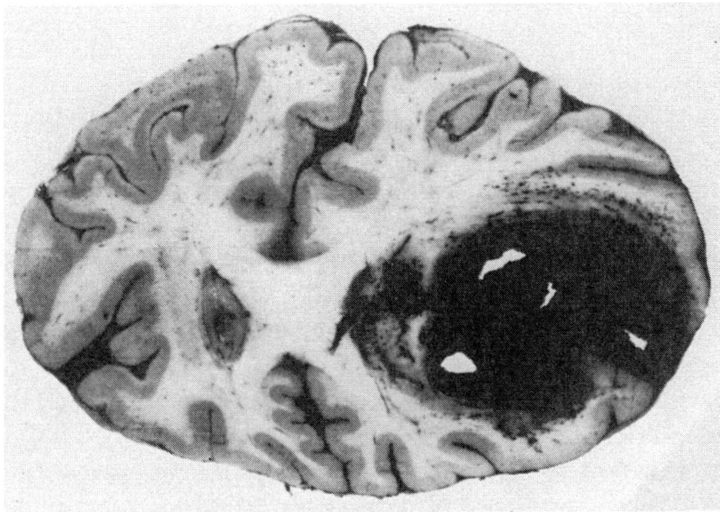

Fig. 112. "Atypical", surgically accessible frontal hemorrhage without topical relation to striatal arteries

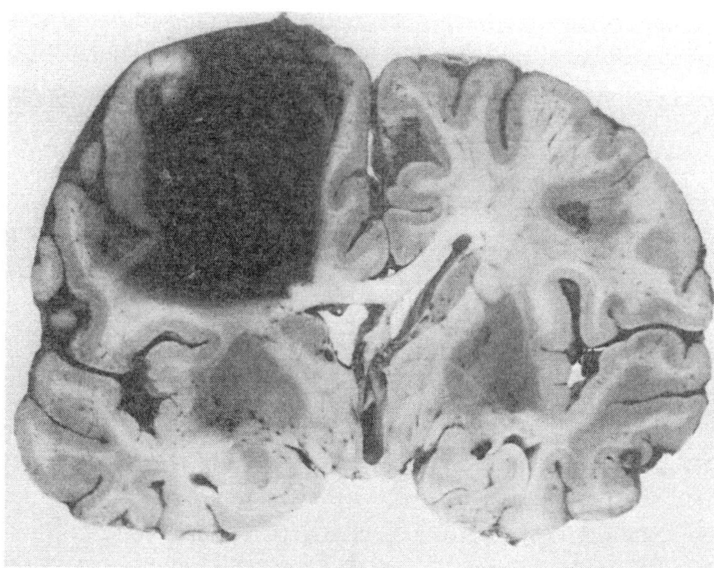

Fig. 113. Atypical, surgically accessible parietal hemorrhage. No relation to the striatal arteries

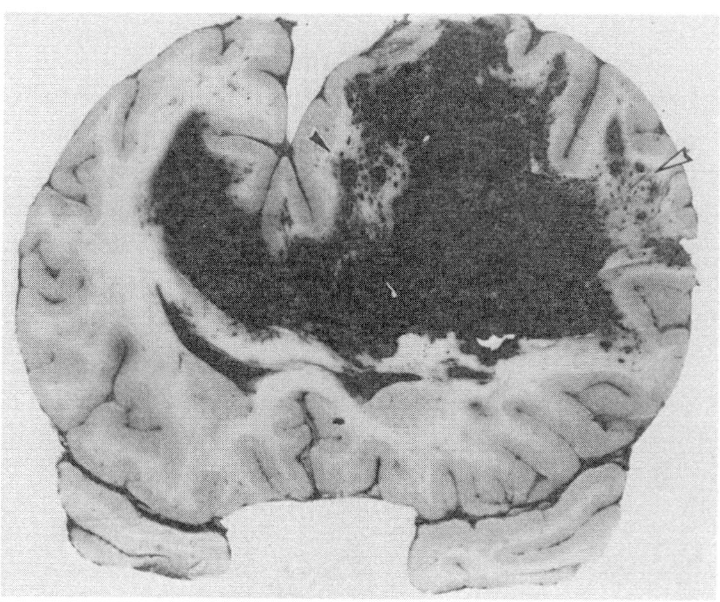

Fig. 114. "Atypical" fronto-parietal hemorrhage with rupture into the contralateral frontal lobe. The basal ganglia are not compromised. Petechiae in the marginal zone *(arrows)*. Not operable

It is of importance to note that the "second" component, the contused brain tissue, is scarce compared with the abundant hemorrhage. Such bleedings may occur anywhere in the brain, however, with some topographical preference. Large hemorrhages into the *frontobasal* brain are not infrequent in case of frontoorbital contusions (Fig. 116). A second predilection seems to be for the *aged* brain, where in the later decades massive bleedings may occur in the white matter, again without a previously larger contusion, the so-called Schwarzacher's Markblutungen (SCHWARZACHER, 1924).

Hemorrhages due to natural or iatrogenic disturbances of the coagulation system. Other causes of hemorrhages must also be mentioned (leukemias; for details see SCHMITT, 1970; see Fig. 117), not forgetting "iatrogenic" hemorrhages. These may follow ischemic vascular lesions, when

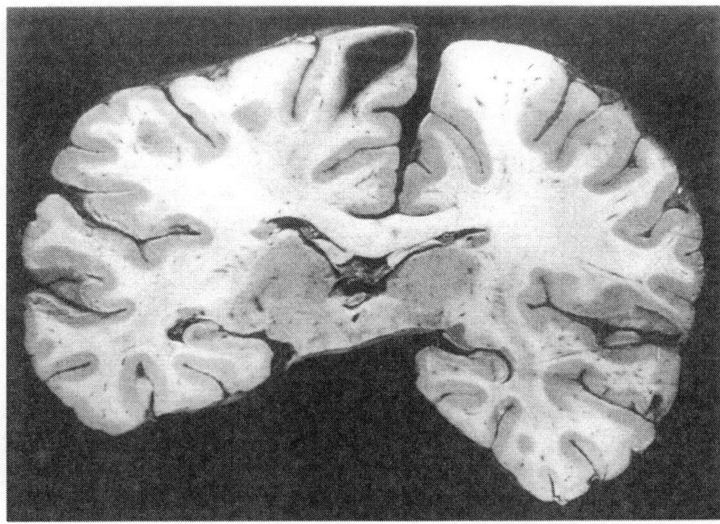

Fig. 115. Small – plum sized – hematoma of unexplained origin arising following an accident not involving the head

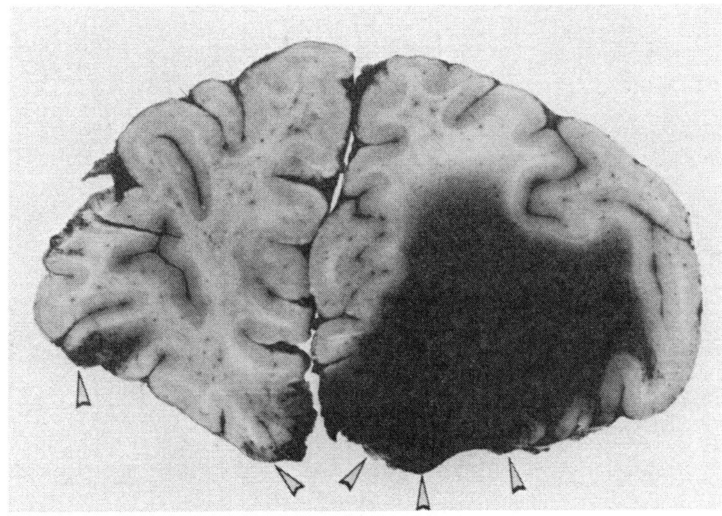

Fig. 116. Massive hemorrhage in right fronto-orbital white substance, in case of typical small cortical (contralateral!) frontoorbital contusions. See also gyrus rectus and lateral edge of surface *(arrows)*

the circulation is "restored" by endarterectomy or thrombectomy into a zone of a white infarct which had been deprived of blood supply (BRUETMAN et al., 1963; WYLIE et al., 1964).

Cerebral hemorrhage resulting from changes in the blood coagulability may occur without site of predilection due to failures or unforeseen accidents in anticoagulation or fibrinolytic (see Fig. 118) (HANAWAY et al., 1976) therapy of thromboses of cerebral or other arteries.

Such bleedings are demonstrated by our own observations (ZÜLCH and KLEIHUES, 1967) during a typical regime of streptokinase, where hemorrhage in the borderline zones of an infarct occurred as a final and fatal complication after thrombosis of the middle cerebral artery. This hemorrhage was located in the frontier zone of the infarct, which very often is already hemorrhagic by nature (Fig. 120) as had been shown earlier by VIRCHOW (1856) for the edge of a renal infarct (Fig. 118).

Still more frequently anticoagulation therapy (Fig. 118) for medical reasons may provoke massive hemorrhages anywhere in the brain (ZUCKSCHWERDT and THIES, 1958).

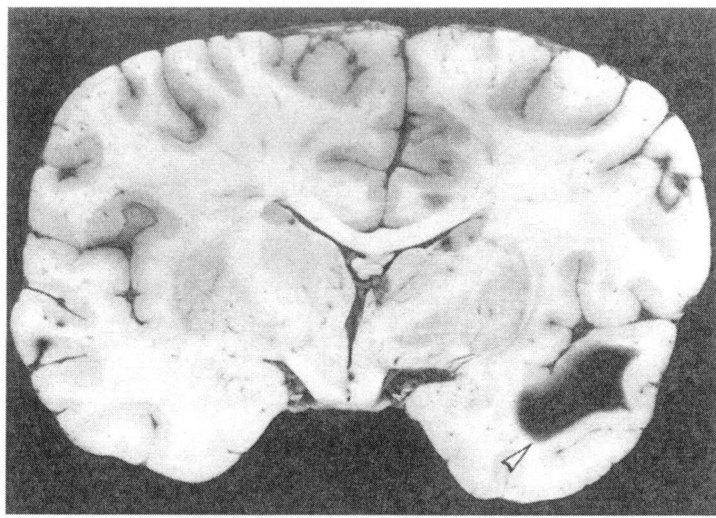

Fig. 117. One larger hemorrhage and some smaller ball-hemorrhages („Kugelblutungen") in leukemia

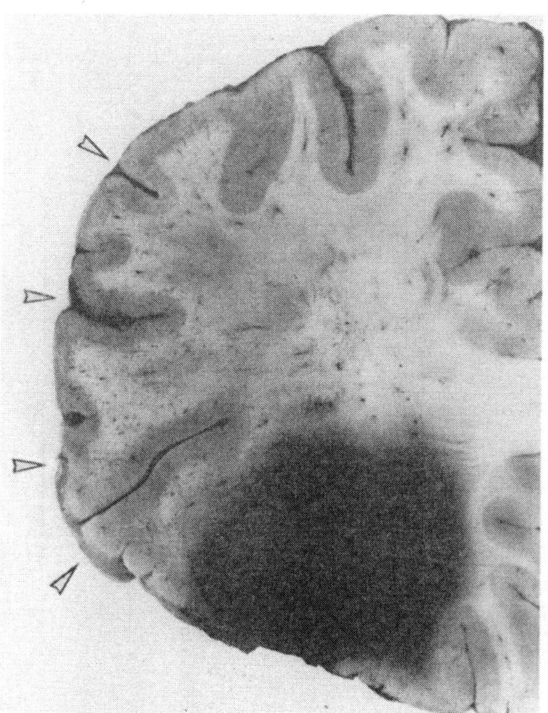

Fig. 118. Mass hemorrhage in the "watershed" zone following fibrinolytic therapy (streptokinase) for thrombosis of a middle cerebral artery with infarction, which is apparent above the hemorrhage *(arrows)*

XII. Clinical Pathology and Pathophysiology of Ischemic Lesions

1. Correlation Between Morphology of Atherosclerosis and Its Clinical Manifestation as "Stroke"

One has to distinguish between the morphological phenomena of atherosclerosis and the clinical symptoms which may ensue. The morphological lesion may precede the cerebrovascular insufficiency for decades or the latter may not occur at all. The incidence of stroke is far easier

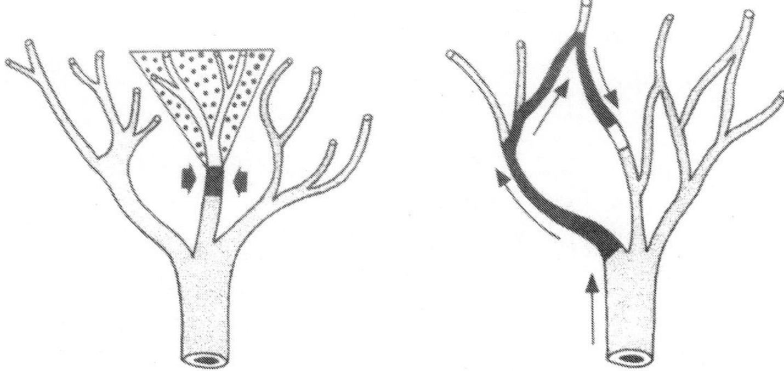

Fig. 119. *Left:* Infarction in case of occlusion of an "end artery". *Right:* No infarction, if anastomoses are functioning adequately

to ascertain than that of atherosclerosis and stroke registries exist in many countries (see for instance RIISHEDE, 1967; WHISNANT et al., 1973; AHO and FOGELHOLM, 1974).

Complete obstruction of an artery does not lead necessarily to total infarction of a supply area (Fig. 119). Formerly, however, the concept that softening of the dependent area followed obstruction by thrombosis was so widely accepted that clinically the terms were used synonymously (i.e. "thrombosis" equal to "softening"). Since then, not only single morphologic observations, but also angiographic studies, have demonstrated frequently the occurrence of infarcts without vascular obstruction (HICKS and WARREN, 1951) and vascular obstructions without infarcts. We not only have to accept this information regarding pathogenesis, but must also note it with emphasis.

Early observations (LECENE and J. LHERMITTE, 1920) had already demonstrated occlusion of the middle cerebral artery and a "missing" infarct and on the other hand an infarct with an open "resource artery".

Moreover, lysis of clots and recanalization of occluded arteries have been demonstrated by CRONQVIST (1969) and recently emphasized by DALAL et al. (1965). Some of the "occluded vessels" turned out to be only secondarily blocked, offering at least a partial explanation for the pathogenesis of an infarct with an "open" supply artery.

Total vascular occlusion caused by thrombosis, embolism or atherosclerosis was found only in 20%–50% of all cases of cerebral infarction, angiographically (GURDJIAN et al., 1961a, b, c; GURDJIAN and THOMAS, 1970; TATELMANN, 1958) and morphologically (BAKER et al., 1963; YATES and HUTCHINSON, 1961).

GURDJIAN et al. (1961a, b, c) in the angiograms of apoplectic patients demonstrated thrombotic occlusion of the internal carotid artery in only 10.5% of the cases, occlusion of the middle cerebral artery in 5%, occlusion of the vertebral or basilar arteries in 2.5% and finally occlusion of the anterior cerebral artery in 7.5% (according to present day experience to provide clear evidence this artery should have been filled by contrast from the other side as well). This means that only 25% of all cerebrovascular accidents had true vascular occlusions in this study while in all other cases only stenosing atherosclerosis was present (see also ALTER et al., 1972). In the review by KLEIHUES et al. (1964) from our Institute, obstruction in the proximal vessel was seen in 106 out of 329 (32%) brain infarcts found at autopsy. HICKS and WARREN (1951) claimed that arterial occlusion is absent in as many as 60% of infarctions (for further references see STEHBENS, 1972; ZÜLCH, 1971a).

BAKER et al. (1963) reported that infarction occurred in 145 cases out of a total of 290 with severe stenosis. Conversely, in 267 other cases, severe stenosis or occlusion was present without gross tissue changes.

In the last two decades it has been shown that the *extracranial* portions (YATES and HUTCHINSON, 1961) of the cerebral vasculature were also important, both with regard to stenosis or occlusion of an artery and also for the formation of an anastomotic supply system (FIELDS, 1969; WEIBEL and FIELDS, 1969; ZÜLCH, 1971c). Other data see p. 8ff.

MOOSSY (1966b) in his study of 204 cases with cerebrovascular atherosclerosis, however, came to the conclusion that one must interpret the pathogenetic significance of an arterial stenosis with great care – as did MILLIKAN (1963) – since it may be demonstrated angiographically even in asymptomatic individuals.

In an Indian sample of 850 patients with cerebrovascular disease (ABRAHAM and DANIEL, 1972) 546 patients were finally classified as having cerebral thrombosis, 48 with cerebral embolism, and 61 with occlusions of the internal carotid artery. However, the system of diagnosis was not very logical (partly pathomorphological, partly symptomatological).

Most of these statistics are valid only for larger vessels and are based either on morphologic or angiographic studies. However, more refined methods of angiographic visualization have convinced us that occlusion of smaller branches is not at all uncommon (in a series of angiograms made in the period 1965 to 1974, WODARZ (1975) in our department found 41 cases of middle cerebral artery branch occlusions). Moreover, it has not been confirmed that the thrombosis which is morphologically demonstrated is always the *cause* of the infarct and not its consequence. It has been shown from clinical observations (ZÜLCH, 1962a, Fig. 17a, b) that the circulatory disorder occurred prior to thrombosis and that the thrombosis developed secondarily.

2. Risk Factors (Myocardial and Brain Infarction)

The following data are derived from clinical studies of stroke patients (abbreviation: *A*therosclerotic *B*rain *I*nfarction = ABI, *M*yocardial *I*nfarction = MI). They can only partly be transposed to the problem of "risk factors for atherosclerosis", the latter being the major cause of ABI (see pp. 50, 98), and may have some similarities to the risk factors in MI.

Factors affecting the risk of either ABI or MI are as follows:

1) Elevated blood pressure is a potent factor in both MI and ABI with a somewhat greater effect in ABI.
2) Cholesterol levels in the blood are important factors for MI in younger subjects, especially in men. Cholesterol level is weakly related to ABI development.
3) Cigarette smoking is similarly of value in predicting MI in younger males, but loses its importance with age. Only a weak relationship can be found between cigarette smoking and ABI.
4) Diabetes is an important factor in both disorders. Certain other relationships are of lesser importance (DAWBER et al., 1977).

Elevated blood pressure, the risk factor "hypertension", is therefore certainly of prime importance for the two types of stroke,

a) cerebral mass hemorrhage (via hyalinosis in striatal arteries etc. see p. 57); and for
b) cerebral infarct, where the influence on the heart and on circulatory hemodynamics is greater than on the intracranial arteries (see p. 119ff).

The different correlations between cerebral atherosclerosis and brain infarct on the one hand and mass hemorrhage on the other are shown in Fig. 101.

In a detailed discussion of the risk factors in ABI and MI (general evaluation see KANNEL et al., 1976), the following data must be discussed:

Myocardial infarction (MI) is rarer in women than in men, but this is not the case in atherosclerotic brain infarction (ABI). This is particularly marked below the age of 50 when the incidence of ABI and MI in women is similar and probably consistent with an equal development of atherosclerosis in both organ vessel systems. There is a suggestion that the blood pressure is more important for ABI than MI. DAWBER et al. (1977) used the following blood pressure values for the Framingham Study: for normotensive 140/90 and for hypertensive patients from 160/95 or higher. Cholesterol level in the blood does not allow a precise prediction, however, it decreases in importance with aging. There is no correlation between cholesterol and hypertension. The importance of serum cholesterol levels alone in MI in men below 40 years of age has been well recognised, whereas any relationship to ABI is still questionable. In women a modest risk with higher cholesterol levels is seen in younger age groups only. Cholesterol levels therefore loose their significance with age (little difference after the age of 65). If cigarette smoking has any effect, its importance is not quantitatively related to the number of cigarettes except in older females above 65 years. Cigarette smoking is highly associated with MI in younger men but the association is entirely lost for men between 50 and 59 years of age. A weak but positive association between cigarette smoking and ABI is observed in men, but as yet has shown no correlation either with MI or ABI in women. MI and ABI have a greater incidence in diabetics, this being more pronounced in women than in men. Uric acid levels seem of less importance. Hematocrit turned out to be of importance in the younger age group but not in the older. Oral contraceptives may play a role in thromboembolism inducing a cerebrovascular attack at a rate of 1:10,000 and resulting in death in 1 in 200,000 (MILLIKAN, 1976).

The *World Health Organization* has given the following summary of the sometimes divergent data: Blacks in the USA have more cerebrovascular disease than Whites; however, the severity and frequency of atherosclerosis are less in Blacks living in Africa even in those who are diabetic and hypertensive, than in both Blacks and Whites in the USA. Epidemiologists advise that hypertension and transient ischemic attack are the principal medical issues on which physicians must focus attention in order to prevent stroke. Both heart disease and diabetes mellitus are also important conditions that require attention. Increased blood lipids do not appear to exert a major influence – as they do in heart disease – except in young men; in young women, the use of oral contraceptives clearly has increased the incidence of stroke. We are well acquainted with stroke in the elderly, but are beginning to recognize that the incidence of cerebrovascular disorders in children and young adults is becoming significant.

For the relationship to disease of heart and aorta see BAKER et al. (1961a) and last but by no means least, the "constitutional" or even "hereditary" factor in the development of atherosclerosis and consequently MI and ABI has to be emphasized.

Studies on the clinical prevention of stroke taking into consideration risk factors have been made by WHISNANT et al., 1972.

For references: Risk factor age: JANAKI et al., 1975; risk factor genetics in carotid occlusion: HENSCH, 1979; risk factor blood pressure: KANNEL et al., 1976; FUJISHIMA et al. 1976; HB: KANNEL et al., 1972; lipids: KANNEL et al., 1974; body weight: KLASSEN et al., 1974; NaCl and cholesterol: NAKAMURA et al., 1975 in the experiment; risk factors in a Mexican population: OLIVARES et al., 1973; general survey: Executive Committee, 1971.

3. Hemodynamics; Topographic Predilection of Infarcts

a) Cerebrovascular Insufficiency

The term of cerebrovascular insufficiency (Mangeldurchblutung) was introduced by CORDAY and ROTHENBERG in 1957 in parallel to the German concept of "coronary insufficiency" (Koronarinsuffizienz) developed by the physiologist REIN (1931, 1936) and the pathologist BÜCHNER (1939, 1964). This concept seemed to be of great importance, replacing the all-or-none law of "total infarction" by the dynamic process of insufficiency for both heart and brain pathophysiology.

Far too little has been discussed about the very simple notion of the fundamental difference between heart and brain circulation. In the heart, insufficiency may arise through an increased demand whilst the blood flow does not increase sufficiently, whereas in the brain, it arises because of insufficiency in the general circulatory supply although the demand is fairly steady.

We have only recently learned that there may be a certain very small regional increase in demand in the brain which, however, does not influence the global cerebral circulation and never reaches a proportion which cannot be easily compensated (INGVAR, 1977, 1979) from the total supply.

In order to understand the modern concepts of the pathogenesis of cerebrovascular disease we should begin with the historical development of the concept of "brain softenings". As always in pathology, classification starts with VIRCHOW (1851), and thereafter ROBERTSON (1900) has to be cited. However, with respect to pathogenesis GRASSET (1906), who called the transient intermittent strokes "claudicatio intermittens cerebralis", is important. Also PAGNIEZ (1902) as well as LECENE and J. LHERMITTE (1920) have the merit of having shown that the entire supply area of the middle cerebral artery was not softened in a case of complete occlusion of this artery.

On the other hand most scientists followed the strict concept of COHNHEIM (1882), namely that all brain arteries were "end arteries" (Fig. 119) and that in an occlusion the entire irrigation area would be softened. COHNHEIM's view prevented a satisfactory theory of infarction for a long time, although at least the French scientists kept well in mind the knowledge about the quasi-experimental work carried out by the elder HEUBNER. He had succeeded in filling all arteries of a human brain with a contrast medium (recently repeated by SZAPIRO and PAKULA, 1963) injected into a single extracranial supply artery. The work of VAN DER EECKEN and ADAMS (1953) opened our minds again towards a more hemodynamic concept, that the brain arteries actually form a "network"-like pattern; the concept of "end-arteries" had to be abandoned thereafter for most cerebral arteries (s. p. 17ff.).

The classic triple-classification of the causes of cerebrovascular insufficiency into "mass hemorrhage", "thrombosis" and "embolism" must be considered unsatifactory today because of the logical changing of basic principles.

It has been emphasized above that hemorrhages must be separated from infarction (softenings, necroses) since it finally has been proven that mass hemorrhage is *not* the final stage of hemorrhagic infarction (see p. 128ff.).

Infarcts (necroses) follow a nutritional disturbance of the tissue, i.e. an ischemia (J.S. MEYER, 1958) caused by an *insufficient blood supply* which may – or may not – be of correct composition or contain enough oxygen. This disturbance would be quantitative but could also be qualitative. In the foreground of morphological and pathophysiologic interest in the past were the quantitative alterations of circulation (DENNY-BROWN and J.S. MEYER, 1957). Today changes in this concept have become apparent.

Three main groups of vascular insufficiency can be differentiated according to their cause; they can originate from 1) "embolic", 2) "thrombotic" and 3) "atherosclerotic" arterial occlusion or stenosis.

α) Different Sizes and Locations as a Function of Collateral Supply and the Laws of Unequal Distribution of Blood

Size and location of an infarct depend on the involvement of the responsible artery and the presence and action of anastomoses (see pp. 8, 11). For those inexperienced in this field of cerebrovascular pathology the problem of occurrence and great variation in the origin of cerebral infarcts seems to be of little importance. However, it may be basic for the clinician and neuroradiologist, particularly since the introduction of computed tomography.

We have emphasized the hemodynamic origin of most infarcts and stressed, that there is no *simple* correlation between occlusion of a cerebral artery and an infarct. Such a correlation is valid far more commonly for the coronary arteries where the differences in site and size of infarcts are therefore limited (ROBERTS, 1977). The blood supply to the brain is in fact far more complex and the interarterial ("meningeal") anastomoses on the surface of the brain are physiologically more evident than in the heart. Within as short a time as 30 sec (DENNY-BROWN and J.S. MEYER, 1957) collateral pathways in the brain begin to open through the various anastomoses, a phenomenon which is seen rarely in coronary pathophysiology.

Site of infarct and involvement of irrigating vessels. Cerebral infarcts have a certain topographic predilection in relation to the supply arteries and are of various sizes due to an extensive collateral support as will be described in the next chapter.

The topographic localization of these infarcts including the exact site and extent, is important information for the clinician.

"Classical" neurology, in particular the French (FOIX and HILLEMAND, 1925a, b; FOIX and LEY, 1927) and German (BÖHNE, 1927, 1931a, b) schools has described in an excellent manner the supply territories in case of occlusion of each specific artery.

One of the best survey articles about the achievements of the French school of FOIX and co-workers has been written by W. MISCH (1929) in which the state of knowledge about the vasculature, the type of ensuing infarcts and the clinical syndromes are excellently described.

The unequal distribution of blood in cases of insufficiency. A great number of curiously situated infarcts could not be explained by the classical principle of the blocking of "end arteries", even when taking into account collateral supply systems. It was not until Max SCHNEIDER developed his theory of the "last field" in order to explain some previously unaccounted physiological phenomena that a real new era began.

The theory was initiated by an observation of EICH and WIEMERS (1950) in the Institute of Max SCHNEIDER that after experimental induction of total brain ischemia and subsequent Evans blue injection, the dye could be least washed out in the ring-like frontier (-watershed) zones between the great cerebral arteries. They came to the conclusion that there had been an insufficient circulation in this region resulting in an alteration of the blood-brain barrier. Apart from the observations of EICH and WIEMERS (1950) Max SCHNEIDER (1951, 1952, 1953) tried to explain some vascular phenomena in the terminal zones of a supply territory by the "law of compromise of the last field" in cases of general insufficiency. This law was applied instantaneously by ZÜLCH (1953) to explain processes in the spinal cord where the involvement of critical segments as well as critical zones within the segments, could now be understood hemodynamically (ZÜLCH, 1953, 1954b, 1961a, 1964, 1979). Furthermore, he believed that a longer survival of "deep" cerebral structures could only be explained by the fact that in the case of general vascular insufficiency "last fields" were formed in the circulation of the surface (ZÜLCH, 1953, 1954b) as well as the depth.

Such phenomena as a ring-like "scarred" zone have been observed for a long time by morphologists as a sequel to a "changed" circulation between the middle cerebral artery on one side and the anterior and posterior on the other (see Figs. 64, 65). PENTSCHEW (1934), LINDENBERG and SPATZ (1940) had described granular atrophy in these frontier zones in thromboangiitis obliterans and J.E. MEYER (1948, 1953) in neonatal asphyxia. They are also not uncommon in atherosclerotic vascular diseases.

By knowing this "last field" concept of M. SCHNEIDER (1951), when studying the hemodynamics of cerebral infarction, we were able to define a whole system of "superficial" and "deep" infarctions (according to this law of the "last field" or the "watersheds" ZÜLCH, 1954, 1977a).

Eventually, after many discussions the basic value of such concepts has been accepted (see the report of ROMANUL and ABRAMOWICZ, 1964; GASTAUT et al., 1971).

We must describe now the main types of infarction explainable on such grounds, e.g. to *discuss the concept of the unequal distribution of the circulation in case of a cerebrovascular insufficiency.*

1) Border-zone (watershed) infarcts. These infarcts are localized at the distant frontiers of the blood supply (or the "watersheds") of two supply systems (Figs. 65, 139, 145). Typical infarcts of this pathogenesis are seen:

a) As acute and subacute ring-like (circular) infarcts on the cortical-*surface* of the brain following the margins of the irrigation area of the middle cerebral artery. This infarction is observed particularly in the second frontal convolution and in the upper parietal lobe at the watershed between the anterior and the middle cerebral arteries; finally in the parieto-occipital and the upper temporal lobes at the watershed between the middle and the posterior cerebral arteries (ZÜLCH, 1961b). These corrrespond to what have been described by GASTAUT and his school (GASTAUT and NAQUET, 1966; GAUSTAUT et al., 1971) as the "extraterritorial" zones (Colloque de Marseille à Cologne, 1964).
b) As an infarcted area which borders the three irrigation zones of the anterior, the middle and the posterior cerebral arteries. This also belongs to the group of surface infarcts and can be named as the three territory infarct ("Dreiländereck"-Infarkt; see Figs. 148, 149). It corresponds functionally to the last arterial branches seen in the lateral angiogram at the beginning of the capillary phase (DECKER, 1958, 1960/66; see also the "parietal syndrome", Colloque de Marseille à Cologne, 1964, and GASTAUT et al., 1971).

c) Typical infarcts in the depth of the brain occur in the basal ganglia between the area supplied by the *deep arteries* (Heubner's artery, the lenticulostriate, and the anterior chorioidal artery) on one side and the *superficial* cortical irrigation supplied by the middle cerebral artery (Figs. 130 and 142) on the other. The corresponding *hemorrhagic* infarct passes mostly through the head of the caudate nucleus and the putamen (the internal capsule remaining *anemic*; see Fig. 142).

2) "Proximal" infarcts within an irrigation zone. In an occlusion of the middle cerebral artery the dorsal, posterior or basal parts of the irrigation area may be supplied by the anterior or posterior cerebral arteries (Fig. 139). If the collateral supply is very large a so-called minimal infarct may develop which is located near the obstructed stem of the artery (so-called stump-near infarct).

3) Infarcts in the "center of a supply area". If an artery is only stenosed the proximal zone may be sufficiently nourished, but the distal areas, still supplied within its irrigation territory, are endangered. If the collateral blood supply is further reduced this endangered area concentrically shrinks and an infarct in the "center of a supply area" may result (Fig. 139). This type of infarction is most often found in the territory of the middle cerebral artery and is then characteristically located (Figs. 132 and 133) in the frontal operculum and the insular cortex. When the dominant hemisphere is compromised including most of "Broca's" speech area an isolated motor (expressive) dysphasia may follow; or it may also occur as a small infarction in the "central" part of the posterior cerebral artery territory, which may then affect the primary visual centers of the calcarine region (see page 154 and Figs. 109, 110, 129) and appropriate hemianopic visual field defects may ensue (KLEIHUES and HIZAWA, 1966).

4) "Terminal" infarcts within an irrigation area. Such "terminal" infarcts are typically found in the brain in the form of circumscribed cysts in the centrum semiovale. They commonly occur in association with another "terminal" infarct of similar pathogenesis in the supply area of the striatal vessels (within the corpus nuclei caudati) according to the pattern of a "last field" (see Figs. 129, 151). A third "terminal" infarct occurring in a peculiar location may show the value of a hemodynamic interpretation of cerebral vascular insufficiency. This infarction is a small necrosis or cyst regularly localized in the subependymal basal region of the trigonum. It is commonly observed in a frontal section running through the splenium of the corpus callosum (Figs. 150, 151). Our hemodynamic interpretation is that these are infarcts at the terminal supply area of the *anterior chorioidal artery* (KRIBS and KLEIHUES, 1971). They occur in cases of proximal stenosis or occlusion if there is insufficient collateral supply from the posterior chorioidal artery.

β) Extension of an Infarct Beyond the Anatomical Borders of the Vascular Supply Area

The extent of an infarct may decrease or the margin be shifted to the "center" as we have shown. But an infarct may also extend beyond the borders of the normal supply territories (Fig. 120). This may be explained by the following example. If there is a marked stenosis of the anterior cerebral artery the supply territory of the middle cerebral artery is extended into the territory of the anterior cerebral artery and then if there is a later thrombosis of the middle cerebral artery, an infarct of supernormal size results (ZÜLCH and KLEIHUES, 1967).

γ) Symmetrical Infarcts in Both Hemispheres

Interpretations of infarcts on a hemodynamic basis – as attempted above – are sometimes difficult. Vascular obliteration of minor arteries cannot always be excluded, but if one can demonstrate symmetrical bilateral infarcts in both hemispheres the assumption of a simultaneous block of two identical vessels at symmetrical points does not seems reasonable. The common occurrence of bilateral simultaneous infarcts in the posterior lobes is understandable. This happens because the areas are supplied by the single midline basilar artery. If the basilar or either one

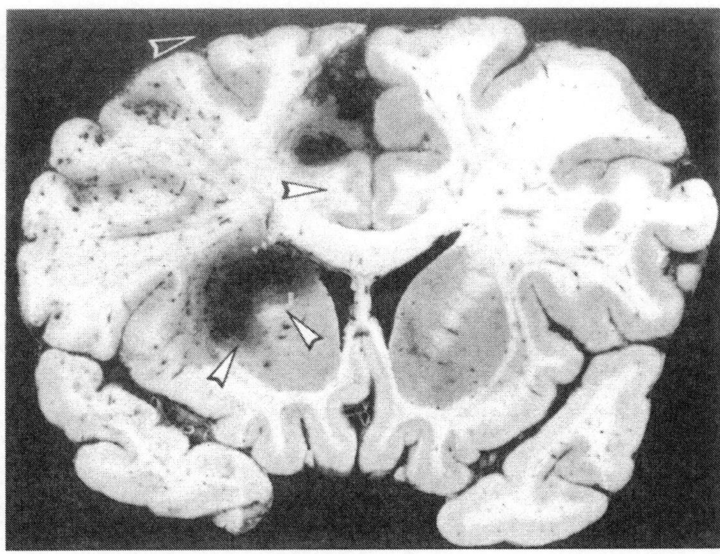

Fig. 120. Embolic occlusion with subsequent ischemic infarct. It is hemorrhagic at the deep border; extension of supply territory of middle cerebral artery towards the anterior cerebral artery following marked stenosis of the anterior cerebral artery. The cingulate gyrus is supplied by the spracallosal anastomosis from the posterior cerebral artery

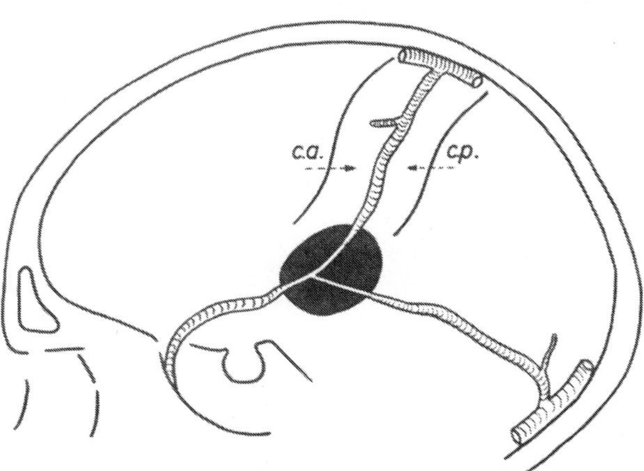

Fig. 121. Area of insufficient blood supply in a case of venous obstruction, e.g. thrombosis of sinuses (venous "last meadow")

of the vertebral arteries is stenosed or occluded, *bilateral posterior cerebral artery* infarcts *may* follow.

In strangulation of the posterior cerebral artery by transtentorial herniation into the cisterna ambiens, a typical infarct in the calcarine region occurs (MOORE and STERN, 1938; RIESSNER and ZÜLCH, 1938, 1939); it may be even bilateral (see Fig. 85, ZÜLCH 1959; ZÜLCH et al., 1974b).

δ) "Last Meadows" in Venous Irrigation

The concept of a "last meadow" can also be applied to the venous system (ZÜLCH, 1966a) to explain in sinus thrombosis what has been called by Sir CHARLES SYMONDS (1937, 1942) the "brachio-facial" syndrome. Insufficient venous drainage by the sinuses seems to provoke a swamping of venous blood around the center of the "tristar" formed by the veins of Trolard, Labbé and the Sylvian veins. This territory corresponds to a cortical area which must necessarily – as deduced from the brachio-facial symptomatology – be compromised (see Fig. 121). Very frequently in such cases "venous criblures" are observed predominantly in the temporal lobe (Figs. 122 and 123).

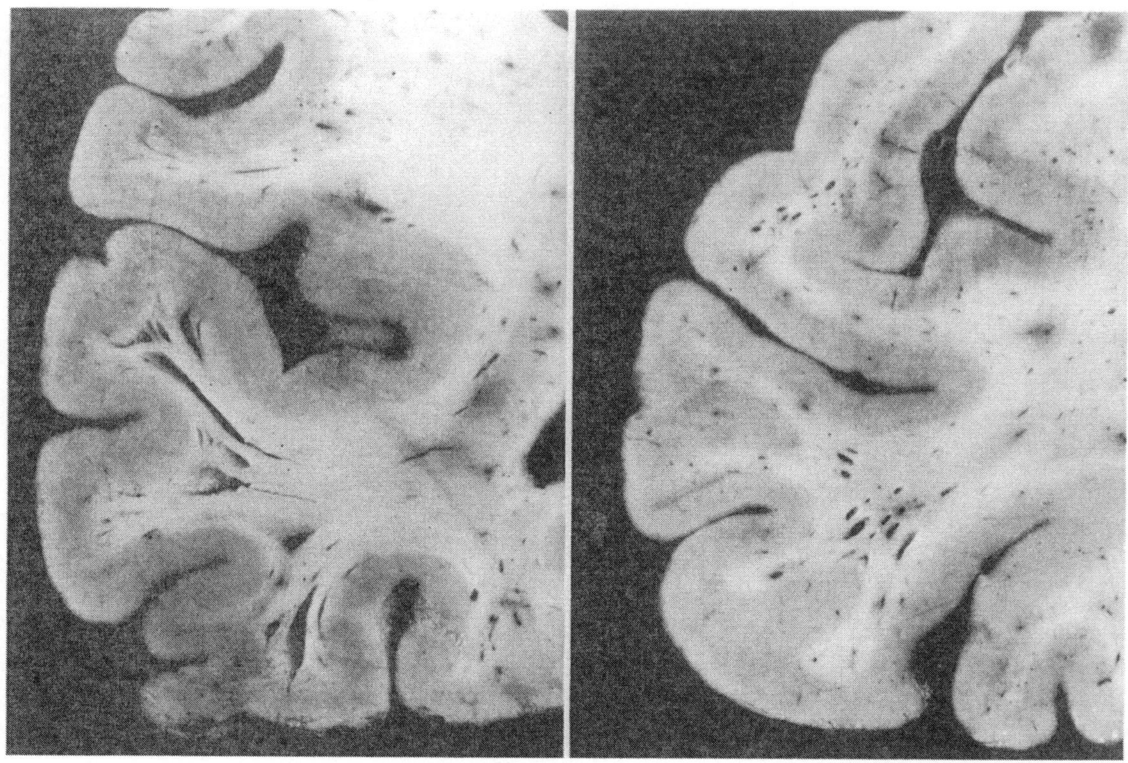

Fig. 122. Venous "criblures" probably arising after prolonged venous hyperemia

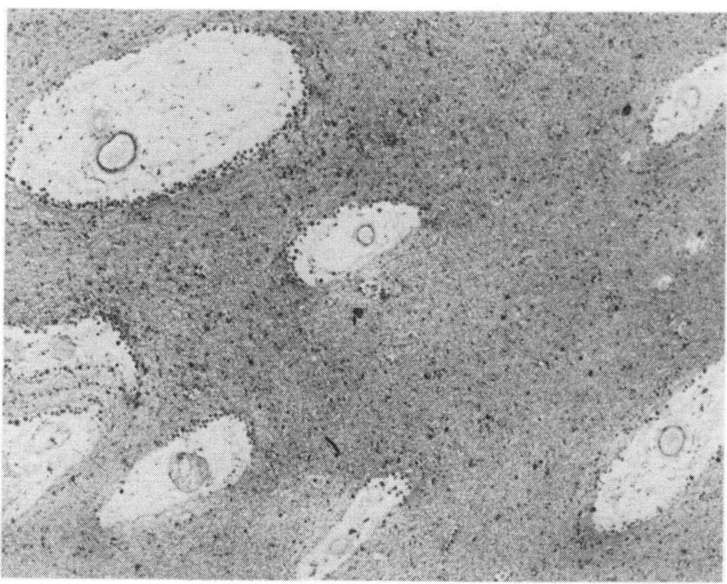

Fig. 123. Peculiar vacuolation of white matter around deep veins of left temporal lobe (sieve-like perforation); probably remnant of venous hyperemia with edema due to subacute venous back pressure. Numerous corpora amylacea

ε) *Hemodynamic Implications of Anastomotic Systems: the Steal Syndromes*

Cerebral angiography has made us understand many hemodynamic disturbances, for which the patterns were formerly not comprehensible merely from morphological data. This occurred, for instance, in cases in which the morphological changes were seen on the "wrong" side, i.e. after occlusion of one carotid artery, some – even major – atrophic changes were noted also in the contralateral hemisphere. It had been difficult in the past to reconstruct the active collateral pathways but the anastomoses were easily demonstrated in serial angiography as for example in the "subclavian steal" syndrome. However, it was not angiography which provided the answers to similar – recently observed – phenomena within the cranial cavity but the ingenious method of Xenon rCBF measurements developed by LASSEN (1959, 1966, 1968, 1969a, b) and LASSEN and INGVAR (1969). The different values of the actual circulation in the border-zones of a regional cerebrovascular insufficiency gave rise to such investigations. It was found that blood was drained into the focus of insufficiency from the neighboring systems via Heubner's "meningeal anastomoses" as shown angiographically and by the new method of rCBF. In some cases, however, rCBF measurements demonstrated that blood flowed from the endangered or infarcted zone paradoxically into the surrounding "normal" tissue ("reverse" or "counter" steal). Such curious hemodynamic phenomena were not encountered only in one cerebral hemisphere but also between the two hemispheres, as first shown by LOEB and FAVALE (1962) in cases of arteriovenous malformation. Peculiarly, the EEG focus was developed not over the arteriovenous malformation but rather in the contralateral hemisphere even though this was detrimental to its own circulation. These observations in the "altruistic" or "donor" hemisphere were enlarged and described in more detail by FAZIO (1964) and FAZIO et al. (1966, 1971; see also ZÜLCH and ESCHBACH, 1972).

The factors operating in the "distribution" and "redistribution" of the blood in the compromised area are characterized today mostly as the phenomena active in "autoregulation" of the brain circulation.

It is surprising to see that such a contribution by anastomotic systems supplies the endangered hemisphere to such a degree that undoubtedly deficiency symptoms arise in the contralateral ("wrong") hemisphere (see LAVY et al., 1975). Similar *interhemispheric* steal phenomena were observed by VAN DER DRIFT and KOK (1970, 1972) both in the angiogram and the EEG when working up 700 cases of primary or secondary cerebrovascular insufficiency. In 3 of 45 patients with occlusion of one carotid the EEG findings or the neurological deficit were not detected in correct correlation but rather on the contralateral side. They suggested a steal from the opposite side via the anterior communicating artery. Moreover, the vertebro-basilar system was drained in some cases to enlarge the circulation of the endangered hemisphere, whenever the posterior communicating artery anastomosis was morphologically sufficient. The "foci" may give rise to neurological symptoms, EEG delta foci, positive scans, angiographic phenomena etc.

Such cases of "interhemispheric steal" were described also by ZÜLCH and ESCHBACH (1972). It is, however, not well understood yet from the hemodynamic standpoint, why a "donor" hemisphere would deprive itself of its necessary supply by such an exaggerated contribution to its endangered partner. Why does the intra-arterial perfusion pressure locally decrease to such a degree as to provoke this phenomenon? And why does not the intra-arterial pressure in the donor hemisphere decrease at once when symptoms of vascular insufficiency appear, so that the regional blood is directed sufficiently once again into its old channels? One can speak here not only of a "steal" phenomenon, but even of "draining", almost by "suction" (see ZÜLCH, 1969d, pp. 80, 106), a terminology used by BIER (1906).

As early as 1906 the German general surgeon BIER in his book on "Hyperemia as a cure" discussed similar phenomena of "hyperemia as a tool for treatment" in the extremities, and he also discussed a "suction" of the blood into the compromised muscle tissue, yet could not find any rational explanation at that time.

Angiographic examination and rCBF measurements will be necessary possibly together with experimental observations on the monkey, to make these curious phenomena in the anastomotic systems better understood from the point of view of hemodynamics.

XIII. Clinical Phenomena: Classification of Cerebrovascular Accidents (CVA)

Classification of cerebrovascular disease (CVD) can be based on a variety of points of view.

If the time course is taken, the following table may be used:
1) impending – incipient stroke or stroke in evolution (stroke in the first phase),
2) progressing stroke (deterioration continues under observation),
3) completed (stabile) stroke (no further worthening in the acute situation),
4) transient ischemic attacks (TIAs) last not more than 24 h and are fully reversible, and
5) PRIND: more prolonged but reversible ischemic neurological defects.

The *morphological* classifications of stroke are based on the *cause* and show the subgroups of
1) mass hemorrhages into the cerebral tissue (see pp. 75, 84),
2) infarcts due to
   a) thrombo-embolism or primary thrombosis (see pp. 69, 72),
   b) stenosis plus cardiovascular insufficiency (see p. 120),
   c) stenosis plus final thrombosis,
   d) atherosclerotic occlusion.

Most cases of the second large group of infarcts (softenings) if caused by hemodynamic factors show:
1) Local alterations of the arteries from atherosclerosis (or from other causes which produce arterial narrowing or widening or, in rare cases, compression of one or both carotid arteries by strangulation etc.). A smaller number have no local alterations of the arteries.
2) Usually in these cases there is a "general factor" influencing the circulation, e.g., cardiac disturbances ranging from insufficiency to arrest or a loss of a resistance in the peripheral arterial systems (shock etc.).

In addition to these ischemic foci originating from obstruction of the arterial supply, there are, less commonly, tissue alterations originating from the obstruction of the venous drainage system (thromboses of veins and sinuses, see p. 128).

Clinical viewpoints were emphasized in a personal classification. Over the past few decades we have tried to correlate biographic particularities with the hemodynamic pathogenesis of stroke of individual patients (ZÜLCH, 1962b, 1963a). We differentiated five main types of cerebral vascular insufficiency which are characterized by the patient's historical cardiovascular situation.

Of these the types 1–4 are probably associated with a "hypotensive" crisis while type 5 is related to a "hypertensive" crisis in the circulation (see p. 119). In analysing the patient's situation at and before stroke we have distinguished:

1) The "lesion at rest" ("midnight stroke"), which is observed in the morning on waking and develops probably after a critical fall in blood pressure which may have occurred shortly after midnight. Serial blood pressure measurements on our patients through the night have shown convincingly a midnight fall (ZÜLCH, 1962b; ZÜLCH and V. HOSSMANN, 1967) in the blood pressure that correlates easily with the onset of cerebrovascular insufficiency (V. HOSSMANN, 1969; V. HOSSMANN and ZÜLCH, 1979).
2) The "stress" lesion. Physical exertion together with an acute decompensation of the heart's action may lead to cerebral blood flow insufficiency and cerebral infarction.
3) The "relaxation" (detention) lesion can occur as a result of an acute collapse or over a period of several hours of more gradual general relaxation usually after antecedent stress. In such a case, among other factors, an acute or subacute fall in blood pressure may be catastrophically effective in causing infarction particularly if the fall in pressure *coincides* with the circadian (nycthemeric) "physiological" falls of pressure in the early afternoon or at midnight (see above 1).
4) The "primary cardiogenic" type of cerebrovascular insufficiency following a primary organic lesion of the heart. It has been known for a long time that a myocardial infarction which

causes an acute vascular insufficiency may induce a secondary cerebral lesion (cerebrocoronary syndrome of the Italian School (DOZZI, 1939; FAZIO, 1949; see also BODECHTEL, 1974).

5) The hypertensive insult due to acute excitation etc. From clinical observations we believe that in about 3%–5% of cases (ZÜLCH, 1962b) the infarctions occur at the height of an attack of increased blood pressure, the effect of which may be angiospasm. In physiological terms this spastic narrowing corresponds to the Bayliss effect (BYROM, 1954; ZÜLCH, 1957–1963). We have published a series of clinical observations of this type.

As a consequence of sudden hypertensive attacks (hypertensive crises) vasoconstriction (angiospasm) and vasodilatation have been observed experimentally with a consequent "break through" of the blood-brain barrier (see p. 75). According to our experience such lesions are less likely to be reversible than "hypotensive" insults.

The prognosis after hypo- or hypertensive episodes has been discussed by FUJISHIMA et al. (1976) and of TIAs by GOLDNER et al. (1971).

1. General Circulatory Factors, a Cause of Infarction

We have emphasized the importance of the "vis a tergo", of the general circulation in the pathogenesis of infarction and mentioned in particular acute or subacute rises and falls of blood pressure leading to regional cerebrovascular insufficiency. We must now critically discuss these possibilities.

a) Hypertension

Hypertension may in three ways participate in a cerebrovascular attack (CVA):
1) chronic hypertension as contributory factor to atherosclerosis (see p. 50),
2) the acute elevation of blood pressure (the hypertensive crisis; see above) and
3) acute lowering of chronic hypertensive pressure values to "normal" or "hypotensive" levels.

The last-mentioned phenomenon is certainly *very common in stroke*. It forms the transition to the group of normotensive patients who suffer a "hypotensive" crisis.

The second phenomenon merits further comment. It is well known that acute hypertension leads to cerebrovascular insufficiency during "hypertensive encephalopathy", in acute eclampsia and in association with pheochromocytomas. Physiologically this was explained by the Bayliss principle in which constriction of an artery occurs after abrupt tension from inside (as in sudden elevation of blood pressure). Early experiments of BYROM (1954) proved this interpretation as well as more recent experimental results (see pages 59, 75).

b) Experiments on Induced Hypertension

In induced hypertension was an associated decrease in diameter of the small arteries and a decrease in arteriovenous transit time (RUSSELL et al., 1970).

Blood pressure = O_2 (KOGURE et al., 1970) apart from CO_2 (HARPER and GLASS, 1965; FIESCHI et al., 1969) is also one of the factors regulating local circulation (autoregulation see JOHANSSEN, 1964; HARPER, 1966; HOEDT-RASMUSSEN, 1969).

Since 1957 we have postulated the existence of stroke after an acute hypertensive insult (hypertensive crisis) as first time conceived 125 years ago by the German clinician TRAUBE (1855) and used as a basic concept by the German School of v. BERGMANN (1932) and Friedrich KAUFFMANN (1925; "angiospastischer Insult"). However, this theory was expanded far too much and was rightly attacked by DENNY-BROWN (1951). Since then the possibility of "vasospasm" as a cause of acute cerebrovascular insufficiency has been rejected. I have cited many clinical examples in 1962b and counted 3%–5% probably angiospastic (hypertensive) insults. Since then angiospasm (see ZÜLCH, 1959; LECHTAPE-GRÜTER and ZÜLCH, 1971) has not only been seen experimentally following mechanical lesions of arteries [and "chemical" (?) in SAH], but also broadly investigated in the experimental laboratory. Angiospasm has been seen not only alternating with vasodilatation and its effect on circulation measured, but also an action on the blood-brain barrier ("break through") has been proven (see PAULSON, 1970; HÄGGENDAL and JOHANSSON, 1971/1972; PANNIER and LEUSEN, 1975; STRANDGAARD et al., 1976; K.-A. HOSSMANN and SCHUIER, 1979). The evidence for our position that a minor group of strokes is caused by hypertensive crisis is increasing steadily.

It has, however, to be distinguished from MARSHALL's (1971, 1977) discussion of the importance of hypertension as a risk for stroke. This concept corresponds, according to my understanding, to the group (2) mentioned in the beginning, i.e., the cerebrovascular insufficiency arising in the hypertensive individual following an acute fall of blood pressure.

The correlation between hypertension and the origin of TIA's is discussed by WHISNANT (1974; see pp. 122, 124). Experimentally comparison has been made between hypertensive strokes in animals and in humans (YAMORI et al., 1976). KIMURA's (1977) statement that the incidence of hypertension among the Japanese population is not high enough to explain the frequency of strokes is interesting.

The pathogenesis of angiospasm has been discussed since FORBES and COBB (1938), FOG's (1939) and BROMAN'S (1940) experiments. This discussion is reinforced after the angiographic and intraoperative observation of angiospasm in subarachnoid hemorrhage. The innervation and thus the possibility of a neurally induced "spasm" has been investigated. Lately OWMAN et al. (1978; see also EDVINSSON and OWMAN, 1979) have proved adrenergic innervation of the cerebrovascular bed (originating in the superior cervical ganglion). The pial circulation in contrast receives cholinergic fibers as well as vasodilatory peptidergic nerve fibers. Pharmacological experiments are said to have proved in detail which specific receptors mediate the contractile and dilatory responses; even sympathetic nerve stimulation reduces the regional cerebral blood flow by 15%–20% (see also D'ALECY and FEIGL, 1972).

c) Hypotension

We have frequently mentioned a fall of blood pressure (acute or subacute hypotensive crisis) as a cause of cerebrovascular insufficiency.

In discussing elevated blood pressure we have to emphasize strongly, that only a blood pressure "profile" (reading at least every hour or thirty minutes) can provide sufficient information apart from 1) frequent blood pressure recordings by the practitioner, 2) observation of a "left heart hypertrophy".

Single values – for instance during the first hours in the hospital – will not rectify such a statement, because they may be a sequel of the "stroke".

Moreover attention has to be paid to the fact that relaxation, the circadian rhythms, the "biographic" situation – acute stress? anxiety? affect? – or on the other hand orthostatic attitude may influence the blood pressure values (see below and pp. 120, 121).

It may even be that a sensitive carotid sinus produces several asystoles of six to ten seconds, which lead to poststenotic regional insufficiency. Or perhaps a severely stenosed internal carotid or middle cerebral artery gets occluded during night by appositional thrombosis following sludging subsequent to acute hypotension.

However, it has been already an old notion of the French school of neurologists (VINCENT and DARQUIER, 1923; WORMS, 1931) that many clinical entities leading to fall of blood pressure such as postoperative or traumatic hemorrhages, blood donation etc. can provoke stroke. The same has been observed in association with the first total or subtotal sympathectomies in the thorax and abdomen (so-called operation of WHITE and SMITHWICK) and cardiac surgery (STOCKARD et al., 1974).

RIISCHEDE (1957) emphasized correctly the dependence of the cerebral circulation on the general circulation. His monograph is filled with examples of gross neurological deficits after sudden hypotension from various causes (his pages 98/99). He reports in detail one of these examples in which the symptoms of facial paresis, clumsy right hand movements with paresthesias and motor aphasia occurred in direct relation to a fall in the blood pressure (critical levels between 160 and 190 systolic). We have observed the same pattern in a patient with stenosis of one paramedian pontine artery where the critical level for his spastic paraparesis was around 180 mmHg. Also DENNY-BROWN (1951) in his remarkable attack on angiospasm as the cause of the majority of strokes cited similar examples.

Later investigations have given some authors, doubts as to the validity of the theory of the hemodynamic pathogenesis by a hypotensive crisis. KENDELL and MARSHALL (1963) deliberately lowered the blood pressure to the point of syncope in 37 patients currently experiencing transient ischemic attacks. Transient ischemic attacks were not produced prior to the development of generalized cerebral ischemia. The same results were reported by F. LHERMITTE (personal communication). For information about the EEG after profound hypotension see GAMACHE et al. (1975)

These authors do not deny that a sudden profound fall of blood pressure may lead to cerebral infarction but they do not ascribe the majority of cases of cerebral infarction to this mechanism. In their opinion acute hypotension applies only to a small minority of cases.

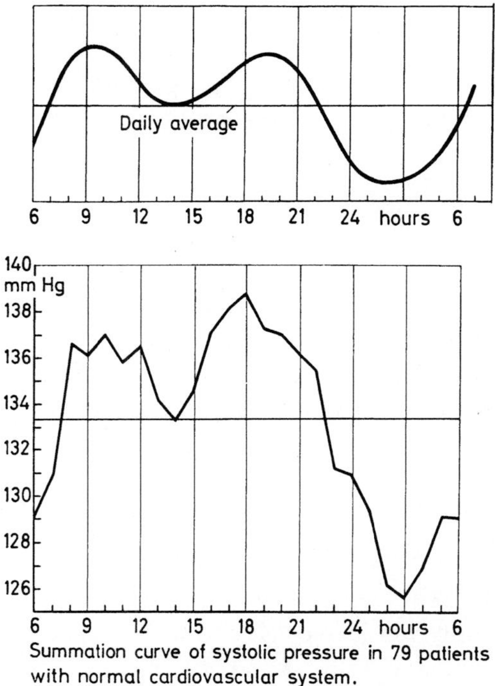

Fig. 124. Curve of normal regulations of the autonomous system with regard to physiological efficiency and alertness. (After GRAF, 1955, Fig. 3)

It is not the goal of this discussion to mention all the possibilities of acute hypotension from orthostasis (THULESIUS, 1977; J.S. MEYER et al., 1973), shock, cardiac insufficiency, and all other forms of medical or postsurgical sequelae (STOCKARD et al., 1974) as a cause of brain infarct (TORVIC and SKULLERUD, 1976). However, two entities will have to be discussed here, because too little attention has been paid to them in the past.

a) Even in cases where these is a rhythmic cardiac action during day arrhythmias have been shown to occur during the "circadian" (nykthemeric) changes at midnight (V. HOSSMANN, 1969; see also "midnight stroke", p. 121).
b) The influence of the "circadian" (nykthemeric) changes on the autonomic nervous system and consequently on the blood pressure has been emphasized in our wards (Fig. 124) for long (ZÜLCH, 1967; ZÜLCH and V. HOSSMANN, 1967; V. HOSSMANN, 1969; V. HOSSMANN et al., 1974). V. HOSSMANN and ZÜLCH (1979) showed in particular the influence on the initiation of cerebrovascular insufficiency and stroke, a concept recently accepted also by MARSHALL (1977). Angina pectoris may occur at the same time, probably for the same reason.

One of the most illustrative examples of this phenomenon is the history of the "first case" of endarterectomy (EASTCOTT et al., 1954) where nocturnal (2 o'clock) arrhythmias led to transient angina and later aphasia 33 times. His blood pressure was 240/150. After endarterectomy the nocturnal attacks of angina remained, but cerebral symptoms did not recur. Blood pressure changes following vascular diseases in the brainstem have been recently discussed (ITO et al., 1973).

Recently a peculiar syndrome of degeneration of cells in the autonomic nervous system is described to lead to hypotension (Shy-Drager Syndrome; see J.S. MEYER et al., 1973).

d) Microcirculation

We have discussed our concept of the hypotensive crisis repeatedly, although I do not believe that hypotension is always the *sole cause* of diminished blood flow through the brain. I would like to refer here to the experimental results of BARTSCH and SWANK (1967) who concluded that in an (induced) hypotensive crisis in the dog there were changes in viscosity which they could measure by the screen-filtration method. I believe that in a human with such an attack – the hallmark of which is a fall in blood pressure – far more changes are set in operation also than simply a possible "diminished blood flow". There are probably also disturbances of the microcirculation (ZÜLCH, 1967).

The logical conclusion is that one must postulate a "multiple factor theory" (ZÜLCH, 1962b, 1967, Fig. 1) as I have exemplified with numerous case histories. I showed at that time a diagrammatic scheme with wheels in which rotation of one of them caused all the others to change.

This discussion is valid particularly for the major forms of stroke. Recently the observations during amaurosis fugax (transient monocular blindness) and transient ischemic attacks (TIA's) in the brain have stimulated the discussion of other forms of pathogenesis in cerebrovascular insufficiency.

e) Viscosity, Sludging and Other Intrinsic Factors of the Blood

We have emphasized above a "multifactor" theory of stroke and mentioned the changes in microcirculation induced by acute hypotension. Modern research supposes that far more intrinsinc factors than previously considered, play an important role. Fibrinogens and their products apparently are important (see FLETCHER et al., 1976; V. HOSSMANN, 1977) in the course and prognosis of hemodynamic disturbances and infarction (OTT et al., 1974). Hypercoagulability may be one of the manifestations (ETTINGER, 1974).

Moreover, all the other discussions on these subjects at the "Brain and Heart Infarct" Symposium in Cologne 1976 have to be taken into account. This went so far that ROBERTS (1977) emphasized that coronary thromboses are rare in a fatal myocardial event and are not therefore the triggering cause. He supported this concept by citing 5 factors (ROBERTS, 1977, p. 297), similar to the discussion emphasized by ZÜLCH (1961, 1967).

f) Microembolic Theory

Since it has been demonstrated that in amaurosis fugax microemboli can frequently be observed in the retina (RUSSELL, 1961, 1963, 1968, 1971; RUSSELL et al., 1970), the concept has been developed that "sloughing off" of microemboli from ulcerated plaques in the cervical carotid bifurcation (MCDONALD, 1967) into the blood stream also causes cerebral "transient ischemic attacks" (TIA's) mainly in the carotid territory (HEYMAN et al., 1974). However, C.M. FISHER (1952, 1959) in his first report on transient monocular blindness ("amaurosis fugax") considered an hypotensive event as one of the possible causes. I have opposed personally the validity of this concept of "microembolism" (ZÜLCH, 1961a, b, 1967) and explained it again on the basis of a suitable case from another standpoint (ZÜLCH, 1977a, 1979). In one patient "amaurosis fugax" persisted even after occlusion of the carotid and disappeared at once only after an extracranial-intracranial bypass (ECIC) on the occluded side (see also ANDERSEN et al., 1977) had been performed. For References see: amaurosis fugax: MARSHALL and MEADOWS, 1968; TIAs: JANEWAY and TOOLE, 1972; ZIEGLER and HASSAWEIN, 1973; WHISNANT et al., 1973; WHISNANT, 1974; GRINDAL and TOOLE, 1974; TOOLE et al., 1975; TOOLE, 1975, 1976; YARNELL et al., 1975.

2. Pathophysiological and Clinical Pathogenesis of Infarction

Damage inflicted upon the brain by ischemia is the result of two different mechanisms: one directly related to the breakdown of energy-dependent biochemical and neurophysiological functions during ischemia, the other a sequel to events occurring during recirculation after ischemia.

Clinically a clear distinction between the two phases is generally not possible because ischemic, oligemic and normemic episodes may occur alternately depending on the particular hemodynamic situation. The pathophysiological and pathobiochemical mechanisms of ischemic brain damage, therefore, are more easily understood in animal experiments in which cerebral blood flow can be arrested and restored at will.

Experiments to elucidate the pathomechanism of cerebral infarction have been performed since the early fifties patterned after some interesting ligations of arteries and veins which had been performed in cats and rabbits by H. BECKER (1939) who emphasized the importance of the collaterals when ligating more then one of the four arteries. THOMPSON and RHODE (1950) showed the importance of a sufficient blood pressure, DENNY-BROWN and J.S. MEYER (1957) the operation of the meningeal anastomoses. More recently the experimental design has been more sophisticated and a transorbital approach with ligature of the middle cerebral artery in the cat been used (SYMON et al., 1974; WALTZ et al., 1967; HEISS et al., 1977).

It has been proved that at the edge of the "occluded" (infarcted) area there is hyperemia and an increase of arteriovenous transit-time (ROSS RUSSELL et al., 1970).

A whole new field has been opened to the pathometabolism of infarction by the "prolonged ischemia" model usually performed in the cat (KLATZO, 1967; K.-A. HOSSMANN and SATO, 1970; K.-A. HOSSMANN et al., 1973; BRIERLY, 1973; K.-A. HOSSMANN and KLEIHUES, 1973; KLEIHUES et al., 1974; ITO et al., 1975; K.-A. HOSSMANN and V. HOSSMANN, 1977) or the monkey (HOSSMANN and OLSSON, 1970; K.-A. HOSSMANN and ZIMMERMANN, 1975). New and basic knowledge has been brought up by these experiments with "global" brain ischemia.

Complete interruption of the cerebral blood flow in the intact animal can be produced by various methods, for instance by clamping the arterial blood supply to the brain (K.-A. HOSSMANN, 1971, 1977; K.-A. HOSSMANN and KLEIHUES, 1973) and cardiac arrest (V. HOSSMANN and K.-A. HOSSMANN, 1973). By this method, cerebral blood flow is instantaneously interrupted, causing an almost immediate loss of the electrophysiological functions of the brain.

The metabolic response of the brain during ischemia depends on the completeness of cerebral circulatory arrest. When blood flow is completely interrupted, the available energy stores are used up within 5 min (NORDSTRÖM and SIESJÖ, 1978; NORDSTRÖM et al., 1978). "Trickling" blood flow provides a continuous supply of glucose which is sufficient to maintain some anaerobic glycolysis. This leads to excessively high lactate levels and to much more severe tissue acidosis than in complete ischemia. It is possible that this is one reason why incomplete ischemia is less well tolerated than complete ischemia (K.-A. HOSSMANN and KLEIHUES, 1973).

Much of the ischemic damage occurs after and not during ischemia. Factors such as a postischemic increase in intracranial pressure, increase in blood viscosity due to platelet aggregation, postischemic disseminated intravascular coagulation, and postischemic hypotension seem to be of greater importance. The "no-reflow phenomenon" can be effectively prevented even after 1 h of ischemia by recirculating the ischemic brain at elevated blood pressure, by osmotherapy for the treatment of brain swelling, and by improving the rheological properties of the blood, e.g. with dextran (K.-A. HOSSMANN, 1977). Under these circumstances, progressive signs of biochemical and functional recovery of the brain have been observed after ischemic periods up to 1 h.

Considerable experimental evidence concerning the "hypotensive", carbon-monoxic/anoxic or ischemic changes in the brain has been gained by the group of R.E. MYERS (MYERS, 1973; GINSBERG and MYERS, 1974a, b, c; MYERS, 1975a, b, c, d; BRANN and MYERS, 1975; GAMACHE and MYERS, 1975).

Clinical implications. Over the last few decades, much research has been carried out into the clinical manifestations of neuronal ischemia. However, the position of the clinician at the bedside is far removed from that of the experimentalist whose clear interpretations we have just demonstrated. The clinician is still faced with the critical time of 8–10 min of ischemia for revival and at present there is no hope of recirculating the brain after a more prolonged period of ischemia. In spite of all attempts at treatment, many progressive cerebrovascular attacks (stroke) lead to irreversible necrosis, e.g., brain infarcts, and we are in the position of not knowing which patient will recover and which not, and why. (First experiences with flow measurements during computed tomography see Traupe et al., 1979.) At the bedside, it is still as impossible to gain sufficient knowledge about the hemodynamics during stroke and the ensuing state of recirculation, as it is to obtain some insight into a temporarily existent collateral circulation. In many cases of stroke in man the pathogenesis remains unclear.

Ethical restrictions may prevent the clinician from applying the usual diagnostic methods and we are often reluctant to perform angiography because of the age or general condition of the patient.

At this point the value of the clinical methods available for diagnosis should be described. Two questions about stroke have to be answered: a) its location and b) the degree of ischemic neuronal damage, e.g., the reversibility.

The following techniques are available for the analysis of stroke:

1) A good history of the cardiovascular system of the patient including the "biographical" situation before and during the stroke.
2) Examination of the actual state of the cardiovascular and cerebrovascular systems.
3) The EEG, preferably with frequency analysis.
4) Computed tomography (CT) can give very precise information about the localization and even, to a certain degree, about the extent of the lesions (edema formation!) at the end of the first 24 h. However, CT is not always available.
5) Technetium scanning can be very informative on the 4th to 5th day, but occasionally gives false-negative results.
6) Angiography is applied (with the above-mentioned restrictions) and can show arterial stenosis and/or occlusion as the cause of the stroke. Collateral pathways may point to existing occlusions which are not demonstrated on a particular X-ray film. It has always to be borne in mind, however, that angiography is an "invasive" method.
7) rCBF measurement can help in the diagnostic process, although it can be useful only for the territory of the middle cerebral artery. It is still an "invasive" method, but may be possible soon routinely by i.v. injections or inhalation.
8) Measuring blood flow during the intravenous application of technetium. This is a simple, though not often practiced, method which can give information about flow in the major supply areas of the intracranial vessels.
9) Rheography, Doppler methods, ophthalmodynamography, spinal tap with bicarbonate analysis, blood chemistry, gas analysis and viscosity measurement rarely help to solve the problem of pathogenesis, but may provide a basis for particular therapeutic procedures.
10) The neurological examination is the easiest and quickest approach to establishing localization, however, may be also entirely uninformative.

In the application of these methods *localization* of the neuronal lesions is our first goal, evaluation of the *degree* and *reversibility*, the second, whereas the first information may be obtained, the second is more problematic, because the degree of an ischemic attack, e.g. the problem of the reversibility of a neuronal lesion is more difficult to solve. We are met with the greatest amount of uncertainty. Was there an arrest of the circulation or was there a residual blood flow? One cannot answer this and other questions in very many cases.

The clinician can try to classify the attack according to its course. A transient ischemic attack (TIA) is supposed to be totally reversible in 24 h. Longer lasting ischemic neuronal disease may also recover without residual deficit (PRIND). However, which symptoms arising from a neuronal lesion can provide clues to a prognosis in the first 24 h or in the first few days? We cannot establish in man whether the neurological deficit is due, in the case of a stenosing arterial lesion, to primary ischemia after a heart attack or, in the case of an occlusion, to a deficiency in a collateral circulation hitherto sufficient. Whether an acute onset was due to embolism or to the acute onset of cardiac insufficiency in Stokes-Adams syndrome remains unanswered. Was the neuronal lesion ischemic or hypoxic in the case of pulmonary deficiency? Is the neuronal lesion primarily due to ischemia/anoxia or is it secondary to postischemic edema? Has recirculation after the event been sufficient? Is a progressive course a sign of an appositional thrombosis leading to occlusion? Is there a postischemic hyperemia and does it suggest recovery? Does a breakdown in autoregulation give any information?

The clinician encounters still more problems in deducing the primary lesion from the neurological symptoms (ZÜLCH, 1977b). The brain is – as once described by Sir Henry HEAD – overwired. This means that we do not know how many of the neurons are actually necessary for maintaining function and how many may be irreversibly destroyed without producing a noticeable neurological deficit.

Since the experiments of OPITZ and SCHNEIDER (1950) we know that a decrease of the circulation to 50% of the normal triggers the first neurological symptoms, yet only a fall beyond 15% to 20% produces irreversible morphological changes, e.g., infarction. There is a 30% "safety mantle" (ZÜLCH, 1962b) in which the circulation defect is still reversible.

Moreover, the problem of "diaschisis", e.g. a functional but merely temporary failure of the neuron, complicates diagnosis. Finally "plasticity" may lead to "recovery" of function; in this case the primary neurons originally responsible for function are deficient, and others have assumed the function. All this shows the degree of uncertainty and the dilemma of not being able to define the degree of reversibility of the neuronal change in "stroke".

3. "Cerebral Death"

The human brain after a critical, 6–8 min period of anoxia or total global ischemia begins to swell to such a volume, that the ensuing intracranial pressure exceeds any possible perfusion pressure. Histological examination shows that all cells, but predominantly astroglia and endothelial cells of the capillaries, swell by "intracellular edema" to such an extent, that the capillary microcirculation is blocked. Arterial blood can therefore not progress in the vessels and in case of angiography contrast medium is seen only outside the cranial cavity. Functionally the brain is "dead", i.e. the EEG shows electrical silence ("flattening"). (Complete discussion see KRÖSL and SCHERZER, 1973; A.E. WALKER, 1977). K.-A. HOSSMANN's experiments (K.-A. HOSSMANN and KLEIHUES, 1973) showed that in the experimental animal (cat or rhesus monkey) recirculation after prolonged ischemia of 1 h is possible in around two third of the cases, as well as a restoration of most functions as EEG, protein metabolism etc. Why is this not possible in the human? Apart from the fact that also in the animal recirculation will succeed only under particular conditions including elevated blood pressure and prevention of aggregation, furthermore the prolonged ischemia must start abruptly and be total, i.e. no rest flow may be present. Most frequently the condition in man is not "experimental" and therefore the necessary measures for recirculation may not be possible *rapidly* enough before the critical time has passed.

It is interesting that total global ischemia is tolerated longer and recirculation possible later, when barbiturate loading is induced at once, but a dose is required which necessitates the use of artificial respiration (NEMOTO, 1977; SAFAR et al., 1979).

In summary, the clue to successful recirculation in man after ischemia has not been found yet and the experience with global total ischemia has not provided hints toward a successful treatment of regional ischemia, e.g., infarction in the human.

4. Epidemiology of Cerebrovascular Disease

In PAUL's (1966) definition epidemiology is the field "concerned with measurement of the circumstances under which diseases occur, where diseases tend to florish and where they do not" (see KURTZKE, 1969). We have indicated above the epidemiology of atherosclerosis as the leading predisposition of a *morphological* lesion for stroke. Different from it is the *clinical* entity of a cerebrovascular insult. We have to discuss here, whether there are particular epidemiologic phenomena for its clinical manifestation and its particular geographical and ethnic distribution. The data about this subject which have been critically collected by KURTZKE (1969; see also page 49) cannot be repeated here in detail. Suffice it to repeat only the much discussed examples of cerebrovascular disease among American Blacks and Japanese in their homeland. It is not doubted that Blacks generally exceed Whites in mortality rate in "hemorrhages and other cerebrovascular disease" but KURTZKE believes that "the best explanation for the high death rate among Blacks would appear to be the scarcity of medical facilities". In the other example, cerebral hemorrhage in Japan has been reported far in excess of Western experience since 1900. KURTZKE's (1969) interpretation of this alledged very elevated incidence of cerebral hemorrhage is that it is the result of an artefact of diagnostic fashion in Japan and that there is no racial predilection for stroke. However recent very precise investigations do not prove that (see KANAYA, 1979). On the contrary, a high incidence of hypertension is probably the leading cause.

In conditions associated with stroke one has to point to some factors operating in some regions or populations such as hypertension in Finland which naturally influences secondarily the incidence of stroke. In the USA hypertension seems to be most common risk factor – in "the obese, the Black and those with a familial history" (see also OLIVARES et al., 1973: Mexico; AHO and FOGELHOLM, 1974: Finland; RIISHEDE, 1967: Denmark; ALTER and KLUZNIK, 1972: Israel). For further elucidation of this discussion one is referred to a most exact general population risk survey about stroke in Rochester/Minnesota 1945–1954 (WHISNANT et al., 1972) about the following years 1955–1969 (MATSUMOTO et al., 1973).

It would appear therefore, that (a) statistics change rapidly due to improved treatment of hypertension and (b) many earlier supposed fact are apparently artefacts due to racial, sociologic, or national peculiarities. Only a careful analysis of the underlying factors allows one to make deductions valuable for *epidemiologic* analysis of stroke.

5. Morphology of Infarction

A very fresh infarct can best be felt with the finger (as a "softening" of the tissue). After a short time, it retracts slightly and its map-like margins can be easily recognized after drying the cut surface and viewing under oblique illumination. The white matter appears slightly grey but is sometimes bluish. The fresh focus can hardly be described better than with NEUBUERGER's (1930) words: "The fresh, few-hours-old focus has a jelly-like consistency, is deliquescent, sometimes more meaty and sharply outlined, more voluminous than the area would be normally. Its color is white to light yellow."

This stage usually lasts 1–2 days; thereafter the tissues of the infarct become softer and retract slightly; "after 2–3 days another change in consistency sets in; the infarct becomes soft but at the same time brittle, crumbly, sticky, fatty". In general, any larger focus becomes sequestrated, then liquefied, and broken down into fatty substances to be resorbed (Fig. 135).

SPIELMEYER (1922, page 389ff.), among others, pointed out that in rare cases the tissue does not become liquefied (according to NEUBUERGER, 1930, this occurs more frequently than is assumed). It remains in the state of primary coagulation as a sequester and is broken down slowly from the outside ("coagulating necrosis"). Histologically, often foci with needles of cholesterin and foreign body giant cells or foam cell granulomas remain in the center for a long time.

GUIZETTI (1897), SPIELMEYER (1922), J. LHERMITTE (1928), NEUBUERGER (1930), HASSIN (1948) differentiate four phases: 1) normal appearance, 2) demarcation, 3) transitional phase, and 4) softening. SPATZ (1936, 1939) recognized three phases of softening: 1) the phase of necrosis lasting until the end of the first week when gitter ("scavenger") cells appear in larger numbers, 2) the phase of resorption when the dead tissue is removed by scavenger cells, the latter being moved along vessels or remaining within the lime-water-like content of larger lesions, and 3) the final or third phase in which there is a terminal cystic defect (formation of a porus).

Summary of microscopic changes. The resorptive stage begins after 2–4 days by a disintegration of the nervous tissue after anoxia and edema. Fibroblasts are formed by the capillaries and swarm out into the tissue and are transformed into gitter cells. Microglia, if not destroyed, further this resorption process. Scavenger cells are transported into the capillaries or stay within the fine mesh of the infarcted and mean while liquified area. Later these infarcted areas begin to shrink by resorption. Liquified regions may become scarred and gliotic by proliferation of astroglia (see below). The ependymal and marginal pial tissues may survive this process and remain as an internal and external fine membrane of the infarction cyst (for details see below).

During the first years of life, practically always the complete softening leads to resorption of an infarct or necrosis (SPATZ, 1921). Cyst formation as described above is then called "porencephaly". But sometimes the softening is incomplete or spotty as mentioned above (see also SPATZ, 1936, 1939). In these cases, the incompletely destroyed brain tissue is transformed into scars, i.e., the nerve cells die, part of the macroglia is preserved and shows progressive changes, e.g. macrogliosis, the capillaries begin to proliferate and phagocytes transformed into gitter cells penetrate the tissues from within. Instead of a cyst, a glial-mesodermal scar tissue is formed. Such a transformation is particularly common in hemorrhagic infarcts and also in embolic microinfarcts (see also "granular atrophy", pp. 62, 63).

6. Detailed Histology of Infarction

Chronological course: Histologically, an anemic necrosis after 7 h, will exhibit a karyorrhexis of the glia, after 12–15 h fatty degeneration may occur, after 7–12 h glial proliferation in the white matter and after 24–30 h large plasmatic glial cells appear which may increase in number during the following 24 h. At the same time, the mesenchymal proliferation at the capillary walls increases starting from the second or third day (first signs of proliferation in 6–8 h according to NISSL). From our experiments on embolic microinfarcts in the cat we may make the following statements as to the time course of events (ZÜLCH, 1971b):

30 min: Spongy enlargement of pericellular and pericapillary spaces, e.g., intracellular edema; in larger infarcts mainly in the marginal zone (visible with Masson's stain).

1 h: Accentuation of edematous (spongy) changes with increased stainability (Hematoxylin-eosin, Masson) of the infarcted area. – Onset of "coagulation" in center.

2 h: Beginning of pallor of the infarct with Nissl stain. Intracellular swelling of capillary endothelial cells. First signs of "ischemic change" (SPIELMEYER, 1922) in nerve cells.

$3^1/_2$ h: Most neurons show "ischemic change"; swelling of oligodendroglia and astroglia and beginning of clasmatodendrosis.

5 h: The process of intracellular edema, having involved at first only the marginal zones, now extends through the whole infarct if the latter is small. Should it be larger, the inner zones may become "coagulated" (SPIELMEYER's "coagulation necrosis") the outer show a zone of intracellular edema. The first signs of extracellular – perivenous – edema are observed.

9 h: Proliferation of vascular endothelial cells at the margins. The nerve cells of the edematous zone begin to disintegrate, the granules are loosened but in the coagulated centers they are pyknotic and hyperchromatic. Numerous white thrombi are seen in veins.

16 h: Leukocytes emigrate diffusely from thrombosed veins into the tissue. Fibroblasts develop and swarm out from capillary walls.

30 h: The infarct is now sharply demarcated. Edematous zone of margin most marked by perivenous and diffuse extracellular edema. Karyorrhexis of neurons in inner portions commences. Endothelial and microglial mitoses occur; microgranulomas on proliferated vessels begin to show up.

57 h: First "gitter" (scavenger) cells in the zone of disintegration.

74 h: Pronounced gitter cell activity. Marginal extracellular edema beginning in the first 4 h which, depending on the size of the infarct, may increase in some cases to an enormous extent, even leading to real "edema lakes" in the white matter.

Later: Rarely there are calcifications or pseudocalcifications in larger parts of a vascular infarct; more often single nerve cells of the marginal zone may appear as "calcified".

A general analysis of the ischemic process shows that a recent infarct has a larger volume than the destroyed brain tissue due to edema in the cells of the marginal zone and within the lesion. This is visible macroscopically as a result of flattening of the convolutions, from the narrowing of the ventricles, and by mass shifting (including not infrequently the pineal gland, as can be seen on X-rays up to the 18th day). Edema is now convincingly demonstrated by hypodense zones seen in computed tomography. This, however, has not the typical pattern of "three finger edema".

7. Red and White Infarcts (Hemorrhagic and Anemic Necroses) and Their Pathogenesis

Cerebral infarcts may be of different pathogenesis and also of different color namely "red" or "white". They may also be either arterial and restricted mainly to the grey matter, or venous and located predominantly in the subcortical white matter (see Fig. 125). The red (hemorrhagic; Figs. 126–128) arterial infarct differs from the white (ischemic; Fig. 153) one by fine, punctate hemorrhages (speckled appearance) in the infarcted *cortex* or *grey nuclei* which often coalesce so much that they cannot be differentiated by the naked eye from a real hemorrhage. The question why, in a given case, one of the two types develops and not the other, has not always been fully explained. However, from experimental observations, some circumstances favoring the development of hemorrhagic infarct are known:

Red infarction always develops after complete regional ischemia when circulation is *reestablished* before the tissues are completely necrotic.

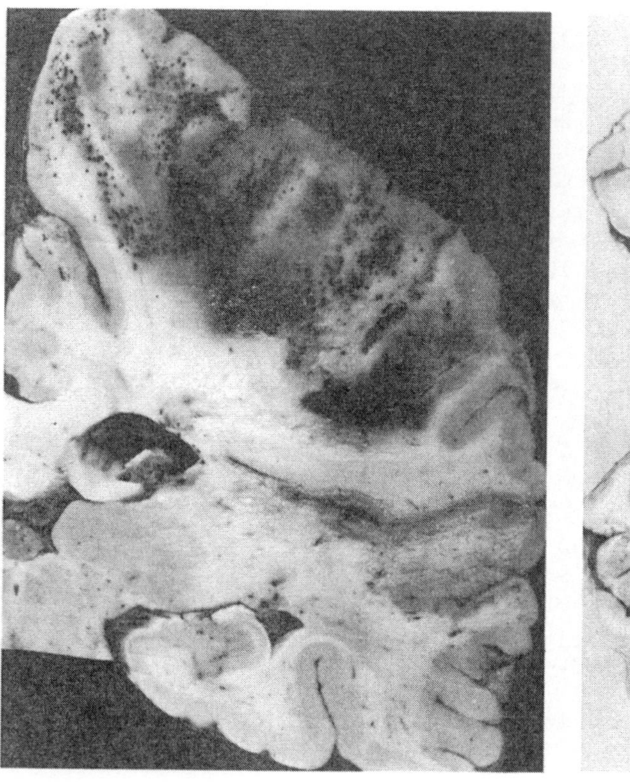

Fig. 125

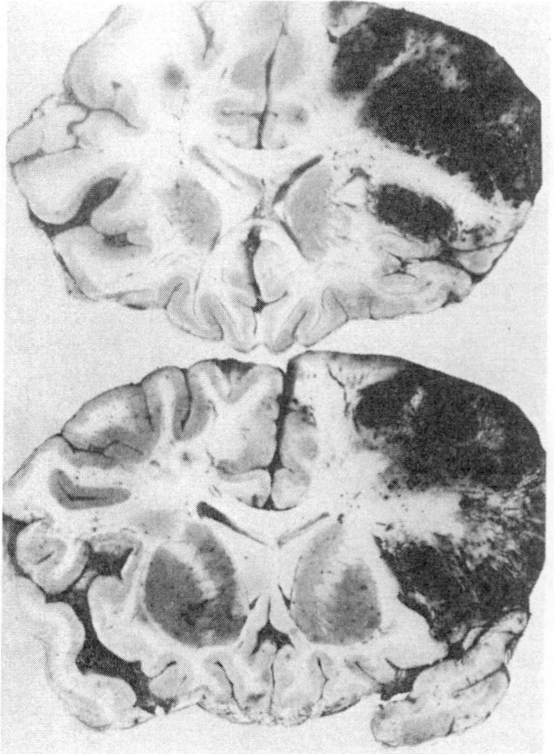

Fig. 126

Fig. 125. *Venous* infarct of the cerebral territories adjoining the sagittal sinus. This red-hemorrhagic infarct resembles only superficially the typical *arterial* infarcts. In contrast the main changes consisting of "perivenous" hemorrhages are situated predominantly in the white matter, less so in the cortex

Fig. 126. Red – hemorrhagic – infarct in the total cortical supply territory of the middle cerebral artery

However, 1) if the circulation stops completely ("ischemia") for long time, anemic necrosis always develops, but the marginal zones may in this case become hemorrhagic due to collateral supply (as in a renal infarct, for which Virchow was the first to demonstrate the effectiveness of collateral marginal circulation).

Occasionally, after a short period of severe ischemia, *collateral blood supply* may develop through the leptomeningeal or other arteries. If the parenchyma is irreparably damaged, the collateral supply is not able to reduce the area of the infarction. The typical result is a diapedetic hemorrhage into the border zone of a brain infarct (Fig. 144), e.g., again a "marginal" red infarction.

2) The probability of the development of an hemorrhagic infarct is large if some blood *near the critical level* of 15% of the normal circulation (see p. 125) is still circulating or the level of actual circulation undulates. There will be initial damage to the vascular endothelium, especially in the oxygen-deprived grey matter (which for this reason is highly capillarized). Diapedesis of erythrocytes will then occur.

3) *Intermittent decrease in circulation* may lead also to hemorrhagic infarcts, as is well known in neurosurgery, in the form of occipital infarcts following temporal hernias (or "tentorial pressure cones").

4) A short-lasting insufficient or arrested circulation may cause damage of the endothelium – but not necrosis – which furthers a diapedesis of erythrocytes into the impaired tissues after restoration of the circulation. A red infarct may ensue.

5) According to the literature, a red infarct is supposed to occur more frequently after embolism, when the embolus is splitting up. The anemic infarct more commonly follows thrombosis.

The concept of the Boston school (C.M.FISHER and ADAMS, 1951) seems plausible as one possible explanation of red infarction. However, the reverse conclusion *that every red infarct is embolic is certainly not legitimate.* Of their 373 cases of infarcts 123 had embolism, 89 a thrombosis and in 161 the cause was unknown. 66 of the infarcts were hemorrhagic.

The embolus often is supposed to be brittle and to split up thereby progressing further and further into the peripheral circulation. This has been actually proved by angiography for larger emboli (see Fig. 124, KAUTZKY, ZÜLCH et al., 1977).

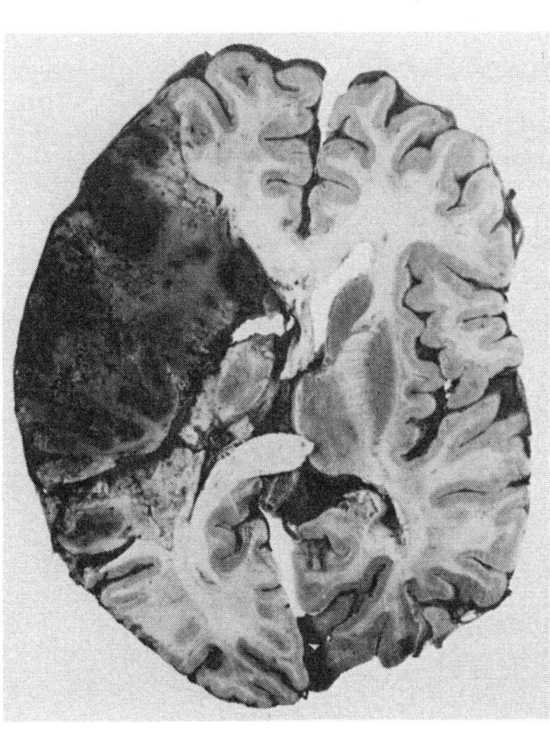

Fig. 127

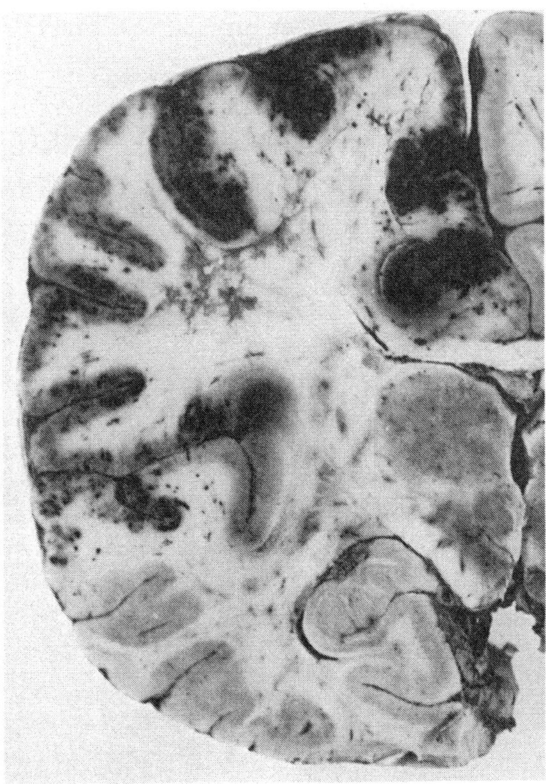

Fig. 128

Fig. 127. "Total" hemorrhagic infarction of the middle cerebral artery seen in a horizontal plane

Fig. 128. Large hemorrhagic infarct in the total supply of the anterior cerebral and the upper part of the middle cerebral supply territory

6) There is also a certain statistical relationship between the development of hemorrhagic infarcts and transient alternating crises of high blood pressure during which the infarcts occurred. This is a statistical correlation (BOTTON, 1955b) for which an actual pathogenesis is not clarified. It could be possible that true angiospastic insults occur after increase in blood pressure leading to short lasting insufficiencies (see p. 119). An interesting clue may be found in the paper of STRANDGAARD et al. (1976), who reported after abrupt experimental hypertension a hyperemia in half of their animals probably due to overstretching of the arteriolar walls.

If anticoagulant or fibrinolytic therapy is used, the marginal zone of erythrodiapedesis (red infarct) can be transformed into a massive hemorrhage (Fig. 118). This is shown in one of our cases where, similar to VIRCHOW's concept, the marginal zone of an infarct gave rise to a arterial rupture and mass hemorrhage.

In summarizing, a brain infarct may be hemorrhagic:

a) if there are cerebrovascular insufficiencies of an intermittent character,
b) if a vessel is occluded over a period close to the time limit of survival of the brain tissue and circulation is then reopened,
c) probably – although not yet fully proved – in any case of a cerebrovascular insufficiency near the quantitative limit of 15% of normal circulation,
d) if an embolus disintegrates and is again given free access to the circulation,
e) after hypertensive crisis where infarcts are (statistically!) more frequently "red",
f) in the marginal zones of an anemic ("white") infarct following establishment of collateral circulation.

It must be added that an infarct morphologically may be:

1) Totally hemorrhagic (Fig. 126–128)
2) Hemorrhagic in the margins (Fig. 144; see also p. 128)
3) In spots only of hemorrhagic appearance having a predilection for the cortex surrounding the bottom of a sulcus.

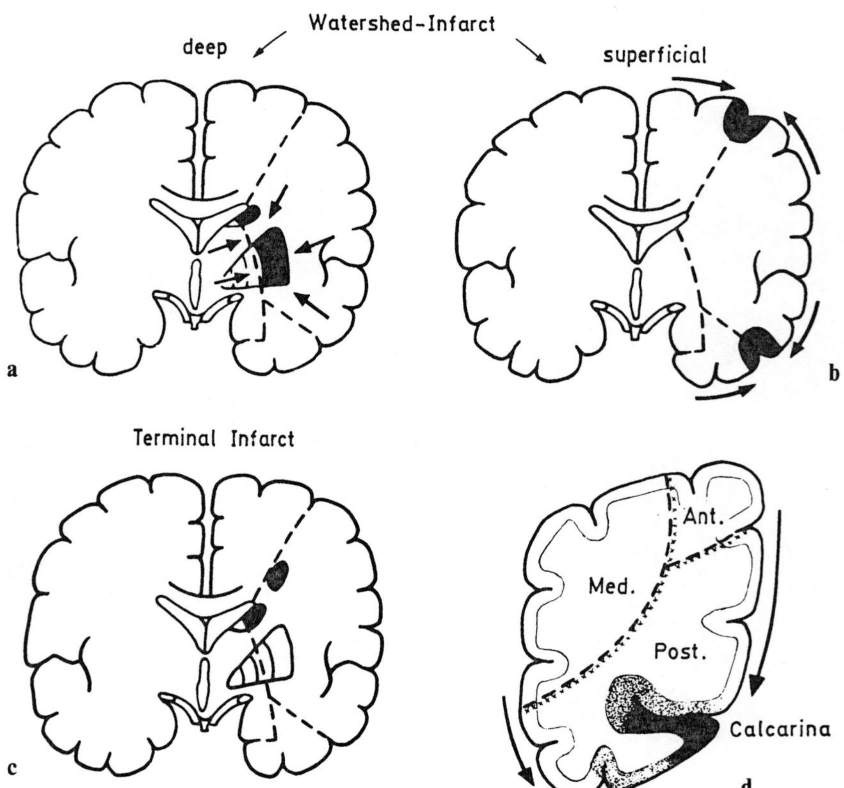

Fig. 129. a Deep borderline infarcts. **b** Superficial borderline infarcts. **c** Deep terminal infarcts. **d** Infarct in the center of the supply area of the posterior cerebral artery

8. Infarcts in the Carotid System

The carotid supply system has been the main subject of all infarct studies because of the perspicuous pattern of its vasculature and the excellent visibility in angiography (see the illuminating chapter in SALAMON, 1973) on the history of the cerebrovascular studies (see also SALAMON and HUANG, 1976). It has also been subject of many symposia (see GERAUD et al., 1973). Vascular surgery mainly deals with the extracranial part of the artery.

Carotid stenosis or thrombosis is one of the main causes of the "carotid syndrome" (ZÜLCH, 1973a; see also p. 68ff).

Our morphological studies of infarcts in the carotid system are based on an investigation of 664 cases of cerebrovascular disease with 700 subsequent infarcts (ZÜLCH and GESSAGA, 1972). The following infarcts may be regarded as typical (Figs. 129, 130) and their gross frequency is shown in Fig. 131.

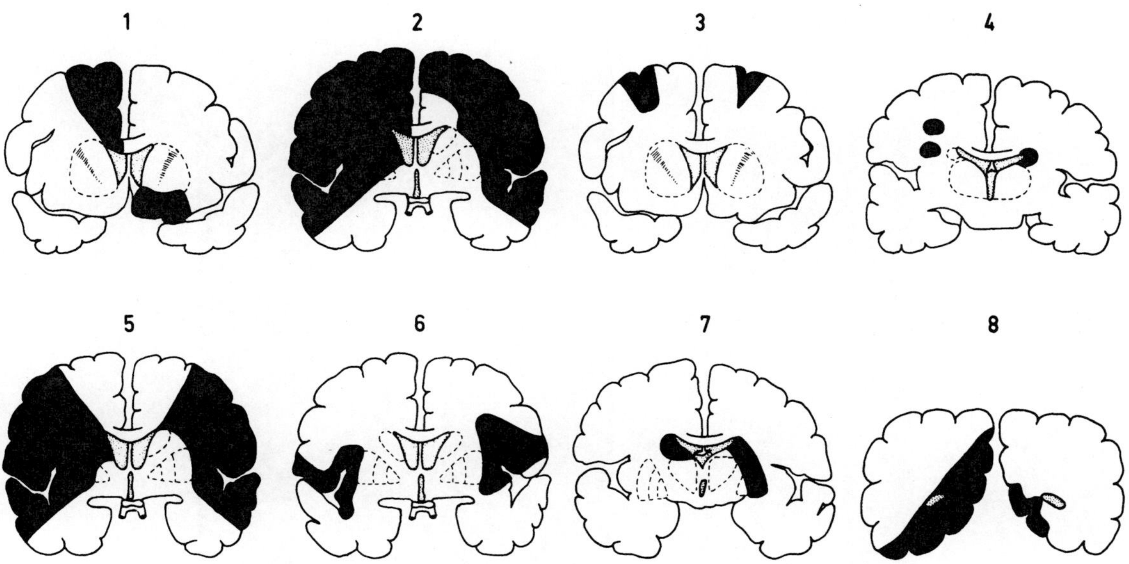

Fig. 130. The site and form of the common and typical supratentorial infarcts in 700 cases

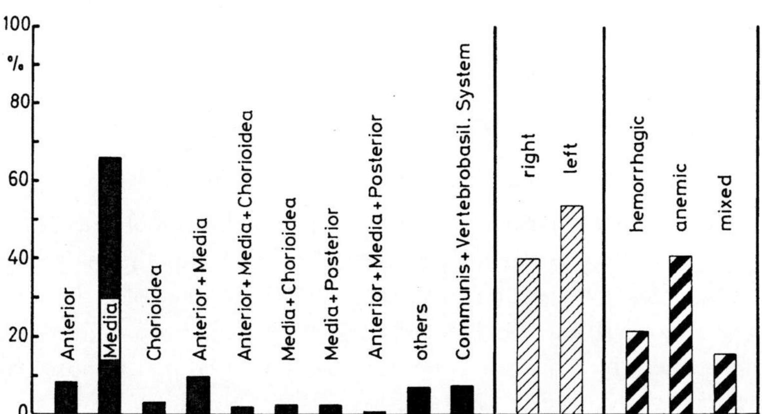

Fig. 131. Mean representation of cerebral arteries in the process of atherosclerotic and/or thrombotic occlusions; also percentage of "red" and "white" infarctions

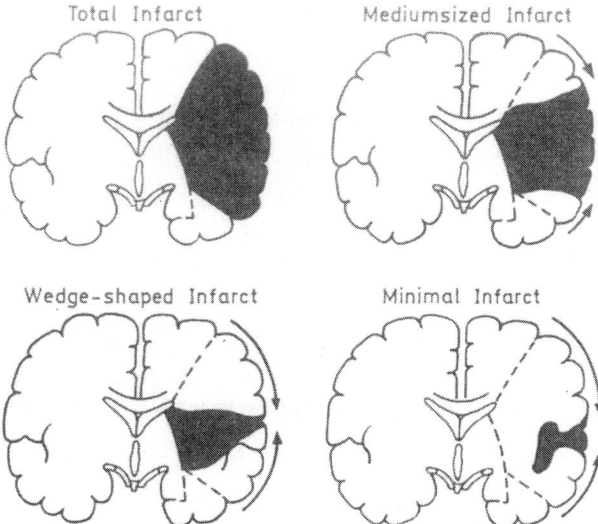

Fig. 132. Various types – e.g. sizes – of infarction in different hemodynamic patterns

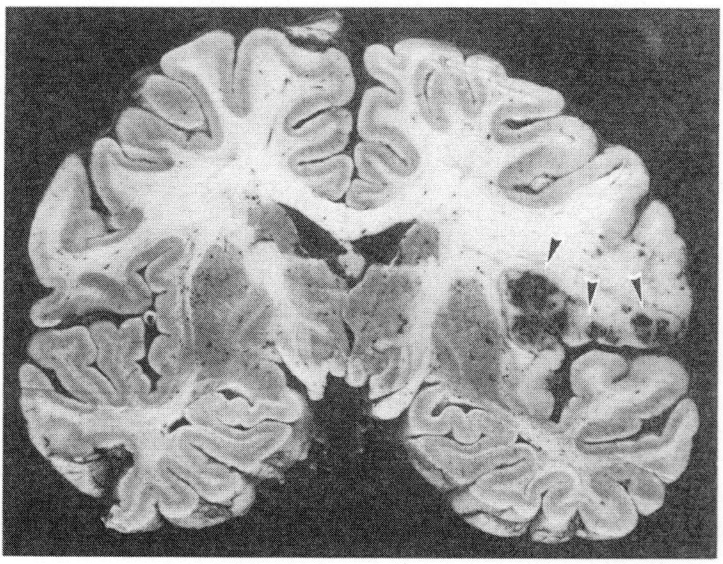

Fig. 133. Minimal infarct in the lower lip of the third frontal convolusion (Broca's area) and the upper insular cortex *(arrows)*. Hemodynamic interpretation see Fig. 139

a) Infarcts in the Middle Cerebral Artery Territory

α) Total or Subtotal Superficial Infarcts

They occur in the *superficial supply territory* of the middle cerebral artery, i.e. the cortical branches of the Sylvian vessels, usually after "distal" occlusion of the main trunk (Figs. 51, 68, 129a). Four different sizes may occur (Figs. 129a–d, 132), a) the total infarct, b) the medium sized, c) the wedge shaped (Figs. 129, 132–138) and d) the minimal infarct, depending on the supply of the outer zones which may be supported by meningeal anastomoses from the anterior and posterior cerebral arteries (see p. 13ff. and Fig. 137).

Of these, the "minimal" infarct can have two sites: either it occurs near the stump of the occluded middle cerebral artery or it corresponds to the infarct "in the center of a supply territory" (see Fig. 139); where the proximal parts are still partly supplied by the middle cerebral

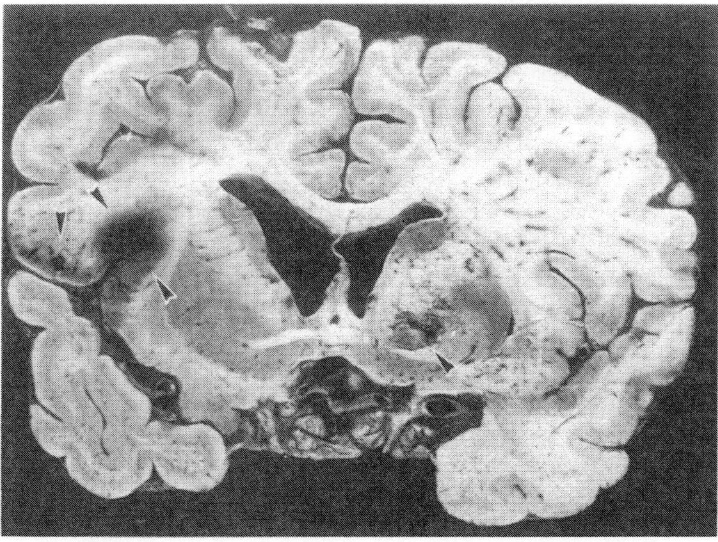

Fig. 134. Hemorrhagic infarct in the center of supply area of middle cerebral artery (Broca's territory). Infarction of the anterior choroidal artery on the contralateral side *(arrows)*

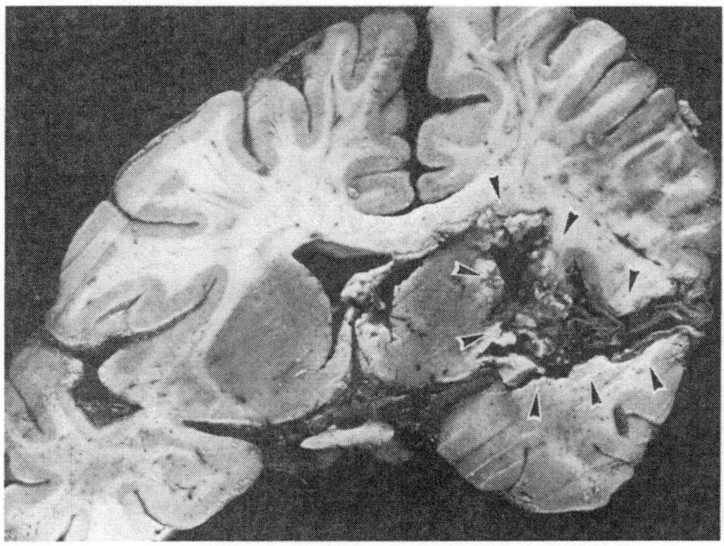

Fig. 135. Typical wedge shaped infarct (*arrows*; see Figs. 136 and 137)

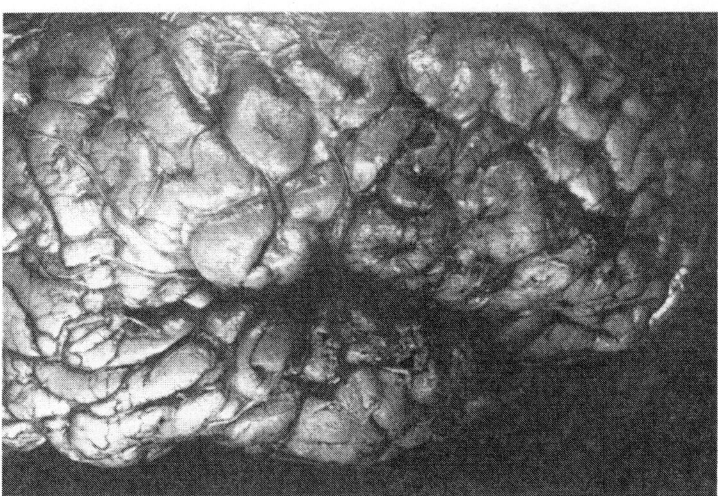

Fig. 136. Outer view on a wedge-shaped infarct (see Fig. 135). The hemodynamics are explained in Fig. 137

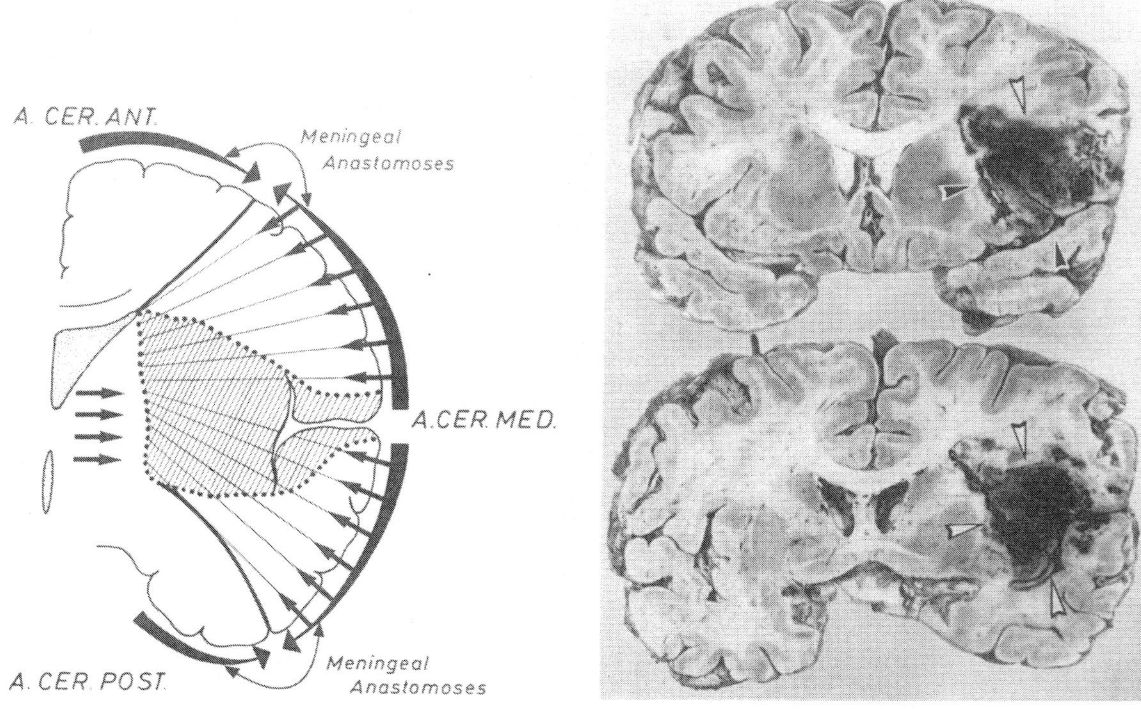

Fig. 137 Fig. 138

Fig. 137. Hemodynamic interpretation of "wedge" – form of infarct in the territory of middle cerebral artery

Fig. 138. Relatively fresh hemorrhagic wedge-shaped infarct of the middle (*arrows*) cerebral artery (see Figs. 135 and 136)

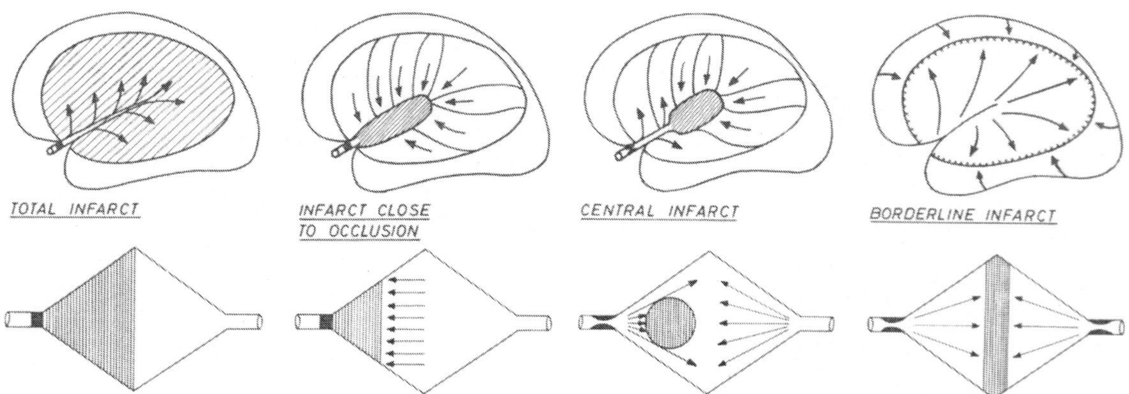

Fig. 139. Hemodynamic interpretation of various infarcts in the supply territory of the middle cerebral artery

artery itself since only a severe stenosis and not an occlusion is the cause of the cerebrovascular insufficiency while the lateral and distal zones are still adequately supplied through the neighboring meningeal anastomoses.

For a full understanding of the various types of middle cerebral artery infarction described below, we have to recall the predilection sites of occlusion or stenosis of the vessel (Fig. 51).

The different types of middle cerebral artery occlusion:

There are four different predilection sites for occlusion or stenosis (see Fig. 51) namely a) the "proximal" directly at the stump, the striatal vessels being uninvolved, b) the "intermediate" type where medial striatal arteries are included into the thrombosis, c) the "proximal complete"

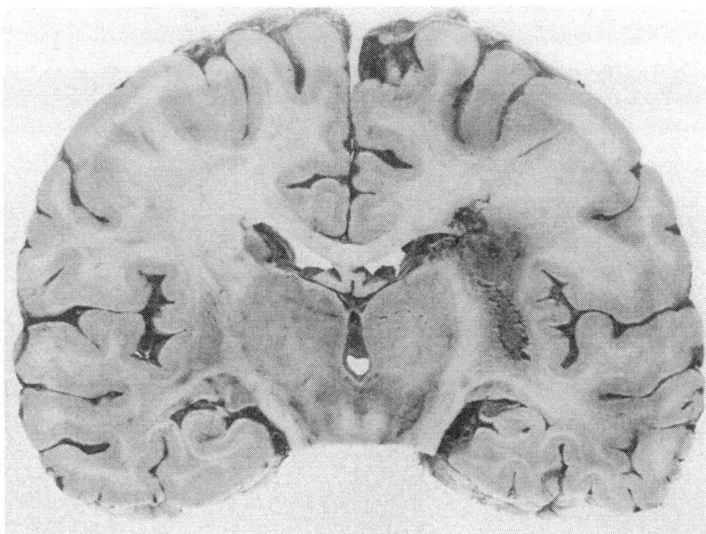

Fig. 140. For comparison with Figs. 142 and 144: Old hemorrhagic infarction after embolism to lenticulo-optic artery. Note the extension into the white matter (VAN DEN BERGH, 1969, Fig. 3-1)

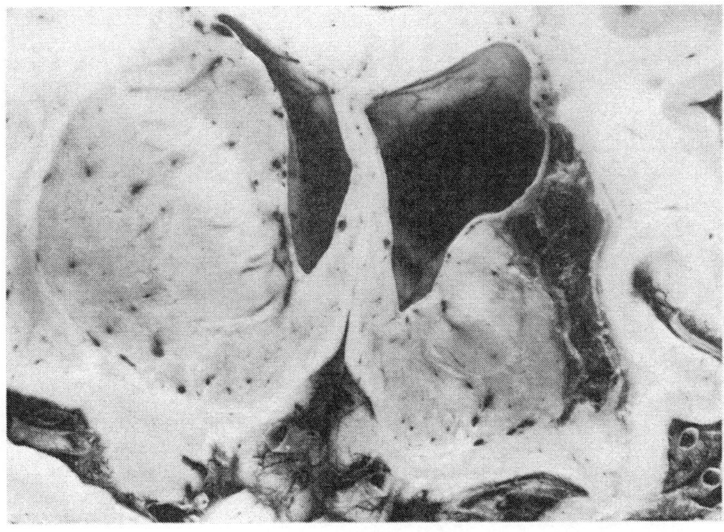

Fig. 141. Old cystic infarct in the territory of the lateral striatal arteries after thrombosis

occlusion where all the arteries to the basal ganglia are compromised, d) the "distal" type beyond the origin of the striatal vessels, e.g., shortly before the branching into the "candelabra". In the latter, clinically significant neurological symptoms and signs may completely disappear (GUIOT and LE BESNERAIS, 1955; SCHÜRMANN and DIETZ, 1961; LASCELLES and BARROWS, 1965; ZÜLCH et al., 1973).

β) Deep Middle Cerebral Artery Infarcts

The second main type of *middle cerebral artery total or subtotal infarction is seen when the deep branches of* the supply territory of the middle cerebral artery (medial and lateral, striatal vessels) are involved (lenticulo-striate and -optic arteries; Figs. 140, 141). This infarct follows type c) – as mentioned above – occlusion with involvement of the orifices of the basal ganglia arteries. The distal segments of the sylvian arteries (see type a) are supplied by retrograde

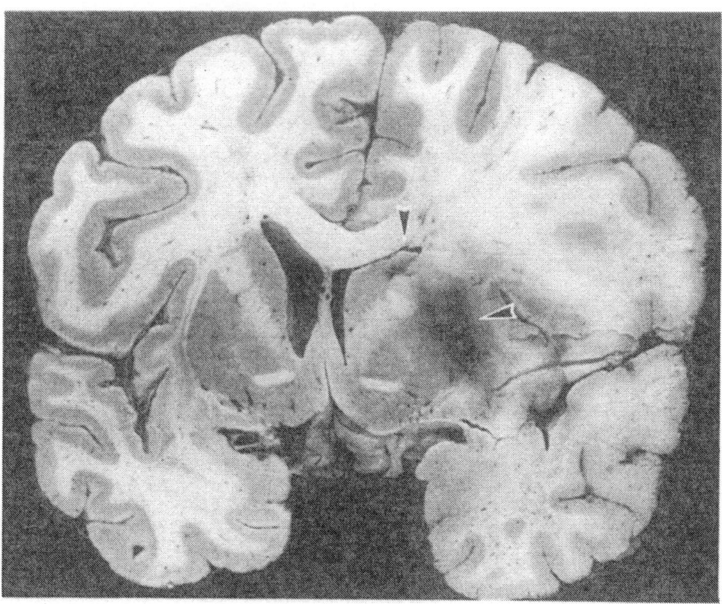

Fig. 142. Hemorrhagic infarction at the watershed between "deep" (Heubner's arising from anterior cerebral artery) and "superficial" (cortical, middle cerebral artery) supply. A white infarct in the middle cerebral artery is visible *(arrows)*. Massive shift

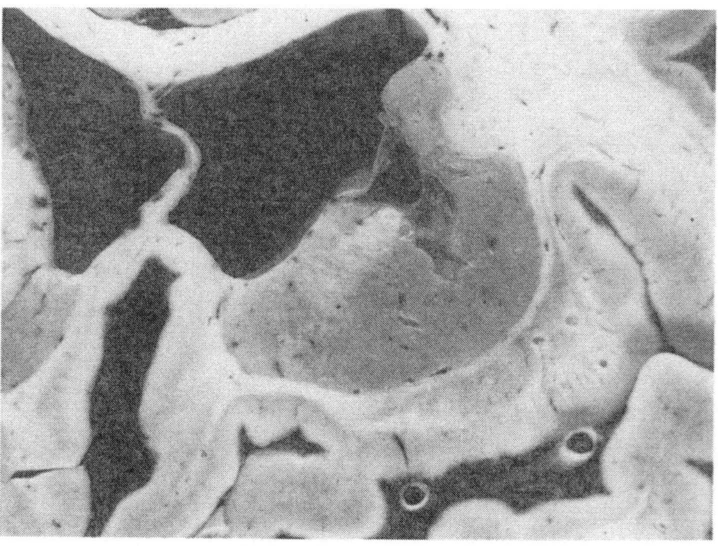

Fig. 143. Old partially cystic infarct in the watershed between deep and superficial blood supply (see Fig. 139)

flux via the meningeal anastomoses. These infarcts in the lenticulostriate/lenticulooptic territory may be partial and only situated in the most distal part of the supply zone near the caudate nucleus (Fig. 152), depending from the degree of compromise.

γ) Total Superficial and Deep Middle Cerebral Artery Infarcts

They comprise the infarcts described under α) and β) which develop when the occlusion of the middle cerebral artery is proximal and when hemodynamic or other causes, prevent retrograde anastomotic supply from the anterior and posterior cerebral arteries via the meningeal anastomoses or when the thrombosis has propagated far into the periphery of the artery (Fig. 130/5).

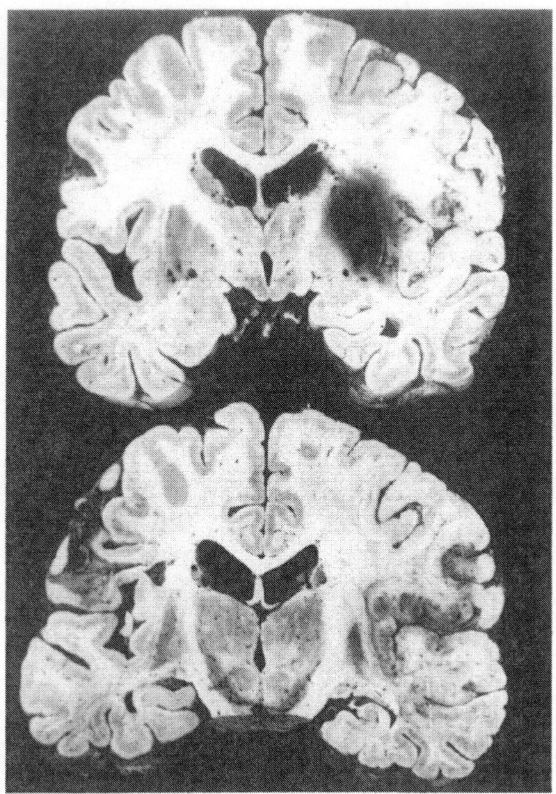

Fig. 144. Middle-sized infarction in the territory of the middle cerebral artery. It is hemorrhagic at the deep "watershed" and in the insular cortex (see Fig. 142)

δ) Deep "Frontier" ("Watershed") Infarcts

These infarcts developing between the superficial and deep branches of the middle cerebral artery (see Figs. 129, 142, 143) are observed in the caudate nucleus, putamen and internal capsule. They follow the hemodynamic law of the endangering of marginal zones between two supply territories. Most commonly they are hemorrhagic (Fig. 142) and not unfrequently part of a larger middle cerebral infarction (Figs. 120, 144).

ε) Superficial Semicircular "Frontier" ("Watershed") Infarcts

These infarcts occurs when a deficient circulation develops in the frontier ("watershed") area (Figs. 145–147) for instance between the middle cerebral artery on one side and the posterior and anterior arteries on the other. They may be old ("resembling the granular atrophy" in v. Winiwarter-Buerger's disease (see Fig. 183) but caused in this instance by diffuse atherosclerosis), or fresh and either uni- or bilateral (Figs. 145–147).

ζ) Superficial Frontier ("Watershed") Infarct in the "Dreiländereck"

These are (Figs. 148 and 149) caused by a deficient blood supply in the terminal zones of the three supply territories of the middle, the anterior and the posterior arteries. Again this infarct often may be old and occur either uni- or bilaterally (Fig. 149).

This type first seen by J.E. Meyer (1953, 1958), has been redescribed by us (Zülch, 1961b, Fig. 16) and was the subject of the EEG Colloque de Marseille à Cologne in 1964. At that meeting Naquet reported EEG changes in that particular region after experimental air embolism (Naquet et al., 1966) and Gastaut et al. (1971) discussed similar phenomena in man.

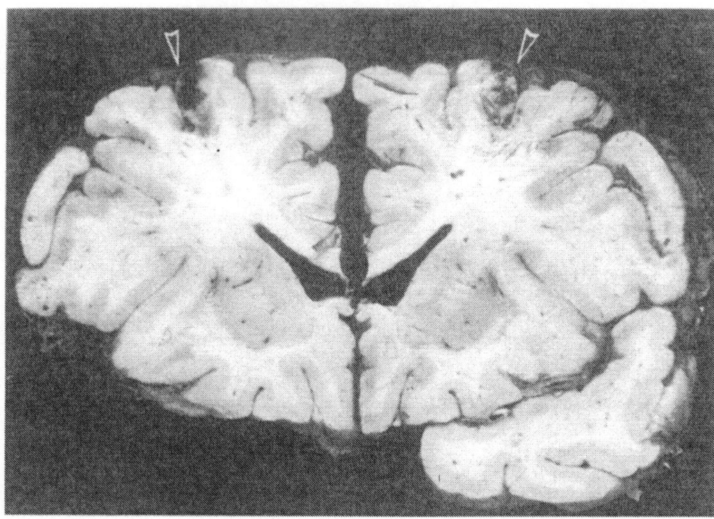

Fig. 145. Bilateral hemorrhagic infarction of the "border-line" between anterior and middle cerebral artery supply territory (*arrows*; see Fig. 146)

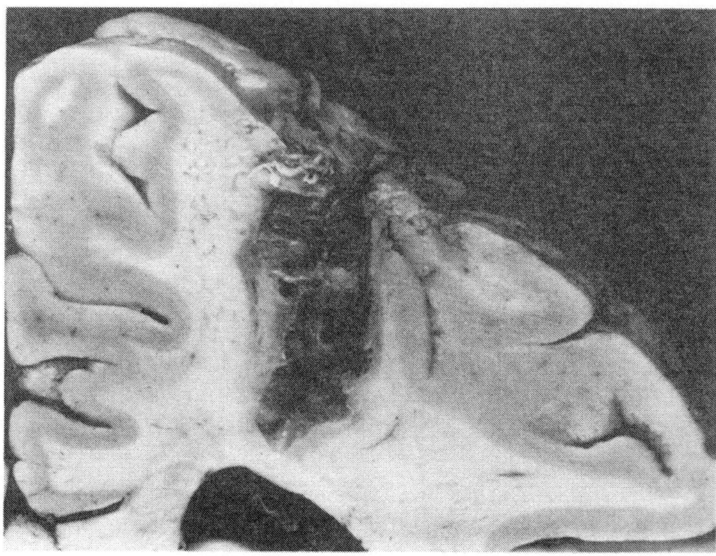

Fig. 146. Old deep cystic hemorrhagic infarct in the "border-line" between anterior and middle cerebral arteries supply territories (see Fig. 145)

η) Anterior Chorioidal Artery Infarcts

The infarct of the anterior chorioidal artery may be different in size and is usually observed in the posterior part of the internal capsule, part of the pallidum and thalamus, the corpus geniculatum and not infrequently also (Fig. 150) in the optic radiation lateral to the trigonum of the lateral ventricle (KLEIHUES, 1966b). Branches from the posterior chorioidal artery can act as collaterals.

The anterior chorioidal artery infarct has had a particular interest after surgical clamping (MORELLO and COOPER, 1955; COOPER, 1956). There are multifold variations in the origin of this artery, which comes from the internal carotid in 77% of cases. It may also originate from middle cerebral artery or posterior communicating artery (CARPENTER et al., 1954). Occlusions are not common (POPPI, 1928; ABBIE, 1933; HANSEN and PETERS, 1940; FURLANI, 1973). In older times syphilitic occlusions have been described (KOLISKO, 1891).

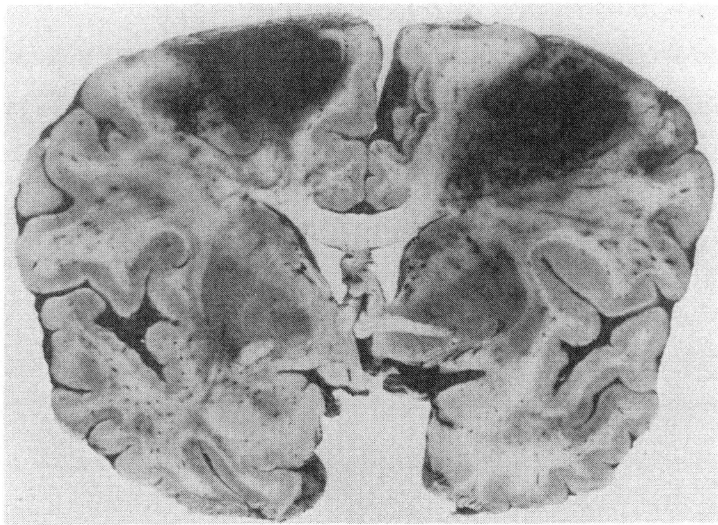

Fig. 147. Bilateral symmetrical border zone infarcts with hemorrhages between the supply areas of anterior and middle cerebral artery

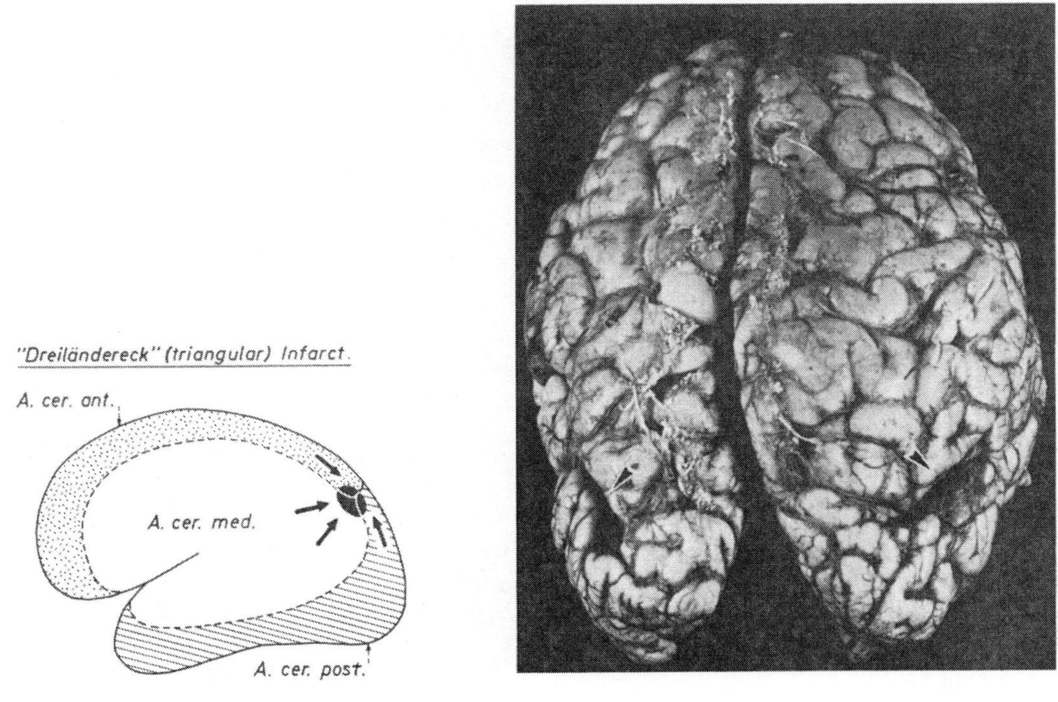

Fig. 148 **Fig. 149**

Fig. 148. Hemodynamic interpretation of the "Dreiländereck" infarct

Fig. 149. Deep crater-like old infarcts in the "Dreiländereck" (triangular) zone between anterior, posterior and middle cerebral arteries (*arrows*)

ϑ) *Terminal Infarcts*

Terminal infarcts between the superficial cortical and the deep branches of the middle cerebral arteries consists of two cysts in the centrum semiovale (Figs. 151, 152), and the terminal district of the lenticulo-striate and -optic arteries (Fig. 140) where they swing around the upper outer rim of the ventricle (see VAN DEN BERGH, 1961, 1969; VAN DEN BERGH and PLETS, 1970).

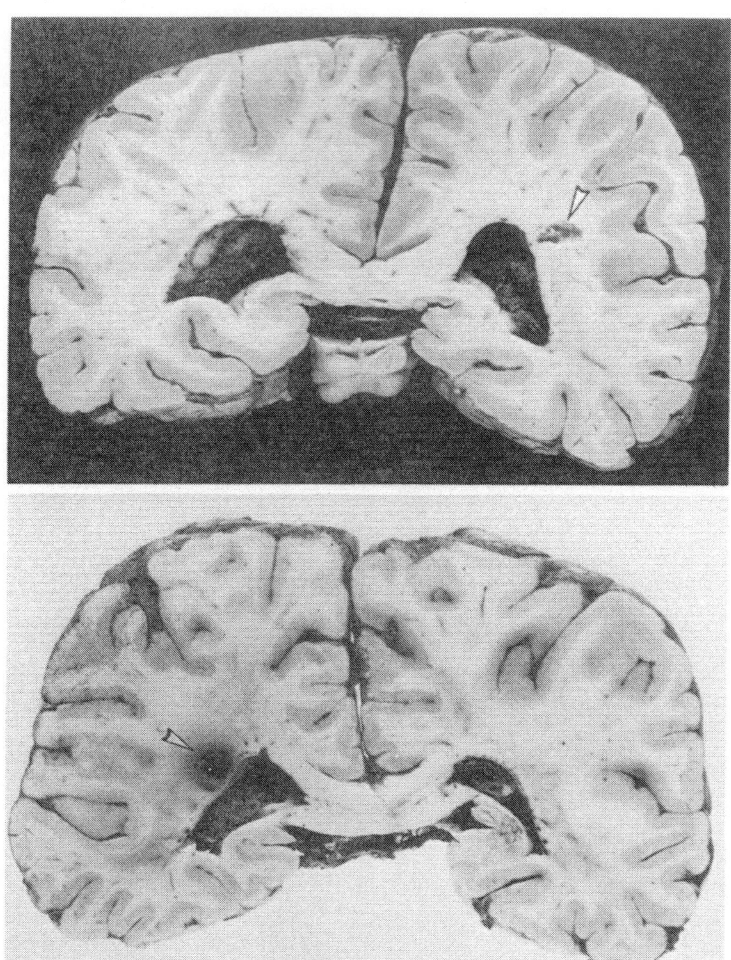

Fig. 150. Isolated infarcts in the optic radiation (terminal supply area of the anterior chorioidal artery; *above:* old and cystic; *below:* hemorrhagic in a case of fibrinolytic therapy

b) Infarcts of Anterior Cerebral Artery

The main causes are stenosis and occlusion with a predilection in the course around the corpus callosum (see pp. 42, 43, Figs. 46–49) caused by atherosclerotic plaques and also rarely by the thrombosis of an aneurysm of the anterior communicating artery with subsequent spasm. Strangulations in herniations under the falx cerebri have been described (ZÜLCH, 1963b; SOHN and LEVINE, 1972). Consequences of surgical clamping have been observed after DANDY (1930, 1946) and by many other neurosurgeons (FALCONER, 1958; MCCARTY and COOPER, 1951; GURDJIAN and WEBSTER, 1953) and neurologists (FOIX and HILLEMAND, 1925a; CRITCHLEY, 1930; ZÜLCH and KLEIHUES, 1967).

1. *Frontobasal – Heubner's – subtotal infarcts.* These subtotal (proximal) infarcts occur usually in the territory of the recurrent branch of HEUBNER (1872, see also Fig. 130/1), where it may be situated typically on the medial supraorbital convolutions and the adjacent more frontal parts of the basal ganglia (striatum). They are rare (see KAPLAN et al., 1954; KAPLAN, 1956; LAZORTHES et al., 1956; LAZORTHES, 1961; KRIBS and KLEIHUES, 1971).

2. *Total (proximal) infarcts.* The infarcts in the proximal part of the supply territory of the anterior cerebral artery (Fig. 153) are most commonly total and observed in the area as those of Heubner's artery, in the poles of the frontal lobe and the paramedian parts of the frontal and parietal lobes, including the corpus callosum up to the midline.

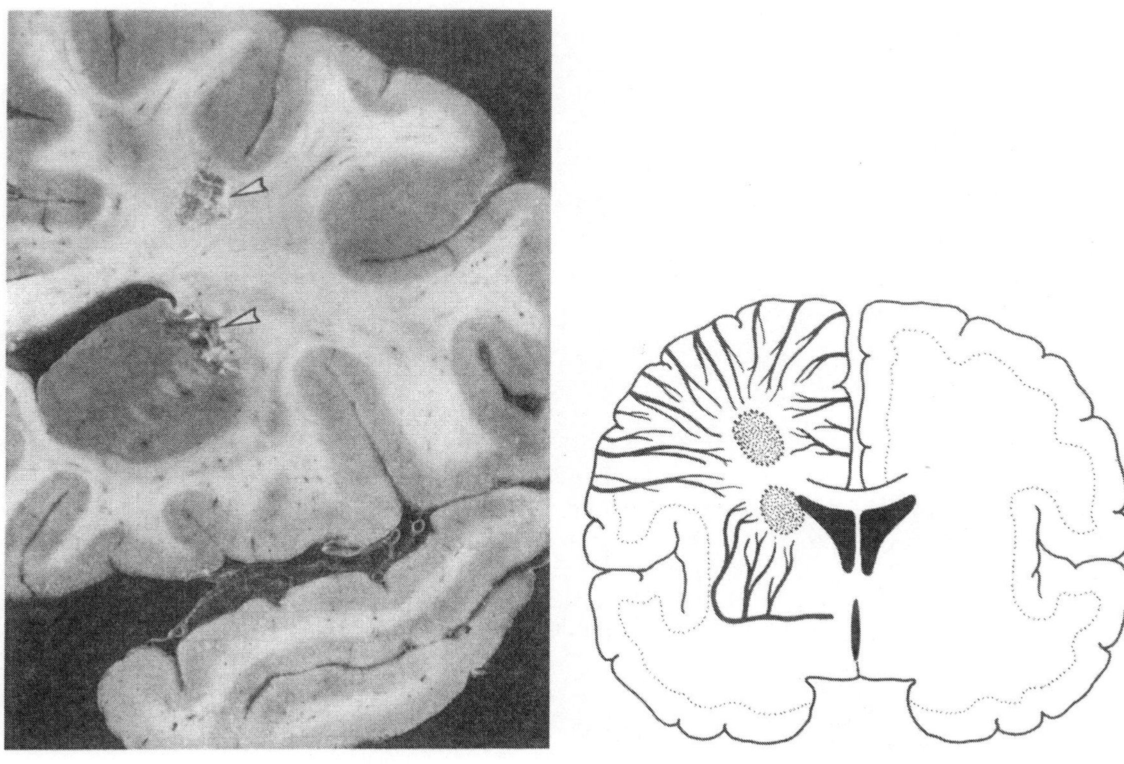

Fig. 151 Fig. 152

Fig. 151. Two softening cysts in typical location: 1. in centrum semiovale, 2. at outer surface of head of caudate nucleus and putamen. Cysts are results of infarcts caused by insufficient supply of terminal ramifications of cortical penetrating branches and of striolenticular artery (*arrows;* see Fig. 152)

Fig. 152. The hemodynamic interpretation of the infarcts of Fig. 151 as "terminal" infarcts

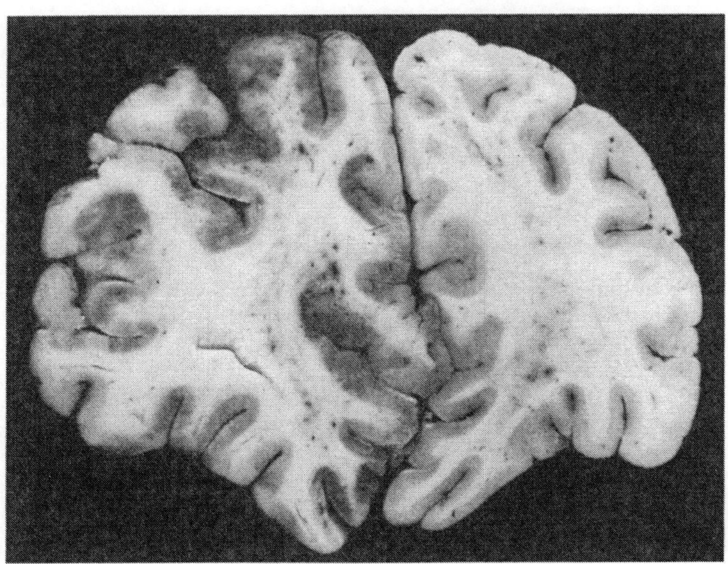

Fig. 153. Total, partly hemorrhagic total infarction of anterior frontal lobe (anterior cerebral artery)

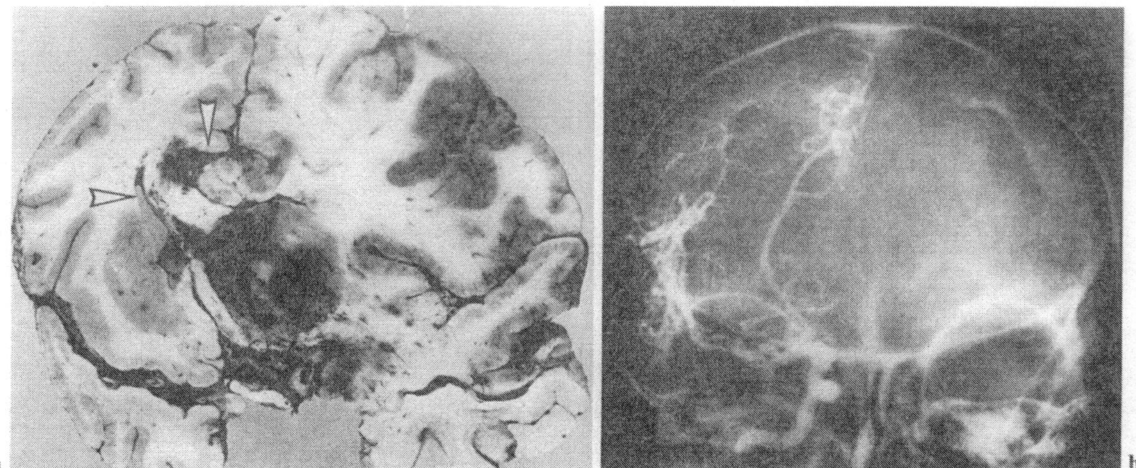

Fig. 154a and b. Extreme cerebral edema on the third day after an infarct in the territory of the anterior and middle cerebral arteries with marked mass shift towards the opposite side. **a** Brain section with a partly hemorrhagic infarct. **b** "Negative angiogram" of tissue displacements. Angiography was performed on the wrong side for the exclusion of a subdural hematoma because of the "wrong", homolateral neurological signs produced by pressure against the opposite tentorial edge (c.f. Fig. 24)

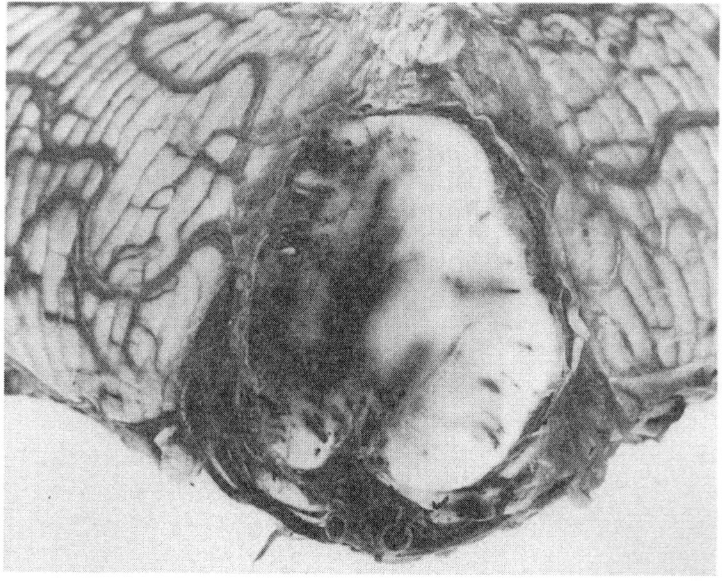

Fig. 155. Hemorrhagic compression of midbrain by large tentorial pressure cone following unusually large supratentorial infarction (c.f. Fig. 95)

They may become *subtotal* by a collateral action of the meningeal anastomoses from the middle cerebral artery; this, however, predisposes that the thrombotic occlusion is restricted to the anterior cerebral artery and spares the middle cerebral artery.

Furthermore transverse interhemispheric supracallosal arteries may be present sometimes (Fig. 14; see also ZÜLCH et al., 1964), acting in an "interhemispheric" collateral supply, and, finally and most commonly, the "epicallosal anastomosis" from the posterior to the anterior cerebral artery (FISCHER-BRÜGGE, 1949; Fig. 1) may preserve the corpus callosum and the region of the cingulate gyrus.

Infarcts of the anterior cerebral arteries may also be *bilateral* when they are usually preferentially situated in the frontal segment of the supply territory. They are then often spotty (Fig. 154).

Combined infarcts of the *anterior and middle cerebral arteries* occur in occlusion of the internal carotid artery and can consist of infarcts of any size: *total* (Fig. 128) or *minimal*. Total infarcts may introduce a catastrophic situation (see Fig. 154) whereby shift to the opposite site produces a peduncular (KERNOHAN's) notch and a homolateral symptomatology may ensue (Fig. 155).

c) Infarcts of the Posterior Cerebral Artery

Infarcts in this area have at least to be mentioned in this chapter on the carotid supply areas since in around 20% of cases, the posterior cerebral artery originates from the carotid system (so-called "embryonic type"; see also MONIZ, 1940; ALPERS et al., 1959); such infarcts are described more fully on p. 154ff. and Figs. 168–171.

9. Carotid Stenosis or Occlusion as Cause of Insufficiency and Infarctions

The internal carotid artery supplies two (three) large territories, i.e. anterior and middle, and in 20% also the posterior cerebral arteries. One may then speak of a ("posterior") "trifurcation" of that artery. Since not infrequently the anterior cerebral artery of the contralateral side is also mainly irrigated in these cases we can speak of an "anterior" trifurcation. The efficacy of the anterior communicating artery may be tested in cases where the anterior cerebral artery is not visualised in the carotid angiogram ("cross filling" of the anterior after compression of carotid). Because of its many extra- and intracranial anastomoses an involvement of the internal carotid may not introduce any clinical or morphological symptoms (see HULTQVIST, 1942, for autopsy; ZÜLCH and HERBERG, 1949; PETERSON et al., 1960; MARSHALL, 1966 and ZÜLCH, 1973a for clinical observations).

These authors have emphasized that in acute ligations of the carotid, generally one third of patients will have very severe symptoms, one third symptoms of middle degree and one third minor or no symptoms at all.

The consequences of carotid stenosis, or occlusion depend on the various, very extensive possibilities of collateral supply, various anastomoses (see pp. 8, 11 and Figs. 5–7 and 14) e.g. they may be lacking or they may lead to any type of cerebrovascular insufficiency and infarction in the supply territory. This depends largely on the hemodynamic situation. It also depends naturally on the site of involvement, e.g. in the neck, in the siphon etc. We will therefore enumerate the *correlations between infarction and changes within the carotid system* (BLADIN, 1964; LHERMITTE et al., 1966; CASTAIGNE et al., 1970; GAUTIER et al., 1975; ZÜLCH, 1973a).

Acute or subacute atherosclerotic occlusion of one carotid artery in the cervical segment or siphon may be the most frequent cause of "carotid infarction".

Occlusion may be:

a) *Embolic* (merely);
b) *Thrombotic* (primary) (see p. 67ff.) or atherosclerotic stenosis plus thrombosis, probably the most frequent event.
c) *Atherosclerotic* (merely; see DEI POLI and ZUCHA, 1940; HULTQVIST, 1942; YATES and HUTCHINSON, 1961; SCHWARTZ and MITCHELL, 1961; CASTAIGNE et al., 1970; ZÜLCH, 1961a, 1973a); it may be not infrequent.
d) *Hemodynamic* by coiling or kinking (see pp. 55, 56; WEIBEL and FIELDS, 1965; DESAI and TOOLE, 1975) where in patients under 50 years around 3%–6% are unilateral; tortuosity may be of lesser importance;
e) *Traumatic*: blunt trauma may play a role (contusion because of proximity of a gunshot wound, choking, blow in motorcycle accident or in boxing (see also ZÜLCH and HERBERG, 1949;

VIGOUROUX and LAVILLE, 1962, with extensive literature: from a total of 34 cases, 26 cases of acute thromboses localized in the neck region and the remainder after skull fracture in the intracranial portion, usually at the siphon). The cavernous sinus fistula may follow atherosclerosis or trauma. Dissecting aneurysms (see p. 24) are more common at the middle cerebral artery (see Fig. 24; and also SORGO, 1939; C.M. FISHER, 1954).

f) *Inflammatory*: earlier (as well as atherosclerosis) it was a main factor in the development of occlusion of the carotid artery.

g) For the significance of *fibromuscular hyperplasia* see RINALDI et al., 1976; ERICSON and METTINGER, 1977; see also p. 74).

h) Iatrogenic (surgical) occlusion.

Clinical syndrome. Clinical syndromes can be very characteristic even for a detailed diagnosis, e.g. for instance for "stenosis of the carotid at the neck", when transient ischemic attacks start with, or alternate with ipsilateral amaurosis fugax. The latter symptom is commonly interpreted as being due to microemboli from an ulcerated carotid plaque (C.M. FISHER, 1959, 1961; R. RUSSELL, 1971) but also it may be hemodynamic (ZÜLCH, 1967, 1979).

A differential diagnosis of the carotid versus the vertebrobasilar syndrome is given in the following table.

Differential diagnosis between the syndrome of the

	Carotid	Basilar
Amaurosis fugax		
monocular	frequent	never
binocular	very infrequent	frequent
Hemianopsia	uncommon	frequent
Diplopia	never	frequent
Alternat. right/left-sided paresis	infrequent	more frequent
Paralysis upper extremities	pronounced distally	pronounced proximally
Perioral paresthesia	never	not infrequent
Dissociated sensations	never	occasional (Wallenberg-S.)
Dysarthria	never	frequent
Aphasia	very frequent	never
Nystagmus	never	not infrequent
Persistent vomiting	infrequent	frequent
Neck stiffness and pain	never	not infrequent

We will not further enumerate in detail (see ZÜLCH, 1973a) the variety of motor sensory, or neuropsychologic syndromes associated with carotid stenosis or occlusion. Only the fact has to be noted that they may begin – paradoxically with a paresis of the leg instead of arm.

However, there exists, albeit rarely, a group of patients with "pure sensory stroke involving face, arm and leg", as described by C.M. FISHER (1965b) which we have also observed several times. We agree with FISHER's concept that a thalamic vascular lesion (hypertension with hyalinosis and lacunae? atherosclerosis?) causes these symptoms in the form of sensory defects, which can also be induced by vertebrobasilar insufficiency. Also "pure motor" hemipareses or hemiplegias may be due to capsular lesions as well as to medial pontine ("basis pontis") infarcts as C.M. FISHER et al. (1965b) described; this concept again corresponds to our own observations. We have, however, made the special observation that mediobasal pontine infarcts lead to a "paradox" syndrome of purely motor hemiparesis, the pareses being more pronounced in the proximal muscles (ZÜLCH, 1975c, page 35 and Fig. 1), whereas isolated finger movement is preserved.

Auscultation of the cervical carotid arteries led in 57% of cases to the detection of a carotid stenosis in the neck by atherosclerotic plaques and also in the vertebral arteries in 40% (GILROY and MEYER, 1962). There are, however, many false positive and negative findings. In a normal general population bruits occur only in 1%, but in up to 20% in children.

A bruit has been heard in up to 60% (80/132) of cases with carotid artery stenoses and in more than 75% (60/84) of cases when stenoses were more than 75% of the lumen (GAUTIER et al., 1975). There is a general consensus that a bruit in the neck does not necessarily indicate an extracranial stenosis, which has to be operated (McDOWELL and EJRUP, 1966).

The interest in intracranial stenoses at the siphon (THOMSON, 1963; SILVERSTEIN and HOLLIN, 1963; see also KAUTZKY, ZÜLCH et al., 1976; Fig. 100–103) arose with the introduction of the transossal anastomoses (temporal superficial artery implanted into large branch of middle cerebral artery).

10. Transient Ischemic Attacks (TIAs)

The TIAs (see pp. 122, 124) are most frequently observed in stenoses of the carotid artery in the neck. In a fifteen year study of the community of Rochester, Minnesota (population increase from 32,600 to 52,629) altogether 777 persons had a first episode of cerebral infarction, from whom 73 (around 9%) previously had TIAs (WHISNANT et al., 1973). TIAs occurred in 1976 with a frequency of 1.24% in Zagreb/Yugoslavia and similarly in Split (FERKOVIC et al., 1977).

Whereas the statistical correlation between carotid stenoses and TIAs is high, fibromuscular dysplasia (see p. 74) or a "narrow carotid artery" triggered TIAs in only 4 out of 48 cases (MILLIKAN, 1976).

70 (8,2%) patients of our series of 850 patients were found to have TIAs of which, however, only 50 (5.9%) of the total series had their final stroke in the same vascular territory in which presumably the TIA occurred. Regarding the neurological syndromes after stroke 30 (60%) came from the carotid, 20 (40%) from the vertebrobasilar territory. In 17 (34%) of the investigated patients no vascular occlusion was found. In 8 (16%) the occlusion was intra-, in 7 (14%) extracranial, in one (2%) combined intra- and extracranial and in one (2%) there were multiple occlusions. Furthermore in the 34 patients with angiography only 7 cases showed marked stenosis of a major vessel, whereas 16 patients had various other changes, particularly marked atherosclerosis.

11. Transient Monocular Blindness – Amaurosis Fugax

After SIEGRIST in 1900 had described the dangers for the eye and brain of ligation of the carotid artery, C.M. FISHER in 1952 turned his attention to a syndrome of transient monocular blindness as a precursor of subsequent hemiplegia or emphasized that it might be associated with it. At that time the concept that vasospasm or vasoconstriction had to be incriminated, was still discussed.

As a proof of this statement the following data are presented: in the series of MARSHALL and MEADOWS (1968) of 27 patients with amaurosis fugax in whom angiography had been performed, 16 had stenosis or occlusion of the carotid artery.

Tragically this transient symptom can become permanent when in rare cases of atherosclerotic occlusion of the internal carotid artery ipsilateral blindness may ensue due to progression of the thrombosis into the retinal artery whilst collaterals fail to be formed (SUGAR et al., 1950).

The prognosis in carotid syndromes depends on the kind and extent of the disturbance of circulation or the ensuing infarct (ZÜLCH, 1961b, 1970). It has been subject of recent studies (GRILLO and PATTERSON, 1975; WALTIMO et al., 1976).

The following conclusions can be drawn from our own observations (HENSCH, 1979). The mortality is increased when the collateral supply is poor. Diabetes and left heart hypertrophy induce a poor prognosis. Likewise EKG changes and hypertension augment the mortality to 50%.

12. Infarcts in the Vertebrobasilar System

The clinical syndrome of "vertebro-basilar insufficiency" (MILLIKAN and SIEKERT, 1955) is derived from the description of a large series of morphologically controlled (SOLBERG, 1962) clinical descriptions, which have been recently summarized in a brief monograph by C. LOEB and J.S. MEYER (1965). Vertebral or basilar thrombosis or stenosis was usually the cause of this insufficiency (for the most important papers see HAYEM, 1868; EISENLOHR, 1879; LEYDEN, 1882; KUBIK and ADAMS, 1946; BIEMOND, 1951; DENNY-BROWN, 1953; CRAVIOTO, 1958; FISHER et al., 1961); mechanical involvement by hyperextension (OKAWARA and NIBBELINK, 1974), head turning (JANEWAY et al., 1966) or impression by the megadolichobasilar artery have also been reported to occur (ESCHBACH and ZÜLCH, 1969, Fig. 2a, b). Cerebrovascular insufficiency may be caused by mechanical factors, for instance by the osteochondrotic rims at the uncovertebrate joints (SHEEHAN et al., 1960; ZÜLCH, 1970, Fig. 19) or even basilar impression (JANEWAY et al., 1966).

Traumatic vascular lesions are rarer with the vertebral artery although they may be associated with fracture-luxations. Even thromboses following chiropractic therapy have been described (PRATT-THOMAS and BERGER, 1947; KUNKLE et al., 1952; FORD and CLARK, 1956; "hind-brain stroke" after trauma to the vertebral artery: FRASER and ZIMBLER, 1975).

The morphological substratum of this vertebro-basilar insufficiency syndrome as the typical area of ischemia has not yet been sufficiently defined and cited, although one recognises certain stereotyped patterns in the cases described in the literature and correspondingly from our own observations. It is for instance proved by our own observation that in one sided vertebral thrombosis 7 different levels may be compromised according to the "last field" concept (Figs. 139, 156), which may explain the "variegated" picture of the vertebrobasilar syndrome.

The vertebrobasilar system somewhat lacks the classical detailed work that has been carried out for the cerebral arteries stemming from the carotid by the French and German classics (references see STEPHENS and STILWELL, 1969), and this is further tempered by the fact that angiographic control or additional information is almost lacking in this region owing to its small nutritional vessels.

Moreover, until very recently even the excellent morphological descriptions of the vasculature, which now are at hand, were not available (STEPHENS and STILWELL, 1969; SALAMON, 1973). Therefore for the bulbar region the discrepancies in the literature concerning the actual supply territories of the arteries are particularly distressing (DURET, 1873; STOPFORD, 1915; FOIX and HILLEMAND, 1925a, b; LAZORTHES et al., 1958; LAZORTHES, 1961; GILLILAN, 1964; SALAMON, 1971; SALAMON and HUANG, 1976; HELMS, 1978). Disregarding this, we point to the dominance of descriptions of the dorsolateral infarcts in the medulla oblongata (Wallenberg's syndrome) in all the series described in the literature.

Basal necroses in the pyramids, for instance, are a rarity (here we have observed only one little grain-like cyst in our extensive collection of vascular cases), this may be due to the additional supply to this region by the anterior spinal artery.

a) Dorsolateral Infarcts of the Medulla (Posterior Inferior Cerebellar Arteries – Wallenberg's Arteries)

The typical infarct (Fig. 157) may involve the sector of the medulla oblongata defined basally by the upper border of the inferior olive and dorsally by a line somewhere below the fourth ventricles or it may even reach the ventricular floor itself.

This typical infarct, thought to be the substratum of the "Wallenberg"-syndrome occurred only rarely in our autopsy series of vertebro-basilar artery thrombosis (METZINGER and ZÜLCH, 1971), although C.M. FISHER et al. (1961) were able to describe 16 cases from the Massachusetts General Hospital series, all in cases of vertebral artery thrombosis (see also BAKER, 1961). Also

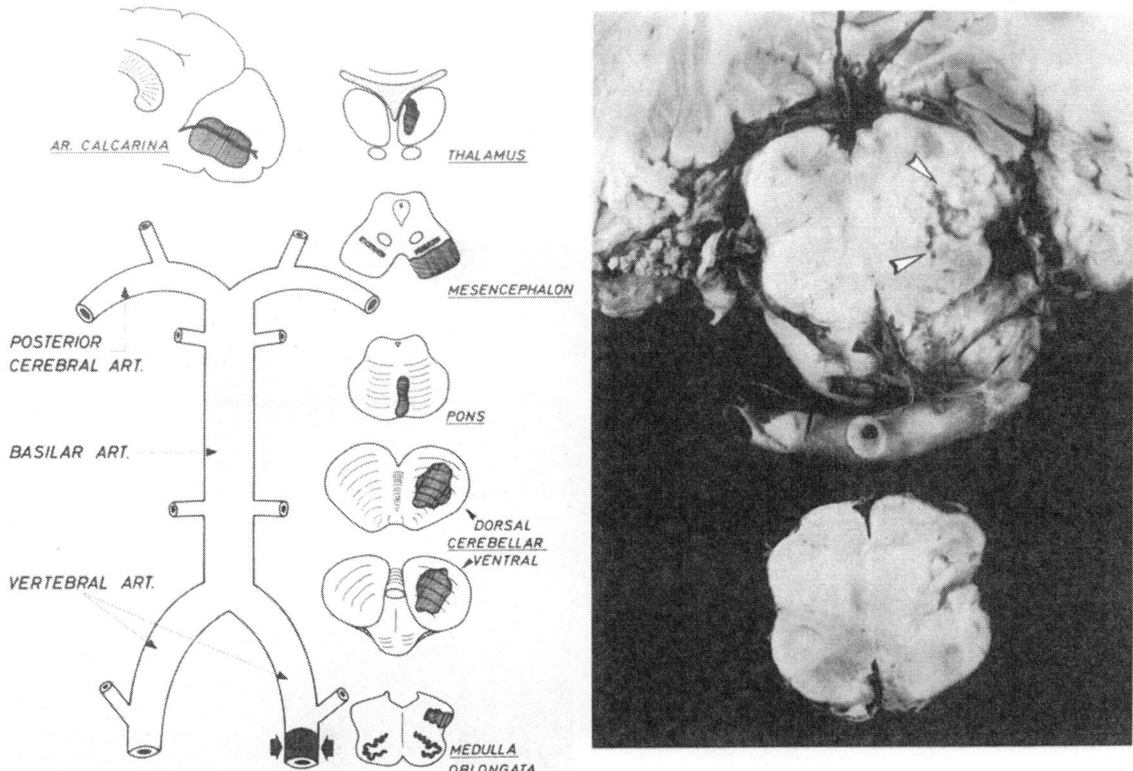

Fig. 156

Fig. 157

Fig. 156. Schematic drawing to show 7 different levels of infarction in case of occlusion of one vertebral artery

Fig. 157. Typical dorso-lateral infarct of the medulla oblongata *(arrows)* usually the cause of Wallenberg's syndrome

Krayenbühl and Yasargil (1957, 1965) correctly emphasized the fact that this infarct may be caused by various vascular lesions arising from the variability of the arterial pattern of this region, because a typical posterior inferior cerebellar artery branching from the vertebral artery is not always seen. In fact, sometimes the posterior cerebellar artery may originate from the basilar artery and it can also arise, as we have observed from our own dissections, as two separate branches (medullary and cerebellar). Also branches of the vertebral or basilar arteries may contribute to the vascular supply of this area (Stephens and Stilwell, 1969).

Variations in size of this infarct are probably due to the differences in the efficiency of meningeal anastomoses between the supplying cerebellar arteries, as shown in Fig. 11 of Loeb and Meyer (1965).

b) Paramedian Pontine Infarcts (Paramedian Pontine Arteries)

In our series this *most frequent infarct* was located in the paramedian segment of the pons (Figs. 158, 159). This infarct was either "total" or "incomplete", and then either more basally or dorsally situated, the other parts of the supply territory being spared, or the infarct was narrower than the whole supply zone. Sometimes it was bilateral and rarely combined with other pontine infarcts (Fig. 160).

Usually the infarct was caused by a basilar artery thrombosis or was due to a local stenosing atherosclerosis of a paramedian pontine artery. In some cases, the cause could not be clarified (for detailed literature see Loeb and J.S. Meyer, 1965, their Table 5, p. 86).

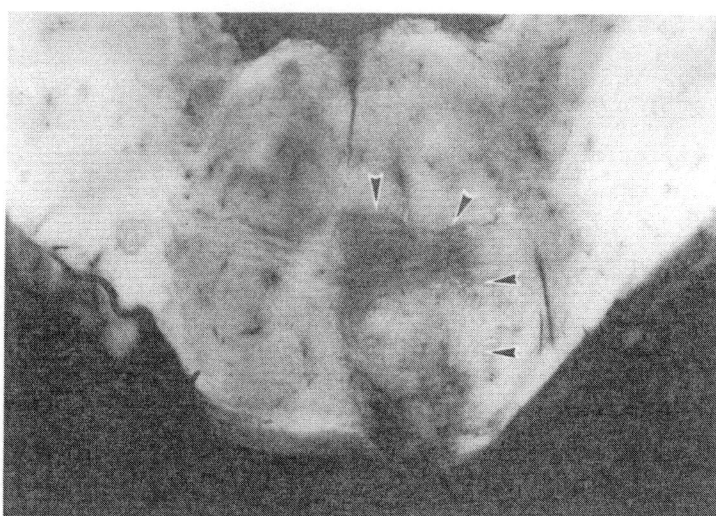

Fig. 158. The most common type is the unilateral "paramedian" infarct of the pons wich is here hemorrhagic at the base *(arrows)*

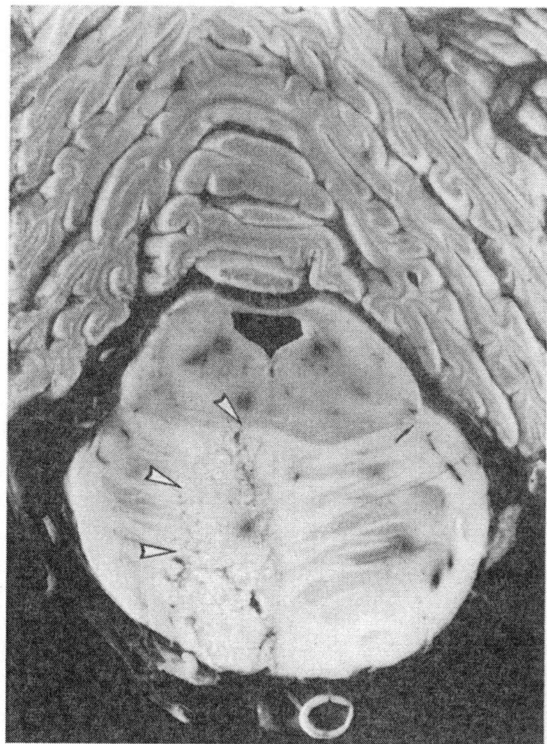

Fig. 159. Unilateral "paramedian" infarct of the pons *(arrows)*

Apparently there are very different hemodynamic patterns which lead to paramedian pontine infarcts. They may depend on the peripontine network of "meningeal anastomoses" although there is very sparse information about this particular anastomotic system.

Clinically, the paramedian pontine infarct is particularly important in the differential diagnosis of the supratentorial (cortical or capsular) hemisyndromes. For instance, ZÜLCH (1967, 1975c, Fig. 1) pointed to the fact that since paramedian pontine infarcts are the most common, the pontine motor hemisyndromes are typically characterised by "proximal" pareses or paralyses,

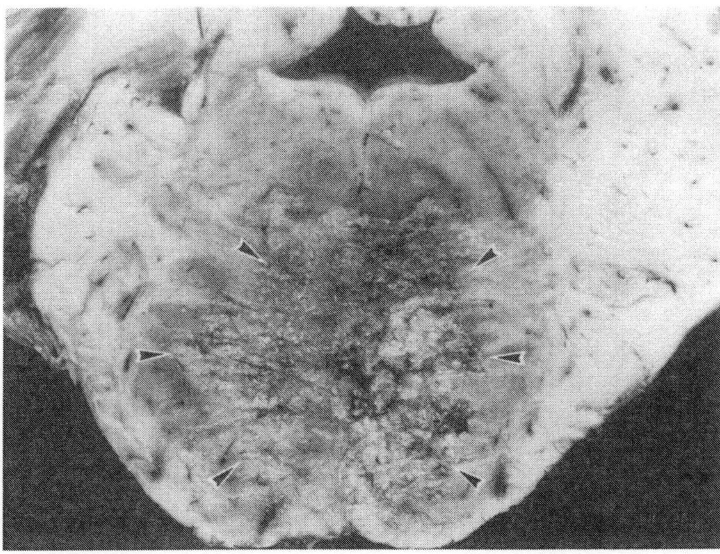

Fig. 160. Bilateral total paramedian infarction of the pons *(arrows)*

the distal extremities being excluded or less severely affected (necessary to test isolated movements of the fingers or toes!).

This is probably due to a dissociation of the pyramidal fibers in the pons, where the bundles for the proximal and distal muscles of the extremities must have different locations, the proximals being situated more medially, the distal ones more laterally. This corresponds to the general pattern of distribution of pyramidal fibers and nuclei. For instance, in the spinal segments, the groups of anterior horn cells for proximal muscles are "centrally", and those for distal muscles "peripherally" located (experiences with acute poliomyelitis!).

c) Laterobasal Pontine Infarcts

More rarely, infarcts in the pons occur in the latero-basal parts supplied by the short circumferential arteries (Fig. 161). According to some authors these are branches of the basilar artery in the rostral third, while according to others, they are supposed to stem from the superior cerebellar artery.

The hemodynamic situation is even less well understood in "pontovascular" insufficiency. This is best shown if we try to analyse, for instance, the extension of the various pontine infarcts in the series of KUBIK and ADAMS (1946). One does not find the clue to the analysis of these patterns even if one considers the action of Heubner's meningeal anastomoses (p. 13ff.) and perhaps also Schmidt's arachnoidal rings (p. 15), which otherwise seem to have no great importance in the pathology of infarcts (see p. 61ff.).

The borders of this infarct in the territory of the short circumferential ("intermediate") arteries are defined by the lateral three fifths of the pons (Fig. 161), a territory which includes some of the pontine nuclei, the lateral borders of the pyramidal pathways and the medial lemniscus, the trigeminal and facial nuclei and the middle cerebellar peduncle. Latero-basal pontine infarcts may be combined with paramedian infarcts.

d) Laterodorsal Pontine Infarcts

These infarcts (Fig. 162) are laterodorsally located in the pons and their borders are the tegmental area and the upper and middle cerebellar peduncles. They are thought to be the sequelae of an occlusion or insufficiency in the long circumferential ("lateral") arteries which are assumed

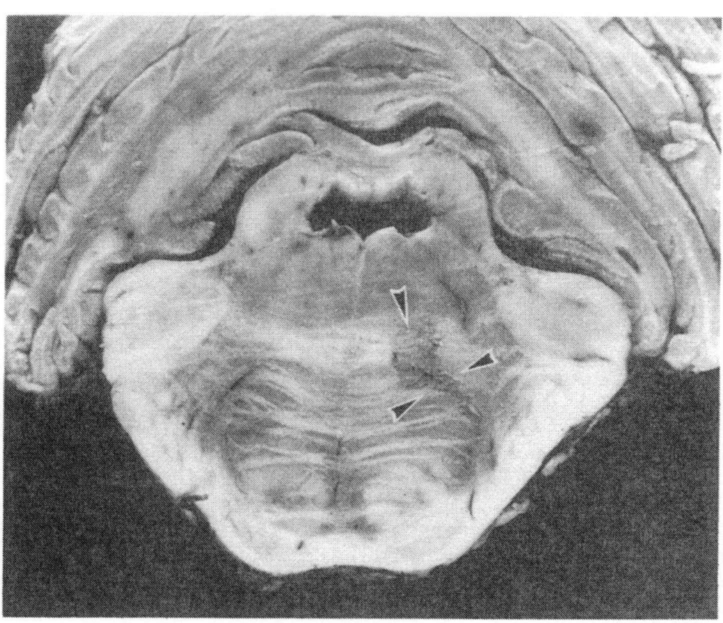

Fig. 161. Latero-basal infarct in the supply territory of a short circumferential artery *(arrows)*

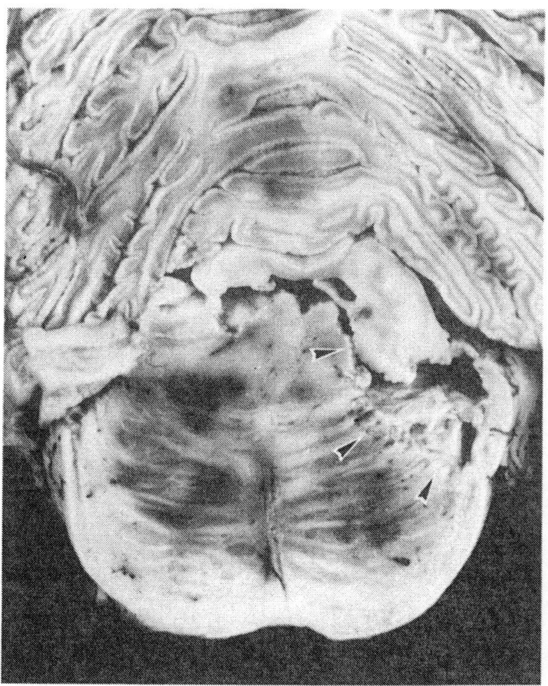

Fig. 162. Latero-dorsal infarct in the territory of a long circumferential artery *(arrows)*

to arise from the superior or from the anterior inferior cerebellar artery. Actually these send some branches to the tectal and tegmental regions.

The variations in the vascular supply are so remarkable that the studies using good injection specimens have not clarified the question as to where they originate in the *majority* of cases. Latero-dorsal infarcts can occur combined with paramedian infarcts.

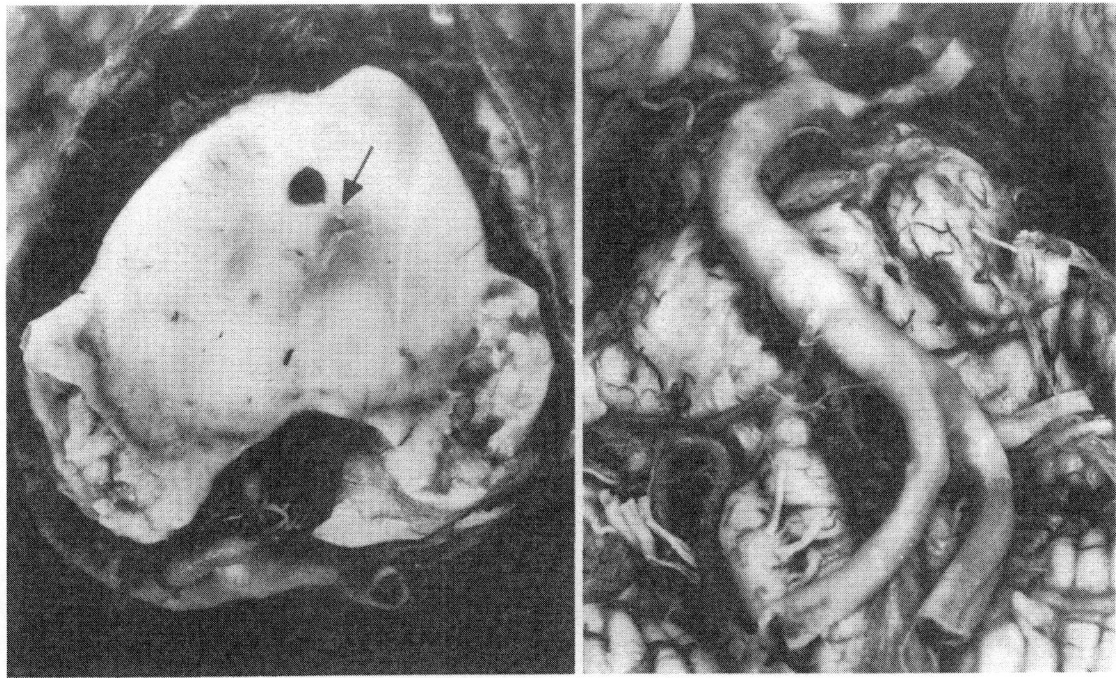

Fig. 163. Thrombosis of a highly atherosclerotic basilar artery with consequent bilateral softenings of the pedunculi (quadruplegia!). Small infarct below the aqueduct in the periaqueductal grey matter *(arrow)*

e) Mesencephalic (Midbrain) Infarcts

These infarcts show total destruction of the peduncular region (Fig. 163), usually bilaterally, whereas the tegmental and tectal segments are spared. Sometimes an extension of the softening into the substantia nigra occurs. Exceptionally rare is a partial infarct in the substantia nigra without basal peduncular involvement. In some cases the infarct may be "partial" and only the medial third of the peduncles on one side necrotic.

A (rare) infarct occurs in the periaqueductal grey (Fig. 163). The zone of destruction in our cases was more frequently bordered dorsally by an *intact* substantia nigra. This may be explained by the differences in the vascular supply, the ventral mesencephalon being supplied by short ("paramedian") branches from the basilar and the proximal part of the posterior artery while the dorsolateral and tectal regions are probably supplied from the superior cerebellar artery. This latter vessel may still have a collateral supply by reflux via the meningeal anastomoses in case of basilar occlusion. However, the relative integrity of the dorsal parts in our cases remains surprising, particularly when compared with the cases of Kubik and Adams (1946) where most destructions extended into the tegmental or tectal parts; if one considers the volume of the destroyed and preserved segments of the mesencephalon, an enormous collateral supply must be presumed in our cases, operating due to favourable general hemodynamics.

On the other hand, cases with an infarct only of the medial third of the peduncles are easily explained because the medial supplying vessels arise from the basilar artery, whereas the lateral perforating rami usually come from the posterior cerebral artery. When, as is often the case, the basilar thrombosis extends into the posterior cerebral artery only for one or two centimeters (Fig. 164), the blood may enter the distal part as well from the "anterior" supply, i.e. the anterior and middle cerebral arteries via Heubner's meningeal anastomoses, as also arise directly from the posterior communicating artery. Hence the lateral parts will be preserved, whereas the medial supply is blocked by the thrombosis of the basilar artery. Moreover, in 20% the "embryonic" pattern guarantees an undisturbed supply through a carotid origin of the posterior cerebral artery.

f) Thalamic Infarcts (Thalamoperforate-Thalamogeniculate Arteries)

If the thalamic region is involved by vascular insufficiency, one cannot expect that *one* typical "thalamic infarct" will ensue. As in the literature our cases were then of different locations;

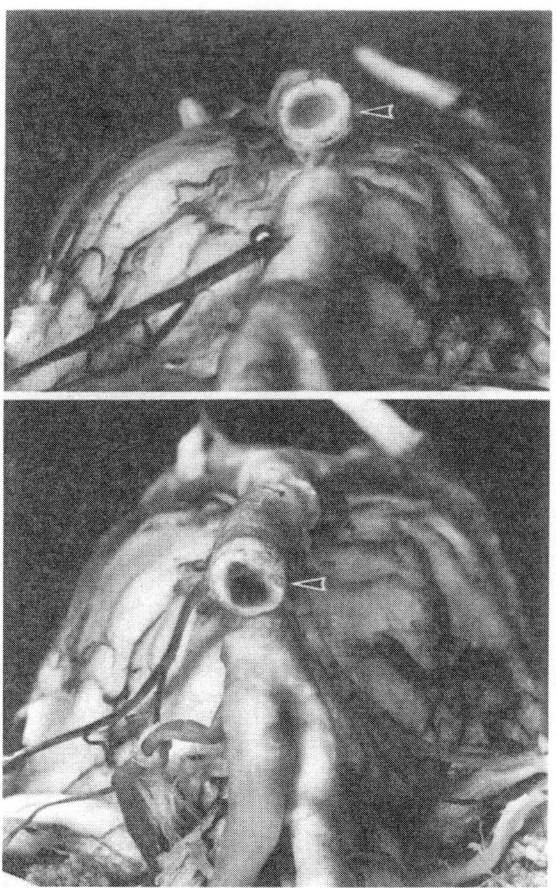

Fig. 164. Total occlusion of the basilar artery by old organized thrombosis (birch-bark type of atherosclerosis, *arrow*)

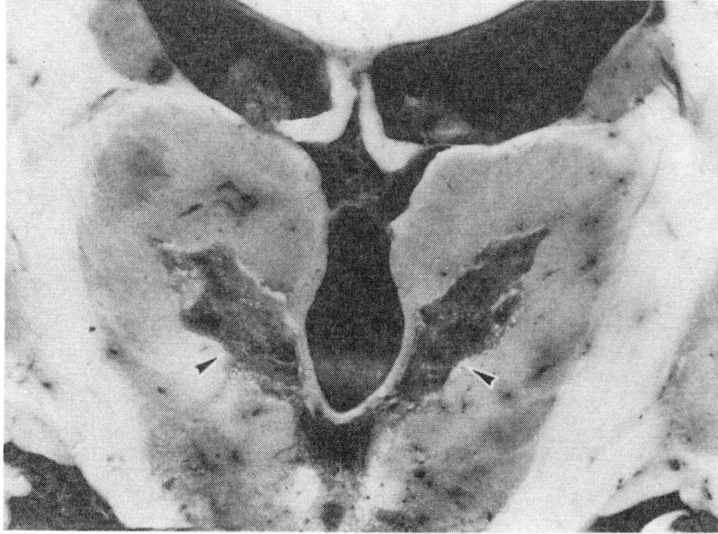

Fig. 165. Bilateral large cystic infarctions in the territory of the thalamoperforate arteries *(arrows)*

however, two typical infarcts can be described, namely when the "thalamoperforate" artery was in the location of the infarct or the "thalamogeniculate" artery. Curiously enough in none of our cases did we see infarcts in another supply areas as, for instance, in that of the posterior

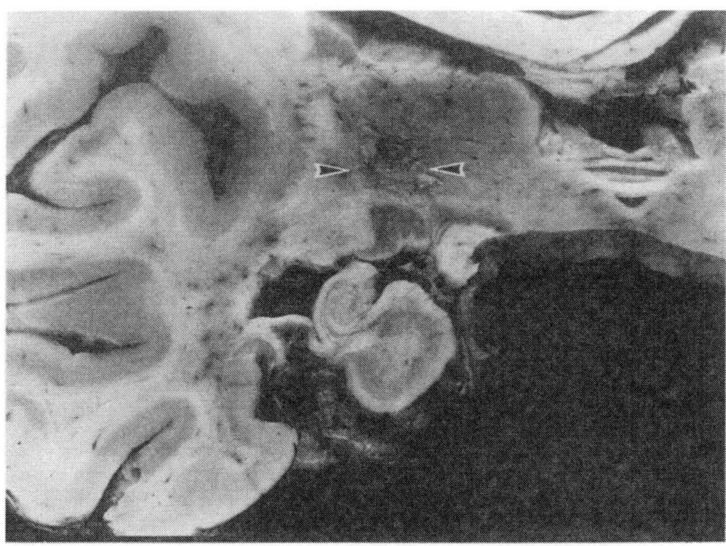

Fig. 166. Infarct in the territory of the thalamogeniculate artery *(arrows)*

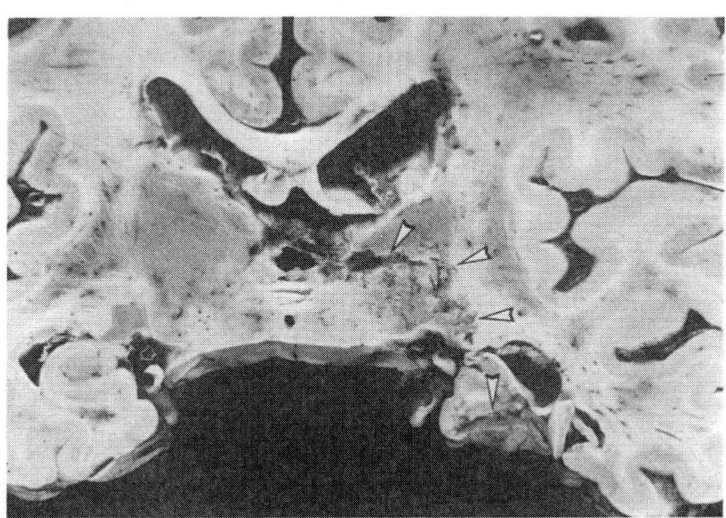

Fig. 167. Infarction within the territory of the thalamoperforate and -geniculate arteries and the temporal branch of the posterior cerebral artery *(arrows)*

chorioidal artery. Most infarcts (see Figs. 165–168) were smaller than the total vascular supply area described in text books or other publications.

A similar problem arises here as with the pontine infarcts. Why, in a particular case, is only *one artery* of the complex supply system compromised by an insufficiency with subsequent necrosis and why in this particular region? This can hardly be the consequence of the meningeal anastomoses, at least if we follow our traditional concept about the *action* of these vessels. This is particularly true if we deny – as we have done up to now and with justification (see ZÜLCH, 1969b) – any great influence of the intracerebral capillary anastomotic bed in this type of vascular disturbance of the brain.

The curious selection of 1) the different levels, 2) the particular arteries involved in vertebrobasilar insufficiency will be discussed later, where we show in one case of occlusion of one vertebral artery, the following insufficiencies or infarcts: medulla oblongata, pons, mesencephalon, thalamus, ventral and dorsal cerebellum and temporo-occipital lobe. All infarcts were partial and understandable by the hemodynamic laws of the "last meadows" or the "watersheds" (Fig. 156).

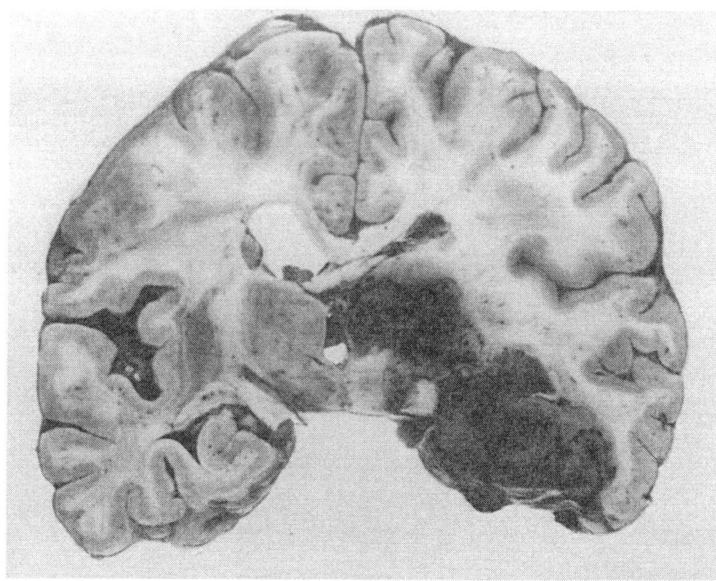

Fig. 168. Typical hemorrhagic infarction in the territory of the posterior cerebral artery with involvement of the thalamus (thalamogeniculate and -perforate arteries)

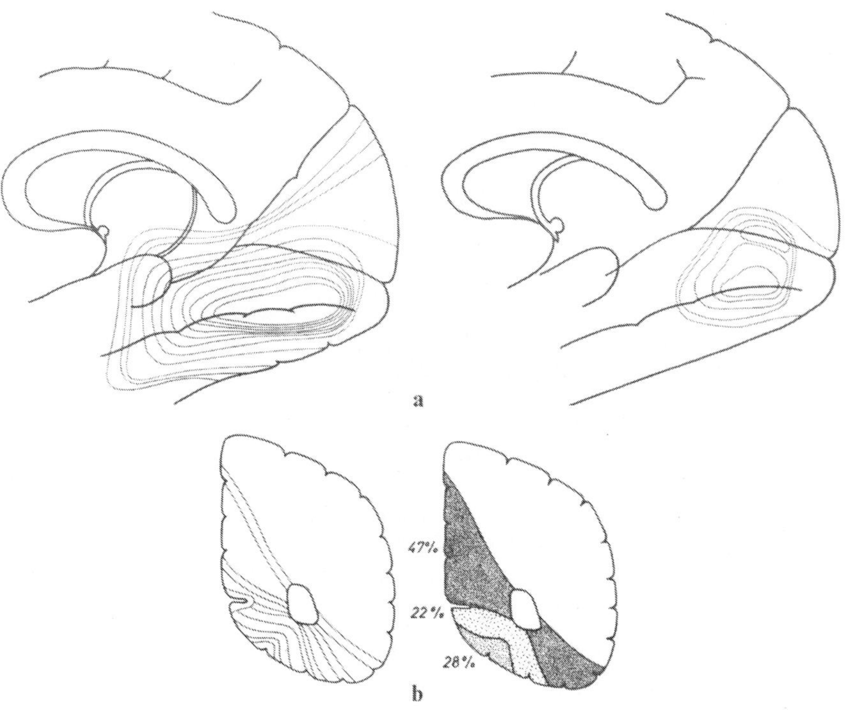

Fig. 169a and b. Extension and topography of posterior cerebral artery infarcts, **a** on a mediobasal view (each line represents two infarcts) and **b** in frontal slices. (From: ZÜLCH and KLEIHUES, 1967)

g) Occipital Lobe Infarcts (Infarcts of the Posterior Cerebral Arteries)

These infarcts may occur as uni- or bilateral necroses of varying location or extent in the supply area of the posterior cerebral artery (Figs. 169–174). We have to emphasize here the different supply to the posterior cerebral artery which may come from the carotid ("embryonal"; 15–25%, see ALPERS et al., 1959) or the basilar artery or in different contributions by both of them.

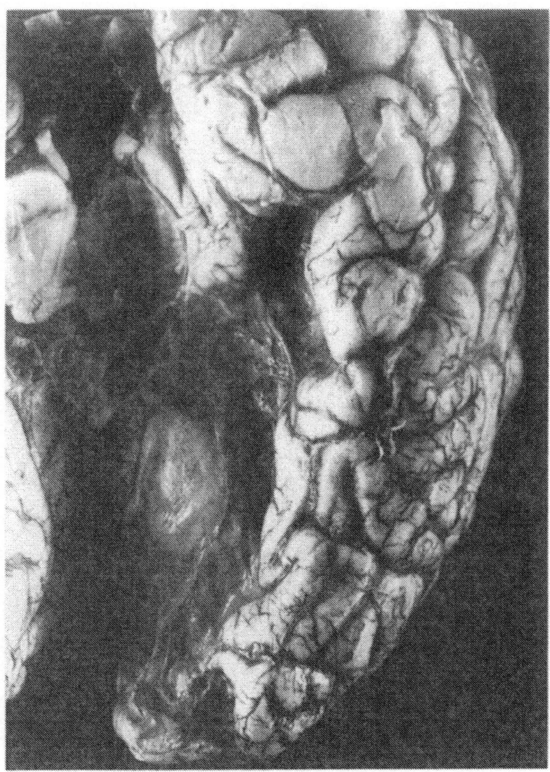

Fig. 170. Almost total infarction of the territory of the posterior cerebral artery in a case of proximal occlusion: rostrally, partial necrosis of lateral thalamus, partial necrosis of Ammon's horn and a large occipital infarction including the lower "lip" of the calcarine fissure and the occipitale pole

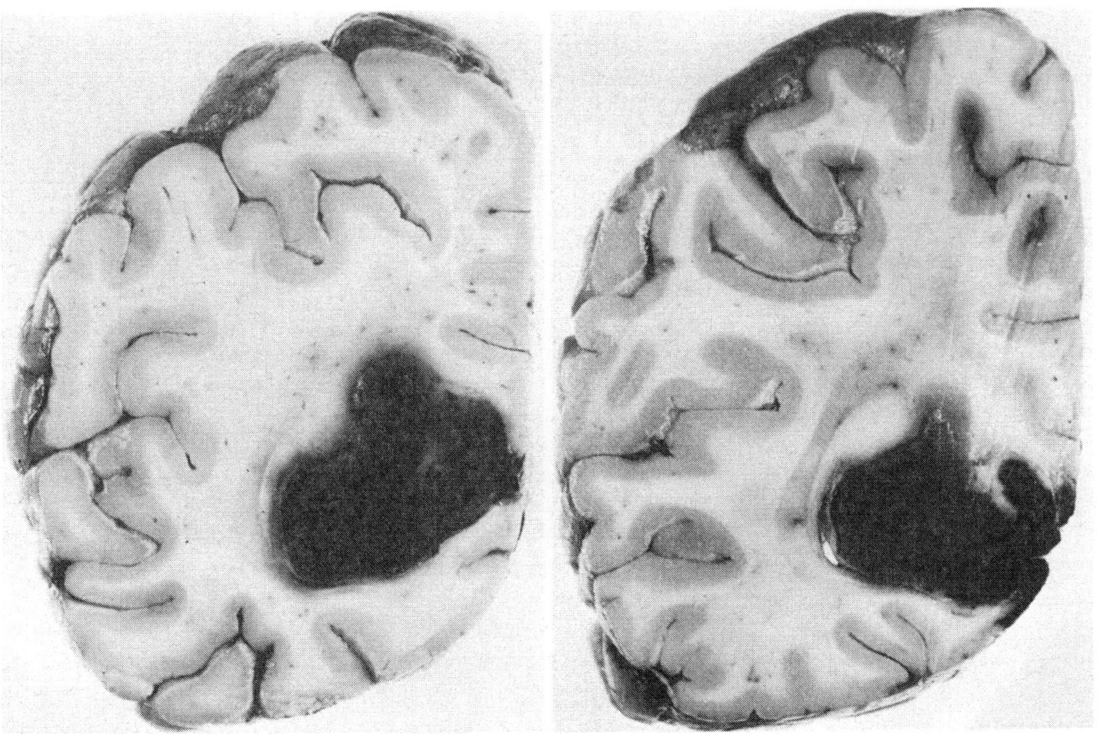

Fig. 171. Typical site and size of a hemorrhagic infarct near the calcarine fissure associated with a tentorial pressure cone

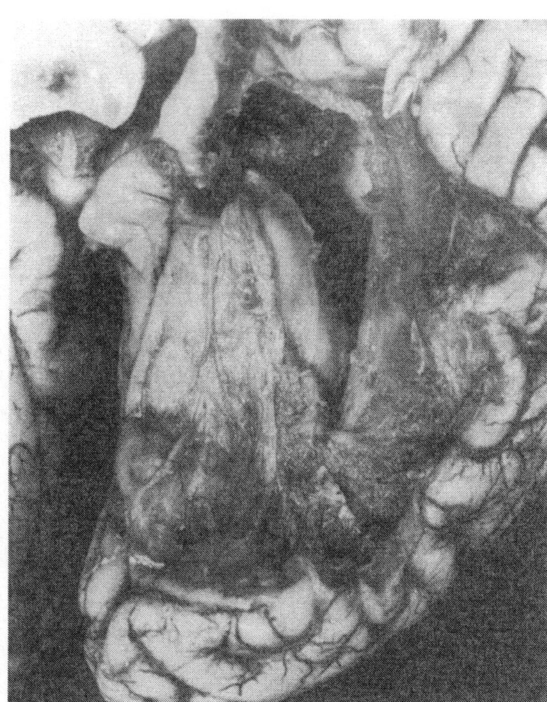

Fig. 172. Almost total – old – proximal infarct in the territory of the posterior cerebral artery

These have been the subject of recent investigations in our laboratory by KLEIHUES (1966a, b) and KLEIHUES and HIZAWA (1966), who extended some theoretical considerations, as published previously by ZÜLCH (1961a, 1962a) to their pathogenesis.

ZÜLCH (1959, Fig. 84; ZÜLCH et al. 1974b, Fig. 41, 42) had described a particular partial ("centrally" located) hemorrhagic infarct as caused by strangulation of the posterior cerebral artery by a trans-tentorial pressure cone (Fig. 171; see also RIESSNER and ZÜLCH, 1939; ZÜLCH, 1961a, b) and later a similarly located infarct as a special form of a hemodynamic disorder, i.e., 1) the occipital "infarct in the center of a supply area" (which corresponded to the lower parts of the calcarine fissures and led to appropriate hemianopic visual field defects) and 2) to the infarcts in the terminal zone of the posterior cerebral artery (Figs. 129 and 169a, b).

The topography of 35 infarcts in the territory of the posterior cerebral artery was determined on frontal sections, and on the mediobasal surfaces of the brain by ZÜLCH and KLEIHUES (1967, Fig. 10, 11). They made a schematic drawing of the localization and extention of all these infarcts so that each line represents the common border of two or three neighbouring softenings. It was not possible to join all the border lines of the infarcts into a single drawing; often the lines crossed. This led them (Fig. 169) to the assumption that the pathogenesis of these infarcts may be different and correspond to the two hemodynamic types described above (ZÜLCH, 1961a). According to the below-mentioned authors, the lower portions of the visual cortex were more frequently compromised (KLEIHUES and HIZAWA, 1966).

The occipital pole, i.e., the cortical representation of the central parts of the visual field, was completely infarcted in only 20%, and partially in 11% of these cases. A complete sparing of the visual cortex occurred in 28% of the cases. The infarcts in the "center of the territory" of the posterior cerebral artery had the tendency to extend more into the basal regions with the collateral sulcus as their central point. The lower border of the calcarine fissure was more often affected than the upper border (Fig. 169).

Hemodynamically this particular infarct occurred when only the posterior artery was stenosed and the bordering parts of the supply territory were supplied by meningeal anastomoses (see Figs. 42 and 44 in ZÜLCH, 1961a). These forms could be hemodynamically explained only by an abundant collateral supply from the large neighboring meningeal anastomoses. Incidentally, a "central" (hemorrhagic) infarct is the typical "occipital" infarct associated with transtentorial herniation (Fig. 171). For references see KLEIHUES (1966a, b) and KLEIHUES and HIZAWA (1966).

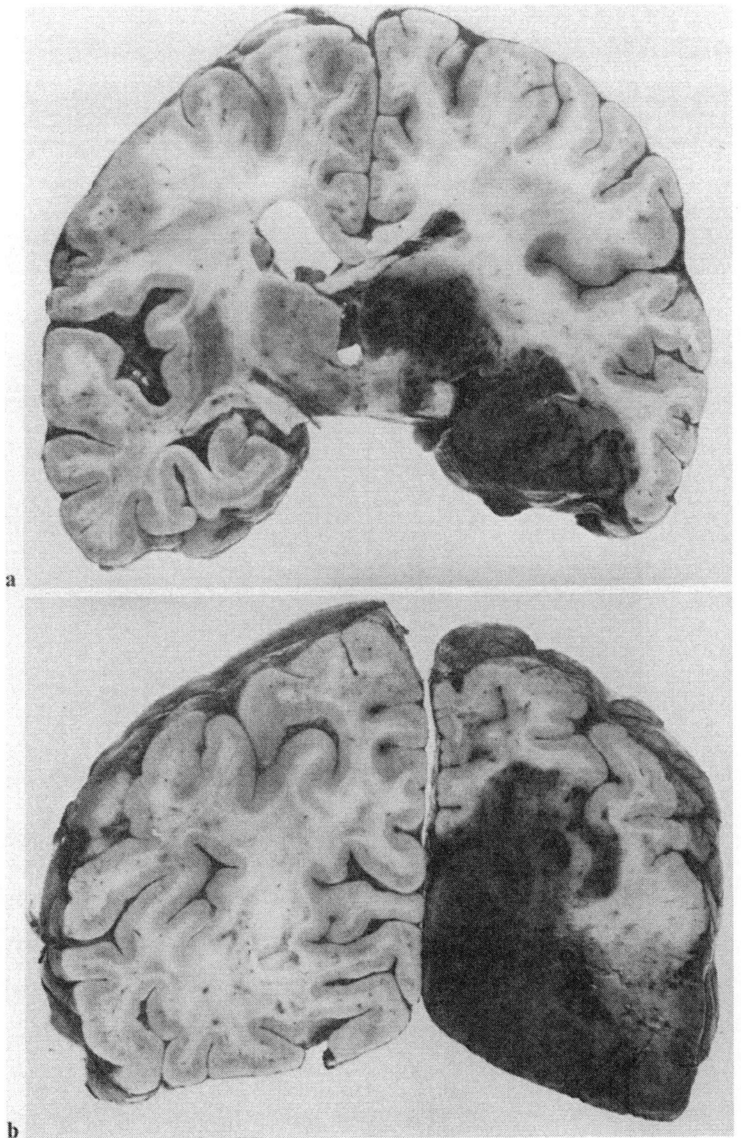

Fig. 173a and b. Complete hemorrhagic infarction of the supply territory of the posterior cerebral artery including the entire thalamus

h) Cerebellar

In the literature and from our observations, two prominent types of infarcts occurred in the cerebellum, namely, the "ventral" and the "dorsal" necroses depending from the main supply territories of the "posterior inferior" (p.i.c.a.) and the "superior" cerebellar arteries (s.c.a.).

The typical "dorsal" infarcts (Figs. 175, 176) were only rarely situated in the entire supply area in the more distal territory of the superior cerebellar artery and they usually varied in size. Commonly a typical case shows when fresh (Figs. 176–179), a mostly hemorrhagic, or if old, deeply scarred infarct which is more often located in the distal part of the supply area of the superior cerebellar artery (Fig. 175). It was stated above that none of them was

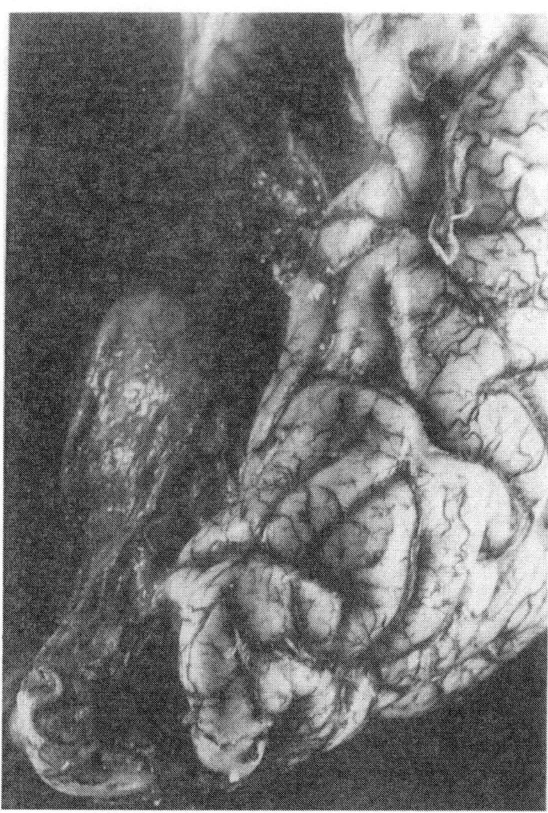

Fig. 174. Large shrunken infarct in the right mediobasal occipital lobe sparing the pole

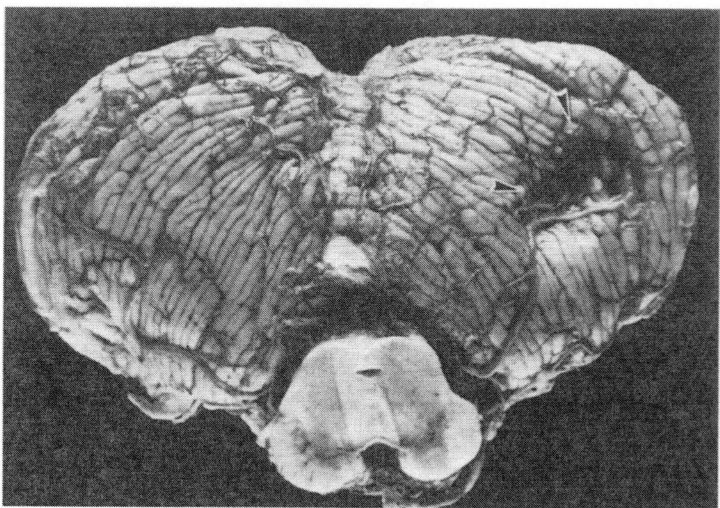

Fig. 175. Small "dorsal" cerebellar infarct *(arrows)*

"total" or *reached far into the* depth, i.e., into the white substance including the dentate nucleus. The supply by the meningeal anastomoses interconnecting the superior and inferior cerebellar arteries (Fig. 15) must be far greater than assumed. Sometimes the dorsal infarcts were combined with ventral infarcts while the lateral segments of the cerebellar hemispheres remained – curiously enough – mostly free of necroses.

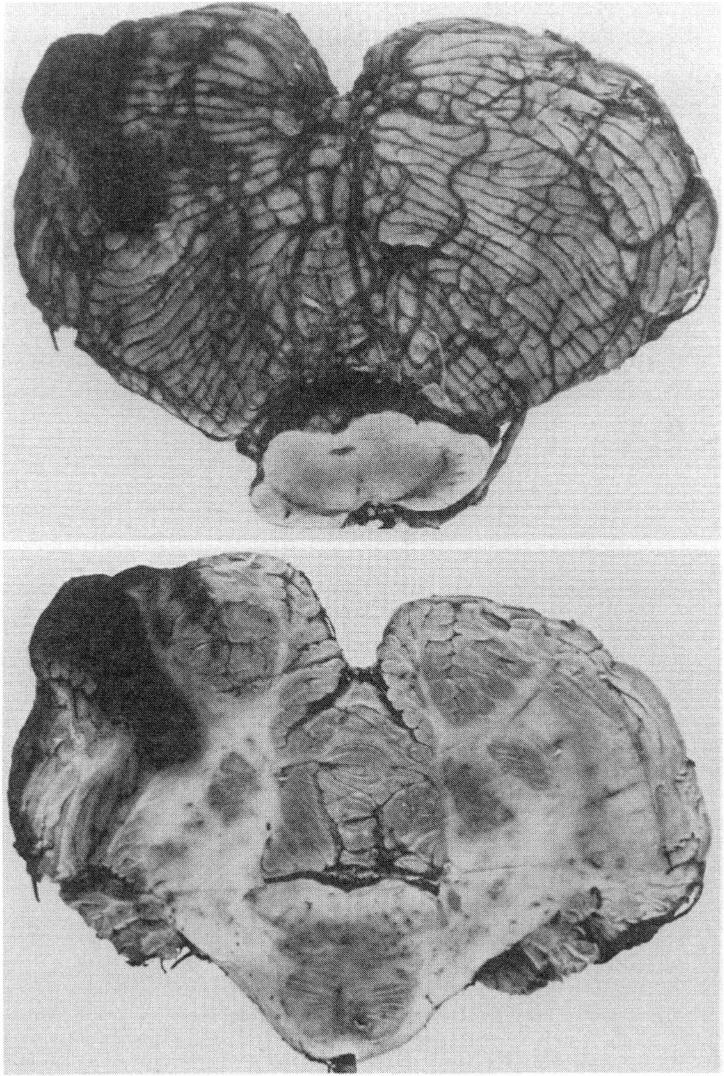

Fig. 176. Small hemorrhagic infarct in the borderline territory between superior and anterior inferior cerebellar arteries

The limited extension of these infarcts on the dorsal surface of the cerebellum can only be explained by the apparent rich collateral network of meningeal anastomoses covering the convexity of the cerebellum, the anastomotic function of which is well proved also neuroradiologically (Fig. 15, see also FIELDS et al., 1965; WEIBEL and FIELDS, 1969).

The "ventral" infarcts (Fig. 180), on the other hand, were usually larger though again usually not "total". In our series the majority of infarcts were old, i.e., scarred (as observed at autopsy) and consisted – of shallow crater-like grooves located more often in the proximal supply territory (and this was to be expected owing to the good anastomotic distal supply) (Figs. 181, 182).

There were variations in the site and extension of these cerebellar infarcts (Figs. 176–178) which were hard to explain, namely when the usual supply territory was unaffected and the main extension occurred (Figs. 176, 177) "laterally". We were not able to detect whether these and some other of the "atypical" infarcts were located in "frontier zones" or "watershed" areas of the three large cerebellar arteries, but we consider this to be likely. Some cases showed multiple necrotic foci in the area of the posterior inferior cerebellar artery or occurred in combination with "dorsally" located necroses.

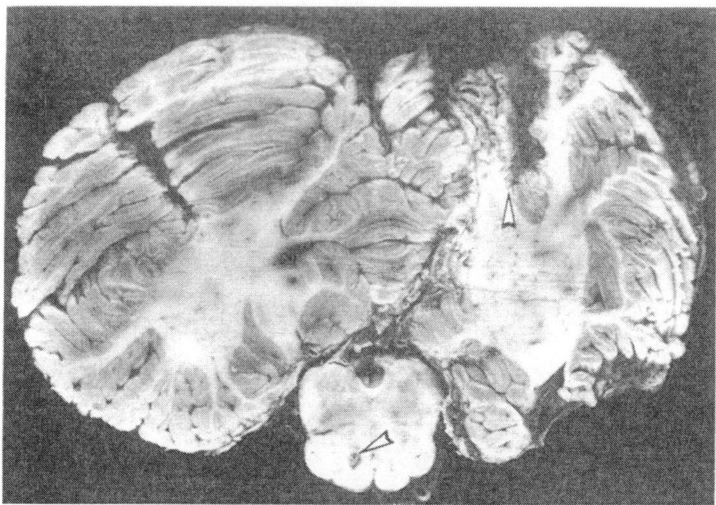

Fig. 177. Left-sided infarction on ventral aspect of the cerebellum; borderline old cystic infarct in right cerebellum (see Fig. 176); one very small cystic infarct between pyramid and inferior olive on the right *(arrows)*

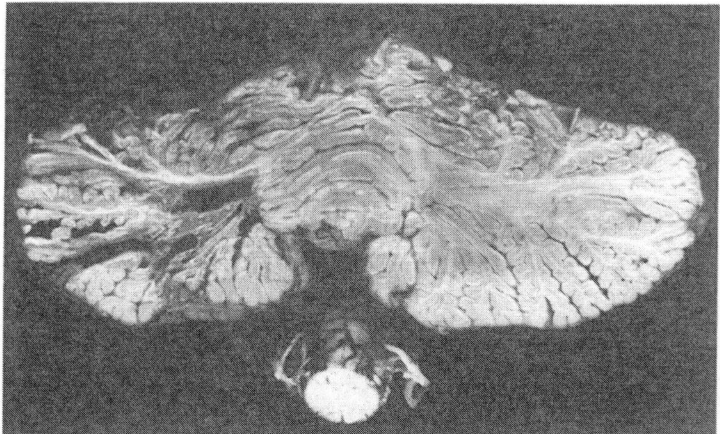

Fig. 178. Infarction following compromised flow in the superior and anterior inferior cerebellar arteries with only the posterior inferior being spared

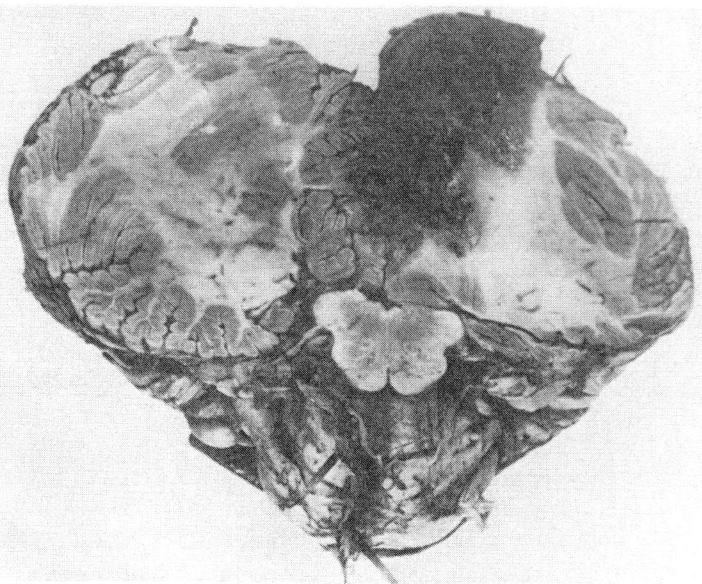

Fig. 179. Large right superior cerebellar infarct (medial branch of superior cerebellar artery)

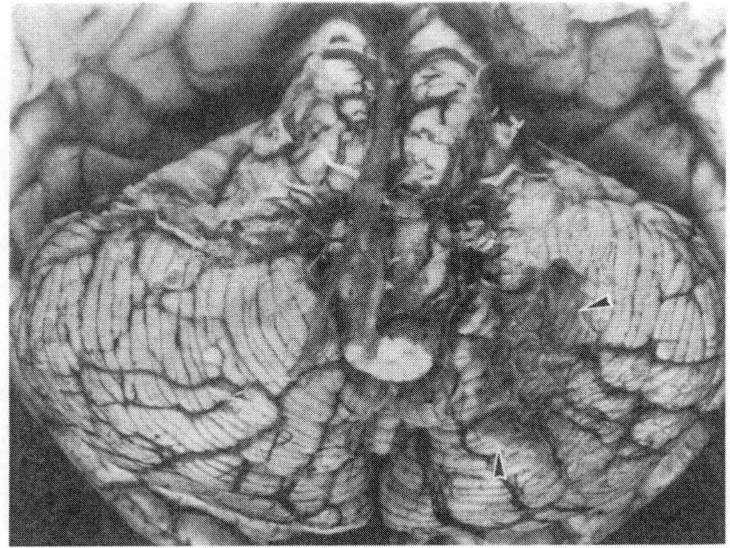

Fig. 180. Median sized "ventral" cerebellar infarct *(arrows)*

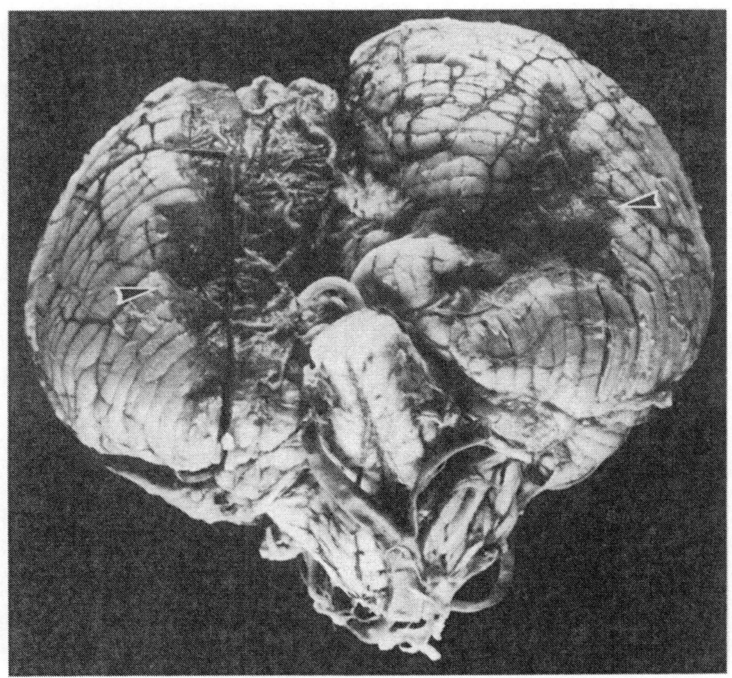

Fig. 181. Large bilateral ventral cerebellar infarcts (within the territory of the posterior inferior cerebellar arteries; *arrows*)

We only can emphasize again the fact that infarction within the vertebro-basilar territory is often patchy and that we do not as yet, sufficiently understand the hemodynamic laws of the involvement of the various contributing arteries (Fig. 176).

In summarizing we should emphasize *that correlative studies on the pathology, pathogenesis and clinical syndromes of vertebrobasilar disease are still needed* and are of great importance because the correlation between the neurological syndromes, the vascular pathogenesis and the ensuing pathology are not yet sufficiently elucidated (Loeb and Meyer, 1965; Metzinger, 1971; Metzinger and Zülch, 1971).

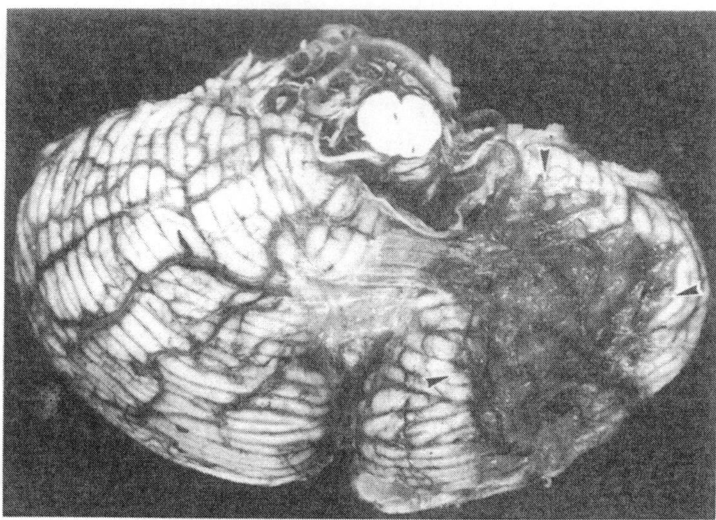

Fig. 182. Large ventral cerebellar infarct in the territory of both the anterior inferior and posterior inferior cerebellar arteries (lateral branches; *arrows*)

13. Symptomatology of Vertebrobasilar Insufficiency

The syndrome of basilar thrombosis (LEYDEN, 1882; KAPLAN, 1951; FREEMAN et al., 1953; DENNY-BROWN, 1953; SIEKERT and MILLIKAN, 1956; WILLIAMS and WILSON, 1962; FISHER and CAPLAN, 1971). The "full blown" clinical syndrome is so characteristic that the diagnosis of occlusion may be made at once (tetraplegia, flaccid or spastic pareses or paralyses of lower cranial nerves with preservation of the eye muscles, signs of decerebration etc.). However, *the syndromes may vary according to the extent of involvement* (Fig. 156). Even akinetic mutism (KEMPER and ROMANUL, 1967) or dementia (RIVERA et al., 1974) may follow after vertebral artery impairment.

The paradox motor syndrome of the paramedian infarct of the pons: see p. 148.

14. Syndrome of the Dorsolateral Medulla Oblongata (Wallenberg-Syndrome)

Again the symptoms are very indicative of an insufficiency or occlusion within the posterior inferior cerebellar artery or dorsolateral infarction of the medulla oblongata (ipsilateral paralysis of the tongue and soft palate, or even more oral cranial nerves, ipsilateral trigeminal analgesia and contralateral analgesia in the lower parts of the body, varying patterns of sensory changes in the uncrossed sensory modalities).

For differential diagnosis between the syndromes of the carotid and basilar artery: see p. 144.

In summary, we would like to emphasize that the data in the vertebrobasilar supply area are so scanty, because none of the available diagnostic tools provide sufficient information of the anatomic lesions. The radionuclide scan, computed tomography (because of the many artefacts in that region!) and even magnification angiography are not able to analyse satisfactorily the regions of vascular insufficiency or necrosis in the posterior fossa.

15. Infarcts Leading to Increased Intracranial Pressure and Mass Movements

The fundamental rules regarding to increased intracranial pressure and local space-occupying lesions (including intra- and extracellular edema, mass movements, hernias etc.) have been sufficiently described elsewhere (ZÜLCH, 1956a, 1959; ZÜLCH et al., 1974b). These rules are valid for any volume increase in the "watertight box" of the intracranial cavity. Suffice it to emphasize here that any ischemia localized or generalized usually produces intra- and extracellular edema, and that this increase in volume may lead to shifts which can, under special conditions, provoke the complications of mass movements, such as are well known in tumor pathology, although generally supposed not to occur in a cerebrovascular infarct. Thus *cerebral edema* may arise to such a degree that the shift towards the opposite hemisphere leads to a herniation of the cingulate gyrus under the falx or even to a temporal pressure cone which compromizes the opposite pedunculus by the sharp edge of the tentorium and produces neurologically a false (because homolateral) symptomatology (Figs. 154, 155; see ZÜLCH, 1968). Experimental edema has supported the observations in man (O'BRIEN and WALTZ 1973). Also cerebellar pressure cones occur (PERRET, 1940). The raised pressure in cerebellar hemorrhages may indicate surgical decompression (IVAMOTO et al., 1974).

XIV. Cerebral Atrophic Processes

Atrophic processes of the brain may follow any circumscribed or diffuse tissue damage and are well described in the textbooks (PETERS, 1970; BLACKWOOD and CORSELLIS, 1976). They are rarely subject to angiographic investigations and are more commonly defined and detected by computed tomography. Global atrophies of one hemisphere with involvement of both the grey and white substance may follow carotid occlusion and also it may be in rare cases bilateral; if occurring perinatal they cause porencephaly. There may be spotty atrophy of brain tissue (Fig. 183) in case of stenosis of single branches for instance within the system of the Sylvian vessels. In rare cases even "granular atrophy" (see pp. 63, 64, Fig. 183) in a ring-like zone may ensue as a result of general disturbance of circulation. Sclerosis and atrophy of grey and white matter of one hemisphere can follow chronic subdural hematomas.

"Granular atrophy" is also observed in asphyxiated children after delivery (J.E. MEYER, 1948, 1953, 1958). The granular atrophy in thromboangiitis obliterans is described on page 64.

A particular form of regional or halfsided cerebral damage is "lobar" or "hemispheric" sclerosis. A rare vascular disease is "Binswanger's cerebral atrophy" (see p. 67), which is associated

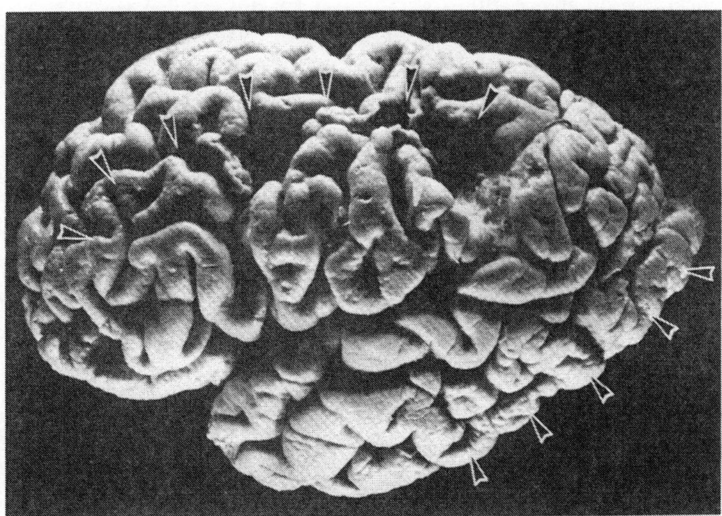

Fig. 183. General cortical atrophy indicated by enlargement of the arachnoidal spaces, however with an addition of two particular lesions: 2 shrunken and circumscribed cortical infarcts (one at "Dreiländereck"), a ring-like zone of cortical "granular atrophy" as usually seen in thromboangiitis obliterans (arrows! see Fig. 64)

with arteriolar atherosclerotic involvement. It consists of diffuse lesions, predominantly in the white matter, which probably start by "perivenous" demyelination (see ZÜLCH, 1973b). The lesions after carbon monoxide poisoning – atrophy of globus pallidus, cortical lesions, white matter atrophy – are related not mainly to hypoxia, but crucially determined by other factors (GINSBERG and MYERS, 1974a, b; GINSBERG et al., 1974).

The interesting question whether Parkinson's disease may be related to cerebrovascular insufficiency ("atherosclerotic" Parkinsonism) has been investigated by KLUGER (1979). In his series the latter group of patients with labile blood pressures has a higher age of manifestation in 2/3 of the cases, the other types of Parkinsonism correspond in their vascular patterns to the various age groups of the normal population.

For references and detailed description of other non vascular forms of brain atrophy see Chapters of: F. SCHOB (1930), J. HALLERVORDEN (1930), E. GRÜNTHAL (1930), H. SPATZ, 1938, A.v. BRAUNMÜHL (1957), G. PETERS (1970), W. BLACKWOOD and J.A.N. CORSELLIS (1976).

References

ABBIE, A.A.: The clinical significance of the anterior chorioidal artery. Brain **56**, 233–246 (1933)

ABRAHAM, J., DANIEL, M.V.: Aspects of cerebrovascular disease in India. Madras: Diocesan Press 1972

ADAMKIEWICZ, A.: Die Blutgefäße des menschlichen Rückenmarkes. I. Teil: Die Gefäße der Rückenmarkssubstanz. S.ber. Akad. Wiss. Wien, Math.-naturw. Kl., Abt. III, 84, 469–502 (1881)

ADAMKIEWICZ, A.: Die Blutgefäße des menschlichen Rückenmarkes. II. Teil: Die Gefäße der Rückenmarksoberfläche. S.ber. Akad. Wiss. Wien, Math.-naturw. Kl., Abt. III, 85, 101–130 (1882)

ADAMS, J.H., GRAHAM, D.I.: Twelve cases of fatal cerebral infarction due to arterial occlusion in the absence of atheromatous stenosis or embolism. J. Neurol. Neurosurg. Psychiatry **30**, 479–488 (1967)

ADAMS, R.D.: Pathology of cerebral vascular diseases. B. Cranial cerebral lesions. In: Cerebral vascular diseases, 2nd Princeton Conference 1957. MILLIKAN, C.H. (ed.), pp. 23–39. New York, London: GRUNE & STRATTON 1958

ADAMS, R.D., FISHER, C.M.: Pathology of cerebral arterial occlusion. In: Pathogenesis and treatment of cerebrovascular disease. FIELDS, W.S. (ed.), pp. 126–150. Springfield: THOMAS 1961

ADAMS, R.D., VAN DER EECKEN, H.M.: Vascular disease of the brain. Ann. Rev. Med. **4**, 213–252 (1953)

ADLER, E.: Stroke in Israel 1957–1961: Epidemiological, clinical, rehabilitation and psycho-social aspects. Jerusalem: Polypress 1969

AHO, K., FOGELHOLM, R.: Incidence and early prognosis of stroke in Espoo-Kauniainen area, Finland, in 1972. Stroke **5**, 658–661 (1974)

ALBERTINI, A. v.: Pathologische Anatomie der Endangiitis obliterans. Schweiz. Arch. Neurol. Psychiatrie **57**, 393 (1946)

ALBUS, G.: Über die Verteilung der Arteriosklerose an den extra- und intrakraniellen Hirnarterien. Doktor-Dissertation, Universität Köln 1970

ALLBUTT, C.: Diseases of the arteries including angina pectoris. Vol. I. London: MCMILLAN 1915

ALPERS, B.J., BERRY, R.G.: Circle of Willis in cerebral vascular disorders. Arch. Neurol. **8**, 398–402 (1963)

ALPERS, B.J., BERRY, R.G., PADDISON, R.M.: Anatomical studies of the circle of Willis in normal brain. Arch. Neurol. **81**, 409–418 (1959)

ALTER, M., KLUZNIK, J.: Genetics of cerebrovascular accidents. Stroke **3**, 41–48 (1972)

ALTER, M., KIEFFER, ST., RESCH, J., ANSARI, K.: Cerebral infarction. Clinical and angiographic correlations. Neurology (Minneap.) **22**, 590–602 (1972)

ALVAREZ, W.C.: The little strokes. J. Am. Med. Assoc. **157**, 1199–1204 (1955)

ALZHEIMER, A.: Die arteriosklerotische Atrophie des Gehirns. Neurol. Zbl. **13**, 765–767 (1894). Z. Psychiatrie **51**, 809 (1895)

ANDERS, H.E., EICKE, W.J.: Über die Veränderungen an Hirngefäßen bei Hypertonie. Z. gesamte Neurol. Psychatrie **167**, 562–575 (1939)

ANDERS, H.E., EICKE, W.J.: Die Gehirngefäße beim Hochdruck. Arch. Psychiatr. Nervenkr. **112**, 1–44 (1940)

ANDERSEN, CH.A., RICH, N.M., COLLINS, G.J., MCDONALD, P.T.: Unilateral internal carotid arterial occlusion: Special considerations. Stroke **8**, 669–671 (1977)

ANDERSON, F.H., DUNCAN, G.W.: Sturge-Weber disease with subarachnoid hemorrhage. Stroke **5**, 509–511 (1974)

ANDRIOLI, G.C., MARIN, G., CARTERI, A.: Considerazioni sull'ipoplasia della carotide interna associata a pseudoangiomatosi cerebrale. Atti del 2. Simposio Internazionale di Neurochirurgia, Acquaviva dell Fonti 1971

ARENDT, A., BACHMANN, P.: Intracerebrale Gefäßwandveränderungen bei hypertonischer Hirnmassenblutung. Acta Neuropathol. (Berl.) **7**, 79–85 (1966)

ARING, Ch.D., MERRITT, H.H.: Differential diagnosis between cerebral hemorrhage and cerebral thrombosis. Arch. Intern. Med. **56**, 438–456 (1935)

ARMSTRONG, M.L., WARNER, E.D., CONNOR, W.E.: Regression of coronary atheromatosis in rhesus monkeys. Circ. Res. **27**, 59–67 (1970)

ARONSON, St.M.: Intracranial vascular lesions in patients with diabetes mellitus. J. Neuropathol. Exp. Neurol. **32**, 183–196 (1973)

ASCHOFF, L.: Über Atherosklerose. Vorträge über Pathologie. Jena 1925

ASCHOFF, L.: Über Arteriosklerose. Z. gesamten Neurol. Psychiatrie **94**, 344–345 (1939)

ASKENASY, H.M., KOSARY, I.Z., BRAHAM, J.: Thrombosis of the longitudinal sinus. Neurology (Minneap.) **12**, 288–292 (1962)

ATKINSON, W.J.: Anterior inferior cerebellar artery: Its variations, pontine distribution, and significance in surgery of cerebello-pontine angle tumors. J. Neurol. Neurosurg. Psychiatry **12**, 137–151 (1949)

AURELL, M., HODD, B.: Cerebral haemorrhage in a population after a decade of active antihypertensive treatment. Acta Med. Scand. **176**, 377–383 (1964)

AZUMA, T., FUKUSHIMA, T.: Turbulence generation in stenotic blood vessel models. In: Brain and heart infarct. ZÜLCH, K.J., KAUFMANN, W., HOSSMANN, K.-A., HOSSMANN, V. (eds.), pp. 57–71. Berlin, Heidelberg, New York: Springer 1979

BAILEY, O.T.: Thrombosis of dural sinuses and meningeal veins. In: Pathology of the nervous system. MINCKLER, J. (ed.), Vol. 2, chapter 114, pp. 1537–1543. New York: McGraw-Hill Book 1971

BAILLIE, M.B.: London, 1761–1823

BAKER, A.B.: Cerebrovascular disease. IX. The medullary blood supply and the lateral medullary syndrome. Neurology (Minneap.) **11**, 852–861 (1961)

BAKER, A.B., IANNONE, A.: Cerebrovascular disease: I. The large arteries of the circle of Willis. Neurolgy (Minneap.) **9**, 321–332 (1959a)

BAKER, A.B., IANNONE, A.: Cerebrovascular disease: II. The smaller intracerebral arteries. Neurology (Minneap.) **9**, 391–396 (1959b)

BAKER, A.B., IANNONE, A.: Cerebrovascular disease: III. The intracerebral arterioles. Neurology (Minneap.) **9**, 441–446 (1959c)

BAKER, A.B., IANNONE, A., KINNARD, J.: Cerebrovascular disease. VI. Relationship to disease of the heart and the aorta. Neurology (Minneap.) **11**, 63–70 (1961a)

BAKER, A.B., KINNARD, J., IANNONE, A.: Cerebrovascular disease. VIII. Role of nutritional factors. Neurology (Minneap.) **11**, 380–389 (1961b)

BAKER, A.B., DAHL, E., SANDLER, B.: Cerebrovascular Disease. Etiologic factors in cerebral infarction. Neurology (Minneap.) **13**, 445–454 (1963)

BAKER, A.B., FLORA, G.C., RESCH, J.A., LOEWENSON, R.B.: The geographic pathology of atherosclerosis: a review of the literature with some personal observations on cerebral atherosclerosis. J. Chronic Dis. **20**, 685–706 (1967)

BAKER, A.B., RESCH, J.A., LOEWENSON, R.B.: Hypertension and cerebral atherosclerosis. Circulation **39**, 701–710 (1969)

BAKER, A.B., RESCH, J.A., LOEWENSON, R.B.: Cerebral atherosclerosis in European populations: A preliminary report. Stroke **4**, 898–903 (1973)

BALBO, R.J., SARIAN, L., SPERLESCU, A., RIBEIRO, L.A.O.: Doença oclusiva progressiva das arterials cerebrais ("Moya-Moya"). Seara Med. Neuroc. (Sao Paulo) **1**, 166–173 (1972)

BAPTISTA, A.G.: Studies on the arteries of the brain. II. The anterior cerebral artery. Some anatomic features and their clinical implications. Neurology (Minneap.) **13**, 825–835 (1963)

BARTSCH, W., SWANK, R.L.: Der Effekt von Herzleistung und Blutdruck auf die Hämodynamik der spinalen Durchblutung. Verh. dtsch. Ges. inn. Med. **72**, 1105–1110 (1967)

BATTACHARJI, S.K., HUTCHINSON, E.C., MCCALL, A.J.: The circle of Willis – the incidence of developmental abnormalities in normal and infarcted brains. Brain **90**, 747–758 (1967)

BAYLISS, W.M.: On the local reactions of the arterial wall to changes of internal pressure. J. Physiol. (Lond.) **28**, 220–231 (1902)

BECKER, H.: Experimentelle Verschlüsse von Arterien und Venen und ihre Einwirkung auf das Gewebe. Z. ges. Neurol. Psychiatrie **167**, 546–553 (1939)

BEEVOR, Ch.E.: The cerebral arterial supply. Brain **30**, 403–425 (1907)

BEHREND, R.Ch., GASTAUT, H.: Pathophysiologie und Differentialdiagnose der synkopalen Anfälle. Verh. dtsch. Ges. inn. Med. **68**, 71–87 (1962)

BEHREND, R.Ch., ZÜLCH, K.J., KLEIHUES, P., KALM, H., SCHULTZE-BERGMANN, G., WACK, H.-O.: La clinique des sténoses carotidiennes et la portée du traitement médical. Rev. Neurol. **115**, 627–640 (1966)

BEITZKE, H.: Zur Entstehung der Atherosklerose. Virchows Arch. pathol. Anat. **267**, 625–647 (1928)

BELL, E.T.: Primary hypertension; a clinical and pathological study of 1.520 cases with especial reference to renal arteriosclerosis. Proc. A. Life Insur. M. Dir. Am. 1939, 26; 1940, 269

BERGMANN, G.v.: Funktionelle Pathologie. Kap. 12: Die Lehre von der Apoplexie. Berlin: Springer 1932

BERGSTRAND, H., OLIVECRONA, H., TÖNNIS, W.: Gefäßmißbildungen und Gefäßgeschwülste des Gehirns. Leipzig: Thieme 1936

BERNSMEIER, A.: Die zirkulatorisch bedingten Krankheitsbilder des Gehirns. In: Differentialdiagnose neurologischer Krankheitsbilder. G. BODECHTEL (Hrsg.), 2. Aufl. Stuttgart: Thieme 1963

BETHKE, C.C.: Über Schlagflüsse und Lähmungen oder Geschichte der Apoplexie, Paraplegie und Hemiplegie. Leipzig: Fleischer, Jr. 1797

BETZ, E., SCHLOTE, W.: Development and regression

of experimental local carotid atheromatosis in rabbits. In: Brain and heart infarct. ZÜLCH, K.J., KAUFMANN, W., HOSSMANN, K.-A., HOSSMANN, V. (eds.), pp. 50–56. Berlin, Heidelberg, New York: Springer 1979

BIEMOND, A.: Thrombosis of the basilar artery and the vascularization of the brain stem. Brain **74**, 300–317 (1951)

BIER, A.: Hyperämie als Heilmittel. Leipzig: Vogel 1906

BIZZOZERO, J.: Über einen neuen Formbestandteil des Blutes und dessen Rolle bei der Thrombose und der Blutgerinnung. Virchows Arch. pathol. Anat. **90**, 261–332 (1882)

BLACKBURN, J.W.: Anomalies of the encephalic arteries among the insane. J. Comp. Neurol. **17**, 493–517 (1907)

BLACKWOOD, W.: Vascular disease of the central nervous system. In: Greenfield's neuropathology. BLACKWOOD, W., MCMENEMY, W.H., MEYER, A., NORMAN, R.M., RUSSELL, D.S. (eds.), p. 71. London: Arnold 1963

BLACKWOOD, W., CORSELLIS, J.A.N.: Greenfield's Neuropathology, 3rd ed. London: Arnold 1976

BLACKWOOD, W., DODDS, T.C., SOMMERVILLE, J.-C.: Atlas of Neuropathology. Edinburgh: Livingstone 1949

BLADIN, P.F.: A radiologic and pathologic study of embolism of the internal carotid – middle cerebral arterial axis. Radiology **82**, 615–625 (1964)

BLANKENHORN, D.H.: Angiographic evidence of atherosclerosis regression in man. In: Atherosclerosis IV. SCHETTLER, G., GOTO, Y., HATA, Y., KLOSE, G. (eds.), pp. 414–421. Berlin, Heidelberg, New York: Springer 1977

BLAUMANIS, O.: Morphology and hemodynamic consequences of vasospasm. 11th Princeton Conference on Cerebral Vascular Disease 1978. (in press) (1979)

BLOOR, B.M.: Cerebral hemodynamics. The critical closing pressure. Bull. Soc. Int. Chir. **31**, 311–317 (1972)

BLUMENTHAL, H.T., HANDLER, F.P., BLACHE, J.O.: The histogenesis of arteriosclerosis of the larger cerebral arteries, with an analysis of the importance of mechanical factors. Am. J. Med. **17**, 337–347 (1954)

BODECHTEL, G.: Differentialdiagnose neurologischer Krankheitsbilder. 2. Aufl. Stuttgart: Thieme 1963

BÖHNE, C.: Beiträge zum Problem der apoplektischen Hirnblutung. Beitr. pathol. Anat. allg. Pathol. **78**, 260–282 (1927)

BÖHNE, C.: Beiträge zum Problem der apoplektischen Hirnblutung. Beitr. pathol. Anat. allg. Pathol. **86**, 566–612 (1931a)

BÖHNE, C.: Kompakte apoplektische Hirnblutung und hämorrhagische Hirnerweichung (Klinik, Pathologie, Pathogenese). Z. klin. Med. **117**, 31–54 (1931b)

BÖHNE, C.: Über die Bedeutung der Hirnerweichung in der Pathogenese der kompakten apoplektischen Hirnblutung. Z. gesamten Neurol. Psychiatrie **137**, 610–620 (1931c)

BOERI, R., PASSERINI, A.: The megadolichobasilar anomaly. J. Neurol. Sci. **1**, 475–484 (1964)

BÖTTCHER, C.J.F.: Chemische Aspekte der Atherosklerose. Arbeitsgemeinschaft für Forschung des Landes Nordrhein-Westfalen, Heft 164, S. 7–24. Köln, Opladen: Westdeutscher Verlag 1965

BÖTTCHER, C.J.F., WOODFORD, F.P., TER HAAR ROMENY,, C.Ch., BOELSMA, E., VAN GENT, C.M.: Composition of lipids isolated from the aorta, coronary arteries and circulus Willisii of atherosclerotic individuals. Nature **183**, 47–48 (1959)

BOTTON, J.: L'artériosclérose cérébrale au niveau du polygone de Willis. Etude anatomo-clinique et statistique. Encéphale **44**, 350–396 (1955a)

BOTTON, J.: Artériosclérose cérébrale. Etude anatomo-clinique et statistique. Thèse de Genève. Paris: Doin 1955b

BRANN, A.W., MEYERS, R.E.: Central nervous system findings in the newborn monkey following severe in utero partial asphyxia. Neurology (Minneap.) **25**, 327–338 (1975)

BRAUNMÜHL, A. v.: Alterserkrankungen des Zentralnervensystems. Senile Involution. Senile Demenz. Alzheimersche Krankheit. In: Handbuch der speziellen pathologischen Anatomie und Histologie. LUBARSCH, O., HENKE, F., RÖSSLE, E. (Hrsg.), Band XIII, Teil 1A. S. 337–539. Berlin, Göttingen, Heidelberg: Springer 1957

BREDT, H.: Morphologie und Pathogenese der Arteriosklerose. In: Arteriosklerose. Ätiologie, Pathologie, Klinik und Therapie. SCHETTLER, G. (Hrsg.), S. 1–46. Stuttgart: Thieme 1961

BREIG, A., EKBOM, K., GREITZ, T., KUGELBERG, E.: Hydrocephalus due to elongated basilar artery. A new clinicoradiological syndrome. Lancet (1967) I, 874–875

BRICE, J.G., DOWSETT, D.J., LOWE, R.D.: The effect of constriction on carotid blood-flow and pressure gradient. Lancet (1964) I, 84–85

BRIERLEY, J.B.: Pathology of cerebral ischemia. In: Cerebral vascular diseases. MCDOWELL, F.H., BRENNAN, R.W. (eds.), pp. 59–75. New York: Grune & Stratton 1973

BROBEIL, A.: Hirndurchblutungsstörungen. Ihre Klinik und arteriographische Diagnose. Stuttgart: Thieme 1950

BROMAN, T.: Über cerebrale Circulationsstörungen. Tierexperimentelle Untersuchungen über Mikroembolien, Schädigungen der Gefäßpermeabilität und Blutungen verschiedener Art. Acta Pathol. Microbiol. Scand., Supp. 42 (1940)

BRUETMAN, M.E., FIELDS, W.S., CRAWFORD, E.St., DEBAKEY, M.E.: Cerebral hemorrhage in carotid artery surgery. Arch. Neurol. **9**, 458–467 (1963)

BRUETSCH, W.L.: Arteriosclerotic occlusion of cerebral arteries: mechanism and therapeutic considerations. Circulation **11**, 909–913 (1955)

BRUETSCH, W.L., WILLIAMS, C.L.: Embolic cerebral sequel in rheumatic mitral stenosis precipitating senile mental deterioration. Am. J. Psychiatry **116**, 364–365 (1959)

BÜCHNER, F.: Die Coronarinsuffizienz. Dresden: Steinkopff 1939

BÜCHNER, F.: Spezielle Pathologie, 3. Aufl. München, Berlin: Urban & Schwarzenberg 1960

BÜCHNER, F.: Struktur, Stoffwechsel und Funktion in der modernen Pathologie. Vorträge und Vorlesungen in Japan, München, Berlin: Urban & Schwarzenberg 1964

BUERGER, L.: The circulatory disturbances of the extremities. Philadelphia: Saunders 1924

BUERGER, L.: Thrombangiitis obliterans concepts of pathogenesis and pathology. J. Int. Chir. **4**, 399–426 (1939)

BURGER, P.C., BURCH, J.G., KUNZE, U.: Subcortical arteriosclerotic encephalopathy (Binswanger's disease). A vascular etiology of dementia. Stroke **7**, 626–631 (1976)

BURMESTER, K., STENDER, A.: Zwei Fälle von einseitiger Aplasie der Arteria carotis interna bei gleichzeitiger Aneurysmabildung im vorderen Anteil des Circulus arteriosus Willisi. (Zur Frage der Kombination von sackförmigen Aneurysmen der Hirnarterien mit anderen Fehlbildungen). Acta Neurochir. (Wien) **9**, 367–378 (1961)

BYROM, F.B.: The pathogenesis of hypertensive encephalopathy and its relation to the malignant phase of hypertension. Experimental evidence from the hypertensive rat. Lancet (1954) II, 201–211

CAIRNEY, J.: Tortuosity of the cervical segment of the internal carotid artery. J. Anat. **59**, 87–96 (1924)

CARPENTER, M.B., NOBACK, C.R., MOSS, M.L.: The anterior choroidal artery. Its origin, course distribution and variations. Arch. Neurol. Psychiatry **71**, 714–722 (1954)

CARTER, A.B.: Cerebral infarction. Oxford, London, Edinburgh, New York, Paris, Frankfurt: Pergamon Press 1964

CASTAIGNE, P., LHERMITTE, F., GAUTIER, J.C., ESCOUROLLE, R., DEROUESNE, C.: Internal carotid artery occlusion. A study of 61 instances in 50 patients with post-mortem data. Brain **93**, 231–258 (1970)

CATOLA, G.: Etude clinique et anatomo-pathologique sur les lacunes de désintegration cérébrale. Rev. Méd. (Paris) **24**, 778–809 (1904)

CHANSON, J.L., LANDERS, J.W., SWANSON, R.E.: Cotton fiber embolism. A frequent complication of cerebral angiography. Neurology (Minneap.) **13**, 558–560 (1963)

CHARCOT, J.M.: Über die Localisationen der Gehirn-Krankheiten. Vorlesungen. Stuttgart: Verlag von Adolf Bonz 1878

CHARCOT, J.M., BOUCHARD, C.: Nouvelles recherches sur la pathogénie de l'hémorragie cérébrale. Arch. physiol. norm. et pathol. (Paris) **1**, 110–127, 643–675, 725–734 (1868)

CHOROBSKI, J., PENFIELD, W.: Cerebral vasodilator nerves and their pathway from the medulla oblongata with observations on the pial and intracerebral vascular plexus. Arch. Neurol. Psychiatry **28**, 1257–1289 (1932)

COHEN, ST.I., ARONSON, St.M.: Secondary brain stem hemorrhages. Arch. Neurol. **19**, 257–263 (1968)

COHNHEIM, J.: Vorlesungen über allg. Pathologie, 2. Aufl., Vol. I. Berlin: Hirschwald 1882

COLE, F.M., YATES, P.: Intracerebral microaneurysms and small cerebrovascular lesions. Brain **90**, 759–767 (1967)

CONNET, M.C., LAUSCHE, J.M.: Fibromuscular hyperplasia of the internal carotid artery. Report of a case. Ann. Surg. **162**, 59–62 (1965)

CONSTANTINIDIS, J.: L'incidence familiale des lésions cérébrales vasculaires et dégénératives de l'âge avancé. Encéphale **54**, 204–239 (1965)

COOK, T.A., YATES, P.O.: A histometric study of cerebral and renal arteries in normotensive and chronic hypertensives. J. Pathol. Bacteriol. **108**, 129–135 (1972)

COOPER, I.S.: The neurosurgical alleviation of Parkinsonism. Springfield: Thomas 1956

CORDAY, E., ROTHENBERG, S.F.: The clinical aspects of cerebral vascular insufficiency. Ann. Intern. Med. **47**, 626–639 (1957)

CORNING, H.K.: Lehrbuch der topographischen Anatomie. München: Bergmann 1949

COURVILLE, C.B.: Pathology of the central nervous system. Mountain View/California: Pacific Press 1937

COURVILLE, C.B.: Subdural empyema secondary to purulent frontal sinusitis. A clinicopathologic study of forty-two cases verified at autopsy. Arch. Otolaryngol. **39**, 211–230 (1944)

COURVILLE, C.B.: Intracranial complications of otitis media and mastoiditis in the antibiotic era. Laryngoscope **65**, 31–46 (1955)

CRAVIOTO, H.: Occlusion of the basilar artery. A clinical and pathologic study of 14 autopsied cases. Neurology (Minneap.) **8**, 145–157 (1958)

CRAWFORD, J.V., RUSSELL, D.S.: Cryptic arteriovenous and venous hamartomas of the brain. J. Neurol. Neurosurg. Psychiatry **19**, 1–11 (1956)

CRITCHLEY, M.: The anterior cerebral artery and its syndromes. Brain **53**, 121–162 (1930)

CROMPTON, M.R.: The pathogenesis of cerebral infarction following the rupture of cerebral berry aneurysm. Brain **87**, 491–510 (1964)

CRONQVIST, St.: Transitory hyperemia in focal cerebral ischemic lesions. In: Research on the cerebral circulation, III. Int. Salzburg Conference. MEYER, J.S., LECHNER, H., EICHHORN, O. (eds.), pp. 71–82. Springfield/Ill.: Thomas 1969

CRONQVIST, S., EKBERG, R., INGVAR, D.H.: Regional cerebral blood flow related to neuroradiological findings. Acta Neurol. Scand. **41**, Suppl. 14, 176–178 (1965)

CRUVEILHIER, J.: Anatomie pathologique du corps humain ou descriptions avec figures lithographieés et coloriées des diverses altérations morbides dont le corps humain est susceptible. Paris: Baillière 1829a

CRUVEILHIER, J.: Apoplexie. Dictionnaire de médecine et de chirurgie pratiques, Tome III. Paris: Baillière 1829b

DALAL, P.M., SHAH, P.M., SHETH, S.C., DESHPANDE, C.K.: Cerebral embolism. Angiographic observations on spontaneous clot lysis. Lancet (1965), 61–64

D'ALECY, L.G., FEIGL, E.O.: Sympathetic control of cerebral blood flow in dogs. Circ. Res. **31**, 267–283 (1972)

DANDY, W.E.: Changes in our conceptions of localization of certain functions in the brain. Am. J. Physiol. **93**, 643–658 (1930)

DANDY, W.E.: Surgery of the brain. In: Lewis' practice of surgery. Vol. XII, pp. 1–682. Hagerstown/Maryland: Prior 1932

DANDY, W.E.: Location of consciousness center in brain: Corpus striatum. Bull. Johns Hopk. Hosp. **79**, 34–58 (1946)

DAOUD, A.S., GOODALE, F., FLORENTIN, R., BEADENKOPF, W.G.: Chemicoanatomic studies in geographic pathology. Arch. Pathol. **73**, 74–81 (1962)

DAOUD, A.S., JARMOLYCH, J., FRITZ, K., AUGUSTYN, J.: Regression of advanced atherosclerosis in swine. Circulation **49** and **50**, Suppl. III, 92 (1975)

DAVID, N.J., KLINTWORTH, G.K., FRIEDBERG, S.J., DILLON, M.: Fatal atheromatous cerebral embolism associated with bright plaques in the retinal arterioles. Report of a case. Neurology (Minneap.) **13**, 708–713 (1963)

DAWBER, T.R.: Risk factors for atherosclerotic disease. Current concepts, pp. 1–36. Kalamazoo/Minn.: Institute of Imployment Research 1975

DAWBER, T.R., WOLF, Ph.A., COLTON, Th., NICKERSON, R.J.: Risk factors: comparison of the biological data in myocardial and brain infarctions. In: Brain and heart infarct. ZÜLCH, K.J., KAUFMANN, W., HOSSMANN, K.-A., HOSSMANN, V. (eds.), pp. 228–252. Berlin, Heidelberg, New York: Springer 1977

DECKER, K.: Der Schlaganfall als neuroradiologisches Problem. Dtsch. med. Wochenschr. **83**, 205–210 (1958)

DECKER, K.: Klinische Neuroradiologie. Stuttgart: Thieme 1960

DECKER, K.: Clinical Neuroradiology. New York: McGraw-Hill 1966

DEI POLI, G., ZUCHA, J.: Beiträge zur Kenntnis der Anomalien und der Erkrankungen der Arteria carotis interna. Zentralbl. Neurochir. **5**, 209–238 (1940)

DELACHAUX, A.: L'ictus apoplectique, problème de gérontologie. Schweiz. med. Wochenschr. **89**, 223–227 (1959)

DELONG, W.B.: Anatomy of the middle cerebral artery: the temporal branches. Stroke **4**, 412–418 (1973)

DENNY-BROWN, D.: The treatment of recurrent cerebrovascular symptoms and the question of "vasospasm". Med. Clin. North Am. **35**, 1457–1474 (1951)

DENNY-BROWN, D.: Basilar artery syndromes. Bull. New Engl. Med. Cent. **15**, 53–60 (1953)

DENNY-BROWN, D.: Recurrent cerebrovascular episodes. Arch. Neurol. **2**, 194–210 (1960)

DENNY-BROWN, D., MEYER, J.S.: The cerebral collateral circulation. II. Production of cerebral infarction by ischemic anoxia and its reversibility in early stages. Neurology (Minneap.) **7**, 567–579 (1957)

DESAI, B., TOOLE, J.F.: Kinks, coils, and carotids: A review. Stroke **6**, 649–653 (1975)

DILENGE, D., FISCHGOLD, H., DAVID, M.: L'artère ophthalmique. Aspects angiographiques. Neurochirurgie **7**, 249–257 (1961)

DJINDJIAN, M.: Les malformations arterio-veineuses de la moëlle épinière e leur traitement. Thèse pour le doctorat, Univ. Paris 1976

DJINDJIAN, R., HOUDART, R., HURTH, M.: Les angiomes de la moëlle. Paris: Sandoz 1976

DÖRFLER, J.: Ein Beitrag zur Frage der Lokalisation der Arteriosklerose der Gehirngefäße mit besonderer Berücksichtigung der A. carotis interna. Arch. Psychiatr. Nervenkr. **103**, 180–190 (1935)

DOERR, W.: Gangarten der Arteriosklerose. S.-B. Akad. Wiss. Heidelberg, math.-nat. Kl. Heidelberg: Springer 1964

DONIGER, D.E.: Bilateral complete carotid and basilar artery occlusion in a patient with minimal deficit. Neurology (Minneap.) **13**, 673–678 (1963)

DOW, D.R.: The incidence of arteriosclerosis in the arteries of the body. Br. Med. J. **2**, 162–163 (1925)

DOZZI, D.L.: Unsuspected coronary thrombosis in patients with hemiplegia; a clinical study. Ann. Intern. Med. **12**, 1991–1995 (1939)

DROPMANN, K.: Über die Prädilektionsstellen der Atherosklerose und die hämodynamischen Verhältnisse in Krümmerstrecken und an Teilungsstellen. Z. Kreisl. Forsch. **52**, 171–183 (1963)

DUGUID, J.B.: Thrombosis as a factor in the pathogenesis of aortic atherosclerosis. J. Pathol. Bacteriol. **60**, 57–61 (1948)

DUGUID, J.B.: Mural thrombosis in arteries. Br. Med. Bull. **11**, 36–38 (1952)

DUGUID, J.B., ANDERSON, G.S.: The pathogenesis of hyaline arteriosclerosis. J. Pathol. Bacteriol. **64**, 519–526 (1952)

DUMAN, S., STEPHENS, J.W.: Posttraumatic middle cerebral artery occlusion. Neurology (Minneap.) **13**, 613–616 (1963)

DUMAS, M., GIRARD, P.L, COLLOMB, H.: Occlusions bilatérales de la carotide interne associée à une circulation de suppléance cortico-corticale, transdurale, et du type "Moya-Moya" chez l'enfant noir. J. Neurol. Sci. **16**, 1–25 (1972)

DURAND-FARDEL, M.: Traité clinique et pratique des maladies des vieillards. Paris: 1854

DURET, H.: Sur la distribution des artères nourricières du bulbe rachidien. Arch. Physiol. (Paris) **5**, 97 (1873)

EASTCOTT, H.H.G., PICKERING, G.W., ROB, C.G.: Reconstruction of internal carotid artery in a patient with intermittent attacks of hemiplegia. Lancet (1954) **II**, 994–996

EDVINSSON, L., OWMAN, C.: Neurovascular aminergic and peptidergic functions in brain and the possible pathophysiological role in cerebral vasospasm. In: Brain and heart infarct. ZÜLCH, K.J., KAUFMANN, W., HOSSMANN, K.-A., HOSSMANN, V. (eds.), pp. 140–156. Berlin, Heidelberg, New York: Springer 1979

EEG-COLLOQUE DE MARSEILLE A COLOGNE, 1964 (unpublished)

EICH, J., WIEMERS, K.: Über die Permeabilität der Bluthirnschranke gegenüber Trypanblau, speziell im akuten Sauerstoffmangel. Dtsch. Z. Nervenheilkd. **164**, 537–559 (1950)

EICKE, W.J.: Gehirngefäßveränderungen bei Hypertonie. Atti del Primo Congresso Internationale di Istopathologia del Sistema Nervoso, Roma 1952, pp. 249–257. Torino: Rosenberg & Sellier 1952

EICKE, W.J.: Die Endangiitis obliterans der Hirngefäße. In: Handbuch der speziellen pathologischen Anatomie und Histologie. LUBARSCH, O., HENKE, F., RÖSSLE, R. (Hrsg.), Band XIII, Teil 1 B, S. 1536–1575. Berlin, Göttingen, Heidelberg: Springer 1957

EINSIEDEL-LECHTAPE, H., KLEIHUES, P.: Pathology of cerebral vascular insufficiency. In: Radiology of the skull and brain. Anatomy and pathology. HEWTON, Th.H., POTTS, D.G. (eds.), Vol. III, pp. 3173–3196. St. Louis: Mosby 1977

EISENLOHR, L.: Über Bulbär- und Ponsaffektionen. Arch. Psychiatr. Nervenkr. **9**, 1–48 (1879)

EKSTRÖM-JODAL, B., HÄGGENDAL, E., LINDER, L.-E., NILSSON, N.J.: Cerebral blood flow autoregulation at high arterial pressures and different levels of carbon dioxide tension in dogs. Eur. Neurol. **6**, 6–10 (1971/1972)

EKSTRÖM-JODAL, B., HÄGGENDAL, E., JOHANSSON, B., LINDER, L.-E., NILSSON, N.J.: Acute arterial hypertension and the blood brain barrier: An experimental study in dogs. In: Cerebral circulation and metabolism. LANGFITT, T.W., MCHENRY, L.C. jr., REIVICH, M., WOLLMAN, H. (eds.), pp. 7–9. Berlin, Heidelberg, New York: Springer 1975

ELLINGTON, A.L.: The smaller intracerebral vessels. Stroke **1**, 128–134 (1970)

ELLIS, A.G.: The pathogenesis of spontaneous cerebral hemorrhage. Proc. Pathol. Soc. Philad. **12** (New Series) **3**, 197–239 (1909)

ELVIDGE, A.R., WERNER, A.: Hemiplegia and thrombosis of the internal carotid system. Arch. Neurol. **66**, 752–782 (1951)

EPPINGER, H.: Pathogenesis (Histogenesis und Aetiologie) der Aneurysmen. Langenbecks Arch. klin. Chir. **35**, Supplementum, (1887)

EPPINGER, H.: Die miliaren Hirnarterienaneurysmen (Charcot-Bouchard). Virchows Arch. pathol. Anat. **111**, 405–414 (1888)

EPSTEIN, F.H.: Die Epidemiologie des Hochdrucks. Verh. Dtsch. Ges. inn. Med. **80**, 36–42 (1974)

EPSTEIN, F.H.: Highlights of epidemiological research in western countries. In: Atherosclerosis IV. SCHETTLER, G., GOTO, Y., HATA, Y., KLOSE, G. (eds.), pp. 471–478. Berlin, Heidelberg, New York: Springer 1977

EPSTEIN, F.H., ECKHOFF, R.D.: The epidemiology of high blood pressure – geographic distribution and etiological factors. In: Epidemiology of hypertension. STAMLER, J., STAMLER, R. (eds.), p. 155. New York: Grune & Stratton 1967

ERICSON, K., METTINGER, K.L.: Fibromuscular dysplasia (FMD). A neglected risk factor for stroke before 55? In: 11th World Congress of Neurology, Amsterdam, Sept. 11–16, 1977, p. 48. Amsterdam, Oxford: Excerpta Medica 1977

EROS, G.: Observations on cerebral arteriosclerosis. J. Neuropathol. Exp. Neurol. **10**, 257–294 (1951)

ESCHBACH, O., ZÜLCH, K.J.: Seltene angiographische Befunde bei cerebro-vasculärer Insuffizienz. Radiologe **9**, 415–418 (1969)

ESCOLA, J.: Die Gewebsveränderungen bei Thrombosen der Sinus und cerebralen Venen. Arch. Psychiatr. Nervenkr. **203**, 342–357 (1962)

ETTINGER, M.G.: Thromboelastographic studies in cerebral infarction. Stroke **5**, 350–354 (1974)

Executive Committee of the Council on Cerebral Vascular Disease of the American Heart Association: Risk factors in stroke due to cerebral infarction. Stroke **2**, 423–428 (1971)

FAHR, Th.: Apoplexie und Erweichung. Vergleichende statistische Untersuchungen. Zentralbl. allg. Pathol. pathol. Anat. **66**, 84–93 (1937)

FALCONER, M.A.: Surgical treatment of spontaneous intracerebral hemorrhage. Br. Med. J. **1**, 790–792 (1958)

FANG, H.C.H., FOLEY, J.M.: Hypertensive hemorrhages of the pons and cerebellum. Trans. Am. Neurol. Assoc. **79**, 126–130 (1954)

FANKHAUSER, R., LUGINBÜHL, H.: Pathologische Anatomie des zentralen und peripheren Nervensystems der Haustiere. Berlin, Hamburg: Pary 1968

FANKHAUSER, R., LUGINBÜHL, H., MCGRATH, J.T.: Cerebrovascular disease in various animal species. Ann. N.Y. Acad. Sci. **127**, 817–860 (1965)

FASANO, V.A., BROGGI, G.: Aspect clinique et chirurgical de l'hémorragie cérébrale. Neurochirurgie **2**, 357–387 (1956)

FAWCETT, E., BLACKFORD, J.V.: The circle of Willis: an examination of 700 specimens. J. Anat. **40**, 63–71 (1906)

FAY, T.: The cerebral vasculature. J. Am. Med. Assoc. **89**, 1727–1730 (1925)

FAZIO, C.: Betrachtungen zur Frage des assoziierten Coronar- und Gehirnsyndroms. Schweiz. med. Wochenschr. **79**, 1108–1109 (1949)

FAZIO, C.: Observations sur la pathogénèse de l'infarctus cerebral. In: Der Hirnkreislauf in Forschung und Klinik. 2. Int. Salzburg Conference

1964. EICHHORN, O., LECHNER, H., AUELL, K.-H. (Hrsg.), S. 117–123. Wien: Brüder Hollinek 1964

FAZIO, C., FIESCHI, C., AGNOLI, A., BUGIANI, O., GOTTLIEB, A.: Fréquence et rôle des anomalies du polygone de Willis et de l'artériosclérose dans l'apoplexie cérébrale. In: Symposium International sur la Circulation Cérébrale, Paris, 15–16 Octobre 1965, p. 225–236. Paris: Sandoz 1966

FAZIO, C., FIESCHI, C., AGNOLI, A.: The "intracerebral steal": a phenomenon in the pathogenesis of focal brain ischemia. In: Cerebral circulation and stroke. ZÜLCH, K.J. (ed.), pp. 143–147. Berlin, Heidelberg, New York: Springer 1971

FEINLEIB, M.: The epidemiology of coronary heart disease. In: Brain and heart infarct. ZÜLCH, K.J., KAUFMANN, W., HOSSMANN, K.-A., HOSSMANN, V. (eds.), pp. 4–19. Berlin, Heidelberg, New York: Springer 1979

FERKOVIĆ, M., POLJAKOVIĆ, Z., DOGAN, S., UGLESIC, B., REIC, P.: Transient ischemic attacks (TIA): Epidemiological and geomedical study. In: 11th World Congress of Neurology, Amsterdam, September 11–16, 1977. DEN HARTOG JAGER, W.A., BRUYN, G.W., HEIJSTEE, A.P.J. (eds.), Abstracts, p. 53. Amsterdam, Oxford: Excerpta Medica 1977

FETTERMAN, G.H., MORAN, T.J.: Anomalies of the circle of Willis in relation to cerebral softening. Arch. Pathol. **32**, 251–257 (1941)

FIELDS, W.S.: Stenosis of internal carotid artery. (Abstract). Int. Congr. Ser. No. 193, p. 11. Amsterdam-Oxford: Excerpta Medica 1969

FIELDS, W.S., CRAWFORD, E.S., DEBAKEY, M.E.: Surgical considerations in cerebral arterial insufficiency. Neurology (Minneap.) **8**, 801–808 (1958)

FIELDS, W.S., BRUETMAN, M.E., WEIBEL, J.: Collateral circulation of the brain. Monogr. Surg. Sci. **2**, 183–259 (1965)

FIELDS, W.S., MASLENIKOV, V., MEYER, J.S., HASS, W.K., REMINGTON, R.D., MACDONALD, M.: Joint study of extracranial arterial occlusion. V. Progress report of prognosis following surgery or nonsurgical treatment for transient cerebral ischemic attacks and cervical carotid artery lesions. J. Am. Med. Assoc. **211**, 1993–2003 (1970)

FIELDS, W.S., NORTH, R.R., HASS, W.K., GALBRAITH, J.G., WYLIE, E.J., RATINOV, G., BURNS, M.H., MACDONALD, M.C., MEYER, J.S.: Joint study of extracranial arterial occlusion as a cause of stroke. I. Organization of study and survey of patient population. J. Am. Med. Assoc. **203**, 955–960 (1968)

FIESCHI, C., AGNOLI, A., PRENCIPE, M., BATTISTINI, N., BOZZAO, L., NARDINI, M.: Impairment of the regional vasomotor response of cerebral vessels to hypercarbia in vascular diseases. Eur. Neurol. **2**, 13–30 (1969)

FINKEMEYER, H.: Zur Diagnose und Behandlung der extracraniellen Aneurysmen der A. carotis interna. Zentralbl. Neurochir. **10**, 210–214 (1950)

FISCHER-BRÜGGE, E.: Der persistierende Hirnprolaps nach Schußverletzungen. Zentralbl. Neurochir. **9**, 18–45 (1949)

FISHER, A.G.T.: A case of complete absence of both internal carotid arteries, with a preliminary note on the developmental history of the stapedial artery. J. Anat. **48**, 37–46 (1913)

FISHER, C.M.: Transient monocular blindness associated with hemiplegia. Arch. Ophthalmol. **47**, 167–203 (1952)

FISHER, C.M.: Occlusion of the carotid arteries. Further experiences. Arch. Neurol. **72**, 187–204 (1954)

FISHER, C.M.: Cerebral thrombangiitis obliterans. Medicine (Baltimore) **36**, 169–209 (1957)

FISHER, C.M.: Observations of the fundus oculi in transient monocular blindness. Neurology (Minneap.) **9**, 333–347 (1959)

FISHER, C.M.: The pathology and pathogenesis of intracerebral hemorrhage. In: Pathogenesis and treatment of cerebrovascular disease. FIELDS, W.S. (ed.), pp. 295–311. Springfield/Ill.: Thomas 1961

FISHER, C.M.: Pure sensory stroke involving face, arm and leg. Neurology (Minneap.) **15**, 76–80 (1965a)

FISHER, C.M.: Lacunes: small deep cerebral infarcts. Neurology (Minneap.) **15**, 774–784 (1965b)

FISHER, C.M.: The circle of Willis: Anatomical variations. Vasc. Dis. **2**, 99–105 (1965c)

FISHER, C.M.: A lacunar stroke. The dysarthria-clumsy hand syndrome. Neurology (Minneap.) **17**, 614–617 (1967)

FISHER, C.M.: The arterial lesions underlying lacunes. Acta Neuropathol. (Berl.) **12**, 1–15 (1969)

FISHER, C.M.: Pathological observations in hypertensive cerebral hemorrhage. J. Neuropathol. Exp. Neurol. **30**, 536–550 (1971)

FISHER, C.M., ADAMS, R.D.: Observations on brain embolism with special reference to the mechanism of hemorrhagic infarction. J. Neuropathol. Exp. Neurol. **10**, 92–93 (1951)

FISHER, C.M., CAPLAN, L.R.: Basilar artery branch occlusion: a cause of pontine infarction. Neurology (Minneap.) **21**, 900–905 (1971)

FISHER, C.M., KARNES, W.E., KUBIK, C.S.: Lateral medullary infarction. – The pattern of vascular occlusion. J. Neuropathol. Exp. Neurol. **20**, 323–379 (1961)

FISHER, C.M., GORE, J., OKABE, N., WHITE, P.D.: Atherosclerosis of the carotid and vertebral arteries – extracranial and intracranial. J. Neuropathol. Exp. Neurol. **24**, 455–476 (1965a)

FISHER, C.M., PICARD, E.H., POLAK, A., DALAL, P., OJEMANN, R.G.: Acute hypertensive cerebellar hemorrhage: diagnosis and surgical treatment. J. Nerv. Ment. Dis. **140**, 38–57 (1965b)

FLETCHER, A.P., ALKJAERSIG, N., DAVIES, A., LEWIS, M., BROOKS, J., HARDIN, W., LANDAU, W., RAICHLE, M.E.: Blood coagulation and plasma fibrinolytic enzyme system pathophysiology in stroke. Stroke **7**, 337–348 (1976)

FLORA, G.C., BAKER, A.B., KLASSEN, A.C.: Age and cerebral atherosclerosis. J. Neurol. Sci. **6**, 357–372 (1968a)

FLORA, G.C., BAKER, A.B., LOEWENSON, R.B., KLASSEN, A.C.: A comparative study of cerebral atherosclerosis in males and females. Circulation **38**, 859–869 (1968b)

FLORY, C.M.: Arterial occlusions produced by emboli from eroded aortic atheromatous plaques. Am. J. Pathol. **21**, 549–565 (1945)

FOG, M.: Cerebral circulation: II. Reaction of pial arteries to increase in blood pressure. Arch. Neurol. **41**, 260–268 (1939)

FOIX, Ch., HILLEMAND, P.: Le syndrome de l'artère cérébrale antérieure. Encéphale **20**, 209–232 (1925a)

FOIX, Ch., HILLEMAND, P.: Les artères de l'axe encéphalique jusqu'au diencéphale inclusivement. Rev. Neurol. **2**, 705–739 (1925b)

FOIX, Ch., LEY, J.: Contribution à l'étude du ramollissement cérébral envisagé au point de vue de sa fréquence, de son siège et de l'état anatomique des artères du territoire nécrosé. J. Neurol. (Bux.) **27**, 658–684 (1927)

FOIX, Ch., HILLEMAND, P., LEY, J.: Relativement au ramollissement cérébral, à sa fréquence, à son siège, et à l'importance relative des oblitérations artérielles complètes ou incomplètes dans sa pathogénie. Bull. Soc. Méd. Paris **43**, 189–199 (1927)

FORBES, H.S., COBB, St.S.: Vasomotor control of cerebral vessels. Res. Publ. Assoc. Nerv. Ment. Dis. **18**, 201–217 (1938)

FORBES, H.S., WOLFF, H.G.: Cerebral circulation: III. The vasomotor control of the cerebral vessels. Arch. Neurol. **19**, 1057–1086 (1928)

FORD, F.R., CLARK, D.: Thrombosis of basilar artery with softenings in cerebellum and brain stem due to manipulation of neck; report of 2 cases with one post-mortem examination. Bull. Johns Hopk. Hosp. **98**, 37–42 (1956)

FOSTER, J.H.: Blood pressure of foreigners in China. Arch. Intern. Med. **40**, 38–45 (1927)

FOWLER, N.O.: Thromboembolism: a survey of the recent literature. Angiology **1**, 257–287 (1950)

FRANTZEN, E., JACOBSEN, H.H., THERKELSEN, J.: Cerebral artery occlusions in children due to trauma to the head and neck. A report of 6 cases verified by cerebral angiography. Neurology (Minneap.) **11**, 695–700 (1961)

FRASER, R.A.R., ZIMBLER, S.M.: Hindbrain stroke in children caused by extracranial vertebral artery trauma. Stroke **6**, 153–159 (1975)

FREEMAN, J., ELLIS, W.R., KOX, L.J.: Occlusion of the basilar artery. Neurology (Minneap.) **3**, 154–157 (1953)

FREITAG, E.: Fatal hypertensive intracerebral haematomas: a survey of the pathological anatomy of 393 cases. J. Neurol. Neurosurg. Psychiatry **31**, 616–620 (1968)

FRIEDE, R.L.: Zur Pathogenese des Hirnschadens nach cerebraler Blutung. Schweiz. med. Wochenschr. **82**, 1257–1259 (1952)

FRIEDE, R.L.: An enzyme histochemical study of cerebral arteriosclerosis. Acta Neuropathol. (Berl.) **2**, 58–72 (1962)

FRIEDE, R.L., ROESSMANN, U.: The pathogenesis of secondary midbrain hemorrhages. Neurology (Minneap.) **16**, 1210–1216 (1966)

FRIEDLANDER, W.J.: About three old men: an inquiry into how cerebral arteriosclerosis has altered world politics. Stroke **3**, 467–473 (1972)

FUJISHIMA, M., OMAE, T., TAKEYA, Y., TAKESHITA, M., OGATA, J., UEDA, K.: Prognosis of occlusive cerebrovascular diseases in normotensive and hypertensive subjects. Stroke **7**, 472–476 (1976)

FUKUSCHIMA, K., UENO, A., SAITO, K.: Relationship between Takayasu's arteritis and giant-cell arteritis. Folia Angiol. (Pisa) **23**, 68–71 (1975)

FURLANI, J.: The anterior choroidal artery and its blood supply to the internal capsule. Acta Anat. **85**, 108–112 (1973)

GÄNSHIRT, H.: Die Sauerstoffversorgung des Gehirns und ihre Störung bei der Liquordrucksteigerung und beim Hirnödem. Monographien a. d. Gesamtgebiete der Neurologie und Psychiatrie, Heft 81. Berlin, Göttingen, Heidelberg: Springer 1957

GÄNSHIRT, H.: Der Hirnkreislauf. Physiologie, Pathologie, Klinik. Stuttgart: Thieme 1972

GALLIGIONI, F., ANDRIOLI, G.C., MARIN, G., BRIANI, S., IRACI, G.: Hypoplasia of the internal carotid artery associated with cerebral pseudoangiomatosis. Am. J. Roentgenol. **112**, 251–262 (1971)

GAMACHE, F.W., MYERS, R.E.: Effects of hypotension on rhesus monkeys. Arch. Neurol. **32**, 374–380 (1975)

GAMACHE, F.W., DOLD, G.M., MYERS, R.E.: Changes in cortical impedance and EEG activity induced by profound hypotension. Am. J. Physiol. **228**, 1914–1920 (1975)

GARCIN, R., PESTEL, M.: Thrombophlébites cérébrales. Paris: Masson 1949

GARDNER, W.J.: Traumatic subdural hematoma with particular reference to the latent interval. Arch. Neurol. **27**, 847–858 (1932)

GARDNER, W.J.: Traumatic subdural hematoma; report of 22 cases. Ohio State Med. J. **31**, 660–665 (1935)

GASTAUT, H., BEHREND, R.Ch.: Die klinische und elektroencephalographische Differentialdiagnostik der fokalen und generalisierten epileptischen und ischämischen Anfälle. Acta Neuroveg. (Wien) **23**, 137–153 (1961)

GASTAUT, H., NAQUET, R.: Colloque de Marseille à Cologne. (unpublished) (1964)

GASTAUT, H., NAQUET, R.: Etude électroencéphalographique de l'insuffisance circulatoire cérébrale. In: Symposium international sur la circulation cérébrale, Paris 1965, p. 163–191. Paris: Sandoz 1966

GASTAUT, H., NAQUET, R., VIGOUROUX, R.A.: The vascular syndrome of the parieto-temporo-occipital "triangle" based on 18 cases. In: Cerebral circulation and stroke. ZÜLCH, K.J. (ed.), pp. 82–92. Berlin, Heidelberg, New York: Springer 1971

GAUTIER, J.-C., ROSA, A., LHERMITTE, F.: Auscultation carotidienne. Corrélations chez 200 patients avec 332 angiographies. Rev. Neurol. **131**, 175–184 (1975)

GEJROT, T., LAUREN, T.: Retrograde venography of the internal jugular veins and transverse sinuses; Technique and anatomy. Acta Otolaryngol. (Stockh.) **57**, 556–610 (1964)

GERAUD, J., LAZORTHES, G., BES, A.: L'ischémie cérébrale dans le territoire carotidien. Journées Internationales de Circulation Cérébrale, Toulouse 1972. Suppl. à la Revue de Médecine de Toulouse, Juin 1973

GERLACH, J., JENSEN, H.P.: Die intracerebralen Haematome bei Mikroangiomen. Acta Neurochir. (Wien), Suppl. **7**, 367–373 (1961)

GERLACH, J., JENSEN, H.: Mikroangiome des Gehirns. Langenbecks Arch. klin. Chir. **293**, 481–493 (1965)

GERLACH, J., JENSEN, H.-P., KOOS, W., KRAUS, H.: Pädiatrische Neurochirurgie. Stuttgart: Thieme 1967

GIERTSEN, J.C.: Atherosclerosis in an autopsy series: 6. Relation of cerebral atherosclerosis to age and sex. Acta Pathol. Microbiol. Scand. **65**, 329–339 (1966)

GILLILAN, L.A.: Significant superficial anastomoses in the arterial blood supply to the brain. J. Comp. Neurol. **112**, 55–74 (1959)

GILLILAN, L.A.: The correlation of the blood supply to the human brain stem with clinical brain stem lesions. J. Neuropathol. Exp. Neurol. **23**, 78–108 (1964)

GILROY, J., MEYER, J.S.: Auscultation of the neck in occlusive cerebrovascular disease. Circulation **25**, 300–310 (1962)

GILROY, J., MEYER, J.S.: Medical neurology. London: Macmillan 1969

GINSBERG, M.D., MYERS, R.E.: Fetal brain damage following maternal carbon monoxide intoxication. An experimental study. Acta Obstet. Gynecol. Scand. **53**, 309–317 (1974a)

GINSBERG, M.D., MYERS, R.E.: Experimental carbon monoxide encephalopathy in the primate. I. Physiologic and metabolic aspects Arch. Neurol. **30**, 202–208 (1974b)

GINSBERG, M.D., MYERS, R.E., MCDONAGH, B.F.: Experimental carbon monoxide encephalopathy in the primate. II. Clinical aspects, neuropathology, and physiologic correlation. Arch. Neurol. **30**, 209–216 (1974)

GLOBUS, J.H., EPSTEIN, J.A.: Massive cerebral hemorrhage: spontaneous and experimentally induced. J. Neuropathol. Exp. Neurol. **12**, 107–131 (1953)

GLYNN, A.A.: Vascular diseases of the nervous system, a series of 315 cases. Br. Med. J. **1**, 1216–1219 (1956)

GOFMAN, J.W., JONES, H.B., STRISOWER, B., TRAMPLIN, A.R.: Evaluation of serum lipoproteins and cholesterol measurements as predictors of clinical complications of atherosclerosis. Report of a cooperative study of lipoproteins and atherosclerosis. Appendix A. Circulation **14**, 725–731 (1956)

GOLDNER, J.C., WHISNANT, J.P., TAYLOR, W.F.: Long-term prognosis of transient cerebral ischemic attacks. Stroke **2**, 160–167 (1971)

GOMENSORO, J.B., MASLENIKOV, V., DE BONI, J.A., LAGUARDIA DE PEREZ, G., PURRIEL, J., MEDOC, J., RODRIGUEZ BARRIOS, R., ABO, J.C., TENYI, A., AZAMBUJA, N.: Ulcerated atheromatous plaques of the carotid artery bifurcation. Stroke **4**, 912–916 (1973)

GORE, I., TEJADA, C.: The quantitative appraisal of atherosclerosis. Am. J. Pathol. **33**, 875–884 (1957)

GOUAZE, A., LAZORTHES, G., SANTINI, J.-J.: Les anastomoses artérielles corticales. Evolution morphologique et physiologique. In: L'ischémie cérébrale dans le territoire carotidien. GERAUD, J., LAZORTHES, G., BES, A. (eds.), pp. 17–23. Toulouse: Suppl. à la Revue de Médecine de Toulouse 1973

GOWERS, W.R.: Handbuch der Nervenkrankheiten. Bonn: Cohen 1892

GRAF, O.: Physiologische Leistungsbereitschaft und nervöse Belastung. In: Jb. 1954 der Max-Planck-Ges., S. 97–123. Göttingen: Hubert 1955

GRASSET, J.: La claudication intermittente des centres nerveux. Rev. Neurol. **14**, 433–440 (1906)

GREENFIELD, J.C. jr., TINDALL, G.T.: Effect of acute increase in intracranial pressure on blood flow in the internal carotid artery of man. J. Clin. Invest. **44**, 1343–1351 (1965)

GREITZ, T.: A radiological study of the brain circulation by rapid serial angiography of the carotid artery. Acta Radiol. [Suppl.] (Stockh.), **140**, 1–123 (1956)

GREITZ, T.: Angiography in the investigation of patients with stroke. In: Stroke. Thule Int. Symp. 1966. ENGEL, A., LARSSON, T. (eds.), pp. 159–165. Stockholm: Nordiska Bokhandelns Förlag 1967

GREITZ, T., LÖFSTEDT, S.: The relationship between the third ventricle and the basilar artery. Acta Radiol. (Stockh.) **42**, 85–100 (1954)

GRESHAM, G.A.: Atherosklerose: ihre Ursachen und potentielle Reversibilität. Triangel **15**, 39–43 (1976)

GRILLO, P., PATTERSON, R.H.: Occlusion of the carotid artery: prognosis (natural history) and the possibilities of surgical revascularization. Stroke **6**, 17–20 (1975)

GRINDAL, A.B., TOOLE, J.F.: Headache and transient ischemic attacks. Stroke **5**, 603–606 (1974)

GRÜNTHAL, E.: Die pathologische Anatomie der senilen Demenz und der Alzheimerschen Krankheit. (Mit besonderer Berücksichtigung der Beziehungen zur Klinik). In: Handbuch der Geisteskrankheiten, Bd. XI, Teil VII: Die Anatomie der Psychosen. BUMKE, O. (Hrsg.), S. 638–672. Berlin: Springer 1930

GUIOT, G., LE BESNERAIS, Y.: Oblitérations de l'artère cérébrale moyenne sans séquelles neurologiques.

Remarques sur les facteurs influençant l'efficacité des anastomoses périphériques. Neurochirurgie **1**, 287–291 (1955)

Guizetti, P.: Contributo sperimentale alla conoscenza dell'istogenesi del ramollimento cerebrale ischemico. Arch. Sci. Med. **21**, 1 (1897)

Gunning, A.J., Pickering, G.W., Robb-Smith, A.H., Russell, R.W.R.: Mural thrombosis of the internal carotid artery and subsequent embolism. Q. J. Med. **33**, 155–195 (1964)

Gurdjian, E.S., Thomas, L.M.: Operative neurosurgery, 3rd ed. Baltimore: Williams & Wilkins 1970

Gurdjian, E.S., Webster, J.E.: Stroke resulting from internal carotid artery thrombosis in the neck. J. Am. Med. Assoc. **151**, 541–545 (1953)

Gurdjian, E.S., Hardy, W.G., Lindner, D.W.: The surgical considerations of 258 patients with carotid artery occlusion. Surg. Gynecol. Obstet. **110**, 327–338 (1960)

Gurdjian, E.S., Hardy, W.G., Lindner, D.W., Thomas, L.M.: Analysis of occlusive disease of carotid artery and the stroke syndrome. J. Am. Med. Assoc. **176**, 194–204 (1961a)

Gurdjian, E.S., Lindner, D.W., Hardy, W.G., Thomas, L.M.: "Completed stroke" due to occlusive cerebro-vascular disease. An analysis of 409 cases. Neurology (Minneap.) **11**, 724–733 (1961b)

Gurdjian, E.S., Lindner, D.W., Hardy, W.G., Thomas, L.M.: Incidence of surgically treatable lesions in cases studied angiographically. Neurology (Minneap.) **11**, 150–152 (1961c)

Gurdjian, E.S., Portnoy, H.D., Hardy, W.G., Lindner, D.W., Thomas, L.M.: Evaluation of tortuosity of extracranial vessels. Angiology **6**, 261–272 (1964a)

Gurdjian, E.S., Hardy, W.G., Lindner, D.W., Thomas, L.M.: Four-vessel-angiography: experiences with three hundred consecutive cases. Clin. Neurosurg. **10**, 251–274 (1964b)

Hacker, H.: Abflußwege der Sylvischen Venengruppe. Radiologe **8**, 383–387 (1968)

Häggendal, E., Johansson, B.: Pathophysiological aspects of the blood brain barrier change in acute arterial hypertension. Eur. Neurol. **6**, 24–28 (1971/1972)

Haferl, A.: Lehrbuch der topographischen Anatomie. Berlin, Göttingen, Heidelberg: Springer 1953

Hallervorden, J.: Die extrapyramidalen Erkrankungen. In: Handbuch der Geisteskrankheiten, Band XI, Teil VII: Die Anatomie der Psychosen. Bumke, O. (Hrsg.), S. 996–1062. Berlin: Springer 1930

Hanau, J., Redondo, A.: Anatomie pathologique de l'ischémie cérébrale compliquant les ruptures des anévrismes sus-tentoriels. In: L'ischémie cérébrale dans le territoire carotidien. Geraud, J., Lazorthes, G., Bes, A. (eds.), pp. 77–79. Toulouse: Suppl. à la Revue de Médecine de Toulouse 1973

Hanaway, J., Torack, R., Fletcher, A.P., Landau, W.M.: Intracranial bleeding associated with urokinase therapy for acute ischemic hemispheral stroke. Stroke **7**, 143–146 (1976)

Handa, J., Handa, H.: Progressive cerebral arterial occlusive disease: analysis of 27 cases. Neuroradiology **3**, 119–133 (1972)

Handa, H., Tani, E., Handa, J., Kondo, A., Kikuchi, H., Sato, K.: Idiopathic occlusive arterial disorders in the cervical region and the main trunks of the cerebral arteries in Japan. In: A disease with abnormal vascular network – spontaneous occlusion of the circle of Willis. Kudo, T. (ed.), pp. 83–88. Tokyo: Igaku Shoin 1967

Hannah, J.B.: Civilization, race, and coronary atheroma with particular reference to its incidence and severity in copperbelt Africans. Cent. Afr. J. Med. **4**, 1 (1958)

Hansen, K., Peters, E.: Symptomatologie und Pathogenese eines Falles von migraine ophthalmique associée (Charcot): Syndrom der A. chorioidea anterior. Klin. Monatsbl. Augenheilkd. **105**, 521–542 (1940)

Harper, A.M.: Autoregulation of cerebral blood flow: Influence of the arterial blood pressure on the blood flow through the cerebral cortex. J. Neurol. Neurosurg. Psychiatry **29**, 398–403 (1966)

Harper, A.M., Glass, H.I.: Effect of alterations in the arterial carbon dioxide tension on the blood flow through the cerebral cortex at normal and low arterial blood pressures. J. Neurol. Neurosurg. Psychiatry **28**, 449–452 (1965)

Harris, L.S., Roessmann, U., Friede, R.L.: Bursting of cerebral ventricular walls. J. Pathol. Bacteriol. **96**, 33–38 (1968)

Harvey, J., Rasmussen, T.: Occlusion of the middle cerebral artery: An experimental study. Arch. Neurol. Psychiatry **66**, 20–29 (1951)

Hass, W.K., Fields, W.S., North, R.R., Kricheff, I.I., Chase, N.E., Bauer, R.B.: Joint study of extracranial arterial occlusion. II. Arteriography, techniques, sites and complications. J. Am. Med. Assoc. **203**, 961–968 (1968)

Hasse, K.E.: Über Verschliessung der Hirnarterien als nächste Ursache einer Form der Hirnerweichung. Z. ration. Med. **4**, 91–111 (1846)

Hasse, K.E.: Krankheiten des Nervensystems. In: Handbuch der speziellen Pathologie und Therapie, 1. Abt. Virchow, R. (Hrsg.), Band 4, S. 1–686. Erlangen: Enke 1855

Hasselbach, H.v.: Die Endangiitis obliterans. Stuttgart: Thieme 1939

Hassin, G.B.: Histopathology of the peripheral and central nervous system, 3rd ed. Hamilton/Ill.: Hamilton Press 1948

Hassler, O.: Morphological studies on the large cerebral arteries; with reference to the aetiology of subarachnoid haemorrhage. Acta Psychiatr. Scand. **36**, Suppl. **154** (1961)

Hayem, G.: Sur la thrombose artérielle du tronc basilaire comme cause de mort rapide. Arch. Physiol. norm. Pathol. **1**, 270–289 (1868)

Heberer, G., Rau, G., Schoop, W.: Angiologie, Grundlagen, Klinik und Praxis, 2. Aufl. Stuttgart: Thieme 1974

Heidrich, R.: Die subarachnoidale Blutung. Leipzig: Thieme 1970

Heidrich, R.: Subarachnoid haemorrhage. In: Handbook of Clinical Neurology, Vinken, P.J., Bruyn, G.W. (eds.), Vol. 12, pp. 68–204. Amsterdam: North-Holland, New York: American Elsevier 1972

Heiss, W.-D.: Relationship of cerebral blood flow to neurological deficit and to long-term prognosis of stroke. In: Brain and Heart Infarct. Zülch, K.J., Kaufmann, W., Hossmann, K.-A., Hossmann, V. (eds.), pp. 280–292. Berlin, Heidelberg, New York: Springer 1979

Heiss, W.-D., Waltz, A.G., Hayakawa, T.: Microflow and unit activity in the cerebral cortex following ligation of the middle cerebral artery. In: Brain and heart infarct. Zülch, K.J., Kaufmann, W., Hossmann, K.-A., Hossmann, V. (eds.), pp. 137–149. Berlin, Heidelberg, New York: Springer 1977

Helms, J.: Die Gefäße der hinteren Schädelgrube. Anatomie, Pathophysiologie, Klinik – eine Übersicht. Arch. Otorhinolaryngol. **219**, 179–196 (1978)

Hensch, U.: Carotis-Interna-Verschluß im Halsteil. 135 Fälle. Doktor-Dissertation, Universität Köln 1979

Herxheimer, G.: Über Arteriolonekrose der Nieren. Virch. Arch. pathol. Anat. **251**, 709–717 (1924)

Heubner, O.: Zur Topographie der Ernährungsgebiete der einzelnen Hirnarterien. Zentralbl. med. Wiss. **10**, 817–821 (1872)

Heubner, O.: Die luetische Erkrankung der Hirnarterien. Leipzig: Vogel 1874

Heyman, A., Leviton, A., Millinkan, C.H., Nefzger, M.D., Ostfeld, A.M., Sahs, A.L., Stallones, R.A., Whisnant, J.P.: Transient focal cerebral ischemia: Epidemiological and clinical aspects. Stroke **5**, 277–287 (1974)

Hicks, S.P., Warren, S.: Infarction of the brain without thrombosis. An analysis of 100 cases with autopsies. Arch. Pathol. **52**, 403–412 (1951)

Hiller, Fr.: Circulationsstörungen im Gehirn, eine klinische und pathologisch-anatomische Studie. Arch. Psychiatr. Nervenkr. **103**, 1–53 (1935)

Hiller, Fr.: Die Zirkulationsstörungen des Gehirns und Rückenmarks. In: Handbuch der Neurologie, Bumke, O., Foerster, O. (Hrsg.), Band XI, S. 178–465. Berlin: Springer 1936

Hiller, Fr.: Aussprachebemerkung zum haemorrhagischen Infarkt. J. Neuropathol. exp. Neurol. **10**, D93–94 (1951)

Hiller, Fr.: The vascular syndromes of the basilar and vertebral arteries and their branches. J. Nerv. Ment. Dis. **116**, 988–1016 (1952)

Hiller, Fr.: Cerebral hemorrhage in hyperergic angiitis. J. Neuropathol. exp. Neurol. **12**, 24–40 (1953)

Hills, J., Sament, S.: Bilateral agenesis of the internal carotid artery associated with cardiac and other anomalies. Neurology (Minneap.) **18**, 142–146 (1968)

Høedt-Rasmussen, K.: Regional variations in cerebral blood flow in cerebrovascular disease studied under variations of blood pressure and arterial pCO_2. In: Research on the cerebral circulation. III. Intern. Salzburg Conference 1966. Meyer, J.S., Lechner, H., Eichhorn, O. (eds.), pp. 223–228. Springfield/Ill.: Thomas 1969

Hoff, H.H.: Human intracranial atherosclerosis. A histochemical and ultrastructural study of gross fatty streak lesions. Am. J. Pathol. **69**, 421–438 (1972)

Holman, R.L., McGill, H.C. Jr., Strong, J.P., Geer, J.C.: The natural history of atherosclerosis. The early aortic lesions as seen in New Orleans in the middle of the 20th century. Am. J. Pathol. **34**, 209–235 (1958)

Horton, B.T., Brown, G.E.: Thrombo-angiitis obliterans among women. Arch. Intern. Med. **50**, 884–907 (1932)

Horton, B.T., Dorsey, A.H.E.: Experimental thrombo-angiitis obliterans. Bacteriologic and pathologic studies. Arch. Pathol. **13**, 910–915 (1932)

Hossmann, K.-A.: Zur Pathogenese des „otitischen Hydrocephalus“. Fortschr. Neurol. **34**, 236–246 (1966)

Hossmann, K.-A.: Cortical steady potential, impedance and exitability changes during and after total ischemia of cat brain. Exp. Neurol. **32**, 163–175 (1971)

Hossmann, K.-A.: Total ischemia of the brain. In: Brain and heart infarct. Zülch, K.J., Kaufmann, W., Hossmann, K.-A., Hossmann, V. (eds.), pp. 107–124. Berlin, Heidelberg, New York: Springer 1977

Hossmann, K.-A., Hossmann, V.: Coagulopathy following experimental cerebral ischemia. Stroke **8**, 249–254 (1977)

Hossmann, K.-A., Kleihues, P.: Reversibility of ischemic brain damage. Arch. Neurol. **29**, 375–384 (1973)

Hossmann, K.-A., Olsson, Y.: Suppression and recovery of neuronal function in cerebral ischemia. Brain Res. **22**, 313–325 (1970)

Hossmann, K.-A., Schuier, F.J.: Pathophysiology of stroke edema. In: Brain and heart infarct. Zülch, K.J., Kaufmann, W., Hossmann, K.-A., Hossmann, V. (eds.), pp. 119–129. Berlin, Heidelberg, New York: Springer 1979

Hossmann, K.-A., Sato, K.: Recovery of neuronal function after prolonged cerebral ischemia. Science **168**, 375–376 (1970)

Hossmann, K.-A., Zimmermann, V.: Cerebral blood flow, brain water, and electrolytes during recovery from one hour's cerebral ischemia. In: Cerebral circulation and metabolism. Langfitt, T.W., McHenry, L.C. Jr., Reivich, M., Wollman, H. (eds.), pp. 173–176. Berlin, Heidelberg, New York: Springer 1975

Hossmann, K.-A., Kobayashi, K., Hossmann, V.,

KLEIHUES, P.: Recovery of cerebral energy metabolism after complete ischemia of one hour's duration. Naturwissenschaften **60**, 53–54 (1973)

HOSSMANN, V.: Der Hirninfarkt und seine Abhängigkeit von exogenen und endogenen Faktoren des Blutdrucks. Doktor-Dissertation, Universität Köln 1969

HOSSMANN, V.: Coagulation disturbances in cerebrovascular disorders. In: Brain and heart infarct. ZÜLCH, K.J., KAUFMANN, W., HOSSMANN, K.-A., HOSSMANN, V. (eds.), pp. 81–90. Berlin, Heidelberg, New York: Springer, 1977

HOSSMANN, V., HOSSMANN, K.-A.: Return of neuronal functions after prolonged cardiac arrest. Brain Res. **60**, 423–438 (1973)

HOSSMANN, V., ZÜLCH, K.J.: Circadian variations of hemodynamics and stroke. In: Brain and heart infarct. ZÜLCH, K.J., KAUFMANN, W., HOSSMANN, K.-A., HOSSMANN, V. (eds.), pp. 171–180. Berlin, Heidelberg, New York: Springer 1979

HOSSMANN, V., LOY, V., ZÜLCH, K.J.: Polygraphic study of eight patients with cerebral stroke. Electroencephalogr. Clin. Neurophysiol. **36**, 89–90 (1974)

HOUSER, O.W., BAKER, H.L. Jr., SANDOK, B.A., HOLLEY, K.E.: Cephalic arterial fibromuscular dysplasia. Radiology **101**, 605–611 (1971)

HSIEH, H.H.: Cerebrovascular disease: A comparative study of cerebral and visceral arteries. Neurology (Minneap.) **17**, 752–762 (1967)

HUANG, Y.P., WOLFF, B.S.: The lateral anastomotic mesencephalic vein and other variations in drainage of the basal central vein. Am. J. Roentgenol. **89**, 411–422 (1963)

HUANG, Y.P., WOLF, B.S.: Angiographic features of the pericallosal cistern. Radiology **82**, 14–23 (1964a)

HUANG, Y.P., WOLF, B.S.: Veins of the white matter of the cerebral hemispheres (the medullary veins). Am. J. Roentgenol. **92**, 739–755 (1964b)

HUANG, Y.P., WOLF, B.S.: The veins of the posterior fossa-superior or galenic draining group. Am. J. Roentgenol. **95**, 808–821 (1965)

HUANG, Y.P., WOLF, B.S.: Precentral cerebellar vein in angiography. Acta Radiol. (Stockh.) **5**, 250–262 (1966)

HUANG, Y.P., WOLF, B.S.: The vein of the lateral recess of the fourth ventricle and its tributaries. Roentgen appearance and anatomic relationship. Am. J. Roentgenol. **101**, 1–61 (1967)

HUANG, Y.P., WOLF, B.S., ANTIN, S.P., OKUDERA, T.: The veins of the posterior fossa-anterior or petrosal draining group. Am. J. Roentgenol. **104**, 36–56 (1968)

HUBER, P., FUCHS, W.A.: Gibt es eine fibromuskuläre Hyperplasie cerebraler Arterien? Fortschr. Röntgenstr. **107**, 119–126 (1967)

HUECK, W.: Anatomisches zur Frage nach Wesen und Ursache der Arteriosklerose. Münch. med. Wochenschr. **67**, 535–539, 573–576, 606–609 (1920)

HULTQUIST, G.T.: Über Thrombose und Embolie der Arteria carotis und hierbei vorkommende Gehirnveränderungen. Pathologisch-anatomische Studie. Jena: Fischer 1942

HUTCHINSON, E.C., YATES, P.O.: The cervical portion of the vertebral artery. A clinico-pathological study. Brain **79**, 319–331 (1956)

HYLAND, H.H.: Prognosis in spontaneous subarachnoid hemorrhage. Arch. Neurol. **63**, 61–78 (1950)

INGVAR, D.H.: Distribution of cerebral blood flow at rest and during mental activation in normals and in patients with brain disorders. In: Brain and heart infarct. ZÜLCH, K.J., KAUFMANN, W., HOSSMANN, K.-A., HOSSMANN, V. (eds.), pp. 167–174. Berlin, Heidelberg, New York: Springer 1977

INGVAR, D.H.: Functional activation in the diseased brain: In: Brain and heart infarct. ZÜLCH, K.J., KAUFMANN, W., HOSSMANN, K.-A., HOSSMANN, V. (eds.), pp. 232–239. Berlin, Heidelberg, New York: Springer 1979

ITO, A., OMAE, T., KATSUKI, S.: Acute changes in blood pressure following vascular diseases in the brain stem. Stroke **4**, 80–84 (1973)

ITO, U., SPATZ, M., WALKER, J.T. jr., KLATZO, I.: Experimental cerebral ischemia in Mongolian gerbils. I. Light microscopic observations. Acta Neuropathol. ((Berl.) **32**, 209–223 (1975)

IVAMOTO, H.S., NUMOTO, M., DONAGHY, R.M.P.: Surgical decompression for cerebral and cerebellar infarcts. Stroke **5**, 365–370 (1974)

JACOB, H.: Zur Genese und Begutachtung der Pachymeningitis haemorrhagica interna. Zentralbl. Neurochir. **10**, 266–279 (1950)

JANAKI, S., BARUAH, J.K., JAYARAM, S.R., SAXENA, V.K., SHARMA, S.R., GULATI, M.S.: Stroke in the young: A four-year study, 1968 to 1972. Stroke **6**, 318–320 (1975)

JANEWAY, R., TOOLE, J.F.: Vascular anatomic status of patients with transient ischemic attacks. Trans. Am. Neurol. Assoc. **97**, 137–141 (1972)

JANEWAY, R., TOOLE, J.F., LEINBACH, L.B., MILLER, H.S.: Vertebral artery obstruction with basilar impression. Arch. Neurol. **15**, 211–214 (1966)

JENSEN, H.P.: Microangiomas and ICH. In: Spontaneous intracerebral hematomas. Workshop, Bad Nauheim/Giessen, Febr. 1–3, 1979 (Proceedings to be published)

JOHANSSON, P.C.: Review of previous studies and current theories of autoregulation. Circ. Res. **15**, 2–9 (1964)

JOHANSSON, S.H., MELIN, H.S.: Spontaneous cerebral haemorrhage and encephalomalacia. A clinicopathological study of 263 cases with special reference to cardiovascular diseases and cerebral atherosclerosis. Acta Psychiatr. Scand **35**, 457–479 (1960)

JOHNSON, H.C., WALKER, A.E.: The angiographic diagnosis of spontaneous thrombosis of the internal and common carotid arteries. J. Neurosurg. **8**, 631–659 (1951)

Jones, R.J.: Atherosclerosis. Proceedings of the 2nd Int. Symp. Chicago 1969. Berlin, Heidelberg, New York: Springer 1970

Kagan, A.R.: Focus on atherosclerosis. A WHO study on atherosclerosis of the aorta and coronary arteries in five towns. WHO Chronicle **13**, 167–174 (1977)

Kagan, A.R., Uemura, K.: Atherosclerosis of the aorta and coronary arteries in five towns. Bull. WHO **53**, 485–645 (1976)

Kalbag, R.M., Woolf, A.L.: Cerebral venous thrombosis. New York, Toronto: Oxford University Press 1967

Kameyama, M., Okinaka, S.: Collateral circulation of the brain. With special reference to atherosclerosis of the major cervical and cerebral arteries. Neurology (Minneap.) **13**, 279–286 (1963)

Kanaya, H.: Epidemiology. In: Spontaneous intracerebral hematomas. Workshop, Bad Nauheim/Giessen, Febr. 1–3, 1979 (Proceedings to be published)

Kane, W.C., Aronson, S.M.: Cerebrovascular disease in an autopsy population. Arch. Neurol. **20**, 514–526 (1969)

Kannel, W.B.: Current status of the epidemiology of brain infarction associated with occlusive arterial disease. Stroke **2**, 295–318 (1971)

Kannel, W.B., Dawber, T.R., Cohen, M.E., McNamara, P.M.: Vascular disease of the brain-epidemiologic aspects: the Framingham study. Am. J. Publ. Health. **55**, 1355–1366 (1965)

Kannel, W.B., Gordon, T., Wolf, Ph.A., McNamara, P.: Hemoglobin and the risk of cerebral infarction: The Framingham study. Stroke **3**, 409–420 (1972)

Kannel, W.B., Gordon, T., Dawber, T.R.: Role of lipids in the development of brain infarction: The Framingham study. Stroke **5**, 679–685 (1974)

Kannel, W.B., Dawber, T.R., Sorlie, P., Wolf, Ph.A.: Components of blood pressure and risk of atherothrombotic brain infarction: The Framingham study. Stroke **7**, 327–331 (1976)

Kaplan, L.A.: Occlusion of the basilar artery. Arch. Neurol. **66**, 389–390 (1951)

Kaplan, H.A.: Arteries of the brain. An anatomic study. Acta Radiol. (Stockh.) **46**, 364–370 (1956)

Kaplan, H.A., Rabiner, A.M., Browder, J.: Anatomical study of blood vessels in the brain: The perforating arteries of the base of the forebrain. Trans. Am. Neurol. Assoc. **79**, 38–40 (1954)

Katsuki, S., Hirota, J.: Recent trends in incidence of cerebral hemorrhage and infarction in Japan. Jpn. Heart J. **5**, 12–36 (1966)

Katsuki, S., Omae, T., Okabe, N., Nishimaru, K., Yamaguchi, T., Kimoto, K., Nishino, Y.: Hypertension and cerebral atherosclerosis in relation to cerebral infarction and cerebral hemorrhage. In: Cerebral circulation and stroke. Zülch, K.J. (ed.), pp. 183–192. Berlin, Heidelberg, New York: Springer 1971

Kauffmann, Fr.: Klinisch-experimentelle Untersuchungen zum Krankheitsbild der arteriellen Hypertension. Z. gesamten exp. Med. **42**, 473–495 (1925); **43**, 141–169 (1925); Z. klin. Med. **100**, H. 3 u. 4 (1925)

Kaunitz, H.: Bedeutung der Nahrungsfette bei der Arteriosklerose: eine überholte Theorie. Münch. med. Wochenschr. **119**, 539–542 (1977)

Kautzky, R.: Zur Kenntnis intracerebraler Verkalkungen. Dtsch. Z. Nervenheilkd. **159**, 490–500 (1948)

Kautzky, R.: Die Bedeutung der Hirnhaut-Innervation und ihrer Entwicklung für die Pathogenese der Sturge-Weberschen Krankheit. Dtsch. Z. Nervenheilkd. **161**, 506–525 (1949)

Kautzky, R., Zülch, K.J., Wende, S., Tänzer, A.: Neuroradiologie auf neuropathologischer Grundlage, 2. neu bearb. erweit. Aufl. Berlin, Heidelberg, New York: Springer 1976

Kemper, Th.L., Romanul, F.C.A.: State resembling akinetic mutism in basilar artery occlusion. Neurology (Minneap.) **17**, 74–86 (1967)

Kendell, R.E., Marshall, J.: Role of hypotension in the genesis of transient focal cerebral ischaemic attacks. Br. Med. J. **2**, 344–348 (1963)

Kikuchi, Y., Yamamoto, H., Nakamura, M.: Cerebral atherosclerosis in Japanese. 3. Predilection site of atherosclerotic lesions. Stroke **4**, 768–772 (1973)

Kimura, N.: Epidemiological studies of atherosclerotic disease in Japan. In: Atherosclerosis IV. Schettler, G., Goto, Y., Hata, Y., Klose, G. (eds.), pp. 461–470. Berlin, Heidelberg, New York: Springer 1977

Klassen, A.C., Loewenson, R.B., Resch, J.A.: Body weight, cerebral atherosclerosis and cerebral vascular disease: An autopsy study. Stroke **5**, 312–317 (1974)

Klatzo, I.: Presidential address: Neuropathological aspects of brain edema. J. Neuropathol. Exp. Neurol. **26**, 1–13 (1967)

Kleihues, P.: Über die doppelseitigen symmetrischen Occipitallappeninfarkte. Pathogenese und klinisch-ophthalmologische Befunde. Dtsch. Z. Nervenheilkd. **188**, 25–52 (1966a)

Kleihues, P.: Isolierte Infarkte in der Sehstrahlung. Graefes Arch. Ophthalmol. **169**, 181–193 (1966b)

Kleihues, P., Hizawa, K.: Die Infarkte der A. cerebri posterior: Pathogenese und topographische Beziehungen zur Sehrinde. Arch. Psychiatr. Nervenkr. **208**, 263–284 (1966)

Kleihues, P., Hossmann, K.-A., Schröder, M.: Morphologische Betrachtung zur Topik und Pathologie der Hirndurchblutungsstörungen. EEG-Colloque de Marseille à Cologne, 1964 (unpublished)

Kleihues, P., Hossmann, K.-A., Zimmermann, V., Kobayashi, K.: Cerebral protein synthesis and polysome profiles after prolonged periods of complete ischemia. In: Pathology of cerebral microcirculation. Cervos Navarro, J. (ed.), pp. 327–332. Berlin: De Gruyter 1974

KLEISS, E.: Die verschiedenen Formen des Circulus arteriosus cerebralis Willisi. Anat. Anz. **92**, 216–230 (1942)

KLUGER, R.: Zur Frage des vaskulär bedingten (sogenannten „arteriosklerotischen") Parkinsonismus. Doktor-Dissertation, Universität Köln 1979

KÖLLIKER, A.: Über blutkörperchenhaltige Zellen. Z. wiss. Zool. **1**, 260–267 (1849)

KÖLLIKER, A.: Handbuch der Gewebelehre des Menschen. Leipzig: Engelmann 1896

KOGURE, K., SCHEINBERG, P., REINMUTH, O.M., FUJISHIMA, M., BUSTO, R.: Mechanism of cerebral vasodilatation in hypoxia. J. Appl. Physiol. **29**, 223–229 (1970)

KOLISKO, A.: Über die Beziehung der Arteria choroidea anterior zum hinteren Schenkel der inneren Kapsel des Gehirns. Wien: Hölder 1891

KRAFKA, J.: The mechanical factors in arteriosclerosis. Arch. Pathol. **23**, 1–19 (1937)

KRAULAND, W.: Über Hirnschäden durch stumpfe Gewalt. Dtsch. Z. Nervenheilkd. **163**, 265–328 (1950)

KRAYENBÜHL, H.: Zur Diagnostik und chirurgischen Therapie der zerebralen Erscheinungen bei der Endangiitis obliterans v. Winiwarter-Buerger. Schweiz. med. Wochenschr. **75**, 1025–1029 (1945)

KRAYENBÜHL, H., RICHTER, H.R.: Die zerebrale Angiographie. Stuttgart: Thieme 1952

KRAYENBÜHL, H., WEBER, G.: Die Thrombose der Arteria carotis interna und ihre Beziehung zur Endangiitis obliterans v. Winiwarter-Buerger. Helv. med. Acta **11**, 289–333 (1944)

KRAYENBÜHL, H., YASARGIL, M.G.: Die vaskulären Erkrankungen im Gebiet der Arteria vertebralis und Arteria basilaris. Stuttgart: Thieme 1957

KRAYENBÜHL, H., YASARGIL, M.G.: Das Hirnaneurysma. Documenta Geigy: Series chirurgica, Nr. 4 (1958)

KRAYENBÜHL, H., YASARGIL, M.G.: Die zerebrale Angiographie, 2. Aufl. Stuttgart: Thieme 1965

KRIBS, M., KLEIHUES, P.: The recurrent artery of Heubner. A morphological study of the blood supply of the rostral basal ganglia in normal and pathological conditions. In: Cerebral circulation and stroke. ZÜLCH, K.J. (ed.), pp. 40–56. Berlin, Heidelberg, New York: Springer 1971

KRÖSL, W., SCHERZER, E.: Die Bestimmung des Todeszeitpunktes. Wien: Maudrich 1973

KRUEGER, D.E., WILLIAMS, J.L., PAFFENBARGER, R.S. jr.: Trends in death rates from cerebrovascular disease in Memphis, Tennessee, 1920–1960. J. Chronic Dis. **20**, 129–137 (1967)

KUBIK, CH.S., ADAMS, R.D.: Occlusion of the basilar artery. – A clinical and pathological study. Brain **69**, 73–121 (1946)

KUDO, T.: Juvenile occlusion of the circle of Willis. Clin. Neurol. (Tokyo) **5**, 607–627 (1965)

KUDO, T.: Juvenile occlusion of the circle of Willis. Proc. 8th Int. Congr. Neurol. **4**, 503 (1966)

KUNKLE, E.C., MULLER, J.C., ODOM, G.L.: Traumatic brainstem thrombosis: report of case and analysis of mechanism of injury. Ann. Intern. Med. **36**, 1329–1335 (1952)

KURLAND, L.T.: The frequency of intracranial and intraspinal neoplasms in the resident population of Rochester, Minnesota. J. Neurosurg. **15**, 627–641 (1958a)

KURLAND, L.T.: Descriptive epidemiology of selected neurologic and myopathic disorders with particular reference to a survey in Rochester, Minnesota. J. Chronic. Dis. **8**, 378–418 (1958b)

KURLAND, L.T.: Discussion, In: Cerebral Vascular Diseases. MILLIKAN, C.H., SIEKERT, R.G., WHISNANT, J.P. (eds.), p. 77, New York, London: Grune & Stratton 1966

KURLAND, L.T.: Introduction to vascular disorders. In: The pathology of the nervous system. MINCKLER, J. (ed.), Vol. 2, pp. 1420–1423. New York: McGraw-Hill 1971

KURTZKE, J.F.: Epidemiology of cerebrovascular disease. Berlin, Heidelberg, New York: Springer 1969

LABAUGE, R., THEVENET, A., CROUZET, G.: Les hémodétournements dans les artères du cou à destinée encéphalique. Rev. Neurol. **116**, 5–30 (1967)

LAMPERT, H., MÜLLER, W.: Bei welchem Druck kommt es zu einer Ruptur der Gehirngefäße? Frankfurt. Z. Pathol. **33**, 471–477 (1926)

LANCET: Leading articles: Intracerebral haemorrhage and microaneurysms. London, 25 November, 1967

LANDAU, B., RANSOHOFF, J.: Prolonged cerebral vasospasm in experimental subarachnoid hemorrhage. Neurology (Minneap.) **18**, 1056–1065 (1968)

LANGE-COSACK, H.: Anatomie und Klinik der Gefäßmißbildungen des Gehirns und seiner Häute. In: Handbuch der Neurochirurgie, OLIVECRONA, H., TÖNNIS, W. (Hrsg.), Band IV/Teil 2, S. 1–145. Berlin, Heidelberg, New York: Springer 1966

LANZA, G.: Studio sistematico sull' arteriosclerosi del cervello e del midollo spinale. Arch. ital. Anat. Istol. pat. **9**, 259–336 (1938)

LASCELLES, R.G., BURROWS, G.: Occlusion of the middle cerebral artery. Brain **88**, 85–96 (1965)

LASSEN, N.A.: Cerebral blood flow and oxygen consumption in man. Physiol. Rev. **39**, 183–238 (1959)

LASSEN, N.A.: The luxury-perfusion syndrome and its possible relation to acute metabolic acidosis localised within the brain. Lancet (1966) II, 1113–1115

LASSEN, N.A.: On the regulation of cerebral blood flow in diseases of the brain with special regard to the "luxury perfusion syndrome" of brain tissue, i.e. a syndrome characterized by relative hyperemia or absolute hyperemia of the brain tissue. In: Cerebral circulation. LUYENDIJK, W. (ed.), Vol. 30, pp. 121–124. Amsterdam, London, New York: Elsevier 1968

LASSEN, N.A.: Clinical implications of cerebral blood flow studies. In: Cerebral blood flow. Clinical and experimental results. BROCK, M., FIESCHI, C., INGVAR, D.H., LASSEN, N.A., SCHÜRMANN, K. (eds.), pp. 278–285. Berlin, Heidelberg, New York: Springer 1969a

LASSEN, N.A.: Abolition of normal regulation of cerebral blood flow after anoxia and trauma ("luxury perfusion syndrome"). In: 9th Int. Congr. of Neurology, New York 1969. DRAKE, Ch.G., DUVOISIN, R. (eds.), Int. Congr. Ser. No. 193, Abstracts, p. 10. Amsterdam: Excerpta Medica 1969

LASSEN, N.A., INGVAR, D.H.: Regional cerebral blood flow in apoplexy: studies of its pathophysiology, using 8 to 16 external detectors with the xenon 133 method. In: Research on the cerebral circulation. III. Intern. Salzburg Conference 1966. MEYER, J.S., LECHNER, H., EICHHORN, O. (eds.), pp. 96–107. Springfield/Ill.: Thomas 1969

LASSEN, N.A., INGVAR, D.H., SKINHOJ, E.: Brain function and blood flow. Sci. Am. **239**, 50–59 (1978)

LAUDA, E.: Physiologische Druckschädigungen und Arteriosklerose der Duralgefäße. Beitr. pathol. Anat. **68**, 180–184 (1921)

LAVY, S., MELAMED, E., PORTNOY, Z.: The effect of cerebral infarction on the regional cerebral blood flow of the contralateral hemisphere. Stroke **6**, 160–163 (1975)

LAZORTHES, G.: L'hemorragie cérébrale vue par le neuro-chirurgien. Vol. I. Paris: Masson 1956

LAZORTHES, G.: Vascularisation et circulation cérébrales. Paris: Masson 1961

LAZORTHES, G., POULHES, J., ESPAGNO, J.: Les artères du cervelet. 37e Réunion Ass. des Anat. Louvain 1950. C.R. Ass. Anat. III, 279–288 (1951)

LAZORTHES, G., GAUBERT, J., POULHES, J.: La distribution centrale et corticale de l'artère cérébrale antérieure. Etude anatomique et incidences neurochirurgicales. Neurochirurgie **2**, 237–253 (1956)

LAZORTHES, G., PUOULHES, J., BASTIDE, G., ROULLEAU, J.: Les territoires artèriels du tronc cérébral. Press. méd. **91**, 2048–2051 (1958)

LEARY, T.: Atherosclerosis. Arch. Pathol. **21**, 419–462 (1936)

LECENE, B., LHERMITTE, J.: Une observation anatomoclinique d'un cas de ramollissement cérébral consécutif à l'obliteration de l'artère sylvienne gauche par embolie métallique. Rev. Neurol. **27**, 1116–1121 (1920)

LECHTAPE-GRÜTER, H., ZÜLCH, K.J.: Gibt es einen Spasmus der Hingefäße? Radiologe **11**, 429–435 (1971)

LECHTAPE-GRÜTER, R.: Die Verschlüsse der A. cerebri posterior. Klinische, angiographische, szintigraphische und elektroencephalographische Korrelation. Doktor-Dissertation, Universität Köln 1978

LEE, M.L.K., CHEUNG, E.M.T.: Moyamoya disease as a cause of subarachnoid haemorrhage in Chinese. Brain **96**, 623–628 (1973)

LEEDS, N.E., ABBOTT, K.H.: Collateral circulation in cerebrovascular disease in childhood via rete mirabile and perforating branches of anterior choroidal and posterior cerebral arteries. Radiology **85**, 628–634 (1965)

LENIGER-FOLLERT, E., HOSSMANN, K.-A.: Simultaneous measurements of microflow and evoked potentials in the somatomotor cortex of the cat brain during specific sensory activation. Pflügers Arch. **380**, 85–89 (1979)

LETTERER, E.: Allgemeine Pathologie (Grundlagen und Probleme). Stuttgart: Thieme 1959

LEYDEN, E.: Über die Thrombose der Basilar-Arterie. Z. klin. Med. **5**, 165–185 (1882)

LHERMITTE, J.: Les idées nouvelles sur la genèse de l'hémiplégie transitoire et du ramollissement cérébral. Encéphale **23**, 27–39 (1928)

LHERMITTE, F., GAUTIER, J.-C., DEROUESNE, C.: Anatomopathologie et physiopathologie des sténoses carotidiennes. Rev. Neurol. **115**, 641–672 (1966)

LHERMITTE, F., GAUTIER, J.C., DEROUESNE, C., GUIRAUD, B.: Ischemic accidents in the middle cerebral artery territory. A study of the causes in 122 cases. Arch. Neurol. **19**, 248–256 (1968)

LICHTENSTEIN, R.S.: Spontaneous cerebellar hematomas: a report of three operated cases and review of the literature. Bull Johns Hopk. Hosp. **122**, 319–328 (1968)

LIE, T.A.: Congenital anomalies of carotid arteries (angiographic study and review of the literature). Academisch Proefschrift, Amsterdam 1968

LIE, T.A.: Congenital malformations of the carotid and vertebral arterial systems, including the persistent anastomoses. In: Handbook of clinical neurology, VINKEN, P.J., BRUYN, G.W. (eds.), Vol. 12, pp. 289–339. Amsterdam: North Holland; New York: American Elsevier 1972

LIEBEGOTT, G.: Hochdruck und periphere Arteriosklerose. Dtsch. med. Wochenschr. **84**, 1697–1703 (1959)

LINDEMANN, H.: Die Hirngefäße in apoplektischen Blutungen. Virch. Arch. pathol. Anat. **253**, 27–44 (1924)

LINDENBERG, R.: Die Gefäßversorgung und ihre Bedeutung für Art und Ort von kreislaufbedingten Gewebsschäden und Gefäßprozessen. In: Handbuch der speziellen pathologischen Anatomie und Histologie, LUBARSCH, O., HENKE, F., RÖSSLE, R. (Hrsg.), Band XIII, 1. Teil B, S. 1071–1164. Berlin, Göttingen, Heidelberg: Springer 1957

LINDENBERG, R.: Gefäßsyndrome bei intrakranieller Drucksteigerung. Acta Neurochir. (Wien), Suppl. 7, 430–436 (1961)

LINDENBERG, R., SPATZ, H.: Über die Thromboendarteriitis obliterans der Hirngefäße (cerebrale Form der v. Winiwarter-Buergerschen Krankheit). Virch. Arch. pathol. Anat. **305**, 531–557 (1940)

LINK, K.H.: Traumatische sub- und intradurale Blutung – Pachymeningitis haemorrhagica. Jena: Fischer 1945

LINK, K.H.: Zur Pathogenese des subduralen Hämatoms und der Pachymeningitis haemorrhagica interna. Zentralbl. Neurochir. **10**, 264–265 (1950)

LIPPMANN, H.J.: Cerebrovascular thrombosis in patients with Buerger's disease. Circulation **5**, 680–692 (1952)

LLAVERO, F.: Thromboendangiitis obliterans des Gehirns. Basel: Schwabe 1948

LOCKSLEY, H.B.: Report on the cooperative study of intracranial aneurysms and subarachnoid hemorrhage, section V, part I and II: Natural history of subarachnoid hemorrhage, intracranial aneurysms and arteriovenous malformations. Based on 6368 cases in the cooperative study. J. Neurosurg. **25**, 219–239, 321–368 (1966)

LOEB, C., FAVALE, F.: Contralateral EEG abnormalities in intracranial arteriovenous aneurysms. Arch. Neurol. **7**, 121–128 (1962)

LOEB, C., MEYER, J.S.: Strokes due to vertebro-basilar disease. Infarction, vascular insufficiency and hemorrhage of the brain stem and cerebellum. Springfield, Ill.: Thomas 1965

LOEW, F., WÜSTNER, S.: Diagnose, Behandlung und Prognose der traumatischen Hämatome des Schädelinnern. Acta Neurochir. (Wien), Suppl. VIII (1960)

LÖWENFELD, L.: Studien über Ätiologie und Pathogenese der spontanen Hirnblutungen. Wiesbaden: Bergmann 1886

LUGINBÜHL, H.: Spontaneous atherosclerosis in swine: Symposium on swine in biomedical research. Richland, Washington: Battelle-Northwest 1966

LYAGER, T.: Dødsarsager ved apoplexia cerebri. Nordisk Medicin **54**, 1315–1317 (1955)

MAKI, Y., NAKATA, Y.: An autopsy case of hemangiomatous malformation of bilateral internal carotid artery at the base of brain. Brain Nerve (Tokyo) **17**, 764–766 (1965)

MARCHAND, L.: Über das Gehirngewicht des Menschen. Abhandlungen der Sächsischen Gesellschaft der Wissenschaften 1902

MARIE, P.: Des foyers lacunaires de désintégration et de différents autres états cavitaires du cerveau. Rev. Méd. (Paris) **21**, 281 (1901)

MARKS, J.S.: Apoplectic death due to intracerebral haemorrhage. An anatomic study. Neurology (Minneap.) **10**, 278–280 (1960)

MARSHALL, J.: The management of occlusion and stenosis of the internal carotid artery. Neurology (Minneap.) **16**, 1087–1093 (1966)

MARSHALL, J.: Hypertension: Permanent or temporary cause of cerebral infarction and insufficiency. In: Cerebral circulation and stroke. ZÜLCH, K.J. (ed.), pp. 175–182. Berlin, Heidelberg, New York: Springer 1971

MARSHALL, J.: Familial incidence of cerebral hemorrhage. Stroke **4**, 38–41 (1973)

MARSHALL, J.: Diurnal variation in occurrence of strokes. Stroke **8**, 230–231 (1977)

MARSHALL, J., MEADOWS, S.: The natural history of amaurosis fugax. Brain **91**, 419–434 (1968)

MARTIN, M.J., WHISNANT, J.P., SAYRE, G.P.: Occlusive vascular disease in the extracranial cerebral circulation. Arch. Neurol. **3**, 530–538 (1960)

MARX, F.: An arteriographic demonstration of collaterals between internal and external carotid arteries. Acta Radiol. (Stockh.) **31**, 155–160 (1949)

MASTRI, A.R., SILVERSTEIN, P.M., GOLD, L., ESELIUS, E.P.: Multiple progressive intracranial arterial occlusions. Stroke **4**, 380–386 (1973)

MATSUMOTO, N., WHISNANT, J.P., KURLAND, L.T., OKAZAKI, H.: Natural history of stroke in Rochester, Minnesota, 1955 through 1969: An extension of a previous study, 1945 through 1954. Stroke **4**, 20–29 (1973)

MATSUOKA, SH.: Histopathological studies on the blood vessels in apoplexia cerebri. Atti del Primo Congresso Internazionale di Histopathologia del Sistema Nervoso, Roma 1952, Vol. III, pp. 221–231. Torino: Rosenberg & Sellier 1952

MATUOKA, S.: Studien über Hirnblutung und -erweichung (III. Mitt.). Über kleine Aneurysmen in den Gehirnen ohne Blutung bzw. mit blutungsfreien Hirnpartien. Trans. Soc. pathol. jap. **29**, 449–455 (1939)

MCCARTY, C.S., COOPER, J.S.: Neurologic and metabolic effects of bilateral ligation of the anterior cerebral arteries in man. Proc. Mayo Clin. **26**, 185–190 (1951)

MCCORMICK, W.F.: The pathology of vascular ("arteriovenous") malformations. J. Neurosurg. **24**, 807–816 (1966)

MCCORMICK, W.F., NOFZINGER, J.D.: "Cryptic" vascular malformations of the central nervous system. J. Neurosurg. **24**, 865–875 (1966)

MCCORMICK, W.F., ROSENFIELD, D.B.: Massive brain hemorrhage: A review of 144 cases and an examination of their causes. Stroke **4**, 946–954 (1973)

MCCULLOUGH, A.W.: Some anomalies of the cerebral arterial circle (of Willis) and related vessels. Anat. Rec. **142**, 537–543 (1962)

MCDONALD, W.I.: Recurrent cholesterol embolism as a cause of fluctuating cerebral symptoms. J. Neurol. Neurosurg. Psychiatry **30**, 489–496 (1967)

MCDONALD, C.A., KORB, M.: Intracranial aneurysms. Arch. Neurol. **42**, 298–328 (1939)

MCDOWELL, F., EJRUP, B.: Arterial bruits in cerebrovascular disease. A follow-up study. Neurology (Minneap.) **16**, 1127–1129 (1966)

MCGILL, H.C. Jr.: The geographic pathology of atherosclerosis. Lab. Invest. **18**, 463–653 (1968)

MCHEDLISHVILI, G.I.: Vascular mechanisms of the brain. New York: Plenum Press 1972

MCHEDLISHVILI, G.I., KOMETIANI, P.A., ORMOTSADZE, L.G.: On the mechanism of spasm of the internal carotid artery. Biochim. Biol. Sperim. **9**, 231–240 (1970–1971)

MCKISSOCK, W., PAINE, K.W.E.: Subarachnoid haemorrhage. Brain **82**, 356–366 (1959)

MCKISSOCK, W., PAINE, K., WALSH, L.: Further observations on subarachnoid hemorrhage. J. Neurol. Neurosurg. Psychiatry **21**, 239–248 (1958)

MCMAHAN, C.A.: Age-Sex distributions of selected groups of human autopsied cases. Arch. Pathol. **73**, 52–59 (1962)

MERRITT, H.H.: cited by SUZUKI, J., TAKAKU, A. (as written communication 1968). Arch. Neurol. **20**, 288 (1969)

METTINGER, K.L., ERICSON, K., LARSSON, S.: A model for non-invasive screening of ulcerous plaques in the carotid arteries using isotope labelled blood elements. In: 11th World Congress of Neurology: Abstracts. DEN HARTOG JAGER, W.A., BRUYN, G.W., HEIJSTEE, A.P.J. (eds.), pp. 48–49. Amsterdam, Oxford: Excerpta Medica 1977

METTLER, F.A., COOPER, I., LISS, H., CARPENTIER, M., NOBACK, CH.: Patterns of vascular failure in the central nervous system. J. Neuropathol. Exp. Neurol. **13**, 528–539 (1954)

METZ, H., MURRAY-LESLIE, R.M., BANNISTER, R.G., BULL, J.W.D., MARSHALL, J.: Kinking of the internal carotid artery in relation to cerebrovascular disease. Lancet (1961) **I**, 424

METZINGER, H.: Über die Basilaris- und Vertebralis-Insuffizienz unter besonderer Berücksichtigung der Thrombosen dieser Arterien. Doktor-Dissertation, Universität Köln 1971

METZINGER, H., ZÜLCH, K.J.: Vertebro-basilar occlusion and its morphological sequelae. In: Cerebral circulation and stroke. ZÜLCH, K.J. (ed.), pp. 67–81. Berlin, Heidelberg, New York: Springer 1971

MEYER, J.E.: Studien zur cerebralen Thrombangiitis obliterans. Arch. Psychiatr. Nervenkr. **180**, 647–680 (1948)

MEYER, J.E.: Über die Lokalisation frühkindlicher Hirnschäden in arteriellen Grenzgebieten. Arch. Psychiatr. Nervenkr. **190**, 328–341 (1953)

MEYER, J.E.: Zur Lokalisation arteriosklerotischer Erweichungsherde in arteriellen Grenzgebieten des Gehirns. Arch. Psychiatr. Nervenkr. **196**, 421–432 (1958)

MEYER, J.S.: Importance of ischemic damage to small vessels in experimental cerebral infarction. J. Neuropathol. Exp. Neurol. **17**, 571–585 (1958)

MEYER, J.S., FANG, H.C., DENNY-BROWN, D.S.: Polarographic study of cerebral collateral circulation. Arch. Neurol. **72**, 296–312 (1954)

MEYER, J.S., GOTOH, F., TAZAKI, Y.: Circulation and metabolism following experimental cerebral embolism. J. Neuropathol. Exp. Neurol. **21**, 4–24 (1962)

MEYER, J.S., OHUCHI, T., OKAMOTO, S., KOTO, A., ERICSSON, A.D.: Cerebral dysautoregulation in central neurogenic orthostatic hypotension (Shy-Drager syndrome). Neurology (Minneap.) **23**, 262–273 (1973)

MEYER, W.W.: Cholesterinkrystallembolie kleiner Organarterien und ihre Folgen. Virchows Arch. pathol. Anat. **314**, 616–638 (1947)

MEYER, W.W.: Einführung in die Pathomorphologie der Arterien. In: Angiologie (begründet von M. Ratschow), 2. neu bearb. Aufl. HEBERER, G., RAU, G., SCHOOP, W. (Hrsg.), S. 54–60. Stuttgart: Thieme 1974a

MEYER, W.W.: Spezielle Pathologie der Arterien. In: Angiologie, 2. neu bearb. Aufl. HEBERER, G., RAU, G., SCHOOP, W. (Hrsg.), S. 60–103. Stuttgart: Thieme 1974b

MILLIKAN, C.H.: Perplexities in cerebrovascular disease (Editorial). Ann. Intern. Med. **58**, 191–192 (1963)

MILLIKAN, C.H.: Strokes in women age 15 to 45. In: Maladies vasculaires cérébrales (cerebrovascular diseases). Conférences de la Salpêtrière 1975. Paris: Baillière 1976

MILLIKAN, C.H., SIEKERT, R.G.: Studies in cerebrovascular disease; syndrome of intermittent insufficiency of basilar arterial system. Proc. Mayo Clin. **30**, 61–68 (1955)

MISCH, W.: Die cerebralen Gefäßverschlüsse und ihre klinischen Syndrome. Zentralb. gesamten Neurol. Psychiatrie **53**, 673–784 (1929)

MITTERWALLNER, F.v.: Variations-statistische Untersuchungen an den basalen Hirngefäßen. Acta Anat. (Basel) **24**, 51–58 (1955)

MIZUKAMI, M., KIN, H., ARAKI, G., MIHARA, H., YOSHIDA, Y.: Surgical treatment of primary intracerebral hemorrhage. Part 1: New angiographical classification. Stroke **7**, 30–40 (1976)

MÖNCKEBERG, J.G.: Mediaverkalkung und Atherosklerose. Virchows Arch. pathol. Anat. **216**, 408–416 (1914)

MOLINARI, G.F.: Septic cerebral embolism. Stroke **3**, 117–122 (1972)

MONAKOW, C.v.: Gehirnpathologie. Wien: Hoelder 1897

MONIZ, E.: L'angiographie cérébrale. Paris: Masson 1934

MONIZ, E.: Die cerebrale Arteriographie und Phlebographie. In: Ergänzungsband II zum Handbuch der Neurologie. BUMKE, O., FOERSTER, O. (Hrsg.). Berlin: Springer 1940

MONTGOMERY, P.O.B., MUIRHEAD, E.E.: A characterization of hyaline arteriolar sclerosis by histochemical procedures. Am. J. Pathol. **30**, 521–531 (1954)

MONTRIEUL, B., JANNY, P.: Contribution à l'étude angiographique des thromboses veineuses cérébrales. Neurochirurgie **8**, 175–188 (1962)

MOORE, M.T., STERN, K.: Vascular lesions in brainstem and occipital lobe occurring in association with brain tumors. Brain **61**, 70–98 (1938)

MOOSSY, J.: Development of cerebral atherosclerosis in various age groups. Neurology **9**, 569–574 (1959)

MOOSSY, J.: Cerebral infarction and intracranial arterial thrombosis. Necropsy studies and clinical implications. Arch. Neurol. **14**, 119–123 (1966a)

MOOSSY, J.: Cerebral infarcts and the lesions of intracranial and extracranial atherosclerosis. Arch. Neurol. **14**, 124–128 (1966b)

MOOSSY, J.: Morphology, sites and epidemiology of cerebral atherosclerosis. Assoc. Res. Nerv. Dis. Proc. **41**, 1–22 (1966c)

MOOSSY, J.: Cerebral atherosclerosis: intracranial and extracranial lesions. In: Pathology of the nervous system. MINCKLER, J. (ed.), Vol. II, pp. 1423–1432. New York: McGraw-Hill 1971

MOREL, F., WILDI, E.: Examen anatomique du polygone de Willis et de ses anomalies. Etude statistique. V. Congrès Neurologique International, Lisbonne 1953, Vol. II. Lisboa: Tip. Severo-Freitas-Mega 1953

Morello, G., Borghi, G.P.: Cerebral angiomas. A report of 154 personal cases and a comparison between the results of surgical excision and conservative management. Acta Neurochir. (Wien) **28**, 135–155 (1973)

Morello, A., Cooper, I.S.: Visual field studies following occlusion of the anterior chorioidal artery. Am. J. Ophthalmol. **40**, 796–801 (1955)

Morgagni, J.B.: The seats and causes of diseases investigated by anatomy. London: 1769. Repr. New York: Hafner 1960

Moschcowitz, E.: The cause of arteriosclerosis. Am. J. Med. Sci. **178**, 244–267 (1929)

Moser, M., Goldman, A.G.: Hypertensive vascular disease. Philadelphia: Lippincott 1967

Mossakowski, M.J., Krasnicka, Z., Iwanowski, L.: Atheroma of the larger arteries of the brain in a Polish population: A study of 600 cases. J. Neurol. Sci. **1**, 13–23 (1964)

Mount, L.A., Taveras, J.M.: A study of the collateral circulation of the brain following ligation of the internal carotid artery. Trans. Am. Neurol. Assoc. **78**, 47–49 (1953)

Müller, H.R., Wüthrich, R., Wiggli, U., Hünig, R., Elke, M.: The contribution of computerized axial tomography to the diagnosis of cerebellar and pontine hematomas. Stroke **6**, 467–475 (1975)

Muirhead, E.E., Turner, L.B., Grollman, A.: Hypertensive cardiovascular disease. Nature and pathogenesis of the arteriolar sclerosis induced by bilateral nephrectomy as revealed by a study of its tinctorial characteristics. Arch. Pathol. **52**, 266–279 (1951)

Murray, J.F.: Types and effects of heart disease in cerebrovascular disorders. Stanf. Med. Bull. **15**, 78–82 (1957)

Myers, R.E.: The clinical and pathological effects of asphyxiation in the fetal rhesus monkey. In: Diagnosis and treatment of fetal disorders. Adamsons, K. (ed.), pp. 226–249. Berlin, Heidelberg, New York: Springer 1969

Myers, R.E.: Threshold values of oxygen deficiency leading to cardiovascular and brain pathologic changes in term monkey fetuses. In: Oxygen transport to tissue: instrumentation, methods and physiology. Bruley, D.F., Bicher, H.I. (eds.), Vol. 37B, pp. 1047–1054. New York: Plenum Press 1973

Myers, R.E.: Fetal asphyxia due to umbilical cord compression. Metabolic and brain pathologic consequences. Biol. Neonate **26**, 21–43 (1975a)

Myers, R.E.: Four patterns of perinatal brain damage and their conditions of occurrence in primates. Advances in Neurology 10. Meldrum, B.S., Marsden, C.D. (eds.), pp. 223–234. New York: Raven Press 1975b

Myers, R.E.: Maternal psychological stress and fetal asphyxia: A study in the monkey. Am. J. Obstet. Gynecol. **122**, 47–59 (1975c)

Myers, R.E.: Perinatal asphyxia: The neurologist's viewpoint. In: Preventability of perinatal injury. Adamsons, K. (ed.), pp. 59–93. New York: Liss 1975d

Nakamura, M., Murakami, H., Shigemi, U.: Effects of excess NaCl intake on blood pressure and cholesterol-induced atherosclerosis in the monkey. Stroke **6**, 9–16 (1975)

Nakamura, M., Imaizumi, K., Kikuchi, Y., Kanaide, H.: Cerebral atherosclerosis in Japanese. Part 4: Relationship between lipid content and macroscopic severity of atherosclerosis. Stroke **7**, 591–594 (1976a)

Nakamura, M., Imaizumi, K., Shigemi, U., Nakashima, Y., Kikuchi, Y., Tanaka, K.: Cerebral atherosclerosis in Japanese. Part 5: Relationship between cholesterol deposition and glycosaminoglycans. Stroke **7**, 594–598 (1976b)

Nakayama, Y.: Epidemiological research in Japan on smoking and cardiovascular diseases. In: Atherosclerosis IV. Schettler, G., Goto, Y., Hata, Y., Klose, G (eds.), pp. 149–156. Berlin, Heidelberg, New York: Springer 1977

Naquet, R.: L'importance du carrefour parieto-temporo-occipital dans la pathologie épileptique d'origine vasculaire. Brux. méd. **45**, 378–384 (1965)

Naquet, R., Vigouroux, R.P.: Embolies expérimentales par voie carotidienne chez le babouin (Papio papio). Rev. Neurol. **114**, 339–360 (1966)

Naquet, R., Arfel, G., Choux, M., Dubois, D.: Etude expérimentale de l'embolie gazeuse par voie carotidienne chez le chat. Electroencephalogr. Clin. Neurophysiol. **20**, 181–196 (1966)

Nedwich, A., Haft, H., Tellem, M., Kauffman, L.: Dissecting aneurysm of cerebral arteries; review of the literature and report of a case. Arch. Neurol. **9**, 477–484 (1963)

Nelson, E., Rennels, M.: Innervation of intracranial arteries. Brain **93**, 475–490 (1970)

Nemoto, E.M.: Postischemic amelioration of brain damage. In: Brain and heart infarct. Zülch, K.J., Kaufmann, W., Hossmann, K.-A., Hossmann, V. (eds.), pp. 73–80. Berlin, Heidelberg, New York: Springer 1977

Neubuerger, K.T.: Arteriosklerose. In: Handbuch der Geisteskrankheiten, Bumke, O. (Hrsg.), Band XI, Teil VII, S. 570–637. Berlin: Springer 1930

Nishimoto, A., Sugiu, R.: Hemangiomatous malformation of bilateral internal carotid artery at the base of brain. Preliminary report. Proc. Annu. Meeting Neuroradiological Assoc. Jpn, No. 5, pp. 2–9, Tokyo: 1964

Nishimoto, A., Takeuchi, S.: Cerebral basal rete mirabile. In: A disease with abnormal intracranial vascular network. – Spontaneous occlusion of the circle of Willis. Kudo, T. (ed.), pp. 56–59. Tokyo: Shoin 1967

Nishimoto, A., Takeuchi, S.: Abnormal cerebrovascular network related to the internal carotid arteries. J. Neurosurg. **29**, 255–260 (1968)

NOETZEL, H.: Die Pathologie des Nervensystems. In: Spezielle Pathologie. 4. neubearb. erweit. Aufl. BÜCHNER, F. (ed.), pp. 470–579. München, Berlin: Urban & Schwarzenberg 1965

NOETZEL, H., JERUSALEM, F.: Die Hirnvenen- und Sinusthrombosen, unter besonderer Berücksichtigung der Topographie der hämorrhagischen Infarkte. Monogr. Ges. Gebiet Neurol. Psychiatrie (Berl.) **106**, 1–63 (1965)

NORDSTRÖM, C.-H., SIESJÖ, BO K.: Effects of phenobarbital in cerebral ischemia. Part I: Cerebral energy metabolism during pronounced incomplete ischemia. Stroke **9**, 327–335 (1978)

NORDSTRÖM, C.H., REHNCRONA, ST., SIESJÖ, BO K.: Effects of phenobarbital in cerebral ischemia. Part II: Restitution of cerebral energy state, as well as of glycolytic metabolites, citric acid cycle intermediates and associated amino acids after pronounced incomplete ischemia. Stroke **9**, 335–343 (1978)

NUUTILA, M.: Atherosclerosis of the circle of Willis and the adjoining arteries in a Finnish medicolegal autopsy material. Acta Pathol. Microbiol. Scand. [A] **235**, Suppl., 1–58 (1973)

OBERNDORFER, S.: Beitrag zur Frage der Lokalisation arteriosklerotischer Prozesse in den peripheren Arterien. Dtsch. Arch. klin. Med. **12**, 515–519 (1911)

O'BRIEN, M.D., WALTZ, A.G.: Intracranial pressure gradients caused by experimental cerebral ischemia and edema. Stroke **4**, 694–698 (1973)

OJEMANN, R.G., FISHER, C.M., RICH, J.CH.: Spontaneous dissecting aneurysm of the internal carotid artery. Stroke **3**, 434–440 (1972)

OKAWARA, S., NIBBELINK, D.: Vertebral artery occlusion following hyperextension and rotation of the head. Stroke **5**, 640–642 (1974)

OKONEK, G.: Spätergebnisse nach operativer Behandlung des subduralen Hämatoms. Zentralbl. Neurochir. **10**, 279–280 (1950)

OLIVARES, L., CASTANEDA, E., GRIFE, A., ALTER, M.: Risk factors in stroke: A clinical study in Mexican patients. Stroke **4**, 773–781 (1973)

OLIVECRONA, H., LADENHEIM, J.: Congenital arteriovenous aneurysms of carotid and vertebral arterial systems. Berlin, Göttingen, Heidelberg: Springer 1957

OONEDA, G., YOSHIDA, Y., SUZUKI, K., SHINKAI, H.: Plasmatic arterionecrosis and its thrombotic occlusion. Thromb. Res. **8**, Suppl. II, 357–364 (1976)

OPITZ, E., SCHNEIDER, M.: Über die Sauerstoffversorgung des Gehirns und den Mechanismus von Mangelwirkungen. Ergeb. Physiol. **46**, 126–260 (1950)

OPPENHEIM, H.: Lehrbuch der Nervenkrankheiten. Berlin: Karger 1908

OPPENHEIM, F.: Review of one hundred autopsies of Shanghai Chinese. China Med. J. **39**, 1067 (1925)

OTT, E.O., LECHNER, H., ARANIBAR, A.: High blood viscosity syndrome in cerebral infarction. Stroke **5**, 330–333 (1974)

OWMAN, CH.: Innervation and receptor sites of intracranial vessels and its relation to spasm. 11th Princeton Conference on Cerebral Vascular Disease 1978. (in press) (1979)

OWMAN, C., EDVINSSON, L., HARDEBO, J.E.: Pharmacological in vitro analysis of amine-mediated vasomotor functions in the intracranial and extracranial vascular beds. Blood Bessels **15**, 128–147 (1978)

PABELICK, W.-H.: Die Veränderungen der Hirnarterien bei den Massenblutungen im Striatum. Klinische und pathologisch-anatomische Untersuchungen an 70 Fällen. Doktor-Dissertation, Universität Köln (1967)

PADGET, D.H.: The circle of Willis: its embryology and anatomy. In: Intracranial arterial aneurysms. DANDY, W.E. (ed.), p. 67. Ithaca, New York: Comstock 1944

PADGET, D.H.: Development of the cranial arteries in the human embryo. Contrib. Embryol. Carneg. Inst. **32**, 205–262 (1948)

PADGET, D.H.: The cranial venous system in man in reference to development, adult configuration, and relation to the arteries. Am. J. Anat. **98**, 307–355 (1956)

PADGET, D.H.: The development of the cranial venous system in man, from the viewpoint of comparative anatomy. Contrib. Embryol. Carneg. Inst. **36**, 79–140 (1957)

PAGET, J.: Fatty degeneration of the small blood vessels of the brain and its relation to apoplexy. Lond. Med. Gaz. **10**, 229 (1850)

PAGNIEZ, P.: Oblitération complète d'une branche de la sylvienne. Rétablissement de la circulation par des anastomoses. Rev. Neurol. **10**, 543 (1902)

PAKARINEN, S.: Incidence, aetiology, and prognosis of primary subarachnoid haemorrhage. A study based on 589 cases diagnosed in a defined urban population during a defined period. Acta Neurol. Scand **43**, Suppl. **29** (1967)

PANNIER, J.L., LEUSEN, I.: Cerebral blood flow in cats after an acute hypertensive insult with damage to the blood-brain barrier. Stroke **6**, 188–198 (1975)

PARISOT, J., CORNIL, L.: Troubles vaso-moteurs. In: Nouveau traité de médecine. Fasc. XXI: Nerfs.-Sympathique. Névroses. ROGER, G.-H., WIDAL, F., TEISSIER, P.-J. (eds.), pp. 457–501. Paris: Masson 1927

PATERSON, J.H., MCKISSOCK, W.: A clinical survey of intracranial angiomas with special reference to their mode of progression and surgical treatment: A report of 110 cases. Brain **79**, 233–266 (1956)

PAUL, R.C.: Clinical epidemiology. Chicago: University of Chicago Press 1966

PAULLIN, J.E., BOWCOCK, H.M., WOOD, R.H.: Complications of hypertension. Am. Heart J. **2**, 613–618 (1926/27)

PAULSON, O.B.: Regional cerebral blood flow in apoplexy due to occlusion of the middle cerebral artery. Neurology (Minneap.) **20**, 63–77 (1970)

PENRY, J.K., NETSKY, M.G.: Experimental embolic

occlusion of a single leptomeningeal artery. Arch. Neurol. **3**, 391–398 (1960)
PENTSCHEW, A.: Die granuläre Atrophie der Großhirnrinde. Arch. Psychiatr. Nervenkr. **101**, 80–136 (1934)
PERNKOPF, E.: Topographische Anatomie des Menschen. Band IV/1: Der Kopf. München, Berlin, Wien: Urban & Schwarzenberg 1957
PERRET, G.E.: Experimentelle Untersuchung über Massenverschiebungen und Formveränderungen des Gehirns bei raumbeengenden Prozessen. Zentralbl. Neurochir. **5**, 5–29 (1940)
PESTALOZZI, R.: Über Aneurysmata spuria der kleinen Gehirnarterien und ihren Zusammenhang mit der Apoplexie. Dissertation. Würzburg: Thein 1849
PETERS, G.: Trauma und Pachymeningitis haemorrhagica interna. Zentralbl. Neurochir. **10**, 280–283 (1950)
PETERS, G.: Die Pachymeningitis haemorrhagica interna, das interdurale Hämatom und das chronische subdurale Hämatom. Fortschr. Neurol. Psychyatrie **19**, 485–542 (1951)
PETERS, G.: Klinische Neuropathologie. Spezielle Pathologie der Krankheiten des zentralen und peripheren Nervensystems, 2. Aufl. Stuttgart: Thieme 1970
PETERS, H.J., CHANDLER, A.B.: Thrombotic atherosclerosis of human cerebral arteries. In: Pathology of the nervous system. MINCKLER, J. (ed.), Vol. 2, pp. 1432–1436. New York: McGraw-Hill 1971
PETERSON, R.E., LIVINGSTON, K.E., ESCOBAR, A.: Development and distribution of gross atherosclerotic lesions at cervical carotid bifurcation. Neurology (Minneap.) **10**, 955–959 (1960)
PFEIFER, R.A.: Anastomosen der Hirngefäße, dargestellt am asphyktisch-hyperämischen Kindergehirn. J. Psychol. Neurol. (Leipzig) **42**, 1–173 (1931)
PFEIFER, R.A.: Grundlegende Untersuchungen über die Angioarchitektonik des menschlichen Gehirns. Berlin: Springer 1930
PICARD, L., LEVESQUE, M., CROUZET, G., SIMON, J., ANDRE, J.M.: Le syndrome "moyamoya". J. Neuroradiol. **1**, 47–144 (1974)
PICK, L.: Über die sogenannten miliaren Aneurysmen der Hirngefäße. Berl. klin. Wochenschr. **47**, 325–329, 382–386 (1910)
PICKERING, G.W.: Transient cerebral paralysis in hypertension and in cerebral embolism. With special reference to the pathogenesis of chronic hypertensive encephalopathy. J. Am. Med. Assoc. **137**, 423–430 (1948)
POLLAK, E., REZEK, PH.: Studien zur Pathologie der Hirngefäße. II. Mitteilung: Die Blutgefäße bei der Hirnpurpura. Virchows Arch. pathol. Anat. **269**, 254–279 (1928)
POOL, J.L., POTTS, D.G.: Aneurysms and arteriovenous anomalies of the brain. New York: Harper & Row 1965
POOR, GY.: Über hypertonische Kleinhirnblutungen. Acta Med. Acad. Sci. Hung. **24**, 81–88 (1967)
POPPER, L.: Die cerebralen Insulte. Wien. Z. inn. Med. **30**, 1–19 (1949)
POPPI, U.: La sindrome anatomo-clinica consequente a lesione dell'arteria corioidea anteriore. Rev. Neurol. **1**, 466–475 (1928)
PRATT-THOMAS, H.R., BERGER, K.E.: Cerebellar and spinal injuries after chiropractic manipulation. J. Am. Med. Assoc. **133**, 600–603 (1947)
PRIBRAM, H.F.W.: Angiographic appearances in acute intracranial hypertension. Neurology (Minneap.) **11**, 10–21 (1961)
PRIBRAM, H.F.W.: Angiography in cerebrovascular disease. J. Neurosurg. **20**, 34–40 (1963)
PRINEAS, J., MARSHALL, J.: Hypertension and cerebral infarction. Br. Med. J. **1**, 14–17 (1966)
PUTNAM, T.J., CUSHING, H.: Chronic subdural hematoma; its pathology, its relation to pachymeningitis hemorrhagica, and its surgical treatment. Arch. Surg. **11**, 329–393 (1925)
QUANDT, J., SOMMER, H.: Die zerebrale Form der Endangiitis obliterans. In: Die zerebralen Durchblutungsstörungen des Erwachsenenalters, 2. Aufl. QUANDT, J. (Hrsg.), S. 735–752. Stuttgart, New York: Schattauer 1969
RALSTON, B., RASMUSSEN, T.B., KENNEDY, T.: Occlusion of middle cerebral artery under normotension, and anemically induced and chemically induced hypotension. J. Neurosurg. **12**, 26–33 (1955)
RASCHER, W.: ICH in hypertensive rats. In: Spontaneous intracerebral hematomas. Workshop, Bad Nauheim/Giessen, Febr. 1–3, 1979 (Proceedings to be published)
RATSCHOW, M.: Angiologie. Stuttgart: Thieme 1959
RAUBER-KOPSCH: Rauber's Lehrbuch der Anatomie des Menschen, Bd. II, neubearb. u. herausgeg. von KOPSCH, FR. Leipzig: Thieme 1948
REIN, H.: Die Physiologie der Coronardurchblutung. Verh. Dtsch. Ges. inn. Med. **43**, 247–262 (1931)
REIN, H.: Einführung in die Physiologie des Menschen. Berlin: Springer 1936
REISNER, H.: Die Klinik und Therapie der cerebralen Gefäßerkrankungen des höheren Lebensalters. Wien. Z. Nervenheilkd. **9**, 92–108 (1954)
RESCH, J.A.: The geographic pathology of cerebral atherosclerosis. In: Research on the cerebral circulation. 5th Int. Salzburg Conference. MEYER, J.S., REIVICH, M., LECHNER, H., EICHHORN, O. (eds.), pp. 43–60. Springfield/Ill.: Thomas 1972
RESCH, J.A., BAKER, A.B.: Etiologic mechanisms in cerebral atherosclerosis. Preliminary study of 3.839 cases. Arch. Neurol. **10**, 617–628 (1964)
RESCH, J.A., OKABE, N., LOEWENSON, R.B., KIMOTO, K., KATSUKI, S., BAKER, A.B.: Pattern of vessel involvement in cerebral atherosclerosis. A comparative study between a Japanese and Minnesota population. J. Atheroscl. Res. **9**, 239–250 (1969)
RESCH, J.A., LOEWENSON, R.B., BAKER, A.B.: Physical factors in the pathogenesis of cerebral atherosclerosis. Stroke **1**, 77–85 (1970)

REY-BELLET, J.: Cerebellar hemorrhage: a clinicopathologic study. Neurology (Minneap.) **10**, 217–222 (1960)

RIBBERT, H.: Fettembolie. Korresp.-Bl. schweiz. Ärz. 1894, Nr. 24; 1900, Nr. 7

RICHARDSON, J.C., HYLAND, H.H.: Intracranial aneurysms. Medicine (Baltimore) **20**, 1–83 (1941)

RIECHERT, T.: Die Arteriographie der Hirngefäße. München, Berlin: Lehmanns 1943

RIESSNER, D., ZÜLCH, K.J.: Paper read at "Bucher Tag", November 1938 (published in 1939, see below)

RIESSNER, D., ZÜLCH, K.J.: Über die Formveränderungen des Hirns (Massenverschiebungen, Zisternenverquellungen) bei raumbeengenden Prozessen. Dtsch. Z. Chir. **253**, 1–61 (1939)

RIGGS, H.E., RUPP, C.: Variation in form of circle of Willis. The relation of the variations to collateral circulation: anatomic analysis. Arch. Neurol. **8**, 8–14 (1963)

RIISHEDE, J.: Cerebral apoplexy. An arteriographical and clinical study of 100 cases. Acta Psychiat. Scand. **32**, Suppl. **118** (1957)

RIISHEDE, J.: Cerebral apoplexy: statistical and diagnostic considerations. Can. Med. Assoc. J. **97**, 151–160 (1967)

RINALDI, I., HARRIS, W.O., KOPP, J.E., LEGIER, J.: Intracranial fibromuscular dysplasia: Report of two cases, one with autopsy verification. Stroke **7**, 511–516 (1976)

RING, B.A.: Occlusio supra occlusionem: Intracranial occlusions following carotid thrombosis as diagnosed by cerebral angiography. Stroke **2**, 487–493 (1971)

RING, B.A., WADDINGTON, M.: Ascending frontal branch of middle cerebral artery. Acta Radiol. [Diagn.] (Stockh.) **6**, 209–220 (1967)

RIVERA, V.M., MEYER, J.S., BAER, P.E., FAIBISH, G.M., MATHEW, N.T., HARTMANN, A.: Vertebrobasilar arterial insufficiency with dementia. Controlled trials of treatment with betahistine hydrochloride. J. Am. Geriatr. Soc. **22**, 397–406 (1974)

ROBERTS, J.C., JR., MOSES, C., WILKINS, R.H.: Autopsy studies in atherosclerosis. I. Distribution and severity of atherosclerosis in patients dying without morphologic evidence of atherosclerotic catastrophe. Circulation **20**, 511–519 (1959a)

ROBERTS, J.C., JR., WILKINS, R.H., MOSES, C.: Autopsy studies in atherosclerosis. II. Distribution and severity of atherosclerosis in patients dying with morphologic evidence of atherosclerotic catastrophe. Circulation **20**, 520–526 (1959b)

ROBERTS, W.C.: Role of thrombus in causing atherosclerosis and fatal coronary heart disease. In: Brain and heart Infarkt. ZÜLCH, K.J., KAUFMANN, W., HOSSMANN, K.-A., HOSSMANN, V. (eds.), pp. 297–308. Berlin, Heidelberg, New York: Springer 1977

ROBERTS, W.C.: Die Koronararterien bei der ischämischen Herzerkrankung. Tatsachen und Meinungen. Triangel **16**, 77–92 (1977)

ROBERTS, W.C., JONES, A.A., VIRMAN, R.: Quantitation of coronary arterial luminal narrowing in coronary heart disease. In: Brain and heart infarct. ZÜLCH, K.J., KAUFMANN, W., HOSSMANN, K.-A., HOSSMANN, V. (eds.), pp. 34–38. Berlin, Heidelberg, New York: Springer 1979

ROBERTSON, E.G.: Cerebral lesions due to intracranial aneurysms. Brain **72**, 150–185 (1949)

ROBERTSON, W.F.: A text-book of pathology. In relation to mental diseases. Edinburgh: Clay 1900

ROCHOUX, J.A.: Recherches sur l'apoplexie, 2nd ed. Paris: Béchet 1833

ROER, H.: Luftembolie des Herzens – die akute Gefahr des Schädelbasisbruches und der Thoraxkompression. Zentralbl. Neurochir. **9**, 237–248 (1949)

ROKITANSKI, C. v.: Über eine der wichtigsten Krankheiten der Arterien. Wien: Kaiserliche Hof- u. Staatsdruckerei 1852

ROKITANSKI, C. v.: Lehrbuch der pathologischen Anatomie, Bd. I u. II, 3. umgearb. Aufl. Wien: Braunmüller 1856

ROMANUL, F.C.A., ABRAMOWICZ, A.: Changes in brain and pial vessels in arterial border zones. Arch. Neurol. **11**, 40–65 (1964)

ROSE, W.M.: Survival period of patients with cerebral hemorrhage dying in hospital. Lancet (1948) **II**, 561–563

ROSEGAY, H., WELCH, K.: Peripheral collateral circulation between cerebral arteries. A demonstration by angiography of the meningeal arterial anastomoses. J. Neurosurg. **11**, 363–377 (1954)

ROSENBERG, E.F.: Brain in malignant hypertension. Arch. Intern. Med. **65**, 545–586 (1940)

ROSENBLATH: Über die Entstehung der Hirnblutung bei dem Schlaganfall. Dtsch. Z. Nervenheilkd. **61**, 10–143 (1918)

ROSENBLATH: Über die apoplektiforme, nicht embolische und vorwiegend unblutige Hirnerweichung und über „arteriocapillary-fibrosis". Z. klin. Med. **106**, 482–527 (1927)

ROSS, R., GLOMSET, J.A.: Atherosclerosis and the arterial smooth muscle cell. Science **180**, 1332–1339 (1973)

ROSS, R., HARKER, L.A., GLOMSET, J.: The pathogenesis of the lesions of atherosclerosis. In: Brain and heart infarkt. ZÜLCH, K.J., KAUFMANN, W., HOSSMANN, K.-A., HOSSMANN, V. (eds.), pp. 20–26. Berlin, Heidelberg, New York: Springer 1979

ROTHEMUND, E., FRISCHE, M.: Klinisch-pathologische Studie zur Entstehung der intracerebralen Gefäßhyalinose bei Hypertonie. Arch. Psychiatr. Nervenkr. **217**, 195–206 (1973)

ROTTER, W.: Über die Bedeutung der Ernährungsstörung, insbesondere des Sauerstoffmangels für die Pathogenese der Gefäßveränderungen mit besonderer Berücksichtigung der „Endarteriitis obliterans" und der „Arteriosklerose". Beitr. pathol. Anat. **110**, 46–102 (1949)

Roux, W.: Über die Verzweigungen der Blutgefäße des Menschen. Doktor-Dissertation, Universität Jena 1878

Rühl, A.: Arteriosklerotische Gefäßruptur oder Spasmus als Ursache der apoplektischen Gehirnblutung? Beitr. pathol. Anat. **78**, 160–186 (1927)

Russell, D.S.: Discussion: The pathology of spontaneous intracranial hemorrhage. Proc. R. Soc. Med. **47**, 689–693 (1954)

Russell, R.W.R.: Atheromatous retinal embolism. Lancet (1963) **II**, 1354–1356

Russell, R.W.R.: Arterial thrombosis and microembolism. In: Cerebral circulation and stroke. Zülch, K.J. (ed.), pp. 193–197. Berlin, Heidelberg, New York: Springer 1971

Russell, R.W.R., Simcock, J.P., Wilkinson, I.M.S., Frears, C.C.: The effect of blood pressure changes on the leptomeningeal circulation of the rabbit. Brain **93**, 491–504 (1970)

Ruysch, F.: Epistola anatomica, problematic, duodecima, authore Mich. Ernesto Ettmullero, etc. ad virum clarissimum Fredericum Ruys, etc. de cerebri corticali substantia. Amsterdam: 1699

Sachs, E. jr.: Arteriographic demonstration of collateral circulation through ophthalmic artery in internal carotid artery thrombosis. Report of 2 cases. J. Neurosurg. **11**, 405–409 (1954)

Sacks, J.G., Lindenberg, R.: Dolicho-ectatic intracranial arteries: Symptomatology and pathogenesis of arterial elongation and distention. Johns Hopkins Med. J. **125**, 95–106 (1969)

Safar, P., Bleyaert, A., Nemoto, E.M., Moossy, J., Stezoski, W.S., Snyder, J.V.: Cerebral resuscitation after global ischemic anoxia. In: Brain and heart infarct. Zülch, K.J., Kaufmann, W., Hossmann, K.-A., Hossmann, V. (eds.), pp. 251–268. Berlin, Heidelberg, New York: Springer 1979

Sako, Y.: Effects of turbulent blood flow and hypertension on experimental atherosclerosis. J. Am. Med. Assoc. **179**, 134–138 (1962)

Salamon, G.: Atlas de la vascularisation artérièlle du cerveau chez l'homme. Paris: Sandoz 1971, 1973

Salamon, G., Huang, Y.P.: Radiologic anatomy of the brain. Berlin, Heidelberg, New York: Springer 1976

Sano, K.: Cerebral juxta-basal telangiectasia. Brain Nerve (Tokyo) **17**, 748–750 (1965)

Sarkari, N.B., Holmes, J.M., Bickerstaff, E.R.: Neurological manifestations associated with internal carotid loops and kinks in children. J. Neurol. Neurosurg. Psychiatr. **33**, 194–200 (1970)

Satinsky, V.P., Braslow, N.: Experimental cerebral hypertension. Circulation **39** and **40**, Suppl. III, 176 (1969)

Saunders, R.L. de C.H., Bell, M.A.: X-ray microscopy and histochemistry of the human cerebral blood vessels. J. Neurosurg. **35**, 128–139 (1971)

Saweliew, N.: Gehirnembolie. Virchows Arch. pathol. Anat. **135**, 112–135 (1894)

Sayre, G.P., Siekert, R.G.: Thrombosis of the basilar artery with infarction of the brain stem. J. Neuropathol. Exp. Neurol. **15**, 221–223 (1956)

Sayre, G.P., Campbell, D.C.: Multiple peripheral emboli in atherosclerosis of the aorta. Arch. Intern. Med. **103**, 799–806 (1959)

Schechter, M.M., Zingesser, L.H.: The anterior spinal artery. Acta Radiol. [Diagn.] (Stockh.) **3**, 489–496 (1965)

Schechter, M.M., Zingesser, L.H.: The spinal arteries. Acta Radiol. [Diagn.] (Stockh.) **5**, 1124–1131 (1966)

Scheid, W.: Lehrbuch der Neurologie. Stuttgart: Thieme 1963; 3. überarb. Aufl. 1968

Scheinker, J.M.: Neurosurgical Pathology. Springfield/Ill.: Thomas 1948

Schettler, G.: Arteriosklerose. Ätiologie, Pathologie, Klinik und Therapie. Stuttgart: Thieme 1961

Schlierf, G.: Gibt es eine Regression der Atherosklerose beim Menschen? Triangel **15**, 71–76 (1976)

Schmidt, H.W.: Über Arterienkreise in der Pia mater des Menschen. Dtsch. Z. Nervenheilkd. **172**, 526–530 (1955a)

Schmidt, H.W.: Über Embolien in den Arterienkreisen der Pia mater. Z. gesamten Exp. Med. **125**, 401–408 (1955b)

Schmitt, R.: Pathologisch-anatomische Untersuchungen über neurologische Veränderungen bei akuten und chronischen Leukosen. Doktor-Dissertation, Universität Köln 1970

Schneider, M.: Kreislauf und Gehirn. Dresden, Leipzig: Steinkopf 1951

Schneider, M.: Chemie und Stoffwechsel der Nervengewebe. Mosbacher Coloquium. Berlin, Göttingen, Heidelberg: Springer 1952

Schneider, M.: Durchblutung und Sauerstoffversorgung des Gehirns. Verh. dtsch. Ges. Kreisl. Forsch. **19**, 3–25 (1953)

Schneider, M.: Die Wiederbelebungszeit verschiedener Organe nach Ischämie. Arch. klin. Chir. **308**, 253–265 (1964)

Schob, F.: Pathologische Anatomie der Idiotie. In: Handbuch der Geisteskrankheiten, Bumke, O. (Hrsg.), Band XI, Teil VII, S. 779–995. Berlin: Springer 1930

Scholz, W., Nieto, D.: Studien zur Pathologie der Hirngefäße. I. Fibrose und Hyalinose. Z. gesamten Neurol. Psychiatrie **162**, 676–693 (1938)

Schoop, W.: Frühdiagnose stenosierender Arterienveränderungen. Dtsch. med. Wochenschr. **92**, 1723–1726 (1967)

Schürmann, K.: Darstellung der A. vertebralis und ihrer Äste im Angiogramm von der A. carotis externa aus. Zentralbl. Neurochir. **14**, 362–365 (1954)

Schürmann, K., Dietz, H.: Die cerebrovasculären Erkrankungen aus neurochirurgischer Sicht. Zentralbl. Neurochir. **21**, 107–126 (1961)

Schuier, F.J., Vise, W.M., Hossmann, K.-A., Zülch, K.J.: Cerebral microembolization. II. Morphological studies. Arch. Neurol. **35**, 264–270 (1978)

Schultz, A.: Pathologie der Blutgefäße. In: Ergebnisse der allg. Pathologie u. pathologischen Anatomie des Menschen und der Tiere, OSTERTAG, R. v., FREI, W. (Hrsg.) Band **23**, S. 471–501. München: Bergmann 1930

SCHULZE, H.A.F., SAUERBREY, A.: Zur Frage der Anastomosen zwischen der A. vertebralis und der A. occipitalis. Zentralbl. Neurochir. **16**, 76–80 (1956)

SCHWARTZ, C.J., MITCHELL, J.R.A.: Observations on localization of arterial plaques. Circ. Res. **11**, 63–73 (1962)

SCHWARTZ, PH.: Die Arten der Schlaganfälle des Gehirns und ihre Entstehung. Berlin: Springer 1930

SCHWARTZ, PH.: Cerebral apoplexy. Types, causes, pathogenesis. Springfield/Ill.: Thomas 1961

SCHWARTZ, PH., GOLDSTEIN, K.: Typen und Lokalisation der apoplektischen Hirnblutungen Erwachsener. Verh. dtsch. Ges. Pathol. **20**, 400–403 (1925)

SCHWARZACHER, W.: Über traumatische Markblutungen des Gehirns. Jb. Psychiatr. Neurol. **43**, 113–164 (1924)

SHEEHAN, S., BAUER, R.B., MEYER, J.S.: Vertebral artery compression in cervical spondylosis. Arteriographic demonstration during life of vertebral artery insufficiency due to rotation and extension of the neck. Neurology (Minneap.) **10**, 968–986 (1960)

SHINKAI, H., YOSHIDA, Y., OONEDA, G.: An electron microscopic study of plasmatic arterionecrosis in the human cerebral arteries. Virchows Arch. pathol. Anat. **369**, 181–190 (1976)

SIEGRIST, A.: Die Gefahren der Ligatur der großen Halsschlagadern für das Auge und das Leben des Menschen. Graefes Arch. Ophthalmol. **50**, 511–646 (1900)

SIEKERT, R.G., MILLIKAN, C.H.: Syndrome of intermittent insufficiency of the basilar arterial system. Collected papers of the Mayo-Clinic and Mayo-Foundation **47**, 539–542 (1956)

SILBERMAN, J., CRAVIOTO, H., FEIGEN, I.: Foreign body emboli following cerebral angiography. Arch. Neurol. **3**, 711–717 (1960)

SILVERSTEIN, A.: Primary pontile hemorrhage. A review of 50 cases. Confin. Neurol. (Basel) **29**, 33–46 (1967)

SILVERSTEIN, A., HOLLIN, S.: Occlusion of the supraclinoid portion of the internal carotid artery. Neurology (Minneap.) **13**, 679–685 (1963)

SIMEONE, F.: Current concepts in the management of vasospasm. 11th Princeton Conference on Cerebral Vascular Disease 1978. (in press) (1979)

SJÖSTRÖM, L., METTINGER, K.L., SÖDERSTRÖM, C.E.: Intracerebral haemorrhage. A study of risk-profile, diagnosis and prognosis in a well-defined material. In: 11th World Congress of Neurology, Amsterdam 1977. Abstracts. DEN HARTOG JAGER, W.A., BRUYN, G.W., HEIJSTEE, A.P.J. (eds.), p. 51. Amsterdam, Oxford: Excerpta Medica 1977

SMITH, D.E., ODEL, H.M., KERNOHAN, J.W.: Causes of death in hypertension. Am. J. Med. **9**, 516–527 (1950)

SMITH, K.R. jr., NELSON, J.S., DOOLEY, J.M. jr.: Bilateral "hypoplasia" of the internal carotid arteries. Neurology (Minneap.) **18**, 1149–1156 (1968)

SOBOTTA, J.: Atlas der deskriptiven Anatomie des Menschen. Band III. Berlin, München, Wien: Urban & Schwarzenberg 1948

SOHN, D., LEVINE, S.: Frontal lobe infarcts caused by brain herniation. Arch. Pathol. (Chic.) **84**, 509–512 (1972)

SOKOLOW, M., PERLOFF, D.: The prognosis of essential hypertension treated conservatively. Circulation **23**, 697–713 (1961)

SOLBERG, L.A.: A method for postmortem dissection of the vertebral arteries. World Neurol. **3**, 765–768 (1962)

SOLBERG, L.A.: Cerebral infarction, hemorrhage and atherosclerosis. In: Atherosclerosis IV. SCHETTLER, G., GOTO, Y., HATA, Y., KLOSE, G. (eds.), p. 91. Berlin, Heidelberg, New York: Springer 1977

SORGO, W.: Über den durch Gefäßprozeß bedingten Verschluß der A. carotis interna. Zentralbl. Neurochir. **4**, 161–179 (1939)

SPATZ, H.: Über die Vorgänge nach experimenteller Rückenmarksdurchtrennung mit besonderer Berücksichtigung der Unterschiede der Reaktionsweise des reifen und des unreifen Gewebes, nebst Beziehungen zur menschlichen Pathologie (Porencephalie und Syringomyelie). Histologische und histopathologische Arbeiten über die Großhirnrinde mit besonderer Berücksichtigung der pathologischen Anatomie der Geisteskrankheiten. NISSL, F., ALZHEIMER, A. (Hrsg.), Ergänzungsband, S. 51–367. Jena: Fischer 1921

SPATZ, H.: Über die Beteiligung des Gehirns bei der v. Winiwarter-Buergerschen Krankheit (Thromboendangiitis obliterans). Dtsch. Z. Nervenheilkd. **136**, 86–130 (1935)

SPATZ, H.: Grundriß der pathologischen Anatomie der Geisteskrankheiten. In: Lehrbuch der Geisteskrankheiten, 4. Aufl. BUMKE, O. (Hrsg.), S. 338–613. Berlin: Springer 1936

SPATZ, H.: Die „systematischen Atrophien“. Eine wohlgekennzeichnete Gruppe der Erbkrankheiten des Zentralnervensystems. Arch. Psychiatr. Nervenkr. **108**, 1–18 (1938)

SPATZ, H.: Pathologische Anatomie der Kreislaufstörungen des Gehirns. Z. gesamten Neurol. Psychiatrie **167**, 301–357 (1939)

SPATZ, H.: Pathologisch-anatomische Befunde bei den Psychosen des Rückbildungs- und Greisenalters. In: Lehrbuch der Geisteskrankheiten. 5. Aufl. BUNKE, O. (Hrsg.), S. 456–479. München: Bergmann 1942

SPIELMEYER, W.: Allgemeine Histopathologie des Nervensystems. Band I: Allgemeiner Teil. Berlin: Springer 1922

STAEMMLER, M.: Über Veränderungen der kleinen Hirngefäße in apoplektischen und traumatischen Erweichungsherden und ihre Beziehungen zur traumatischen Spätapoplexie. Beitr. pathol. Anat. **78**, 408–429 (1927)

STAEMMLER, M.: Zur Lehre von der Entstehung des Schlaganfalles. Klin. Wochenschr. **15**, 1300–1306 (1936)

STAEMMLER, M.: Die Kreislauforgane. In: Lehrbuch der speziellen pathologischen Anatomie. KAUFMANN, E., STAEMMLER, M. (Hrsg.), S. 1–380. Berlin: de Gruyter 1955

STAEMMLER, M.: Kreislaufstörungen und Gefäßerkrankungen des Zentralnervensystems mit Hirnödem und Hirnschwellung. In: Lehrbuch der speziellen pathologischen Anatomie, Band III, Teil 1. KAUFMANN, E., STAEMMLER, M. (Hrsg.), S. 271–342. Berlin: de Gruyter 1958

STEHBENS, W.E.: Turbulence of blood flow. J. Exp. Physiol. **44**, 110–117 (1959)

STEHBENS, W.E.: Intimal proliferation and spontaneous lipid deposition in the cerebral arteries of sheep and steers. J. Atheroscler. Res. **5**, 556–568 (1965)

STEHBENS, W.E.: Pathology of the cerebral blood vessels. St. Louis: Mosby 1972

STEHBENS, W.E.: Local factors contributing to the pathogenesis of atherosclerosis. In: Brain and heart infarct. ZÜLCH, K.J., KAUFMANN, W., HOSSMANN, K.-A., HOSSMANN, V. (eds.), pp. 27–33. Berlin, Heidelberg, New York: Springer 1979

STEIMLE, R., ROYER, J., ACHARD, M., SAINT-HILLIER, Y.: Agénésie de la carotide interne. Neurochirurgie **15**, 147–152 (1969)

STEIN, B.M., MCCORMICK, W.F., RODRIGUEZ, J.N., TAVERAS, J.M.: Postmortem angiography of cerebral vascular system. Arch. Neurol. **7**, 545–559 (1962)

STEINMETZ, E.F., CALANCHINI, PH.R., AGUILAR, M.J.: Left atrial myxoma as a neurological problem: A case report and review. Stroke **4**, 451–458 (1973)

STEPHENS, R.B., STILWELL, D.L.: Arteries and veins of the human brain. Springfield/Ill.: Thomas 1969

STERN, K.: The pathology of apoplexy. J. Neurol. Neurosurg. Psychiatry **23**, 26–37 (1938)

STOCHDORPH, O., MEESSEN, H.: Die arteriosklerotische und die hypertonische Hirnerkrankung. In: Handbuch der speziellen pathologischen Anatomie und Histologie, Teil 1B, LUBARSCH, O., HENKE, F., RÖSSLE, R. (Hrsg.), Band XIII, S. 1465–1510. Berlin, Göttingen, Heidelberg: Springer 1957

STOCKARD, J.J., BICKFORD, R.G., MYERS, R.R., AUNG, M.H., DILLEY, R.B., SCHAUBLE, J.F.: Hypotension-induced changes in cerebral function during cardiac surgery. Stroke **5**, 730–746 (1974)

STOPFORD, J.S.B.: The arteries of the pons and medulla oblongata, Part I and II. J. Anat. Physiol. (Lond.) **50**, 131–164, 255–279 (1915)

STRANDGAARD, S., MACKENZIE, E.T., JONES, J.V., HARPER, A.M.: Studies on the cerebral circulation of the baboon in acutely induced hypertension. Stroke **7**, 287–290 (1976)

STRONG, J.P.: Unexplained variability in extent of atherosclerosis in homogenous human populations. In: Atherosclerosis IV. SCHETTLER, G., GOTO, Y., HATA, Y., KLOSE, G. (eds.), pp. 671–674. Berlin, Heidelberg, New York: Springer 1977

STRONG, J.P., MCGILL, H.C. jr.: The pediatric aspects of atherosclerosis. J. Atheroscler. Res. **9**, 251–265 (1969)

SUGAR, H.S., WEBSTER, J.E., GURDJIAN, E.S.: Ophthalmologic findings in spontaneous thrombosis of the carotid arteries. Arch. Ophthalmol. **44**, 823–832 (1950)

SUZUKI, J., KODAMA, N.: Cerebrovascular "moyamoya" disease. Second Report: Collateral routes to forebrain via ethmoid sinus und superior nasal meatus. Angiology **22**, 223–236 (1971)

SUZUKI, J., TAKAKU, A.: Cerebrovascular "moyamoya" disesase. A disease showing abnormal netlike vessels in base of brain. Arch. Neurol. **20**, 288–299 (1969)

SUZUKI, J. et al.: A study on disease showing singular cerebroangiographical findings which seemed to be due to new collateral circulation, read before the 22nd meeting of the Japan Neurosurgical Society, September 1963

SWANK, R.L., HAIN, F.: The effect of different sized emboli of the vascular system and parenchyma of the brain. J. Neuropathol. Exp. Neurol. **11**, 280–299 (1952)

SYMON, L.: Experimental study of cerebral arterial spasm. 3rd Eur. Congr. of Neurosurg., Madrid 1967. Int. Congr. Ser. No.139. Amsterdam: Excerpta Medica 1967

SYMON, L., PASZTOR, E., BRANSTON, N.M.: The distribution and density of reduced cerebral blood flow following acute middle cerebral artery occlusion: An experimental study by the technique of hydrogen clearance in baboons. Stroke **5**, 355–364 (1974)

SYMONDS, CH.: Hydrocephalic and focal cerebral symptoms in relation to thrombophlebitis of the dural sinuses and cerebral veins. Brain **60**, 531–550 (1937)

SYMONDS, CH.: Intracranial thrombophlebitis. Ann. R. Coll. Surg. Engl. **10**, 347–356 (1942)

SYMONDS, CH.: The circle of Willis (Harveian oration)! Br. Med. J. **1**, 119–124 (1955)

SZAPIRO, J., PAKULA, H.: Anatomical studies of the collateral blood supply to the brain and the retina. J. Neurol. Neurosurg. Psychiatry **26**, 414–417 (1963)

TAKEUCHI, K.: Occlusive diseases of the carotid artery. Especially on their surgical treatment. Shinkei Kenkyu no Shinpo **5**, 511–543 (1961)

TAMURA, M., ZÜLCH, K.J.: Experimental microembolism of the brain. Neurosurg. Rev. **1**, 111–117 (1978)

TATELMANN, M.: The angiographic evaluation of cerebral atherosclerosis. Radiology **70**, 801–810 (1958)

TAVERAS, J.M., WOOD, E.H.: Diagnostic neuroradiology. Baltimore: Williams & Wilkins 1964

TEAL, J.S., RUMBAUGH, C.L., BERGERON, R.T., SEGALL, H.D.: Congenital absence of the internal carotid artery associated with cerebral hemiatrophy, absence of the external carotid artery, and persistence of the stapedial artery. Am. J. Roentgenol. **118**, 534–545 (1973)

TESTUT, L., LATARJET, A.: Traité d'anatomie humaine. 8e éd. Paris: Doin 1929

TEXON, M.: Hemodynamic concept of atherosclerosis with particular reference to coronary occlusion. Arch. Intern. Med. **99**, 418 (1957)

TEXON, M.: Hemodynamic concept of atherosclerosis. Am. J. Cardiol. **5**, 291–294 (1960)

TEXON, M.: The role of vascular dynamics in the development of atherosclerosis. In: Atherosclerosis and its origin. SANDLER, M., BOURNE, G.H. (eds.), pp. 167–196. New York, London: Academic Press 1963

TEXON, M., IMPARATO, A.M., LORD, J.W. jr.: The hemodynamic concept of atherosclerosis. The experimental production of hemodynamic arterial disease. Arch. Surg. **80**, 47–53 (1960)

THIENEMANN, H.H.: Atypische intrakranielle Blutungen aus sogenannten Mikroangiomen. Doktor-Dissertation, Universität Köln 1975

THOMA, R.: Die Gestalt der Gefäßlichtung bei der diffusen und knotigen Arteriosklerose. Virchows Arch. pathol. Anat. **216**, 314–320 (1914)

THOMA, R.: Über die Störung des Blutes in der Gefäßbahn und die Spannung der Gefäßwand; ihre Bedeutung für das normale Wachstum, für die Blutstillung und für die Angiosklerose. Beitr. pathol. Anat. **66**, 377–432 (1920)

THOMA, R.: Über die Genese und die Lokalisation der Arteriosklerose. Virchows Arch. pathol. Anat. **245**, 78–122 (1923)

THOMAS, A.: Pathologie du Cervelet. In: Nouveau traité de Médecine. ROGER, G.H., WIDAL, F., TEISSIER, P.-J. (eds.), pp. 755–980. Paris: Masson 1925

THOMAS, C.B., COHEN, B.H.: Familial occurrence of hypertension and coronary artery disease, with observations concerning obesity and diabetes. Ann. Intern. Med. **42**, 90–127 (1955)

THOMPSON, R.K., RHODE, C.M.: Effects of anterior cerebral circulation occlusion with varying levels of blood pressure in the macaque. J. Nerv. Ment. Dis. **112**, 58–65 (1950)

THOMSON, J.L.G.: Stenosis of the carotid siphon. Acta Radiol. [Diagn.] (Stockh.) **1**, 481–484 (1963)

Thule International Symposia: "Stroke", April 19–21, 1966. ENGEL, A., LARSSON, T. (eds.). Stockholm: Nordiska Bokhandelns Förlag 1967

THULESIUS, O.: Hypotension as a risk factor. In: Brain and heart infarct. ZÜLCH, K.J., KAUFMANN, W., HOSSMANN, K.-A., HOSSMANN, V. (eds.), pp. 197–199. Berlin, Heidelberg, New York: Springer 1977

TINDALL, G.T., ODOM, G.L., DILLON, M.L., CUPP, H.B. jr., MAHALEY, M.S. jr., GREENFIELD, J.C. jr.: Direction of blood flow in the internal and external carotid arteries following occlusion of the ipsilateral common carotid artery. J. Neurosurg. **20**, 985–994 (1963)

TÖNDURY, G.: Angewandte und topographische Anatomie. 2. erw. Aufl. 1959. Stuttgart: Thieme 1951

TÖNNIS, W., SCHIEFER, W.: Zirkulationsstörungen des Gehirns im Serienangiogramm. Berlin, Göttingen, Heidelberg: Springer 1959

TÖNNIS, W., SCHIEFER, W., WALTER, W.: Zur Differentialdiagnose intrakranieller Blutungen (unter Ausschluß der neuroradiologischen Methoden). Dtsch. Z. Nervenheilkd. **176**, 666–692 (1957)

TÖNNIS, W., SCHIEFER, W., WALTER, W.: Signs and symptoms of supratentorial arteriovenous aneurysms. J. Neurosurg. **15**, 471–480 (1958)

TOOLE, F.J.: Diagnostic techniques in the medical evaluation and treatment of transient ischemic attacks. Clin. Neurosurg. **22**, 148–162 (1975)

TOOLE, J.F.: Management of transient ischemic attacks. In: Cerebrovascular diseases. SCHEINBERG, P. (ed., pp. 23–30. New York: Raven Press 1976

TOOLE, J.F., PATEL, A.N.: Cerebrovascular disorders, 2nd ed. New York: McGraw-Hill 1974

TOOLE, J.F., JANEWAY, R., CHOI, K., CORDELL, R., DAVIS, C., JOHNSTON, F., MILLER, H.S.: Transient ischemic attacks due to atherosclerosis. Arch. Neurol. **32**, 5–12 (1975)

TORRES, N.V.J.: Medicamentos utilizados en los accidentes vasculares cerebrales. 3rd Symposium Internacional Sobre Accidentes Vasculares Transitorios (AIT), Valencia 1977, pp. 243–251. Valencia: Semana Grafica 1977

TORVIK, A., SKULLERUD, K.: How often are brain infarcts caused by hypotensive episodes? Stroke **7**, 255–257 (1976)

TOURNADE, A., MAILLOT, CL., KORITKE, J.G.: Les veines superficielles du tronc cérébral chez l'homme. Essai de systematisation. Arch. Anat. Histol. Embryol. **55**, 233–281 (1972)

Transient Ischemic Attacks. III. Symp. Internacional Sobre Accidentes Vasculares Transitorios (AIT), Valencia 1977. Valencia: Semana Grafica 1977

TRAUBE, J. (ed.): cit. by HASSE, K.E.: Handbuch der speziellen Pathologie und Therapie, Band IV, Teil 1, S. 517. Erlangen: Enke 1855

TRAUPE, H., HEISS, W.-D., HACKER, H., ZÜLCH, K.J., HOEFFKEN, W.: Time controlled angio-computertomography in cerebro-vascular ischemia. In: Cerebral blood flow and metabolism. GOTO, F., NAGAI, H., TAZAKI, Y. (eds.), pp. 414–415. Copenhagen: Munksgaard 1979 (Acta Neurol. Scand. **60**, Supp. 72)

TRAUPE, H., HEISS, W.-D., HOEFFKEN, W., ZÜLCH, K.J.: Hyperfusion and enhancement in serial computed tomography of ischemic stroke patients. J. Computer Assisted Tomogr. (in press) (1979)

TROTTER, W.: Chronic subdural haemorrhage of traumatic origin, and its relation to pachymeningitis haemorrhagica interna. Br. J. Surg. **2**, 271–291 (1914)

TURNBULL, I.: Agenesis of the internal carotid artery. Neurology (Minneap.) **12**, 588–590 (1962)

VAERNET, K.: Collateral ophthalmic artery circulation in thrombotic carotid occlusion. Neurology (Minneap.) **4**, 605–611 (1954)

VAN DEN BERGH, R.: La vascularisation artérielle intracérébrale. Acta Neurol. Belg. **61**, 1013–1031 (1961)

VAN DEN BERGH, R.: Einige Besonderheiten der intracerebralen Gefäßordnung. Zentralbl. Neurochir. **25**, 180–197 (1965)

VAN DEN BERGH, R.: The periventricular intracerebral blood supply. In: Research on the cerebral circulation. 3rd Int. Salzburg Conference 1966. MEYER, J.S., LECHNER, H., EICHHORN, O. (eds.), pp. 52–65. Springfield/Ill.: Thomas 1969

VAN DEN BERGH, R., PLETS, C.: The blood supply and angioarchitecture of corpus callosum. In: Research on the cerebral circulation. 4th Int. Salzburg Conference 1968. MEYER, J.S., LECHNER, H., REIVICH, M., EICHHORN, O. (eds.), pp. 5–16. Springfield/Ill.: Thomas 1970

VAN DER DRIFT, J.H.A., KOK, N.K.D.: "Intracerebral steal" in cerebrovascular occlusion, vascular malformation, and brain tumor: Clinical EEG, angiographic, and circulatory findings. In: Research on the cerebral circulation. 4th Int. Salzburg Conference 1968. MEYER, J.S., REIVICH, M., LECHNER, H., EICHHORN, O. (eds.), pp. 60–75. Springfield/Ill.: Thomas 1970

VAN DER DRIFT, J.H.A., KOK, N.K.D.: The EEG in cerebro-vascular disorders in relation to pathology. In: Handbook of electroencephalography and clinical neurophysiology, VAN DER DRIFT, J.H.A. (ed.), Vol. 14A, Part A, pp. 13–64. Amsterdam: Elsevier 1972

VAN DER EECKEN, H.M.: The anastomoses between the leptomeningeal arteries of the brain. Springfield/Ill.: Thomas 1959

VAN DER EECKEN, H.M., ADAMS, R.D.: The anatomy and functional significance of the meningeal arterial anastomoses of the human brain. J. Neuropathol. Exp. Neurol. **12**, 132–157 (1953)

VIGOUROUX, R., LAVIELLE, J.: Les thromboses post-traumatiques de la carotide interne. Neurochirurgie **8**, 115–142 (1962)

VINCENT, CL., DARQUIER, J.: Les dangeurs de la grande saignée chez les hypertendus. Sci. méd. (Paris) 1923

VIRCHOW, R.: Über die Erweiterung kleinerer Gefäße. Virchows Arch. pathol. Anat. **3**, 442 (1851)

VIRCHOW, R.: Phlogose und Thrombose im Gefäßsystem. Thrombose und Embolie. In: Gesammelte Abhandlungen zur wissenschaftlichen Medizin, S. 219–380. Frankfurt: Meidinger Sohn 1856

VISE, W.M., SCHUIER, F.J., HOSSMANN, K.-A., TAKAGI, S., ZÜLCH, K.J.: Cerebral microembolization. I. Pathophysiological studies. Arch. Neurol. **34**, 660–665 (1977)

VITEK, J.J., HALSEY, J.H., MCDOWELL, H.A.: Occlusion of all four extracranial vessels with minimal clinical symptomatology. Case report. Stroke **3**, 462–466 (1972)

VOGT, C., VOGT, O.: Zur Kenntnis der pathologischen Veränderungen des Striatum und des Pallidum und zur Pathophysiologie der dabei auftretenden Krankheitserscheinungen. S.-B. Heidelberger Akad. Wiss. math.-nat. Kl., Abt. B, Abh. **14**, 1–56 (1919)

WALKER, A.E.: Cerebral death. The professional information. Dallas/Texas: Library 1977

WALTIMO, O., KASTE, M., FOGELHOLM, R.: Prognosis of patients with unilateral extracranial occlusion of the internal carotid artery. Stroke **7**, 480–482 (1976)

WALTZ, A.G., SUNDT, T.M. jr., OWEN, C.A. jr.: Effect of middle cerebral artery occlusion on cortical blood flow in animals. Neurology (Minneap.) **16**, 1185–1190 (1967)

WANSCHER, O., CLEMMESEN, J., NIELSEN, A.: Negative correlation between atherosclerosis and carcinoma. Br. J. Cancer **2**, 172–174 (1951)

WARTMAN, W.B.: The incidence and severity of arteriosclerosis in the organs from five hundred autopsies. Am. J. Med. Sci. **186**, 27–35 (1933)

WEIBEL, J., FIELDS, W.S.: Tortuosity, coiling, and kinking of the internal carotid artery. Neurology (Minneap.) **15**, 7–18, 462–468 (1965)

WEIBEL, J., FIELDS, W.S.: Atlas of arteriography in occlusive cerebrovascular disease. Stuttgart: Thieme 1969

WEIDNER, W., HANAFEE, W., MARKHAM, C.H.: Intracranial collateral circulation via leptomeningeal and rete mirabile anastomoses. Neurology (Minneap.) **15**, 39–47 (1965)

WEPFER, J.T.: Observationes anatomicae ex cadaveribus eorum, quos sustulit apoplexia, cum exercitatione de ejus loco affecto. Schaffhusii: Suter 1658

WESOLOWSKI, S.A., FRIES, C.C., SABINI, A.M. et al.: The significance of turbulence in hemic systems and in the distribution of the atherosclerotic lesion. Surgery **57**, 155–162 (1965)

WESSLER, S., MING, S., GUREWICH, V., FREIMAN, D.G.: A critical evaluation of thromboangiitis obliterans. N. Engl. J. Med. **262**, 1149–1160 (1960)

WESTPHAL, K.: Über die Entstehung des Schlaganfalles. II. Klinische Untersuchungen zum Problem der Entstehung des Schlaganfalles. Dtsch. Arch. klin. Med. **151**, 31–95 (1926a)

WESTPHAL, K.: Über die Entstehung des Schlaganfalles. III. Experimentalle Untersuchungen zum Apoplexieproblem. Dtsch. Arch. klin. Med. **151**, 96–109 (1926b)

WESTPHAL, K., BAER, R.: Über die Entstehung des Schlaganfalls. Dtsch. Arch. klin. Med. **151**, 1–30 (1926)

WHISNANT, J.P.: Epidemiology of stroke: Emphasis on transient cerebral ischemic attacks and hypertension. Stroke **5**, 68–70 (1974)

WHISNANT, J.P., MARTIN, M.J., SAYRE, G.P.: Atherosclerotic stenosis of cervical arteries. Arch. Neurol. **5**, 429–432 (1961)

WHISNANT, J.P., ANDERSON, E.M., ARONSON, ST.M., HARRISON, C.E., HAYNES, M.A., KURTZKE, J.F.,

LINDSEY, W.H., OSTFELD, A.M., RENTZ, L.E., SUNDT, T.S.: Report of the Joint Committee for Stroke Facilities. V. Clinical prevention of stroke. Stroke **3**, 806–825 (1972)

WHISNANT, J.P., MATSUMOTO, N., ELVEBACK, L.R.: Transient cerebral ischemic attacks in a community. Rochester, Minnesota, 1955 through 1969. Proc. Mayo Clin. **48**, 194–198 (1973)

WHITE, R.: Multiple origins of cerebral vasospasm. 11th Princeton Conference on cerebral vascular disease 1978. (in press) (1979)

WHITE, R.P., HAGEN, A.A., MORGAN, H., DAWSON, W.N., ROBERTSON, J.T.: Experimental study on the genesis of cerebral vasospasm. Stroke **6**, 52–57 (1975)

WIENER, L.W., BERRY, R.G., KUNDIN, J.: Intracranial circulation in carotid occlusion. Arch. Neurol. **11**, 554–561 (1964)

WILLIAMS, A.O., LOEWENSON, R.B., LIPPERT, D.M., RESCH, J.A.: Cerebral atherosclerosis and its relationship to selected diseases in Nigerians: A pathological study. Stroke **6**, 395–401 (1975)

WILLIAMS, C.L., SCOTT, S.M., TAKARO, T.: Subclavian steal. Circulation **28**, 14–19 (1963)

WILLIAMS, D., WILSON, T.G.: The diagnosis of the major and minor syndromes of basilar insufficiency. Brain **85**, 741–774 (1962)

WILLIS, G.C.: Localizing factors in atherosclerosis. Can. Med. Assoc. J. **70**, 1–9 (1954)

WINDLE, B.C.A.: On arteries forming the circle of Willis. J. Anat. **22**, 289 (1887)

WINIWARTER, F. v.: Über eine eigentümliche Form von Endarteriitis und Endophlebitis mit Gangrän des Fußes. Langebecks Arch. klin. Chir. **23**, 202–262 (1879)

WIRTZ, H.: Die disseminierten Erweichungsherde des Hypertonikergehirns und ihre pathogenetische Bedeutung für die große Hochdruckblutung. Beitr. pathol. Anat. **97**, 219–232 (1936)

WISSLER, R.W.: Development of the atherosclerotic plaque. In: Myocardium: Failure and infarction. BRAUNWALD, E. (ed.), pp. 155–166. New York: Hospital Practice 1974

WISSLER, R.W.: Coronary atherosclerosis and ischemic heart disease. In: Brain and heart infarct. ZÜLCH, K.J., KAUFMANN, W., HOSSMANN, K.-A., HOSSMANN, V. (eds.), pp. 206–223. Berlin, Heidelberg, New York: Springer 1977

WODARZ, R.: Mediaastverschlüsse – 41 Fälle mit angiographischer, szintigraphischer und elektroenzephalographischer Korrelation zum klinischen Befund. Doktor-Dissertation, Universität Köln 1975

WOLFE, H.R.J.: Spontaneous subarachnoid haemorrhage. A surgical challenge. Br. J. Surg. **40**, 319–325 (1953)

WOLFF, K.: Grundlagen zu dem Problem der spontanen apoplektischen Hirnblutungen. Beitr. pathol. Anat. **89**, 249–512 (1932)

WOLMAN, L.: Cerebral dissecting aneurysms. Brain **82**, 276–291 (1959)

World Federation of Neurology: Collaborative study of epidemiological factors in cerebrovascular disease. Coding Guide. Antwerpen: Buschmann 1959

World Health Organization: Epidemiological and vital statistics. Reports, Vol. I–III. Geneva 1947–1950

World Health Organization: Classification of atherosclerotic lesions. Report of a study group. WHO techn. Rep. Ser. **143**, 3–20 (1958)

World Health Organization: Maladies cérébro-vasculaires: prévention, traitement et réadaptation. WHO techn. Rep. Ser. **469**, 1–63 (1971)

World Health Organization: Atherosclerosis of Aorta. World Health Bull., Geneva 1976

World Health Organization: The application of advances in neurosciences for the control of neurological disorders. WHO techn. Rep. Ser. **629**, 1–83 (1978)

WORM, R.: Les accidents nerveux consécutifs aux pertes de sang. Paris: Doin 1931

WRIGHT, J.S., MARPLE, C.D., BECK, D.F.: Myocardial infarction: A study of 1031 cases. New York: Grune & Stratton 1954

WÜLLENWEBER, G.: Fortdauer des Lebens bei doppelseitigem vollständigem Verschluß der Aa. carotides internae. Dtsch. Z. Nervenheilkd. **105**, 283–288 (1928)

WYLIE, E.J., HEIN, M.F., ADAMS, J.E.: Intracranial hemorrhage following surgical revascularization for treatment of acute strokes. J. Neurosurg. **21**, 212–215 (1964)

YAMORI, Y., HORIE, R., HANDA, H., SATO, M., FUKASE, M.: Pathogenetic similarity of strokes in stroke-prone spontaneously hypertensive rats and humans. Stroke **7**, 46–53 (1976)

YARNELL, PH.R., EARNEST, M.P., SANDERS, B., BURDICK, D.: The "hot stroke" and transient vascular occlusions. Stroke **6**, 517–520 (1975)

YATES, P.O.: Changing pattern of cerebrovascular disease in the United Kingdom. In: 5th Princeton Conference on Cerebral Vascular Disease. MILLIKAN, C.H., SIEKERT, R.G., WHISNANT, J.P. (eds.), pp. 67–82. London: Grune & Stratton 1966

YATES, P.O.: Epidemiology of cerebral haemorrhages. In: Maladies vasculaires cérébrales. Cerebrovascular diseases. Conférences de la Salpêtrière 1975, pp. 29–37. Paris: Baillière 1976

YATES, P.O., HUTCHINSON, E.C.: Cerebral infarction: The role of stenosis of the extracranial cerebral arteries. Spec. Rep. Ser. Med. Res. Counc., No. 300. London: Her Majesty's Stationery Office 1961

ZEHNDER, M.: Die subduralen Hämatome. Zentralbl. Neurochir. **1/2**, 339–353 (1937)

ZENKER, F.A.Z.: Über die Pathogenese der spontanen Hirnhämorrhagien. Verh. Naturforsch. Ges. Leipzig: 1872

ZERVAS, N.: Cerebral vasospasm. Introduction, definition and overview. In: 11th Princeton Conference on Cerebral Vascular Diseases 1978. (in press) (1979)

ZIEGLER, D.K., HASSAWEIN, R.S.: Prognosis in patients with transient ischemic attacks. Stroke **4**, 666–673 (1973)

ZIEGLER, D.K., ZOSA, A., ZILELI, T.: Hypertensive encephalopathy. Arch. Neurol. **12**, 472–478 (1965)

ZIMMERMAN, H.B., FARELL, W.-I.: Cervical vertebral erosion caused by vertebral artery tortuosity. Am. J. Roentgenol. **108**, 767 (1970)

ZIMMERMAN, H.M.: Cerebral apoplexy: mechanism and differential diagnosis. N.Y. State J. Med. **49**, 2153 (1949)

ZUCKSCHWERDT, L., THIES, H.A.: Die Thromboembolie. Dtsch. med. Wochenschr. **83**, 1001–1007 (1958)

ZÜLCH, K.J.: Vegetative und psychische Symptome bei umschriebenen traumatischen Zwischenhirnschäden und ihre Beurteilung im Gutachten. Zentralbl. Neurochir. **10**, 73–97 (1950)

ZÜLCH, K.J.: Neue Befunde und Deutungen aus der Gefäßpathologie des Hirns und Rückenmarks. Zentralbl. allg. Pathol. pathol. Anat. **90**, 402 (1953)

ZÜLCH, K.J.: Betrachtungen über die Entstehung der frühkindlichen Hirnschäden aufgrund der klinischen und morphologischen Befunde. Arch. Kinderheilkd. **149**, 3–27 (1954a)

ZÜLCH, K.J.: Mangeldurchblutung an der Grenzzone zweier Gefäßgebiete als Ursache bisher ungeklärter Rückenmarksschädigungen. Dtsch. Z. Nervenheilkd. **172**, 81–101 (1954b)

ZÜLCH, K.J.: Biologie und Pathologie der Hirngeschwülste. In: Handbuch der Neurochirurgie, Band III. OLIVECRONA, H., TÖNNIS, W. (Hrsg.). Berlin, Göttingen, Heidelberg: Springer 1956a

ZÜLCH, K.J.: Histologische Untersuchungen bei chronischem subduralem Hämatom. Hefte Unfallheilkd. **55**, 121–123 (1956b)

ZÜLCH, K.J.: Störungen des intrakraniellen Druckes. In: Handbuch der Neurochirurgie, Band I, 1. Teil. OLIVECRONA, H., TÖNNIS, W. (Hrsg.), S. 208–303. Berlin, Göttingen, Heidelberg: Springer 1959

ZÜLCH, K.J.: Die Pathogenese von Massenblutung und Erweichung unter besonderer Berücksichtigung klinischer Gesichtspunkte. Acta Neurochir. (Wien), Suppl. VII, 51–117 (1961a)

ZÜLCH, K.J.: Über die Entstehung und Lokalisation der Hirninfarkte. Zentralbl. Neurochir. **21**, 158–178 (1961b)

ZÜLCH, K.J.: The pathogenesis of disturbances of cerebral blood flow. Int. J. Neurol. **3**, 464–482 (1962a)

ZÜLCH, K.J.: Neuere Anschauungen über die Entstehung der cerebralen Insulte. Acta Med. Belg. 1962b, 890–904

ZÜLCH, K.J.: Zur Pathogenese des cerebrovasculären Insultes. Internist (Berl.) **4**, 64–70 (1963a)

ZÜLCH, K.J.: Les déplacements en masse dans le processus cérébraux expansifs et leurs rapports avec le siège et le genre de la tumeur. – La classification des tumeurs cérébrales. – Les altérations dues à l'hypertension intracranienne. – Le«gonflement» et l'oedème cérébral. Acta Neurochir. (Wien) **11**, 161–193 (1963b)

ZÜLCH, K.J.: Neurologische Diagnostik bei endokraniellen Komplikationen von oto-rhinologischen Erkrankungen. Arch. Ohr.-, Nas.-, u. Kehlk.-Heilkd. **183**, 1–85 (1964)

ZÜLCH, K.J.: Brain tumors. Their biology and pathology, 2nd ed. New York: J. Springer Publ. Comp. Inc. 1965

ZÜLCH, K.J.: La circulation cérébrale: Étude physiopathologique. In: Symposium international sur la circulation cérébrale, Paris 1965, pp. 121–146. Paris: Sandoz 1966a

ZÜLCH, K.J.: Les sténoses carotidiennes. Rev. Neurol. **115**, 627–640 (1966b)

ZÜLCH, K.J.: Morphology and pathogenesis of cerebral infarction. Symposium Int. de Investigaciones Neurologicas, Lima 1967, pp. 255–265. Anales del XII Congreso Latinoamericano de Neurocirugia 1967

ZÜLCH, K.J.: Neuropathology of intracranial haemorrhage. Prog. Brain Res. **30**, 151–165 (1968a)

ZÜLCH, K.J.: The morphologic basis of the abnormal echo-encephalogramm. In: Proceedings in echoencephalography. KAZNER, E., SCHIEFER, W., ZÜLCH, K.J. (eds.), pp. 12–24. Berlin, Heidelberg, New York: Springer 1968b

ZÜLCH, K.J.: The cerebral form of v. Winiwarter-Buerger's disease, does it exist? Angiology **20**, 61–69 (1969a)

ZÜLCH, K.J.: Allgemeine Prinzipien bei der Entstehung der Kollateralkreisläufe der Hirnarterien. Radiologe **9**, 396–406 (1969b)

ZÜLCH, K.J.: Reconsiderations of the clinical problem of cerebrovascular insufficiency. In: Research on the cerebral circulation. 3rd Int. Salzburg-Conference 1966. MEYER, J.S., LECHNER, H., EICHHORN, O. (eds.), pp. 1–41. Springfield/Ill.: Thomas 1969c

ZÜLCH, K.J.: Discussion. In: Research on the cerebral circulation. 3rd Int. Salzburg Conference 1966. MEYER, J.S., LECHNER, H., EICHHORN, O. (eds.), pp. 80, 106. Springfield/Ill.: Thomas 1969d

ZÜLCH, K.J.: Angiographische Befunde zur Pathogenese der Hirndurchblutungsstörungen. Zentralbl. Neurochir. **31**, 1–25 (1970)

ZÜLCH, K.J.: Pathological aspects of cerebral accidents in arterial hypertension. Acta Neurol. Belg. **71**, 196–220 (1971a)

ZÜLCH, K.J.: Hemorrhage, thrombosis, embolism. In: Pathology of the nervous system. MINCKLER, J. (ed.), Vol. 2, pp. 1499–1536. New York: McGraw-Hill 1971b

ZÜLCH, K.J.: Quelques observations sur l'artériosclérose intracranienne en Allemagne de l'ouest. Afr. J. med. Sci. **2**, 301–318 (1971c)

ZÜLCH, K.J.: Some basic patterns of the collateral circulation of the cerebral arteries. In: Cerebral circulation and stroke. ZÜLCH, K.J. (ed.), pp. 106–122. Berlin, Heidelberg, New York: Springer 1971d

ZÜLCH, K.J.: Die Karotis-Insuffizienz. Folia angiol. (Pisa) **21**, 47–62 (1973a)

Zülch, K.J.: Differentialdiagnose zwischen Krampfschäden und anderen Arten frühkindlicher Hirnschäden. In: Die neuropathologische Problematik der Hirngewebsveränderungen nach spontanen und therapeutischen Krämpfen. Beihefte zur Z. Psychiatrie, Neurologie und Medizinische Psychologie, Heft 17/18. Quandt, J., Sommer, H. (Hrsg.), pp. 65–73. Leipzig: Hirzel 1973b

Zülch, K.J.: Atlas of gross neurosurgical pathology. Berlin, Heidelberg, New York: Springer 1975a

Zülch, K.J.: Cerebrovasculäre Insuffizienz. Langenbecks Arch. klin. Chir. **339**, 161–167 (1975b)

Zülch, K.J.: Pyramidal and parapyramidal motor systems in man. In: Cerebral localization. Zülch, K.J., Creutzfeldt, O., Galbraith, G.C. (eds.), pp. 32–47. Berlin, Heidelberg, New York: Springer 1975c

Zülch, K.J.: Pathogenetic and clinical observations in spinovascular insufficiency. Zentralbl. Neurochir. **37**, 1–13 (1976)

Zülch, K.J.: Transient ischemic attacks (TIA). In: III. Symp. Internacional sobre Accidents Vasculares Transitorios (A.I.T.), Valencia 1977, pp. 177–189. Valencia: Semana Grafica 1977a

Zülch, K.J.: Clinical ischemia: Brain infarcts. In: Brain and heart infarct. Zülch, K.J., Kaufmann, W., Hossmann, K.-A., Hossmann, V. (eds.), pp. 288–296. Berlin, Heidelberg, New York: Springer 1977b

Zülch, K.J.: Predilection of cerebral atherosclerotic stenosis: A morphological and radiologic demonstration. In: Brain and heart infarct. Zülch, K.J., Kaufmann, W., Hossmann, K.-A., Hossmann, V. (eds.), pp. 39–49. Berlin, Heidelberg, New York: Springer 1979

Zülch, K.J., v. Einsiedel-Lechtape, H.: Thrombosis and embolism as a cause of ischemic cerebrovascular disturbances. Analysis from a series of 1000 patients. In: Platelet aggregation in the pathogenesis of cerebrovascular disorders. Agnoli, A., Fazio, C. (eds.), pp. 64–74. Berlin, Heidelberg, New York: Springer 1977

Zülch, K.J., Eschbach, O.: The interhemispheric steal syndromes. Neuroradiology **4**, 179–184 (1972)

Zülch, K.J., Gessaga, E.: Infarcts in the carotid system. Vasc. Surg. **6**, 114–119 (1972)

Zülch, K.J., Herberg, H.-J.: Das klinische Bild der akuten Blutsperre der A. carotis. Dtsch. Z. Nervenheilkd. **160**, 38–79 (1949)

Zülch, K.J., Hossmann, V.: Über die 24-Stunden-Rhythmik des menschlichen Blutdrucks. Dtsch. med. Wochenschr. **92**, 567–572 (1967)

Zülch, K.J., Kleihues, P.: Neuropathology of cerebral infarction. In: Thule International Symposia: "Stroke", 19–21. April 1966. Engel, A., Larsson, T. (eds.), pp. 57–75. Stockholm: Nordiska Bokhandelns Förlag 1967

Zülch, K.J., Tzonos, T.: Transsudationsphänomene an den tiefen Hirnvenen nach Blockade von Arteriolen oder Kapillaren der Rinde durch Mikroembolien. Naturwissenschaften **51**, 539–540 (1964)

Zülch, K.J., Tzonos, T.: Transsudation phenomena at the deep veins after blockage of arterioles and capillaries by micro-emboli. Bibl. Anat. (Basel) **7**, 279–284 (1965)

Zülch, K.J., Kleihues, P., Gabe, D.: Die aktuelle Problematik auf dem Gebiet der Pathogenese, Klinik und Therapie der Hirndurchblutungsstörungen. In: Der Hirnkreislauf in Forschung und Klinik. 2nd Int. Salzburg Conference 1964. Wien: Brüder Hollinek 1964 (see also: Wien. med. Wochenschr. **116**, 494–503, 1966)

Zülch, K.J., Einsiedel-Lechtape, H., Hartmann, W.: Der Mediahauptstamm-Verschluß. Klinisch-angiographische Korrelation. In: Fisiopatologia clinica e terapia del circolo. Atti delle Giornate Mediche Triestine 1972, pp. 117–124. Trieste: Tipografia Gaetano Coana 1973

Zülch, K.J., Dreesbach, H.A., Eschbach, O.: Occlusion of the middle cerebral artery with the formation of an abnormal arterial collateral system – moyamoya type – 23 months later. Neuroradiology **7**, 19–24 (1974a)

Zülch, K.J., Mennel, H.D., Zimmermann, V.: Intracranial hypertension. In: Handbook of clinical neurology, Vinken, P.J., Bruyn, G.W. (eds.), Vol. 16, pp. 89–149. Amsterdam: North Holland 1974b

Zülch, K.J., Creutzfeldt, O., Galbraith, G.C.: Cerebral localization. Berlin, Heidelberg, New York: Springer 1975

Zülch, K.J., Pakula, H., Schuier, F.: Distant perivenous demyelination after microembolization of the brain. Neuropathol. Appl. Neurobiol. **2**, 163 (1976)

Physiologie und Pathophysiologie der Gehirndurchblutung

Von

E. Betz

Mit 37 Abbildungen und 5 Tabellen

A. Historische Einleitung

Die Bedeutung der Halsschlagadern für die mentalen Funktionen hatten schon die Griechen erkannt, die deshalb den Halsschlagadern den Namen Karotiden (von griech. *καρος*) gaben, das soviel wie „Betäubung" heißt. Daß die Herzaktionen und die Durchblutung des Gehirns etwas miteinander zu tun haben müßten, ist von R.C. Colombo (1516–1559) erkannt worden, der beschrieb, daß die Pulsationen des Herzens und der Arterien mit denen des Gehirns synchron waren. Vesalius (1514–1564) beschreibt im 7. Buch von „De humanis corporis fabrica" das Gefäßsystem des Gehirns und zeichnet eine breite Verbindung zwischen den zuführenden Halsgefäßen und dem Venensinus, was zwar nicht richtig ist, aber der damaligen Annahme entsprach, daß das Blut aus den inneren Halsschlagadern in die großen Venen entleert wird. Durch Untersuchungen von William Harvey (1578–1657), der das Experiment in die Erforschung des Kreislaufs einführte, kam die funktionelle Betrachtungsweise stärker in das Gesichtsfeld der Forschung. Thomas Willis (1621–1675) hat bei seinen Beschreibungen der Gehirngefäße die wichtigsten Grundlagen für die Erkennung einer kollateralen Versorgung des Gehirns geschaffen. Alexander Monro der Jüngere (1733–1817) ist derjenige Forscher gewesen, der durch seine „Observations on the structure and function of the nervous system" über viele Jahre die Meinung festigte, daß die knöcherne Schädelkapsel des Gehirns eine rein druckpassive Gehirndurchblutung bewirke. Als Grund hierfür wurde angegeben, daß das Gehirn – ganz ähnlich wie andere feste Bestandteile des Körpers – inkompressibel ist. 1837 bestätigte Kellie zu Leith die druckpassive Durchblutung, und diese Auffassung ging als Monro-Kellie-Doktrin in die Literatur ein; dies, obwohl schon 1846 Burrows feststellte, daß der Liquorgehalt des Gehirns keineswegs konstant sei. Zwei wichtige Probleme beschäftigten dann auch einige Forscher im 18. und 19. Jahrhundert: Der Ursprung der Gehirnpulsationen und die Frage nach den motorischen Reaktionen der Muskulatur der Gehirngefäße. Ridley (1700) war einer der ersten, der eine systematische Studie der Gehirnpulsationen durchführte, und er stellte – ähnlich wie Haller (1755) – fest, daß die Arterien die Ursache dieser Pulsationen waren. Haller war der erste, der Bohrlöcher im menschlichen Schädel anbrachte, um die Schädelpulsationen genauer beobachten zu können. Durch Donders (1850) wurde dieses Untersuchungsverfahren dahingehend modifiziert, daß er luftdichte Fenster in das Bohrloch einsetzte und beobachtete, daß dann, wenn alle Luft aus dem Bohrloch verschwunden war, die Gehirnpulsationen nicht mehr auftraten. Er schloß daraus, daß die früheren Beobachter Artefakte beschrieben hatten, weil die Pulsationen des Gehirns nur dann möglich waren, wenn das Gehirn sich ausdehnen und Liquor verschwinden konnte. Leyden (1866) träufelte während der Beobachtung der Gehirnoberfläche Medikamente auf das Gehirn und beobachtete durch das Schädeldachfenster die Weitenänderungen der Piagefäße. Auch in der Folgezeit waren

Beitrag abgeliefert 1976, ergänzt 30. 5. 1978

die direkten Beobachtungen der Piagefäße eine der erfolgreichsten Methoden bei der Beurteilung des Gehirnkreislaufs. Von HENLE (1841) stammt der Begriff der „vasomotorischen Nerven", die die Muskelfasern in der Media der Arterien versorgen. NOTHNAGEL (1867) untersuchte mit der Methode der Schädeldachfensterung Fragestellungen, die auch heutzutage noch aktuell sind. So hat er bei Reizung des Nervus suralis am wachen Tier deutliche Verengerungen der Piagefäße beobachtet und Untersuchungen zur Rolle von Nerven bei der Gehirngefäßkonstriktion und -dilatation vorgenommen. Angeregt durch die Untersuchungen von CLAUDE BERNARD (1851) hat DONDERS (1851) seine ersten Experimente zum Zusammenhang der Asphyxie mit der zerebralen Gefäßweite durchgeführt. Auch zeigte er, daß bei Reizungen des Halssympathikus Piagefäße auf der Seite der Reizung verengert wurde. BRACHET hatte schon 1837 festgestellt, daß nach Durchtrennung des Sympathikus eine Blutansammlung im Gehirn auftrat und er war damit derjenige, der die zahlreichen Untersuchungen über die Wirkung des Sympathikus auf die Gehirngefäßdurchblutung einleitete. SCHULTZ beschrieb 1866 spontane Weitenänderungen von Piagefäßen und SCHÜLLER (1874) untersuchte die Wirkungen von Chloroform auf die Gehirngefäßweite bei Tieren und am Patienten und leitete damit die Fragestellungen nach der Rolle der Anaesthesie bei der Gehirndurchblutung ein. Nachdem von HALES (1733) die ersten Blutdruckmessungen beschrieben wurden, sind auch die Beziehungen zwischen Blutdruck und Gehirnzirkulation untersucht worden (FRANCOIS-FRANCK, 1887; HÜRTLE, 1889). GÄRTNER und WAGNER (1887a u. b) stellten fest, daß der Anstieg des Aortendrucks zu einer Erhöhung der Durchflußmenge durch das Gehirn führt. Die Gehirndurchblutung wurde dabei erstmalig quantitativ bestimmt, indem das aus dem lateralen Sinus ausfließende Blut gemessen wurde. Man hat später festgestellt, daß die Gärtner- und Wagnerschen Untersuchungen nicht zu richtigen Resultaten führten, weil relativ große Volumina aus extrakraniellen Quellen dem ausfließenden Blut zuströmten. COOPER hat nach HEGELMAIR (1859) als erster den Zusammenhang zwischen Liquordruck und Blutgehalt des Gehirns demonstriert, indem er durch eine Trepanlücke im Schädel einen Druck auf das Gehirn ausübte. Am Menschen hat als erster MOSSO (1881) systematische Untersuchungen der Änderungen des Gehirnvolumens durchgeführt. Er fand enge Beziehungen zwischen den Druckabläufen im Liquorraum und der Atmung und stellte fest, daß die Venen durch Änderungen der Thoraxweite beeinflußt werden. Druckmessungen in den Jugularvenen sind von CRAMER (1873) durchgeführt worden und KNOLL (1866) beschrieb, daß ein Druck auf den Bulbus zu einer Erhöhung des Druckes im Liquorraum führte. Ähnlich wie CRAMER verwendeten auch ROY und SHERRINGTON (1890) Onkometer. Diese Geräte registrieren die vertikalen Schwankungen des Gehirns am offenen Schädel. Mit diesem Gerät wurden zahlreiche Untersuchungen zur Blutfüllenänderung im Gehirn bei sehr unterschiedlichen Reizungen festgestellt. Bei den Messungen des Zustroms benutzte CYBULSKI (1891) ein Photohämotachometer, das die Blutstromstärke in der Arteria carotis interna unter verschiedenen experimentellen Bedingungen registrierte. Das Vierordtsche Hämotachometer (1877) ist eine Fortentwicklung dieses Gerätes und es kann mit diesem Gerät – ähnlich wie mit der von LUDWIG (1885) entwickelten Stromuhr – der Einstrom in die Karotis als Strömungsgeschwindigkeit festgestellt werden. Alle diese letzteren Meßmethoden wurden im Tierexperiment verwendet. HILL (1896) und BAYLISS und HILL (1895) registrierten gleichzeitig Aortendruck, zentralvenösen Druck, Venendruck und intrakraniellen Druck. Bei der damals noch bestimmenden Monro-Kellie-Doktrin wurde aus den Druckdifferenzen die Gehirndurchblutung errechnet. Aus Temperaturmessungen im Gehirn hat MOSSO 1881 die ersten systematischen Ergebnisse der Änderung des Gehirnstoffwechsels gewonnen. Er verwendete ein Quecksilberthermometer, das in seinen Formen so ausgestaltet war, daß es die Oberflächentemperatur des Gehirns recht gut erfaßte. Aus seinen Untersuchungen zog er die Schlußfolgerung, daß im Schlaf und in Narkose eine Verminderung des Stoffwechsels im Gehirn besteht; bei hoher psychischer Aktivität fand er eine leichte Temperaturerhöhung. Die Untersuchungen führte er an Patienten mit Schädeldachdefekten durch. ALEXANDER und RÉVÉSZ (1912) fanden Zusammenhänge zwischen optischen Reizen und Erhöhung des Gehirnstoffwechsels. Das Ficksche Prinzip

(1870) der Bestimmung des Energiestoffwechsels eines Organs aus der arteriovenösen Sauerstoffdifferenz wurde von Lennox und Gibbs (1932) für das Gehirn eingeführt. Bei diesen Messungen wurde vorausgesetzt, daß der Sauerstoffverbrauch des Gehirns während der gesamten Meßzeit konstant blieb. Es hat sich später erwiesen, daß die Voraussetzungen eines konstant angenommenen Sauerstoffverbrauchs in manchen Fällen nicht zutraf, daß aber gewisse Näherungen bei einem Steady-state der Durchblutung angenommen werden können. Ferris (1941) gab eine auf der Monro-Kellie-Doktrin beruhende Methode an, mit der er bei Verschluß beider Jugularvenen aus der Liquordruckänderung einen Index des arteriellen Einstroms zu gewinnen versuchte. Die bei dieser Meßtechnik ermittelten Durchblutungswerte lagen unter denen, die mit anderen Methoden gemessen werden konnten. Das beruhte darauf, daß durch Verschluß der Jugularvenen nicht der gesamte venöse Rückstrom unterbrochen wurde. 1933 entwickelte F.A. Gibbs eine Methode, die eine fortlaufende thermoelektrische Registrierung der Blutstromgeschwindigkeit in der Jugularvene des Menschen erlaubte. Ein entscheidender Durchbruch der Durchblutungsmessung gelang, als Kety und Schmidt (1948a) ihre Meßtechnik publizierten und anstatt der arteriovenösen Sauerstoffdifferenz die Differenz der Sättigung des Blutes mit einem inerten Fremdgas (N_2O) als Indikator für Durchblutungsmessungen verwendeten. Seit der Einführung dieser Technik haben sich Clearance-Messungen sehr stark in den Vordergrund geschoben.

B. Messungen der Gesamtdurchblutung des Gehirns

Neben der weitverbreiteten Methode der Angiographie zur Untersuchung der Gehirndurchblutung gibt es eine Reihe von Meßverfahren, mit denen die Gesamtdurchblutung des Gehirns quantitativ erfaßt werden kann. Andere Techniken ermöglichen fortlaufende Registrierungen der regionalen Durchblutung, wieder andere Methoden geben Hinweise auf den Durchstrom durch einzelne Gefäße. Schließlich gibt es Durchblutungsmeßverfahren, z.B. die Szintigraphie, welche die Folgen von Durchblutungsstörungen erfassen. Der Angiographie und der Szintigraphie sind besondere Kapitel dieses Buches gewidmet, so daß der folgende methodische Abschnitt diese Meßtechniken nicht behandelt.

I. Künstliche Perfusion des Gehirns

Finesinger und Putnam (1933) durchströmten eine Arteria carotis mit Blut konstanten Drucks und registrierten den Einstrom. Gleichzeitig beobachteten sie die Piagefäßweite, wobei sie feststellten, daß eine Reizung der zervikalen sympathischen Nerven eine Verminderung der Durchblutung und eine Konstriktion der Piagefäße erzeugte. Der Vorteil einer solchen isolierten Perfusion besteht darin, daß sie den Untersucher in die Lage versetzt, ohne Änderung des arteriellen Systemdrucks die Wirkungen eines Reizes auf den Gefäßwiderstand zu untersuchen. Die Technik weist jedoch einige Schwierigkeiten auf, denn das Gehirn ist ja mit einer Reihe von Zuflüssen versehen. Von Hill (1896) und Ferris (1941) wurde über Untersuchungen berichtet, bei denen alle Arterien bis auf eine zuführende Arterie unterbunden waren und dann der Einstrom durch diese eine Arterie gemessen wurde. Der venöse Ausstrom aus dem Sinus transversus wurde fortlaufend registriert. Von Geiger und Magnes (1947) sind mit dieser Methode Durchblutungswerte von mehr als 1 $ml \cdot g^{-1} \cdot min^{-1}$ gemessen worden. Diese sehr hohen Durchblutungswerte weisen darauf hin, daß bei solchen Experimenten wahrscheinlich keine Normalbedingungen des Gehirns vorlagen. Für die Problematik des Stoffwechsels in Cerveau-isolé-Präparaten sind jedoch diese Untersuchungen von grundlegender Bedeutung. Sie werden in ähnlicher Weise auch jetzt noch durchgeführt. Bei den Versuchen der Durchströmung des isolierten Gehirns durch ein einzelnes Gefäß fanden Sagawa und Guyton (1961) zahlreiche Anastomosen zwischen der intrakraniellen und extrakraniellen Zirkulation, die bei den einzelnen Versuchstieren verschieden ausgeprägt waren, wie das auch vorher schon Batson (1940, 1944), Holmes et al. (1958a u. b) und Jewell (1952) gesehen hatten. Das liegt daran, daß die Versuchstiere z.T. ein ausgedehntes Rete mirabilis besitzen, über das diese Verbindungen möglich werden.

Bei derartigen großen Operationen kommt es nicht selten vor, daß die Beziehung zwischen Durchblutung und Perfusionsdruck im physiologischen Bereich kein Plateau mehr zeigt, d.h. daß die Autoregulation der Durchblutung aufgehoben wird. Die künstliche Perfusion hat eine weitere Schwierigkeit: Wie Held et al. (1971) zeigten, ist bei längerer künstlicher Perfusion auch mit Blut der Durchblutungswert relativ niedrig. Experimente von Rapport et al. (1948) bestätigen diese niedrigen Durchblutungswerte. Die Ursache wird z.T. darin gesehen, daß durch die Perfusionspumpen Störungen verursacht werden. Dadurch werden vasoaktive Stoffe, z.B. 5-HT (Hydroxytryptamin, Serotonin) freigesetzt, oder das Fehlen der pulsatilen Änderungen bewirkt diese Störungen der Durchblutung (Held et al., 1971).

II. Stickoxydulmethode

Die in der Vergangenheit am häufigsten angewendete Methode zur Untersuchung der Durchblutung des Gesamthirns ist die von Kety und Schmidt (1948a) in Einzelheiten beschriebene Stickoxydulmethode (Kety, 1948, 1951). Sie ermöglicht bei einer Durchblutungskonstanz über die gesamte Meßzeit von 10–15 min pro Einzelmessung eine Bestimmung der Durchblutung in ml Blut/100 g Gewebe · min. Als diffusibler Indikator dient N_2O, dessen arterielle und gehirnvenöse Konzentration (Messung im Bulbus venae jugularis) über die Meßzeit (Aufsättigungszeit oder Entsättigungszeit) bestimmt wird. Wird der Sauerstoffgehalt im arteriellen und gehirnvenösen Blut mitgemessen, so kann aus Durchblutungsgröße und *a-v*-Sauerstoffdifferenz gleichzeitig der O_2-Verbrauch des Gesamtgehirns errechnet werden.

Die Stickoxydulmethode beruht auf dem Fickschen Prinzip, welches besagt, daß eine Menge (Q) einer Substanz (S), z.B. inertes Gas im Blut, das in ein homogenes Gewebe eintritt, gleich ist der vom Gewebe aus dem Blut aufgenommenen Menge von S plus der Menge, die sich noch im ausströmenden Blut befindet. Die Menge von S der vom Gewebe aufgenommenen Substanz sei $Q_{\text{aufgen.}}$. Während einer kurzen (infinitesimalen) Zeit dt ist die in das Gewebe eintretende Menge (dQ_a) im arteriellen Einstrom dem infinitesimalen Blutvolumen, das ins Gewebe eintritt ($F \cdot dt$) multipliziert mit der Konzentration von S im einströmenden Blut (C_a) gleich.

$$dQ_a = F \cdot dt\, C_a. \tag{1}$$

Hierbei ist der Fluß (F) = Volumen/Zeit. C_a ist die Konzentration im arteriellen Blut. Die Menge von S, die das Gewebe durch das venöse Blut verläßt, beträgt:

$$dQ_{\text{ven}} = F \cdot dt \cdot C_{\text{ven}} \tag{2}$$

C_{ven} ist die venöse Konzentration.
Die Menge der Substanz S, die aus dem Blut durch das Gewebe aufgenommen wird ($dQ_{\text{aufgen.}}$), beträgt:

$$dQ_{\text{aufgen.}} = V \cdot dC_{\text{Gewebe}}. \tag{3}$$

Hierbei ist C_{Gewebe} die Konzentration im Gewebe und V bedeutet Volumen. Von Kety und Schmidt (1948a) und anderen Untersuchern wird häufig anstelle des Gewebsvolumens V das

Gewicht G verwendet. In diesem Fall muß das spezifische Gewicht des Gewebes berücksichtigt werden.

Nach dem Fickschen Prinzip ist:

$$dQ_a = dQ_{\text{aufgen.}} + dQ_{\text{ven}}. \tag{4}$$

Wenn man die aus den Gleichungen 1 bis 3 gewonnenen Werte in Gleichung 4 einsetzt, so ergibt sich:

$$F \cdot dt\, C_a = V \cdot dC_{\text{Gewebe}} + F \cdot dt\, C_{\text{ven}}. \tag{5}$$

Will man die Menge der Substanz *S*, die vom Gewebe pro Zeiteinheit aufgenommen wurde, beschreiben, so wird:

$$dQ_{\text{aufgen.}}/dt = V \cdot dC_{\text{Gewebe}}/dt = F(C_a - C_{\text{ven}}). \tag{5a}$$

Bei Verwendung eines Atemgases mit 10% N_2O zur Messung der Gehirndurchblutung wurden von KETY und SCHMIDT folgende Voraussetzungen als erfüllt betrachtet:

1. Arterieller Einstrom = venöser Ausstrom.
2. Das Blut im Bulbus venae jugularis superior ist das aus dem Gehirn ausströmende Blut.
3. Die Verteilung des Gases aus dem Blut in das Gewebe erfolgt in der Weise, daß $C_{\text{Gewebe}} = \lambda \cdot C_{\text{ven}}$ ist. λ ist der Verteilungskoeffizient des Gases Gewebe/Blut. Er beträgt 1, wenn N_2O als Meßgas verwendet wird.

Für die Messung der Gehirndurchblutung wird die Gleichung 5a bis zum Ende der Meßzeit *T* integriert, nachdem beide Seiten der Gleichung mit *dt* multipliziert wurden.

$$\int_0^{Q_{\text{gesamt}}} dQ_{\text{aufgen.}} = V \int_0^{C_{\text{Ende}}} dC_{\text{Gewebe}} = F \int_0^T (C_a - C_{\text{ven}})\, dt \tag{6}$$

$$Q_{\text{gesamt}} = V C_{\text{Ende}} = F \int_0^T (C_a - C_{\text{ven}})\, dt. \tag{7}$$

Bei Annahme eines Gleichgewichtszustandes am Ende der Meßzeit *T* also $\lambda \cdot C_{\text{ven}} = C_{\text{Ende}}$ wird die Gleichung 7 zu:

$$V\lambda C_{\text{ven}} = F \int_0^T (C_a - C_{\text{ven}})\, dt. \tag{8}$$

Wird die Gleichung 8 nach F/V aufgelöst, so ergibt sich:

$$F/V = \frac{C_{\text{ven}} \cdot \lambda}{\int_0^T (C_a - C_{\text{ven}})\, dt}. \tag{9}$$

Eine typische Kurve der arteriellen (a) und hirnvenösen N_2O-Konzentrationen bei Atmung von 10% N_2O ist in Abb. 1 dargestellt. Der Nenner der Gleichung 9 entspricht der Fläche der arteriovenösen Differenz (schraffiert) in Abb. 1.

Aus Gründen der Zweckmäßigkeit wird die Durchflußmenge oft auf 100 g (oder ml) Hirngewebe bezogen. Der Zähler der Gleichung 9 muß dann mit 100 multipliziert werden.

BERNSMEIER und SIEMONS (1953) modifizierten die KETY-SCHMIDTsche Methode in der Weise, daß nach einer Blutgasanalyse vor N_2O-Atmung und während der 10minütigen Atmung des N_2O-O_2-Gasgemisches mit einer motorgetriebenen Absaugspritze fortlaufend 1,6 ml Blut/min abgesaugt wurde. In den erhaltenen 16 ml arteriellen bzw. venösen Blut wird die mittlere N_2O-Konzentration art(m) und ven(m) ermittelt. Unmittelbar nach Beendigung dieser Entnahme wird die arterielle und venöse Endkonzentration gemessen.

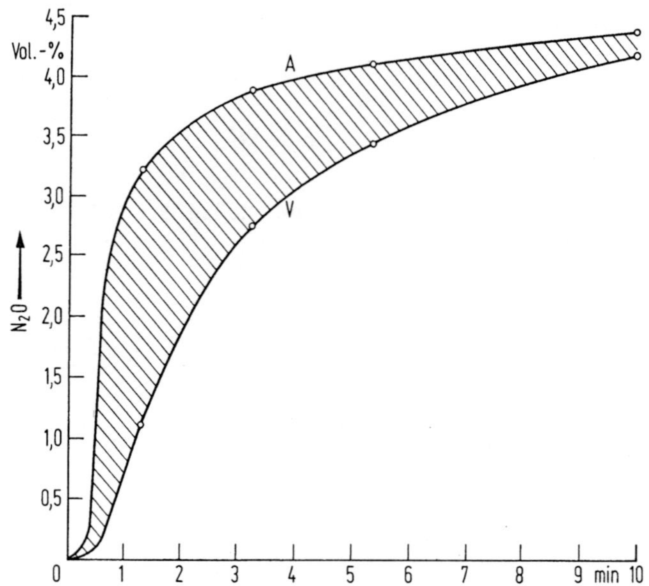

Abb. 1. Typische N_2O-Aufsättigungskurve des arteriellen (*A*) und gehirnvenösen (*V*) Bluts (Bulbus venae jugularis) zur Messung der Durchblutung des gesamten Gehirns (entspr. Gleichung 9)

Damit wird die Durchblutung $F/V = \frac{100 \cdot C_{ven} \cdot \lambda}{(C_{art(m)} - C_{ven(m)}) \cdot T}$.

Für die Brauchbarkeit der Methode wird vorausgesetzt, daß bei Ende der N_2O-Inhalation ein Gleichgewicht zwischen Blut und Gewebe eingetreten ist. Wenn der arterielle vom venösen Endwert der N_2O-Konzentration um mehr als 0,5 Vol% differiert, so wird die Messung als unbrauchbar für eine quantitative Auswertung betrachtet. Diese Art der Messung erlaubt nämlich keine Extrapolation der Meßkurve. Der Vorteil dieser Modifikation ist, daß nur eine relativ geringe Blutmenge zur Bestimmung der Durchblutung benötigt wird, s. Tab. 1.

Es besteht bei ausgedehnten einseitig lokalisierten Durchblutungsstörungen die Möglichkeit von Fehlmessungen mit der N_2O-Methode, denn Untersuchungen des venösen Ausstroms aus den Jugularvenen ergaben, daß etwa $^2/_3$ des Blutes in jedem Bulbus venae jugularis superior ipsilateraler Herkunft sind und etwa $^1/_3$ von der Gegenseite kommt (SHENKIN et al., 1948). Zwischen rechter und linker Hemisphäre fanden sich bei normalen wachen oder narkotisierten Menschen keine signifikanten Unterschiede (GIBBS et al., 1945; HIMWICH et al., 1947; KETY u. SCHMIDT, 1948a u. b; SCHEINBERG, 1950; BROBEIL, 1950; WECHSLER et al., 1951).

Im Prinzip kann anstelle von N_2O auch H_2 als Indikator verwendet werden (MEYER et al., 1968). Hierbei besteht ein gewisser Vorteil gegenüber der N_2O-Methode, denn der H_2-Druck kann fortlaufend mit wasserstoffempfindlichen Platinelektroden in der A. carotis und dem Bulbus venae jugularis registriert werden. Größere Blutentnahmen sind nicht notwendig. Bei Verwendung radioaktiver Edelgase als Indikatoren sind die erforderlichen Blutmengen ebenfalls klein. Die bisher erwähnten Methoden erlauben eine quantitative Registrierung der Gesamthirndurchblutung in ml Blut · ml Gewebe^{-1} · min^{-1}.

III. Farbstoffverdünnungsmethoden

Eine Indikatorverdünnungsmethode zur Durchblutungsmessung, bei welcher als Indikator eine nicht aus den Gefäßen diffundierende Substanz verwendet wurde, beruht auf dem von STEWART (1890) und HAMILTON et al. (1928) angegebenen Prinzip. Wird bei Injektion einer derartigen Substanzmenge (I) in die Gefäße, die ausschließlich das Gehirn versorgen, der Farbstoff vollständig mit dem fließenden Blut durchmischt, während er durch den Meßbereich fließt, dann kann aus der Änderung der gehirnvenösen Blutkonzentration des Farbstoffs die Durchblutung berechnet werden. Die Indikatormenge, die bei Integration des zeitlichen Konzentrationsanstiegs wie -abfalls des Farbstoffs bei konstanter Durchblutung während der Meßzeit nach schneller Injektion des Farbstoffs im venösen Blut erscheint, entspricht der injizierten Indikatormenge und beträgt

$$I = \int_0^\infty c(t) \cdot \dot{Q} \cdot dt.$$

$\dot{Q}$ ist hierbei die Durchblutung (gemessen in ml Blut $\cdot$ min^{-1}), $c(t)$ ist die zeitlich veränderliche Farbstoffkonzentration.

Unter der Voraussetzung, daß der Durchfluß konstant bleibt, kann $\dot{Q}$ vor das Integral gebracht werden

$$I = \dot{Q} \int_0^\infty c(t) \cdot dt.$$

Durch Umformung ergibt sich

$$\dot{Q} = \frac{I}{\int_0^\infty \cdot c(t) \cdot dt}.$$

Die Konzentrationen von geeignetem Farbstoff (z.B. Cardiogreen) können photometrisch leicht bestimmt werden. Um nur kleine Farbstoffmengen anwenden zu müssen, soll

1. der verwendete Farbstoff für die Messung ein charakteristisches und deutliches Absorptionsmaximum besitzen, so daß kleine Konzentrationsdifferenzen schon zu deutlich unterscheidbaren Meßsignalen führen,
2. Eine Änderung der O_2-Sättigung die Meßsignale nicht beeinflussen,
3. der Indikator das Gefäßsystem während der Meßzeit nicht verlassen, er muß aber schnell ausgeschieden werden.
4. der Indikator nicht toxisch sein und die Durchblutung nicht beeinflussen.

Cardiogreen erfüllt diese Bedingungen weitgehend. Von GROTE und KREUSCHER (1967) sowie GROTE et al. (1973) sind mit dieser Methode zahlreiche Gehirndurchblutungsmessungen bei narkotisierten Hunden vorgenommen worden. Die Tiere waren mit N_2O narkotisiert. Es wurden Durchblutungswerte von etwa 60 ml Blut $\cdot$ (100ml Gewebe)$^{-1}$ $\cdot$ min^{-1} gefunden.

Die bei der Stickoxydultechnik erforderlichen größeren Blutentnahmen entfallen bei dieser Technik vollständig. Ein gewisser Nachteil der Farbstoffverdünnungsmethode ergibt sich aber daraus, daß man sicher sein muß, daß das Gefäß, in welches man den Farbstoff injiziert, lediglich das Gehirn versorgt. Bei Messungen an Hunden besteht dabei die Notwendigkeit, bei der Injektion der Substanz durch Unterbinden von Ästen der A. carotis communis dafür zu sorgen, daß der Farbstoff lediglich in die A. carotis interna gelangt. Das venöse Blut wird von den genannten Autoren aus dem Sinus confluens entnommen. Die Dauer einer Einzelmessung liegt zwischen 20–40 s, so daß die Konstanz der Durchblutung während dieser Zeit häufig als gegeben betrachtet werden darf.

IV. Bestimmung der Zirkulationszeit

Die Geschwindigkeit des Durchstroms von Blut durch das Gehirn kann mit unterschiedlichen Techniken gemessen werden. Wenn die verwendeten Indikatoren nicht in die Gewebe diffundieren, so lassen sich sowohl Farbstoffe als auch radioaktiv markierte Substanzen verwenden. Durch die Entwicklung der Röntgentechnik werden heutzutage die Zirkulationszeitmessungen in der Regel mit Röntgenuntersuchungen kombiniert, so daß Veränderungen der Zirkulationszeit durch das Gehirn mit der Darstellung der Gehirngefäße in Beziehung gesetzt werden können. Von HEDLUND et al. (1966), OLDENDORF (1964), WILCKE (1969) wird angenommen, daß Verringerungen des Durchstromvolumens durch das Gehirn (Hirnminutenvolumen) mit Verlängerungen der Zirkulationszeit durch das Gehirn verbunden sind. Eine einigermaßen zuverlässige Bestimmung der zerebralen arteriovenösen Zirkulationszeit setzt eine Reihe von Vorbedingungen voraus:

Der Indikator sollte gleichmäßig und schlagartig in das Gehirn eintreten und eine Messung des Indikators nach Möglichkeit fortlaufend erfolgen können. Bei der Zirkulationszeitbestimmung mit radioaktiven Isotopen kann durch entsprechend abgeschirmte Szintillationszähler das Auftreten der radioaktiven Strahlung über den großen Blutleitern des Gehirns erfaßt werden und die Zeit vom Erscheinen der Radioaktivität bis zum Verschwinden registriert werden. Die Szintillationszähler eignen sich vorwiegend zur Bestimmung von Gamma-Strahlungen, weshalb vorwiegend ^{131}J, ^{51}Cr, ^{24}Na und ^{64}Cu zur Bestimmung der zerebralen Zirkulationszeit verwendet wurden. Bei Messungen in Blutproben hat sich ^{32}P als geeignet erwiesen, das von EICHHORN (1959, 1966) durch Registrierung der Bremsstrahlung bei intravenöser Dosis von 45 μCi/kg Körpergewicht mittels eines auf den Confluens sinuum aufgesetzten Szintillationszählers erfaßbar war. Weiche Bremsstrahlung ist bei dieser Anordnung noch gut meßbar und es sind keine besonderen Abschirmvorrichtungen, wie bei der Verwendung energiereicher Gammastrahler, notwendig. Bei den erhaltenen Kurven wird der aufsteigende initiale Schenkel als arterielle Phase gedeutet. Dieser hat in der Regel in der Mitte einen Knick, der als kapillärer Knick – nach Passage der großen Arterien – der diffusen Verteilung des Indikators in den Hirnkapillaren zugeordnet wird. Der absteigende Schenkel entspricht der venösen Abflußphase. Bei gefäßgesunden normalen Versuchspersonen betrug die Zirkulationszeit der arteriellen Phase 2,5–3 s, die der kapillären Phase 1,0–1,5 s und die der venösen Phase 3,0–4 s. Bei Patienten mit Hirntrauma, diffuser Gefäßsklerose und manchen anderen Gefäßerkrankungen des Gehirns, wurden Verlängerungen der Zirkulationszeit nachgewiesen.

C. Messung der regionalen und lokalen Gehirndurchblutung

I. Isotopenclearance

In zahlreichen Fällen – zum Beispiel bei Hirninfarkten – gibt die Globalmessung keine wesentliche Information über die Durchblutungsstörung, so daß hierbei lokale Durchblutungsmessungen von wesentlich höherer Bedeutung sind.

Dabei haben sich Durchblutungsmessungen mit Hilfe von Indikatoren ebenfalls bewährt. Sie haben mittlerweile eine ähnlich große Bedeutung für lokale Durchblutungsmessungen erlangt wie die N_2O-Technik für die Gesamt-Gehirndurchblutungsmessung. Wegen ihrer relativ einfachen Anwendungsmöglichkeit werden beim Menschen vorzugsweise radioaktive Indikatoren zur Messung verwendet. LEWIS et al. (1960) haben diese Technik im Prinzip eingeführt, die 1961 von LASSEN und INGVAR für lokale Messungen am Menschen modifiziert wurde. Die Autoren lösten ^{85}Kr in isotoner Kochsalzlösung und injizierten eine kleine Menge davon in die A. carotis. Mit Geiger-Müller-Rohren wurde die β-Aktivität über dem exponierten Kortex registriert und die Clearancerate mit einem Ratemeter erfaßt. Da etwa 95% der β-Emission des ^{85}Kr aus einer Tiefe bis zu 1 mm unterhalb der Cortexoberfläche stammt, kann diese Meßtechnik für lokale Messungen der Kortexdurchblutung angewandt werden. Hierbei wird ^{85}Kr-haltige NaCl-Lösung so lange in die A. carotis infundiert bis eine konstante Radioaktivität des kortikalen

Gewebes besteht. Dann wird die Infusion schlagartig gestoppt und der darauf folgende Abfall der Aktivität kontinuierlich aufgezeichnet. Hierzu können zahlreiche kleine Geiger-Müller-Rohre über dem Kortex angebracht werden, so daß die Durchblutung vieler Regionen gleichzeitig und getrennt erfaßt wird. Die Berechnung der Durchblutung ist eine Modifikation der N_2O-Durchblutungsmessung. Es werden deshalb im Folgenden auch die Symbole dieser oben beschriebenen Berechnung verwendet. Aus Gleichung 5a folgt nach Umformung:

$$\frac{dC_{\text{Gewebe}}}{dt}=\frac{F}{V\cdot\lambda}\,(\lambda\cdot C_a-C_{\text{Gewebe}}). \tag{10}$$

Dabei ist $F/(V\cdot\lambda)$ der Fluß pro Einheit des Gewebevolumens, d.h. die Durchblutung.

Wenn man einen Zustand betrachtet, in dem die Edelgaskonzentration im Gewebe, im Folgenden kurz $C_g(t)$ genannt, zur Zeit $t=0$ den Wert $C_g(0)$ hat, außerdem die Durchblutung durch den betrachteten Gewebsbereich homogen und konstant ist und zudem keine Rezirkulation stattfindet, d.h. $C_a=0$, dann wird die Entsättigung des Gewebes durch eine Gleichung beschrieben, die sich aus der Lösung der Gleichung 10 ergibt:

$$C_g(t)=C_g(0)\cdot\exp(-f\cdot t/\lambda).$$

Hierbei ist $f=F/V$ (Fluß pro Volumen).

Die übliche Form der Auswertung einer Clearance-Kurve besteht darin, die Gewebskonzentration $C_g(t)$ auf halblogarithmischem Papier gegen die Zeit (linear) aufzutragen. Dabei soll ein linearer Abfall der Kurve erkennbar sein. Diese Funktion ist demnach eine Entsättigungsfunktion eines diffusiblen Stoffes in einem homogen durchbluteten Gewebe. Weil jedoch die einzelnen Gewebsteile nicht homogen durchblutet sind, mußte eine Lösung für heterogen durchblutete Gewebsareale gefunden werden. INGVAR und LASSEN (1962) nahmen eine mittlere Isotopenkonzentration $\bar{C}_g(t)$ unter der Voraussetzung von gleichem f/λ in den unterschiedlichen Kompartimenten an. Dabei wird

$$\bar{C}_g(t)=\frac{1}{\sum V_i}\sum_i\,[V_i\cdot C_{g,i}(0)\cdot\exp(-f\cdot t/\lambda)]. \tag{11}$$

Konzentrationen, Volumina und Durchblutungen der verschiedenen Kompartimente sind mit dem Index i bezeichnet.

Nimmt man an, daß die Aufsättigungszeit so lange dauert, daß ein vollständiges Gleichgewicht zwischen den verschiedenen Kompartimenten besteht, daß keine Rezirkulation auftritt und die initialen Konzentrationen $C_g, i,$ (0) bei Clearancebeginn alle den gleichen Wert $C_g(0)$ haben, dann erhält man die relative mittlere Gewebskonzentration:

$$\bar{C}_g(t)/C_g(0)=\frac{1}{\sum V_i}\sum V_i\cdot\exp(-f_i\cdot t/\lambda)$$

In dieser Gleichung wurde f_i anstelle von f geschrieben. Damit ist eine etwas unterschiedliche Durchblutung in den einzelnen Kompartimenten berücksichtigt.

Die logarithmische Auftragung von $\bar{C}_g(t)/C_g(0)$ gegen die Zeit (linear) ergibt eine in ihrem Anfangsteil linear abfallende Kurve. Diese wird nun als $y_0(t)$, ihre Steigung als $y'_0(t)$ bezeichnet. Wegen des linearen Abfalls ist $y'_0(t)=\text{konstant}\equiv y'_0$ (der Index „Null“ kennzeichnet den Anfangsteil der Kurve). Für diesen initialen Abfall (initial slope) gilt

$$y'_0=\frac{1}{\sum V_i}\sum V_i\cdot f_i/\lambda. \tag{12}$$

Da $(1/\sum V_i)\cdot(\sum V_i\cdot f_i)=\sum F_i/(\sum V_i)=\bar{f}$ ist, wobei $\bar{f}$ die durchschnittliche Durchblutung (mittlere Durchblutung) bedeutet, wird die Gleichung (12)

$$y_0'=\frac{\bar{f}}{\lambda} \quad \text{oder} \quad \bar{f}=y_0'\cdot\lambda.$$

Im Normalfall genügt eine Aufsättigungszeit von 5–6 min, um etwa gleich hohe Konzentrationen in allen Gewebskompartimenten zu erhalten. Da die Rezirkulation nur bis zu 10% beträgt, kann sie meist vernachlässigt werden.

Es gibt noch eine andere Art der Auswertung der logarithmischen Auftragung von $\bar{C}_g(t)/C_g(0)$ gegen die Zeit (linear). Der lineare Anfangsteil dieser Kurve kann als

$$\ln y_0(t)=-f^*\cdot t/\lambda$$

beschrieben werden, wobei $-f^*/\lambda$ den Abfall (Steigung) dieses linearen Kurventeils bedeutet. Diese Gleichung ist gleichbedeutend mit der folgenden Schreibweise:

$$y_0(t)=y_0(0)\cdot\exp(-f^*\cdot t/\lambda), \tag{12a}$$

wobei $y_0(0)$ den (extrapolierten) Wert der Funktion $y_0(t)$ zur Zeit $t=0$ bedeutet. Ermittelt man aus der graphischen Aufzeichnung der Funktion $y_0(t)$ diejenige Zeit $T_{1/2}$, nach der $y_0(t)$ auf die Hälfte des Anfangswertes, also auf $y_0(0)/2$ abgefallen ist, so erhält man aus Gleichung (12a)

$$\tfrac{1}{2}=\exp(-f^*\cdot t/\lambda) \quad \text{oder nach Logarithmieren dieser Gleichung}$$
$$f^*=\frac{\lambda\cdot 0{,}693}{T_{1/2}} \quad (\text{da } \ln 2=0{,}693). \tag{13}$$

Da für die Auswertung der Messung der Abfall der initialen Aktivität verwendet wird, wurde diese Meßtechnik als „initial slope" Methode nach kontinuierlicher Infusion von NaCl-Lösung, die radioaktives Edelgas enthielt, bezeichnet. Für die praktische Auswertung bedeutet das, daß die beiden ersten Minuten der Aufzeichnung zur Auswertung verwendet werden.

Ein anderes Auswertverfahren einer Isotopenclearance, das nach HUTTEN et al. (1969) etwas unterschiedliche Resultate ergibt, wurde von ZIERLER (1965) eingeführt. Bei diesem Meßverfahren wird, wie vorher beschrieben, ein radioaktives Edelgas (^{85}Kr oder ^{133}Xe in 0,9% NaCl-Lösung) verwendet. Eine kleine Menge davon wird schlagartig in eine das Gehirn versorgende Arterie (z.B. eine A. carotis) injiziert. Für eine richtige Anwendung muß vorausgesetzt werden, daß die maximale Höhe, die die Aktivität in der Meßregion erreicht, die Gesamtmenge des Indikators repräsentiert, d.h. daß noch kein Indikator aus dem Venensystem abgeströmt ist und auch kein Indikator aus dem arteriellen System zuströmt. Der radioaktive Indikator wird in der auf diesen Zustand folgenden Zeit durch das nachströmende Blut, welches frei von radioaktivem Indikator ist, allmählich aus dem Gewebe „ausgewaschen". Um den theoretischen Erfordernissen zur richtigen Auswertung zu entsprechen, muß deshalb die Injektion in Form einer Deltafunktion (d.h. schlagartig) erfolgen. Daher wird dieses Verfahren auch „Durchblutungsmessung durch Slug-Injektion" genannt.

Nimmt man an, daß das kleine ^{133}Xe- oder ^{85}Kr-haltige Flüssigkeitsvolumen wie ein kurzer Pfropf durch die zuführenden Gefäße ins Gewebe gelangt sei, und sich dort verteilt habe, daß aber noch kein Abstrom erfolgt sei, so erfaßt das Geiger-Müller-Rohr bzw. der Scintillationskristall die gesamte Radioaktivität des Bolusteils, der sein Meßgebiet erreicht hat und der Q_0 Teilchen enthalte. Von diesem Zeitpunkt Null an verlassen dh Indikatorteilchen dieses Gewebegebiet mit dem Blutstrom. Der Teilchenmenge Q_0 zum Zeitpunkt Null entspricht eine maximale Aktivitätshöhe H. Die Teilchenmenge, die das betrachtete Gewebsvolumen zwischen den Zeitpunkten t und $t+dt$ verläßt, ist das Produkt der aus dem Meßbereich abströmenden Blutmenge während dieser Zeit $(F\cdot dt)$ sowie der Konzentration im ausströmenden Blut $C\,(t)$.

Das Meßinstrument erfaßt die einzelnen radioaktiven Teilchen des Edelgases gerade so lange wie sie sich im Meßfeld aufhalten. Die Teilchenmenge, die die Meßregion zwischen t und $t+dt$ verläßt, beträgt $Q_0 \cdot h(t) \cdot dt$. Hierbei ist $h(t)$ die Wahrscheinlichkeitsdichte der radioaktiven Teilchen während der Passagezeit. Der mittlere Wert aller Passagezeiten t kann errechnet werden, wenn t als eine Funktion der Aktivitätshöhe betrachtet wird, zu der alle einzelnen radioaktiven Teilchen des Meßbereichs einen Beitrag leisten.

$$\bar{t} = \frac{\int_0^H t(h)\,dh}{\int_0^H dh}. \tag{14}$$

Da $\int_0^H dh$ gleich der initialen Aktivitätshöhe H ist und $\int_0^H t(h)\,dh$ die Fläche A unter der Clearance-Kurve (Abb. 2) wird $\bar{t} = A/H$. Die mittlere Passagezeit des radioaktiven Edelgases in der Meßregion ist gleich dem Verhältnis seines Verteilungsraumes V und des Blutflusses F

$$\bar{t} = V/F. \tag{15}$$

Formt man die Gleichung 15 um und definiert als Durchblutung f den Durchstrom pro Volumeneinheit ($f = F/W$), so wird

$$f = V/(W \cdot \bar{t})[\text{ml Verteilungsraum} \cdot \text{ml Gewebevolumen}^{-1} \cdot \text{min}^{-1}]. \tag{16}$$

Setzt man die aus Gl. 14 gewonnenen Symbole ein und definiert λ als das Verhältnis des Verteilungsraums V zum Gewebsvolumen V_{gewebe}, so wird aus Gl. 16

$$f = \lambda \cdot \frac{H}{A} \text{ml} \cdot \text{g}^{-1} \cdot \text{min} \tag{17}$$

wobei üblicherweise anstelle des Gewebsvolumens die Gewebsmasse eingesetzt wurde (INGVAR u. LASSEN, 1962). Abb. 2 zeigt ein Beispiel.

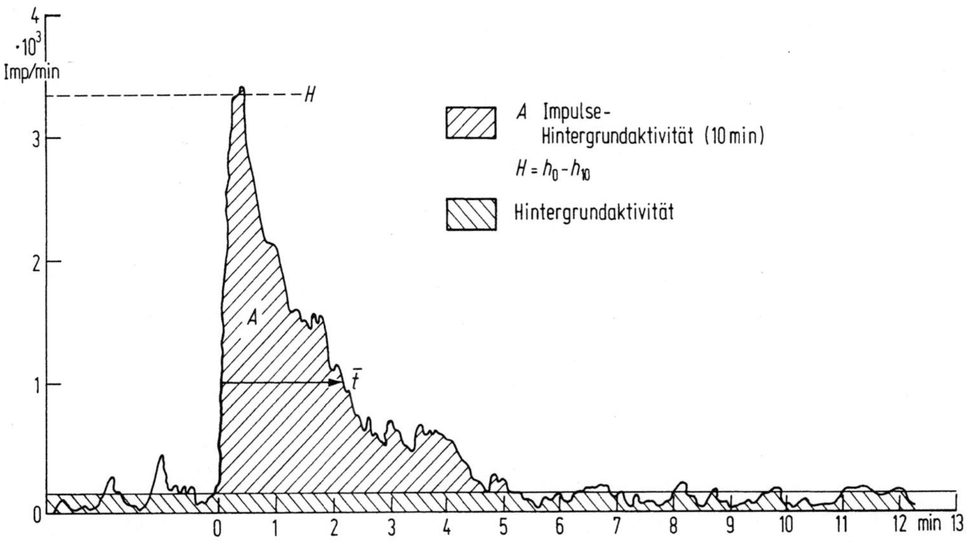

Abb. 2. Clearance-Kurve von ^{85}Kr aus der Gehirnrinde nach Injektion von 0,2 ml ^{85}Krypton-gesättigter NaCl-Lösung in die A. Carotis eines Versuchstiers. Die Errechnung der Durchblutung erfolgt entsprechend Gleichung (17). $\lambda = 0{,}95$

Bei der Registrierung der Clearancekurve wird diese so lange aufgezeichnet, bis die Radioaktivität des Edelgases die Hintergrundaktivität erreicht. Im normalen Gehirn dauert dies 10–20 min.

Mathematische Analysen zur Berechnung der lokalen Durchblutung mit der slug-injection-Technik sind von Zierler (1965) und Reivich et al. (1969a, b) durchgeführt worden.

Eine halblogarithmische Aufzeichnung der Aktivitätsänderungen nach Injektion des Isotops beim Patienten wurde zuerst von Glass u. Harper (1963) vorgenommen. Sie verwendeten ^{133}Xe und registrierten die γ-Strahlung mit einem Detektor, den sie über dem intakten Schädel anbrachten, Lassen et al., die 1963 ebenfalls Patienten mit dieser Technik untersuchten, registrierten anstatt der β-Strahlung die γ-Strahlung von ^{85}Kr (s. auch Agnoli et al., 1969c; Harper, 1965a; Lassen, 1964; Rosendorff u. Cranston, 1969).

II. Wärme als Indikator

Seit der Einführung der fortlaufenden Durchblutungsmessung, mit Hilfe geheizter Thermoelemente von Gibbs 1933, wird auch Wärme als Indikator für lokale Durchblutungsmessungen verwendet. Gibbs hatte die in einer Nadel untergebrachten Lötstellen eines Thermoelementes, von denen eine Lötstelle heizbar war, in das Gewebe eingestochen und die Temperaturdifferenz zwischen geheizter und nicht geheizter Lötstelle fortlaufend registriert. Unter der Voraussetzung, daß die Wärmeleitfähigkeit des Gewebes und damit der konduktive Wärmeabtransport vom aufgeheizten Gewebspunkt konstant bleibt (d.h., daß sich bei undurchblutetem Gewebe eine stationäre Temperaturdifferenz einstellt), waren die Änderungen des stationären Zustands durch Änderungen des konvektiven Wärmeabtransports (d.h. durch Durchblutungsänderungen) bedingt. Diese Methode hat gegenüber anderen u.a. folgende Vorteile: Es wird nur ein minimaler Gewebsdefekt verursacht. Die Methode kann angewendet werden, um den Durchfluß durch relativ unzugängige Strukturen zu studieren. Es ist möglich, qualitative Änderungen der Gewebsdurchblutung zu messen, ohne daß das zuführende oder ableitende Gefäß kanalisiert werden muß.

Die Meßmethode ist in der Folgezeit mehrfach modifiziert worden (Schmidt u. Pierson, 1934; Noyons et al., 1936; Norcross, 1938; Lubsen, 1940a; Hensel, 1953/54, 1958/59; Ludwigs, 1954; Carlyle u. Grayson, 1956; Sugano u. Inanaga, 1961; Kanzow, 1961). Mit Wärmeleitsonden, die von Betz und Hensel (1962) für Messungen der Gehirndurchblutung eingerichtet wurden, konnten fortlaufende Registrierungen der lokalen Durchblutung nicht nur am narkotisierten Tier, sondern auch über sehr lange Zeiten bei frei beweglichen Tieren vorgenommen werden (Betz, 1964). Die Sonden erlaubten bei geeigneter Anwendung auch Messungen der Gehirndurchblutung an Patienten, an denen neurochirurgische Eingriffe ausgeführt wurden (Betz u. Wüllenweber, 1962; Wüllenweber, 1965a, b). Meßelemente zur Durchblutungsregistrierung gibt es sowohl für Messungen auf der Gehirnoberfläche als auch für Messungen im Inneren der Gewebe. Eine zusammenfassende Übersicht über die Durchblutungsmessung mit Wärmeleitelementen wurde von Golenhofen et al. (1963) gegeben. Grayson (1952) registrierte diejenige Heizstromstärke, die zur Aufrechterhaltung einer Temperaturdifferenz von 1 °C zwischen der geheizten Lötstelle eines ins Gewebe implantierten Thermoelements und der Vergleichslötstelle notwendig war, wobei die Wärmeleitfähigkeit des Gewebes, sowie eine Konstante k berücksichtigt wurden. Hensel registrierte hingegen fortlaufend die Temperaturdifferenz zwischen geheizter und nicht geheizter Lötstelle eines ins durchblutete Gewebe implantierten Thermoelements bei konstantem Heizstrom (I) und Heizwiderstand (R) und berechnete daraus die Wärmeleitfähigkeit.

$$K = \frac{k \cdot I^2 \cdot R}{\vartheta}. \tag{18}$$

Die Wärmeleitfähigkeit wird üblicherweise in $\mathrm{cal \cdot cm^{-1} \cdot s^{-1} \cdot {}^\circ C^{-1}}$ angegeben.

Durch fortlaufende Registrierung konnte die Durchblutung nur als relative Änderung der Wärmeleitfähigkeit erfaßt werden. Mit kombinierten Messungen der ^{85}Krypton-Clearance und fortlaufender Registrierung des Wärmeabtansports mit Hilfe geheizter Thermoelemente an der gleichen Gewebsstelle, an welcher auch die ^{85}Krypton-Clearance gewonnen wurde, war eine Eichung der Wärmeleitfähigkeit auf absolute Durchblutungswerte [ml/g·min] möglich (BETZ et al., 1966a). Die Standardisierung durch intermittierende ^{85}Krypton-Clearance-Messungen ist dann schwierig, wenn geheizte und nicht geheizte Lötstelle eines Thermoelements in unterschiedlich hoch durchbluteten Bereichen liegen. Solche Situationen kommen z.B. bei lokalen Durchblutungsstörungen vor.

In gewisser Analogie zur ^{85}Krypton-Clearance wurde daher ein Verfahren entwickelt, das allein mit Hilfe von Wärme eine Durchblutungsmessung in ml Blut/g Gewebe·min erlaubt. Hierbei können geheizte Lötstellen von Thermoelementen als auch heizbare Mikrothermistoren verwendet werden. Man erhält nach Aufheizung oder Abheizung eine Wärmeclearancekurve. Im Prinzip wurden zwei Meßmöglichkeiten angegeben (MÜLLER-SCHAUENBURG et al., 1975; MÜLLER-SCHAUENBURG u. BETZ, 1969):

1. Eine Aufheizung, bei der die Heizzeit im Vergleich zur Meßzeit extrem kurz ist.
2. Die Durchblutungsmessung mittels plötzlicher Aufheizung z.B. des implantierten Mikrothermistors und Aufzeichnung der entstehenden Aufheizkurve oder eine Registrierung der lokalen Temperatur nach plötzlichem Abschalten des Heizstroms eines vorher konstant aufgeheizten Gewebsbezirks.

Das Meßprinzip basiert auf der Beobachtung, daß die Temperaturänderung nach lokaler, kurzer Aufheizung des Gewebes (=Wärmeinjektion) am Meßort bei durchblutetem Gewebe von derjenigen des undurchbluteten Gewebes nur durch eine Exponentialfunktion unterschieden ist. Für die stoßförmige, kurze Aufheizung bedeutet dies, daß:

$$\frac{u_{\text{slug}}(\vec{r}, t, \Phi/\lambda)}{u_{\text{slug}}(\vec{r}, t, 0)} = \exp(-(\Phi/\lambda)\cdot t). \tag{20}$$

u bedeutet die Übertemperatur der geheizten Gewebsstelle, gemessen in einem (kleinen) konstanten Abstand $|\vec{r}|$ von der Wärmequelle. Der Nullpunkt des Koordinatensystems liege in der Wärmequelle, der Vektor $\vec{r}$ geht von dieser aus und ist zum Temperaturmeßpunkt hin gerichtet. Die Betragsstriche $|\ \ |$ kennzeichnen die Entfernung. u_{slug} beschreibt die zeitabhängige Änderung dieses Übertemperaturfeldes nach der zur Zeit $t=0$ erfolgten Wärme-„Stoßinjektion". u_{slug} hängt außerdem von der Durchblutung Φ sowie von dem Wärmeverteilungsquotienten λ zwischen Gewebe und Blut ab. $\Phi=0$ bedeutet Durchblutungsstillstand. Wenn anstelle der stoßförmigen Aufheizung die Temperaturänderung des Thermistors nach länger dauernder Aufheizung als Meßprinzip verwendet wird, so muß man statt u die zeitliche Ableitung $\dot{u}$ zur Errechnung der Durchblutung verwenden.

$$\frac{\dot{u}_{\text{on}}(\vec{r}, t, \Phi/\lambda)}{\dot{u}_{\text{on}}(\vec{r}, t, 0)} = \exp(-(\Phi/\lambda)\cdot t). \tag{21}$$

Zur Bestimmung der Durchblutung aus Abkühlungskurven (=Abheizkurven) wird zunächst der Thermistor aufgeheizt, bis sich stationäre Bedingungen eingestellt haben. Dann wird die Thermistorheizung abgeschaltet und die Thermistorentemperatur registriert. Es wird:

$$\frac{\dot{u}_{\text{off}}(\vec{r}, t, \Phi/\lambda)}{\dot{u}_{\text{off}}(\vec{r}, t, \Phi/\lambda)} = \exp(-(\Phi/\lambda)\cdot t). \tag{22}$$

In der Gleichung 21 bedeutet $\dot{u}_{\text{on}}$ das Temperaturfeld nach Einschalten des Heizstroms; in Gleichung 22 ist $\dot{u}_{\text{off}}$ das entsprechende Temperaturfeld nach Abschalten der Wärmequelle.

(Die partielle Ableitung von u nach der Zeit wird allgemein durch einen hochgestellten Punkt symbolisiert.) r ist in allen Gleichungen der Ort, $\rightarrow$ ist die Entfernung der Temperaturmeßstelle von Wärmequelle (siehe oben). $\vec{r}$ faßt alle Raumkoordinaten zusammen. Es wurde von Müller-Schauenburg et al. (1975) gezeigt, daß die Durchblutung mit dieser Methode nicht nur im Inneren von Geweben, sondern auch oberflächennah bestimmt werden kann, wenn folgende Randbedingungen eingehalten werden können:

1. konstante Oberflächentemperatur
2. Wärmeisolierung oder
3. Wärmeabstrahlung proportional zur lokalen Übertemperatur.

An der Gehirnoberfläche können diese Randbedingungen hinreichend gut eingehalten werden. Wird eine punktförmige Heizquelle, z.B. ein Mikrothermistor, im Gewebe durch eine kleine Heizspirale für kurze Zeit aufgeheizt, so tritt Wärme in Form eines Wärmestoßes in das Gewebe ein. Analog zur Messung mit radioaktivem Edelgas ist dies als „slug injection" von Wärme aufzufassen. Von Perl (1962) wurde zur Beschreibung des Wärmetransports die folgende Differentialgleichung verwendet:

$$\dot{u}_{\text{slug}} = \frac{1}{\rho c} \operatorname{div}(K \cdot \operatorname{grad} u_{\text{slug}}) - \frac{\Phi}{\lambda} u_{\text{slug}} + \frac{1}{\rho c} \cdot \text{Wärmestoßdichte}(\vec{r}) \cdot \delta(t). \tag{23}$$

Es ist dabei

$c =$ spezifische Wärme bei konstantem Druck ($\text{cal} \cdot \text{g}^{-1} \cdot {}^\circ\text{C}^{-1}$)

$\rho =$ Dichte ($\text{g} \cdot \text{cm}^{-3}$)

$\lambda/\Phi =$ Zeitkonstante der effektiven Durchblutung, d.h. Φ/λ ist der reziproke Wert der Zeit, in welcher ein Gewebsvolumen von einem Blutvolumen durchströmt wird, wobei Gewebe und Blut die gleiche Wärmekapazität haben. $\delta(t)$ stellt die Deltafunktion dar.

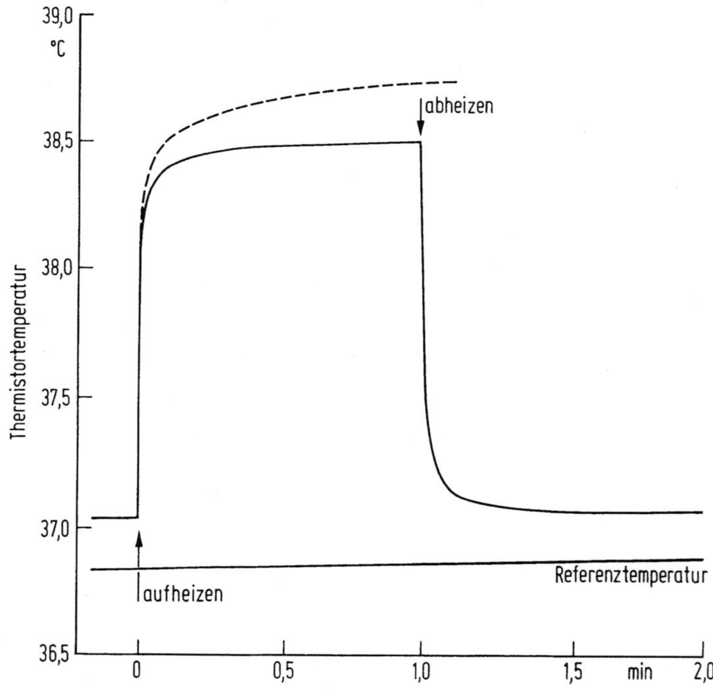

Abb. 3. Aufheizkurven zur Errechnung der regionalen Gehirndurchblutung mit Hilfe der quantitativen Wärme-clearance. Aufheizung bewirkt einen Temperaturanstieg. Durchgezogene Linie: Messung der Temperaturänderung im Thalamus eines wachen Tiers; gestrichelt gezeichnete Linie: Messung am gleichen Meßort des toten, nicht durchströmten Gehirns bei gleichhoher Ausgangstemperatur. Die Referenz-Temperatur ist nicht abszissenparallel, so daß der Temperaturtrend bei der Auswertung mit berücksichtigt werden muß. (Nach Müller-Schauenburg et al., 1975)

Bei Wärmeclearancemessung wird in der Praxis meist nicht eine kurzzeitige Wärmeinjektion, sondern eine plötzlich einsetzende Aufheizung (s. Gl. 21) oder nach konstanter Aufheizung die Abkühlungskurve (s. Gl. 22) verwendet. In einem solchen Fall (z.B. Aufheizung) gilt für die Beschreibung des Wärmetransports folgende Differentialgleichung:

$$\dot{u}_{\text{on}} = \frac{1}{\rho c} \operatorname{div}(K \cdot \operatorname{grad} u_{\text{on}}) - \frac{\Phi}{\lambda} \cdot u_{\text{on}} + \frac{1}{\rho c} \cdot \text{Heizdichte}(\vec{r}) \cdot \Theta(t). \tag{24}$$

$\Theta(t)$ bedeutet die Funktion des Einheitssprungs. In der Praxis sind folgende Meß- bzw. Rechenschritte zur Ermittlung der Durchblutung erforderlich:

1. Registrierung der Temperaturänderung nach Einschalten (bzw. Ausschalten) der Thermistorenheizung im nichtdurchbluteten Gewebe ($u_0(r, t)$)
2. Registrierung der Temperaturänderungen im durchbluteten Gewebe ($u_\Phi(\vec{r}, t)$)
3. Errechnung der differentiellen Temperaturänderung im Meßpunkt des Temperaturfeldes [Diff $u_\Phi(\vec{r}, t)$ und Diff $u_0(\vec{r}, t)$, wobei $\partial u/\partial t \equiv \dot{u} = \tan\alpha$]. $\tan\alpha$ ist der Anstieg der Kurve zu verschiedenen Zeitpunkten.
4. Errechnung von $\ln \dot{u}_\Phi - \ln \dot{u}_0 \equiv -(\Phi/\lambda) \cdot t$

Man sieht, daß das Ergebnis $-((\Phi/\lambda) \cdot t)$ die gesuchte Meßgröße enthält und daß die Durchblutung bei bekanntem Verteilungskoeffizienten (für das Gehirn beträgt dieser 0,995) ermittelt werden kann. Abb. 3 zeigt ein Beispiel.

III. Messung der Mikrozirkulation mit Hilfe der Wasserstoffclearance

Bei Untersuchungen der Mikrozirkulation haben Lübbers u. Stosseck (1970) eine Methode angegeben, die die Wasserstoffclearance zur Durchblutungsmessung einsetzt. Hierbei wurde folgende Meßanordnung verwendet: auf die Gehirnoberfläche wurde ein gasundurchlässiges (gläsernes) Plättchen mit einer eingeschmolzenen Platinelektrode aufgelegt. Die Platinelektrode hatte einen Durchmesser von 100 oder 200 µm. Durch diese Elektrode wird an der Oberfläche Wasserstoff generiert, der in das Gewebe diffundiert. Als Referenzelektrode für den Stromkreis dient eine 2–3 cm von der Wasserstoffgeneratorelektrode auf der Gehirnoberfläche aufliegende Ag/AgCl-Elektrode. Die Stromstärke wurde zwischen 0,3 und 1,0 µA variiert. In einem Abstand von etwa 300 µm von der wasserstoffgenerierenden Elektrode wird ein weiterer Platindraht, der 15 µm Durchmesser hat, durch die Glasoberfläche hindurch auf die Gehirnoberfläche aufgelegt. Diese Elektrode dient als Meßelektrode und kann den diffundierenden Wasserstoff polarographisch messen. Diese zweite Elektrode kann auch kleiner gewählt und in das Gewebe eingestochen werden.

Unter der Voraussetzung, daß an jedem Ort des Meßbereichs immer die Wasserstoffmenge, die vom Blut wegtransportiert wird, dem Partialdruck des Wasserstoffs proportional ist, kann das H_2-Druckfeld nach der Erzeugung mit der Generatorelektrode durch folgende partielle Differentialgleichung beschrieben werden.

$$\alpha_t \frac{\partial p(\vec{r}, t)}{\partial t} = \alpha_t \cdot D \cdot \Delta \cdot p(\vec{r}, t) - \alpha_b \cdot f \cdot p(\vec{r}, t) + Q(\vec{r}, t). \tag{25}$$

Hierbei kennzeichnet $p(\vec{r}, t)$ den Wasserstoffpartialdruck am Punkt $\vec{r}$ im Gewebe; t ist die Zeit; Δ ist der Laplace-Operator, α_t ist der Löslichkeitskoeffizient von H_2 im Gewebe (einschließlich der blutgefüllten Kapillaren); α_b entspricht dem Löslichkeitskoeffizienten im Blut und $Q(\vec{r}, t)$ ist die Menge von H_2, die pro Zeit- und Volumeneinheit am Ort $\vec{r}$ und zur Zeit t generiert wird. Der Term $-\alpha_b \cdot f \cdot p(\vec{r}, t)$ beschreibt den Abtransport von H_2 durch das Blut (obige Annahmen vorausgesetzt), f ist dabei die Durchblutung. Ist der Abstand von der H_2 erzeugenden Elektrode und der Meßelektrode konstant (d.h. für einen festen Wert von $\vec{r}$) so folgt aus der Lösung der Gleichung (25):

$$\ln \frac{p_0(t)}{p(t)} = -\frac{f}{\lambda}(t) + d(t)$$

λ ist wie in Gleichung (9) der Verteilungskoeffizient von H_2; p_0 (t) ist der H_2-Druck bei undurchblutetem Gewebe; $p(t)$ ist der H_2-Druck bei durchblutetem Gewebe, t ist die Zeit. $d(t)$ ist eine Korrekturfunktion, die bei der Auswertung als Konstante verwendet wird.

Bei der Auswertung solcher Kurven wird der Wert von $\ln \frac{p_0(t)}{p(t)}$ gegen die Zeit aufgetragen. Die Steigung dieser Geraden beträgt $(-f/\lambda)$, woraus die Durchblutung f berechnet werden kann. Die Auswertung der bisher gemessenen Kurven zeigte, daß es zweckmäßig ist, den Wasserstoff für eine Sekunde Dauer mit einer Stromstärke von $0{,}5-1\,\mu A$ zu erzeugen und den Abstand von H_2 generierender Elektrode und Meßelektrode zwischen 250 und $350\,\mu m$ zu wählen. Mit dieser Technik wird das Meßsignal nur durch die Durchblutung eines Gewebsvolumens von ca. $6\,mm^3$ (maximal) beeinflußt, wenn die Durchblutung nahe Null ist. Da bei Erhöhung der Durchblutung der lokale H_2-Druck schneller abfällt, wird bei hoher Durchblutung auch das erfaßte Gewebsvolumen geringer. Von STOSSECK et al. (1974) wird angegeben, daß bei normaler Gehirndurchblutung von $1{,}2\ \mu l \cdot min^{-1} \cdot \mu l^{-1}$ das durch die Messung erfaßte Gewebsvolumen maximal $2\,mm^3$ beträgt. Mit dieser Methode wurden im zerebralen Kortex sehr große lokale Durchblutungsdifferenzen an den verschiedenen Meßorten bestimmt. Auffällig waren die z.T. sehr hohen Meßwerte an einzelnen Meßorten, die bis zu 5 ml Blut/g · min betrugen. WODICK (1973), der der Frage nachging, warum solche hohen Werte gehäuft auftraten, sah sich bei der Definition der Durchblutung im Mikrobereich mit der Frage der Dimensionierung der Durchblutung konfrontiert. Es ergeben sich sowohl von theoretischen als auch von praktischen Gesichtspunkten her Schwierigkeiten, wenn in solch kleindimensionierten Gewebsbezirken die Durchblutung als Fluß je Volumeneinheit bestimmt werden soll. Wird nämlich bei einer Messung nur ein Gewebsbereich erfaßt, in welchem sich eine geringe Zahl von Kapillaren befindet, so „sieht" die Elektrode die an ihr vorbeiströmende H_2-Konzentration in Form einer H_2-Druck/Zeit-Beziehung. Nimmt man z.B. an, daß eine Elektrode sich im Zentrum von 20 Kapillaren befände, die an ihr vorbeizögen, wovon 5 von rechts nach links und 15 von links nach rechts ziehen mögen, so würde mehr Gas von links nach rechts transportiert als in umgekehrter Richtung, wenn die anderen Richtungen des Raumes einmal unberücksichtigt bleiben. Zwischen den Kapillaren kann das Meßgas hin und her diffundieren (entsprechend der Druckdifferenzen), aber im Endeffekt wird das Blut und damit H_2 von der in einer Flußrichtung überwiegenden Kapillarenzahl abtransportiert. Es tritt eine Vorzugsrichtung des Wasserstoffabstroms durch die betrachtete Meßfläche auf; dies auch bei einer dreidimensionalen Betrachtung. (Die Kapillaren sind hier nicht anatomisch definiert, sondern müssen als enge Kanäle, die durch das Gewebe ziehen und die das Gewebe drainieren, verstanden werden.) Nimmt man an, diese Kapillaren seien 10 cm lang und seien in einem Querschnitt von $10\,mm^2$ gleichmäßig verteilt, so wäre das Gewebsvolumen, das sie versorgen, grade $1000\,mm^3$. Wenn aus der Gesamtheit dieser Kapillaren 0,1 ml Blut/min ausströmte, so betrüge die Durchblutung $0{,}1\ ml \cdot cm^{-3} \cdot min^{-1}$. Wenn die Kapillaren aber nur 1 cm lang wären, so wäre bei gleichem Durchstrom die Durchblutung $1{,}0\ ml \cdot cm^{-3} \cdot min^{-1}$. Sind die Kapillaren aber nur 0,1 cm lang, so errechnet sich die Durchblutung auf $10{,}0\ ml \cdot cm^{-3} \cdot min^{-1}$. Die Definition hängt also in einem solchen Fall von der betrachteten Kapillarlänge ab. Als zusätzliche Schwierigkeit tritt auf, daß eine gewisse Willkür angewendet werden muß, wenn die zu berücksichtigenden interkapillären Gewebe hinsichtlich ihres Einflusses auf die Diffusion des Gases mit berücksichtigt werden sollen. WODICK (1973) hat das Problem dadurch gelöst, daß er beim Auswaschvorgang nicht den Wasserstofftransport/Volumen Gewebe betrachtet, sondern den Durchtritt durch eine Fläche, in die die Kapillaren von der einen oder anderen Seite eintreten. Es wird angenommen, daß die Fläche senkrecht zur resultierenden mittleren Flußrichtung steht. Trägt man den gemessenen H_2-Druck am Meßort multipliziert mit $t^{3/2}$ und einer Konstanten, also $p(\vec{r}, t) \cdot t^{3/2} \cdot k$ gegen die Meßzeit t auf, so zeigt die resultierende Kurve ein Maximum: t_{max}. Die Durchblutung (Fluß je Fläche) ist dann die Blutmenge $\bar{v}$, die in der Zeiteinheit (t) je Flächeneinheit (s) fließt. Sie beträgt nach WODICK (1973):

$$\bar{v} = \frac{\bar{a}}{t_{max}};$$

$\bar{a}$ ist bei dieser einfachen Formel zur Auswertung des Flusses/Fläche der mittlere Abstand der H_2-Quelle zur Meßelektrode. t_{max} ist die Zeit des Maximums einer Darstellung der H_2-Clearance-Kurve, wenn der am Meßort gemessene H_2-Druckverlauf p (t) mit $t^{3/2}$ multipliziert wird. WODICK (1973) gibt eine ausführliche theoretische Herleitung dieser Formel an. Werden vier Meßelektroden an den Ecken eines Quadrates angeordnet und befindet sich im Schnittpunkt der Diagonalen dieses Quadrates die H_2-erzeugende Meßelektrode, dann können mit dieser Meßmethode auch Aussagen über den Gegenstromanteil der Mikrozirkulation gemacht werden und es kann die mittlere Flußrichtung errechnet werden, auch wenn eine stark anisotrope Gefäßanordnung existiert Bereiche des Schädels fließen kann. Es wird zwischen den Elektroden ein elektrisches Feld aufgebaut in nichtdurchbluteten Geweben kann die normale Diffusionskonstante bestimmt werden, so daß es möglich wird, die beiden Transportphänomene, welche beim Gastransport durch das Gewebe eine Rolle spielen und bei der Herleitung der Auswertformel benutzt werden: mittlere Drift von H_2 im Gewebe um den Scheindiffusionstensor zu errechnen.

IV. Messung der Durchblutung mit Impedanzmethoden

Beim Durchgang eines elektrischen Stroms durch den Schädel und das Gehirn wird dem Stromdurchgang ein Widerstand entgegengesetzt, der sich aus einem relativ konstanten Teilwiderstand durch das Gehirngewebe und einem variablen Teilwiderstand zusammensetzt, der durch die pulssynchronen Änderungen der Blutfülle im Gehirn bedingt ist. Die Technik der Messung dieses Widerstands geht auf Versuche von CREMER (1907) zurück, der die Kapazität eines Plattenkondensators registrierte, wenn zwischen den Platten ein Froschherz schlug. Die Kondensatorkapazität änderte sich dabei im Rhythmus des Herzschlags. Von MEYER wurden 1921 Widerstandsmessungen im Gehirngewebe durchgeführt, POLZER und SCHUHFRIED (1950) berichteten erstmalig über die Anwendung der Impedanzmessung in Form einer Rheographie am Schädel. Von KAINDL et al. (1956) wurde die Rheographie weiterentwickelt und sie ist vor allem von LECHNER u. RODLER (1961, RODLER (1960), LECHNER et al. (1968) und LECHNER (1972) ausführlich behandelt und zu einer am Patienten anwendbaren Methode weiterentwickelt worden (LECHNER u. RODLER, 1961; MARTIN et al., 1964; RODLER, 1960). Bei dieser Methode wird von einem Konstant-Stromgenerator mittels zweier am Schädel anliegender Elektroden ein konstanter elektrischer Strom durch den Schädel geschickt. Die Elektroden sind so angelegt, daß der elektrische Strom durch tiefe Bereiche des Schädels fließen kann. Es wird zwischen den Elektroden ein elektrisches Feld aufgebaut und dieses ist durch die Widerstandsverhältnisse im Innern des Schädels beeinflußt. Von der Schädeloberfläche werden mit Hilfe kleiner bipolarer Meßelektroden Spannungen abgegriffen. Die Technik erlaubt multiple Spannungsabgriffe ähnlich wie bei der EEG-Technik. Durch entsprechende Verstärkung und Anpassung können die zeitlichen Impedanzänderungen fortlaufend registriert werden. Nach LECHNER (1972) ist es möglich, durch entsprechendes Anlegen der Elektroden die Kopfschwartendurchblutung weitgehend zu eliminieren. Bei Messungen des rheographischen Leitwertes mit solchen Methoden zeigt sich, daß es bei Bewegung des Blutes in einem elektrischen Feld zu Änderungen des Leitwertes kommt (GEYER et al., 1965; GUTMAN et al., 1968; LECHNER u. RODLER, 1961; LECHNER et al., 1965), so daß die gemessenen Werte nicht reine plethysmographische Änderungen des Schädelvolumens darstellen. Der rheographische Leitwert ist von der Durchstromgeschwindigkeit durch den Meßbereich sowie auch von der Art der strömenden Flüssigkeit (zelluläre Elemente) abhängig. Die Leitwertänderung ist nur bei vollwertigem Blut, nicht aber bei hämolysiertem Blut oder Serum erkennbar (LECHNER, 1972).

Besonderen Wert gewinnt die Methode bei Rechts-Links-Vergleichen. Es zeigt sich, daß bei Änderungen der Durchblutung (z.B. bei Karotisverschlüssen) deutliche Differenzen zwischen beiden Seiten auftreten. Es ist aber auch erkennbar, daß sich mit zunehmendem Alter die Kurvenform verändert, indem die initialen Anstiege steiler werden. Weiterhin zeigen sich bei Erhöhungen von CO_2 Zunahmen der Amplitude des Rheogramms; bei Hypoxien wird nach anfänglicher Abnahme der Amplitude eine starke Zunahme beobachtet. Die Methode, die klinisch häufig verwertet wird, bietet allerdings keine Möglichkeiten zur Quantifizierung der Gehirndurchblutung.

D. Normalwerte der Durchblutung und des zerebralen Sauerstoffbedarfs

I. Gesamtgehirn

Von verschiedenen Autoren sind Normwerte der Durchblutung des Gesamtgehirns angegeben worden. Sie betragen beim wachen, liegenden, gesunden und erwachsenen Menschen zwischen 52 und 60 ml pro 100 g Gehirngewebe und Minute, wenn der Kohlendioxyddruck des arteriellen Blutes 40 mm Hg (5,3 k Pa) beträgt. In der Tabelle 1 ist eine Übersicht über Normwerte, die mit der N_2O-Methode gewonnen wurden, dargestellt. Als Gesamtwiderstand des Gehirngefäßsystems ergeben sich Werte zwischen 1,69 und 1,3 mm Hg · cm^{-3}(100 g · min). Wird ein mittleres Gehirngewicht von ca. 1500 g angenommen, so beträgt die Gesamtgehirndurchblutung ca. 750 ml/min (KETY u. SCHMIDT, 1948a u. b; KETY, 1950; LASSEN u. MUNCK, 1955; NOVACK et al., 1953; SCHMIDT, 1961). Das sind rund 15% des Herzminutenvolumens. Der O_2-Verbrauch errechnet sich nach Tabelle 1 für das Gesamtgehirn, bei einem Hirngewicht von 1400 g auf ca. 47 ml/min. Durchblutungsmessungen mit ^{32}P-markierten Erythrozyten (NYLIN et al., 1961 a, b) an 24 Männern im Alter von 25 bis 50 Jahren ergaben einen Mittelwert der Durchblutung von 846 ml/min, d.h. ca. 11,4% des Herzminutenvolumens. Das Gehirngefäßvolumen betrug nach diesen Berechnungen ca. 100 ml.

Tabelle 1. Ergebnisse von Durchblutungs- und Sauerstoffverbrauchsmessungen am Gesamthirn von normalen Menschen

	Durchblutung $ml \cdot 100\ g^{-1} \cdot min^{-1}$	O_2-Verbrauch $ml/100\ g^{-1} \cdot min^{-1}$
1) KETY u. SCHMIDT (1945, 1948a und b)	54,0 ± 12,0	3,3 ± 0,4
2) SCHEINBERG u. STEAD (1949)	64,7 ± 12,1	3,8 ± 0,6
3) BERNSMEIER u. SIEMONS (1953)	58,3 ± 6,6	3,7 ± 0,4
4) BROBEIL et al. (1954)	67,0 ± 9,0	4,7 ± 0,8
5) LINDEN (1955)	54,5 ± 9,7	3,9 ± 0,6
6) LASSEN u. MUNCK (1955)	52,0 ± 8,6	3,4 ± 0,6
7) GÄNSHIRT u. TÖNNIS (1956)	55,7 ± 6,8	3,5 ± 0,5
8) KENNEDY u. SOKOLOFF (1957)	60,1 ± 2,6	4,2 ± 0,5
9) GERAUD et al. (1963)	53,4 ± 1,9	3,3 ± 0,2
10) GOTTSTEIN et al. (1963)	55,1 ± 6,1	3,7 ± 0,5

Mit einer Farbstoffverdünnungsmethode hatten GIBBS et al. (1947) Durchblutungswerte von 600 ml Blut·min^{-1}·(100 g)$^{-1}$ gefunden. Die Blutentnahme erfolgte aus einer Jugularvene und es war nicht sicher, ob nicht doch eine Zumischung von extrazerebralem Blut erfolgt war. Die in Tabelle 1 erkennbaren Unterschiede der Durchblutung können z.T. dadurch bedingt sein, daß die Alterszusammensetzung der Kollektive unterschiedlich ist. Da die Untersuchungen an wachen Menschen vorgenommen wurden, kann außerdem angenommen werden, daß die innere Anspannung der Untersuchten verschieden war. Angst vor diagnostischen Eingriffen kann die Hirndurchblutung verändern (BETZ, 1975).

Die mittlere Zirkulationszeit (OLDENDORF u. KITANO, 1964, 1965) beträgt bei Menschen unter 40 Jahren 6–11 s. Bei Personen, die über 40 Jahre alt waren, wurde eine höhere Zirkulationszeit von durchschnittlich 9,5 s beobachtet (OLDENDORF, 1964; WILCKE, 1969).

Von den meisten Autoren, die die N_2O-Methode verwenden, wird betont, daß die Durchblutung des Gesamthirns einer Einzelperson außerordentlich konstant ist. Auch im Schlaf oder bei Kopfrechnen werden mit integrierend messenden Methoden keine signifikanten Durchblutungsänderungen gemessen (GIBBS et al., 1935; SOKOLOFF et al., 1955; MANGOLD et al., 1955).

II. Die regionale Durchblutung

1. Örtliche Durchblutungsunterschiede

LASSEN et al. (1963) fanden bei den Clearance-Kurven von ^{85}Kr, daß sich der Auswaschvorgang des Edelgases durch das Blut in zwei Exponentialfunktionen zerlegen ließ (Abb. 4), die als zwei Durchblutungskomponenten aufgefaßt wurden. Die schnelle Komponente soll die Durchblutungswerte der grauen Substanz, die langsame Komponente die der weißen Substanz widerspiegeln. Die Zwei-Kompartiment-Analyse ist Gegenstand zahlreicher Diskussionen und Symposien gewesen (EICHHORN et al., 1964; INGVAR u. LASSEN, 1965a, b; INGVAR et al., 1968; LUYENDIJK, 1968; BAIN u. HARPER, 1968; MEYER et al., 1969a; BROCK et al., 1969; BETZ u. WÜLLENWEBER, 1969; ROSS-RUSELL, 1971; TISSEYRE, 1973; LANGFITT et al., 1975).

Die Durchblutungswerte des menschlichen Kortex betragen nach Messungen mit dieser Methode etwa 80 ml/100 g·min. Temporale Rindenabschnitte haben nach INGVAR et al. (1965) eine niedrigere Durchblutung (ca. 70 ml/100 g·min). Andere Untersucher fanden niedrigere mittlere kortikale Durchblutungswerte von etwa 50–60 ml/100 g·min (WOLLMAN et al., 1965; VEALL u. MALLETT, 1965; UEDA et al., 1965).

Die Durchblutungswerte der weißen Substanz wurden von INGVAR et al. (1965) mit ca. 21 ml/100 g·min, von AUSTIN et al. (1936) mit 25±2 ml/100 g·min angegeben, von WOLLMAN et al. mit 16 ml/100 g·min. Beim Hund wurden von HÄGGENDAL (1965) Werte zwischen 6 und 20 ml/100 g·min gemessen.

Wie aus der Abb. 4 hervorgeht, kann aus der schnellen Komponente des Aktivitätsabfalls schon nach 2–3 min ein Durchblutungswert mit ausreichender Genauigkeit abgelesen werden, und der 2-Minuten-Index wird neuerdings oft für die Bestimmung kurz dauernder Durchblutungsänderungen angewendet. Aber auch bei dieser Auswertungsform ist während der Meßzeit eine konstante Durchblutung erforderlich, und diese kann mit der Isotopentechnik allein nicht kontrolliert werden.

Die technische Entwicklung der Messung der regionalen Gehirndurchblutung mit Scintillationszählern erlaubt inzwischen, die Durchblutung an zahlreichen Stellen gleichzeitig zu messen (BARKER et al., 1975). Abb. 5 zeigt ein Beispiel einer derartigen lokalen Durchblutungsmessung an 11 Gehirnstellen gleichzeitig (HERRSCHAFT et al., 1975). Von SVEINSDOTTIR u. LASSEN (1975) sind synchrone Messungen an 254 Stellen mit verschiedenen Detektoren durchgeführt worden. Die Entwicklung der Meßtechniken mit der γ-Kamera erlaubt Messungen durch bis zu 1600 Kanäle (HEISS et al., 1968, 1972).

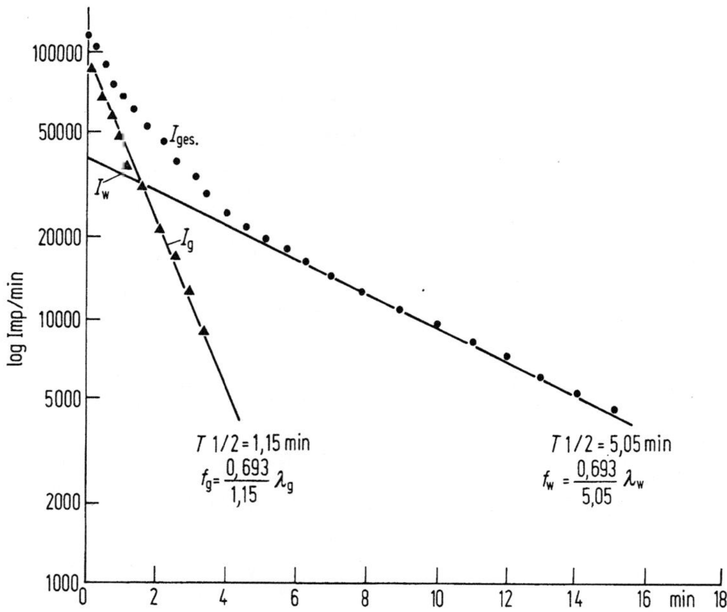

Abb. 4. Analyse der Clearance eines radioaktiven Indikators (^{133}Xe) zur Messung der Durchblutung (f) der grauen Substanz (f_g) und der weißen Substanz (f_w). Bei halblogarithmischer Auftragung kann die Clearance-Kurve (I_{ges}) in zwei e-Funktionen zerlegt werden, die einem gering durchbluteten (I_w) und einem stark durchbluteten (I_g) Gewebsanteil entsprechen, λ=Verteilungskoeffizient des radioaktiven Indikators (für ^{133}Xe beträgt er 1,3), t=Zeit. (Modifiziert nach HØEDT-RASMUSSEN et al., 1966)

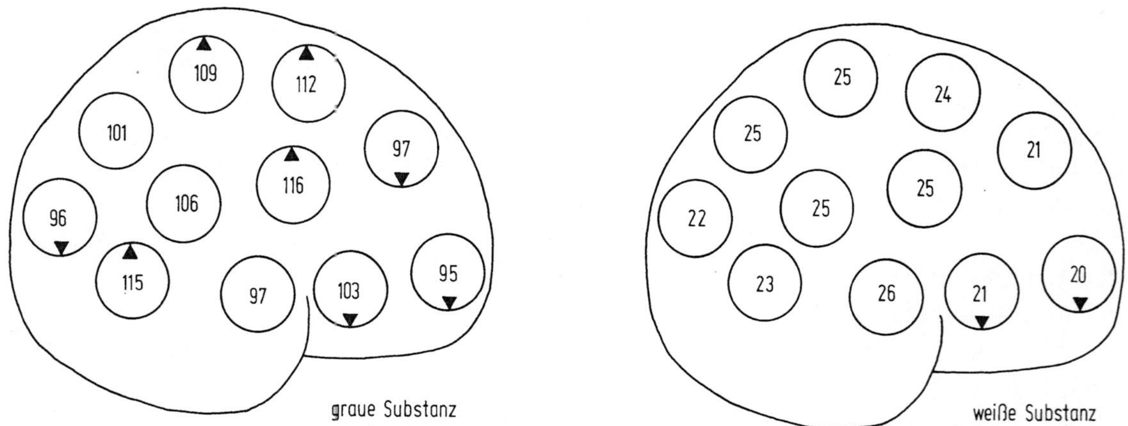

Abb. 5. Normalwerte der lokalen Gehirndurchblutung eines erwachsenen Menschen (gemessen mit der ^{133}Xe-Clearance). Die Werte sind Mittelwerte von 20 Menschen und auf einen arteriellen CO_2-Druck von 40 mm Hg korrigiert. Die Dreiecke kennzeichnen die Orte, an denen die Meßwerte gegenüber dem Mittel aus allen Werten signifikant unterschiedlich waren (Dreiecke mit Spitze nach oben = Erhöhung gegenüber dem Mittelwert, Spitze nach unten = Verminderung). (Nach HERRSCHAFT et al., 1975)

Beim Vergleich der Durchblutung einzelner Hirnregionen können beträchtliche Differenzen in der Durchblutungshöhe gefunden werden. Diese Unterschiede zeigen sich nicht nur zwischen grauer und weißer Substanz, sondern auch in verschiedenen Anteilen der grauen Substanz.

Von LANDAU et al. (1955) und SOKOLOFF (1961) wurden ein Isotop des Trifluorjodmethans ($CF_3{}^{131}J$) als diffusibler Indikator zur Anreicherung der Indikatorsubstanz im Gewebe verwendet und von REIVICH et al. (1969a) C^{14}-Antipyrin. Eine definierte Zeit nach Injektion des Indikators wurden die Versuchstiere durch Dekapitation getötet und aus der Radioaktivität von Gehirnschnitten die lokale Durchblutung bestimmt (Einzelheiten zur Methode: siehe REIVICH, 1972).

Tabelle 2. Die regionale Gehirndurchblutung wacher (1. und 2. Spalte) und thiopental-narkotisierter (3. Spalte) Katzen. Die Meßwerte der 1. Spalte wurden mit der ^{131}J-Trifluorjodmethantechnik gewonnen, die Werte der 2. und 3. Spalte sind mit ^{14}C-Antipyrin gemessen worden. Die Reduzierung der Durchblutung bei den narkotisierten Tieren tritt hauptsächlich im Cortex und subcorticalen Kernen auf. In der weißen Substanz ist eine Verminderung kaum oder gar nicht nachweisbar (Durchblutungswerte in ml Blut · g Gewebe^{-1} · min^{-1}.)

	1 LANDAU et al. (1955) 10 wache Katzen	2 REIVICH et al. (1969) 6 wache Katzen	3 SOKOLOFF (1961) 11 Katzen mit Thiopental narkotisiert
	Oberflächliche Gehirnstrukturen		
Kortex			
Sensomotorische Rinde	1,38 × 0,12	1,09 × 0,04	0,65 × 0,07
Hörrinde	1,30 × 0,05	1,22 × 0,11	0,72 × 0,07
Sehrinde	1,25 × 0,06	1,17 × 0,04	0,77 × 0,09
Assoziationsgebiete	0,88 × 0,04	0,81 × 0,05	0,67 × 0,06
Riechhirn	0,77 × 0,06	0,74 × 0,05	0,62 × 0,07
Weiße Substanz	0,23 × 0,02	0,21 × 0,01	0,26 × 0,04
	Tiefe Gehirnstrukturen		
Corpus geniculatum mediale	1,22 × 0,04	1,43 × 0,11	0,81 × 0,09
Corpus geniculatum laterale	1,21 × 0,08	1,64 × 0,14	0,79 × 0,07
Nucleus caudatus	1,10 × 0,08	1,02 × 0,07	0,91 × 0,11
Thalamus	1,03 × 0,05	1,06 × 0,06	0,71 × 0,09
Hypothalamus	0,84 × 0,05	0,68 × 0,06	0,55 × 0,06
Basalganglien	0,75 × 0,03		0,58 × 0,05
Corpora amygdala		0,54 × 0,03	
Hippocampus	0,61 × 0,03	0,62 × 0,04	0,59 × 0,04
Tractus opticus	0,27 × 0,02	0,20 × 0,01	0,22 × 0,08
	Mittelhirn und Brücke		
Colliculus inferior	1,80 × 0,11	1,74 × 0,08	1,41 × 0,14
obere Olive	1,17 × 0,13	1,08 × 0,07	1,56 × 0,27
Colliculus superior	1,15 × 0,07	1,10 × 0,16	0,82 × 0,10
untere Olive		0,75 × 0,03	
Formatio reticularis	0,59 × 0,05	0,65 × 0,03	0,49 × 0,06
	Kleinhirn und Medulla		
Kleinhirn			
Kerne	0,79 × 0,05	0,84 × 0,03	0,56 × 0,08
Kortex	0,69 × 0,04	0,83 × 0,03	0,57 × 0,05
weiße Substanz	0,24 × 0,01	0,24 × 0,01	0,29 × 0,06
Medulla oblongata			
Vestibulariskerne	0,91 × 0,04	0,92 × 0,03	0,84 × 0,10
Kochleakerne	0,87 × 0,07	0,95 × 0,11	0,99 × 0,14
Pyramiden	0,26 × 0,02	0,22 × 0,02	0,28 × 0,03

Diese Art der Bestimmung der Durchblutungshöhe ergibt ein Bild der Durchblutung einzelner Gehirnstrukturen. Die Methode erlaubt jedoch keine Wiederholung der Messungen am gleichen Tier. Die Tabelle 2 zeigt die gewonnenen Meßergebnisse verschiedener Untersucher.

Durchblutungsunterschiede ähnlicher Art wurden auch von FIESCHI (1967, 1968), FIESCHI et al. (1968a, c), HEISS et. al. (1969, 1971), SVEINSDOTTIR et al. (1969, 1971/72), WILKINSON et al. (1969), IWABUCHI et al. (1971), OLESEN (1971), MCHENRY et al. (1971), SOKOLOFF et al. (1971/72), BROWN u. DONALDSON (1971/72), RISBERG und INGVAR (1971/72), INGVAR und FRANZEN (1973) sowie von SVEINSDOTTIR und LASSEN (1973) gefunden.

Tabelle 3. Prozentuales Kapillarvolumen, Menge und Dichte der Kapillaren in verschiedenen Hirnregionen des Menschen (Nach LIERSE: Acta anat. *54*, Tabelle 10, 1963)

Region	Vol %	Z	a (μ)	Region	Vol %	Z	a (μm)
Fornix	0,3	0,7	117,8	Nucl. olivae	1,4	3,5	53,2
Zentrales Höhlengrau	0,5	1,2	90,1	Nucl. N. XII	1,4	3,5	53,2
Pyramidenbahn	0,5	1,2	90,1	Thalamus	1,5	3,8	51,0
Tractus long. med.	0,5	1,2	90,1	Nucl. term. spin. N. V	1,5	3,8	51,0
Chiasma	0,6	1,6	80,6	Hippocampus	1,5	3,8	51,0
Nucl. centr. sup.	0,7	1,9	73,5	Nucl. term. N. IX, X	1,6	4,2	49,0
Nucl. pontis	0,8	2,1	69,4	Nucl. ambiguus	1,6	4,2	49,0
Cerebellum, Mark	0,9	2,4	64,1	Calcarinarinde	1,6	4,2	49,0
Nucl. arcuatus				Inselrinde	1,6	4,2	49,0
Med. oblongata	0,8	2,2	68,0	Nucl. med. fasc. dors.	1,6	4,2	49,0
Frontalrinde	1,0	2,6	62,1				
Formatio reticul.	1,0	2,6	62,1				
Nucl. niger	1,0	2,6	62,1	N. cochleae	1,7	4,4	47,8
Nucl. caudatus	1,1	2,8	59,9	Calcarinarinde Lam. IV	2,0	5,2	43,9
Colliculus inf.	1,1	2,8	59,9	Cerebellum,			
Gyrus dentatus	1,2	3,1	57,1	Hemisphäre,			
Calcarinarinde				Strat. moleculare	2,1	5,4	43,1
Lam. I, II, III	1,2	3,1	57,1	Putamen	2,4	6,2	40,2
Cerebellum, Vermis				Cerebellum,			
Strat. moleculare	1,3	3,4	54,1	Hemisphäre,			
Gyrus praecentral.	1,3	3,4	54,1	Strat. granulosum	3,3	8,5	34,2

Vol % = prozentuales Volumen der Kapillaren; Z = Kapillarzahl/10000 μ^2; a = mittlerer Kapillarabstand in μm

Wie Tabelle 2 zeigt, sind die regionalen Durchblutungsdifferenzen bei wachen Tieren sehr viel deutlicher ausgeprägt als beim narkotisierten Tier. Bei Narkose wird die Durchströmung von stark durchbluteten Bereichen besonders deutlich reduziert.

Da die graue Substanz in der Regel höher durchblutet ist als die weiße Substanz, so bedeutet dies, daß die durch die Narkose verursachte Flußminderung vorwiegend auf Kosten der grauen Hirnsubstanz geschieht.

Es ist eine z.Z. noch nicht ganz gelöste Frage, ob die lokale Durchblutung mit der Kapillardichte in einzelnen Gefäßabschnitten übereinstimmt. Nach LIERSE (1963) sowie LIERSE u. HORSTMANN (1965) ist die Kapillarisierung außer vom Sauerstoffbedarf auch von anderen Faktoren abhängig – zumindest beim erwachsenen Menschen. Tabelle 3 zeigt das prozentuale Volumen der Kapillaren, die Kapillarzahl/10000 μ^2 und den mittleren Kapillarabstand in verschiedenen Hirnregionen von erwachsenen Menschen. Ein Vergleich von Tabelle 2 und Tabelle 3 läßt erkennen, daß die Kapillardichten und die gemessenen Durchblutungen in einzelnen Gehirnregionen nicht völlig übereinstimmen. Allerdings muß einschränkend gesagt werden, daß die Kapillardichten beim Menschen gemessen wurden, während die Flußmessungen im Tierexperiment durchgeführt wurden.

2. Zeitliche Änderungen der regionalen, spontanen Gehirndurchblutung

Im Gegensatz zu den sehr konstanten Meßwerten der Durchblutung des Gesamtgehirns mit Methoden, die den Durchstrom über mehrere Minuten integriert messen, findet man mit kontinuierlich registrierenden Meßmethoden spontane Variationen der lokalen Durchblutung. Sie können in allen Hirnteilen nachgewiesen werden; sie sind manchmal, aber nicht immer synchronisiert. Mit geheizten Thermoelementen hat schon GIBBS (1933) lokale spontane Variationen der Durchblutung registriert. Die Frequenzen dieser Oszillationen können eingeteilt werden in:

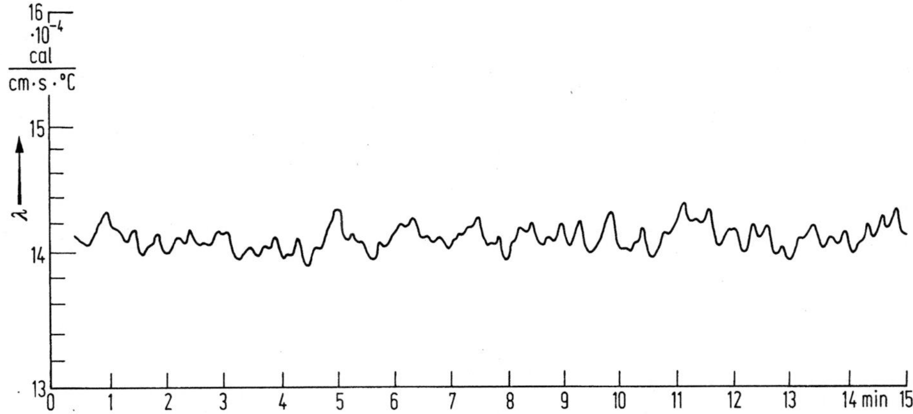

Abb. 6. Originalregistrierung der lokalen Durchblutung im Thalamus bei einer ruhig liegenden Katze mit spontanen Durchblutungsschwankungen (gemessen mit einer chronisch implantierten Wärmeleitsonde, BETZ, 1967)

1. pulssynchrone Schwankungen, die an den großen Hirnarterien besonders deutlich registrierbar sind,

2. atemsynchrone Schwankungen (sie sind sowohl bei Messungen der Durchströmung der Jugularvenen (BETZ, 1972), als auch bei Messungen des Liquordrucks deutlich nachweisbar),

3. Spontanschwankungen einer Periodendauer von über 5–60 s. Bei tief narkotisierten Tieren sind Spontanschwankungen einer Periodendauer von mehr als 30 s oft regelmäßig ausgeprägt. Bei tief narkotisierten Tieren waren darüber hinaus keine Spontanschwankungen erkennbar, wenn der arterielle P_{O_2} und der P_{CO_2} konstant blieben. Die Periodendauer der, in tiefer Narkose meßbaren, sehr regelmäßigen Oszillationen der Durchblutung betrug meist 50–60 s und war von gleichartigen regelmäßigen Schwankungen des O_2-Drucks auf der Gehirnoberfläche begleitet. Bei wachen, frei beweglichen Tieren sind die spontanen Durchblutungsvariationen meist unregelmäßig und weisen unterschiedlich hohe Amplituden auf (BETZ, 1967). Die Abb. 6 zeigt die Originalregistrierung solcher spontanen Durchblutungsschwankungen im Thalamus. Die Messung wurde am wachen Tier, einige Wochen nach Implantation des Meßelements, vorgenommen. Im Gegensatz zum narkotisierten Tier waren die Durchblutungsoszillationen nicht mit gleichgerichteten Blutdruckschwankungen gekoppelt. Abb. 7 zeigt ein Häufigkeitsspektrum von Durchblutungsänderungen beim Tier, bei welchem die Verteilung von Durchblutungsperioden zwischen 3 und 30 s dargestellt ist (atem- und pulssynchrone Schwankungen fehlen). Beim wachen Menschen wurden von WÜLLENWEBER (1963), WÜLLENWEBER et al. (1967) ähnliche Befunde mitgeteilt.

4. Bei wachen Individuen sind darüber hinaus Durchblutungsänderungen mit längerer Periodendauer, die von den frequenteren Schwankungen überlagert sind, zu registrieren. Deren Häufigkeitsverteilung ist in der Abb. 8 dargestellt.

Die Amplituden aller dieser Änderungen waren klein im Verhältnis zu zahlreichen reaktiven Änderungen (etwa bei Inhalation von 6% CO_2). Sie betrugen durchschnittlich bis $\pm 20\%$ der Ausgangswerte. In Ruhe und im Schlaf sind sie ausgeprägter als bei wachen und aufmerksamen Tieren.

Die kurz dauernden spontanen Oszillationen sind nicht immer mit Änderungen des EEG verbunden (KANZOW u. KRAUSE, 1962; KANZOW et al., 1962; KRUPP, 1966), jedoch sind Aktivitätssteigerungen (wie Arousal-Reaktionen) oft mit Durchblutungserhöhungen gekoppelt (KANZOW et al., 1961).

Bei fortlaufender Registrierung der lokalen Durchblutung über mehrere Tage und Nächte zeigte sich, daß der Mittelwert der Durchblutung bei Ruhe konstant blieb, daß aber zu Zeiten erhöhter Aktivität die Durchblutung stärker schwanken konnte und über mehrere Minuten andauernde Anstiege aufwies. Verminderungen unter den Ruhewert waren meist kürzer dauernd,

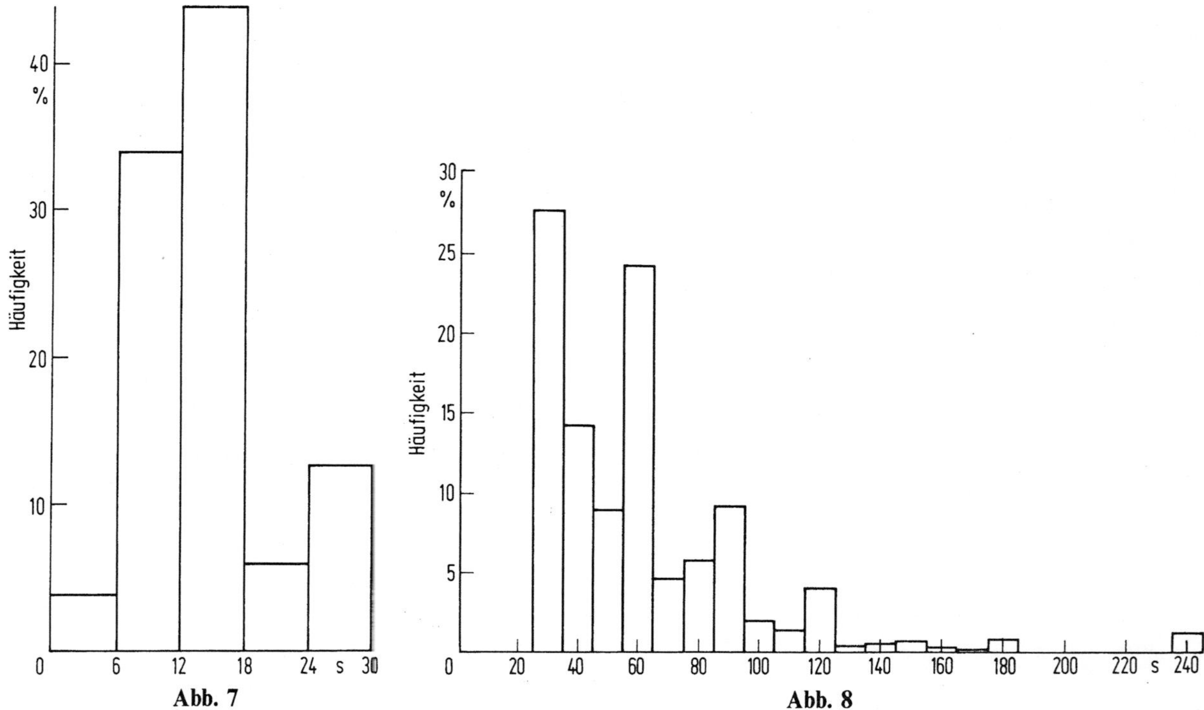

Abb. 7. Prozentuale Verteilung der Häufigkeit von 3000 spontanen Oszillationen der lokalen Gehirndurchblutung, Schwingungsdauern von weniger als 30 s, pulssynchrone und atemsynchrone Oszillationen sind nicht dargestellt. (Nach BETZ, 1963)

Abb. 8. Spontane periodische Änderungen der lokalen Gehirndurchblutung von wachen Katzen (1500 Meßwerte). Es sind prozentuale Häufigkeiten von solchen Durchblutungsperioden dargestellt, die eine Dauer von mehr als 30 s haben. (Nach BETZ, 1967)

kamen aber ebenfalls vor (BETZ, 1967). Wurde die Durchblutung mit implantierten Meßelementen mehrere Wochen lang täglich fortlaufend gemessen und die Mittelwerte von jeweils 1 Std Meßdauer bei ruhig liegenden Tieren gegen die Zeit aufgetragen, so zeigten sich lediglich in den ersten Tagen nach der Operation Schwankungen der Durchblutungshöhe. Später blieben die Mittelwerte konstant.

Aus diesen Befunden ergibt sich, daß die regionale Gehirndurchblutung um einen Mittelwert, der relativ konstant gehalten wird, schwankt.

3. Einfluß des Lebensalters auf die Gehirndurchblutung

In der Tabelle 3 ist dargestellt, daß die Kapillardichte in verschiedenen Gehirnregionen unterschiedlich ist. Bei Untersuchung der Änderungen der Kapillarzahl pro Volumeneinheit Gehirn zeigt sich, daß nicht nur örtliche, sondern auch zeitliche Unterschiede der Dichte der kleinen Arterien und der Kapillaren zu erkennen sind. Im Fetalleben ist die Kapillarisierung des Gehirns geringer als kurz nach der Geburt. Sie steigt dann zwischen dem vierten und sechsten Monat steil an und erreicht etwa im fünften Lebensjahr den endgültigen Wert, der auch beim Erwachsenen nachweisbar ist (LIERSE, 1963a, b; HARNARINE-SINGH u. HYDE, 1970; Abb. 9).

DIEMER (1968) gibt an, daß beim neugeborenen Kind 98,4 Kapillaren/mm^2, beim Erwachsenen dagegen 290 Kapillaren/mm^2 vorkommen. Die Anstiege der Kapillardichten nach der Geburt sind nach seiner Ansicht deutlich von der Sauerstoffversorgung des Kindes abhängig. In Untersuchungen an hypoxischen Kindern hat sich gezeigt, daß der Anstieg der Kapillardichte hier sehr viel steiler verläuft als bei normalen Kindern. Abhängigkeit der Kapillardichte im Gehirngewebe von

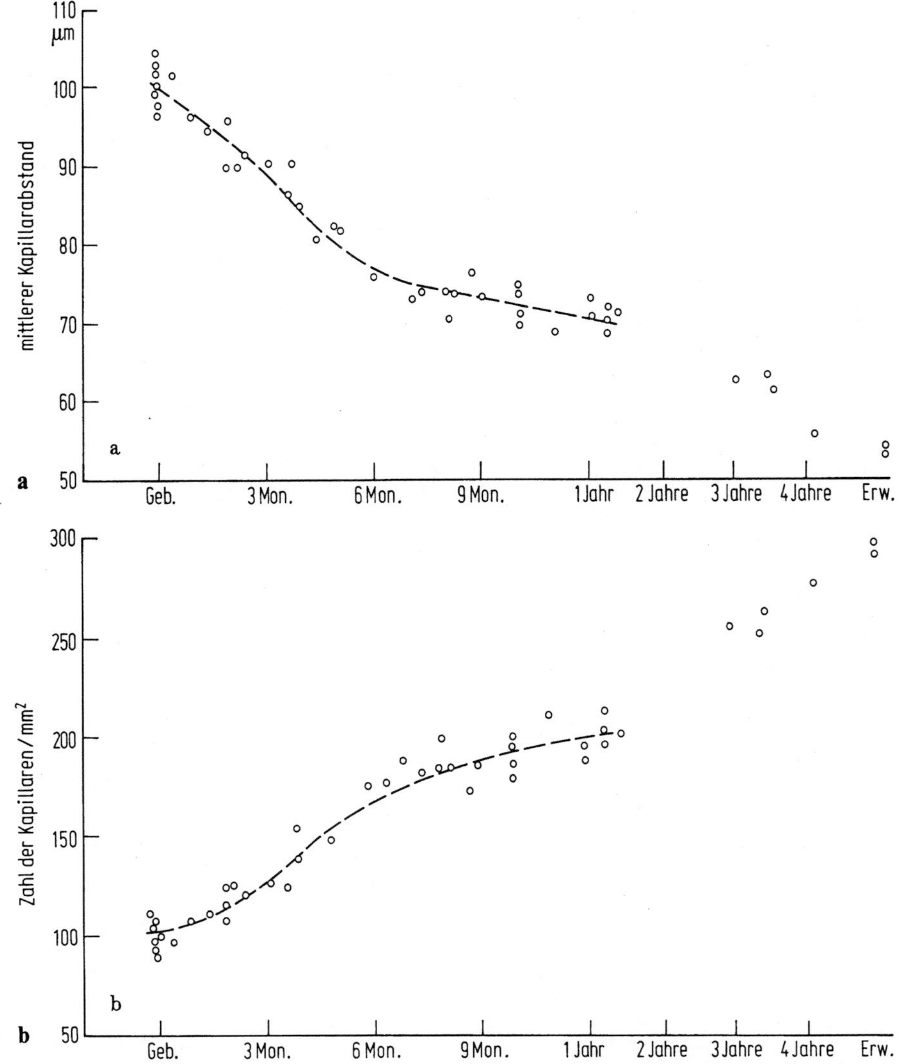

Abb. 9a u. b. Postnatale Entwicklung der Kapillarabstände (**a**) und der Kapillardichte (**b**) in der Rinde des menschlichen Frontalhirns. (Nach DIEMER aus LÜBBERS et al., 1968)

der Sauerstoffversorgung des Organismus wurde früher schon von OPITZ und PALME (1944), DIEMER (1964), DIEMER und HENN (1965) mitgeteilt. Daß hierbei der Sauerstoffdruck nicht die allein entscheidende Rolle spielt, ergibt sich aus einer Untersuchung von RAO (zit. nach CRAIGE, 1928), der bei neugeborenen Ratten ein Auge entfernte und, trotz normaler Sauerstoffversorgung, eine starke Verzögerung der Kapillarentwicklung im korrespondierenden Colliculus superior und im posterioren Kern des Corpus geniculatum laterale beobachtete. Diese Untersuchungen zeigen, daß die zeitliche Entwicklung der Kapillarisierung des Gehirns nach andern funktionellen Anforderungen des Gewebes geschehen kann. Nach BÄR und WOLFF (1975) besteht kein Zusammenhang von Gefäßwachstum und O_2-Mangel bei erwachsenen Tieren.

Systematische Durchblutungsmessungen jenseits des fünften Lebensjahres lassen erkennen, daß Durchblutung und Sauerstoffverbrauch des kindlichen Gehirns höher liegen als beim Erwachsenen (KENNEDY u. SOKOLOFF, 1957; BERNSMEIER u. GOTTSTEIN, 1958). Nach Abb. 10 sinken beide Parameter regelmäßig im späteren Lebensalter weiter ab. Es gibt allerdings viele Ausnahmen von dieser Regel, wie die Abb. 11 erkennen läßt. SCHEINBERG et al. (1953), BROBEIL (1954), KETY (1956), SOKOLOFF (1959) u.a. stellten fest, daß mit fortschreitendem Lebensalter die Hirndurchblutung statistisch signifikant abnimmt und der zerebrale Gefäßwiderstand anwächst. Auch der mittlere Sauerstoffverbrauch des Gehirns, der bei Personen zwischen 30 und 50 Jahren etwa

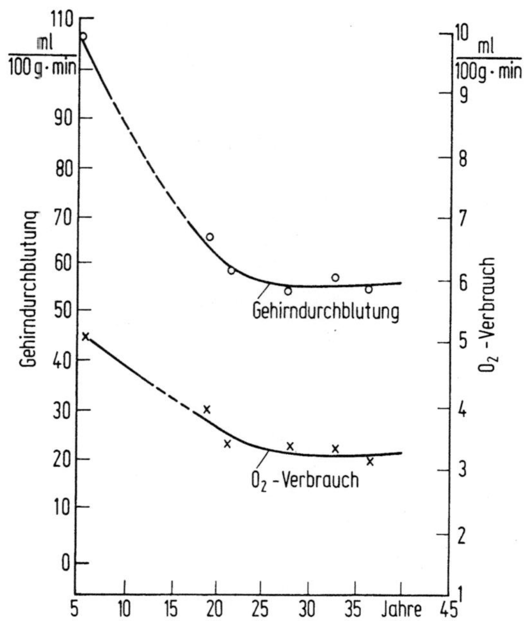

Abb. 10. Die Entwicklung der Gehirndurchblutung und des Sauerstoffverbrauchs des Gehirns vom 5. bis zum 40. Lebensjahr. (Etwas modifiziert nach KENNEDY und SOKOLOFF sowie BERNSMEIER und GOTTSTEIN aus HIRSCH und SCHNEIDER: Durchblutung und Sauerstoffaufnahme des Gehirns. In: Hdb. der Neurochirurgie, Bd. I/2, Hrsg.: OLIVECRONA et al., 1968)

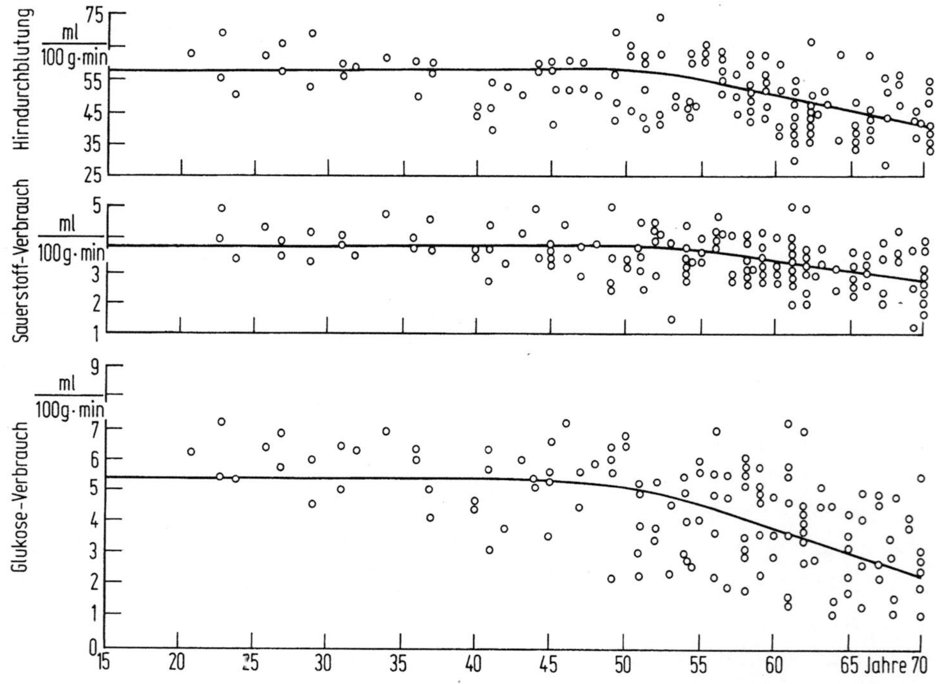

Abb. 11. Altersabhängigkeit von Gehirndurchblutung, Sauerstoffverbrauch und Glukoseverbrauch. (Nach GOTTSTEIN, 1969)

4 ml O_2/min · 100 g Hirngewebe beträgt, nimmt statistisch signifikant ab. Bei 17 Personen zwischen 56 und 79 Jahren wurde z.B. ein Sauerstoffverbrauch von nur 3,32 ml O_2/100 g Hirngewebe pro min gemessen (KETY, 1956). Auch im deutschen Schrifttum sind von BERNSMEIER u. GOTTSTEIN (1958) ähnliche Ergebnisse publiziert worden, wobei die Gehirndurchblutung einen Mittelwert von etwa 58 ml Blut/min · 100 g Hirngewebe zwischen dem 15. und 20. Lebensjahr aufweist. Diese Durchblutungsgröße bleibt etwa bis zum 50.–60. Lebensjahr gleich. Bei Untersuchungen an Patien-

ten, bei denen eine Arteriosklerose mit seniler Psychose diagnostiziert wurde, kam es zu einem signifikanten Abfall der Gehirndurchblutung und des zerebralen Sauerstoffverbrauchs unter die physiologischen Werte (FREYHAN et al., 1951; SOKOLOFF, 1959). Auch bei Kranken mit kardialer Dekompensation sinkt die Gehirndurchblutung, und da sich unter diesen Kranken in größerer Zahl ältere Menschen befinden, muß die kardiale Insuffizienz als auslösender Mechanismus für die Erniedrigung der Gehirndurchblutung bei älteren Menschen mitbedacht werden. BERNSMEIER et al. (1962) und BERNSMEIER und GOTTSTEIN (1963) fanden bei 26 kardial dekompensierten Patienten eine Hirndurchblutungsgröße von im Mittel 38 ml Blut/min · 100 g Hirngewebe, was einer Verminderung von 20 ml Blut/min · 100 g Hirngewebe gegenüber Normalen entspricht. Ähnliche Ergebnisse berichten auch MEYER et al. (zit. nach BERNSMEIER u. GOTTSTEIN, 1958). Aus umfangreichen Untersuchungen von HERRMANN (1964) ist erkennbar, daß mit dem Absinken der Gehirndurchblutung angiographisch deutlich nachweisbare Gefäßveränderungen einhergehen, wobei allerdings lediglich die großen Arterien beurteilbar sind. Alle erwähnten quantitativen Durchblutungsmessungen sind mit Methoden gewonnen worden, die über das gesamte Gehirn mitteln; dabei wurde die KETY-SCHMIDTsche Technik angewendet.

Der zerebrale Sauerstoffverbrauch, der eine gewisse Parallelität zur Kapillarisierung des Gehirns zeigt, ändert sich im Verlauf des Lebens ebenfalls. Während er bei sechsjährigen Kindern noch etwa 50% des Grundumsatzes eines Menschen beträgt (KETY, 1955), sinkt er im Verlauf des Lebens auf Werte unter 4 ml Sauerstoff/min · 100 g (Abb. 11). Bei Messungen der regionalen Sauerstoffaufnahme kann nach Untersuchungen von LÜBBERS et al. (1964) angenommen werden, daß sie im Bereich der Gehirnrinde ca. 8 ml Sauerstoff/100 g · min beträgt, wenn im flachnarkotisierten Zustand von Hunden gemessen wird. Bei Messungen im Wachzustand wurden sogar Werte bis zu 12 ml/100 g · min gefunden. Es gibt bisher noch keine systematischen Untersuchungen zur Sauerstoffaufnahme einzelner Gehirnstrukturen in Abhängigkeit vom Lebensalter. Da bei alten Menschen die Erkrankungen des Zentralnervensystems infolge von Arteriosklerose zahlreicher werden, ist es nicht verwunderlich, daß die Sauerstoffaufnahme des Gehirns bei derartigen pathologischen Zuständen geringer wird. In der Tabelle 4 sind bei einer Reihe von Erkrankungsbildern des höheren Lebensalters die O_2-Aufnahmen dargestellt, bei denen klar erkennbar wird, daß sie geringer sind als bei jugendlichen Menschen.

Tabelle 4. Sauerstoffverbrauch des Gehirns bei einer Reihe von Gehirnerkrankungen des höheren Lebensalters

O_2-Verbrauch/100 ml · min (Mittelwerte)			
Hirnarteriosklerose	Störungen verschiedenen Grades	< 3,0	LASSEN, MUNCK u. TOTTEY (1957)
	Störungen verschiedenen Grades	2,7	BERNSMEIER u. GOTTSTEIN (1958)
	Störungen verschiedenen Grades	2,7	BODECHTEL (1928)
	Störungen verschiedenen Grades	2,9	SCHEINBERG et al. (1953)
	Störungen verschiedenen Grades	1,8–2,8	BROBEIL et al. (1957)
Senile Demenz	dement	2,8	SCHIEVE u. WILSON (1953)
	dement	1,6–2,8	LASSEN, MUNCK u. TOTTEY (1957)
	dement	2,7	FREYHAN, WOODFORD u. KETY (1951)

E. Die Gehirndurchblutung bei emotionalen und psychischen Reizen

Bei der Festlegung von Normwerten der lokalen Gehirndurchblutung können Meßmethoden, die Schmerz oder Aufregungen des Patienten bewirken, nur mit großer Vorsicht verwendet werden. Im Tierexperiment haben schon 1867 NOTHNAGEL und 1871 RIEGEL und JOLLY beobachtet, daß bei Tieren, die schmerzhaften Reizen ausgesetzt wurden, Änderungen der Durchmesser kortikaler und pialer Gefäße auftraten. Durch physiologische Reize optischer, akustischer oder taktiler Art werden Synchronisierungen des EEG bewirkt, die gewöhnlich mit mäßigen Steigerungen der Gehirndurchblutung verbunden sind (INGVAR, 1958, 1969; KANZOW et al., 1961; KANZOW u. KRAUSE, 1962; MOLNAR, 1967; KRUPP, 1966; BETZ u. HENSEL, 1962; BETZ, 1963, 1965a). Versucht man, diese Einflüsse durch Narkose auszuschalten, so muß man feststellen, daß durch die Wirkung der Narkotika selbst Änderungen der Gehirndurchblutung bewirkt werden können (siehe weiter unten). An Patienten mit Schädeldefekten fand MOSSO (1881) mit einem Plethysmographen eine Zunahme des Gehirnvolumens und der Gehirnpulsation bei verschiedenen Sinneseindrücken, beim Kopfrechnen und bei Denktätigkeiten. Emotionelle Erregungen lösten besonders starke Änderungen aus. Die Durchblutung wird durch Schmerz (HERRMANN, 1968), Furcht oder andere emotionale Reize verändert (KETY, 1950, 1952; RISBERG u. INGVAR, 1968). Bei Rechentests wurden unterschiedliche Ergebnisse gesehen. LENNOX (1931), ALLWOOD et al. (1959), RISBERG u. INGVAR (1971/72, 1973a, b) sahen deutliche Anstiege, während SOKOLOFF et al. (1955) keine signifikanten Änderungen der Gehirndurchblutung erkannten. SCHEINBERG und STEAD (1949) konnten auch bei Schmerzen und visuellen Reizen keine Durchblutungsänderung erkennen. Diese Diskrepanz der Reaktionen mag z.T. daran liegen, daß die Untersucher, die mit integrierenden Techniken gemessen haben, die lokalen Unterschiede nicht erfassen konnten, während SEM-JAKOBSEN et al. (1969) und RISBERG und INGVAR (1973a, b) mit zahlreichen Szintillationszählern, die über dem Kopf angeordnet waren, beim Menschen deutliche Durchblutungsmusteränderungen erkannten. Hierbei war auffällig, daß bestimmte Gehirnregionen im Bereich des Frontalhirns besonders deutliche Erhöhungen zeigten, wenn eine geistige Leistung verlangt wurde. Bei Emotionen stieg dagegen der Durchstrom im gesamten corticalen Bereich an. Die Lokalisierung bei willkürlichen Bewegungen ist inzwischen so weit geklärt, daß eine deutliche Beziehung zwischen Durchblutungsänderung in kortikalen Projektionsfeldern und bewegten Gliedmaßen als gesichert bezeichnet wurde (RISBERG u. INGVAR, 1973b; INGVAR, 1975). Bei gleichzeitigen Messungen der Gehirnperfusion, des EEG's und des Sauerstoffdrucks auf dem Kortex sowie des arteriellen Blutdrucks konnte schon 1964 gezeigt werden (LÜBBERS et al.), daß bei kontinuierlichen Messungen dieser Größen die Beziehungen zwischen dem Grad der EEG-Aktivität und der Durchblutung deutlich sind (s. auch BALDY-MOULINIER u. INGVAR, 1965). In der Regel kommt es bei emotionsauslösenden Reizen, z.B. Schmerzreizen, sowohl zu Durchblutungssteigerungen als auch zu Blutdruckerhöhungen. Beim völlig wachen Tier zeigt sich eine deutliche Situationsabhängigkeit vom dargebotenen Reiz. Durchblutungsänderungen im Thalamus oder Hypothalamus von Katzen waren immer dann beobachtbar, wenn der Reiz für das Tier einen Aufforderungscharakter (KATZ, 1933) besaß. Der gleiche Reiz bewirkt also nicht immer Durchblutungsänderungen. An einem typischen Beispiel möge das erläutert werden: sieht eine Katze eine Maus, und ist die Katze hungrig, so steigt die Gehirndurchblutung an. Ist die Katze dagegen gesättigt, so bewirkt der gleiche Reiz keine Reaktion oder nur einen geringen Anstieg. Allerdings wird in diesem Fall ein Lärmreiz oder ein Reiz, durch den sich die Katze in irgendeiner Weise betroffen fühlt, zu einer Steigerung der Durchblutung führen (BETZ, 1975). KANZOW u. REICHEL (1967) bezeichnen diese Reaktion als Aufmerksamkeitsreaktion oder als apperzeptiv-affektive Gehirngefäßreaktion. Es fällt bei der Betrachtung solcher Reaktionen auf, daß die Durchblutungssteigerung sowohl im Bereich der Gehirnrinde als auch im Bereich tieferer Strukturen außerordentlich schnell auftritt. In einer Zeit von weniger als 10 Sekunden steigt sie stark an und erreicht bisweilen schon während dieser Zeit ihren Gipfelwert. Derartige Steigerungen treten häufig mit steilen Blutdruckanstiegen gekoppelt auf; es kommt jedoch auch vor, daß der arterielle Blutdruck nicht wesentlich ansteigt. Die Steigerungen geschehen auch bei konstant gehaltenem CO_2- und Sauerstoffdruck.

Beim Menschen verursacht auch belästigender Lärm Erhöhungen der Gehirndurchblutung, vor allem, wenn der Lärm (weißes Geräusch) eine Lautstärke von etwa 100 Phon erreicht. Kopfschmerzen und Störung des Wohlbefindens sind die Folge (MIYAZAKI, 1972). Es wird geschlossen, daß schwerer und wiederholter Lärm Abnormalitäten der zerebralen Zirkulation verursachen kann. Wenn bei Hunden der Plexus des Nervus tympanicus aber nicht die Rezeptoren einer Hemisphäre gereizt werden, kommt es zu einem deutlichen Anstieg der Durchblutung in der Arteria carotis interna der gereizten Körperseite. Auf der gereizten Seite steigt der Tonus der Vertebralarterien an, auf der Gegenseite wird er vermindert. Der arterielle Blutdruck fällt dabei ab (ROMANOV u. GAEVYI, 1971).

Derartige emotionsauslösende Reize haben Ähnlichkeit mit Durchblutungsanstiegen bei der Stimulation der Formatio reticularis im Gehirnstamm (BENETATO et al., 1958; MOLNAR u. SZANTO, 1964; BAUST, 1967; SHALIT et al., 1967b; VYSHATINA, 1970; CZOPF u. MOLNAR, 1970). MEYER et al. (1969a, b) demonstrierten, daß parallel mit der ansteigenden Gehirndurchblutung die zerebrale Sauerstoffaufnahme ansteigt, wenn das EEG eine Desynchronisation aufweist. Ein Anstieg der Durchblutung um 10% war von einem Anstieg der Sauerstoffaufnahme von über 7,7% begleitet. Ein ähnlicher Effekt konnte beim Menschen beobachtet werden, wenn eine Arousal-Reaktion durch einen schmerzhaften Reiz hervorgerufen war (MEYER et al., 1966; KRUPP, 1966).

F. Habituationsphänomene

Bei wachen, frei beweglichen Tieren konnte gezeigt werden (BETZ, 1965b, 1975), daß bei Fortdauer eines Lärmreizes, der beim Tier initial starke Gehirndurchblutungssteigerungen auslöst, die Durchblutung wieder in Richtung Ausgangswert zurückkehrt (gemessen im Thalamusbereich und in einigen Kortexregionen). Setzt man das Tier wiederholten Lärmperioden von einer halben bis einer Minute Dauer (90–110 Phon, weißes Geräusch) aus und legt Pausen von jeweils einer Minute zwischen die einzelnen Lärmserien, so kommt es während des Reizes jeweils zu steilen und kurzdauernden Durchblutungsanstiegen. Nach einer Reihe von Lärmserien am gleichen Tag reduziert sich die Durchblutungssteigerung und verschwindet schließlich. Wird der gleiche Versuch

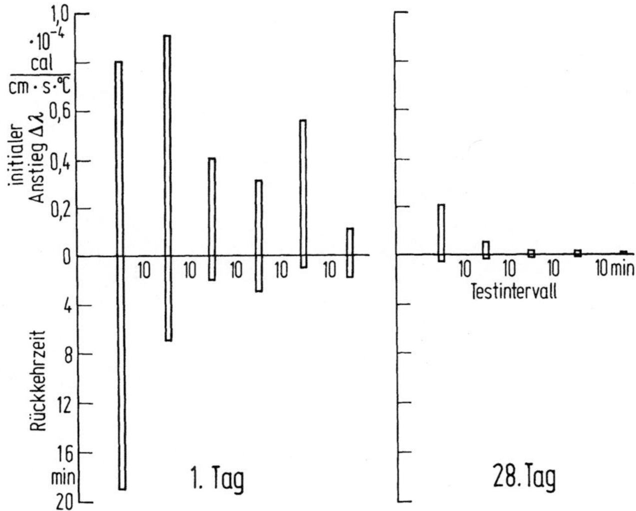

Abb. 12. Die Wirkung von Lärmreizen (90–110 Phon) auf die Durchblutung im Thalamus bei einer wachen Katze; fortlaufende Durchblutungsregistrierung mit implantiertem Wärmeleitelement. In der Ordinate sind nach oben die maximalen Steigerungen der Durchblutung bei mehrfach wiederholten Lärmreizen aufgetragen. Nach unten sind die Zeiten aufgetragen, die anzeigen, wann nach einer Reizserie die Durchblutung wieder auf den Ausgangswert zurückgekehrt ist. Jeweils 10 min später wurde mit der nächsten Reizserie begonnen. Auf der Abszisse sind die Reaktionen während des ersten Tages und des 28. Tages einer täglich gleichartigen Lärmreizserie dargestellt. (Nach BETZ in: Brain Work, 1975)

über einen Monat täglich vorgenommen, so bleibt die Durchblutungssteigerung schließlich auch schon beim ersten Lärmreiz aus (Abb. 12).

Der Verlauf der Gehirndurchblutung ist typisch für ein Habituationsphänomen, welches demjenigen anderer Funktionen (z.B. der Herzfrequenz) ähnlich ist. HEUSER und LENZI (1975, unveröffentl.) haben inzwischen nachgewiesen, daß bei elektrischer β-Stimulation peripherer, afferenter Nerven, im Bereich des Nucleus Cuneatus, die Wasserstoffionenkonzentration initial stärker ansteigt als bei Fortdauer des Reizes, was bestätigt, daß Habituationen auch im Bereich des Stoffwechsels einzelner Gehirnstrukturen ihr Korrelat haben. Bei Durchblutungsmessungen an Menschen zeigten sich ebenfalls Habituationserscheinungen in der Gehirndurchblutung (BETZ u. HERRMANN, 1966). Wird bei einem Patienten, bei dem eine flexible Wärmeleitsonde in den Bulbus venae jugularis eingeschoben wurde, eine ihn betreffende Unterhaltung geführt, so steigt in der Regel die Gehirndurchblutung deutlich an. Diese Steigerung ist meist vorübergehender Natur, und noch während der Unterhaltung geht sie wieder langsam auf den Ausgangswert zurück. Als Beispiel einer Störung dieser Verhaltensweise und der damit gekoppelten Durchblutungsreaktion dient Abb. 13. Hier wurde bei einem Kranken eine Durchstrommessung im Bulbus venae jugularis vorgenommen, und der Patient ängstigte sich vor einer Infusion, die im Untersuchungsraum vorbereitet wurde, aber gar nicht für ihn vorgesehen war. Die Gehirndurchblutung stieg sofort steil an. Es kam zu einer psychomotorischen Störung des Kranken, die mit mäßigem Schweißausbruch verbunden war und zu einer Steigerung der Herzfrequenz, aber zu kaum einer Steigerung des arteriellen Blutdrucks, führte. Obgleich der Patient über seine irrtümliche Annahme aufgeklärt wurde, blieb die Durchblutung zunächst hoch. Erst verbale Suggestion des behandelnden Arztes beruhigte den Patienten, und es kam schließlich zur Normalisierung der Gehirndurchblutung, und der Patient schlief ein.

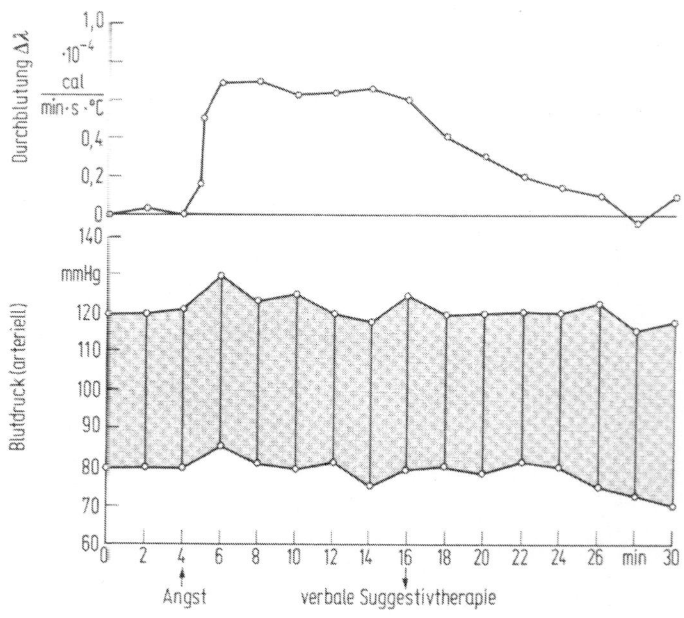

Abb. 13. Durchstromänderung durch den Bulbus venae jugularis bei einem Patienten, der irrtümlich annahm, es solle bei ihm eine intravenöse Infusion einer größeren Menge Flüssigkeit vorgenommen werden. Die Durchblutung wurde mit einer, längere Zeit vorher, in den Bulbus venae jugularis implantierten flexiblen Wärmeleitsonde als Wärmetransportzahländerung fortlaufend registriert. Die Sonde behinderte den Patienten nicht. Die Durchblutung kehrte nach Beruhigung des Patienten wieder auf den Ausgangswert zurück, s. Text. (Aus BETZ, in: Brain Work, 1975)

G. Narkose und Gehirndurchblutung

In den beiden vorhergehenden Abschnitten kommt zum Ausdruck, daß eine enge Interaktion zwischen der funktionellen Aktivität des Gehirns und dem Hirnkreislauf besteht. Schon SCHMIDT (1949) stellte fest, daß

a) der zerebrale Sauerstoffbedarf in vivo direkt von der funktionellen Aktivität des Gehirns abhängt, und

b) der Tonus der zerebralen Arterien direkt an die metabolischen Erfordernisse und entsprechend an die Aktivität des Gehirns angekoppelt ist.

Eine Reihe von Untersuchungen unterstützen diese Hypothese: SUZUKI und TUKAHARA (1965) untersuchten gleichzeitig die lokale Durchblutung und die elektrische Aktivität im Thalamus und im Kortex während elektrischer Reizung der mesenzephalen retikulären Strukturen. Bei wachen Tieren verursachte eine derartige Stimulation eine deutliche Arousal-Reaktion und einen signifikanten Anstieg der Durchblutung im Thalamus-Bereich (mit Wärmeleitsonden registriert). 5 Minuten nach der Injektion von 20 mg/kg Pentobarbital waren die Gefäßeffekte und die EEG-Antworten leicht reduziert. Weitere Injektionen von Pentobarbital, die die elektrische Aktivität deutlich erniedrigten, führten zum Verschwinden sowohl des EEG als auch von vaskulären Reaktionen. Erneute Stimulation der gleichen Region führte zum Auftreten von EEG-Spindeln, aber zu keiner Steigerung der Gehirndurchblutung. Sehr hohe Dosen von Pentobarbital unterdrückten die EEG-Aktivität vollständig, jedoch sank zunächst die Gehirndurchblutung nicht unter einen bestimmten Wert ab. KRUPP (1966) fand ebenfalls Anstiege der intrazerebralen Durchblutung, wenn die Aktivität durch exterozeptive Reize erhöht wurde. Die Durchblutungsreaktionen verschwanden nach Blockierung der EEG-Aktivität durch Barbitursäure-Injektionen. Eine signifikante Korrelation zwischen der mittleren EEG-Frequenz und der Durchblutungshöhe wurde von INGVAR (1969) und FREEMAN und INGVAR (1968a und b) bei normalen und anaesthesierten Tieren gefunden. Sie war dann am deutlichsten zu sehen, wenn die Durchblutung und das EEG von der gleichen Gehirnregion registriert wurden. Bei diesen Untersuchungen waren die Kontrollwerte bei künstlich beatmeten Katzen unter Stickoxydul-Anaesthesie gewonnen worden. Die regionale Gehirndurchblutung wurde mit der ^{85}Kr-Clearance gemessen, die EEG-Spektren durch manuelle Frequenzanalyse gewonnen. Die kortikale Aktivität wurde zunächst durch geringe Dosen von Thiopental (5 mg/kg) vermindert. Durch Injektion von Pentetrazol (6–10 mg/kg) konnte sie wieder erhöht werden. Bei dieser Dosis traten noch keine Konvulsionen auf. Niedrige Durchblutungswerte waren in der Regel bei gehäuftem Auftreten langsamer Frequenzen im EEG zu erkennen. Diese Befunde unterstützen die These, daß die Gehirndurchblutung lokal an die funktionelle Aktivität des Gehirns gekoppelt ist, wobei von BALDY-MOULINIER (1971) eine besonders enge Beziehung zu dem Frequenzmuster des EEG gefunden wurde. Untersuchungen von KRUPP (1966) und KRUPP und CARPI (1964) konnten allerdings auch zeigen, daß eine Aktivierung des EEG nicht immer mit einer Steigerung der Gehirndurchblutung gekoppelt ist. Eine sich verstärkende Hemmung des dilatierenden Effektes von CO_2 trat bei ansteigenden Dosen von Pentobarbital, Hexobarbital und Butethal auf. Pentobarbital führte zu einer gleichzeitigen Verminderung der elektrischen Hirnaktivität. Hexobarbital beeinflußte nur wenig die CO_2-induzierte zerebrale Vasodilatation, hemmte jedoch deutlich die elektroencephalographische Reaktion, ohne daß deren Antwort auf CO_2-Erhöhung ausblieb. Aus diesen Untersuchungen schloß KRUPP, daß *keine* kausale Abhängigkeit der Gehirndurchblutung von der elektrischen Hirnaktivität besteht. FREEMAN und INGVAR (1968a, b) betonten, daß die Korrelation zwischen EEG-Muster und Gehirndurchblutung auch während und nach einer Hypoxie aufgehoben ist. Die unterschiedlichen Narkotika haben auf die Gehirndurchblutung z.T. gegensätzliche Wirkung (Übersichten zu diesem Problem, s. BETZ, 1972a, b). Viele dieser Substanzen verursachen sowohl eine Verminderung der Gehirndurchblutung als auch der Sauerstoffaufnahme des Gehirns (BERNSMEIER, 1959; DAweke et al., 1959; Fieschi, 1967; Gottstein et al., 1961; Himwich et al., 1947; Homburger et al., 1946; Kety et al., 1948b; McCall u. Taylor, 1952; Novack et al., 1963; Pierce et al., 1962; Rosomoff, 1965; Schmidt et al., 1945; Taylor u. McCall, 1951). Diese Parallelität findet sich nicht gleichmäßig in allen Gehirnstrukturen, denn wie Sokoloff 1963 nachwies, sinkt unter Barbituratnarkose die Durchblutung und der Sauerstoffverbrauch in der grauen Substanz stärker ab als in der weißen Substanz, so daß die normalerweise unterschiedliche Durchblutung einzelner Gehirnbezirke nivelliert und im Ganzen auf ein tieferes Niveau gesenkt wird. Andere Injektionsnarkotika, wie Urethan oder Morphin bewirken, bei Konstanz des Säure-Basen-Haushalts, ebenfalls Verminderungen der Gehirndurchblutung. Gasförmige Narkotika hingegen wirken anders. So werden nach Äthergaben häufig Anstiege oder keine Änderungen der Hirndurchblutung berichtet (Literatur s. Betz, 1972a, b). Zyklopropan oder Stickoxydul haben diesbezüglich nur geringe Wirksamkeit, wohingegen deutliche Dilatationen der Gehirngefäße, bei Halothan-Narkose auftreten (Literatur s. Betz, 1972b).

Eine proportionale Verminderung von Sauerstoffverbrauch und Hirndurchblutung ist demnach kein charakteristisches Kennzeichen aller narkotischer Substanzen. Halothan z.B. oder Chloroform bewirken zwar eine Verminderung der Sauerstoffaufnahme, aber eine deutliche Steigerung der Gehirndurchblutung. Bei Anwendung narkotisch wirksamer Substanz muß außerdem bedacht werden, daß in den verschiedenen Stadien der Narkose die Durchblutung sehr unterschiedlich sein kann. So fand sich bei Gaben verschiedener Inhalationsnarkotika nicht selten in der Excitationsphase eine Steigerung der Durchblutung, in der späteren narkotischen Phase ein Rückgang auf den Ausgangswert oder eine weitere Verminderung, wenn mit fortlaufend registrierenden Methoden gemessen wurde (Betz et al., 1965; Hadji-Dimos et al., 1969; Birzis u. Tachibana, 1964).

Es ist aus dem Gesagten klar, daß eine Übertragung der Ergebnisse von durchblutungsändernden Reizen bei narkotischen Tieren auf den Wachzustand, d.h. den physiologischen Zustand, nicht ohne weiteres möglich ist.

H. Die Hämodynamik der Gehirndurchblutung

I. Die Bedeutung von Blutdruck und Gefäßwiderstand

Im Prinzip kann jede Veränderung der Gehirndurchblutung auf drei hämodynamisch wirksame Komponenten zurückgeführt werden: Den effektiven Blutdruck, den Gefäßwiderstand und die Fließeigenschaften des Blutes. Alle wirksamen durchblutungsändernden Reize bewirken schließlich eine Veränderung der Beziehung von effektivem Blutdruck (d.h. dem Druckgefälle zwischen dem arteriellen Einstrom und venösen Ausstrom der Gehirngefäße) und dem zerebralen Gefäßwiderstand. Die Abb. 14 zeigt in einer schematischen Übersicht eine Reihe von Faktoren, die bei dieser Gesetzmäßigkeit die Gehirndurchblutung beeinflussen können. In Abweichung von vielen anderen Organen ist das Gehirn insofern in einer besonderen Situation, als es sich in einer geschlossenen Kapsel befindet. Der Druck, der in dieser Kapsel herrscht, wirkt sich auf den Perfusionsdruck des Gesamtgehirns zusätzlich aus. Vor allem der venöse Druck wird durch den intrakraniellen Druck verändert. Eine Steigerung des intrakraniellen Drucks muß bei gleichbleibendem arteriellen Druck zu einer Verminderung des wirksamen Perfusionsdrucks führen. Dies ist in einem späteren Kapitel noch eingehender dargestellt.

Der zerebrale Gefäßwiderstand selbst wird durch den arteriellen Einstromdruck variiert. Der Gefäßwiderstand steigt an, wenn der arterielle Druck ansteigt und fällt ab, wenn der arterielle Druck vermindert wird. Als Ergebnis dieses Mechanismus bleibt die Durchblutung relativ kon-

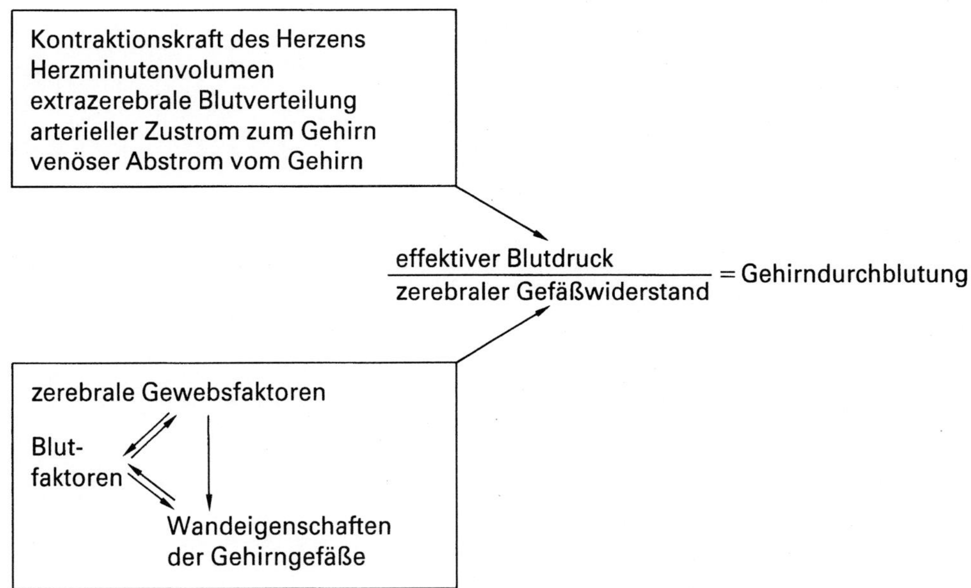

Abb. 14. Schematische Darstellung von Faktoren, die über den effektiven Blutdruck und den Gehirngefäßwiderstand die Durchblutungshöhe des Gehirns bestimmen

stant. Die dieser Konstanz zugrundeliegenden Phänomene werden als Autoregulation der Durchblutung zusammengefaßt. Die autoregulatorischen Mechanismen werden unwirksam, sobald der mittlere arterielle Blutdruck unter einen Wert von etwa 80 mm Hg absinkt, denn jetzt vermag das Gehirngefäßsystem sich nicht weiter auszudehnen. Das Wirksamwerden autoregulatorischer Mechanismen der Gehirndurchblutung hängt von zahlreichen Komponenten ab. Wird der arterielle Blutdruck schlagartig vermindert, so resultiert sofort ein Abfall, auch der Gehirndurchblutung. Der verminderte Durchstrom bleibt jedoch nicht auf einem erniedrigten Niveau sondern es kommt wegen der, nach einer zeitlichen Latenz wirksam werdenden, autoregulatorischen Gehirngefäßdilatation, zu einem Wiederanstieg der Durchblutung. Fog (1937, 1938, 1939) stellte fest, daß die Piagefäße dilatieren, wenn der arterielle Druck momentan vermindert wurde. Diese Dilatation erreichte etwa 1–2 min nach dem Abfall des arteriellen Blutdrucks ihr Maximum. Bei fortlaufender Registrierung der lokalen Gehirndurchblutung (Betz u. Schmahl, 1966; Betz, 1969a; Kanzow, 1969; Capon, 1969) sowie bei intermittierender Messung (Rapela u. Green, 1964; Ekström-Jodal, 1970) wurden Zeitkonstanten der autoregulatorischen Durchblutungsantwort gemessen, die zwischen 30 s und 2 min betrugen. Hirsch und Körner (1964) fanden etwas längere Zeiten. Sie entsprechen etwa dem Wiederanstieg der zerebral-venösen Sauerstoffsättigung nach derartig schnellen Blutdruckabfällen. Diese Reaktionen zeigten, daß die Regulation der Gehirndurchblutung bei arteriellen Blutdruckänderungen nicht dem Poiseuilleschen Gesetz, das von Hagen näher untersucht wurde, gehorcht, sondern dadurch modifiziert ist, daß jede Druckerhöhung nicht nur das Blut vorantreibt, sondern auch als dehnende Kraft auf die Gefäßwand wirkt (Wezler u. Sinn, 1953). Die Reaktion der Gehirngefäße ist – wie in anderen Organen – jedoch nicht allein eine Funktion der bei Druckänderungen auftretenden myogenen Reaktionen, sondern auch der elastischen Verhältnisse der Gefäßwände. Die Antwort auf Dehnungsreize, wie sie Druckänderungen darstellen, wird daher bei verschieden elastischen Gefäßen unterschiedlich sein.

Die zerebrale Autoregulation wird in der Regel als Diagramm dargestellt, in dem der arterielle Blutdruck und die Gehirndurchblutung einander zugeordnet sind (Abb. 15). Von Lassen (1959) ist die Bedeutung dieser Kurven für die zahlreichen Gefäßerkrankungen des Menschen ausführlich diskutiert worden. Beim normalen Menschen oder beim normalen Tier wird eine relativ konstante Durchblutung zwischen arteriellen Mitteldruckwerten von 70–80 mm Hg und einer oberen Grenze

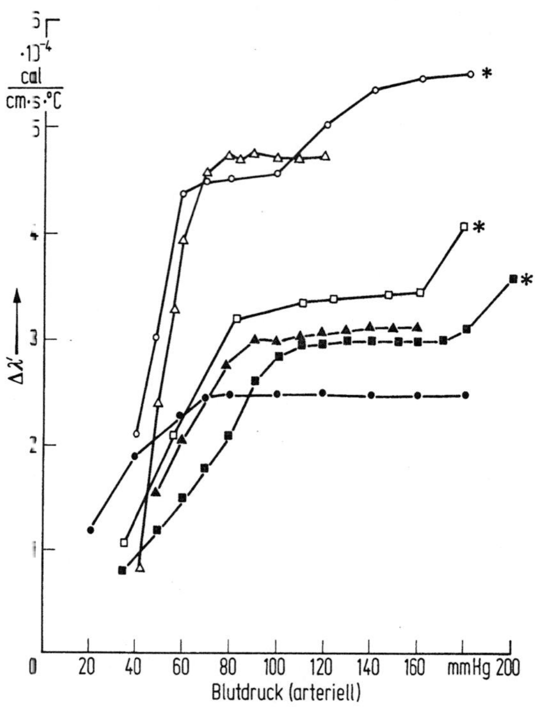

Abb. 15. Gleichzeitige Registrierung von mittlerem arteriellem Blutdruck und lokaler Gehirndurchblutung in unterschiedlichen Gehirnregionen bei Blutdruckänderung. Die Durchblutungsmessungen sind mit implantierten Wärmeleitsonden vorgenommen worden. Als Meßwert wurde jeweils die Änderung der Wärmetransportzahl $\lambda'[10^{-4}\,\mathrm{cal\cdot cm^{-1}\cdot s^{-1}\cdot {}^{\circ}C^{-1}}]$ verwendet. (Implantationsstellen: Großhirnrinde, Thalamus, Hypothalamus, Basalganglien bei Katzen.) Bei den mit einem Stern (*) bezeichneten Versuchen konnten starke Blutdrucksteigerungen kurzfristig ermöglicht werden. Die Durchblutung stieg kurzzeitig über die obere autoregulatorische Grenze an. (Nach BETZ in: Handbuch exp. Pharmakol. XVI, Teil 3, 1975)

von 150–170 mm Hg gesehen. Ein Abfall unter 70 mm Hg verursacht gewöhnlich eine druckpassive Verminderung, schnelle Anstiege über den kritischen oberen Wert nicht selten einen Anstieg der Durchblutung. Dieser obere, kritische Wert ist nicht konstant, sondern hängt von lokalen metabolischen Bedingungen und von den Gefäßwandeigenschaften selbst ab. Bei Individuen mit langandauernden Erhöhungen des arteriellen Blutdrucks wird auch die untere Schwelle der Autoregulation erhöht. Es kann daher bei solchen Patienten schon zu Blutversorgungsstörungen kommen, wenn der erhöhte Blutdruck rasch auf Werte unter 120 mm Hg (Mitteldruck) gesenkt wird.

II. Die Autoregulation und ihre Störungen

1. Mechanismen

Sowohl im Tierexperiment als auch bei Patienten kommt es vor, daß die Autoregulation vollständig aufgehoben wird. Das ist z.B. der Fall während und kurz nach schwerer Hypoxie. Auch bei starker Azidose zeigt sich dies Verhalten (Abb. 16) (RAPELA u. GREEN, 1964; INGVAR, 1967, 1968, 1969; FREEMAN u. INGVAR, 1968a, b; HÄGGENDAL, 1968; LASSEN u. PAULSON, 1969). Bei Hunden fanden RAPELA u. GREEN (1964) auch nach einem schweren Operationstrauma eine blutdruckpassive Reaktion der Gehirndurchblutung. Der Verlust der Autoregulation nach zerebralem Trauma wurde auch von REIVICH et al. (1969c) gesehen. Starke, nervöse Reize können die Schwelle der Autoregulation verschieben. Die Abb. 15 zeigt typische Beispiele von Druck/Flußbeziehungen bei einer Anzahl von Katzen in verschiedenen Gehirnregionen, wobei bei drei Tieren, deren Säure-Basenstatus normal war und die im Normbereich mit einer Autoregulation reagierten,

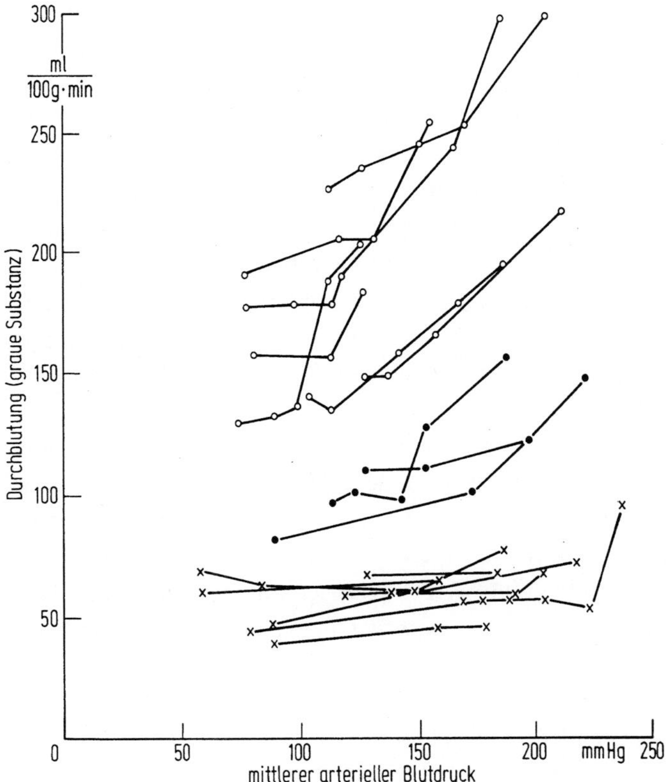

Abb. 16. Beziehungen zwischen mittlerem arteriellem Blutdruck und Durchblutung der grauen Substanz (in ml/100 g·min). Die untere Kurvenschar ×–×–× ist bei unbeeinflußten Individuen (mit normalem pCO_2), die mittlere Kurve ●–●–● bei leicht erhöhtem CO_2, die obere Kurvenschar o–o–o bei Tieren unter CO_2-bedingter Azidose gewonnen worden (Autoregulation aufgehoben). Es ist erkennbar, daß die obere autoregulatorische Grenze bei höheren CO_2-Drucken in Richtung zu niedrigeren Blutdruckwerten verschoben ist. (Nach Ekström-Jodal et al., 1971/72)

bei starker, schneller Steigerung des arteriellen Blutdrucks die autoregulatorische Grenze durchbrochen wurde. Die Hypothesen, die zur Erklärung des Phänomens der Autoregulation herangezogen werden und die in einem späteren Kapitel noch einmal diskutiert werden, sind folgende:

1. Die myogene Hypothese, welche besagt, daß trotz Ausschaltung nervöser Verbindungen der Tonus der zerebralen Gefäßarterien bei ansteigendem Blutdruck größer wird.
2. Die metabolische Hypothese. Sie besagt, daß bei einem kurzdauernden initialen druckpassiven Anstieg der Durchblutung eine gefäßdilatierende Effektorsubstanz ausgewaschen wird, so daß eine konstriktorische Komponente übrig bleibt. Hierbei wird angenommen, daß Metabolite, die normalerweise als Dilatatoren wirken, durch die initiale Durchblutungssteigerung verschwinden. Verminderungen des Druckes bewirken andererseits, daß sich dilatatorisch wirksame Stoffe anhäufen.
3. Die Gewebsdruckhypothese. Entsprechend dieser Hypothese steigt der perivaskuläre Druck an, wenn die Durchblutung ansteigt. Daraus resultiert, daß in Organen mit einer festen Kapsel, wie der Schädelkapsel, der Gefäßwiderstand ansteigen muß.

Die Autoregulation durch myogene Mechanismen wird folgendermaßen erklärt: Anstiege des intravaskulären Drucks dehnen die Gefäßmuskelzellen der zerebralen Arterien aus. Einige dieser Zellen depolarisieren und leiten den Reiz entlang der übrigen Muskelzellen des Gefäßes. Solche Schrittmacherzellen bewirken Änderungen im Membranpotential der benachbarten Muskelzellen und erregen diese. Die Erregung breitet sich sowohl in distaler als auch in proximaler Richtung entlang der Gefäßwand aus. Nach Held et al. (1969) spielt dabei die pulsatorische Dehnung der Gefäßwand eine wichtige Rolle. Während pulsatorischer Perfusion ist nämlich die Autoregulation deutlicher ausgeprägt als bei nicht pulsierender Strömung, wenn der Blutdruck dem Mitteldruck bei kontinuierlicher Pulsation entspricht. In welcher Weise der mechanische Reiz das Membranpotential der zerebralen Gefäßmuskelzellen ändert, ist noch unklar. Daß dabei Ionen eine wesentliche Rolle spielen wird in Kap. K näher erörtert. Die myogene Theorie, die erstmals durch BAYLISS (1902) aufgestellt wurde, hat durch die Untersuchung von FOLKOW (1949) eine starke Stütze erhalten. Dieser zeigte, daß sich nach weitgehender Ausschaltung des Einflusses neuraler Faktoren das Gefäßkaliber in entgegengerichteter Weise zum intravasalen Druck verändert. Ähnliches zeigten auch GASKELL und BURTON (1953), sowie JOHANSSON u. BOHR (1966). Nach diesen Befunden würde bei intaktem Gefäßsystem eine Gefäßkonstriktion infolge von Blutdruckanstieg eine weitere Erhöhung des Gefäßwiderstandes verursachen, was wiederum einen Blutdruckanstieg bewirkt, so daß eine Art von positivem Rückkopplungsmechanismus entsteht. FOLKOW (1964) versuchte das darin liegende Problem durch die Konzeption einer pulsierenden Spannungsänderung der Gefäßwand zu lösen.

Rhythmische Kontraktionen der Gefäßmuskulatur treten auch spontan auf. Diese haben gewisse Ähnlichkeiten mit den phasischen Änderungen glatter Muskulatur im intestinalen Bereich (BÜLBRING, 1962). SIEGEL et al. (1972) fanden in ihren Untersuchungen von Natrium- und Natrium$^{24}_{11}$-und Kalium$^{42}_{19}$-bewegungen durch die Membranen von glatten Muskelzellen isolierter Carotisarterien, daß die Natrium- und Kaliumverschiebungen rhythmisch auftreten. Sie schlossen daraus, daß langsame Schwankungen der Ionenbewegungen durch rhythmische Tätigkeit von aktiven Ionenpumpen an den Zellmembranen geschehen. Die Frequenz dieser Schwankungen war etwa ähnlich groß wie die bei spontan auftretenden zerebralen Durchblutungsoszillationen (BETZ, 1967). WEISS und THIEMANN (1973) zeigten in einem Modell, daß nach einer schrittweisen Erhöhung des Gefäßinnendrucks aufgrund von Synchronisationsphänomenen Oszillationen der Gefäßdurchmesser auftreten können und haben damit das myogene Verhalten von Gefäßen bei der Autoregulation erklärt. Die myogene Theorie der Durchblutungsregulation erklärt jedoch die autoregulatorischen Einstellungen des Gehirngefäßsystems nicht vollständig. RAPELA und GREEN (1964) zeigten, daß diese Hypothese nur einen von mehreren Mechanismen betrifft. In der Regel muß eine beträchtliche Änderung des transmuralen Drucks auftreten, um eine myogene Antwort der Gehirngefäße auszulösen. Bei den Untersuchungen zur metabolischen Theorie, auf die noch einzugehen sein wird, ergaben Messungen des lokalen Gewebs-pH oder des CO_2-Drucks im Gewebe eine hohe Geschwindigkeit von Konzentrationsänderungen derjenigen Metaboliten, die die Gefäßmuskelkontraktion beeinflussen können. Während eines plötzlichen Anstiegs des Blutdrucks wird die Durchblutung für eine kurze Zeit passiv erhöht. Da der CO_2-Druck im arteriellen Blut niedriger ist als im Gewebe, wird Kohlendioxyd aus den Gefäßwänden ausgewaschen, und es entsteht dort eine Alkalose. Diese Verschiebung des Gefäßwand-pH, die durch Perfusion mit Blut eines erniedrigten CO_2-Drucks bewirkt werden kann, ist ein konstriktorischer Reiz, ähnlich dem einer durch Hypokapnie verursachten Änderung. Da der Organismus dazu tendiert, das perivaskuläre pH relativ konstant zu halten, kann durch Reduktion der Durchblutung infolge einer Vasokonstriktion die Konstanz der Wasserstoffionenkonzentration, nach initialer blutdruckbedingter Durchblutungserhöhung, wieder hergestellt werden. Es erscheint daher plausibel, auch diesen Mechanismus als Komponente der zerebralen Autoregulation zu betrachten (Literatur s. PURVES, 1972; BETZ, 1969b, 1972b, c; INGVAR et al., 1968).

Änderungen der Autoregulation lassen sich auch zeigen, wenn Tiere wiederholt hohen CO_2-Konzentrationen der Atemluft ausgesetzt werden, die eine deutliche Gefäßdilatation und einen Anstieg des Flüssigkeitsgehalts im Gehirngewebe bewirken. Nach Beendigung einer CO_2-Inhalationsperiode von 10–15 min jeweils 6–8% CO_2 sank in der Regel die lokale Gehirndurchblutung unter den Ausgangswert. Dieser Effekt kann nicht durch einen sekundären Anstieg des Liquor-pH oder eine sekundäre Verminderung des CO_2-Drucks erklärt werden, da pCO_2 nur auf den Ausgangswert zurückgeführt wurde. In einigen Fällen bewirken solche wiederholten Steigerungen des CO_2 ein Gehirnödem (BETZ u. KOZAK, 1967) mit einer begleitenden Verminderung der Gehirndurchblutung bei gleichbleibendem Blutdruck.

2. Schwellenphänomene

Das Unterschreiten der unteren Schwelle der Autoregulation kann eine große Anzahl von Ursachen haben, die z.T. gar nicht in den Eigenschaften des Gehirngefäßsystems selbst begründet sind. Störungen der Kontraktilität des Herzens, starke Verminderung des Herzminutenvolumens, Störungen der extrazerebralen Blutverteilung, Verminderung des arteriellen Blutzustroms zum Gehirn oder des venösen Abstroms vom Gehirn, kann den wirksamen Blutdruck unter die kritische Schwelle absinken lassen und Minderdurchblutungen des Gehirns verursachen. Überschreitungen der oberen Schwelle der Autoregulation sind in der letzten Zeit häufiger beschrieben worden (Ekström-Jodal et al., 1971/1972, 1975). Sie fanden sich besonders dann, wenn bereits starke Blutdruckerhöhungen bestanden und zusätzlich plötzliche weitere Druckanstiege nicht verhindert werden konnten. Die Autoren beschrieben, daß nach Rückgang der Druckspitzen die Durchblutung unter den Ausgangswert abfiel und durch die resultierenden Störungen der Blut-Hirn-Schranke ein lokales Hirnödem auftrat.

3. Herzminutenvolumen und Autoregulation

Bei normalen Menschen bleibt bei Steigerung des Herzminutenvolumens z.B. durch körperliche Arbeit, die Autoregulation erhalten (Hedlund et al., 1962). Die Gehirndurchblutung wird demnach relativ unabhängig vom Herzminutenvolumen konstant gehalten (Gottstein et al., 1960). Pichlmayr (1969) fand jedoch bei Patienten mit Herzblock oder mit implantierten elektrischen Schrittmachern eine deutliche Abhängigkeit der Hirndurchblutung vom Herzminutenvolumen. Ob die nach Implantation des elektrischen Schrittmachers auftretende Steigerung der Gehirndurchblutung allein auf die Erhöhung und Normalisierung des arteriellen Mitteldrucks zurückzuführen ist (Held et al., 1968), kann noch nicht sicher gesagt werden.

III. Die Blutstromverteilung im Gehirn

1. Der Gefäßwiderstand

Wie aus der schematischen Übersicht (Abb. 14) hervorgeht, wird die Durchblutung des Gehirns außer vom Blutdruck durch den zerebralen Gefäßwiderstand geregelt. Bei normalem Blutdruck beträgt der Gesamtströmungswiderstand des Gehirnkreislaufs bei normaler Viskosität und normaler Gehirndurchblutung zwischen 1,5 und 2,0 mm $Hg \cdot ml^{-1}$ (100 g·min) (Sokoloff et al., 1955; Gottstein, 1965). Bei der Gehirnstrombahn handelt es sich um ein Netz von Strömungswiderständen, bei denen Parallelschaltungen mit Hintereinanderschaltungen kombiniert sind. Die Anteile der in Serie geschalteten einzelnen Gefäßabschnitte am Gesamtströmungswiderstand sind außerordentlich unterschiedlich. Söderberg u. Weckmann (1959) untersuchten die Rolle von zerebralen und extrazerebralen Anteilen des Gefäßsystems bei der Regulation des zerebralen Gefäßwiderstands von Katzen. Sie fanden einen bemerkenswerten Einfluß des Widerstandes der großen Arterien auf den gesamten zerebralen Gefäßwiderstand. Bei Messungen von Blutdruckwerten entlang der extrazerebralen Arterien wurde ein Druckabfall bis zur Arteria basilaris auf 70–90% des aortalen Blutdrucks gemessen. Unter normalen Bedingungen werden beim Menschen die Anteile des Gefäßwiderstandes von der Aorta bis zum Circulus Willisi auf Werte bis zu 10% des Gesamtwiderstandes geschätzt (Woodhall et al., 1952; Symon, 1967). In der Klinik spielen wegen der zahlreichen Erkrankungen der großen, zuführenden Gefäße deren Widerstandsveränderungen eine nicht unbeträchtliche Rolle, wie bei der Störung der Blutverteilung beschrieben ist (S. 231). Kanzow u. Dieckhoff (1969), Kanzow et al. (1971) ermittelten bei der Katze nach dem Landisschen Gegendruckverfahren die intravasalen Drucke entlang der intrazerebralen Arterien und fanden, daß bei normalem Aortendruck der Druckabfall bis zur Arteria cerebri media in der Nähe des Circulus Willisi und seiner großen Zweige ungefähr 20% betrug. In den kleineren Ästen der Arteria cerebri media war der relative Druckabfall ebenfalls etwa 20% groß. Bei Arteriendurchmessern von 80–120 µm betrug er 30% und er erreichte Werte von etwa 40%, wenn bis zu Arteriolen von 30–40 µm ∅ gemessen wurde. Es wurde errechnet, daß bei etwa 100 mm Hg Aortendruck 42% des Gesamtwiderstandes durch arterielle Gefäße bis herab auf 30–40 µm ∅ verursacht wurden. Zu ähnlichen Schlußfolgerungen gelangten bei ihren Untersuchungen STROMBERG und FOX (1972). Bei höheren Aortendrucken war der Anteil der Arterien am Gesamtwiderstand größer.

2. Arterienverschlüsse und arterielle Kollateralen

Es ist ein den praktischen Ärzten wohlbekanntes Phänomen, daß der Verschluß eines einzelnen Gehirngefäßes bei Patienten außerordentlich variable Symptome hervorruft. In einer Anzahl von Fällen verursacht ein extrazerebraler Verschluß eines einzelnen Gehirngefäßes keine Störung. Dagegen sieht man in anderen Fällen schwerste Ausfälle von Funktionen oder Strukturen. Im Tierexperiment (Katzen) wird nach Verschluß einer einzelnen Arteria carotis nur selten eine bleibende Störung von Gehirnfunktionen beobachtet. Die an der Gehirnbasis ringförmig zusammengeschlossenen Arterien sind eine wichtige Ursache für die manchmal geringen Auswirkungen von Verschlüssen, die vor dem Circulus Willisi lokalisiert sind. Durchblutungsmessungen in verschiedenen Gehirnregionen haben seit vielen Jahren bestätigt, daß nicht nur dort ausgeprägte arterielle Kollateralfunktionen existieren, sondern auch in anderen Bereichen des Gehirnkreislaufs (SHENKIN et al., 1951; RICHTER, 1953; DENNY-BROWN u. MEYER, 1957; MEYER u. DENNY-BROWN, 1957; SYMON, 1960; FIELDS et al., 1965; BETZ, 1969a; SYMON u. ROSS-RUSSEL, 1971). Die Untersuchungen zeigen jedoch auch, daß eine erhebliche interindividuelle Variabilität solcher Anastomosen besteht. Nach Verschluß eines Gehirngefäßes sind im wesentlichen drei Faktoren für das Schicksal des Gehirngewebes determinierend:

1. Der effektive Blutdruck (CORDAY et al., 1956),
2. die Anzahl und die Weite der präformierten Kollateralen,
3. ein Zeitfaktor, der für die Entwicklung von entsprechend weiten Kollateralkanälen nach Gefäßverschluß oder Gefäßverengerung notwendig ist, um eine ausreichende Blutversorgung wieder in Gang zu bringen.

Es ist daher nicht verwunderlich, daß experimentell bei nacheinander durchgeführten Verschlüssen kleiner Gefäße des Gehirns, die präinformierten Kollateralen allmählich weiter werden und es zu einer relativ guten Versorgung auch letztlich bei Verschluß mehrerer Gefäße kommt. So hat BUNCE (1960) eine oder zwei Karotiden sowie eine oder beide Vertebralarterien bei Hunden ligiert und festgestellt, daß die Tiere länger als drei Monate überleben konnten. Das stimmte mit Untersuchungen überein, die 1936 EVANS und SAMAAN durchführten. Bei den Tieren, bei denen in einem größeren zeitlichen Abstand nur die Karotiden oder die Vertebralarterien unterbunden wurden, waren keine wesentlichen Abweichungen vom Normalverhalten erkennbar, während bei denjenigen, bei denen kurz nacheinander sowohl die Karotiden als auch die Vertebralarterien unterbunden waren, Störungen zahlreicher zerebraler Funktionen erkennbar wurden. Ähnliche Ergebnisse wurden auch von ANTHONY et al. (1963) mitgeteilt. SYMON und ROSS-RUSSELL (1971), die solche Experimente bei Affen durchführten, fanden, daß einige Monate nach Gefäßunterbindungen der initial deutlich abgefallene Blutdruck in der Arteria Ophthalmica wieder langsam in Richtung Ausgangswert anstieg. In der Regel sieht man bei akutem Verschluß initial einen starken Abfall der Durchblutung im versorgten Gewebsbezirk, jedoch beginnt schon kurze Zeit nach Bestehen einer Ligatur die Durchblutung wieder in Richtung Ausgangswert anzusteigen (BETZ u. SCHMAHL, 1966).

Neumann et al. (1970) haben bei Messungen des kortikalen Sauerstoffdrucks mit feinen Mehrdrahtplatinelektroden festgestellt, daß während und nach Verschluß einer Arteria cerebri media der Sauerstoffdruck im Versorgungsbereich dieser Arterie abfällt. Die Sauerstoffdruckminderungen waren jedoch nicht gleichmäßig verteilt, sondern zeigten innerhalb des insgesamt erniedrigten Sauerstoffdruckfeldes einzelne Punkte, bei denen der Sauerstoffdruck normal war, so daß angenommen werden kann, daß aus dem umgebenden Gewebe einzelne Kollateralgefäße mit relativ hoher Sauerstoffkonzentration in das insgesamt schlecht versorgte Gewebe hineinzogen. Diese Heterogenität der Ausfallserscheinungen zeigt sich auch bei lokalen Durchblutungsmessungen mit der Antipyrinmethode (Fieschi, 1966; Fieschi et al., 1968a, b). Ist die Verschlußzeit eines Gefäßes sehr kurz, dann tritt nach dessen Wiedereröffnung eine reaktive Hyperämie auf. Häufig sieht man in den hyperämischen Regionen, daß das abfließende venöse Blut einen relativ hohen Sauerstoffgehalt hat (Feindel, 1968; Feindel et al., 1966, 1967, 1968; Høedt-Rasmussen et al., 1967; Yamamoto et al., 1969; Blair u. Waltz, 1970). Bei langdauernden Gefäßverschlüssen werden häufig derartige hyperämische Regionen in der Umgebung der Bezirke mit stark erniedrigter Durchblutung beobachtet. Neben den verschlossenen und z.T. thrombosierten Gefäßen existieren auch sehr weite Gefäße, wobei von fokaler Vasoparalyse mit Luxusperfusion gesprochen wird (Paulson, 1968, 1971; Paulson et al., 1970; Lassen, 1966). Die örtlichen Störungen bestehen also in Veränderungen der Blutverteilung mit lokalen hyperämischen Herden neben lokalen ischämischen Herden und lokaler Vasoparalyse (Heppner, 1961). Die Autoregulation der Gefäße ist in diesen Regionen in der Regel aufgehoben oder gestört (Lassen u. Paulson, 1969; Rees et al., 1971; Symon et al., 1971; Fein, 1973; Sengupta et al., 1973). Messungen der regionalen Durchblutung beim Menschen und beim Tier zeigten also, daß im Prinzip ähnliche Verhältnisse vorliegen.

3. Mechanismen der Störungen der Verteilungsregulation

1961 beschrieben Reivich et al., daß bei Einengungen der Strombahnen der Karotis im Bereich des Abgangs von Truncus brachiocephalicus eine Umkehr der Flußrichtung des Blutes durch die Vertebralarterie erfolgen könne. Diese Flußumkehr trat dann auf, wenn mit dem Arm der betroffenen Seite stark gearbeitet wurde. Das Phänomen wurde als Subclavian Stealphänomen oder Subclavian Steal-Syndrom bezeichnet (Fischer, 1962). Es ist seitdem im Tierexperiment vielfach imitiert worden und zeigt, daß der Verschluß der versorgenden Arterie einer Region Auswirkungen auf eine benachbarte Gefäßregion haben kann. Im Prinzip sind ähnliche Veränderungen der Blutverteilung auch innerhalb des Gehirns bei Verschlüssen oder Verengerungen intrazerebraler Gefäße beobachtet worden. (Sie wurden bei gleichzeitigen Messungen in niedrig perfundierten Regionen und deren Umgebung gemessen.) Solche Dysregulationen der Blutstromverteilung sind von wesentlicher Bedeutung bei der Anwendung solcher gefäßaktiven Substanzen, die den zerebralen Gefäßwiderstand vermindern. 1966 wurde gezeigt (Betz u. Schmahl), daß während des Verschlusses einer Karotis die Injektion einer gefäßdilatierenden Substanz zu Verminderungen der Durchblutung im Bereich des bereits schlecht versorgten Bezirks führten, während die Durchblutung in allen übrigen Regionen des Gehirns anstieg. (Diese Reaktion war jedoch nur in einem Drittel der Experimente zu sehen.) Bei den übrigen Experimenten sah man z.T. Durchblutungsanstiege in beiden Bezirken des Gehirns oder man sah im minderversorgten Bereich keine Reaktion. Dieses Verhalten wurde schon 1961 und 1964 bei Verschluß eines Koronargefäßes im Myokard gesehen (Betz et al.) und später bei Patienten als lokales Steal-Phänomen bezeichnet (Lassen u. Palvölgyi, 1968; Symon, 1968, 1969; Paulson, 1968; Neumann et al., 1970; Barnett et al., 1970; Dyken, 1971/72). Die Ursache für das unterschiedliche Verhalten der Blutverteilung nach Applikation vasodilatierender Reize kann darin gesehen werden, daß in einzelnen Fällen das Gefäßsystem im Bereich der minderversorgten Zone noch in der Lage ist, sich zu erweitern, so daß bei nur geringem Abfall des effektiven Blutdrucks eine relativ stärkere Widerstandsverminderung durchblutungserhöhend wirken kann, während in anderen Fällen eine Widerstandsverminderung in der Umgebung der schlecht versorgten Zone nach den Krischoffschen Regeln der Stromverteilung sich so auswirkt, daß eine Verteilungsänderung zugunsten des normal durchbluteten Bereichs auftritt und die Durchblutung im schlecht versorgten Bereich noch weiter vermindert wird. Die erheblichen individuellen Variationen der Reaktionen der lokalen Durchblutung und des lokalen Sauerstoffdrucks entsprechen den Befunden, die während Angiographie beim Menschen beobachtet wurden (Literatur s. HERRMANN, 1964). Sie bewirken, daß die Indikation für die Anwendung von vasoaktiven Substanzen indivudell gestellt werden muß. Es hat den Anschein, daß bei Menschen mit Gefäßverschlüssen und gleichzeitiger Arteriosklerose die Verminderung der Durchblutung im schlecht versorgten Bezirk nach Anwendung von vasoaktiven Substanzen häufiger vorkommt als im Tierexperiment (FIESCHI, 1967; LASSEN u. PALVÖLGYI, 1968; SYMON, 1968; WÜLLENWEBER, 1968). Die Auswirkung der Durchblutungsverminderung auf die Gewebsenergetik ist ähnlich wie diejenige einer Hypoxie, so daß man bei der starken, individuellen Variabilität unterschiedlich starke lokale Verminderungen der energiereichen Substrate im Hirngewebe beobachten kann.

IV. Blutviskosität und Gehirndurchblutung

Untersucht man die Leitfähigkeit von starren Gefäßen für Blut, so ist das Verhältnis Blutkörperchen/Plasma (Hämatokrit) zu berücksichtigen. In einer starren Röhre ist der Plasmafluß Q_p

$$Q_p = G_p \cdot P$$

P ist der wirksame Blutdruck, G_p ist die Strömungsleitfähigkeit für Plasma und steht für den genaueren Ausdruck

$$\pi r^4 / 8\, \eta_p \cdot \eta_w \cdot l$$

(η_p ist die relative Viskosität des Plasmas, η_w ist die absolute Viskosität des Wassers, l ist die Länge der Röhre eines Radius r.)

Man kann die Durchblutung mit Gesamtblut (Q_b) in der Röhre, auch als $Q_b = (G_p/\eta^*) \cdot P$ schreiben, wobei η^* die Scheinviskosität des Blutes in Relation zum Plasma ist. Der Wert für die Scheinviskosität hängt nicht nur vom Hämatokritwert ab, sondern auch von der Scherung, dem Durchmesser der Röhre und anderen Faktoren.

Aus Untersuchungen von WELLS et al. (1961), mit einem Wells-Brookfield-Viskosimeter, geht hervor, daß eine etwa lineare Relation zwischen der Viskosität des gesamten Blutes und dem Hämatokrit über einen Bereich von 35–52% bei drei unterschiedlichen Scherraten besteht. Bei einem Hämatokritwert von 35% war – bei einer Scherrate von $11{,}5\ s^{-1}$ – der Wert 4,5 cP, bei einem Hämatokritwert von 52% betrug der Wert 9,0 cP. Diese Werte stimmen mit denen von HÄGGENDAL und NORBÄCK (1966a) überein. Über die Bedeutung des Hämatokritwertes für die Gehirndurchblutung hat schon KETY (1950) berichtet, der bei Patienten mit lange bestehender Polyzythämie und einem Hämatokritwert von über 65% eine Verminderung der Gehirndurchblutung fand (BURGER et al., 1967). HÄGGENDAL et al. (1966b) variierten den Hämatokritwert zwischen 30 und 60% durch Änderung oder Ersatz des Blutvolumens mit Plasma oder Dextranlösungen hohen oder niedrigen Molekulargewichts. Unterhalb eines Hkt von 30% stieg die Gehirndurchblutung an. Dieser Anstieg wurde auf eine verminderte Sauerstoffkapazität des Blutes zurückgeführt, denn die Durchblutung stieg auch trotz konstantem Hämatokritwert an, wenn eine entsprechend hohe arterielle Carboxy-Hämoglobin-Sättigung verwendet wurde. Eine ähnliche Beziehung wie zwischen dem arteriellen Hämatokrit und der Gehirndurchblutung wurde auch gefunden, wenn nicht der Hämatokritwert des arteriellen Blutes, sondern die Blutviskosität als Maßstab

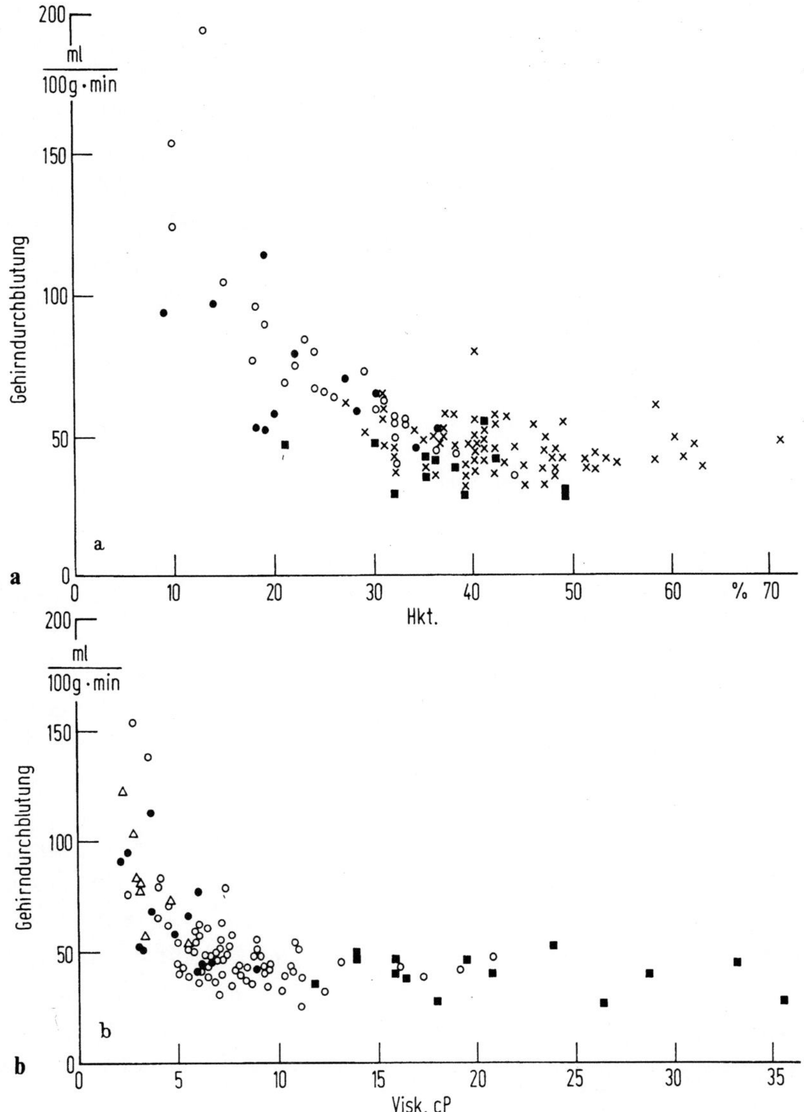

Abb. 17. a Beziehung zwischen Gehirndurchblutung und Hämatokrit. Kontrollen: ×, homologes Plasma: ○, niedermolekulares Dextran: ●, hochmolekulares Dextran: ■. **b** Abhängigkeit der Gehirndurchblutung von der Viskosität der Durchströmungsflüssigkeit, Kontrolle ■, homologes Plasma ○, Humanalbumin △, niedermolekulares Dextran ●, hochmolekulares Dextran □. In allen Versuchen war der arterielle Blutdruck höher als 100 mm Hg, die arterielle Sauerstoffsättigung höher als 85% und der arterielle CO_2-Druck 20–35 mm Hg. (Nach HÄGGENDAR NILSSON und NORBÄCK in: Pharmakologie der lokalen Gehirndurchblutung. Eds.: BETZ u. WÜLLENWEBER, Banaschewski, München 1969, S. 94)

verwendet wurde. Bei Scherraten von 23 s^{-1} war zu erkennen, daß die Änderung der Durchblutung in Abhängigkeit von der Viskosität etwa bei 5 cP auftrat. Die Abb. 17a u. b zeigen die Verhältnisse (HÄGGENDAL u. NORBÄCK, 1966a; HÄGGENDAL et al., 1969). HIRSH (1969a) weist darauf hin, daß bei Hypoxie und nach Ischämien häufig Thrombozytenaggregate auftreten, die zu Veränderungen der Scherraten und des Siebungsdrucks des Blutes führen und deshalb ähnliche Störungen bewirken wie andersartige starke Erhöhungen der Scheinviskosität.

Bezüglich der Probleme der pathologischen Physiologie ist daran zu denken, daß Störungen der Erythrozytenflexibilität die Viskosität ebenfalls stark ansteigen lassen (BRAASCH, 1963). Außer von den erwähnten Faktoren ist die Scheinviskosität des Blutes von der Gefäßweite abhängig. Entsprechend den Untersuchungen von FÅRAEUS und LINDQVIST (1931) sinkt die Scheinviskosität im Kapillarbereich ab und steigt erst dann wieder an, wenn die Kapillaren so eng sind, daß die Erythrozytendurchmesser etwa dem Kapillardurchmesser entsprechen. Bei Gefäßen von 20 µm Durchmesser beträgt die Scheinviskosität ungefähr $^2/_3$ derjenigen in Röhren von etwa 300 µm Durchmesser.

Wegen der speziellen Fließeigenschaften des Blutes ist die Strömungsgeschwindigkeit ein zusätzlicher Faktor zur Veränderung der Fließeigenschaften. In vivo ergibt sich aus der Kombination der Viskositätsänderungen, die durch Blutstromgeschwindigkeit und Gefäßweite bedingt sind, daß die Scheinviskosität von den Arterien bis zu den Kapillaren abfällt und dann wieder ansteigt. Diese Viskositätsänderungen werden bei Strömungsstudien in kleinen Gefäßen oft nur ungenügend berücksichtigt. Bei einer Dilatation kleiner Gehirngefäße steigt nämlich entsprechend dem Abfall des Perfusionsdrucks die Scheinviskosität des Blutes besonders dann, wenn außer der Gefäßerweiterung auch noch eine Verminderung der Strömungsgeschwindigkeit auftritt.

V. Die Rolle intrakranieller Druck- und Volumenänderungen bei der Durchblutungsregulation

In der Übersicht der Abb. 13 ist gezeigt, daß nicht nur diejenigen Kräfte zu Gefäßwiderstandsveränderungen führen, die sich in den Gefäßwänden selbst entwickeln, sondern daß auch von außen auf die Gefäße einwirkender Druck den Widerstand beeinflußt. Hierbei bewirken intrakranielle Volumenänderungen intrakranielle Druckänderungen. Volumenänderungen können durch das Blutvolumen, den Liquor cerebrospinalis, die extracelluläre Flüssigkeit oder die intrazelluläre Flüssigkeit verursacht sein.

Die Zerebrospinalflüssigkeit wird z.T. durch den chorioidalen Plexus gebildet, der in den lateralen Ventrikeln und dem dritten Ventrikel liegt. Zum Teil besteht er aus der interstitiellen Flüssigkeit des Gehirns. Der in den Ventrikeln gebildete Liquor Zerebrospinalis zirkuliert durch das ventrikuläre System, kann dann vom vierten Ventrikel aus in die Cisterna magna, die Cisterna pontis und die Cisterna basalis durch die Foramina Luschkae und Magendie gelangen. Von hier aus fließt er nach oben über die Konvexität des Gehirns oder nach unten in den Subarachnoidalraum des Rückenmarks. In jedem Fall erreicht er schließlich die Arachnoidalzotten, wo er in die venöse Zirkulation absorbiert wird. Diese Absorption wird dadurch erleichtert, daß im Liquor ein etwas höherer Druck herrscht als im venösen Blut. Der Plexus chorioideus besteht aus stark vaskularisiertem Gewebe, das durch die Pia und eine einzelne Lage ependymaler Zellen überzogen ist. (Diese Epithellage setzt sich kontinuierlich über den chorioidalen Plexus fort.) Die Arachnoidalzotten sind Vorsprünge der Arachnoidea in den venösen Sinus, haben die Form von Zapfen und sind von einer dünnen Membran bedeckt (Thomas, 1966). Da mechanische Druckkräfte weitgehend am Abtransport des Liquors beteiligt sind, tritt ein Liquortransport nicht mehr auf, wenn der Liquordruck unter ca. 70 mm H_2O fällt.

Bei Erhöhung des Liquordrucks über 70 mm H_2O ist die Größe der Reabsorption proportional zum Liquordruck (Bering, 1959; Betz et al., 1972).

Der Liquor unterscheidet sich vom Blutplasma u.a. dadurch, daß er nur eine sehr niedrige Proteinkonzentration hat. Die Konzentration von Chlorid ist höher als im Blut, diejenige von Glukose, Harnstoff, Kalium, Kalzium und Phosphat ist niedriger. Die Wasserstoffionenkonzentration bleibt weitgehend konstant, auch bei Änderungen im Blut. Das sind deutliche Hinweise dafür, daß der Liquor Zerebrospinalis nicht ein einfaches Ultrafiltrat des Bluts darstellen kann. Im Verlauf der Passage des Liquors durch die Liquorräume ändert sich seine Zusammensetzung, so daß der ventrikuläre Liquor eine andere Zusammensetzung hat als derjenige in den lumbalen Bereichen. Diese Differenzen setzen voraus, daß Mechanismen in den Wänden der Liquorräume existieren, die eine funktionelle Barriere für bestimmte Substanzen als „Blutliquorschranke" darstellen. Besonders stark machen sich die Durchlässigkeitsveränderungen für lipoidhaltige Lösungen und für ionisierte Stoffe bemerkbar. Die Stoffe erreichen den Liquor einmal durch Sekretion aus dem chorioidalen Plexus, zum zweiten durch die Kapillaren des Gehirns über die Blut-Hirnschranke. Substanzen aus dem Blut erreichen zunächst den Extrazellulärraum des Gehirns und haben dann die Möglichkeit, mit dem Liquor in einen Austausch zu treten. Eine Passagemöglichkeit von Stoffen besteht durch „Poren“ in Kapillarwänden, die allerdings nicht ubiquitär im Gehirn vorhanden sind und auch in bestimmten Bereichen nur zeitweise vorzukommen scheinen (Rapoport, 1973; Rapoport et al., 1972; Rapoport u. Thompson, 1973, 1974).

Die Menge Liquor, die pro Zeiteinheit gebildet werden kann, variiert stark. Beim Menschen rechnet man mit 0,3–0,8 ml/min. Es wird angenommen (Bering, 1965; Davson, 1960), daß etwa die Hälfte aus dem Extrazellulärraum, die andere Hälfte aus dem Plexus chorioideus stammt.

1. Der Liquordruck

Beim Menschen beträgt der Liquordruck zwischen 90–150 mm Wassersäule oder 7–11 mm Quecksilbersäule. Dieser Druck ist ein Wert, der als Resultante des Gleichgewichts von Liquorproduktion und Reabsorption besteht und wird in der Regel in liegender Position gemessen.

Beim Aufrichten in senkrechte Körperhaltung wirkt sich, vorwiegend im unteren Bereich des Liquorraums, die Schwerkraft aus. Die hydrostatisch bedingte Druckerhöhung entspricht jedoch nicht genau der Höhe der gesamten Flüssigkeitssäule in senkrechter Körperhaltung. Der Anteil der durch Gravitation bewirkten Druckerhöhungen beträgt vielmehr nur etwa 100–300 mm Wassersäule, die sich zum normalen Liquordruck hinzuaddiert. Die Ursache für diese nur geringen Druckerhöhungen wird von Davson (1960) dadurch erklärt, daß der Gesamtliquorraum ein geschlossenes Röhrensystem darstellt und daß dann, wenn man ein derartiges Röhrensystem aus horizontaler in vertikale Position bringt, die Flüssigkeit nicht aus dem Röhrensystem herauslaufen kann. Der Flüssigkeitsdruck am unteren Ende wäre bei einer starren Röhre nicht größer als der atmosphärische Druck. Daß ein Druckanstieg im Bereich des Lumbalraums trotzdem auftritt, wird dadurch erklärt, daß das Gesamtsystem, damit auch die obere Begrenzung des Liquorraums, etwas elastisch ist.

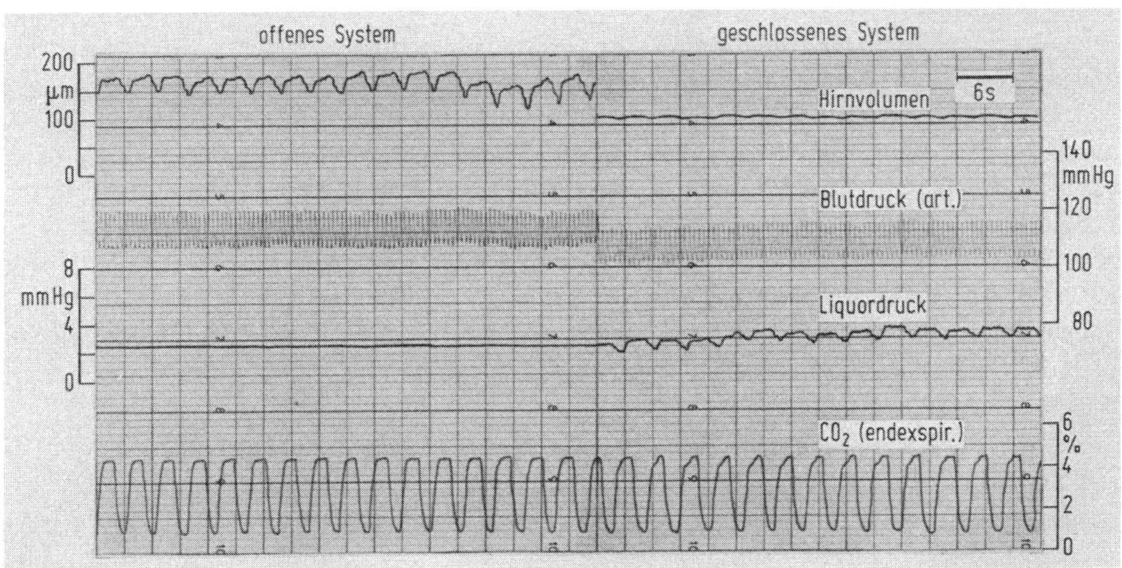

Abb. 18. Spontane Oszillationen von Gehirnvolumen und Liquordruck. Es sind pulssynchrone und atemsynchrone Änderungen erkennbar. Der erste Abschnitt zeigt deutliche atemsynchrone Schwankungen des Gehirnvolumens bei offenem Schädel, die bei Verschluß des Schädels kaum noch nachweisbar sind; dagegen treten bei geschlossenem Schädelraum deutliche Oszillationen des Liquordrucks auf, welche bei geöffnetem Schädelraum nicht vorhanden sein können

Der Liquordruck ist nicht konstant, sondern zeigt, ähnlich wie die Gehirndurchblutung, spontane Variationen, die sich bei kontinuierlicher Messung als aus pulssynchronen und atemsynchronen Schwankungen zusammengesetzt darstellen. In der Abb. 18 ist eine gleichzeitige Registrierung des Liquordrucks und des Gehirnvolumens mit einem Wegeaufnehmer in einem geschlossenen System (zur Methode siehe Betz u. Roos, 1971) sowie einiger anderer für die Registrierung wichtiger Größen dargestellt. Bei der Analyse von Liquordruckmessungen findet man, daß während der Systole des Herzens der Druck in den Hirnventrikeln stärker ansteigt als im Lumbalbereich, während bei der Diastole entgegengerichtete Veränderungen erkennbar sind (Bering, 1965). Die respiratorisch bedingten Durchblutungs- und Druckänderungen verlaufen in der Regel streng parallel.

2. Hirnvolumen, Hirndurchblutung und Liquordruck

Mißt man gleichzeitig mit dem Liquordruck fortlaufend die relativen Änderungen des Gehirnvolumens mit einem Wegeaufnehmer, so sieht man, daß bei den puls- und atemsynchronen Oszillationen das Hirnvolumen parallel zu den Liquordruckänderungen verläuft (Betz u. Roos, 1971). Änderungen des Hirnvolumens können sowohl durch Erhöhung oder Erniedrigung des intravasalen Blutvolumens als auch durch Änderungen des Wassergehaltes in extra- und intrazellulären Räumen bedingt sein. Bei raschen Änderungen des intrakraniellen Blutvolumens tritt eine deutliche Korrelation zwischen dem Liquordruck und dem Blutvolumen auf, auch wenn der arterielle Blutdruck sich nicht wesentlich verändert (Risberg et al., 1969b; Nylin et al., 1956, 1960, 1961a u. b). Diese Korrelation besteht auch zwischen dem lokalen Blutvolumen und der lokalen Durchblutung der gleichen Gehirnregion (Risberg et al., 1969a). Daraus könnte man den Schluß ziehen, daß es auch eine enge Korrelation zwischen zerebralem Blutvolumen, Hirndurchblutung und Liquordruck, gibt. Diese Schlußfolgerung wurde zwar häufig bei schnellen Änderungen der Gehirndurchblutung bestätigt gefunden, wenn die Flußänderungen nur mäßig groß waren, jedoch bei Infusionen von Azetylcholin in die Arteria carotis (Baust et al., 1963) oder nach intravenöser Gabe von Papaverin (Betz u. Roos, 1971) sind die resultierenden Änderungen von Gehirndurchblutung, Gehirnvolumen und Liquordruck oft nicht parallel (Abb. 19). Allerdings ist eine Dissoziation von Gehirnvolumen und Liquordruckänderung nur bei hohen Dosen dieser Pharmaka zu erreichen. Bei relativ niedrigen Dosen verläuft die Gehirndurchblutung entsprechend den Liquordruckänderungen (Goldenson et al., 1951; Ryder et al., 1952a, b; Rich et al., 1953). Bei Messungen von Gesamthirndurchblutung und intrakraniellem Druck fanden Kety et al. (1948a), daß bei langsamen Steigerungen des Liquordrucks bis auf 33 mm Hg keine Änderung der Gehirndurchblutung erfolgte. Verminderungen der Gehirndurchblutung bei ansteigendem Liquordruck wurden von anderen Autoren (Noell u. Schneider, 1942c; Zwetnow et al., 1968; Fitch et al., 1969; Zwetnow, 1970; Miller et al., 1971/72; Lewis u. McLaureen, 1972; Nagai et al., 1972a, b), berichtet. Aus den Messungen geht hervor, daß die Reaktion der Gehirndurchblutung außer von der kritischen, absoluten Höhe des Liquordrucks noch von der Geschwindigkeit der Druckänderungen abhängt. Bei sehr schnellen Steigerungen des Liquordrucks fällt die Gehirndurchblutung steil ab, steigt dann aber wieder an.

Für die Größe der Gehirndurchblutung ist der effektive Perfusionsdruck entscheidend. Die Durchblutung blieb in einigen Fällen erhalten, wenn der wirksame Perfusionsdruck durch Erhöhung des intrakraniellen Drucks auf 35–40 mm Hg gesenkt wurde (Jennett et al., 1971). Sogar bei Perfusionsdrucken von weniger als 10 mm Hg wurde noch ein geringer Durchstrom durch das Gehirn registriert. Rowan et al. (1972) und Johnston et al. (1972) geben an, daß der kritische Druckwert bei einem intrakraniellen Druck von etwa 50 mm Hg liegt. Diesen Wert fanden sie bei Infusionen von künstlichem Liquor in die Cisterna magna. Bei Experimenten an Affen, bei denen der Druck in einem supratentorial, subdural eingelegten Ballon erhöht wurde, fand man noch normale Gehirndurchblutungswerte, wenn der intrakranielle Druck etwa 60 mm Hg

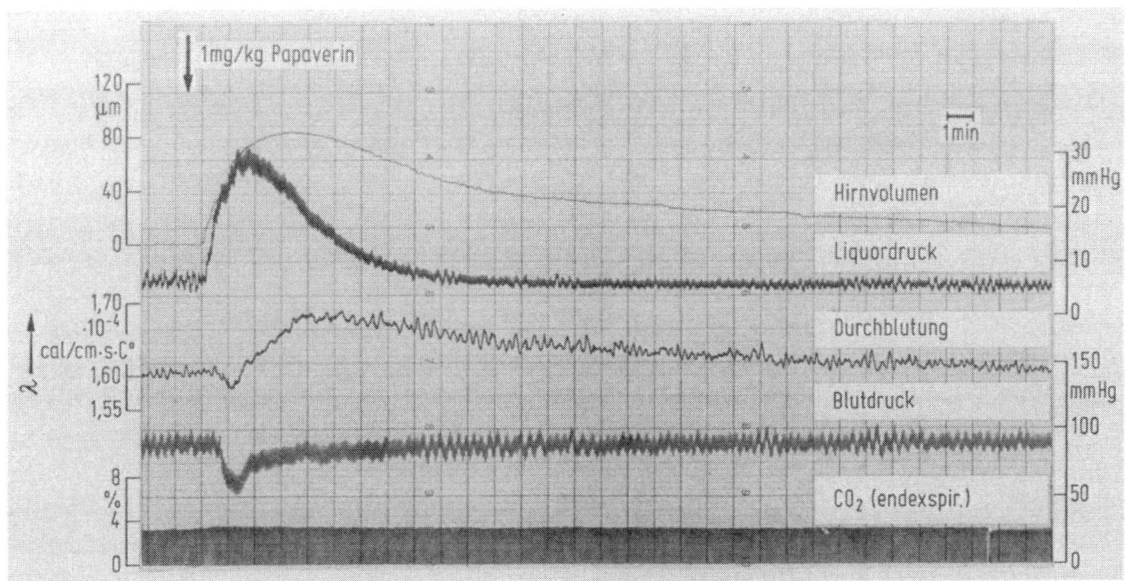

Abb. 19. Die Wirkung einer intravenösen Injektion von Papaverin auf Gehirnvolumen (gemessen als relative Änderung mit einem induktiven Wegeaufnehmer), kortikale Durchblutung (gemessen mit einem Oberflächen-Wärmeleitmesser), mittleren arteriellen Blutdruck (gemessen mit einem Statham-Element) und auf die CO_2-Konzentration in der Ausatemluft, gemessen mit einem Ultrarotabsorber. (Nach BETZ und ROOS in: Brain and Blood Flow. Eds.: ROSS-RUSSEL, PITMAN, Med. and Sci., Publ. Co Ltd. London, 1971, p. 294)

betrug. Allerdings wurden bei diesen Ballonexperimenten sehr starke Änderungen des arteriellen Blutdrucks erzeugt. Diese experimentellen Befunde haben ihre klinische Analogie bei intrakraniellen Hämatomen nach Schädeltraumen, bei denen die Gehirndurchblutung vermindert wird, weil der Druck im Liquorraum über einen kritischen Schwellenwert ansteigt. HEKMATPANAH (1970, 1972) zeigte, daß bei ansteigendem intrakraniellen Druck die Störung der Zirkulation zunächst in Kapillaren und später in größeren Gefäßen auftrat. Nach Normalisierung des intrakraniellen Drucks wurde die Durchblutung nicht in allen Bereichen des Gehirngefäßsystems wieder normal hoch. Das wird als Hinweis darauf gedeutet, daß kapilläre Verschlüsse bestehen bleiben. Wegen dieses Ausmaßes der Abhängigkeit einer zerebralen Zirkulationsstörung vom intrakraniellen Druck, wurde dieser als prognostisches Maß für Patienten mit Schädelhirntraumen verwandt. Von 17 Patienten mit intraventrikulären Drucken über 60 mm Hg starben 14. Bei Patienten, deren intrakranieller Druck unter 30 mm Hg betrug, überlebten die meisten jedoch (KUURNE et al., 1972). Die Wirkung diffuser intrakranieller Hypertension auf die Gehirndurchblutung ist nicht nur von der absoluten Höhe des intrakraniellen Drucks, sondern auch von der Geschwindigkeit seiner Entwicklung abhängig (HEMMER, 1960; LANGFITT et al., 1965a). Bei schnellem Füllen eines intrakraniellen Ballons fällt die Gehirndurchblutung sofort ab. Hingegen ist, bei langsamer Steigerung des intrakraniellen Drucks, die Reduktion der Durchblutung zunächst minimal, wenn er nicht mehr als 35–40 mm Hg erreicht. Diese geringen Änderungen der Hirndurchblutung stehen im Einklang mit Befunden bei Patienten mit Hirntumoren, bei denen trotz hohen Liquordrucks die Gehirndurchblutung im vom Tumor entfernt gelegenen Gehirngewebe noch normal bleibt.

CUSHING (1901, 1902) hatte schon Anstiege des arteriellen Blutdrucks während erhöhtem intrakraniellem Druck beobachtet. Das Ausmaß der Blutdruckerhöhung betrug allerdings meist nur wenige mm Hg (GÄNSHIRT, 1957; LANGFITT et al., 1965a; SCHWARTZ u. ZAREA, 1969). Um Anstiege des Blutdrucks zu erreichen, müssen die Liquordrucke meist stark erhöht werden.

Die Blutdrucksteigerung ist nicht die einzige Reaktion, mit deren Hilfe der Organismus bei Erhöhung des Liquordrucks die Hirndurchblutung konstant zu halten trachtet. Während Liquordrucksteigerung kommt es zu einer Erschlaffung der Gehirngefäße, im Sinne einer Autoregulation. Nach KJÄLLQUIST et al. (1969) scheinen starke Ähnlichkeiten der autoregulatorischen Mechanismen bei Liquordrucksteigerungen mit denen bei andersartig bedingten Perfusionsdruckerniedrigungen zu bestehen. Bei Erhöhung des intrakraniellen Drucks treten Anstiege des Laktatgehaltes im Liquor Zerebrospinalis auf. Die Laktat-Pyruvat-Relation wird erhöht und die Bikarbonatkonzentration fällt ab. Dies weist auf das Auftreten einer Laktazidose im Gehirngewebe hin (ZWETNOW et al., 1968; ZWETNOW, 1970; NAGAI et al., 1972a). Sie wurde nicht nur im Tierexperiment sondern auch bei Patienten mit erhöhtem intrakraniellen Druck gefunden (ZUPPING, 1972). Bei direkter Beobachtung der Piagefäße durch Schädeldachfenster konnte eine Erweiterung gesehen werden, wenn der Liquordruck gesteigert wurde (WOLFF u. FORBES, 1928), was ebenfalls für das Auftreten einer autoregulatorischen Reaktion spricht. Nach langzeitiger intrakranieller Hypertension tritt eine Vasomotorenlähmung der Gehirngefäße auf (LANGFITT et al., 1965b).

Bei Wiedernormalisierung des intrakraniellen Drucks bleiben zunächst die Gefäße weit und die Durchblutung wird hoch. Dies wird häufig als Luxusperfusionsphase beschrieben (MEYER et al., 1969a; HALSEY u. CAPRA, 1971/72). Die Luxusperfusion kann auch dann gesehen werden, wenn das Liquor-pH in der Postdekompressionsphase wieder normalisiert ist. Die Gefäßerweiterung kann demnach nicht als allein durch pH-Erniedrigung ausgelöst erklärt werden. Wenn bei gestörter Autoregulation oder Vasoparalyse der arterielle Blutdruck erhöht wird, kommt es zu einem Anstieg des Wassergehaltes im Gehirngewebe (MEINIG et al., 1971/72, 1972). Die Ausbildung des entstehenden Hirnödems ist zeitabhängig. Je länger die arterielle Hypertension dauert und je höher sie ist, um so stärker steigt der Wassergehalt im Gewebe an (LANGFITT et al., 1971).

3. Hirnödem

Wenn, wie beschrieben, ein Hirnödem auftritt, fällt die lokale Perfusion innerhalb des Ödems ab. Die regionale Gehirndurchblutung ist dann streng mit dem Wassergehalt korreliert (MEINIG et al., 1971/72; BRUCE et al., 1972; MILLER et al., 1973). Mäßige Hypokapnie führt zu einer Erhöhung der lokalen Zirkulation durch das ödematöse Gewebe, dagegen kommt es bei starker Hypokapnie zu einem ungünstigen Effekt auf die Gehirndurchblutung in diesen Regionen (WALLENFANG et al., 1973). Für die Erhöhung des Gefäßwiderstandes im Ödembereich ist nicht unbedingte Voraussetzung, daß die Gefäße sich aktiv verengen. Die Widerstandserhöhung kann z.B. auch durch eine starke Erhöhung des Gewebedrucks verursacht werden. Bei einem bereits bestehenden Ödem kommt es bei CO_2-Atmung nicht zu der gewünschten Erhöhung der Gehirndurchblutung, sondern die Gehirndurchblutung steigt zwar initial geringfügig an, wird aber im Verlauf einer längeren CO_2-Atmung allmählich wieder reduziert. Bei Wiederbeatmung mit normaler Luft fällt sie unter den Ausgangswert ab (BETZ u. KOZAK, 1967).

GROTE et al. (1975) wiesen nach, daß die Gefäße in ödematösen Gehirnbezirken nicht mehr mit Erweiterung reagierten, wenn eine lokale perivaskuläre Azidose erzeugt wurde.

Hirnödeme und zu hoher Liquordruck werden oft mit hyperosmolaren Lösungen behandelt. Steigerung der Osmolarität des Bluts ist nicht nur wegen der daraus resultierenden Wassertransporte, aus dem Gewebe ins Blut, für die Zirkulation wichtig (zusammenfassende Übersicht s. BAKAY u. LEE, 1965; KLATZO u. SEITELBERGER, 1967; BETZ, 1972; BROCK u. DIETZ, 1972), die Steigerung des osmotischen Drucks hat auch eine dilatierende Wirkung auf die glatte Muskulatur der Gehirngefäße (RAPELA u. BUYNISKI, 1969; SCOTT et al., 1970). Der Grad der Durchblutungssteigerung hängt nach WAHL et al. (1973) nicht davon ab, welche Stoffe zur Erhöhung der Osmolarität verwendet werden. Die Endothelien der kapillären Gefäße verlieren bei Erhöhung der Blut-Osmolarität reversibel ihre Schrankenfunktion, so daß auch große Moleküle aus dem Blut in den perivaskulären Raum übertreten können (RAPOPORT, 1972, 1973; PICKARD et al., 1975).

I. Gehirndurchblutung, Atemgase und Energiestoffwechsel des Gehirns

I. Sauerstoff

In den vorangehenden Abschnitten wurde darauf hingewiesen, daß zwischen Sauerstoffverbrauch und Durchblutung des Gehirns eine enge Beziehung herrscht. Bei Ruhebedingungen ist mit $3{,}71 \pm 0{,}53$ ml $O_2/100\,g \cdot min$ der Sauerstoffverbrauch des Gesamthirns relativ konstant. Aus den wenigen bisher vorliegenden Messungen der regionalen Sauerstoffversorgung ergibt sich, daß örtliche Unterschiede im Sauerstoffverbrauch bestehen. DAVIES u. GRENELL (1962), GLEICHMANN et al. (1962a), LÜBBERS (1968) kommen bei ihren Messungen zu dem Ergebnis, daß die Hirnrinde höheren Sauerstoffverbrauch haben muß, als das Mark. Das stimmt mit Meßergebnissen von ELLIOT und HELLER (1957) an Gehirnschnitten des Menschen überein, die den Sauerstoffverbrauch lokaler Strukturen direkt gemessen haben und von RIDGE (1967), der die Zytochromoxydase in verschiedenen Hirnschichten des Kaninchenhirns untersuchte. Nach TOLANI und TALWAR (1963) ist die Aktivität der mitochondrialen Zytochromoxydasen im Kleinhirn am höchsten und im Corpus callosum am geringsten. Dazwischen liegen z.B. Werte für den Thalamus.

Der Sauerstoffverbrauch ändert sich, wie auch die Gehirndurchblutung, mit dem Lebensalter. Mit der Zunahme des Reifegrades nimmt der Sauerstoffverbrauch zu (DIEMER, 1964, 1965a u. b). Auch die bereits erwähnten Messungen von KETY (1956) zeigen die gleiche Tendenz. Im höheren Lebensalter sinkt häufig der Sauerstoffverbrauch des Gehirns beim Menschen wieder ab. Dem entspricht die Durchblutungsverminderung.

1. Sauerstoffdruck und Sauerstoffversorgung des Gehirns bei wechselnden Durchblutungszuständen

Die Sauerstoffversorgung des Gehirns ist ausreichend, wenn der lokale Sauerstoffdruck an den sauerstoffverbrauchenden Mitochondrien so hoch ist, daß deren Bedarf gedeckt werden kann.

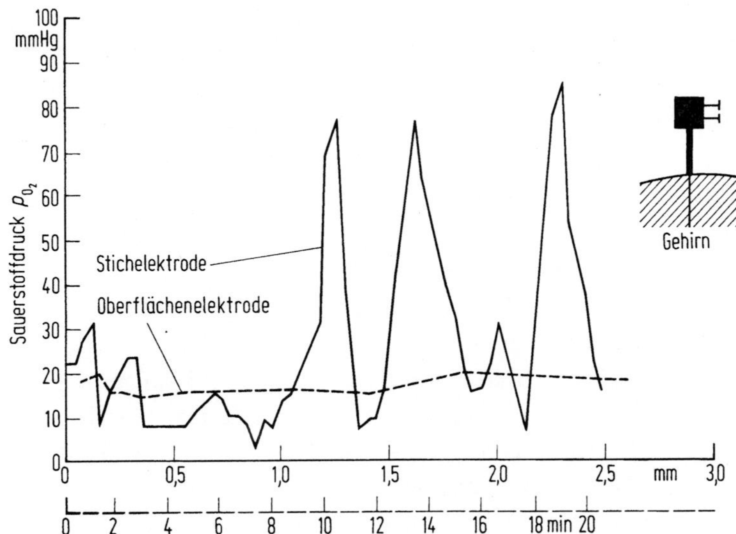

Abb. 20. Sauerstoffdruckwerte, die mit einer dünnen Platinelektrode in der Großhirnrinde eines Meerschweinchens registriert wurden. Die Meßelektrode wurde langsam von der Kortexoberfläche in die Tiefe vorgeschoben. In der Ordinate sind die O_2-Druckwerte aufgetragen. Abszisse: Einstichtiefe. Zur Kontrolle wurde mit einer anderen Elektrode während der gesamten Versuchszeit (zweite Abszisse: Zeit in min) der Sauerstoffdruck auf der Oberfläche des Gehirns gemessen (gestrichelt gezeichnete Linie). (Nach LÜBBERS, in: Der Gehirnkreislauf. Ed.: GÄNSHIRT, Thieme, Stuttgart, 1972, S. 230)

Dies ist abhängig von der Kapillarisierung, vom Transportweg des Sauerstoffs durch Diffusion, von der Höhe des Sauerstoffverbrauchs und vom kritischen mitochondrialen Sauerstoffdruck. Sauerstoffverbrauchswerte sind in den vorhergehenden Kapiteln angegeben worden. Auch über die Kapillarisierung wurden einige Daten mitgeteilt. Beim Vergleich der Kapillardichte des Gehirns mit anderen Organen ähnlich hoher Durchblutung zeigt sich, daß die Kapillardichte des Gehirngewebes relativ niedrig ist. Mißt man den Sauerstoffdruck mit Platinmikroelektroden im Gehirngewebe an verschiedenen Stellen, so findet man, daß eine Sauerstoffdruckverteilung besteht, die deutliche Beziehungen zum Muster der Gefäße im Meßbereich aufweist. Die Abb. 20 zeigt eine derartige Sauerstoffdruckverteilung in der Großhirnrinde eines Meerschweinchengehirns. Für die Theorie der Kapillarversorgung des Gehirns gilt das Zylindermodell nach KROGH (1924) (OPITZ u. SCHNEIDER, 1950) nur in eingeschränkter Form, denn die Kapillaren verlaufen nicht parallel, sondern in der Regel asymmetrisch. Aus den theoretischen Analysen der Sauerstoffversorgung in Geweben mit derartigen Kapillarmustern (DIEMER, 1963; GRUNEWALD, 1968; METZGER, 1972) ergibt sich, daß der Sauerstoffdruck, der im venösen System gemessen wird, beträchtlich höher sein muß als die niedrigsten Werte, die im Gewebe gemessen werden, was den tatsächlichen Meßergebnissen entspricht.

2. Sauerstoffmangel und Gehirndurchblutung

In zahlreichen Lehrbüchern, Übersichten und einzelnen Aufsätzen über die Wirkung der Hypoxie auf das Gehirn, wird mitgeteilt, daß die Hypoxie eine Verringerung des Gehirngefäßwiderstandes bewirkt und daß damit die Gehirndurchblutung ansteigt (CHORNYAK, 1938; KETY u. SCHMIDT, 1948b; SCHMIDT, 1950; SCHNEIDER, 1953, 1961; LASSEN, 1959; WOLF, 1959; GLEICHMANN et al., 1962b; COHEN, 1965; SHIMOJYO et al., 1966; BETZ, 1968b; KOGURE et al., 1970a, b; MANN, 1970; BARTKO, 1971; BAKAY u. KOBAYASHI, 1971; GÄNSHIRT, 1972). Bei anästhesierten Tieren haben NOELL und SCHNEIDER (1942b) gefunden, daß der zerebrale Gefäßwiderstand dann abzusinken und die Gehirndurchblutung anzusteigen beginnt, wenn der Sauerstoff in der eingeatmeten Luft unter 11% abfällt. Bei wachen, frei beweglichen Katzen fand sich jedoch, daß in der thalamischen und hypothalamischen Region die Durchblutung schon anstieg, wenn ein Luft-O_2-Gehalt von etwa 16% erreicht wurde (BETZ, 1965b). Diese Differenz ist wahrscheinlich durch den niedrigeren Sauerstoffverbrauch des Gehirns anästhesierter Tiere im Vergleich zu wachen Tieren verursacht (SOKOLOFF, 1959; MCDOWALL, 1967). Die Beziehung zwischen der Sauerstoffspannung im Blut des Bulbus venae jugularis und der Gehirndurchblutung sieht so aus, daß die Durchblutung des gesamten Gehirns dann ansteigt, wenn der Sauerstoffdruck im Bulbus venae jugularis unter einen Wert von 30–28 mm Hg abfällt (NOELL u. SCHNEIDER, 1942a, b). Die Durchblutung erreicht einen Maximalwert, wenn der hirnvenöse Sauerstoffdruck etwa 20 mm Hg beträgt (NOELL u. SCHNEIDER, 1942b; SCHAERTLIN, 1961; GROTE et al., 1971a, b). Der Anstieg der hypoxisch bedingten Gehirndurchblutung wird höher, wenn gleichzeitig eine respiratorische Azidose besteht. Von KOGURE et al. (1970a, b) wurde berichtet, daß immer dann eine Verminderung des Gehirngefäßwiderstands auftrat, wenn sich eine Gewebsazidose entwickelt hatte.

Die Ursachen einer Hypoxie, die zu Gehirndurchblutungsänderungen führen kann, sind nicht einheitlich. Neben der hypoxischen Hypoxidose, die durch Hypoxämie des arteriellen Blutes bedingt ist, kennen wir die venöse Hypoxidose, die dadurch verursacht wird, daß ein zu hoher Bedarf des Gewebes und damit eine stärkere Ausschöpfung des vorhandenen Blutsauerstoffs besteht. Neben diesen Formen gibt es die ischämische Hypoxidose, durch verminderte Durchblutung verursacht, nutritive Hypoxidosen bei Mangel an Substraten und die histotoxische Hypoxidose durch Vergiftung von Fermenten oder durch Fermentmangel (Einzelheiten der Ursachen und Einteilungen, siehe BETZ, 1968b). Die Änderungen der Energiegehalte im Gewebe sind bei den Hypoxidosen, die durch Reduzierung des Sauerstoffgehalts im Blut oder durch Durchblutungsverminderung bedingt sind, ähnlich. Abb. 21 zeigt den Effekt eines akuten Sauerstoffmangels

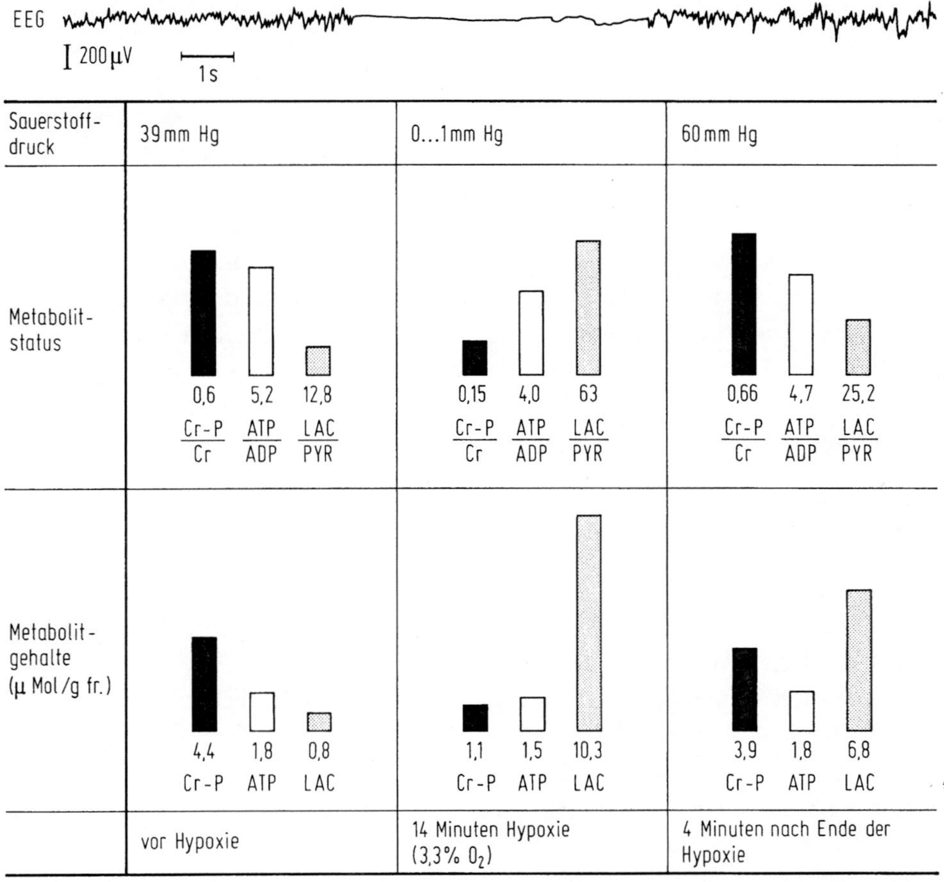

Abb. 21. Die Reaktionen von EEG, kortikalem Sauerstoffdruck (gemessen mit einer 10-Drahtplatinelektrode an mehreren Meßstellen der Großhirnrinde), energiereichen Substraten (in μmol/g Frischgewicht) der Großhirnrinde, Quotienten von CrP/Cr, ATP/ADP und Lactat/Pyruvat bei einer Katze, die einige Minuten 3,3% O_2 in N_2 atmete. Die Gewebsentnahme erfolgte mit einer in flüssiger Luft gekühlten Saugstanze, wenige Sekunden nachdem das EEG isoelektrisch wurde. Die eingerahmten Meßwerte sind Kontrollwerte von 10 Tieren. Die Versuche wurden an Barbiturat-narkotisierten Katzen gewonnen. (Nach SCHMAHL et al., Pflügers Arch. Physiol. **292**, 46, 1966)

auf das EEG, den kortikalen Sauerstoffdruck, das Laktat, Pyruvat sowie auf die energiereichen Phosphate im Kortexgewebe, der, während aufrechterhaltener Zirkulation, durch eine Verminderung der Sauerstoffgehalte im arteriellen Blut auftritt. Es zeigte sich in diesen Experimenten, daß das EEG dann verschwindet, wenn das Kreatinphosphat einen Wert von etwa 1,5 mMol/l im kortikalen Gehirngewebe erreicht. Eine Durchblutung ist zu diesem Zeitpunkt noch nachweisbar. Atmet das Versuchstier anschließend an die Hypoxie ein Atemgemisch mit hoher Konzentration von Sauerstoff, so stellen sich die energiereichen Substrate sehr schnell wieder auf den Ausgangswert ein. Am längsten bleibt Laktat erhöht. Es ist in vielen anderen Experimenten beschrieben worden, daß die Erhöhung von Laktat das erste deutliche Zeichen eines zu niedrigen Sauerstoffdrucks im Blut darstellt, was insofern gut verständlich ist, als das Gehirn im wesentlichen Glukose metabolisiert (s. auch S. 246).

Ob die hypoxisch bedingte Aufhebung der Autoregulation letztlich durch Veränderung der extravaskulären Wasserstoff- oder Kalium-Ionenkonzentration oder durch die Wirkung anderer vasoaktiver Substanzen hervorgerufen wird oder durch die Kombination mehrerer Reize, ist noch nicht ausreichend geklärt (HOSSMANN et al., 1973; HOSSMANN u. KLEIHUES, 1973; ASTRUP et al., 1978).

Beim Sauerstoffmangel wird die intrazelluläre Konzentration der Adeninnukleotide AMP und Adenosin größer, wenn die Resynthese von ATP vermindert wird. Die Erhöhung der

Konzentration des gefäßdilatierend wirkenden Adenosins im Gewebe und in den perivaskulären Räumen wird außer für die hypoxiebedingte Koronargefäßdilatation auch als wichtige Komponente für die hypoxiebedingte Dilatation der Gehirngefäße diskutiert (BERNE et al., 1974). Dilatierende Wirkungen von Adenosin konnten an isolierten kaliumkontrahierten Gehirnarterien von Kaninchen und Menschen nachgewiesen werden (TODA, 1974, WAHL und KUSCHINSKY, 1976).

Von OLSSON et al. (1976) und SCHRADER et al. (1977) wird angenommen, daß freigesetztes Adenosin an Membranrezeptoren von Gefäßmuskelzellen wirkt (untersucht an Koronargefäßen). Möglicherweise bewirkt Adenosin eine Verminderung der Membranpermeabilität für Ca^{++} (HERLIHY et al., 1976), so daß die Dilatation letztlich auf die Veränderung des Ca^{++}-Einstroms in die glatten Muskelzellen zurückzuführen wäre (s. folgende Kapitel). Ob die Geschwindigkeit des Austransports von Adenosin in der erforderlichen Konzentration für die Gefäßdilatation der Gehirngefäße ausreicht und ob die z.T. langdauernden posthypoxischen Hyperämien mit den Konzentrationsänderungen des perivaskulären Adenosins korrelieren, ist noch nicht hinreichend geklärt.

a) Chronischer Sauerstoffmangel

Werden Menschen oder Tiere in große Höhen gebracht oder wird auf künstlichem Wege der Sauerstoffgehalt in der Atemluft über längere Zeit erniedrigt, so reagiert die Gehirndurchblutung in charakteristischer Weise:
Im Anfang des Sauerstoffmangels steigt die Durchblutung in ähnlicher Weise an wie bei den akuten Sauerstoffmangelzuständen beschrieben. Bleibt der Sauerstoffmangel erhalten, so kommt es zu einer allmählichen Verminderung der initialen Durchblutungserhöhung. Diese Anpassungserscheinungen verlaufen relativ schnell. Bei Tieren, bei denen der Sauerstoffgehalt konstant auf Werte von ca. 10% Sauerstoff in der Atemluft erniedrigt wurde, fand sich schon 5–6 Stunden nach Einsetzen des Sauerstoffmangels eine deutliche Tendenz zur Rückkehr in Richtung auf die Ausgangswerte, in einzelnen Fällen waren sie sogar schon wieder erreicht (BETZ u. WÜNNENBERG, 1964). Während dieser kurzen Zeit ist es nicht möglich, daß so viel Erythrozyten neu gebildet werden, daß durch die Entwicklung einer Polyzythämie die Verminderung der anfänglich stark gesteigerten Gehirndurchblutung erklärt werden kann. Welche Mechanismen letztlich für diese schnelle Phase der Anpassung an den Sauerstoffmangel verantwortlich gemacht werden können, ist bisher nicht klar. Die Tiere hyperventilieren und es kommt meist zu einer Alkalose im Blut. Nach Untersuchungen von SEVERINGHAUS et al., 1963, 1966) und SEVERINGHAUS (1964) ist im Liquor cerebrospinalis bei Höhenanpassung jedoch nicht selten eine leichte Azidose zu beobachten. Eine sehr klare Beziehung zum Säure-Basenhaushalt findet sich beim Vergleich von tierexperimentellen Daten und Untersuchungen an Menschen nicht, wenn auch nachweisbar ist, daß bei hypoxiebedingter Gehirngewebsazidose die Durchblutung in der Regel nicht wieder den Ausgangswert erreicht, sondern erhöht bleibt. Wird ein Sauerstoffmangel im Experiment täglich wiederholt und wird die Exposition an den niedrigen Sauerstoffdruck täglich fünf bis sechs Stunden lang durchgeführt, so steigt zehn bis zwölf Tage nach der ersten Exposition an 10% Sauerstoff die Durchblutung auch anfänglich kaum noch an und erreicht schon kurz nach Beginn der Exposition an Sauerstoffmangelgemische, wieder den Ausgangswert (Abb. 22). Bei solchen Anpassungen ändert sich der Gewebsstoffwechsel während der Adaptationsperiode. DAHL und BALFOUR (1964) sahen einen Anstieg der anaeroben Glykolyse bei adaptierten Tieren. DETAR und BOHR (1968), die spiralige Streifen von Kaninchenaorten wiederholt niedrigen Sauerstoffdrucken aussetzten, fanden modifizierte Reaktionen in der Spannungsentwicklung dieser Gefäßstreifen während wiederholter Hypoxie. Sie nehmen an, daß die Änderung der Reaktion in der glatten Muskulatur Manifestationen der Adaptation an die hypoxischen Bedingungen sind. Fügte man den Gefäßstreifen Noradrenalin zu, so entwickelten die adaptierten Muskeln eine höhere Spannung als die nicht adaptierten. Auch das wird von DETAR und BOHR (1968) als Folge einer erhöhten anaeroben Glykolyse betrachtet. Bei vollständig an große Höhe adaptierten Ratten wurden keine signifikanten Änderungen der energiereichen

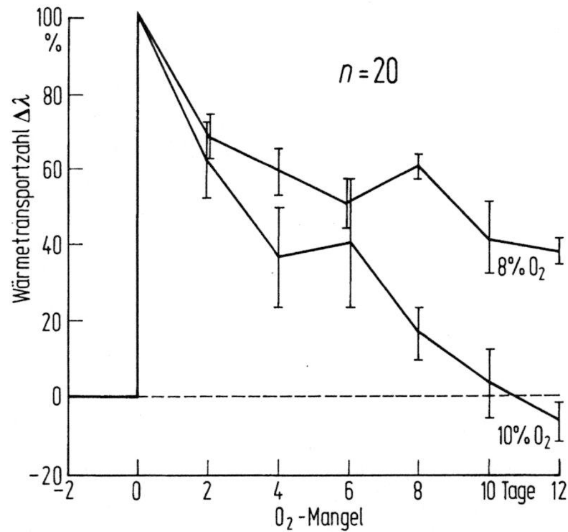

Abb. 22. Die Gehirndurchblutung bei täglich wiederholter 4–6stündiger Exposition an niedrige O_2-Gehalte in der Inspirationsluft (10 Katzen wurden an 8% O_2 in N_2 und 10 Katzen an 10% O_2 in N_2 adaptiert). Die mittlere Durchblutungserhöhung des ersten Expositionstages wurde als 100% gesetzt. Der Ausgangswert (Durchblutungsmittelwert über 1 Std vor Beginn des Experiments) als 0%. Die kontinuierlichen Durchblutungsmessungen wurden an wachen Katzen mit chronisch implantierten Wärmeleitsonden vorgenommen. (Nach BETZ: Acta neurol. Scand, Suppl. **14**, 121, 1965)

Substrate beobachtet (ALBAUM u. CHINN, 1953). Diese Tiere wiesen, wie auch Katzen, die man längere Zeit an niederen Sauerstoffdruck gewöhnte, einen Anstieg des Hämoglobingehaltes auf. Das entspricht den Zuständen, wie man sie bei höhenakklimatisierten Menschen findet. Auffällig war, daß junge Tiere, die aus der Ebene kamen, sich schneller an große Höhen adaptierten als ältere und daß die zerebellare Durchblutung bei den Ratten keine Adaptation zeigte (HAINING et al., 1970). Während langdauernder Hypoxien steigt die Anzahl der Kapillaren im Gehirnkortex im Vergleich zu Normaltieren an (DIEMER u. HENN, 1965), und der mittlere Durchmesser der Arterien wird vergrößert (MERCKER u. SCHNEIDER, 1949). Für diese morphologischen Änderungen ist allerdings eine relativ starke Hypoxie notwendig (DIEMER, 1965b). Diesen Befunden entsprechen neuere Ergebnisse von BÄR et al. (1976) nicht. Wird der Sauerstoffmangel kurzzeitig bis zur Anoxie geführt und werden Tiere wiederholt in kurze anoxische Zustände versetzt, so kommt es zu Gefäßveränderungen in Form subpialer und intrazerebraler, perivaskulärer Hämorrhagien und Koagulationen. Die Gefäßwände zeigen fibröse Umwandlungen. Diese Veränderungen finden sich zusätzlich zu den zellulären, degenerativen Veränderungen im Gehirngewebe (THORNER u. LEWEY, 1940).

b) Anoxie und Ischämie

Wird eine Hypoxie zu einer generellen Anoxie, so verhält sich die Gehirndurchblutung zunächst wie bei der Hypoxie. Sie steigt an und erreicht ein Maximum. Im weiteren Verlauf sinkt sie jedoch wieder ab, weil die arteriellen Blutdruckwerte unter die autoregulatorische Grenze sinken. Es kommt bei Unterschreiten eines kritischen P_{O_2}-Werts (kritische Schwelle) zu Funktionsstörungen der komplex arbeitenden Strukturen des Gehirns, d.h. zunächst zu Störungen der Koordination, dann zu Störungen des Bewußtseins, dann zu Veränderungen der Blut- Hirnschranke und der Mikrozirkulation und schließlich zum Ausfall aller übrigen Gehirnfunktionen und zum Tod. Das Schema in Abb. 23 zeigt die Reihenfolge der auftretenden Störungen bei einer, wie auch immer bedingten, Anoxie. Im postanoxischen Zustand wird die Gehirndurchblutung im Fall einer nicht allzu lange andauernden, vorhergehenden anoxischen Periode stark erhöht. Bei der Ischämie bezeichnet man diese Hyperämie als reaktive, postischämische Hyperämie, bei der Anoxie oder Hypoxie ohne Ischämie als posthypoxische Hyperämie. Die Unterschiede dieser beiden Reaktionsweisen sind im wesentlichen dadurch bedingt, daß bei der posthypoxischen oder postanoxi-

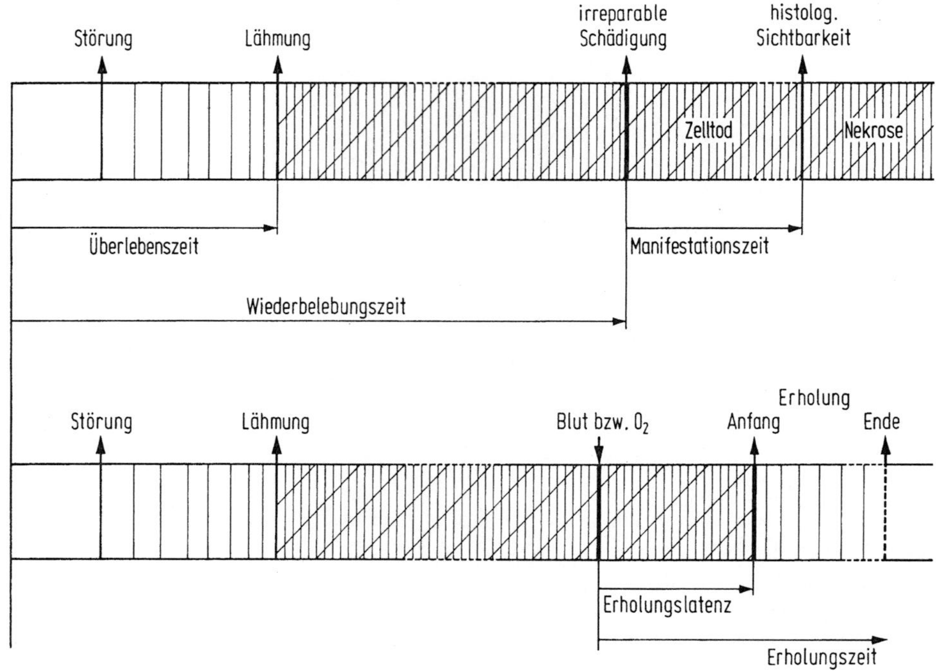

Abb. 23. Obere Reihe. Reihenfolge von Störungen nach Anoxie sowie Definition von Überlebenszeit, Wiederbelebungszeit und Manifestationszeit. Untere Reihe: Postanoxische Wiederherstellung von Funktionen. (Aus REIN u. SCHNEIDER: Physiologie des Menschen, 15. Aufl., Berlin, Göttingen, Heidelberg; Springer, 1964)

schen Hyperämie keine Anreicherung von CO_2 im Gehirn erfolgt, während bei der postischämischen Hyperämie diese durch das angehäufte CO_2 mitbedingt ist. Die Dauer solcher postanoxisch oder postischämisch-hyperämischen Zustände ist sehr unterschiedlich. Bei sehr kurz dauernden (bis zu zwei oder drei Minuten anhaltenden) Gewebshypoxien dauert die hyperämische Periode nur wenige Minuten. Nach länger andauernden Ischämien können hyperämische Zonen über sehr viel längere Zeiten beobachtet werden (PAULSON, 1968, 1971; LASSEN, 1968b). Nach Ischämien kann es zu sekundären Schädigungen des Gehirns kommen, wobei auch das Gefäßsystem mit betroffen wird. (Im Bereich der Kapillaren findet man mikroskopisch z.B. Endothelschwellungen. In anderen Gefäßen kommt es zu Mikrothrombosierungen, perivaskulär zu Ödemen.) Der Ablauf der Störungen während der Ischämie ist im wesentlichen durch den Sauerstoffmangel bedingt. So lange der im Blut vorhandene Sauerstoff noch ausreicht, sieht man keine Störungen (freies Intervall), fünf bis sieben Sekunden später tritt Bewußtseinsverlust und Ausfall anderer Gehirnfunktionen auf, die mit Änderungen der elektrischen Aktivität verbunden sind. Die Zeit bis zum Erlöschen der geprüften Funktionen nach Anoxie wird als Überlebenszeit bezeichnet (SUGAR u. GERARD, 1938). Nach Wiederzufuhr von sauerstoffhaltigem Blut kann es bei nur kurzdauernder Ischämie zu einer völligen Restitution aller Funktionen kommen. Bei längerdauerndem Sauerstoffmangel bleiben Störungen zurück. Dieser Zustand wird als inkomplette Wiederbelebung bezeichnet. Die Zeit, die ein totaler Sauerstoffmangel dauern kann, ohne die Wiederbelebung zu gefährden, wird als Wiederbelebungszeit (SUGAR u. GERARD, 1938) bezeichnet. Die Zeit, die es dauert, bis eine Schädigung auch histologisch sichtbar wird, nennt man Manifestationszeit. Tritt eine irreversible Schädigung nicht ein, so dauert es nach Beseitigung des Sauerstoffmangels eine gewisse Zeit, bis eine Erholung erfolgt. Diese Zeit wird als Erholungszeit bezeichnet. Die Zeitspanne bis zum Auftreten der ersten Zeichen der Erholung heißt Erholungslatenz. Es hat sich bei Untersuchungen von HOSSMANN u. LECHTAPE-GRÜTER (1971/72) sowie HOSSMANN u. KLEIHUES (1973) gezeigt, daß unter bestimmten Bedingungen einer intensiven Therapie der postanoxischen Störungen, auch nach längeren Zeiten als von SUGAR und GERARD (1938) beschrieben, eine inkomplette Wiederbelebung erreichbar ist. Die von HOSSMANN u. LECHTAPE-GRÜTER (1971/72) und HOSSMANN

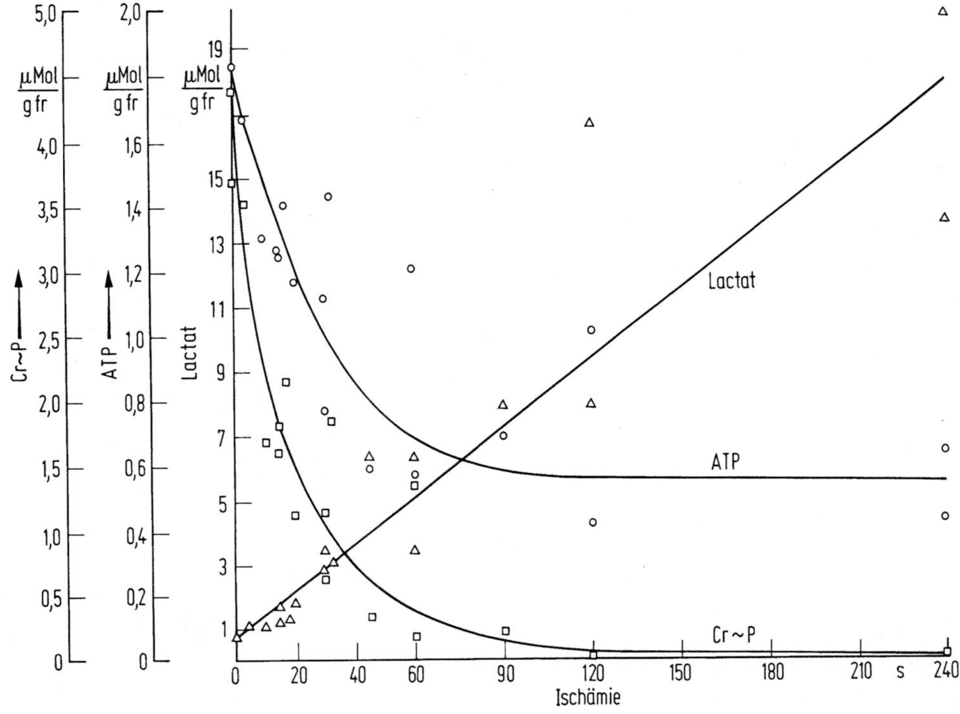

Abb. 24. Änderung der energiereichen Phosphate und des Laktats in der Großhirnrinde bei kompletter Ischämie bis 240 s nach Ischämiebeginn bei Narkose. (Nach SCHMAHL et al., Biochem. Z. **342**, 518, 1965)

et al. (1973) beschriebenen Ergebnisse stehen in einem gewissen Gegensatz zu denen von GÄNSHIRT et al. (1952a, b) SCHNEIDER (1953, 1957, 1958), HIRSCH (1969), HIRSCH et al. (1957, 1961, 1968a u. b), HIRSCH und SCHNEIDER (1968), OBERDÖRSTER et al. (1969). Es kann bisher noch nicht gesagt werden, wieweit aus den von HOSSMANN und LECHTAPE-GRÜTER (1971/72) zunächst ermittelten Daten sich Ansätze für eine erfolgversprechende Therapie postanoxischer Zustände, auch beim Menschen, entwickeln lassen.

3. Durchblutungsverminderung und Gewebsenergetik

Die Änderungen des Energiezustands im Gehirngewebe bei Durchblutungsverminderungen kann wegen der sehr schnellen Veränderungen von Substratkonzentrationen nur im Tierexperiment untersucht werden. Die dramatischsten Effekte einer verminderten Gehirndurchblutung auf die zerebrale Energetik entstehen, wenn der wirksame Blutdruck schlagartig auf Null fällt, z.B. bei Herzstillstand oder plötzlichem Durchblutungsstopp. Die Abb. 24 zeigt, daß innerhalb weniger Sekunden nach einem solchen Ereignis das energetische Potential des Gehirngewebes steil abfällt (THORN u. HEITMANN, 1954; SCHMAHL et al., 1965; MÜLLER et al., 1970a u. b; SIESJÖ u. NILSSON, 1971). Die steilste Verminderung erfährt das Kreatinphosphat, das innerhalb von etwa zwei Minuten praktisch den Nullwert erreicht. Auch im ATP sieht man anfänglich einen steilen Abfall, der sich dann verlangsamt. Die Menge des produzierten Lactats als Ausdruck einer anaeroben Glykolyse beträgt beim anästhesierten Tier etwa 4 μmol/ min · g Kortex (SCHMAHL et al., 1965; DÖRING u. OLBRISCH, 1970). Bei länger dauernder kompletter Ischämie haben HOSSMANN und LECHTAPE-GRÜTER (1971, 1972) und KOBAYASHI et al. (1973) gefunden, daß bei Ischämien von längerer Dauer als fünf Minuten auch das ATP stärker abfällt und schließlich verschwindet (LJUNGREN u. SIESJÖ, 1973). Bei Verschluß eines einzelnen Gefäßes sind die Änderungen des Energiezustands von der Kollateralversorgung abhängig. Da diese individuell stark variiert, sind auch die Änderungen in der Energetik sehr unterschiedlich. Bei Verschluß einer Arteria carotis bei Katzen fanden SCHMAHL et al. (1971, 1972) im Kortexgewebe der ipsilateralen Seite, im Vergleich zur kontralateralen Seite, lediglich Veränderungen des Redox-Verhältnisses, wobei die Steigerung des Gewebslactats mit einer Verminderung des lokalen Gewebs-pH-Wertes verbunden war. HELD et al. (1973) sahen, daß in infarzierten Bereichen, 24 Std nach dem Gefäßverschluß, immer noch ein beträchtlicher Anteil von Kreatinphosphat und ATP vorhanden war. Der Glukosestoffwechsel war nicht nur im infarzierten Bereich sondern auch in der grauen und weißen Substanz nicht infarzierten Gewebes verändert. In der perifokalen Region war ebenfalls eine Verminderung der energiereichen Substrate meßbar. Der Wassergehalt des Gewebes steigt in infarzierten Bereichen an, was bedeutet, daß die Wirkung des Ödems sekundär eine Verminderung der Mikrozirkulation verursacht. Nach Wiederdurchblutung eines 30–60 min lang nicht durchbluteten Gehirns erreichen die energiereichen Substrate rasch wieder die Normalwerte (HINZEN et al., 1972).

4. Glukosebedarf des Gehirns und Durchblutung

Bei ausreichender Sauerstoffzufuhr wird der Energiebedarf des Gehirns durch aeroben Glukoseabbau gedeckt. Normalerweise beträgt die Glukoseaufnahme des menschlichen Gesamtgehirns $5{,}3 \pm 0{,}96$ mg/100 g·min. Bei einer normalen O_2-Aufnahme des Gehirns von $3{,}71 \pm 0{,}53$ ml O_2/100 g·min müßte bei einem RQ von 1, bei vollständiger aerober Glykolyse $1{,}34 \cdot 3{,}71 = 4{,}97$ mg Glukose/100 g·min umgesetzt werden. Der tatsächliche Mehrumsatz von $5{,}3 - 4{,}97 = 0{,}33$ mg Glukose kann dadurch erklärt werden, daß sowohl die arteriovenöse Milchsäuredifferenz als auch die arteriovenöse Brenztraubensäuredifferenz negativ ist. Das heißt beide Stoffe werden von den Zellen des ZNS abgegeben. Aus Bilanzuntersuchungen (GOTTSTEIN et al., 1963, 1964) errechnet sich, daß die Glukose zu 92% aerob und zu 8% anaerob abgebaut wird. Wie aus Abb. 11 hervorgeht, ist die Höhe der Glukoseaufnahme altersabhängig. Bei Messungen der regionalen zerebralen Glukoseutilisation haben SOKOLOFF et al. (1975) und KENNEDY et al. (1975) beträchtliche regionale Unterschiede festgestellt.

Auch die Gehirngefäße sind auf diese Form der Energieverwertung eingestellt. Das zeigt sich bei vergleichenden Untersuchungen der Enzymmuster von Gehirngefäßwänden und der Arteria carotis. Tabelle 5 gibt eine Übersicht über die Aktivität von Enzymen der Glykogenolyse, der Glykolyse, der β-Oxydation von Fettsäuren und des Zitronensäurezyklus glatter Gefäßmuskeln von zerebralen und extra-zerebralen Arterien. Die Werte (Mittelwerte, $N = 4$) sind als Milli-Einheiten pro Gramm Frischgewicht mit den Standardabweichungen angegeben. Die deutlichen Unterschiede der Hexokinase-Aktivitäten weisen darauf hin, daß bei intrazerebralen Gefäßmuskeln die Glykose über die Phosphotransferase-Reaktion der Hexokinase in den Zitronensäurecyclus überführt wird und damit Glukose direkt bevorzugt utilisiert werden kann. Die Enzymaktivitäten sind Indikatoren dafür, daß auch eine β-Oxydation von Fettsäuren in den Muskelzellen der Gefäßwände eine erhebliche Rolle spielt. In den extrazerebralen Gefäßwänden ist dagegen die Aktivität der Enzyme für die anaerobe Energiegewinnung vergleichsweise größer.

Tabelle 5. Enzymaktivitäten in Gefäßwänden von intra- und extrazerebralen Gefäßwänden (s. Text)

	intrazerebral (I) [mU/g Frischgewicht]	extrazerebral (II) [mU/g Frischgewicht]	Signifikanz I/II
Phosphorylase	329 ± 58	320 ± 87	NS
Hexokinase	507 ± 88	295 ± 23	$p < 0{,}05$
Triosephosphatdehydrogenase	22075 ± 2054	24440 ± 7542	NS
Laktatdehydrogenase	11905 ± 3723	21305 ± 10874	NS
β-hydroxyacyl-CoA-dehydrogenase	4128 ± 593	1741 ± 654	$p < 0{,}025$
Zitratsynthetase	1624 ± 187	1101 ± 123	$p < 0{,}05$

Bei experimentellem, insulininduziertem, hypoglykämischem Koma steigt die Gehirndurchblutung an (DELLA PORTA et al., 1964). Diese Anstiege erfolgen, obgleich weder eine Acidose noch Anzeichen eines vermehrten Auftretens von Adenosin erkennbar sind (NORBERG u. SIESJÖ, 1975). Auch sind bei diesen Anstiegen keine Kaliumerhöhungen nachgewiesen worden (ASTRUP et al., 1975, unveröffentlicht). Dieser Befund zeigt, daß bei einem Defizit von Glukose die Gefäße mit einer Widerstandsverminderung reagieren. Zwar ist noch nicht klar, welcher Mechanismus dieser Durchblutungssteigerung zugrunde liegt, jedoch liegt die Vermutung nahe, daß die Besonderheiten des Glukosestoffwechsels der intrazerebralen Gefäßmuskeln mit der hypoglykämischen Dilatation verknüpft sein könnten.

II. Die Gehirndurchblutung bei CO_2-Änderung

1. Hyperkapnie

Außer dem Sauerstoffmangel ist eine Erhöhung des CO_2 im Blut oder Gehirngewebe, nach Meinung vieler Autoren, der adäquate physiologische Reiz zur Steigerung der Gehirndurchblutung (WOLFF u. LENNOX, 1930; BENZINGER et al., 1938; NOELL u. SCHNEIDER, 1944; KETY u. SCHMIDT, 1946, 1948b; SCHIEVE u. WILSON, 1953; SCHNEIDER, 1953; NOVACK et al., 1953; PATTERSON et al., 1955; LASSEN, 1959; BÜHLMANN et al., 1960; MEYER u. GOTOH, 1960; HARPER u. BELL, 1963; MCHENRY et al., 1964; ALEXANDER et al., 1965; HARPER, 1965a, b; HARPER u. GLASS, 1965; HÄGGENDAL u. JOHANSSON, 1966; SHACKELFORD u. HEGEDUS, 1966; SKINHØJ, 1966; FIESCHI, 1967; AGNOLI, 1968; AGNOLI et al., 1969b, c; FENCL et al., 1969; POSNER et al., 1969; RYZHOVA, 1970; HAINING et al., 1970; CRANSTON u. ROSENDORFF, 1971; RAICHLE et al., 1971; GÄNSHIRT, 1972; BETZ, 1973). Die Durchblutungsreaktionen nach CO_2-Atmung in der weißen Substanz sind nicht genau so groß wie in der grauen Substanz (HANSEN et al., 1959). Nach den Untersuchungen von JAMES et al. (1969) steigt bei Kohlendioxyddruckerhöhung von 35 auf 65 mm Hg im arteriellen Blut die Durchblutung der grauen Substanz um etwa 1,4 ml Blut/100 g·min·mm Hg $PaCO_2$ an, während die Durchblutung in der weißen Substanz nur um 0,46 ml/100 g·min·mm Hg $PaCO_2$ ansteigt. Nach den in Tabelle 2 dargestellten sehr unterschiedlichen Durchblutungswerten einzelner Gehirnanteile ist die einfache Untergliederung in graue und weiße Substanz, auch in diesem Falle, eine zu starke Vereinfachung der tatsächlichen Reaktionsmuster (RYZHOVA, 1970). Die CO_2-bedingten Durchblutungsreaktionen hängen vom arteriellen Blutdruck und vom lokalen Gefäßwiderstand ab. Bei arteriellen Blutdruckwerten unter 50 mm Hg war eine Gehirngefäßreaktion auf Kohlendioxyd nicht mehr nachweisbar (HARPER u. GLASS, 1965). Es zeigt sich auch, daß bei einer oberen Konzentration von etwa 10% CO_2 in der Atemluft eine weitere CO_2-Erhöhung nicht zu wesentlich stärkeren Verminderungen des Gehirngefäßwiderstands führt (BETZ, 1965a). Die Reaktionsschwelle für CO_2-bedingte Durchblutungserhöhungen liegt außerordentlich niedrig. Schon bei knapp 1% CO_2-Erhöhung in der Inspirationsluft steigt die Gehirndurchblutung des wachen Tieres (BETZ, 1965a). Zahlreiche Befunde sprechen dafür, daß die Reaktion der Gehirndurchblutung auf CO_2-Erhöhung nicht durch CO_2 per se erfolgt, sondern daß die jede CO_2-Erhöhung begleitende pH-Erniedrigung der Gefäßwand den adäquaten Reiz für die Verminderung des lokalen Gefäßwiderstandes im Gehirn darstellt (Literatur s. INGVAR u. LASSEN, 1965b; LASSEN, 1966; SKINHØJ u. PAULSON, 1969; KOGURE et al., 1970c; PURVES, 1972; BETZ, 1972b; PANNIER u. LEUSEN, 1973). Da jedoch CO_2 auch zu Veränderungen der elektrischen Aktivität der Gehirnzellen führt, ist eine zusätzliche Wirkungskomponente des CO_2, z.B. über nervöse Strukturen möglich (SCHIEVE u. WILSON, 1953; Übersicht BETZ, 1974).

Ähnlich wie beim chronischen Sauerstoffmangel kommt es auch bei langdauernder, mäßiger Erhöhung der Kohlendioxydkonzentration in der Atemluft zur Habituation und Adaptation an die erhöhte CO_2-Konzentration. AGNOLI (1968) und AGNOLI et al. (1969b, c) wiesen nach, daß bei gleichbleibend hoher CO_2-Konzentration und gleichbleibendem CO_2-Druck im Gehirngewebe die Gehirndurchblutung im Verlauf von Stunden bis Tagen wieder in Richtung zum Ausgangswert zurückkehrte, wobei die Blutdruckänderung nicht der entscheidende Parameter war. Die allmähliche Widerstandserhöhung des Gehirngefäßsystems ging mit einem entsprechenden Wiederansteigen des initial erniedrigten Liquor pH-Werts, in Richtung auf den Ausgangswert, einher. Die pH-Erhöhung wird durch einen Anstieg des Bicarbonats im Liquor bedingt. EKSTRÖM-JODAL und HÄGGENDAL (1969) bestätigten diese Reaktionsweise der Gehirndurchblutung auch bei Patienten mit chronischer respiratorischer Insuffizienz. Werden Tiere täglich für sechs bis acht Stunden einer CO_2-Konzentration von 5–6% CO_2 ausgesetzt, so tritt, ähnlich wie bei intermittierender hypoxischer Belastung, eine allmähliche Abflachung der Durchblutungssteigerungen auf (BETZ, 1965b), und man sieht nach einigen Wochen der intermittierenden Exposition kaum noch Anstiege der Gehirndurchblutung, obgleich das pH während jeder Exposition etwas absinkt. Es ist bisher nicht klar, ob außer den von AGNOLI beschriebenen Änderungen des extravaskulären Bicarbonats noch andere Adaptate bei derartigen Anpassungsphänomenen eine Rolle spielen.

2. Hypokapnie

Bei einer akuten Verminderung des CO_2-Gehalts im Blut steigt in der Regel der Gehirngefäßwiderstand an, und die Gehirndurchblutung sinkt ab. Ein Schwellenwert der Durchblutungsänderung durch Hyperventilation läßt sich ebenso schwer ermitteln wie ein Schwellenwert bei CO_2-Anstieg. Von GIBBS et al. (1942) und NOELL u. SCHNEIDER (1944) wurde festgestellt, daß die Gesamtgehirndurchblutung während der Hyperventilation nicht weiter reduziert wird, wenn der Sauerstoffdruck im Bulbus venae jugularis unter 19 mm Hg abfällt. Die maximale Reduktion bei länger dauernder oder starker Hyperventilation erreicht etwa 40% der normalen Gesamtdurchblutung (KETY u. SCHMIDT, 1946, 1948b). Warum die Gehirndurchblutung bei CO_2-Minderung nicht unter einen Grenzwert abfällt, ist bisher nicht endgültig beantwortbar. Wahrscheinlich tritt bei starker Durchblutungsverminderung eine Azidose im Gewebe auf, die eine weitere Durchblutungsminderung verhindert (Abb. 25). Bei Hyperventilation kommt es zu einem Anstieg des Laktats im Gehirngewebe und auch im extrazellulären Raum des Gehirns (ALEXANDER et al., 1965; ELDRIDGE u. SALZER, 1967; GRANHOLM u. SIESJÖ, 1967, 1968, 1969; PLUM u. POSNER, 1967; COHEN et al., 1968; GRANHOLM et al., 1968, 1969). Dieser Laktatanstieg ist ein Anzeichen dafür, daß der Energiestoffwechsel des Gehirns nicht normal ist. Die Quotienten von Kreatin-Phosphat/Kreatin und ATP/ADP bleiben zunächst normal, auch wenn Lactatwerte vom 5fachen der Norm gefunden wurden (WEIDNER, 1969). Das bedeutet, daß ein hypokapniebedingter Abfall der Durchblutung nicht unbedingt auch eine Verminderung der verfügbaren energiereichen Substrate im Gehirn zur Folge hat. Messungen des Sauerstoffdrucks auf der Gehirnoberfläche zeigten (PICKERODT, 1971), daß bei Hyperventilation die lokalen Änderungen des Sauerstoffdrucks so ausgeprägt sein konnten, daß an vielen Orten des Kortex die Sauerstoffdruckwerte bei 0 mm/Hg lagen, obgleich im Sinus sagittalis der Sauerstoffdruck noch etwa 19 mm Hg betrug. Während lang andauernder Hyperventilation bleibt das arterielle pH höher als bei normaler Ventilation. Der pH-Wert im Liquor cerebrospinalis, welcher initial deutlich ansteigt, wird im Verlauf einer länger dauernden Hyperventilation wieder in Richtung auf den Ausgangswert verschoben und kann den Ausgangswert erreichen. Bei schwerer Hyperventilation kann das kortikale pH sogar azidotischer als bei normaler Atmung werden (MCDOWALL u. HARPER, 1968; BETZ, 1969b; LEUSEN, 1972). Die Laktatkonzentration im Gehirngewebe steigt, unabhängig von der pH-Änderung, im extravaskulären kortikalen Raum an, – was zeigt, daß die Laktatkonzentration nicht streng zum Gefäßwiderstand im Gehirn korreliert ist.

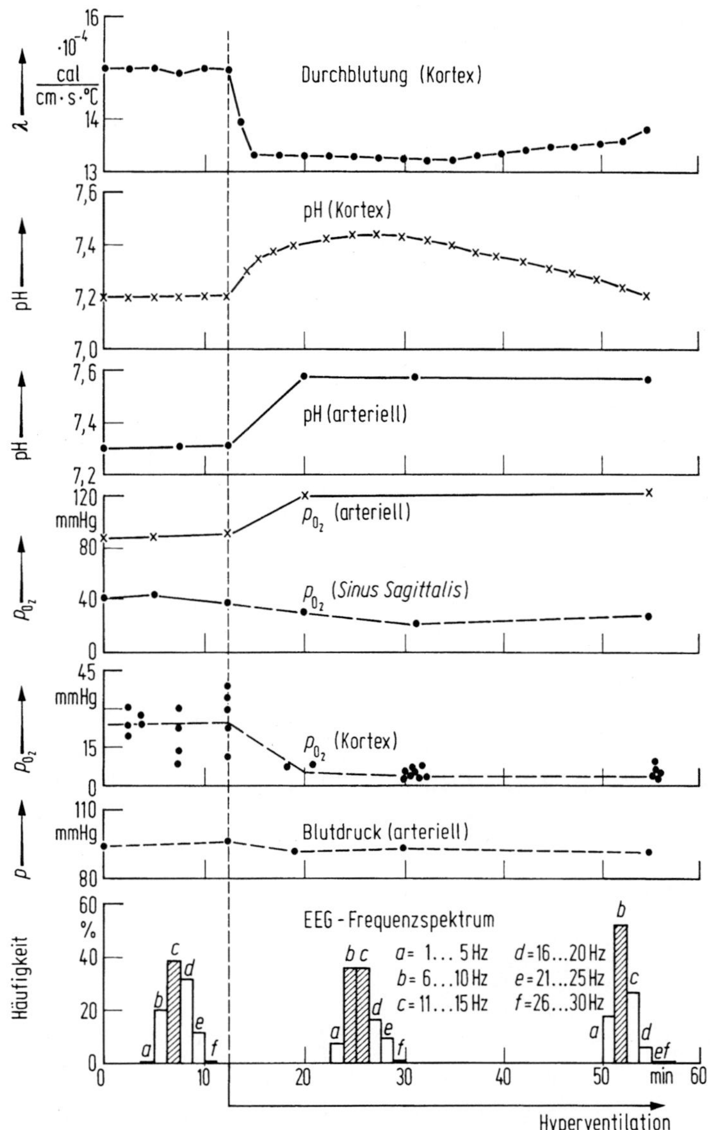

Abb. 25. Sehr starke Hypokapnie durch exzessive künstliche Hyperventilation. Wirkung auf die lokale kortikale Durchblutung (gemessen mit einem Wärmeleitmesser), das kortikale und arterielle pH (gemessen mit Einstab-Glaselektroden), den arteriellen und gehirnvenösen Sauerstoffdruck, sowie den lokalen pO_2 auf der Gehirnrinde und den arteriellen Blutdruck (Mitteldruck). Die Frequenzverteilung im EEG läßt eine deutliche Verschiebung der mittleren EEG-Frequenz mit Bevorzugung langsamer Frequenzen erkennen. (Nach BETZ: Internat. Anaesthesic. Clinics **7**, 525, 1969)

J. Neurogene Einflüsse auf den Gehirnkreislauf

I. Wirkungen von Sympathicus und Vagus

Es gibt zahlreiche Untersuchungen, die den Beweis erbringen, daß die zerebrale Zirkulation durch Änderungen der sympathischen oder parasympathischen Aktivität beeinflußt wird.

Nervenendigungen haben anatomische Kontakte zu den Gefäßen im Bereich des Circulus Willisi, zu den pialen Gefäßen und kleineren arteriellen Gefäßen, die das Gehirnparenchym versorgen. Piale Arterien scheinen am stärksten innerviert zu sein (PEERLESS u. KENDALL, 1976). Die nervale Versorgung der Gehirngefäße ist sowohl mit Hilfe der Lichtmikroskopie als auch der Elektronenmikroskopie nachgewiesen worden (STÖHR, 1921; CHOROBSKY u. PENFIELD, 1932;

McNaughton, 1938; Erkhov, 1965; Nielsen u. Owman, 1967; Nelson et al., 1971; Edvinsson et al., 1972; Cervos-Navarro u. Matakas, 1974; Nielsen et al., 1975). Bei den Nervenendigungen handelt es sich z.T. um solche, die dichte Granula enthalten und solche, die optisch leer sind. Die Nerven, deren Endformationen Vesikel mit Granula enthalten, wurden als noradrenerge, diejenigen, die agranuläre Vesikel enthalten, als acetylcholinerge Nervenendigungen identifiziert (Dahl u. Nelson, 1964; Nelson u. Rennels, 1968).

Eine einheitliche Meinung darüber, wie groß der Abstand der Nervenendigungen von den Gefäßmuskelzellen ist, besteht nicht. Lever et al. (1968) geben an, daß bei glatten Muskeln von intestinalen Gefäßen die Abstände etwa 4000 Å betragen. Spätere Messungen von Nelson et al. (1971) ergaben bei Gehirngefäßen wesentlich geringere Abstände um 1000 Å.

In den Nervenfasern der Adventitia zerebraler Gefäße wurde Noradrenalin nachgewiesen (Boullin, 1965; Falck et al., 1965; Owman et al., 1965; Peerless u. Kendall, 1976; Rosenblum, 1976; Edvinsson u. Owman, 1976). Viele dieser Fasern degenerieren nach einer zervikalen Sympathektomie. Von Forbes u. Cobb (1938) wurde angenommen, daß alle diejenigen Fasern, die nach einer Sympathektomie noch übrig bleiben als cholinerg bezeichnet werden können. Die Fasern begleiten die zerebralen Arterien (Chorobski u. Penfield, 1932; Hagen u. Wittkowski, 1969). In einzelnen Nervenfasern wird Azetylcholinesterase gefunden.

Die Untersuchung der Funktionen der Nervenendigungen hat zahlreiche kontroverse Befunde erbracht, so daß es auch jetzt, trotz einer umfangreichen Literatur, noch nicht möglich ist, eine exakte Übersicht aller nervösen Einflüsse auf die Gehirndurchblutung zu geben (Lit. s. Wolff, 1936; Kety u. McDowall, 1956; Holmquist et al., 1957; Lassen, 1959; Kety, 1961; Molnar, 1967; Mchedlishvili, 1968a, 1972; Lübbers, 1972; Edvinsson et al., 1977; Mendelow et al., 1977; Aubineau u. Sercombe, 1977; Heistad et al., 1977). Die Ursache dieser Schwierigkeiten basiert z.T. darauf, daß Untersuchungen häufig bei tief narkotisierten Individuen durchgeführt wurden und angenommen werden muß, daß die Narkose die Reaktionen auf nervöse Reize verändert.

Bei Untersuchungen der Wirkung einer Exstirpation des oberen zervikalen Ganglions ergab sich, daß diese Maßnahme auf die spontane Gehirndurchblutung nur geringen oder gar keinen Effekt hatte (Forbes u. Wolff, 1928; Fog, 1934; Forbes u. Cobb, 1938; Schmidt u. Hendrix, 1938; Forbes, 1954; Shackelford u. Hegedus, 1966; Waltz et al., 1971; Skinhøj, 1975). Reizung der zervikalen sympathischen Nerven führt in der Regel zu einer Verminderung der Gehirndurchblutung oder zu einer Veränderung der Blutverteilung im Gehirn (Forbes u. Wolff, 1928; Schmidt, 1934, 1936; Forbes et al., 1939; Lubsen, 1940; Ludwigs u. Schneider, 1954; Lluch et al., 1975; Traystman u. Rapela, 1975). Nach D'Alecy und Feigl (1972) kann unter bestimmten experimentellen Bedingungen die Durchblutungserniedrigung nach Sympathikusreizung bis zu 80% betragen, obgleich der Kohlendioxyddruck ansteigt. Ein bei dieser Untersuchung registrierter Anstieg des Liquordrucks während der Reizung ist nicht erklärt. Es gibt auch Untersucher, die keine Konstriktion nachweisen konnten (z.B. Meyer u. Klassen, 1975). Die Reaktion auf eine Sympathikusreizung wird durch Änderung des CO_2-Drucks modifiziert. James et al. (1969); Harper et al. (1970); Stone et al. (1975) fanden bei ihren Untersuchungen einen Verlust der Sensitivität des Gehirngefäßsystems gegenüber CO_2, wenn die beiden oberen Zervikalganglien ausgeschaltet worden waren. Auch bei der Untersuchung der Autoregulation nach zervikaler Sympathektomie werden unterschiedliche Befunde berichtet. James et al. (1969) fanden eine Verschlechterung der autoregulatorischen Antworten, sowohl in der grauen als auch in der weißen Substanz (Abb. 26). Bei Sympathektomie war die untere autoregulatorische Grenze in Richtung höherer Blutdruckwerte verschoben. Hernandez-Perez et al. (1975) fanden dagegen, daß nach Blockierung sympathischer Fasern, die zum Gehirn führen, die Autoregulation voll erhalten blieb.

Usinger et al. (1966) fanden keine Einflüsse der Vagotomie auf die spontanen Änderungen der Gehirndurchblutung. Wenn aber sowohl beide Vagusnerven als auch beide Sinusnerven durchschnitten wurden, kam es zu einer Reduktion der Reaktion des Gehirngefäßsystems auf CO_2,

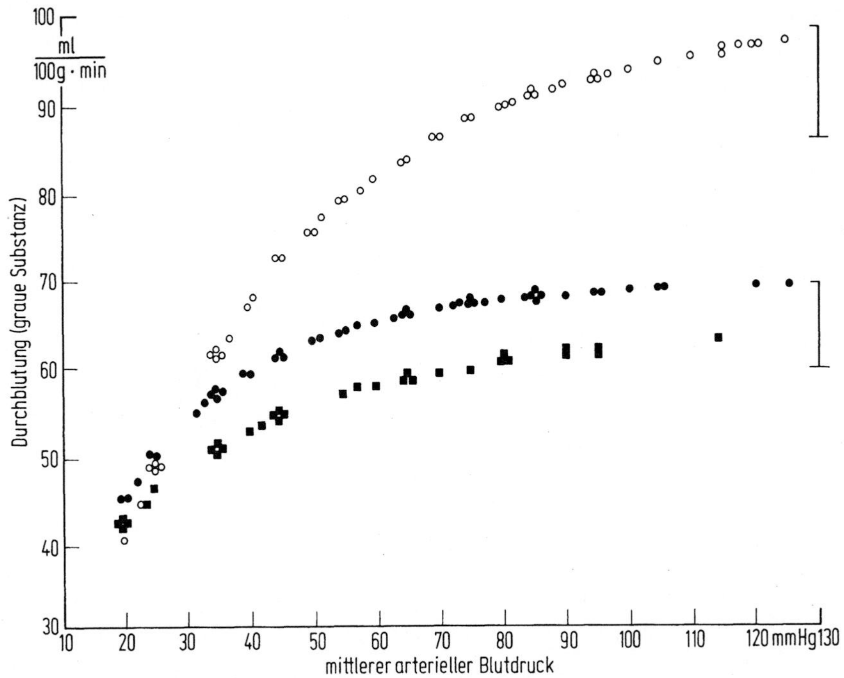

Abb. 26. Beziehung zwischen kortikaler Durchblutung und mittlerem arteriellem Blutdruck bei intaktem sympathischem Nervensystem (Punkte), nach Sympathektomie (offene Kreise) und während Sympathicusreizung (Quadrate). Mittelwerte von 13 Affen. Die vertikalen Linien an der rechten Seite repräsentieren die 95%igen Vertrauensgrenzen der Kurven gegen die oberen Asymptoten der Kurven. (Nach JAMES, MILLAR u. PURVES: Circulat. Res. **25**, 77, 1969)

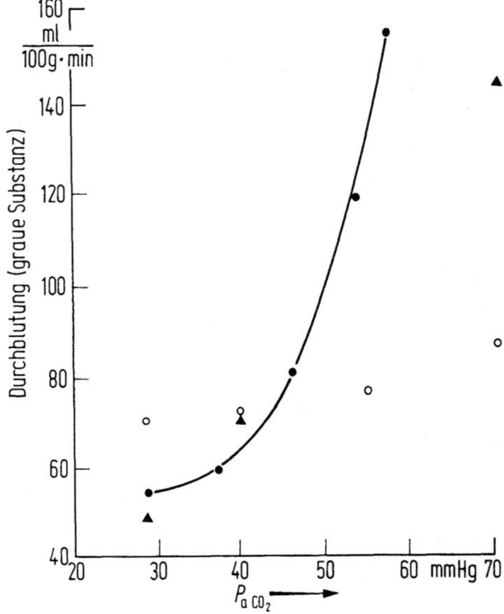

Abb. 27. Beziehung zwischen kortikaler Durchblutung und arteriellem CO_2-Druck (P_aCO_2) bei einem narkotisierten Affen. Ausgefüllte Kreise: bei intakten Nerven. Offene Kreise: nach Vagotomie, ausgefüllte Dreiecke: während Reizung des zentralen Abschnitts des durchtrennten Nervus vagus. (Nach JAMES, MILLAR u. PURVES: Circulat. Res. **25**, 77, 1969, Abb. 8)

was von den Autoren als eine Interaktion von neurogenen und lokalen metabolischen Mechanismen bezeichnet wurde. Von JAMES et al. (1969) wurde gezeigt, daß nach Vagotomie die Reaktion der Gehirndurchblutung bei Erhöhung der CO_2-Konzentration im Blut durch Reizung des zentralen Vagusendes verändert wurde. Aus den aufgezählten Befunden darf daher geschlossen werden, daß sowohl parasympathische als auch sympathische Reize die Gefäßreaktionen nach CO_2-Atmung modifizieren (Abb. 27).

II. Einflüsse zentralnervöser Regionen bei der Regulation der lokalen Gehirndurchblutung

Außer den neuralen Einflüssen über den Halssympathikus oder den Vagus werden Stamm- oder Mittelhirnbereiche als wichtige, durchblutungskontrollierende Strukturen diskutiert. Auch hier sind die Befunde, die über die Auswirkungen von Aktivierungen dieser Regionen auf die Gehirndurchblutung erhoben wurden, nicht einheitlich. FLOREY (1925) reizte das Vasomotorenzentrum elektrisch und fand keine Änderungen der Piagefäßdurchmesser. SPINA (1898, 1900) reizte die Medulla und beobachtete Erweiterungen der Piagefäße. Die genaue Kontrolle der Lokalisation der Reizelektroden ergab (STAVRAKY, 1936), daß eine Konstriktion der Piagefäße dann auftrat, wenn die posteriore Region des Hypothalamus gereizt wurde. Die Konstriktion der Piagefäße war von Anzeichen einer sympathischen Erregung, z.B. Pupillendilatation und Steigerung des arteriellen Blutdrucks begleitet. Die Gefäßkonstriktion war schon nachweisbar, bevor Änderungen im Blutdruck oder in den Blutgaswerten erkennbar waren. Auch BLUM et al. (1977) berichten über blutdruckunabhängige Piagefäßreaktionen bei Hypothalamusreizung.

Reizungen des ventralen Anteils des Hypothalamus verursachte bilaterale Dilatation pialer Gefäße und einen Abfall des Blutdrucks, der mit einer Verminderung der Herzfrequenz kombiniert war. Reizungen im Bereich des Thalamus hatten Dilatation von Piagefäßen zur Folge, die aber keine Beziehung zu den arteriellen Blutdruckänderungen hatte. Die Möglichkeit, daß bestimmte Bezirke des Gehirnstamms in eine reflektorische Regulation der zerebralen Durchblutung eingeschaltet sind, ist auch von SHALIT et al. (1967b, 1969) diskutiert worden. Läsionen im Gehirnstamm hatten eine erhebliche Reduzierung der Gefäßreaktionen auf CO_2 zur Folge (Abb. 28). Wurde die Läsion durch lokale Kühlung hervorgerufen, so trat die veränderte Gefäßreaktion auf CO_2-

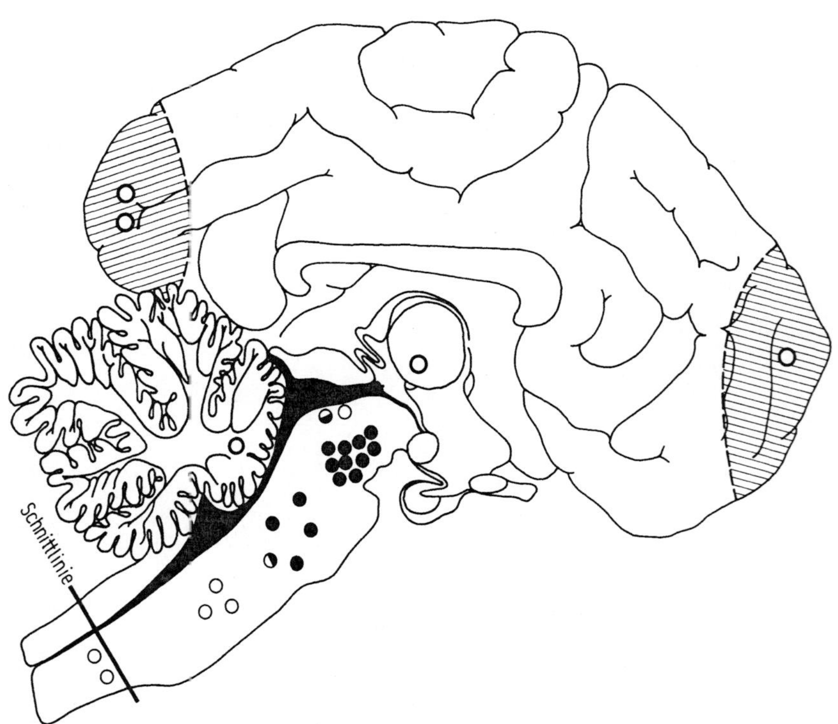

Abb. 28. Verteilung und Wirkung von Läsionen im Gehirn auf die Durchblutung des Gesamttieres bei Änderungen des arteriellen CO_2-Drucks. Die schwarz ausgefüllten Punkte kennzeichnen die Gehirnregionen, deren Schädigung zu einer Reduzierung der CO_2-bedingten Durchblutungsreaktion führte. Die offenen Kreise kennzeichnen Gehirnstrukturen, deren Schädigung zu keiner Veränderung der Gehirndurchblutung führte. Bei Läsionen in den Regionen, die durch halbausgefüllte Kreise gekennzeichnet sind, kam es zu geringen Veränderungen der Reaktivität auf CO_2. Die schraffiert gezeichneten Zonen sind Lobektomien. (Nach SHALIT et al., Acta Neurol. Psychiat. (Chic.) **17**, 337–341, 1967. Abb. 1)

Gabe ebenfalls auf. Bei Wiedererwärmung kam es zu einer Wiederherstellung der normalen Regulation. Auch diese Befunde geben einen Hinweis darauf, daß die Wirkung von CO_2 mit reflektorischen Veränderungen an den Gehirngefäßen gekoppelt ist. Neuere Untersuchungen von HASS et al. (1977) lassen erkennen, daß Änderungen des Energieumsatzes bei bilateralen Läsionen im Bereich der Formatio reticularis mit Durchblutungsänderungen gekoppelt sind. In der Regel werden schon eine Stunde nach bilateralen Läsionen der Formatio reticularis Verminderungen der Sauerstoffaufnahme des Gehirns gesehen und nach etwa 6 Stunden auch deutliche Verminderungen der Gehirndurchblutung.

III. Lokaler Gewebsstoffwechsel und neurogene Einflüsse auf den Gehirnkreislauf

Um die Frage untersuchen zu können, ob lokale Gewebsstoffwechseländerungen in den durch die Reize aktivierten Regionen oder die bei der Reizung freigesetzten Transmitter die Gefäßreaktionen hervorrufen, ist es notwendig, die lokalen Säure-Basen-Parameter und evtl. die die Gefäßreaktionen bestimmenden Faktoren lokal zu kontrollieren, denn HEUSER et al. (1975b) fanden, daß bei elektrischen Reizungen peripherer Nerven und gleichzeitiger Messung der Durchblutung und des pH im Bereich des Nucleus cuneatus mit den reizbedingten Änderungen der Durchblutung in der Regel Azidosen auftraten, die auf den Herd der Durchblutungssteigerung begrenzt waren. Bei Reizungen im Bereich der Formatio reticularis wiesen INGVAR und SÖDERBERG (1956, 1958) nach, daß die regionale Gehirndurchblutung während der Reizung anstieg, wobei im EEG eine Desynchronisierung auftrat. Die Änderung der elektrischen Hirnaktivität veranlaßte INGVAR und SÖDERBERG anzunehmen, daß die primäre Folge einer Gehirnreizung ein Anstieg des Gehirnstoffwechsels sei und daß die Durchblutungsveränderung als Konsequenz dieser Stoffwechselsteigerung betrachtet werden könne. Dagegen scheint zunächst die Geschwindigkeit der Änderung der pialen Gefäßdurchmesser zu sprechen. Es wird von PURVES (1972) mitgeteilt, daß die Änderungen der Piagefäßreaktionen bei nervalen Reizen sehr schnell – in wenigen Sekunden – auftreten, während bei Azidosen, die durch Stoffwechseländerungen bedingt sind, eine Zeit von etwa 20–30 Sekunden nötig wird, um eine Gefäßerweiterung zu bewirken. Bei perivaskulärer Mikroperfusion (durch Umspülen der Gefäße mit azidotischem Liquor erzeugt) ist diese Zeit etwas kürzer (eigene Experimente), so daß das Argument, daß metabolische Änderungen im perivaskulären Raum zur Erzeugung einer Gefäßreaktion eine wesentlich längere Zeit benötigen als die neural vermittelten, mit Wahrscheinlichkeit in der von PURVES formulierten Schärfe nicht zutrifft. Zudem sind letztlich an der Gefäßmuskulatur, die den Widerstand des Gehirngefäßsystems reguliert, Freisetzungen von Transmittern immer mit metabolischen Änderungen an Membranen gekoppelt und es ist nicht unbedingt notwendig, daß die Wasserstoffionen als entscheidende Stellglieder angesehen werden müssen, denn membranbedingte Veränderungen können genau so gut durch Kalziumverschiebungen oder Verschiebungen des Kaliums an der Zellmembran hervorgerufen werden. Im strengen Sinne kann nur schwer zwischen metabolischer Kontrolle und neuraler Kontrolle am Wirkort, d.h. an der glatten Muskelzelle, unterschieden werden. Im folgenden Kapitel wird gezeigt, daß die glatten Muskelzellen auf die Interaktion von Transmittern des vegetativen Systems und lokal entstehende Metaboliten reagieren. Das Problem der neuralen Kontrolle muß daher anders gefaßt werden. Als neurale Kontrolle sollte die Vermittlung von Signalen über eine Nervenbahn an die glatten Muskelzellen verstanden werden, wobei es für die Reaktion in der Muskelzelle unwichtig ist, ob die Nervenbahn aus dem Inneren des Gehirns oder aus Regionen außerhalb des Schädelinnenraums an die Hirngefäße heranzieht. Die am Wirkort freigesetzten Transmitter werden in ihren Effekten durch die lokalen Stoffwechselbedingungen mehr oder weniger stark modifiziert.

Alle nervalen und metabolisch bedingten Reaktionen des Gehirngefäßsystems weisen darauf hin, daß für das Verständnis der Tonusregulation die Notwendigkeit besteht, Untersuchungen an den glatten Muskelzellen der Gehirngefäße selbst durchzuführen. In den folgenden Kapiteln sind daher solche Basismechanismen näher betrachtet, wobei gesagt werden muß, daß bisher relativ geringe Informationen über die Physiologie der Gefäßmuskelzellen des Gehirngefäßsystems vorliegen.

K. Die Rolle der glatten Gefäßmuskulatur bei der Durchblutungsregulation des Gehirns

I. Funktion von Gefäßmuskelzellen

Bei der Autoregulation der Durchblutung, bei der Wirkung von nerval übertragenen Reizen und bei der Übermittlung von Signalen, die die Gefäße über die Erfordernisse des lokalen Hirngewebsstoffwechsels an die Durchblutung informieren, spielen Gefäßmuskeln des Gehirngefäßsystems eine entscheidende Rolle. Sie stellen durch Erweiterung oder Verengerung von Hirngefäßen den lokalen Gefäßwiderstand ein und regulieren die Blutverteilung in den nachgeschalteten Kapillaren. Jeder Reiz, sei er elektrisch, mechanisch, metabolisch oder nervös, führt letzten Endes zu einer Reaktion der kontraktilen oder viskoelastischen Strukturen, d.h., es tritt eine zum Teil kompliziert verknüpfte Kette von Ereignissen auf, die eine Dilatation oder Konstriktion der muskulären Gehirngefäße bewirkt.

Die glatte Muskelzelle unterscheidet sich von der quer gestreiften im wesentlichen dadurch, daß eine regelmäßige Anordnung von dicken und dünnen Filamenten fehlt und daß kein gleichartiges Tubulussystem vorhanden ist. Außerdem ist die Koppelung zwischen der Zellmembran und den kontraktilen Elementen direkter, und die Faserdurchmesser sind dünner. Die Erforschung der glatten Muskelzellen gestalet sich insofern schwierig als ihre Eigenschaften in den verschiedenen glattmuskulären Organen unterschiedlich sind und erhebliche Differenzen bei den untersuchten Spezies bestehen. Da die Eigenschaften der glatten Muskelzellen am Gehirngefäßsystem bisher wenig untersucht wurden, müssen für eine Reihe von Problemen Untersuchungen anderer glattmuskulärer Organe als Modelle dienen. Entsprechend kann daraus oft nur indirekt und mit Vorbehalten auf die Funktionen der Gefäßmuskulatur im Gehirn geschlossen werden.

Bei der Definition des glatt-muskulären Tonus unterscheiden wir zwischen tetanischem Tonus und nichttetanischem Tonus. Beim tetanischen Tonus werden zwei Arten differenziert. Wenn er von der Reizung durch Nerven abhängig ist, spricht man vom neurogenen Tonus, der bei einer Reihe von Gefäßmuskeln wirksam ist (BURNSTOCK, 1969). Der myogene Tonus ist nicht von nervöser Reizung abhängig. Er tritt spontan und in isolierten, nervenfreien Präparationen auf. Typische Beispiele glatter Muskeln, die myogenen Tonus entwikkeln, sind intestinale Muskeln oder der Uterus, aber auch manche Gefäßmuskeln (HOLMAN, 1969; JEWELL u. WILKIE, 1960). Bei dieser Tonusart entsteht die Erregung spontan in einer Gruppe von glatten Muskelzellen, die als Schrittmacherzellen bezeichnet werden und von denen sich Aktionspotentiale auf die umgebenden glatten Muskelzellen durch tight junctions ausbreiten. Die Ausbreitungsgeschwindigkeit der Erregung ist in der Regel langsam. Da die betroffenen Muskelzellen entsprechend der funktionellen Verknüpfung einheitlich reagieren, spricht man auch von einer single unit (BOZLER, 1948), während die neurogen erregten Zellen als multi units funktionieren. In der Aktivierung der Erregung spielt Kalzium eine entscheidende Rolle (Übersichten s. RÜEGG, 1971; HUBBARD, 1973).

Der nichttetanische Tonus tritt auf, wenn Kalzium-Ionen in das Sarkoplasma ohne Membranerregung eingeschleust werden. In diesem Falle ist die Spannungsentwicklung nicht mit der Frequenz oder der Anwesenheit von Aktionspotentialen korreliert. BOHR und UCHIDA (1969) sowie SOMLYO und SOMLYO (1968a) nehmen an, daß sich der nichttetanische Tonus vermittels einer nichtelektrischen Kopplung durch Neurotransmitter ausbreitet. Auch in diesem Fall spielen Kalziumionen bei der Kontraktion eine entscheidende Rolle. Typische Beispiele solcher nichttetanischer Spannungsänderungen sind der plastische Tonus oder der visköse Tonus.

Sowohl bei tetanischem Tonus als auch beim nichttetanischen Tonus ist ein Anstieg des freien intrazellulären Kalziums für die Kontraktion wichtig. Das Kalzium überträgt die Information aus dem Sarkoplasma an jede Myofibrille. Wenn dort das Kalzium gebunden wird, resultiert eine Kontraktion (WEBER, 1966; WEBER u. HERZ, 1963; WEBER u. MURRAY, 1973) und leitet damit eine Steigerung des Energieverbrauchs durch die Kontraktion ein. Die Umsatzrate ist bei langsamen tonischen Kontraktionen geringer als beim Tetanus schneller Muskeln.

II. Die Wirkung von CO_2 und Hypoxie auf die Gefäßmuskulatur

Die CO_2-Wirkung ist, wie aus den vorhergehenden Kapiteln bereits erkenntlich, komplexer Natur. Eine CO_2-Atmung ändert neben dem arteriellen Blutdruck die Aktivität des Gehirns und infolgedessen die Konzentration der an den lokalen Gefäßen direkt angreifenden Stoffwechselprodukte. Sie wirkt zudem auf die Chemorezeptoren und damit auf nervös-metabolischem Wege auf das Gehirngefäßsystem. Ihre Wirkung auf die Nebenniere verursacht eine Änderung der Katecholaminausschüttung. Diese Komplexität der Wirkungen ist eine Ursache dafür, daß bisher nicht entschieden werden kann, ob nur lokal direkte molekulare Wirkungen des Kohlendioxyds auf das Gehirngefäßsystem für CO_2-bedingte Reaktionen wichtig sind. Anhaltspunkte dafür, daß die jede CO_2-Änderung begleitenden pH-Veränderungen eine wichtige Rolle spielen, sind häufig. LASSEN (1968a) nimmt an, daß das extrazelluläre pH an der Gefäßmuskulatur ein Hauptfaktor für die Kontrolle des Gehirngefäßwiderstandes ist.

Wie bereits dargestellt, verursacht eine Atmung von CO_2-angereicherten Gasgemischen eine Dilatation der Gehirngefäße und eine Verminderung des CO_2-Gehalts, eine Konstriktion. Injiziert man jedoch Bikarbonat ins Blut, so steigt der CO_2-Druck im Blut an, gleichzeitig wird das Blut alkalischer. Es erweist sich nun, daß zwischen der Änderung des Blut-pH und der Gehirndurchblutung keine feste Kopplung besteht, denn trotz der Alkalose kommt es sofort nach Injektion zu einer Dilatation der Gehirngefäße (Abb. 29). Diese Dilatation ist dadurch verursacht, daß das CO_2, das bei einer Bikarbonatinfusion den CO_2-Druck im Blut erhöht, sehr schnell durch die Bluthirnschranke diffundiert und im extrazellulären Raum eine Azidose bewirkt, da die Bikarbonationen nicht so schnell durch die Bluthirnschranke zu folgen vermögen. MEYER (1966) teilte mit, daß lokale Applikation von CO_2 auf die Gehirnoberfläche zu einer Dilatation der Oberflächengefäße führte, wobei allerdings nicht entschieden ist, ob CO_2 in molekularer Form oder wegen seiner pH-verändernden Wirkung die Dilatation verursachte.

In welcher Weise eine generelle Hypoxämie auf die Muskulatur des Gehirngefäßsystems wirkt, ist bisher noch nicht ganz geklärt. Man weiß, daß schon bei mäßig ausgeprägten Hypoxien Durchblutungssteigerungen mit Verminderungen der Gefäßwiderstände des Gehirns auftreten. Bei fortlaufender Registrierung der Durchblutung, des Sauerstoffdrucks, des CO_2-Drucks und des pH-Werts auf der Gehirnoberfläche sowie des arteriellen Blutdrucks (BETZ u. HEUSER, 1967) war erkennbar, daß die Reaktion der Gehirndurchblutung schon einsetzt, wenn noch keine Azidose der Gehirnoberfläche nachweisbar ist. Innerhalb der ersten Minute einer Hypoxie steigt die Gehirndurchblutung bereits steil an, wobei es oft zu einer hyperventilatorisch bedingten Verminderung der Wasserstoff-Ionenkonzentration, sowohl im Blut als auch auf der Gehirnoberfläche, kommen kann. Sogar bei künstlicher Beatmung kann initial eine kortikale Alkalose auftreten (ASTRUP et al., 1978). Zwar setzt bei einer schweren Hypoxie nach einer kurzen Latenzperiode die Anreicherung von Wasserstoff-Ionen im Gehirngewebe ein, jedoch ist schwer erklärbar, daß über diesen Weg die initiale Durchblutungssteigerung erfolgt. Es ist auch schlecht vorstellbar, daß schon ein geringfügig erniedrigter, lokaler Sauerstoffdruck in den glatten Muskeln der durchbluteten Widerstandsgefäße die primäre Ursache für die Steigerung der Gehirndurchblutung bei Beginn einer mäßig ausgeprägten Hypoxie ist, denn die Gefäßwände sind in direktem Kontakt mit dem noch sauerstoffreichen arteriellen Blut, während entfernter gelegene Orte im Gewebe bei einer mäßigen Hypoxie eher anoxisch werden, entsprechend den Vorstellungen, die aus den Versorgungsmodellen des Gehirngewebes entwickelt worden sind (THEWS, 1960; LÜBBERS, 1968; GRUNEWALD, 1968; METZGER, 1972). Ob unter O_2-Mangel durch eine andersartige Blutverteilung die

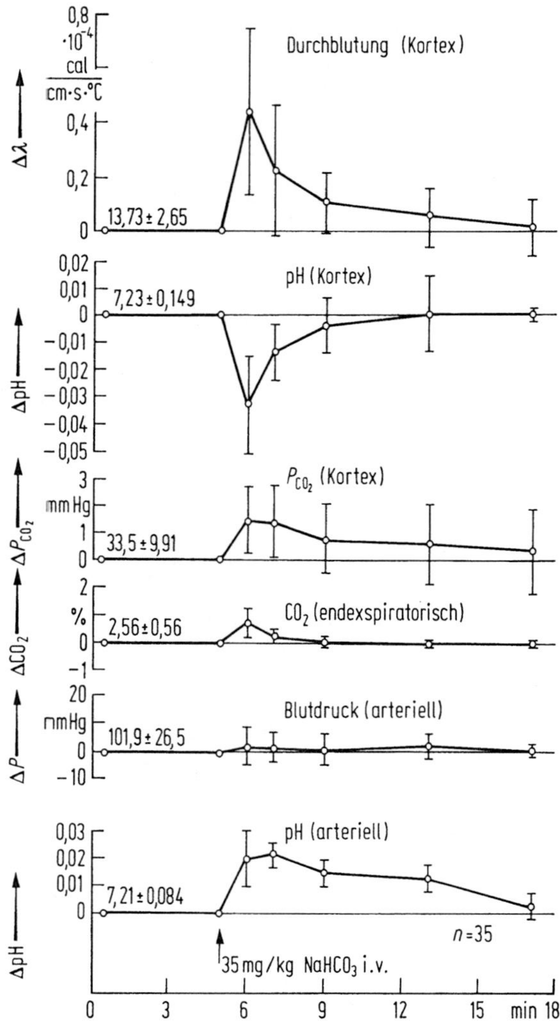

Abb. 29. Änderungen der lokalen kortikalen Durchblutung, des kortikalen pH, des kortikalen P_{CO_2}, der endexspiratorischen CO_2-Konzentration, des mittleren arteriellen Blutdrucks und des arteriellen pH vor sowie 1, 2, 4, 8 und 12 min nach intravenöser Injektion einer Bikarbonatlösung. Mittelwerte von 35 Experimenten. Die Injektion wurde vorgenommen, wenn die Werte wenigstens 8 min vorher konstant geblieben waren. Die mittleren Initialwerte (Absolutwerte) betrugen: Durchblutung: $13{,}8 \pm 2{,}1 \cdot 10^{-4}$ cal·cm^{-1}·s^{-1}·°C^{-1} ≈ 0,96 ml·g^{-1}·min^{-1}. Kortikales pH: 7,23. Kortikaler P_{CO_2}: 33,5 mm Hg. Endexspiratorische CO_2-Konzentration: 2,56. Blutdruck: 101,9 mm Hg. Arterielles pH: 7,21. Diese Werte sind als Zahlenwerte dargestellt. Die Änderungen von den jeweiligen, etwas unterschiedlichen Ausgangswerten sind mit den Standardabweichungen dargestellt. (Nach BETZ u. HEUSER: J. appl. Physiol. **23**, 726, 1967)

höhere Durchströmung erklärbar ist, bedarf noch des Nachweises. Bei Beobachtung der Gefäßmusteränderung auf der Gehirnoberfläche gewinnt man den Eindruck, daß Gefäße eröffnet werden, die vorher so niedrig durchströmt waren, daß eine Blutsäule darin kaum oder gar nicht sichtbar war. Möglicherweise kann ein Übergang von „Plasmaskimming" zu Erythrozytenpassage an diesen Änderungen beteiligt sein (ROSENBLUM, 1972). Es ist von KORNMÜLLER et al. (1941) und SCHAERTLIN (1961) berichtet worden, daß das EEG sich schon verändert, wenn der zerebralvenöse Sauerstoffdruck auf Werte zwischen 29 und 23 mm Hg abfällt. Diese Beziehung zwischen EEG-Veränderungen und zerebralvenösem Sauerstoffdruck ist vor allem bei der Einleitung einer Hypoxie beobachtbar, so daß nicht ausgeschlossen werden kann, daß auch in der steilen ersten Phase eine Beziehung zwischen dem Funktionszustand des Gehirns und der Gehirndurchblutung besteht. Über Transmitteränderungen bei derartigen schnellen Reaktionen ist bisher am Gehirngefäßsystem nichts bekannt. Die Rolle der Adenosinbildung infolge Sauerstoffmangel bei der Regulation der Gehirndurchblutung ist auf S. 242 beschrieben.

Die in den folgenden Kapiteln dargestellten ionalen Interaktionen erklären möglicherweise auch die beim Sauerstoffmangel auftretenden schnellen Gefäßerweiterungen.

HEUSER (1978) konnte zeigen, daß im Gehirngewebe beim Sauerstoffmangel etwa gleichzeitig mit der Erhöhung der lokalen Durchblutung eine Steigerung der Kaliumionenaktivität auftrat.

III. Ionen und Kontraktion glatter Muskeln

Sowohl passive als auch aktive Änderungen von Ionenkonzentrationen an der Membran glatter Muskelzellen können deren Kontraktionszustand beeinflussen (Literatur s. in CASTEELS et al., 1977). Die folgenden Befunde geben nur ein sehr lückenhaftes und unvollständiges Bild dieses in vollem Fluß befindlichen Forschungsgebiets. Es wird auf Übersichten von KURIYAMA et al. (1976), HUDDART und PRICE (1976), SOMLYO und SOMLYO (1976) verwiesen.

Man nimmt an, daß in den Membranen glatter Muskeln Natriumpumpen, Kaliumpumpen und Chloridpumpen existieren. Die Permeabilitätskonstanten der Membran glatter Muskelzellen für Natrium und Kalium sind andere als in der Skeletmuskulatur. Das Verhältnis von P_{Na}/P_K ist für glatte Muskeln höher als für quergestreifte. Als Ruhepotential der Zellen werden Werte zwischen -35 mV und ca. -55 mV angenommen (CASTEELS et al., 1971; SOMLYO u. SOMLYO, 1968a, b). In zerebralen Gefäßmuskeln wurde 35,8 mV gemessen (SIEGEL et al., 1974a, b). Bei den Permeabilitätsänderungen für Natrium und Kalium spielt anscheinend Calcium eine Rolle, wobei angenommen wurde, daß Ca^{++} die Natriumpermeabilität an der Außenseite der Membran beeinflußt. An der Innenseite soll dagegen Kalium die Natriumpermeabilität kontrollieren (BRADING, 1973; BRADING et al., 1969). Die Wirkungen von Kalzium sind komplexer als die der univalenten Ionen. Einige seiner Membranwirkungen resultieren daraus, daß die Permeabilität für andere Ionen (besonders der Kalium- und Natriumionen) modifiziert wird, andere aus kalziumeigenen elektrischen Aktionen.

Hohe Kalziumkonzentration auf der Außenseite steigert die Permeabilität für Kalium und erniedrigt das Verhältnis von P_{Na}/P_K. Aus der Analyse von Kalziumauswaschkurven wurde die Schlußfolgerung gezogen, daß drei Kalziumkompartimente in den Zellen vorliegen. Die schnellste Komponente der Auswaschkurve repräsentiert das extrazelluläre Kalziumkompartiment. Die zweite Komponente repräsentiert wahrscheinlich die Kalziumbindung in den Zellen und Vesikeln der Zellmembranen (GOODFORD u. WOLOWYK, 1972). Das dritte Kompartiment wird als intrazelluläres Kompartiment bezeichnet. Ein Teil davon ist austauschbar, der andere Teil nicht oder jedenfalls nicht in den Zeiten, in denen Auswaschkurven registriert wurden (WEISS u. GOODMAN, 1969). Der Kalziumeinstrom in glatte Muskelzellen wird durch erregende Agentien, die depolarisieren, erhöht. Die Kontraktion braucht Kalzium auf, das durch einen Einstrom aus dem extrazellulären Raum, aus dem in intrazellulären Räumen liegenden Kalzium sowie aus Membranspeichern verfügbar wird.

Die in den glatten Muskeln existierenden Natrium-Kaliumpumpen können durch Stoffwechselhemmstoffe, z.B. DNP, ausgeschaltet werden. Glatte Muskeln variieren hinsichtlich der Bedeutung des Natriumkanals. Nach Ergebnissen von WAHL et al. (1973) führt eine starke Reduktion von Na^+ im perivaskulären Raum zu einer Gefäßkonstriktion. Bei dieser Reduktion wurde allerdings gleichzeitig Cl^- vermindert. Es ist aber nicht klar, ob eine Interferenz zwischen Natrium und Kalzium besteht, d.h. ob Natrium den Kalziumausstrom beeinflußt, ob es parallele Kanäle gibt oder ob beide Ionen um ein gemeinsames Carriermolekül konkurrieren. Auch der Mechanismus der Repolarisationsphase ist unklar. Anhaltspunkte für einen Kaliumeinstrom sind bei einigen Muskeln vorhanden, aber auch Kalziumbindung allein kann eine Repolarisation hervorbringen. Die Chloridpumpe in der Membran glatter Muskeln soll nach CASTEELS et al. (1971) Na/K gekoppelt sein. Das Gleichgewichtspotential des Chlorids glatter Muskelzellen ist geringer als das Gleichgewichtspotential des Chlorids der Skeletmuskelzellen, so daß geschlossen werden kann, daß eine ziemlich hohe Chloridinnenkonzentration gegen ein steiles elektrochemisches Gefälle aufrecht erhalten wird.

IV. Die Wirkungen von Ionen auf die glatte Muskulatur der Gehirngefäße

1. Wasserstoffionen

In früheren Untersuchungen zur Beziehung des Blut-pH-Wertes zur Gehirndurchblutung konnten KETY et al. (1948 b) keine Veränderung der Gehirndurchblutung bei Patienten mit diabetischer Azidose feststellen. SCHIEVE und WILSON (1952, 1953) fanden keine Beziehung von Blutacidose oder -alkalose zur Gehirndurchblutung und HARPER und BELL (1963) zeigten bei Hunden, daß bei arteriellen pH-Änderungen zwischen 6,7 und 7,8 keine Beziehung von Gehirndurchblutung und Plasma-pH nachzuweisen war. Das Fehlen dieser Beziehung wird darauf zurückgeführt, daß zwischen Blut und interstitiellem Raum der Gefäßmuskeln eine Schranke für Wasserstoffionen besteht, die erklärt, daß eine metabolische Acidose oder Alkalose im arteriellen Blut nicht von

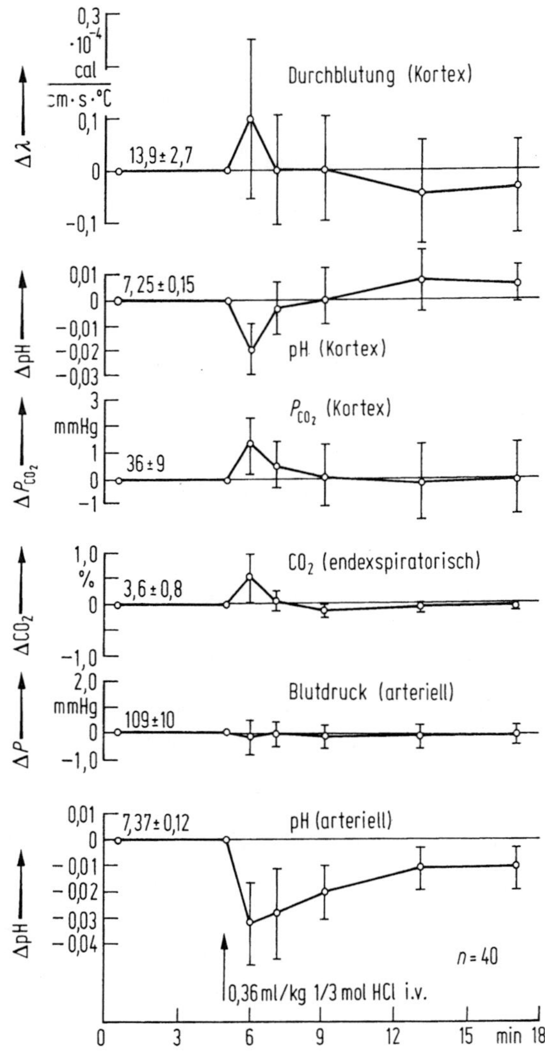

Abb. 30. Die Wirkung von intravenöser Injektion von 0,36 ml/kg $^1/_3$ mol HCl. Die Messungen stellen, wie diejenigen der Abb. 29, Mittelwerte dar (40 Experimente). Die Ausgangswerte in Absolutzahlen sind an den jeweiligen Kurven aufgetragen. Im übrigen gilt die Legende der Abb. 29 entsprechend. (Nach BETZ u. HEUSER: J. appl. Physiol. **23**, 726, 1967)

einer entsprechenden Änderung im extravaskulären Raum begleitet ist. Schon ROBIN et al. (1958) hatten gefunden, daß Säureinjektion ins Plasma sogar von einer paradoxen Reaktion des pH im Liquor cerebrospinalis gefolgt wird. Eigene Untersuchungen (BETZ u. HEUSER, 1967) bestätigen diese Effekte, wobei eine leichte Abweichung von den Befunden von ROBIN erkennbar ist. Die in Abb. 30 dargestellten Reaktionen werden so erklärt, daß nach der Injektion von Säure ins Blut die starke Säure die schwache aus ihren Bindungen verdrängt und dadurch zu einem Freiwerden von CO_2 beiträgt. Das CO_2 vermag schnell in den perivaskulären Raum zu diffundieren, verursacht hier vorübergehend eine CO_2-Erhöhung mit leichter Azidose. Die Durchblutung steigt kurzzeitig an. Gleichzeitig reizt CO_2 jedoch die Chemorezeptoren und es kommt zu einer Hyperventilation. Diese bewirkt, daß CO_2 schnell wieder abgeatmet wird und damit die ursprüngliche Azidose in eine mehr alkalische Richtung umschlägt, so daß in der zweiten Phase dieser Reaktion im Blut zwar eine Azidose bestehen bleibt, im perivaskulären Raum jedoch eine leichte Alkalose auftritt. Diese Veränderungen wurden nur über relativ kurze Zeit verfolgt, da im Verlauf länger dauernder schwerer Azidosen, im Blut sich zusätzliche Veränderungen einstellen, die dieses Phänomen wieder modifizieren. Um die Wirkungen von Wasserstoffionen auf die Gefäßwiderstände direkt zu überprüfen, haben ELLIOT u. JASPER (1949) in die Umgebung von Piagefäßen ungepufferte Säurelösungen gebracht und eine Gefäßerweiterung beobachtet. Die Ergebnisse solcher Experimente wurden später von WAHL et al. (1970), KNABE und BETZ (1972) sowie von BÖNING (1972) bestätigt. Mit Hilfe von Mikropipetten, deren Spitze im perivaskulären Raum kleiner Piagefäße fixiert war, wurden Mikroperfusionen des perivaskulären Raums durchgeführt und das betroffene Gefäß gefilmt oder fotografiert. Änderungen der Gefäßweite konnten so gemessen und dokumentiert werden. Ein charakteristisches Beispiel der dilatierenden Wirkung von Wasserstoffionen auf die glatte Muskulatur einer kleinen Gehirnarterie zeigt die Abb. 31. Kleine Gehirnvenen reagierten unter gleichen Bedingungen kaum oder gar nicht. Bei extrazellulärer Azidose von isolierten Gehirnarterien wurde von SIEGEL et al. (1974a) eine Hyperpolarisation der Membran glatter Muskelzellen gemessen (−4,3 mV bei einem Übergang von pH 7,3 auf 6,8) und bei Alkalose eine Depolarisation (+ 3,4 mV bei Änderung des pH von 7,3 auf 7,8).

Es ist von anderen Muskeln bekannt, daß Erniedrigungen der H^+-Konzentration zu einer Aktivierung von Ca^{++}-aktivierbaren ATP'asen führt (FLECKENSTEIN u. GRÜN, 1972; GRÜN, 1972). Auch wird durch Änderung der Azidität der Dissoziationsgrad von Kalzium beeinflußt. Die Kette der pH-abhängigen, biochemischen Wirkungsmechanismen bei der Kontraktion ist noch hypothetisch.

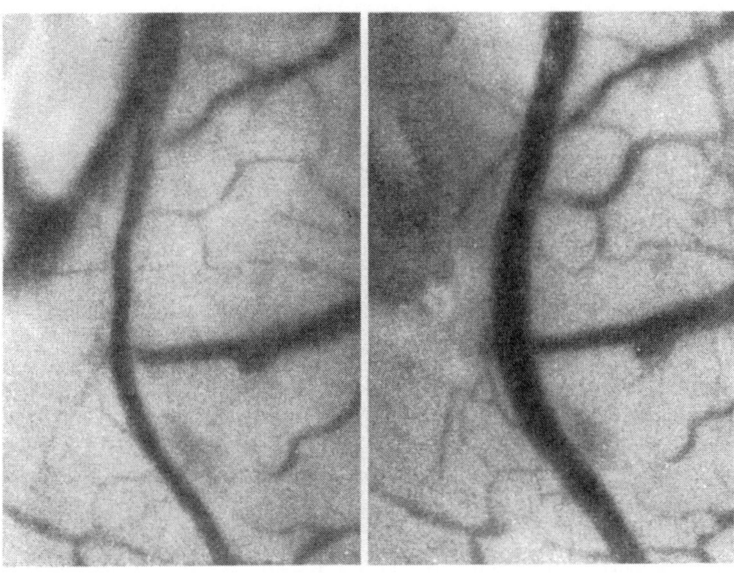

Abb. 31. Die Wirkung einer Änderung der H^+-Ionenaktivität auf eine Piaarterie. Das enger gewordene Gefäß wurde mit Liquor umspült, der ein pH von 8,0 aufwies. Kontrolle pH: 7,23

2. Kaliumionen und Gehirngefäße

SCHINDLER et al. (1973) und SCHINDLER (1974) untersuchten Änderungen der H^+-Aktivität sowie der K^+-Konzentration im Liquor cerebrospinalis bei Katzen mit schwerer Azidose und fanden unter diesen Bedingungen eine Erhöhung der Kaliumgehalte. Die Gefäßmuskulatur in anderen Organen reagiert bei Azidose mit Kaliumeffluxänderungen (CASTEELS, 1970). Zwischen Kaliumänderungen und Wasserstoffionenänderungen besteht also eine Beziehung. Bei Gehirnischämien folgt die Änderung des Kaliumausstroms in den Liquor der Änderung der Wasserstoffionenaktivität in einem gewissen zeitlichen Abstand (HEUSER et al., 1975a).

Aus der Kopplung von Azidosen mit Kaliumänderungen ergibt sich zwangsläufig die Frage, ob Kalium selbst als dilatierendes Agens eine Rolle spielt. KUSCHINSKY et al. (1971/72, 1972), KNABE und BETZ (1972), BÖNING (1972), sowie TODA (1974) haben bei ihren Experimenten gezeigt, daß die Erhöhung der Kaliumkonzentration im extravaskulären Raum eine Erweiterung des Gehirngefäßsystems bewirkt. Systematische Untersuchungen der Wirkung von Kaliumionen auf die Weite von Pia-Arteriolen und kleinen Arterien ergaben, daß es bei Mikroperfusionen des perivaskulären Raums mit leichter Erhöhung der Kaliumkonzentration zu einer Erweiterung, bei Fehlen von K^+ sowie bei sehr starker K^+-Erhöhung zu einer Konstriktion kommt (Abb. 32). Man kann die Ergebnisse aus dieser Abbildung nicht ohne Einschränkung auf künstlich perfundierte Gefäße übertragen, denn bei den in Abb. 31 dargestellten Versuchen ist das Gefäßinnere mit normalem Blut perfundiert und die Änderung der K^+-Aktivität ist auf den perivaskulären Raum beschränkt. Beim Vergleich mit gleichzeitiger perivaskulärer und intravaskulärer Kaliumionenveränderung ergeben sich somit etwas andere Konzentrations-Wirkungsbeziehungen. KONOLD et al. (1968) berichten, daß auch an extrazerebralen Gefäßen hohe K^+-Konzentrationen zu einer Kontraktur führen.

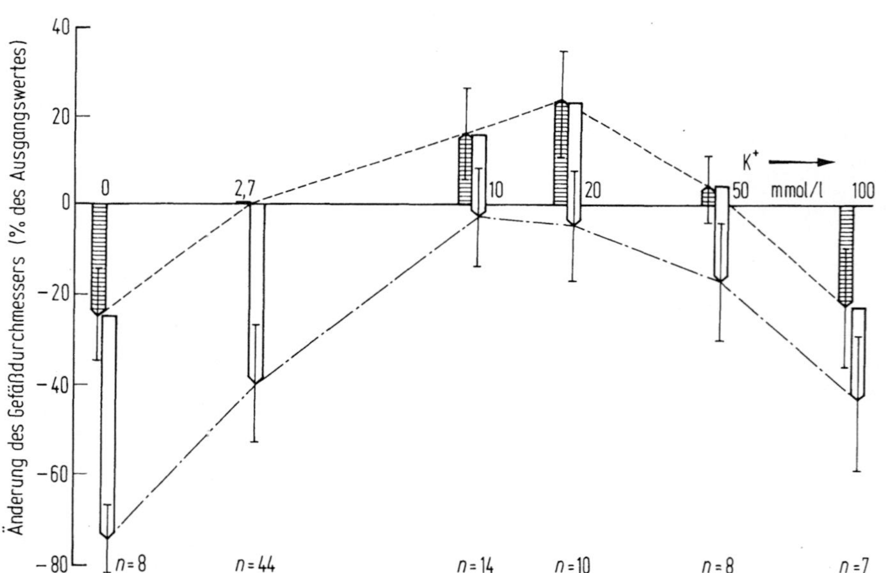

Abb. 32. Die schraffierten Säulen stellen Änderung der Durchmesser von kleinen Piaarterien (Durchmesser zwischen 75–200 μm) bei perivaskulärer Perfusion mit künstlichem Liquor zerebrospinalis dar, dessen K^+-Konzentration verändert wurde (bei sonst normaler Ionenzusammensetzung des Liquors). Positive Werte auf der Ordinate sind Dilatationen, negative Werte sind Konstriktionen. Auf der Abszisse sind die K^+-Konzentrationen dargestellt. Der perivaskuläre Raum kleiner Piagefäße wurde mittels Mikropipetten perfundiert. Die weißen Säulen stellen die lokale Reaktion der durch elektrischen Strom (3 mA, 10 Imp/s, Reizdauer 10 s) gereizten, umspülten Gefäßabschnitte dar. Man erkennt, daß die Gefäße auf elektrischen Reiz mit unterschiedlich starker Konstriktion reagieren, die von der perivaskulären K^+-Konzentration abhängig ist. (Nach BETZ in Hdb. exp. Pharmakol. XVI Teil 3, Heart and Circulation. Eds.: SCHMIER u. EICHLER, 1975, p. 204)

Schon KNABE und BETZ (1972), BETZ (1972b) sowie KUSCHINSKY et al. (1972) haben mitgeteilt, daß zwischen den Effekten von Kalium- und Wasserstoffionenänderungen auf die Gefäßmuskulatur eine Wechselwirkung besteht. Messungen von Membranpotentialen an Gehirngefäßmuskelzellen bestätigen diese Interaktion (SIEGEL et al., 1974a, b). Kaliumbedingte Dilatationen sind weniger stark ausgeprägt, wenn gleichzeitig eine Alkalose vorliegt. Bei einer Azidose bewirkt eine Verminderung der perivaskulären Kaliumaktivität eine schwächere Dilatation des umspülten Gefäßes als bei Verwendung von Liquor cerebrospinalis mit normalem pH.

3. Einfluß von Kalziumionen

Wie in allen erregbaren Strukturen des Organismus spielt das Kalzium auch an der Membran glatter Muskelzellen beim Zustandekommen eines Aktionspotentials eine wichtige Rolle. Darüber hinaus ist es bei der elektromechanischen Kopplung und der Aktin-Myosininteraktion beteiligt, so daß es als ein zentral in die Muskelaktion eingeschaltetes Glied betrachtet werden muß (GRÜN, 1972).

Es besteht eine Parallelität der Verkürzungsgeschwindigkeit der kontraktilen Elemente der glatten Muskelzelle mit der ATPase-Aktivität ihres Aktin-aktivierten Myosins (BARANY, 1967). Das bedeutet für die glatte Muskulatur, daß die Verkürzungsgeschwindigkeit die Aktomyosin-ATPase-Aktivität als begrenzenden Faktor hat. Dies wiederum führt zu einem relativ niedrigen Bedarf an freiem, aktivierendem Kalzium. Von BOHR (1973) wird angenommen, daß die Parallelität zwischen dem Kalziumbedarf für die enzymatische Aktivität und für die physikalische Änderung ein Zeichen dafür ist, daß die physikalische Längenänderung direkt von der enzymatischen Aktivität, welche Energie aus dem ATP freisetzt, abhängig ist.

Beobachtungen von EBASHI und ENDO (1968) liefern Hinweise dafür, daß das Kalzium sich auch in manchen glatten Muskeln mit dem Troponin verbindet, – ähnlich wie im Skelettmuskel. Das Troponin-Tropomyosin-System, das beim Skelettmuskel die ATPase-Aktivität des Aktomyosins verhindert und bei Kalziumeinwirkung diese Aktivität nicht mehr hemmen kann, – was eine Kontraktion des Systems zur Folge hat –, scheint aber nach Untersuchungen von MRWA und RÜEGG (1976) nicht genau in der gleichen Weise zu funktionieren wie am Skelettmuskel. Troponin als für die Kontraktion hemmend wirkende Substanz fehlt in einer Reihe von Arterienwandmuskeln und es wird von den erwähnten Autoren angenommen, daß Kalzium an leichten Ketten des glattmuskulären Myosins angreift und hier seine regulatorischen kontraktilen Wirkungen entfaltet. Das für die Kontraktionslösung notwendige Kalzium wird dadurch bereit gestellt, daß sich freies Kalzium (Aktivator-Kalzium) im intrazellulären Raum anreichert. Wie das Schema in Abb. 33 darstellt, kann dieses aus dem extrazellulären Raum, aus Membranvesikeln, aus intrazellulären Strukturen, z.B. dem sarkoplasmatischen Retikulum wie aus Mitochondrien stammen. Die Konzentration des freien Kalziums ergibt sich aus der Bilanz von Abgabe und Aufnahme durch diese Kompartimente. Es ist aus dem Schema (Abb. 33) ableitbar, daß sowohl Reize, die an der Membran auftreten und die Membranvesikel zur Entleerung von Kalzium veranlassen, als auch experimentelle Erhöhung des extrazellulären Kalziums zum gleichen Effekt, nämlich zu einer Kontraktion führen. Bei diesem in Abb. 33 dargestellten Schema handelt es sich allerdings um ein Schema, bei dem Troponin als Regulatorprotein vorliegt. Es ist also nicht direkt auf alle glatten Muskeln anzuwenden. Eine Übersicht über die elektromechanischen Kopplungen in glatten Muskeln ist von CASTEELS et al. (1977) gegeben worden. In dieser Übersicht (Symposium) ist (S. 155–239) speziell auch die Frage der Rolle der subzellulären Strukturen bei der Kalziumhomöostase diskutiert worden. Aus dem extrazellulären Raum wird in die glatte Muskelzelle um so mehr Kalzium/Zeiteinheit aufgenommen, je höher die extrazelluläre Kalziumkonzentration ist (LÜLLMANN u. SIEGFRIEDT, 1968). Bei diesen Kalziumaufnahmen limitiert extrazelluläres Magnesium deren Geschwindigkeit. Nach den Untersuchungen von HATTINGBERG und KLAUS (1966), SCHATZMANN (1961) sowie Berichten von LÜLLMANN (1970) sind Transmitter, wie Adrenalin oder Azetylcholin, fast ohne Wirkung auf den Kalziumefflux und -influx an glatten Muskelzellen der Taenia coli. Ganz geringe, eben nachweisbare Erhöhungen des Efflux scheinen jedoch vorhanden zu sein.

Bei den bisher vorliegenden Messungen sind bei der Analyse von Kalziumverschiebungen in der Regel Konzentrationsmessungen mit flammenphotometrischen Methoden oder radioaktivem Kalzium durchgeführt worden. Die notwendigen Aktivitätsmessungen sind erst durch die Entwicklung von kalziumionensensitiven Mikroelektroden möglich geworden, die auf dem Ionenaustauscherprinzip beruhen (AMMANN et al., 1976).

Inzwischen liegen auch die ersten Untersuchungen der Beziehung von Gehirndurchblutung zu lokalen Veränderungen der Kalziumionenaktivität vor. Von BETZ und HEUSER (1977) und HEUSER (1978) wurde berichtet, daß bei wenigen Sekunden dauernden elektrischen Reizungen von

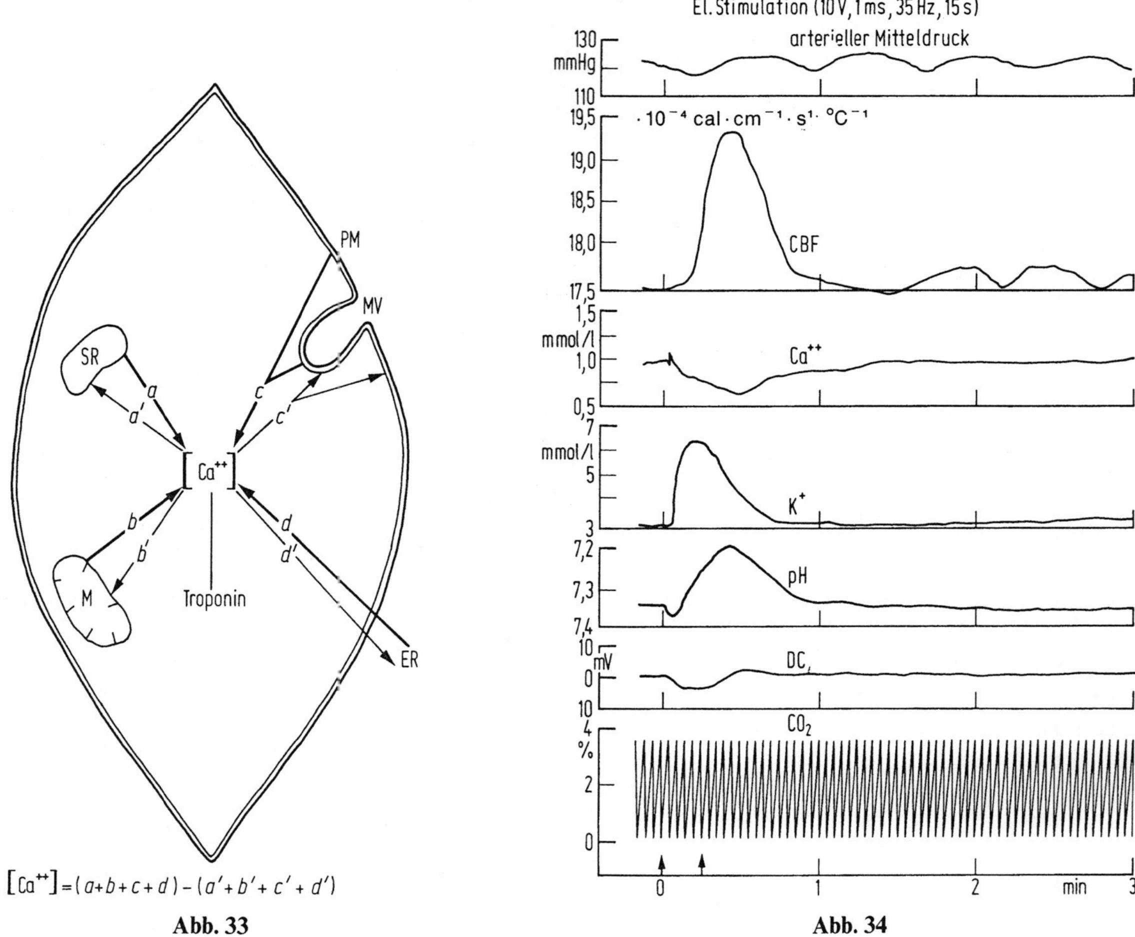

Abb. 33 **Abb. 34**

Abb. 33. Schema der Kalziumbewegungen, die zu Änderungen des aktivierten Ca^{++} am intrazellulären Troponin führen können. Die Ca^{++}-Konzentration kann erhöht werden (dicke Pfeile) durch Abgabe aus dem sarkoplasmatischen Retikulum (*SR*), den Mitochondrien (*M*), der Plasmamembran (*PM*), Vesikeln der Membran (*MV*) oder aus dem Extrazellulärraum (*ER*). Die Verminderung von Ca^{++} (dünne Pfeile) erfolgt durch energiefördernde Transportprozesse in diese Zellbereiche oder durch einen Efflux aus den Zellen entgegen einem hohen Konzentrationsgradienten. (Nach BOHR: Circulat. Res. **32**, 665, 1973, Abb. 1)

Abb. 34. Die Wirkung einer elektrischen Reizung einer umschriebenen Kortexregion (Reizparameter s. obere Zeile) auf den mittleren arteriellen Blutdruck, die mittels Wärmeleitmesser fortlaufend registrierte kortikale Durchblutung innerhalb des gereizten Feldes (Gyrus suprasylvicus der Katze), die Kalziumaktivität im gleichen Feld (gemessen mit einer Ca^{++}selektiven Ionenaustauscher-Mikroelektrode), die Kaliumaktivität ebenfalls im gereizten Areal (gemessen mit einer K^{+}-selektiven Ionenaustauscher-Mikroelektrode) sowie die dort auftretende Änderung der Wasserstoffionenkonzentration (gemessen mit einer miniaturisierten pH-Elektrode). In der vorletzten Reihe ist die Gleichspannungsänderung mitregistriert, die zeigt, daß die Ionenänderungen nicht durch andersartig bedingte Glichspannungsänderungen verursacht sind. Die endexspiratorische CO_2-Konzentration bleibt während der Reizung unverändert. (Nach HEUSER et al., Acta neurol. scand., Suppl. 64, Vol. 56, 216–217, 1977)

Kortexgewebe sofort nach Ende des Reizes eine Verminderung der Kalziumaktivität im extrazellulären Raum des Gehirn auftrat und daß diese Verminderung etwas früher oder gleichzeitig mit der Erhöhung der Durchblutung einherging (Abb. 34). Es muß hier vermerkt werden, daß neben der Calciumverminderung auch eine Kaliumerhöhung auftrat. Möglicherweise wird bei der elektrischen Aktivierung eine erhöhte Menge von Kalziumionen in das Zellinnere der Nervenzellen (Synapsen) transportiert, so daß die ionale Aktivität im extrazellulären Raum vermindert wird. Damit sinkt auch die Ca^{++}-Aktivität an der Außenseite der glatten Muskelzellen und dies wiederum kann die Ursache für die Gefäßdilatation sein.

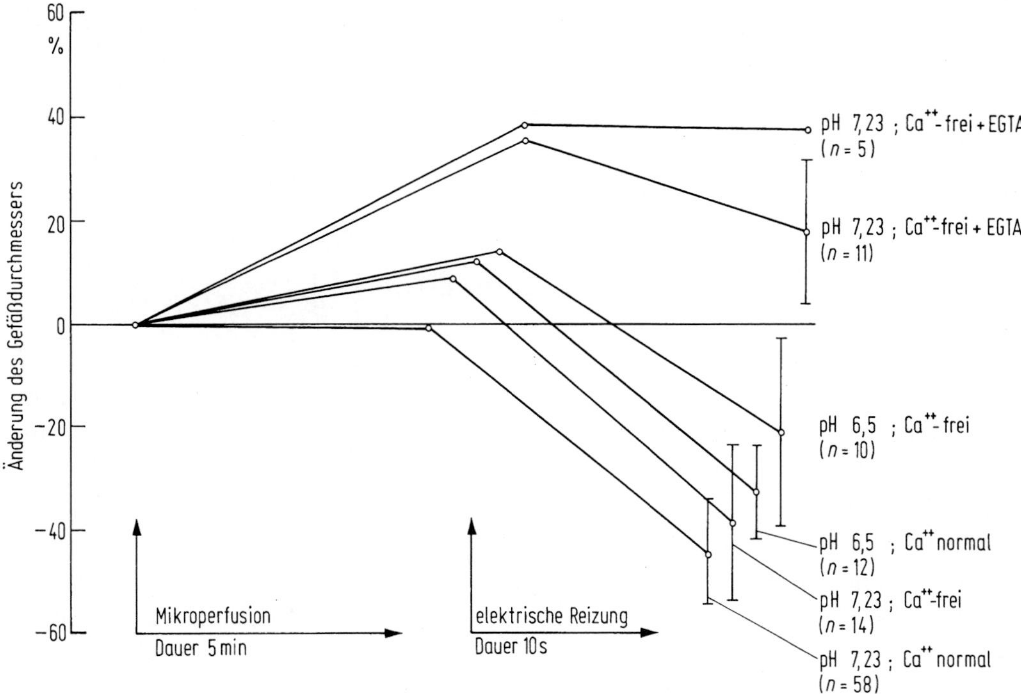

Abb. 35. Perivaskuläre Mikroperfusion (5 min Dauer) und anschließende elektrische Reizung (gleiche Reizparameter wie bei Abb. 32) von kleinen Piagefäßen. Die Mikroperfusionen wurden sowohl mit normalem Liquor als auch mit Liquor veränderter H^+- und Ca^{++}-Konzentration vorgenommen. Es ist zu erkennen, daß Azidosen zu Erweiterung der Gefäße führen. Perivaskulärer Ca^{++}-Mangel führt ebenfalls zur Piagefäßerweiterung, welche bei gleichzeitiger Azidose noch verstärkt wird. Komplexierung von Ca^{++} mit EGTA bewirkt eine sehr starke Dilatation. Lokale elektrische Reizung der vorbehandelten Gefäße führt außer bei EGTA oder EDTA zur lokalen Konstriktion, die bei den erweiterten Gefäßen im Mittel etwas schwächer ausgeprägt ist. (Nach BETZ et al., Pflügers Arch. Physiol. **343**, 79, 1973)

Weitere Resultate, die einen Einblick in die Reaktionen des Gehirngefäßsystems bei Kalziumveränderungen geben, stammen im wesentlichen von Mikroperfusionsexperimenten der perivaskulären Räume. Wird die Kalziumkonzentration in diesen Räumen erhöht (bei gleichbleibendem pH und nahezu gleichbleibender Konzentration der übrigen Ionen), so kommt es erwartungsgemäß zu einer Kontraktion der Gefäße. Bei Fehlen des Kalziums in der umspülenden Flüssigkeit werden die Gehirnarterien und Arteriolen erweitert (VLAHOV u. ENZENROSS, 1973). Es zeigt sich, daß bei einer Blockierung des Kalziums durch Zugabe von z.B. EGTA oder EDTA zum perivaskulären Liquor das umspülte Gefäß weit wird, und daß dieses Gefäß auch die Fähigkeit verliert, auf einen elektrischen Reiz mit einer Kontraktion zu reagieren. Die Abb. 35 zeigt ein Beispiel, aus dem hervorgeht, wie sich Piagefäße bei perivaskulärer Perfusion mit Liquor cerebrospinalis unterschiedlicher Zusammensetzung und vorwiegend wechselnden Kalziumgehalts verhalten, wenn sie elektrisch gereizt werden. Aus der Abbildung geht hervor, daß sowohl bei einer Azidose als auch bei einer Alkalose im perivaskulären Raum eine durch elektrischen Reiz ausgelöste Kontraktion noch möglich ist. Abb. 32 zeigt, daß auch eine Veränderung der Kaliumkonzentration die Reagibilität der Gefäße zwar verschiebt, aber nicht aufhebt. Vollständige Blockierung von Kalzium hebt dagegen in jedem Fall die Kontraktionsfähigkeit der glatten Muskeln der Gehirngefäße auf, so daß hier dem Kalzium mit Recht die zentrale Stellung zugeordnet werden kann.

4. Die Wirkungen von Chloridänderungen auf die Gehirngefäße

In den vorangehenden Kapiteln wurden lediglich die durch Kationen bedingten Reaktionen betrachtet. Änderungen der Anionen zeigen, daß auch diese bei der Einstellung der Piagefäßweite beteiligt sind. Eine Verminderung der Konzentration von perivaskulärem Chlorid bewirkt eine Konstriktion. Es ist bei den Chloridänderungen nicht gleichgültig, welches andere Anion das Chlorid ersetzt. Wird Chlorid durch Azetationen ersetzt, so ist die resultierende Gefäßkonstriktion erheblich stärker als bei Ersatz durch Sulfat oder z.B. durch anorganisches Phosphat (BETZ et al., 1977). Durch Untersuchungen von KARLITZKY (unveröffentlicht) konnte nachgewiesen werden, daß das Phosphat als solches eine dilatierende Wirkung auf konstringierte Gehirngefäße hat.

5. Ionale Interaktionen

Wird die Kalziumkonzentration an der Oberfläche von Piagefäßen erhöht, so steigt die Wandspannung der Gefäße an. Es kommt zu einer Gefäßverengerung. Bei einer gleichzeitigen Erhöhung der Wasserstoffionenkonzentration im perivaskulären Raum wird die allein durch Kalziumionen ausgelöste Kontraktion vermindert, so daß gesagt werden kann, daß die dilatierende Wirkung einer Azidose durch Kalziumerhöhung aufgehoben werden kann. Eine ähnliche Wechselwirkung zeigen Kaliumionen und Kalziumionen (BETZ et al., 1975b; BETZ u. CSORNAI, 1978). Bei Erhöhung von Kalium auf das vierfache der Norm kommt es zu einer Gefäßerweiterung. Wird Kalzium dem Liquor entzogen, so wird die Gefäßerweiterung ausgeprägter. Erhöhung des Kalziums vermindert das Ausmaß der Erweiterung und kann schließlich sogar zu einer Verengerung des Gefäßes trotz hoher Kaliumionenkonzentration führen. Abb. 36 zeigt die Verhältnisse, aus denen zusätzlich

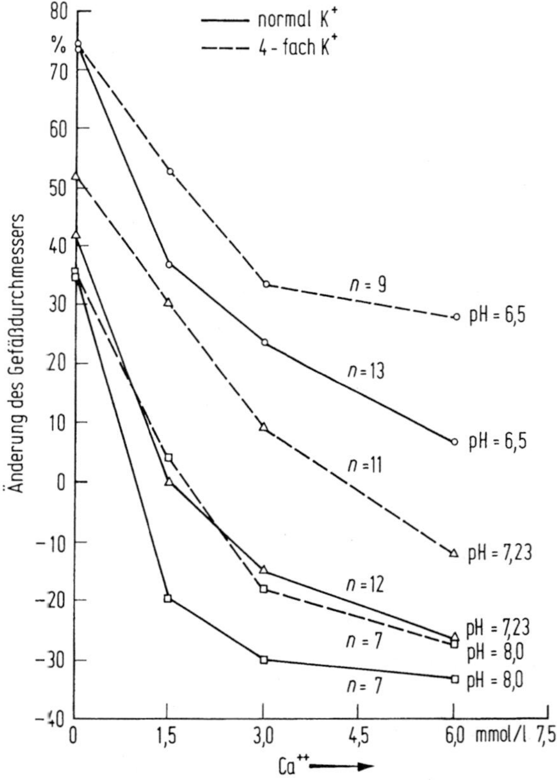

Abb. 36. Der Einfluß veränderter perivaskulärer Kalziumkonzentration (Abszisse) bei gleichzeitiger Veränderung von perivaskulärem pH und perivaskulärem Kalium auf die Durchmesser kleiner Piaarterien von Katzen. Als Ausgangswert wurden 2,6 mM Kalium, 1,5 mM Kalzium und ein perivaskuläres pH von 7,23 angenommen. Der Ausgangswert erhielt infolgedessen auf der Ordinate den Wert 0. Erhöhung der Wasserstoffionenkonzentration bewirkt, daß bei allen gewählten Kalziumkonzentrationen die Gefäße weiter werden als bei normalem oder alkalischem Liquor. Kalziumerhöhung (Abszisse) bewirkt bei gleichbleibendem pH eine konzentrationsabhängige Konstriktion. Bei Vorhandensein von Kalzium wird die dilatierende Wirkung von H^+ bei Erhöhung der perivaskulären Kaliumkonzentration auf das Vierfache der Norm verstärkt. Bei Fehlen von Kalzium im perivaskulären Liquor wird bei Kaliumerhöhung keine zusätzliche Dilatation mehr beobachtet. (Nach CSORNAI und BETZ)

hervorgeht, daß die Aktivitäten von Wasserstoffionen und Kaliumionen sich im Hinblick auf die Gefäßerweiterung addieren, daß aber durch gleichzeitige Erhöhung der Calciumionenaktivität diese Dilatation reduziert werden kann.

Ist das perivaskuläre Perfusat calciumfrei, so wird die Reaktion auf K^+-Änderungen nahezu aufgehoben. Die H^+-bedingten Änderungen bleiben jedoch erhalten (BETZ u. CSORNAI, 1975, 1978). Ob bei diesen Interaktionen von Wasserstoff, Kalium und Kalzium verschiedene Kanäle an der Membran betroffen sind, ist bisher nicht bekannt. Man weiß auch nicht, ob die Änderungen der Kalziumaktivität stets mit einer Veränderung von „second messengers" im Innern der Zelle, z.B. von zyklischem AMP einhergehen und welche Rolle das zyklische AMP bei der Transmission von Signalen über extrazelluläre Ionenaktivitäten spielt. Hier muß auf spezielle Literatur aus dem Bereich der glatten Muskulatur verwiesen werden (z.B. BÜLBRING et al., 1970; RÜEGG, 1971; ANDERSSON et al., 1972). Bei den ionalen Interaktionen spielt auch das Chlorid eine Rolle. So ist nachgewiesen worden, daß eine wasserstoffionenbedingte Dilatation der Gehirngefäße durch eine Verminderung des Chlorids aufgehoben werden kann, ja daß sogar durch eine Reduktion des Chlorids auf die Hälfte der Normalkonzentration die wasserstoffbedingte Dilatation in eine Konstriktion umgewandelt wird. Faßt man die bisherigen bekannten Befunde zusammen, so ist zu erkennen, daß bei den betrachteten Ionenmechanismen zwar das Kalzium im Kontraktionsprozeß eine besondere Rolle spielt, daß aber auch die anderen erwähnten Anionen und Kationen beteiligt sind.

L. Die Wirkung von Transmittern auf die Gehirngefäßmuskulatur

I. Adrenerge Stoffe

Bei der Übertragung von Signalen aus adrenergen Nervenendigungen oder direkt über Katecholamine aus dem perivaskulären Raum auf die glatte Muskulatur werden als Angriffspunkte spezifische Rezeptoren an der Gefäßmuskulatur postuliert, an denen die Signale in energetische Prozesse transformiert werden. So wird z.B. von SUTHERLAND et al. (1968) in einem Review ausführlich dargestellt, daß die Adenylatzyklase, ein membrangebundenes Enzym, die Konversion von ATP in cAMP vollzieht, und daß diese Reaktion durch β-adrenerge Stoffe stimuliert wird. Diese Kette der Umwandlung wird als Teil des β-Rezeptors angesehen. Das zyklische Nucleotid wird dabei durch die Phosphordiesterase zu 5-AMP katabolisiert (ROBINSON et al., 1968).

Bei intravenöser Injektion von Katecholaminen ist die direkte Wirkung von Transmittern auf α- oder β-Rezeptoren der Gehirngefäßmuskulatur schwer nachweisbar, weil die Transmitter auch an anderen Organen Wirkungen entfalten und diese sekundär das Gehirngefäßsystem beeinflussen können. Man denke nur an die Wirkungen von α-Rezeptorenblockern auf den arteriellen Blutdruck und dessen Einfluß auf die autoregulatorische Einstellung der Gehirngefäße oder an Aktionen von Katecholaminen auf den Gewebsstoffwechsel und deren sekundäre Effekte auf die Widerstandsregulation der Gehirngefäße, um zu verstehen, daß nur die Registrierung der direkten Auswirkungen dieser Stoffe auf die Muskulatur des Gehirngefäßsystems genaueren Aufschluß über ihre Aktion auf die Gehirngefäßmuskulatur geben kann. Die Einflüsse der Katecholamine auf die Gefäßmuskulatur zahlreicher Organe wurden in Monographien und Reviews beschrieben (z.B. IVERSEN, 1967; SOMLYO u. SOMLYO, 1968a, b). Spezielle Beobachtungen von Wirkungen auf das Gehirngefäßsystem wurden von SOKOLOFF (1959), BETZ (1972), PURVES (1972), CARPI (1972) in Übersichtsartikeln mitgeteilt. Danach sind bei i.v. Adrenalingaben nur geringe Einflüsse auf die Muskulatur der Gehirngefäße gefunden worden, wohingegen nach Gabe von Noradrenalin eine Konstriktion erfolgt. Die konstriktorische Reaktion der verschiedenen Abschnitte des Gehirngefäßsystems bei Gaben von Noradrenalin ist unterschiedlich stark ausgeprägt. Nach KEATINGE

(1972) und ROACH (1972) reagiert die Arteria carotis auf diese Substanz mit einer starken Konstriktion. In weiter peripher gelegenen Arterien findet man dagegen bei gleichen Transmitterkonzentrationen geringere konstriktorische Effekte. Bei perivaskulärer Mikroperfusion von kleinen Piaarterien müssen hohe Konzentrationen von Noradrenalin im perivaskulären Raum vorhanden sein, um eine Konstriktion auszulösen. Ob die Ursachen der Verschiedenheit der Ansprechbarkeit einzelner Gefäßabschnitte in einer unterschiedlichen Dichte von α-Rezeptoren, in einer unterschiedlichen Aktivität von Aminoxydasen oder -transferasen in den verschiedenen Gefäßabschnitten oder in Unterschieden der Membranpermeabilität für die bei der Rezeptorenerregung beteiligten Ionen zu suchen sind, oder ob die an der Muskulatur endenden Nerven exogen zugeführtes Noradrenalin in besonders starkem Ausmaß aufnehmen und damit die wirksame Konzentration vermindern, kann bisher nicht gesagt werden. Unterschiede der Enzymaktivitäten in der glatten Muskulatur von zerebralen und extrazerebralen Arterien, die von SIEGEL et al. (1974b) beschrieben wurden (Tab. 5), geben einen gewissen Anhaltspunkt dafür, daß auch an den verschiedenen Abschnitten des intrazerebralen Gefäßsystems derartige Unterschiede des Enzymmusters existieren könnten. Für die genauere Analyse der Verschiedenheiten wären vergleichende Messungen der Membranpotentialänderungen einzelner Gehirngefäßabschnitte, entweder mit der Saccharose-Trennwandtechnik oder intracellulärer Ableitung, erforderlich. Solche vergleichenden Messungen gibt es bisher nicht in ausreichendem Maß. Die perivaskuläre Mikroperfusion erlaubt deshalb zur Zeit die weitestgehenden Einblicke in die Wirkungsmechanismen an den verschiedenen Abschnitten des Gehirngefäßsystems. Von WAHL et al. (1972) konnte gezeigt werden, daß konstriktorische Wirkungen von Noradrenalin an Piagefäßen bei Konzentrationen von 10^{-3} mMol/l im perivaskulären Raum eben erkennbar sind und bei ca. 2,5 mMol/l ein Maximum erreichen. FRASER et al. (1971) hatten bei Überströmen der Gehirnrinde von Affen mit Noradrenalin ($2{,}2 \cdot 10^{-6}$ bis $2{,}2 \cdot 10^{-4}$ g/ml) ebenfalls deutliche vasokonstriktorische Effekte beobachtet. Von FRASER et al. (1971), CORBETT et al. (1972), D'ALECY (1973) und MATHEW et al. (1975) werden α-Rezeptoren postuliert, die bei der Noradrenalinwirkung auf die Gehirngefäße beteiligt sind. Bei Mikroperfusionsuntersuchungen haben BETZ et al. (1973) berichtet, daß nach Phentolamingaben die kleinen Piaarterien noch genau so mit einer Konstriktion auf lokale, transmurale, elektrische Reizung reagieren wie vor Applikation. KUSCHINSKY u. WAHL (1975b) haben die Schlußfolgerung gezogen, daß der Ruhetonus der glatten Muskeln der kleinen Piagefäße nicht über α-Rezeptoren aufrecht erhalten wird.

Die Konstriktion der Piaarteriolen bei perivaskulärer Applikation von Noradrenalin hängt vom pH des perivaskulären Raums und damit vom Gewebsstoffwechsel des Gehirns ab. Bei starker Azidose ist die konstriktorische Wirkung des Noradrenalins aufgehoben (in ähnlicher Weise wie bei Serotonin in Abb. 37). Bei Alkalose kann eine zusätzliche Noradrenalinzufuhr in den perivaskulären Raum keine Verstärkung der Konstriktion bewirken (BETZ u. CSORNAI, 1975). Die Ergebnisse dieser Messungen stimmen mit denen überein, die PEIPER u. WENDE (1970) an isolierten Gefäßstreifen der Aorta durchgeführt haben. Diese Autoren fanden auch Wechselwirkungen von Kalium und Noradrenalin bei der Spannungsentwicklung isolierter Gefäßmuskeln (WENDE u. PEIPER, 1970). MITCHELL et al. (1975) nehmen an, daß sowohl α- als auch β-Rezeptoren an Gefäßen im Gehirninnern vorhanden sind und daß diese durch endogen im Gehirn gebildetes Noradrenalin beeinflußt werden. EDVINSSON u. OWMAN (1976) versuchten eine pharmakologische Identifizierung von adrenergen Rezeptoren (α- und β-Rezeptoren). Sie kamen bei ihren Untersuchungen zu dem Schluß, daß es an den Gehirngefäßen α- und β-Rezeptoren gibt.

Die Bedeutung von β-adrenergen Rezeptoren für die Gehirngefäßtonisierung wird sehr unterschiedlich beurteilt. NIELSEN u. OWMAN (1971) fanden unter der Einwirkung von Isoproterenol eine deutliche Verengerung der isolierten Arteria cerebri media. Diese Konstriktion konnte durch den β-Blocker D-INPEA erheblich reduziert werden. WAHL et al. (1974), KUSCHINSKY u. WAHL (1975a) messen der Wirkung von β-Rezeptoren keine oder nur sehr geringe Bedeutung für die Widerstandsregulation von Piagefäßen bei. SEYLAZ et al. (1975) erkennen aus ihren Durchblutungsmessungen bei Gaben von CO_2 und β-rezeptorenerregenden Stoffen Anhaltspunkte dafür, daß regionale Differenzen in der Verteilung von β-Rezeptoren bestehen und postulieren eine regional unterschiedliche Bedeutung dieser Rezeptoren.

Über die Änderung der cAMP-Konzentration in den Muskelzellen der Widerstandsgefäße des Gehirns und die damit gekoppelte Änderung des freien zytoplasmatischen Ca^{++} bei der β-Rezeptorenreizung ist noch nichts bekannt. Befunde über einen konstriktorischen Effekt von Prostaglandinen (YAMAMOTO et al., 1975) weisen allerdings darauf hin, daß über Änderungen der Adenylatzyklaseaktivität in den Membranen von Gehirngefäßen die cAMP-Konzentration verändert wird und daß eine damit gekoppelte Änderung der intrazellulären Ca^{++}-Aktivität bei der Kontraktion eine Rolle spielen könnte. Allerdings geht aus Untersuchungen von WELCH et al. (1974) hervor, daß die Prostaglandine keine einheitliche Wirkung auf die glatte Muskulatur der Gehirngefäße haben. So verursacht $PGF_{1\alpha}$ $PGF_{2\alpha}$ Konstriktion, und PGE_1 Dilatation von Piagefäßen. Über die direkte Wirkung von neurohypophysealen Peptiden und analogen Substanzen sowie körpereigenen Steroiden, Plasmakininen und Polypeptiden auf die isolierten Gehirngefäßmuskeln ist zu wenig bekannt, um als gesichert gelten zu können. Sowohl BOHR u. JOHANSSON (1966) als auch BRANDT et al. (1975) fanden Anhaltspunkte dafür, daß es bisher noch unbekannte Komponenten des Plasmas gibt, die zu Gefäßmuskelkontraktionen führen. HANKO et al. (1977) fanden experimentelle Hinweise darauf, daß an Gehirngefäßen peptiderge Rezeptoren vorkommen.

Über die physiologische und pathophysiologische Bedeutung der durch Transmitterfreisetzung bewirkten nervalen Einflußnahme auf die Gehirngefäße sind in den letzten Jahren einige Arbeiten erschienen. MACKENZIE et al. (1977), BOISVERT et al. (1977) und PEARCE u. D'ALECY (1977) sind gleichermaßen der Meinung, daß vor allem bei schnellen Änderungen des Blutdrucks die an den Gefäßen freigesetzten adrenergen Transmitter eine Überschreitung der autoregulatorischen Schwelle verhindern. Das „Breakthrough"-Phänomen kann nach Meinung der Autoren normalerweise deshalb nicht auftreten, weil die nervalen Einflüsse am Gehirngefäßsystem eine so starke Konstriktion verursachen, daß die Durchblutung im Bereich autoregulatorischer Grenzen gehalten werden kann.

II. Die Wirkung von Serotonin

Serotonin (5-Hydroxytryptamin) hat, wie PAGE (1968) in einer Monographie mitteilt, sowohl dilatatorische als auch konstriktorische Wirkung auf das Gefäßsystem.

Am Gehirngefäßsystem werden vorwiegend konstriktorische Effekte wirksam, wie aus Untersuchungen von KARLSBERG et al. (1963), DESHMUKI u. HARPER (1973), EKSTRÖM-JODAL et al. (1975) (intravenöse Injektionen) oder durch Messung an isolierten Hirnarterien (TODA u. FUJITA, 1973; TODA et al., 1976, ALLEN et al., 1976) oder durch perivaskuläre Mikroperfusion (BETZ u. CSORNAI 1975) nachgewiesen wurde. Von HARPER und MACKENZIE (1977a) wurde allerdings gefunden, daß zwar die großen Gefäße eine starke Konstriktion aufweisen, daß aber die kleinen Piagefäße unter subduraler Gabe von Serotonin dilatieren (HARPER u. MACKENZIE, 1977b). Bei freigelegten Piagefäßen war diese Reaktion jedoch nicht nachweisbar, sondern es kam in der Regel zu Konstriktionen (BETZ u. EITEL, 1978). Möglicherweise erklärt die Interaktion zwischen vom Gewebe freigesetzten Metaboliten und direkter Serotoninwirkung auf die glatte Muskulatur diese etwas divergierenden Befunde. Die physiologische Bedeutung der Serotoninrezeptoren ist noch unklar.

Sowohl die serotoninantagonistische Substanz Methysergid als auch der α-Blocker Phentolamin hatten bei den Untersuchungen von EKSTRÖM-JODAL et al. (1975) keine Wirkung auf die serotoninbedingte Vasokonstriktion von Gehirngefäßen. Antagonistische Wirkungen einer α-Blockade wurden allerdings bei anderen Gefäßgebieten gefunden (Übersicht: SOMLYO u. SOMLYO, 1968b). Auch Atropingaben und Propanolol-Zufuhr veränderten die konstriktorischen Serotoninwirkungen nicht. Bei den Mikroperfusionsexperimenten ergab sich jedoch, ähnlich wie bei den Noradrenalinwirkungen, eine deutliche Abhängigkeit der durch Serotonin verursachten Konstriktionen von

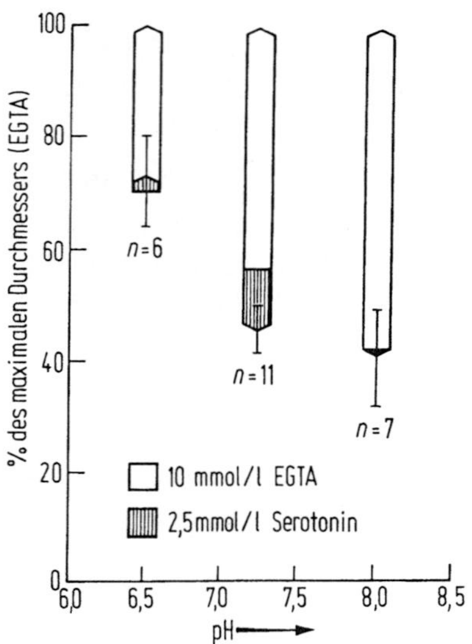

Abb. 37. Die Wirkung von 10^{-3} mM/L perivaskulär an kleine Piaarterien von Katzen gebrachtes Serotonin auf die Änderung der Durchmesser dieser Gefäße bei unterschiedlichem perivaskulärem pH-Wert. Als 100% Dilatation wird die Gefäßweite während Kalziumkomplexierung durch EGTA bezeichnet. Es ist erkennbar, daß bei einem für Katzen normalen pH von 7,23 die durch Serotonin bewirkte Konstriktion stärker ist als diejenige bei Azidose oder Alkalose. Außerdem ist erkennbar, daß eine Azidose von pH=6,5 keine maximale Dilatation der Piagefäße erzeugte, denn EGTA-Zusatz zum perivaskulären Liquor führt zu einer noch beträchtlich stärkeren Dilatation. (Nach CSORNAI)

den perivaskulären pH-Werten. Bei starker Acidose und starker Alkalose waren die Wirkungen nahezu aufgehoben (Abb. 37). Die Abb. läßt erkennen, daß beim Vergleich der maximalen Kontraktions- bzw. Erweiterungsfähigkeit mit der durch Serotonin erreichbaren Weitenänderungen, die stärksten serotoninbedingten Reaktionen verhältnismäßig gering sind.

Injektionen von Serotonin in die Karotiden verursachen besonders starke Konstriktionen der Kortexgefäße bei Affen, wenn diese mit Depot-Östrogen und Progesteron vorbehandelt waren (EIDELMANN et al. 1978).

III. Histaminrezeptoren

Die konstringierende Wirkung von Serotonin auf Gehirngefäße wird durch gleichzeitige Gabe von Histamin potenziert (BEVAN et al., 1975). Auch Noradrenalin oder elektrische Reizung von Gefäßen führt unter Histaminwirkung zu verstärkter Kontraktion der Gehirngefäßmuskeln. BEVAN et al. (1975) nehmen spezifische Histaminrezeptoren an. An extrazerebralen Gefäßen (Ohrgefäßen) wurde nachgewiesen, daß in Gegenwart von erhöhten Kaliumkonzentrationen die potenzierende konstriktorische Wirkung des Histamins auf Serotonin verschwindet. Die vasokonstriktorischen Effekte von Serotonin und Histamin haben bei Gewebsverletzungen oder Hämorrhagien besonders hohe Bedeutung.

Von KUSCHINSKY u. WAHL (1977) wurde an den Piagefäßen nachgewiesen, daß die histamininduzierten Dilatationen vorwiegend über H_2-Rezeptoren vermittelt werden.

IV. Cholinerge Mechanismen

Bei den cholinergen Gefäßrezeptoren werden zwei Typen, der Muskarintyp und der Nikotintyp auch in den Gehirngefäßen unterschieden. Beim Muskarintyp, der wahrscheinlich Vasodilatation unter physiologischen Bedingungen auslöst, kommt es bei hohen Dosen zu einer Konstriktion, während der Nikotintyp der cholinergen Rezeptoren eine Noradrenalinfreisetzung hemmt und dadurch eine Reduktion des sympathischen vaskulären Tonus vermittelt.

Die Bedeutung cholinerger Mechanismen bei der autoregulatorischen Dilatation wurde von LAVRENTEVA et al. (1968), MCHEDLISHVILI u. NIKOLAISHVILI (1970) und von KUSCHINSKY u. WAHL (1975a) betont. Die Wirkung verschwand oder wurde vermindert, wenn der arterielle Druck nach intravenöser Verabreichung von Azetylcholinesteraseblockern gesenkt wurde. Eine Applikation von Azetycholin direkt auf die Oberfläche von Piagefäßen verursachte eine Dilatation dieser Gefäße. Neuere Untersuchungen von ALBORCH et al. (1977) bestätigen die dilatatorische Wirkung von cholinergen Nerven auf das Gehirngefäßsystem.

MCHEDLISHVILI u. KIKOLAISHVILI (1967, 1970) unterbrachen die Fasern, die den zerebralen Kortex mit Piagefäßen verbanden und fanden daraufhin, daß keine funktionelle Dilatation mehr stattfand, die üblicherweise unter den Bedingungen von gesteigerter kortikaler Aktivität auftritt. Aus diesen Befunden schließen sie, daß ein nervöser cholinerger Mechanismus bei der funktionellen Dilatation der Piagefäße beteiligt ist und über diese Fasern vermittelt wird (s. auch MCHEDLISHVILI, 1972). PLETCHKOVA et al. (1969) nehmen an, daß cholinerge Mechanismen auch bei der funktionellen Hyperämie im Bereich des zerebralen Kortex eine Rolle spielen. Nach AUBINEAU u. SERCOMBE (1977) und SHINOHARA et al. (1977) modulieren cholinerge Mechanismen die adrenergen Reaktionen.

Herrn Dr. H. APFEL, Physiologisches Institut Tübingen, danke ich für seine Hilfe bei der Durchsicht der Korrekturen.

Literatur

AGNOLI, A.: Adaptation of CBF during induced chronic normooxic respiratory acidosis. Scand. J. clin. Lab. Invest. Suppl. **102**, VII D (1968)

AGNOLI, A., BATTISTINI, N., NARDINI, M., PASSERO, S., FIESCHI, C.: Lack of adaptation of CBF and CSF pH in hypoxic hypercapnia. In: Cerebral blood flow (BROCK, M., FIESCHI, C., INGVAR, D.H., LASSEN, N.A., SCHÜRMANN, K., eds.). Berlin, Heidelberg, New York: Springer 1969c, pp. 79–81

AGNOLI, A., BOZZAO, L., NARDINI, M., BATTISTINI, N., FIESCHI, C.: Adaptation of cerebral blood flow during induced chronic normoxic respiratory acidosis. In: Pharmakologie der lokalen Gehirndurchblutung (BETZ, E., WÜLLENWEBER, R., eds.). München-Gräfelfing: Banaschewski 1969, pp. 215–220

AGNOLI, A., PRENCIPE, M., PRIORI, A.M., BOZZAO, L., FIESCHI, C.: Measurements of the rCBF by intravenous injection of 133 Xe. A comparative study with the intra-arterial injection method. In: Cerebral Blood Flow (BROCK, M., FIESCHI, C., INGVAR, D.H., LASSEN, N.A., SCHÜRMANN, K., eds). Berlin-Heidelberg-New York: Springer 1969a, pp. 31–34

ALBAUM, H.G., CHINN, H.: Brain metabolism during acclimatization to high altitude. Amer. J. Physiol. **174**, 141–145 (1953)

ALBORCH, E., MARTIN, G., BAGUENA, J.: Influence of cholinergic receptors on cerebral blood flow of the goat. In: Cerebral Function, Metabolism and Circulation (D.H. INGVAR, N.A. LASSEN, eds). Copenhagen: Munksgaard 1977, pp. 298–299

ALEXANDER, F.G., RÉVÉSZ, G.: Über den Einfluß optischer Reize auf den Gaswechsel des Gehirns. Biochem. Z. **44**, 95–126 (1912)

ALEXANDER, S.C., COHEN, P.J., WOLLMAN, H., SMITH, T.C., REIVICH, M., MOLEN, R.A. v.: Cerebral carbohydrate metabolism during hypocarbia in man. Studies during nitrous oxide anesthesia. Anesthesiology **26**, 624–632 (1965)

ALLEN, G.S., GROSS, C.J., HENDERSON, L.M., CHOU, S.N.: Cerebral arterial spasm. Part 4: In vitro effects of temperature, serotonin analogues, large nonphysiological concentrations of serotonin, and extracellular calcium and magnesium on serotonin-induced contractions of the canine basilar artery. J. Neurosurg. **44**, 585–593 (1976)

ALLWOOD, M.J., BARCROFT, H., HAYES, J.P.L.A., HIRSJÄRVI, E.A.: The effect of mental arithmethic on the blood flow through normal, sympathectomized and hyperhidrotic hands. J. Physiol. (Lond.) **148**, 108–116 (1959)

AMMANN, D., BISSIG, R., CIMERMAN, Z., FIEDLER, U., GÜGGI, M., MORF, W.E., OEHME, M., OSSWALD, H., PRETSCH, E., SIMON, W.: Synthetic Neutral Carriers for Cations. In: Ion and Enzyme Electrodes in Biology and Medicine, KESSLER, M., CLARK, L.C., LÜBBERS, D.W., SILVER, I.A., SIMON, W. eds, 22–37, Urban & Schwarzenberg, München, Berlin, Wien 1976

ANDERSSON, R.E., LUNDHOLM, L., MOHME-LUNDHOLM, E., NILSSON, K.: Role of cyclic AMP and Ca^{++} in metabolic and mechanical events in smooth muscle. Advanc. Cycl. Nucl. Res. **1**, 213–229 (1972)

ANTHONY, L.U., GOLDRING, S., O'LEARY, J., SCHWARTZ, H.G.: Experimental cerebrovascular occlusion in dog. Arch. Neurol. **8**, 515–526 (1963)

Astrup, J., Heuser, D., Lassen, N.A., Nilsson, B., Norberg, K., Siesjö, B.K.: Evidence against H^+ and K^+ as main factors for the control of cerebral blood flow: a microelectrode study. Cerebral Vascular Smooth Muscle and its Control. Ciba Foundation Symposium **56**, 313–337 (1978)

Aubineau, P., Sercombe, R.: Evidence for a double cholinergic mechanism capable of reducing the tone of cerebral arteries. In: Cerebral Function, Metabolism and Circulation (D.H. Ingvar, N.A. Lassen, eds). Copenhagen: Munksgaard 1977, pp. 296–297

Austin, G., Laffin, D., Rouhe, S., Hayward, W., Rice-Edwards, M.: Intravenous isotope injection method of cerebral blood flow measurement: Accuracy and reproducibility. In: Cerebral Circulation and Metabolism (T.W. Langfitt, L.C. McHenry, M. Reivich, H. Wollman, eds). New York-Heidelberg-Berlin: Springer 1975, pp. 391–393

Bär, T., Wolff, J.R.: Development and Adult Variations of the Wall of Brain Capillaries in the Neocortex of Rat and Cat. In: The Cerebral Vessel Wall, Cervos-Navarro, J., Betz, E., Matakas, F., Wüllenwber, R. eds, 1–6. Raven Press, New York 1976

Bär, Th., Wolff, J.R., Hunziker, O.H.: Effects of different hemodynamic conditions on brain capillaries: alveolar hypoxia, hypovolemic hypotension and ouabain edema. Adv. Neurosurg., **3**, Brain-Hypoxia-Pain, Ed.: Penzhold, H., Brock, M., Hamer, J., Klinger, M., Spoerri, O. 10–19. Berlin, Heidelberg, New York, Springer, 1975

Bain, W.H., Harper, A.M.: Blood flow through organs and tissues. Edinburgh-London: Livingstone 1968

Bakay, L., Kobayashi, T.: Cerebral isotope uptake in acute experimental hypercapnic hypoxia. Exp. Neurol. **32**, 303–312 (1971)

Bakay, L., Lee, J.C.: Cerebral edema. Springfield, Ill.: Thomas 1965

Baldy-Moulinier, M.: Cerebral reflow after anoxia. In: Brain and Blood Flow (Ross Russell, R.W., ed). London: Pitman Medical and Scientific Publishing Co LTD 1971, pp. 187–190

Baldy-Moulinier, M., Ingvar, D.H.: Regional cortical blood flow and EEG in cat. Electroenceph. clin. Neurophysiol. **19**, 616 (1965)

Barany, M.: ATPase activity of myosin correlated with speed of muscle shortening. J. gen. Physiol. **50**, 197–218 (1967)

Barker, J.N., Youdin, M., Reich, T.: A method and instrumentation for quantitating local cerebral blood flow in 144 subdivisions of human brain, using 133 Xe and a germanium detector array. In: Cerebral circulation and mechanism (Langfitt, W.T. et al., eds). Berlin-Heidelberg-New York: Springer 1975, pp. 413–414

Barnett, H.J.M., Wortzmann, G., Gladstone, R.M., Lougheed, W.M.: Diversion and reversal of cerebral blood flow. Neurology (Minneap.) **20**, 1–14 (1970)

Bartko, D.: Experimental brain hypoxia. Baltimore-London-Tokyo: University Park Press 1971

Batson, O.V.: Function of vertebral veins and their role in spread of metastases. Ann. Surg. **112**, 138–149 (1940)

Batson, O.V.: Anatomical problems concerned in the study of cerebral blood flow. Fed. Proc. **3**, 139–144 (1944)

Baust, W.: Local blood flow in different regions of the brain-stem during natural sleep and arousal. Electroenceph. clin. Neurophysiol. **22**, 365–372 (1967)

Baust, W., Niemczyk, H., Schaefer, H.: Die Beeinflussung des Liquordruckes durch akute hämodynamische Veränderungen. Z. ges. exp. Med. **136**, 619–629 (1963)

Bayliss, W.M.: On the local reaction of the arterial wall to changes of internal pressure. J. Physiol. (Lond.) **28**, 220–231 (1902)

Bayliss, W.M., Hill, L.: On intra-cranial pressure and the cerebral circulation. J. Physiol. (Lond.) **18**, 334–360 (1895)

Benetato, G., Baciu, I., Tomus, L., Benetato, V.: L'effet de l'excitation de la formation réticulaire du tronc cérébral sur la circulation cérébrale. J. Physiol. (Paris) **50**, 903–910 (1958)

Benzinger, Th., Opitz, E., Schoedel, W.: Durchblutung der Arteria carotis interna bei Sauerstoffmangel und Kohlensäureatmung. Luftfahrtmed. **3**, 46–54 (1938)

Bering, E.A., jr.: Cerebrospinal fluid production and its relationship to cerebral metabolism and cerebral blood flow. Amer. J. Physiol. **197**, 825–828 (1959)

Bering, E.A.: The cerebrospinal fluid circulation. In: Cerebrospinal fluid and the regulation of ventilation (Brooks, C., Kao, F.F., Lloyd, B.B., eds). Oxford: Blackwell 1965, pp. 395–412

Bernard, C.: Influence du grand sympathétique sur la sensibilité et sur la calorification. C.R. Soc. Biol. (Paris) **3**, 163–165 (1851)

Berne, R.M., Rubio, R., Curnish, R.R.: Release of adenosine from ischemic brain. Effect on cerebral vascular resistance and incorporat. into cerebral adenine nucleotides. Circulation Res., **35**, 262–271 (1974)

Bernsmeier, A.: Probleme der Gehirndurchblutung. Z. Kreisl.-Forsch. **48**, 278–323 (1959)

Bernsmeier, A., Gottstein, U.: Hirndurchblutung und Alter. Verh. dtsch. Ges. Kreisl.-Forsch. **24**, 248–253 (1958)

Bernsmeier, A., Gottstein, U.: Der Schlaganfall. Kardiale und haemodynamische Faktoren als Ursache der intermittierenden zerebralen Ischaemie. Internist (Berl.) **4**, 55–64 (1963)

Bernsmeier, A., Gottstein, U., Rudolph, W.: Herzkrankheiten als Ursache zerebraler Zirkulationsstörungen. Dtsch. med. Wschr. **87**, 16–22 (1962)

Bernsmeier, A., Siemons, K.: Die Messung der Hirndurchblutung mit der Stickoxydulmethode. Pflügers Arch. ges. Physiol. **258**, 149–162 (1953)

Betz, E.: Die lokale Gehirndurchblutung bei Emotionen. Pflügers Arch. ges. Physiol. **278**, 82–83 (1963)

Betz, E.: Die lokale Gehirndurchblutung im akuten

und chronischen Experiment. Habil.-Schrift Marburg 1964

BETZ, E.: Umstellungsreaktionen der Gehirndurchblutung bei chronischem Lärm. Arch. phys. Ther. (Lpz.) **17**, 61–65 (1965a)

BETZ, E.: Adaptation of regional cerebral blood flow in animals exposed to chronic alterations of PO_2 and PCO_2. Acta neurol. scand. **14**, 121–128 (1965b)

BETZ, E.: Spontane Schwankungen der Gehirndurchblutung in Narkose und im Wachzustand. Ärztl. Forsch. **21**, 88–93 (1967)

BETZ, E.: Zur Pathophysiologie der Sauerstoffversorgung. Z. prakt. Anästh. u. Wiederbelebg. **3**, 261–272 (1968)

BETZ, E.: Die Haemodynamik des Gehirnkreislaufs bei lokalen Gehirndurchblutungsstörungen. Med. Welt **2**, 69–74 (1969a)

BETZ, E.: Influence of cerebrospinal fluid pH on the regulation of cerebral circulation. Internat. Anaesthesiol. Clinics **7**, 525–537 (1969b)

BETZ, E.: Cerebral blood flow: Its measurement and regulation. Physiol. Rev. **52**, 595–630 (1972)

BETZ, E.: Thermische Methoden zur Messung der Gehirndurchblutung. In: Der Hirnkreislauf (GÄNSHIRT, H. Hrsg.), S. 317–324. Stuttgart: Thieme 1972a

BETZ, E.: Pharmakologie des Gehirnkreislaufs. In: Der Hirnkreislauf (GÄNSHIRT, H., Hrsg.), S. 411–440. Stuttgart: Thieme 1972b

BETZ, E.: Central nervous system depressants. In: International encyclopedia of pharmacology and therapeutics. Sect. 33: Pharmacology of the cerebral circulation (CARPI, A., ed). Oxford-New York-Toronto-Sydney-Braunschweig: Pergamon Press 1972c, pp. 149–180

BETZ, E.: The influence of changes of oxygen and carbon dioxide on the EEG, CBF and energy-rich substrates in brain tissue. In: Handbook of electroencephalography and clinical neurophysiology (REMOND, A., ed). Amsterdam: Elsevier 1974, pp. 7B 28–7B 45

BETZ, E.: CBF during emotional stimuli. In: The working brain. Alfred Benzon Symposium VIII 1975 (INGVAR, H., LASSEN, N.A., eds). Copenhagen: Munksgaard 1975, pp. 366–370

BETZ, E.: Ionic and metabolic control of local cerebral blood flow. Acta clin. belg. **32**, 119–128 (1977)

BETZ, E.: Vascular reactivity and ion homeostasis in heart and brain. In: Brain and Heart Infarct (K.J. ZÜLCH, W. KAUFMANN, K.-A. HOSSMANN, V. HOSSMANN, eds). Berlin-Heidelberg: Springer 1977, pp. 10–18

BETZ, E., BRAASCH, D., HENSEL, H.: Messung der Myocarddurchblutung mit der Wärmeleitsonde bei Einwirkung von 2,6-Bis(diaethylamino)-4,8-dipiperidino-pyrimido(5,4-d)pyrimidin (Persantin). Verh. dtsch. Ges. Kreisl.-Forsch. **27**, 321–326 (1961)

BETZ, E., BRANDT, H., CSORNAI, M.: Ionic control of pial arterial resistance. In: Blood flow and metabolisms in the brain (HARPER, A.M., JENETT, W.B., MILLER, J.D., ROWAN, J.O., eds). Edinburgh-London: Livingstone 1975a, pp. 9–12

BETZ, E., CSORNAI, M.: Regulation of pial arteriolar diameters. Pflügers Arch. ges. Physiol. **359**, Suppl. 38 (1975)

BETZ, E., CSORNAI, M.: Ionic actions on cerebral vessels. Int. J. Neurol. **11**, 243–258 (1977)

BETZ, E., CSORNAI, M.: Action and interaction of perivascular H^+, K^+ and Ca^{++} on pial arteries. Pflügers Arch. ges. Physiol. **374**, 67–72 (1978)

BETZ, E., EITEL, W.: Die Wirkung von 2-Äthyl-3-(4-hydroxy-benzoyl)-benzofuran auf die Kontraktion der Piaarterienmuskulatur. Arzneimittel-Forsch. (Drug Res.) **28**, 626–630 (1978)

BETZ, E., ENZENROSS, H.G., VLAHOV, V.: Interaction of H^+ and Ca^{++} in the regulation of local pial vascular resistance. Pflügers Arch. ges. Physiol. **343**, 79–88 (1973)

BETZ, E., ENZENROSS, H.G., VLAHOV, V.: Interactions of ionic mechanisms in the regulation of the resistance of pial vessels. In: Cerebral circulation and mechanism (LANGFITT, T., MCHENRY, L.C., REIVICH, M., WOLLMAN, H., eds). Berlin-Heidelberg-New York: Springer 1975b, pp. 49–51

BETZ, E., HENSEL, H.: Fortlaufende Registrierung der lokalen Durchblutung im Inneren des Gehirns bei wachen, frei beweglichen Tieren. Pflügers Arch. ges. Physiol. **274**, 608–614 (1962)

BETZ, E., HERRMANN, E.: Die fortlaufende Registrierung der Gehirndurchblutung beim Menschen mit flexiblen Wärmeleitsonden. Nervenarzt **37**, 173–175 (1966)

BETZ, E., HEUSER, D.: Cerebral cortical blood flow during changes of acid-base equilibrium of the brain. J. appl. Physiol. **23**, 726–733 (1967)

BETZ, E., HEUSER, D.: Effects of electrical stimulation on vascular walls and perivascular tissue of the arterial brain vessels. Arzneimittel-Forsch. (Drug Res.) **27**, 1510–1519 (1977)

BETZ, E., INGVAR, D.H., LASSEN, N.A., SCHMAHL, F.W.: Regional blood flow in the cerebral cortex, measured simultaneously by heat and inert gas clearance. Acta physiol. scand. **67**, 1–9 (1966a)

BETZ, E., KARLITZKY, G., HEUSER, D.: The effect of pial perivascular chloride on the diameters of small pial arteries. In: Cerebral Function, Metabolism and Circulation (D.H. INGVAR, N.A. LASSEN, eds). Copenhagen: Munksgaard 1977, pp. 390–391

BETZ, E., KOZAK, R.: Der Einfluß der Wasserstoffionenkonzentration der Gehirnrinde auf die Regulation der kortikalen Durchblutung. Pflügers Arch. ges. Physiol. **293**, 56–67 (1967)

BETZ, E., KRUG, A., SCHMAHL, F.W.: Die lokale Myocarddurchblutung bei Ligatur von Koronargefäßen. Verh. dtsch. Ges. Kreisl.-Forsch. **30**, 273–279 (1964)

BETZ, E., OEHMIG, H., WÜNNENBERG, W.: Die Wirkung verschiedener Narkotika auf die lokale Gehirndurchblutung der Katze. Z. Kreisl.-Forsch. **54**, 503–509 (1965)

BETZ, E., ROOS, W.: CBF, brain tissue volume and CSF pressure. In: Brain and blood flow (ROSS RUSSELL, R.W., ed). London: Pitman Medical and Scientific Publishing Co LTD, 1971, pp. 294–297

BETZ, E., ROOS, W., VAMOSI, B., WEIDLER, R.: Subarachnoid pressure dependent drug effects on CSF transport and brain volume. In: Intracranial pressure (BROCK, M., DIETZ, H., eds). Berlin-Heidelberg-New York: Springer 1972, pp. 195–199

BETZ, E., SCHMAHL, F.W.: Durchblutung und Sauerstoffdruck in der Gehirnrinde bei Karotisdrosselung und ihre Beeinflussung durch Pharmaka. Pflügers Arch. ges. Physiol. **287**, 368–384 (1966)

BETZ, E., WÜLLENWEBER, R.: Fortlaufende Registrierung der lokalen Gehirndurchblutung mit Wärmeleitsonden am Menschen. Klin. Wschr. **40**, 1056–1058 (1962)

BETZ, E., WÜLLENWEBER, R.: Pharmakologie der lokalen Gehirndurchblutung. München-Gräfelfing: Banaschweski 1969

BETZ, E., WÜNNENBERG, W.: Anpassungsvorgänge der Gehirndurchblutung an Sauerstoffmangel. Arch. phys. Ther. (Lpz.) **16**, 45–55 (1964)

BEVAN, J.A., DUCKLES, S.P., LEE, T.J.-F.: Histamine potentiation of nerve- and drug-induced responses of a rabbit cerebral artery. Circulat. Res. **36**, 647–653 (1975)

BIRZIS, L., TACHIBANA, S.: The action of stimulant and depressant agents on local cerebral impedance and circulation. Psychopharmacologia (Berl.) **6**, 256–266 (1964)

BLAIR, R.D.G., WALTZ, A.G.: Regional cerebral blood flow during acute ischemia: Correlation of autoradiographic measurements with observations of cortical microcirculation. Neurology (Minneap.) **20**, 802–808 (1970)

BLUM, B., YASHIN, T., BENARY, W., ISRAELI, J., DAVIDOVICH, A.: Responses of the leptomeningeal microcirculation to hypothalamic stimulation. Microvasc. Res. **13**, 283–296 (1977)

BODECHTEL, G.: Befunde am Zentralnervensystem bei Spätnarkosetodesfällen und bei Todesfällen nach Lumbalanästhesie. Z. ges. Neurol. Psychiat. **117**, 366–423 (1928)

BÖNING, U.: Der Einfluß von extrazellulären Kalium-, Calcium- und Magnesiumionen auf den Durchmesser pialer Arteriolen. Med. Dissertation Tübingen 1972

BOHR, D.F.: Vascular smooth muscle updated. Circulat. Res. **32**, 665–672 (1973)

BOHR, D.F., JOHANSSON, B.: Contraction of vascular smooth muscle in response to plasma. Circulat. Res. **19**, 593–601 (1966)

BOHR, D.F., UCHIDA, E.: Myogenic tone in isolated perfused vessels. Circulat. Res. **25**, 549–555 (1969)

BOISVERT, D.P.J., JONES, J.V., HARPER, A.M.: Cerebral blood flow autoregulation to acutely increasing blood pressure during sympathetic stimulation. In: Cerebral Function, Metabolism and Circulation (INGVAR, D.H., LASSEN, N.A., eds). Copenhagen: Munksgaard 1977, pp. 46–47

BOULLIN, D.F.: Effect of divalent ions on release of ^{3}H-noradrenaline by sympathetic nerve stimulation. J. Physiol. (Lond.) **183**, 76–77 (1965)

BOZLER, E.: Conduction, automaticity and tonus in visceral muscles. Experientia (Basel) **4**, 213–218 (1948)

BRAASCH, D.: Verminderte Erythrozytenflexibilität (hervorgerufen durch Barbiturate, Verbrennungen, Hypoxämien) und ihre Wirkung auf den Capillarkreislauf. Pflügers Arch. ges. Physiol. **278**, 130–140 (1963)

BRACHET, J.L.: Recherches experimentales sur les fonctions du systeme nerveux ganglionnaire et son application à la pathologie. Paris: Germer-Baillière 1837

BRADING, A.F.: The role of calcium in cellular function. Ion distribution and ion movements in smooth muscle. Phil. Trans. B **265**, 35–46 (1973)

BRADING, A.F., BÜLBRING, E., TOMITA, T.: The effect of sodium and calcium on the action potential of the smooth muscle of the guinea-pig taenia coli. J. Physiol. (Lond.) **200**, 637–654 (1969)

BRANDT, H., ENZENROSS, H.G., VLAHOV, V.: Piagefäßreaktionen bei Mikrotraumen. Folia angiol. (Pisa) **23**, 42–45 (1975)

BROBEIL, A.: Hirndurchblutungsstörungen. Stuttgart: Thieme 1950

BROBEIL, A.: Beitrag zur Pathogenese des apoplektischen Insultes. Nervenarzt **25**, 154–158 (1954)

BROBEIL, A., HÄRTER, O., HERRMANN, E., KRAMER, K.: Vergleichende Untersuchungen über das Arteriogramm der Hirngefäße und die Gehirndurchblutung beim Menschen nach KETY und SCHMIDT. Klin. Wschr. **32**, 1030–1036 (1954)

BROBEIL, A., HÄRTER, O., HERRMANN, E., NILSSON, N.J.: Messungen von cerebralen Kreislaufzeiten am Menschen und ihre Beziehung zur Gehirndurchblutung. Acta physiol. scand. **40**, 121–129 (1957)

BROCK, M., DIETZ, H.: Intracranial pressure. Berlin-Heidelberg-New York: Springer 1972

BROCK, M., FIESCHI, C., INGVAR, D.H., LASSEN, N.A., SCHÜRMANN, K.: Cerebral blood flow. Berlin-Heidelberg-New York: Springer 1969

BROWN, A.S., DONALDSON, A.A.: Clinical vertebral artery cerebral blood flow measurement. In: Cerebral blood flow and intracranial pressure (FIESCHI, C., ed). Basel-München-Paris-London-New York-Sydney: Karger 1971/72, pp. 274–276. Part I

BRUCE, D.A., VAPALAHTI, M., SCHUTZ, H., LANGFITT, T.W.: rCBF, $CMRO_2$ and intracranial pressures following a local cold injury of the cortex. In: Intracranial pressure (BROCK, M., DIETZ, H., eds). Berlin-Heidelberg-New York: Springer 1972, pp. 85–89

BÜHLMANN, A., HOSSLI, G., HUNZIKER, A.: Respiratorische Acidose und Kreislauf mit besonderer

Berücksichtigung des Gehirnkreislaufes. Schweiz. med. Wschr. **90**, 7–21 (1960)

BÜLBRING, E.: Electrical activity in intestinal smooth muscle. Physiol. Rev. **42**, Suppl. 5, 160–178 (1962)

BÜLBRING, E., BRADING, A.F., JONES, A.W., TOMITA, T.: Smooth muscle. London: Arnold 1970

BUNCE, D.F.M.: Survival of dogs following section of carotid and vertebral arteries. Proc. Soc. exp. Biol. (N.Y.) **103**, 581–585 (1960)

BURGER, T., GALLYAS, F., SZÁNTÓ, J., KESZTHELYI, B., KOPA, J.: Untersuchung des Hirnkreislaufs bei polycythaemia vera. Acta med. Sci. hung. **24**, 21–28 (1967)

BURNSTOCK, G.: Structure of smooth muscle and its innervations. In: Smooth muscle. London: Arnold 1969, pp. 1–69

BURROWS, G.: On disorders of the cerebral circulation and on the connection between affections of the brain and diseases of the heart. London: Longman, Brown, Green and Longmans 1846

CAPON, A.: Variations of cerebral flow in response to rapid increase or decrease in blood pressure. In: Pharmakologie der lokalen Gehirndurchblutung (BETZ, E., WÜLLENWEBER, W., eds). München-Gräfelfing: Banaschewski 1969, pp. 34–36

CARLYLE, A., GRAYSON, J.: Factors involved in the control of cerebral blood flow. J. Physiol. (Lond.) **133**, 10–30 (1956)

CARPI, A.: Pharmacology of the cerebral circulation. (Int. Encyclopedia of pharmacology and therapeutics, Sect. 33, Vol. I). Oxford-New York-Toronto-Sydney-Braunschweig: Pergamon Press 1972

CASTEELS, R.: The relation between the membrane potential and the ion distribution in smooth muscle. In: Smooth muscle (BÜLBRING, E., BRADING, A.F., JONES, A.W., TOMITA, T., eds). London: Arnold 1970, pp. 70–99

CASTEELS, R.: The distribution of chloride ions in smooth muscle cells of the guinea-pigs taemia coli J. Physiol. (Lond.) **214**, 225–243 (1971)

CASTEELS, R., GODFRAIND, T., RÜEGG, J.C. (eds): Excitation-Contraction Coupling in Smooth Muscle. Amsterdam-New York-Oxford: Elsevier/North-Holland 1977

CASTEELS, R., DROOGMANS, G., HENDRIX, H.: Membrane potentials of smooth muscle cells in K-free solution. J. Physiol. (Lond.) **217**, 281–295 (1971)

CERVOS-NAVARRO, J., MATAKAS, F.: Electron microscopic evidence for innervation of intracerebral arterioles in the cat. Neurology (Minneap.) **24**, 282–286 (1974)

CHORNYAK, J.: The structural changes produced in the human brain by oxygen deprivation (anoxemia) and their pathogenesis. Ann Arbor, Mi.: Edwards Brothers 1938, p. 77

CHOROBSKI, J., PENFIELD, W.: Cerebral vasodilator nerves and their pathway from the medulla oblongata. Arch. Neurol. Psychiat. (Chic.) **28**, 1257–1289 (1932)

COHEN, P.J.: The effects of decreased oxygen tension on cerebral circulation, metabolism, and function. In: Proceedings of the International Symposium on the cardiovascular and respiratory effects of hypoxia. Basel-New York: Karger 1965, pp. 81–104

COHEN, P.J., ALEXANDER, S.C., WOLLMAN, H.: Effects of hypocarbia and of hypoxia with normocarbia on cerebral blood flow and metabolism. Scand. J. clin. Lab. Invest. Suppl. 102 IV: A (1968)

COLOMBO, R.C.: De re anatomica libri XV. Venedig 1559

COOPER, A.: Some experiments and observations on tying the carotid and vertebral arteries and the pneumogastric, phrenic and sympathetic nerves. Guy's Hosp. Rep. **1**, 457–475 (1836)

CORBETT, J.L., EIVELMAN, B.H., DEBARGE, O.: Modification of cerebral vasoconstriction with hyperventilation in normal man by thymoxamine. Lancet **2**, 461–463 (1972)

CORDAY, E., ROTHENBERG, S., WEINER, S.M.: Cerebral vascular insufficiency. An explanation of the transient stroke. AMA Arch. int. Med. (Chic.) **98**, 683–690 (1956)

CRAIGE, E.H.: On the relative vascularity of various parts of the central nervous system of the albino rat. J. comp. Neurol. **31/32**, 429–464 (1928)

CRAMER, B.: Experimentelle Untersuchungen über den Blutdruck im Gehirn. 8°. Dorpat 1873

CRANSTON, W.J., ROSENDORFF, C.: Local blood flow, cerebrovascular autoregulation and CO_2 responsiveness in the rabbit hypothalamus. J. Physiol. (Lond.) **215**, 577–590 (1971)

CREMER, H.: Über die Registrierung mechanischer Vorgänge auf elektrischem Wege, speziell mit Hilfe des Saitengalvanometers und Saitenelektrometers. Münch. med. Wschr. **54**, 1629–1630 (1907)

CUSHING, H.: Concerning a definite regulating mechanism of the vasomotor centre which controls blood pressure during cerebral compression. John Hopk. Hosp. Bull. **12**, 290–292 (1901)

CUSHING, H.: Physiologische und anatomische Beobachtungen über den Einfluß von Hirnkompression auf den intrakraniellen Kreislauf und über einige hiermit verwandte Erscheinungen. Mitt. Grenzgeb. Med. Chir. **9**, 773 (1902)

CYBULSKI, O.: O ucisku mózgu. Krakau 1891

CZOPF, J., MOLNÁR, L.: Studies of problems in regulating the cerebral blood flow: II. Effect of cerebral trunk excitation on the blood flow of the stimulated area. Acta physiol. Acad. Sci. hung. **37**, 99–111 (1970)

DAHL, N.A., BALFOUR, W.M.: Prolonged anoxia survival due to anoxia pre-exposure: Brain adenosine triphosphate, lactate, and pyruvate. Amer. J. Physiol. **207**, 452–456 (1964)

DAHL, E., NELSON, E.: Electron microscopic observations on human intercranial arteries: II. Innervation. Arch. Neurol. (Chic.) **10**, 158–164 (1964)

D'ALECY, L.G.: Sympathetic cerebral vasoconstriction

blocked by adrenergic alpha receptor antagonists. Stroke 4, 30 (1973)
D'ALECY, L.G., FEIGL, E.O.: Sympathetic control of cerebral blood flow in dogs. Circulat. Res. **31**, 267–283 (1972)
DAVIES, PH.W., GRENELL, R.G.: Metabolism and function in the cerebral cortex under local perfusion with the aid of an oxygen cathode for surface measurement of cortical oxygen consumption. J. Neurophysiol. **25**, 651–683 (1962)
DAVSON, H.: Intracranial and intraocular fluids. In: American Handbook of Physiology: Neurophysiology (FIELD, J., ed). Washington: American Physiology Society 1960, pp. 1761–1788
DAWEKE, H., HAHN, F., OBERDORF, A.: Einfluß von barbituratantagonistischen Analepticis auf EEG, Sauerstoffaufnahme und Durchblutung des Gehirns bei schwerer Veronalvergiftung des Hundes. Naunyn-Schmiedeberg's Arch. exp. Path. Pharmak. **235**, 247–260 (1959)
DELLA PORTA, P., MAIOLO, A.T., NEGRI, V.U., ROSSELLA, E.: Cerebral blood flow and metabolism in therapeutic insulin coma. Metabolism **13**, 131–140 (1964)
DENNY-BROWN, D., MEYER, J.S.: The cerebral collateral circulation: 2. Production of cerebral infarction by ischemic anoxia and its reversibility in early stages. Neurology (Minneap.) **7**, 567–579 (1957)
DESHMUKI, V.D., HARPER, A.M.: The effect of serotonin on cerebral and extracerebral blood flow with possible implications in migraine. Acta neurol. scand. **49**, 649–658 (1973)
DETAR, R., BOHR, D.F.: Adaptation to hypoxia in vascular smooth muscle. Fed. Proc. **27**, 1416–1419 (1968)
DIEMER, K.: Eine verbesserte Modellvorstellung zur Sauerstoffversorgung des Gehirns. Naturwissenschaften **50**, 617–618 (1963)
DIEMER, K.: Über die Entwicklung der Gefäßversorgung des Gehirns im Säuglingsalter. Mschr. Kinderheilk. **112**, 240–242 (1964)
DIEMER, K.: Über die Sauerstoffdiffusion im Gehirn: I. Mitt. Räumliche Vorstellung, Berechnung der Sauerstoffdiffusion. Pflügers Arch. ges. Physiol. **285**, 99–108 (1965a)
DIEMER, K.: Über die Sauerstoffdiffusion im Gehirn: II. Mitt. Die Sauerstoffdiffusion bei O_2-Mangelzuständen. Pflügers Arch. ges. Physiol. **285**, 109–118 (1965b)
DIEMER, K.: Der Einfluß chronischen Sauerstoffmangels auf die Kapillarentwicklung im Gehirn des Säuglings. Mschr. Kinderheilk. **113**, 281–283 (1965c)
DIEMER, K.: Capillarisation and oxygen supply of the brain. In: Oxygen transport in blood and tissue (LÜBBERS, D.W., LUFT, U.C., THEWS, G., WITZLEB, E., eds). Stuttgart: Thieme 1968, pp. 118–124
DIEMER, K., HENN, R.: Kapillarvermehrung in der Hirnrinde der Ratte unter chronischem Sauerstoffmangel. Naturwissenschaften **52**, 135–136 (1965)
DÖRING, H.J., OLBRISCH, R.R.: Elektrocorticogramm, Bestandspotential des Gehirns und energiereiche Phosphatfraktionen der Hirnrinde bei Narkoticum-Überdosierung, Ischämie und Cyanidvergiftung. Pflügers Arch. ges. Physiol. **319**, 12–35 (1970)
DONDERS, F.C.: Onderzockungen ged. in het physiol. Lab. der Utrechtsche Hoogeschool. 2. Jaar. Schmidts Jb. ges. Med. (1850)
DONDERS, F.C.: Die Bewegung des Gehirns und die Gefäßfüllung der Pia mater auch bei geschlossenem unausdehnbarem Schädel unmittelbar beobachtet. Nederl. Lancet 1850, Abstr. in Schmidts Jb. ges. Med. **69**, 16 (1851)
DYKEN, M.L.: Intracranial "steal" in complete occlusion of the internal carotid artery. In: Cerebral blood flow and intracranial pressure. Proc. 5th int. Symp., Roma-Siena 1971, part I. Europ. Neurol. **6**, 301–305 (1971/72)
EBASHI, S., ENDO, M.: Calcium ion and muscle contraction. In: Progress in biophysics and molecular biology. Vol. 18 (BUTLER, J.A.V., NOBLE, D., eds). Oxford: Pergamon Press 1968, pp. 123–183
EDVINSSON, L., HARDEBO, J.E., OWMAN, C.: Role of perivascular sympathetic nerves in autoregulation of cerebral blood flow and in blood-brain barrier function. In: Cerebral Function, Metabolism and Circulation (INGVAR, D.H., LASSEN, N.A., eds). Copenhagen: Munksgaard 1977, pp. 50–51
EDVINSSON, L., NIELSEN, K.C., OWMAN, C., SPORRONG, B.: Cholinergic mechanisms in pial vessels. Z. Zellforsch. Histochem. electron. Microsc. Pharmacol. **134**, 311–325 (1972)
EDVINSSON, L., OWMAN, C.: Amine receptors in brain vessels. In: The cerebral Vessel Wall (CERVOS-NAVARRO, J., BETZ, E., MATAKAS, F., WÜLLENWEBER, R., eds). New York: Raven Press 1976, pp. 197–206
EDVINSSON, L., OWMAN, C.: Sympathetic innervation and adrenergic receptors in intraparenchymal cerebral arterioles of baboon. In: Cerebral Function, Metabolism and Circulation (INGVAR, D.H., LASSEN, N.A., eds). Copenhagen: Munksgaard 1977, pp. 304–305
EICHHORN, O.: Die Radiocirculographie, eine klinische Methode zur Messung der Hirndurchblutung. Wien. klin. Wschr. **71**, 499 (1959)
EICHHORN, O.: Untersuchungen zur Regulation der Hirndurchblutung. Wien. med. Wschr. **116**, 539–540 (1966)
EICHHORN, O., LECHNER, H., AUELL, K.-H.: Der Hirnkreislauf in Forschung und Klinik. Wien: Hollinek 1964
EIDELMANN, B.H., MENDELOW, A.D., MCCALDEN, T.A., BLOOM, D.S.: Potentiation of the cerebrovascular response to intra-arterial 5-hydroxytryptamine. Amer. J. Physiol. **234**, H 301 (1978)
EKSTRÖM-JODAL, B.: On the relation between blood pressure and blood flow in the canine brain with particular regard to the mechanism responsible for

cerebral blood flow autoregulation. Acta physiol. scand. **350**, Suppl. 5–28 (1970)

EKSTRÖM-JODAL, B., ESSEN, C. VON, HÄGGENDAL, E., ROOS, B.-E.: Effects of norepinephrine, serotonin, and dopamine on the cerebral blood flow in the dog. In: Cerebral circulation and metabolism (LANGFITT, T.W., MCHENRY, JR., REIVICH, M., WOLLMAN, H., eds). Berlin-Heidelberg-New York: Springer 1975, pp. 440–442

EKSTRÖM-JODAL, B., HÄGGENDAL, E.: Cerebral blood flow in patients with chronic respiratory insufficiency, with special regard to induced acute changes of the blood gas situation. In: Cerebral blood flow (BROCK, M., FIESCHI, C., INGVAR, D.H., LASSEN, N.A., SCHÜRMANN, K., eds). Berlin-Heidelberg-New York: Springer 1969, pp. 82–85

EKSTRÖM-JODAL, B., HÄGGENDAL, E., LINDER, L.E., NILSSON, N.J.: Cerebral blood flow autoregulation and high arterial pressures and different levels of carbon dioxide tension in dogs. In: Cerebral blood flow and intracranial pressure. (FIESCHI, C., ed). Proc. 5th int. Symp., Roma-Siena 1971, Part I. Europ. Neurol. **6**, 6–10 (1971/72)

ELDRIDGE, F., SALZER, J.: Effect of respiratory alkalosis on blood lactate and pyruvate in humans. J. appl. Physiol. **22**, 461–468 (1967)

ELLIOT, K.A.C., HELLER, J.H.: Metabolism of neurons and glia. In: Metabolism of the nervous system (RICHTER, D., ed). London: Pergamon Press 1957, pp. 286–290

ELLIOT, K.A.C., JASPER, H.H.: Physiological salt solutions for brain surgery. Studies of local pH and pial vessel reactions to buffered and unbuffered isotonic solutions. J. Neurosurg. **6**, 140–152 (1949)

ERKHOV, I.S.: Material on innervation of the intracerebral vessels. In: Vascular diseases of the brain, Nr. 2. Proc. of the 4th All-Union-Congress of Neuropathologists and Psychiatrists, Vol. 2, Moskau, 333–336 (1965)

EVANS, C., SAMAAN, A.: Simultaneous ligature of the carotid and vertebral arteries in the dog. J. Physiol. (Lond.) **87**, 33-34P (1936)

EVANS, M.C., LINTON, R.A.F., CAMERON, I.R.: The effect of local changes in calcium concentration on hypothalamic blood flow in the anaesthetized rabbit. In: Cerebral Function, Metabolism and Circulation (INGVAR, D.H., LASSEN, N.A., eds). Copenhagen: Munksgaard 1977, pp. 388–389

FÅHRAEUS, R., LINDQVIST, T.: The viscosity of the blood in narrow capillary tubes. Amer. J. Physiol. **96**, 562–568 (1931)

FALCK, B., MCHEDLISHVILI, G.I., OWMAN, C.: Histochemical demonstration of adrenergic nerves in cortex-pia of rabbit. Acta Pharmacol. **23**, 133–142 (1965)

FEIN, J.M.: Focal autoregulatory disturbances in middle cerebral artery vasospasm. Stroke **4**, 333–334 (1973)

FEINDEL, W.: Discussion on cerebral ischemia. In: Cerebral vascular diseases (TOOLE, J.F., SICKERT, R.G., WHISNANT, J.P., eds). New York-London: Grune and Stratton 1968, pp. 120–121

FEINDEL, W., HODGE, CH.P., YAMAMOTO, Y.L.: Epicerebral angiography by fluorescein during craniotomy. Progr. brain Res. **30**, 471–477 (1968)

FEINDEL, W., YAMAMOTO, Y.L., HODGE, CH.P.: The human cerebral microcirculation studied by intraarterial radio-active tracers, coomassie blue and fluorescein dyes. In: 4th Europ. Conf. on Microcirculation, Cambridge 1966, pp. 220–224 (HARDERS, H., ed). Basel-New York: Karger

FEINDEL, W., YAMAMOTO, Y.L., HODGE, CH.P.: Intracarotid fluorescein angiography: A new method for examination of the epicerebral circulation in man. Canad. med. Ass. J. **96**, 1–7 (1967)

FENCL, V., VALE, J.R., BROCH, J.A.: Respiration and cerebral blood flow in metabolic acidosis and alkalosis in humans. J. appl. Physiol. **27**, 67–76 (1969)

FERRIS, E.B. JR.: Objective measurement of relative intracranial blood flow in man with observations concerning the hydrodynamics of the craniovertebral system. Arch. Neurol. Psychiat. (Chic.) **46**, 377–401 (1941)

FICK, A.: Über die Messung des Blutquantums in den Herzventrikeln. S.B. phys. med. Ges. Würzburg 1870

FIELDS, W.S., BRUETMAN, M.E., WEIBEL, J.: Collateral circulation of the brain. In: Monographs in the surgical sciences, Vol. 2. Baltimore: Williams & Wilkins 1965, pp. 183–259

FIESCHI, C.: Iperemia reattiva cerebrale focale nelle lesioni ischemiche. Sist. nerv. **18**, 215–220 (1966)

FIESCHI, C.: Fisiologia della circolazione cerebrale. Soc. ital. Cardiol. **1**, 63–94 (1967)

FIESCHI, C.: Regional cerebral blood flow in apoplexy (acute hemiparesis) without arterial occlusion. Scand. J. clin. Lab. Invest. **102** Suppl. E XVI (1968)

FIESCHI, C., AGNOLI, A., BATTISTINI, N., BOZZAO, L., PRENCIPE, M.: Derangement of regional cerebral blood flow and of its regulatory mechanisms in acute cerebrovascular lesions. Neurology (Minneap.) **18**, 1166–1179 (1968a)

FIESCHI, C., BATTISTINI, N., NARDINI, M.: Experimental cerebral infarction: Focal or perifocal reactive hyperemia and its relationship with the red softening. 4th Int. Symp. of the Research Group on Cerebral Circulation, Salzburg 1968, pp. 25–29, 1968b

FIESCHI, C., ISAACS, G., KETY, S.S.: On the question of heterogeneity of the local blood flow in gray matter of the brain. In: Blood flow through organs and tissues (BAIN, W.H., HARPER, A.M., eds). Edinburgh-London: Livingstone 1968c, pp. 226–231

FINESINGER, J., PUTMAN, T.J.: Cerebral circulation. XXIII. Induced variations in volume flow through the brain perfused at constant pressure. Arch. Neurol. Psychiat. (Chic.) **30**, 775–794 (1933)

FISCHER, C.M.: Concerning recurrent transient cerebral ischemic attacks. J. Canad. med. Ass. **86**, 1091–1099 (1962)

FITCH, W., BARKER, J., MCDOWALL, D.G., JENNETT, W.B.: The effect of methoxyflurane on cerebrospinal fluid pressure in patients with and without intracranial space-occupying lesions. Brit. J. Anaesth. **41**, 564–573 (1969)

FLECKENSTEIN, A., GRÜN, G.: Prinzipielles zur Wirkung von Ca^{++} Antagonisten auf die bioelektrische und mechanische Funktion glatter Muskelzellen. In: Vascular smooth muscle (BETZ, E., ed.). Berlin-Heidelberg-New York: Springer 1972, pp. 62–65

FLOREY, H.: Microscopical observation on the circulation of the blood in the cerebral cortex. Brain **48**, 43–64 (1925)

FOG, M.: Om piaarteriernes vasomotoriske reaktioner. Copenhagen: Munksgaard 1934

FOG, M.: Cerebral circulation. The reaction of the pial arteries to a fall in blood pressure. Arch. Neurol. Psychiat. (Chic.) **37**, 351–364 (1937)

FOG, M.: The relationship between the blood pressure and the tonic regulation of the pial arteries. J. Neurol. Psychiat. **1**, 187–197 (1938)

FOG, M.: Cerebral circulation. II. Reaction of pial arteries to increase in blood pressure. Arch. Neurol. Psychiat. (Chic.) **41**, 260–268 (1939)

FOLKOW, B.: Intravascular pressure as a factor regulating the tone of the small vessels. Acta physiol. scand. **17**, 289–310 (1949)

FOLKOW, B.: Description of the myogenic hypothesis. Circulat. Res. **15**, Suppl. 279–287 (1964)

FORBES, H.S.: Study of blood vessels on cortex of living mammalian brain-description of technique. Anat. Rec. **120**, 309–315 (1954)

FORBES, H.S., COBB, S.S.: Vasomotor control of cerebral vessels. Brain **61**, 221–233 (1938)

FORBES, H.S., SCHMIDT, C.F., NASON, G.I.: Evidence of vasodilatator innervation in the parietal cortex of the cat. Amer. J. Physiol **125**, 216–219 (1939)

FORBES, H.S., WOLFF, H.G.: Cerebral circulation. III. The vasomotor control of cerebral vessels. Arch. Neurol. Psychiat. (Chic.) **19**, 1057–1086 (1928)

FRANCOIS-FRANCK, C.-E.: Sur les fonctions motrices du cerveau. Paris 1887, p. 199

FRASER, R.A.R., STEIN, B.M., POOL, J.L.: Adrenergic blockade of hypocapnic cerebral arterial constriction. Stroke J. cerebr. Circ. **2**, 219–231 (1971)

FREEMAN, J., INGVAR, D.H.: Elimination of the cerebral blood flow – EEG relationship and autoregulation by hypoxia. In: Blood flow through organs and tissues (HARPER, A.M., BAIN, W.H., eds). Edinburgh-London: Livingstone 1968a, pp. 258–259.

FREEMAN, J., INGVAR, D.H.: Elimination by hypoxia of cerebral autoregulation and EEG relationship. Exp. Brain Res. **5**, 61–71 (1968b)

FREYHAN, F.A., WOODFORD, R.B., KETY, S.S.: Cerebral blood flow and metabolism in psychoses of senility. J. nerv. ment. Dis. **113**, 449–456 (1951)

GÄNSHIRT, H.: Die Sauerstoffversorgung des Gehirns und ihre Störung bei der Liquordrucksteigerung und beim Hirnödem. Berlin-Göttingen-Heidelberg: Springer 1957

GÄNSHIRT, H.: Der Hirnkreislauf. Stuttgart: Thieme 1972

GÄNSHIRT, H., DRANSFELD, L., ZYLKA, W.: Das Hirnpotentialbild und der Erholungsrückstand am Warmblütergehirn nach kompletter Ischämie. Arch. Psychiat. Nervenkr. **189**, 109–125 (1952b)

GÄNSHIRT, H., SEVERIN, G., ZYLKA, W.: Die Erholungslatenz des Warmblütergehirns nach kompletter Ischämie. Pflügers Arch. ges. Physiol. **256**, 219–233 (1952a)

GÄNSHIRT, H., TÖNNIS, W.: Durchblutung und Sauerstoffverbrauch des Hirns bei intrakraniellen Tumoren. Dtsch. Z. Nervenheilk. **174**, 305–330 (1956)

GÄRTNER, G., WAGNER, J.: Über den Hirnkreislauf. Wien. med. Wschr. 601–603 (1887a)

GÄRTNER, G., WAGNER, J.: Über den Hirnkreislauf. Wien. med. Wschr. 640–642 (1887b)

GASKELL, P., BURTON, A.C.: Local postural vasomotor reflexes arising from the limb veins. Circulat. Res. **1**, 27–39 (1953)

GEIGER, A., MAGNES, J.: The isolation of the cerebral circulation and the perfusion of the brain in the living cat. Amer. J. Physiol. **149**, 517–537 (1947)

GERAUD, J., BES, A., RASCOL, A., DELPLA, M., MARC-VERGNES, J.P.: Mesure du débit sanguin cérébral au krypton 85. Quelques applications physio-pathologiques et cliniques. Rev. neurol. **108**, 542–557 (1963)

GEYER, N., RODLER, H., LECHNER, H.: Experimentelle Untersuchungen zur Deutung des Rheogramms. In: Rheoencephalographia (MARTIN, E., LECHNER, H., Hrsg.), S. 33–41. Wien: Wiener medizinische Akademie 1965

GIBBS, E.L., LENNOX, W.G., GIBBS, F.A.: Bilateral internal jugular blood: Comparison of arteriovenous differences, oxygen dextrose ratios and respiratory quotients. Amer. J. Psychiat. **102**, 184–190 (1945)

GIBBS, F.A.: A thermoelectric blood flow recorder in the form of a needle. Proc. Soc. exp. Biol. (N.Y.) **31**, 141–146 (1933)

GIBBS, F.A., GIBBS, E.L., LENNOX, W.G.: The cerebral blood flow during sleep in man. Brain **58**, 44–48 (1935)

GIBBS, F.A., MAXWELL, H., GIBBS, E.L.: Volume flow of blood through the human brain. Arch. Neurol. Psychiat. (Chic.) **57**, 137–144 (1947)

GIBBS, F.A., NIMS, L.F., GIBBS, E.L.: Differentiation of the effects of low carbon dioxide on the electrical activity of the cortex. Fed. Proc. **1**, 29–30 (1942)

GLASS, H.J., HARPER, A.M.: Measurement of regional blood flow in cerebral cortex of man through intact scull. Brit. med. J. **1**, 593 (1963)

GLEICHMANN, U., INGVAR, D.H., LASSEN, N.A., LÜBBERS, D.W., SIESJÖ, B.K., THEWS, G.: Regional cerebral cortical metabolic rate of oxygen and carbon dioxide, related to the EEG in the anesthetized dog. Acta physiol. scand. **55**, 82–94 (1962a)

GLEICHMANN, U., INGVAR, D.H., LÜBBERS, D.W., SIESJÖ, K.B., THEWS, G.: Tissue pO_2 and pCO_2 of the cerebral cortex related to blood gas tensions. Acta physiol. scand. **55**, 127–138 (1962b)

GOLDENSON, E.S., WHITEHEAD, R.W., PARRY, T.M., SPENCER, J.H., GROVER, R.F., DRAPER, W.B.: Effect of diffusion respiration and high concentrations of CO_2 on cerebrospinal fluid pressure of anaesthetized dogs. Amer. J. Physiol. **165**, 334–340 (1951)

GOLENHOFEN, K., HENSEL, H., HILDEBRANDT, G.: Durchblutungsmessungen mit Wärmeleitelementen in Forschung und Klinik. Stuttgart: Thieme 1963

GOODFORD, P.J., WOLOWYK, M.W.: Localization of cation interactions in the smooth muscle of the guinea pig taenia coli. J. Physiol. (Lond.) **224**, 521–535 (1972)

GOTTSTEIN, U.: Physiologie und Pathophysiologie des Hirnkreislaufs. Med. Welt **15**, 715–726 (1965)

GOTTSTEIN, U., BERNSMEIER, A., BLÖMER, H., SCHIMMLER, W.: Die cerebrale Hämodynamik bei Kranken mit Mitralstenose und kombiniertem Mitralvitium. Klin. Wschr. **38**, 1025–1030 (1960)

GOTTSTEIN, U., BERNSMEIER, A., LEHN, H., NIEDERMAYER, W.: Hämodynamik und Stoffwechsel des Gehirns bei Schlafmittelvergiftung. Dtsch. med. Wschr. **86**, 2170–2176 (1961)

GOTTSTEIN, U., BERNSMEIER, A., SEDLMEYER, J.: Der Kohlenhydratstoffwechsel des menschlichen Gehirns. I. Untersuchungen mit substratspezifischen enzymatischen Methoden bei normaler Hirndurchblutung. Klin. Wschr. **41**, 943–948 (1963)

GOTTSTEIN, U., BERNSMEIER, A., SEDLMEYER, J.: Der Kohlenhydratstoffwechsel des menschlichen Gehirns. II. Untersuchungen mit substratspezifischen enzymatischen Methoden bei Kranken mit verminderter Hirndurchblutung auf dem Boden einer Arteriosklerose der Gehirngefäße. Klin. Wschr. **42**, 310–313 (1964)

GRANHOLM, L., KAASIK, A.E., NILSSON, L., SIESJÖ, B.K.: The lactate pyruvate ratios of cerebrospinal fluid of rats and cats related to the lactate/pyruvate, the ATP/ADP, and the phosphocreatine/creatine ratios of brain tissue. Acta physiol. scand. **74**, 398–409 (1968)

GRANHOLM, L., LUKJANOVA, L., SIESJÖ, B.K.: The effect of marked hyperventilation upon tissue levels of NADH, lactate, pyruvate, phosphocreatine and adenosine phosphates of rat brain. Acta physiol. scand. **75**, 1–12 (1969)

GRANHOLM, L., SIESJÖ, B.K.: Lactate and pyruvate concentrations in blood, cerebrospinal fluid and brain tissue of the cat. Acta physiol. scand. **70**, 255–256 (1967)

GRANHOLM, L., SIESJÖ, B.K.: Signs of cerebral hypoxia in hyperventilation. Experientia **24**, 337–338 (1968)

GRANHOLM, L., SIESJÖ, B.K.: The effect of hypercapnia and hypocapnia upon the cerebrospinal fluid lactate and pyruvate concentrations and upon the lactate, pyruvate, ATP, ADP, phosphocreatine and creatine concentrations of cat brain tissue. Acta physiol. scand. **75**, 257–266 (1969)

GRAYSON, J.: Internal calorimetry in the determination of thermal conductivity and blood flow. J. Physiol. (Lond.) **118**, 54–72 (1952)

GROTE, J., KREUSCHER, H.: Die Sauerstoffversorgung des Hundegehirns. I. Mitt.: Die zerebrale Durchblutung und Sauerstoffaufnahme. Zool. Anz. **179**, 319–329 (1967)

GROTE, J., KREUSCHER, H., REULEN, H.J., VAUPEL, P., GÜNTHER, H.: Respiratory gas transport in brain under normal and pathological conditions. Advanc. Chem. Ser. **118**, 35–46 (1973)

GROTE, J., KREUSCHER, H., SCHUBERT, R., RUSS, H.J.: New studies on the influence of PaO_2 and $PaCO_2$ on regional and total cerebral blood flow. 6th Europ. Conf. Microcirculation Aalborg 1970. Basel: Karger 1971a, pp. 294–297

GROTE, J., KREUSCHER, H., SCHUBERT, R., RUSS, H.J.: Investigations on the influence of PaO_2 and $PaCO_2$ on the regulation of cerebral blood flow in dogs. In: Brain and blood flow (ROSS RUSSELL, R.W. ed). London: Pitman 1971b, pp. 200–204

GROTE, J., SCHUBERT, R., FENSKE, A.: Cerebral blood flow and oxygen supply during ventricular-cisternal perfusion. Pflügers Arch. **359**, Suppl. R 38 (1975)

GRÜN, G.: Ca^{++}-Antagonismus – ein neu erkanntes Prinzip der Relaxation glatter Muskelzellen. Med. Habil. Freiburg 1972

GRUNEWALD, W.: Theoretical analysis of the oxygen supply in tissue. In: Oxygen transport in blood and tissue (LÜBBERS, D.W., LUFT, U.C., THEWS, G., WITZLEB, E., eds). Stuttgart: Thieme 1968, pp. 100–114

GUTMANN, J., BRÜNDL, G., KACHEL, V., RUHENSTROTH-BAUER, G.: Quantitative Messungen der rheographischen Phänomene. In: Rheoencephalography and plethysmographical methods (LECHNER, H., Hrsg.). Excerpta med. (Amst.) 1968

HADJI-DIMOS, A.A., EKBERG, R., INGVAR, D.H.: Effects of ethyl-alcohol on EEG and cortical blood flow in cat. In: Pharmakologie des Gehirnkreislaufs (BETZ, E., WÜLLENWEBER, R., eds). München-Gräfelfing: Banaschewski 1969, pp. 116–119

HÄGGENDAL, E.: Effects of some vasoactive drugs on the vessels of cerebral gray matter in the dog. Acta physiol. scand. **66**, Suppl. 258, 55–79 (1965)

HÄGGENDAL, E.: Elimination of autoregulation during arterial and cerebral hypoxia. Scand. J. clin. Lab. Invest. Suppl. 102, V:D (1968)

HÄGGENDAL, E., JOHANSSON, B.: Effects of arterial carbon dioxide tension and oxygen saturation on cerebral blood flow autoregulation in dogs. Acty physiol. scand. **66**, Suppl. 258, 27–53 (1966)

HÄGGENDAL, E., NILSSON, N.J., NORBÄCK, B.: Effect of blood corpuscle concentration on cerebral blood flow. Acta chir. scand. Suppl. 364, 3–12 (1966b)

HÄGGENDAL, E., NILSSON, N.J., NORBÄCK, B.: Einfluß von experimentell hervorgerufenen Veränderungen der Blutviskosität auf die Hirndurchblutung beim Hunde. In: Pharmakologie der lokalen Gehirndurchblutung (Betz, E., Wüllenweber, R., Hrsg.), S. 94–97. München-Gräfelfing: Banaschewski 1969

Häggendal, E., Norbäck, B.: Effect of viscosity on cerebral blood flow. Acta chir. scand. Suppl. 364, 13–22 (1966a)

Hagen, E., Wittkowski, W.: Licht- und elektronenmikroskopische Untersuchung zur Innervation der Piagefäße. Z. Zellforsch. **95**, 429–444 (1969)

Haining, J.L., Turner, M.D., Pantall, R.M.: Local cerebral blood flow in young and old rats during hypoxia and hypercapnia. Amer. J. Physiol. **218**, 1020–1024 (1970)

Hales, S.: Statical essays: Vol. 2. Containing haemostatics; or an account of sone hydraulic and hydrostatical experiments made on the blood and blood vessels of animals. London: Innys and Manby 1733

Haller, A. v.: Dissertation on the sensible and irritable parts of animals. London: Nourse 1755, pp. 20–21

Halsey, J.H., Capra, N.F.: Intracranial pressure, luxury perfusion, and progression of experimental cerebral infarction. In: Cerebral blood flow and intracranial pressure. Proc. 5th Int. Symp. Roma-Siena 1971. Europ. Neurol. **6**, 296–300 (1971/72)

Hamilton, W.F., Moore, J.W., Kinsman, J.M., Spurling, R.G.: Simultaneous determination of the greater and lesser circulation times, of the mean velocity of blood flow through the heart and lungs of the cardiac output and an approximation of the amount of blood activeley circulating in the heart and lungs. Amer. J. Physiol. **85**, 377–378 (1928)

Hanko, J., Edvinsson, L., Hakanson, R., Larsson, L.J., Owman, C., Schaffalitzky de Muckadell, O., Sundler, F.: Immunohistochemical demonstration of vasodilatory peptidergic nerves in brain. Acta neurol. scand. Suppl. 64, Vol. 56, 386–387 (1977)

Hansen, D.B., Sultzer, M.R., Freygang, W.H., Sokoloff, L.: Effects of low O_2 and high CO_2 concentrations in inspired air on local cerebral circulation. Fed. Proc. **16**, 54 (1959)

Harnarine-Singh, D., Hyde, J.B.: Post-natal growth of the arterial net in the human cerebral pia mater. Nature **225**, 86–87 (1970)

Harper, A.M.: Physiology of cerebral blood flow. Brit. J. Anaesth. **37**, 225–235 (1965a)

Harper, A.M.: The interrelationship between a pCO_2 and blood pressure in the regulation of blood flow through the cerebral cortex. Acta neurol. scand. Suppl. **14**, 94–103 (1965b)

Harper, A.M., Bell, R.A.: The effect of metabolic acidosis and alkalosis on the blood flow through the cerebral cortex. J. Neurol. Neurosurg. Psychiat. **26**, 341–344 (1963)

Harper, A.M., Glass, H.I.: Effect of alterations in the arterial carbon dioxide tension on the blood flow through the cerebral cortex at normal and low arterial blood pressures. J. Neurol. Neurosurg. Psychiat. **28**, 449–452 (1965)

Harper, A.M., MacKenzie, E.T.: Cerebral circulatory and metabolic effects of 5-hydroxytyptamine in anaesthetized baboons. J. Physiol. **271**, 721–733 (1977a)

Harper, A.M., MacKenzie, E.T.: Effects of 5-hydroxytryptamine on pial arteriolar calibre in anaesthetized cats. J. Physiol. **271**, 735–746 (1977b)

Harper, A.M., Rowan, J.O., Deshmukh, V.D., Jennett, W.B.: Studies on possible neurogenic influences on the cerebral circulation. In: Brain and blood flow (Ross Russell, R.W., ed). London: Pitman 1970, pp. 182–186

Harvey, W.: Exercitatio anatomica de motu cordis et sanguinis in animalibus. Übersetzung: Alliance culturelle du livre. Genève-Paris-Bruxelles: Masson 1962

Hass, W.K., Hawkins, R.A., Ransohoff, J.: Cerebral blood flow, glucose utilization and oxidative metabolism after bilateral reticular formation lesions. In: Cerebral Function, Metabolism and Circulation (D.H. Ingvar, N.A. Lassen, eds). Copenhagen: Munksgaard 1977, pp. 240–241

Hattingberg, H.M., Klaus, W.: Trennung des proteingebundenen vom frei diffusiblen Kalzium im Serum durch Sephadex. Klin. Wschr. **44**, 499–503 (1966)

Hedlund, S., Ljundgren, K., Köhler, V.: Mean cerebral blood transit time obtained by external measurement of an intravenously injected tracer. Acta radiol. (Stockh.) **4**, 581–591 (1966)

Hedlund, S., Nylin, G., Regenström, O.: The behaviour of the cerebral circulation during muscular exercise. Acta physiol. scand. **54**, 316–324 (1962)

Hegelmair, F.: Die Atembewegungen beim Hirndruck 8°. Dissertation Heilbronn 1859

Heistad, D.D., Marcus, M.L., Abboud, F.M.: Effects of sympathetic nerve stimulation on cerebral blood flow. In: Cerebral Function, Metabolism and Circulation (D.H. Ingvar, N.A. Lassen, eds). Copenhagen: Munksgaard 1977, pp. 306–307

Heiss, W.-D., Kvicala, V., Prosenz, P., Tschabitscher, H.: Gamma-camera and multichannel analyser for multilocular rCBF measurement. In: Cerebral blood flow (Brock, M., Fieschi, C., Ingvar, D.H., Lassen, N.A., Schürmann, K., eds). Berlin-Heidelberg-New York: Springer 1969, pp. 29–30

Heiss, W.-D., Prosenz, P., Gloning, K., Tschabitscher, H.: Regional and total cerebral blood flow under vasodilating drugs. In: Brain and blood flow (Ross Russell, R.W., ed). London: Pitman 1971, pp. 270–276

Heiss, W.-D., Prosenz, P., Roszuczky, A.: Technical consideration in the use of a gamma camera 1.600-channel analyser system for the measurement of regional cerebral blood flow. J. nucl. Med. **13**, 534–543 (1972)

HEISS, W.-D., PROSENZ, P., ROSZUCZKY, A., TSCHABITSCHER, H.: Die Verwendung von Gamma-Kamera und Vielkanalspeicher zur Messung der gesamten und regionalen Hirndurchblutung. J. nucl. Med. **7**, 297–318 (1968)

HEKMATPANAH, J.: Cerebral circulation and perfusion in experimental increased intracranial pressure. J. Neurosurg. **32**, 21–29 (1970)

HEKMATPANAH, J.: Irreversible damage and cerebral death in increased intracranial pressure. In: Intracranial pressure (BROCK, M., DIETZ, H., eds). Berlin-Heidelberg-New York: Springer 1972, pp. 149–154

HELD, K., GOTTSTEIN, U., NIEDERMAYER, W.: Cerebral blood flow in non-pulsatile perfusion. In: Cerebral blood flow (BROCK, M., FIESCHI, C., INGVAR, D.H., LASSEN, N.A., SCHÜRMANN, K., eds). Berlin-Heidelberg-New York: Springer 1969, pp. 94–95

HELD, K., JACOBSEN, O., KRAFT, K., BERGHOFF, W.: Regional cerebral metabolism in experimental brain infarction. Stroke **4**, 331 (1973)

HELD, K., NIEDERMAYER, W., GOTTSTEIN, U.: Untersuchungen des menschlichen Hirnkreislaufs bei totalem av-Block und Schrittmacherstimulation. Verh. dtsch. Ges. Kreisl.-Forsch. **34**, 421–424 (1968)

HELD, K., NIEDERMAYER, W., GOTTSTEIN, U.: Die Hirndurchblutung bei nicht pulsierender Perfusion. Z. Kreisl.-Forsch. **60**, 336–346 (1971)

HEMMER, R.: Der Liquordruck. Untersuchungen zur Physiologie, Pathophysiologie und medikamentösen Beeinflussung der Liquordynamik. Stuttgart: Thieme 1960

HENLE, J.: Allgemeine Anatomie. Leipzig: Voss 1841

HENSEL, H.: Fortlaufende Wärmeleitfähigkeits- und Durchblutungsmessung im Gewebe mit einer Differential-Calorimetersonde. Ber. ges. Physiol. **162**, 360 (1953/54)

HENSEL, H.: Meßkopf zur Durchblutungsregistrierung an Oberflächen. Pflügers Arch. ges. Physiol. **268**, 604–606 (1958/59)

HEPPNER, F.: Kapillarmikroskopische Beobachtungen an den Piagefäßen des Großhirns. Acta neurochir. (Wien) Suppl. 7, 303–310 (1961)

HERLIHY, J.T., BOCKMAN, E.L., BERNE, R.M., RUBIO, R.: Adenosine relaxation of isolated vascular smooth muscle. Am. J. Physiol., **230**, 1239–1243 (1976)

HERNANDEZ-PEREZ, M.J., ERICKSON, H.H., FITZPATRICK, E.L.: Autonomic control of cerebral blood flow and autoregulation. In: Cerebral circulation and metabolism (LANGFITT, T.W., MCHENRY, JR., L.C., REIVICH, M., WOLLMANN, H., eds). Berlin-Heidelberg-New York: Springer 1975, pp. 462–465

HERRMANN, E.: Die allgemeinen und die herdförmigen, nicht blutungsbedingten Hirnzirkulationsstörungen. Habil.-Schrift Marburg 1964

HERRMANN, E.: Application of heat clearance for measurements of cerebral blood flow in man. In: Blood flow through organs and tissues (HARPER, A.M., BAIN, W.H., eds). Edinburgh-London: Livingstone 1968, pp. 182–190

HERRSCHAFT, H., GLEIM, F., DUUS, P., SCHMIDT, H.: Heterogeneity of regional cerebral blood flow and regional distribution of relative weights of gray and white matter in normal subjects. In: Cerebral circulation and metabolism (LANGFITT, W.T. et al., eds). Berlin-Heidelberg-New York: Springer 1975, pp. 141–144

HEUSER, D.: The significance of cortical extracellular H^+, K^+ and Ca^{++} activities for regulation of local cerebral blood flow under conditions of enhanced neuronal activity. In: Cerebral Vascular Smooth Muscle and its Control, Ciba Foundation Symposium 56 (New Series). Amsterdam-New York: Elsevier/Excerpta Medica/North-Holland 1978

HEUSER, D., ASTRUP, J., LASSEN, N.A., NILSSON, B., NORBERG, K., SIESJÖ, B.K.: Are H^+ and K^+ factors for the adjustment of cerebral blood flow to changes in functional state: a microelectrode study. In: Cerebral Function, Metabolism and Circulation (D.H. INGVAR, N.A. LASSEN, eds). Copenhagen: Munksgaard 1977, pp. 216–217

HEUSER, D., LENZI, G.L., BATTISTINI, N., FIESCHI, C.: Regional changes of H^+ and K^+ activities in central nervous structures during sensitive activation. Pflügers Arch. ges. Physiol. **359**, Suppl. R 87 (1975a)

HEUSER, D., SCHINDLER, U., HOSSMANN, K.-A., BETZ, E.: The significance of cerebral extracellular H^+ and K^+ activities, brain volume and -metabolism for recovery after prolonge of cerebral ischemia. In: Blood flow and metabolism in the brain (HARPER, A.M., JENNETT, W.B., MILLER, J.D., ROWAN, J.O., eds). Edinburgh-London: Livingstone 1975b

HILL, L.: The physiology and pathology of the cerebral circulation; an experimental research. London: Churchill 1896

HIMWICH, H.E., HIMWICH, W.A., ETSTEN, B.: The functional organization of the central nervous system as observed in pentothal anesthesia. Report of Int. Physiol. Congress Jan. 15, 1947a, 13 p

HIMWICH, W.A., HOMBURGER, E., MARESCA, R., HIMWICH, H.E.: Brain metabolism in man: Unanesthetized and in pentothal narcosis. Amer. J. Psychiat. **103**, 689–696 (1947b)

HINZEN, D.H., MÜLLER, U., SOBOTKA, P., GEBERT, E., LANG, R., HIRSCH, H.: Metabolism and function of dog's brain recovering from longtime ischemia. Amer. J. Physiol. **223**, 1158–1164 (1972)

HIRSCH, H.: Hirndurchblutung und Thrombozytenaggregation. In: Pharmakologie der lokalen Gehirndurchblutung. (BETZ, E., WÜLLENWEBER, R., Hrsg.), S. 90–83. München-Gräfelfing: Banaschewski 1969a

HIRSCH, H.: Über die Abhängigkeit der Gehirndurchblutung von Blutdruck und die Wiederbelebungszeit des Gehirns. In: Diagnostik und Therapie der zerebralen Gefäßverschlüsse (HERRSCHAFT, H., Hrsg.), S. 43–48. Stuttgart: Thieme 1969b

Hirsch, H., Euler, K.H., Schneider, M.: Über die Erholung des Gehirns nach kompletter Ischämie bei Hypothermie. Pflügers Arch. ges. Physiol. **265**, 314–327 (1957)

Hirsch, H., Gleichmann, U., Kristen, H., Magazinovic, V.: Über die Beziehung zwischen O_2-Aufnahme des Gehirns und O_2-Druck im Sinusblut des Gehirns bei uneingeschränkter und eingeschränkter Durchblutung. Pflügers Arch. ges. Physiol. **273**, 213–222 (1961)

Hirsch, H., Körner, K.: Über die Druck-Durchblutungs-Relation der Gehirngefäße. Pflügers Arch. ges. Physiol. **280**, 316–325 (1964)

Hirsch, H., Schneider, M.: Durchblutung und Sauerstoffaufnahme des Gehirns. In: Handb. d. Neurochirurgie, Bd. I/2, S. 434–528 (H. Olivecrona, W. Tönnies, W. Krenkel, Hrsg.). Berlin: Springer 1968

Hirsch, H., Scholl, H., Dickmans, H.A., Eisolt, J., Mann, H., Krankenhagen, B.: Über die kortikale Gleichspannung nach Überschreiten der Wiederbelebungszeit des Gehirns. Pflügers Arch. ges. Physiol. **301**, 351–357 (1968b)

Hirsch, H., Scholl, H., Paschke, K.G., Schmid-Schönbein, H.: Die Veränderung der kortikalen Gleichspannung bei kompletter und inkompletter Ischämie des Gehirns. Pflügers Arch. ges. Physiol. **301**, 334–343 (1968a)

Høedt-Rasmussen, K., Skinhøj, E., Paulson, O., Ewald, J., Bjerrum, J.K., Fahrenkrug, A., Lassen, N.A.: Regional cerebral blood flow in acute apoplexy. The "luxury perfusion syndrome" of brain tissue. Arch. Neurol. (Chic.) **17**, 271–281 (1967)

Holman, M.E.: Electrophysiology of vascular smooth muscle. Ergebn. Physiol. **61**, 137–177 (1969)

Holmes, R.L., Newman, P.P., Wolstencroft, J.H.: The distribution of carotid and vertebral blood in the brain of the cat. J. Physiol. **140**, 236–246 (1958)

Holmes, R.L., Wolstencroft, J.H.: Accessory sources of blood supply to the brain of the cat. J. Physiol. **148**, 93–107 (1959)

Holmquist, B., Ingvar, D.H., Siesjö, B.: Cerebral sympathetic vasoconstriction and EEG. Acta physiol. scand. **40**, 146–160 (1957)

Homburger, W., Himwich, W.A., Etsten, B., York, G., Maresca, R., Himwich, H.E.: Effect of pentothal anesthesia on canine cerebral cortex. Amer. J. Physiol. **147**, 343–345 (1946)

Hossmann, K.-A., Kleihues, P.: Reversibility of ischemic brain damage. Arch. Neurol. (Chic.) **29**, 375–384 (1973)

Hossmann, K.-A., Lechtape-Grüter, H.: Blood flow and recovery of the cat brain after complete ischemia for one hour. Cerebral Blood flow and intracranial pressure. Proc. 5th Int. Symp., Roma-Siena 1971, part I. Europ. Neurol. **6**, 318–322 (1971/72)

Hossmann, K.-A., Lechtape-Grüter, H., Hossmann, V.: The role of cerebral blood flow for the recovery of the brain after prolonged ischemia. Z. Neurol. **204**, 281–299 (1973)

Hubbard, J.I.: Microphysiology of vertebrate neuromuscular transmission. Physiol. Rev. **53**, 674–723 (1973)

Huddart, H., Price, N.R.: Calcium movements during excitation-contraction coupling in smooth muscle cells. Comp. Biochem. Physiol. **54A**, 375–386 (1976)

Hürtle, K.: Beiträge zur Hämodynamik. 3. Abhandlung: Untersuchung über die Innervation der Hirngefäße. Pflügers Arch. ges. Physiol. **44**, 561–618 (1889)

Hutten, H., Schwarz, W., Schulz, V.: Dependence of ^{85}Kr (β)-clearance, rCBF determination of the input function. In: Cerebral blood flow (Brock, M., Fieschi, C., Ingvar, D.H., Lassen, N.A., Schürmann, K., eds). Berlin-Heidelberg-New York: Springer 1969, pp. 1–3

Ingvar, D.H.: Cortical state of excitability and cortical circulation. In: Reticular formation of the brain (Jaspers, H.H., ed). Boston, Mass.: Little & Brown 1958, pp. 381–408

Ingvar, D.H.: The pathophysiology of the stroke related to findings in EEG and to measurements of regional cerebral blood flow. Thule Int. Symp. 19.–21. April, Stroke 1967, pp. 105–122

Ingvar, D.H.: Regional cerebral blood flow in cerebrovascular disorders. In: Cerebral circulation Progr. in brain research, Amsterdam-London-New York 1968, Vol. 30, pp. 57–61

Ingvar, D.H.: Correlation between cerebral function and cerebral blood flow and its disappearance following anoxia. In: Pharmakologie der lokalen Gehirndurchblutung (Betz, E., Wüllenweber, R., Hrsg.), S. 66–70. München-Gräfelfing: Banaschewski 1969

Ingvar, D.H.: Patterns of brain activity revealed by measurements of regional cerebral blood flow. In: Brain work. The coupling of function, metabolism and blood flow in the brain (Ingvar, D.H., Lassen, N.A., eds). Copenhagen: Munksgaard 1975, pp. 397–413

Ingvar, D.H., Cronqvist, S., Ekberg, R., Risberg, J., Høedt-Rasmussen, K.: Normal values of regional cerebral blood flow in man, including flow and weight estimates of gray and white matter. Acta neurol. scand. Suppl. 14, 72–78 (1965)

Ingvar, D.H., Franzen, G.: Abnormalities in chronic schizophrenia with mental deterioration. Stroke **4**, 553 (1973)

Ingvar, D.H., Lassen, N.A.: Regional blood flow of the cerebral cortex determined by Krypton^{85}. Acta physiol. scand. **54**, 325–338 (1962)

Ingvar, D.H., Lassen, N.A.: Methods for cerebral blood flow measurements in man. Brit. J. Anaesth. **37**, 216–224 (1965a)

Ingvar, D.H., Lassen, N.A.: Regional cerebral blood flow. Acta neurol. scand. **41**, Suppl. 14 (1965b)

Ingvar, D.H., Lassen, N.A., Siesjö, B.K., Skinhøj,

E.: CBF and CSF. 3rd Int. Symp. on cerebral blood flow and cerebrospinal fluid. Scand. J. clin. Lab. Invest. Suppl. 102 (1968)

INGVAR, D.H., SÖDERBERG, U.: A new method for measuring cerebral blood flow in relation to the encephalogram. Electroenceph. clin. Neurophysiol. **8**, 403–412 (1956)

INGVAR, D.H., SÖDERBERG, U.: Cortical blood flow related to EEG patterns evoked by stimulation of the brain stem. Acta physiol. scand. **42**, 130–143 (1958)

IVERSEN, L.L.: The uptake and storage of noradrenaline in sympathetic nerves. Cambridge: University Press 1967

IWABUCHI, T., KAWAKAMI, H., UEMURA, K., KUTSUZAWA, T.: Regional cerebral blood flow in apoplexy measured by ^{133}Xe clearance method. Tohoku J. exp. Med. **104**, 1–11 (1971)

JAMES, I.M., MILLAR, R.A., PURVES, M.J.: Observations on the extrinsic neural control of cerebral blood flow in the baboon. Circulat. Res. **25**, 77–93 (1969)

JENNETT, W.B., ROWAN, J.O., HARPER, A.M., JOHNSTON, J.H., MILLER, J.D., DESHMUKH, V.D.: Perfusion pressure and cerebral blood flow. In: Brain and blood flow (ROSS RUSSELL, R.W., ed). London: Pitman 1971, pp. 298–300

JEWELL, B.R., WILKIE, D.R.: The mechanical properties of relaxing muscle. J. Physiol. (Lond.) **152**, 30–47 (1960)

JEWELL, P.A.: The anastomoses between internal and external carotid circulations in the dog. J. Anat. (Lond.) **86**, 83–94 (1952)

JOHANSSON, B., BOHR, D.F.: Rhythmic activity in smooth muscle from small subcutaneous arteries. Amer. J. Physiol. **210**, 801–806 (1966)

JOHNSTON, I.H., ROWAN, J.O., HARPER, A.M., JENNETT, W.B.: Cerebral blood flow in experimental intracranial hypertension. Cerebral blood flow and intracranial pressure. 5th Int. Symp. Roma-Siena 1971, part II. Europ. Neurol. **8**, 57–61 (1972)

KAINDL, F., POLZER, K., SCHUHFRIED, F.: Mehrfach- und Differentialrheographie. Verh. dtsch. Ges. Kreisl.-Forsch. **21**, 451–454 (1956)

KANZOW, E.: Quantitative fortlaufende Messung von Durchblutungsänderungen in der Hirnrinde. Pflügers Arch. ges. Physiol. **273**, 199–209 (1961)

KANZOW, E.: Diskussion. In: Pharmakologie der lokalen Gehirndurchblutung (BETZ, E., WÜLLENWEBER, R., Hrsg.), S. 177. München-Gräfelfing: Banaschewski 1969

KANZOW, E., DIECKHOFF, D.: On the location of the vascular resistance in the cerebral circulation. In: Cerebral blood flow (BROCK, M., FIESCHI, C., INGVAR, D.H., LASSEN, N.A., SCHÜRMANN, K., eds). Berlin-Heidelberg-New York: Springer 1969, pp. 96–97

KANZOW, E., DIECKHOFF, D., HOLZGRAEFE, H.: Pressure drop in cerebral arteries at changes of the cerebrovascular resistance. In: Brain and blood flow (ROSS RUSSELL, R.W., ed). London: Pitman 1971, pp. 309–312

KANZOW, E., GREGL, I.M., HELD, U.P., RICHTERING, I.: Vasomotorische Reaktionen in der Großhirnrinde bei der EEG-Arousal. Pflügers Arch. ges. Physiol. **273**, 288–301 (1961)

KANZOW, E., KRAUSE, D.: Vasomotorik der Hirnrinde und EEG-Aktivität wacher, frei beweglicher Katzen. Pflügers Arch. ges. Physiol. **274**, 447–458 (1962)

KANZOW, E., KRAUSE, D., KÜHNEL, H.: Die Vasomotorik der Hirnrinde in den Phasen desynchronisierter EEG-Aktivität im natürlichen Schlaf der Katze. Pflügers Arch. ges. Physiol. **274**, 593–607 (1962)

KANZOW, E., REICHEL, K.: Apperzeptiv-affective Gefäßreaktionen in der Großhirnrinde. Pflügers Arch. ges. Physiol. **293**, 19–33 (1967)

KARLSBERG, P., ELLIOTT, H.W., ADAMS, J.E.: Effect of various pharmacology agents on cerebral arteries. Neurology (Minneap.) **13**, 772–778 (1963)

KATZ, D.: Zur Grundlegung einer Bedürfnispsychologie. Z. Psychol. **129**, 292–304 (1933)

KEATINGE, W.R.: The role of transmitters and sympathetic innervation in the control of cerebral blood flow. Specific sensitivity of cerebral vessels to pCO_2. Diskussionsbemerkung. In: Vascular smooth muscle (BETZ, E., ed). Berlin-Heidelberg-New York: Springer 1972, p. 131

KELLIE, G.K. zu Leith: Reflections on the pathology of the brain. Sammlung zur Kenntnis d. Gehirn- und Rückenmarkskrankheiten. Hrsg. Nasse, Heft 1, 1837

KENNEDY, CH., DES RODIERS, M., REIVICH, M., SOKOLOFF, L.: Local cerebral glucose utilization in the visual system of the macaque monkey. In: Blood flow and metabolism in the brain (HARPER, A.M., JENNETT, W.B., MILLER, J.D., ROWAN, J.O., eds). Edinburgh-London: Livingstone 1975

KENNEDY, CH., SOKOLOFF, L.: An adaptation of nitrous oxide method to the study of the cerebral circulation in children; normal values for cerebral blood flow and metabolic rate in childhood. J. clin. Invest. **36**, 1130–1137 (1957)

KETY, S.S.: Quantitative determination of cerebral blood flow in man. Meth. med. Res. **1**, 1201 (1948)

KETY, S.S.: Circulation and metabolism of the human brain in health and disease. Amer. J. Med. **8**, 205–217 (1950)

KETY, S.S.: The theory and applications of the exchange of inert gas at the lungs and tissues. Pharmacol. Rev. **3**, 1–41 (1951)

KETY, S.S.: Problems of consciousness. New York: Macy 1952, pp. 26–40

KETY, S.S.: Changes in cerebral circulation and oxygen consumption which accompany maturation and aging. In: Biochemistry of the developing nervous system (H. WAELSCH, ed). New York: Academic Press 1955

KETY, S.S.: Human cerebral blood flow and oxygen

consumption as related to aging. J. chron. Dis. 3, 478–486 (1956)

KETY, S.S.: Cerebral circulation. In: Handbook of physiology. Sect. 1, Vol. 3. Ed. Field, J. Washington: American Physiological Society 1961, pp. 1751–1760

KETY, S.S., MCDOWALL, R.J.S.: The control of the circulation of the blood. London: Dawson 1956

KETY, S.S., SCHMIDT, C.F.: The determination of cerebral blood flow in man by the use of nitrous oxide in low concentrations. Amer. J. Physiol. **143**, 53–66 (1945)

KETY, S.S., SCHMIDT, C.F.: The effects of active and passive hyperventilation on cerebral blood flow, cerebral oxygen consumption, cardiac output and blood pressure of normal young men. J. clin. Invest. **25**, 107–119 (1946)

KETY, S.S., SCHMIDT, C.F.: The nitrous oxide method for the quantitative determination of cerebral blood flow in man: Theory, procedure and normal values. J. clin. Invest. **27**, 476–483 (1948a)

KETY, S.S., SCHMIDT, C.F.: The effects of altered arterial tensions of carbon dioxide and oxygen on cerebral blood flow and cerebral oxygen consumption of normal young men. J. clin. Invest. **27**, 484–492 (1948b)

KETY, S.S., SHENKIN, H.A., SCHMIDT, C.F.: The effects of increased intracranial pressure on cerebral circulatory effects in man. J. clin. Invest. **27**, 493–499 (1948a)

KETY, S.S., WOODFORD, R.B., HARMEL, M.H., FREYHAN, F.A., APPEL, K.E., SCHMIDT, C.F.: Cerebral blood flow and metabolism in schizophrenia: The effects of barbiturate seminarcosis, insulin coma and electro-shock. Amer. J. Psychiat. **104**, 765–770 (1948b)

KJÄLLQUIST, A., SIESJÖ, B.K., ZWETNOW, N.: Effects of increased intracranial pressure on cerebral blood flow and on cerebral venous pO_2, pCO_2, pH, lactate and pyruvate in dogs. Acta physiol. scand. **75**, 345–352 (1969)

KLATZO, J., SEITELBERGER, F.: Brain edema. Proceedings of the Symposium September 11–13 1965, Vienna. Wien-New York: Springer 1967

KNABE, U., BETZ, E.: The effect of varying extracellular K^+-, Mg^{++}- and Ca^{++} on the diameter of pial arterioles. In: Vascular smooth muscle (BETZ, E., ed). Berlin-Heidelberg-New York: Springer 1972, pp. 83–85

KNOLL, PH.: Über die Druckschwankungen in der Zerebrospinalflüssigkeit und den Wechsel in der Blutfülle des centralen Nervensystems. S.-B. Akad. Wiss. Wien, math.-nat. Kl. **93**, 217–252 (1886)

KOBAYASHI, K., KLEIHUES, P., HOSSMANN, K.-A., HOSSMANN, V.: Postischemic recovery of nucleotide metabolism in the cat brain. Stroke **4**, 340 (1973)

KOGURE, K., SCHEINBERG, P., FUJISHIMA, M., BUSTO, R., REINMUTH, O.M.: Effects of hypoxia on cerebral autoregulation. Amer. J. Physiol. **219**, 1393–1396 (1970b)

KOGURE, K., SCHEINBERG, P., REINMUTH, O.M., FUJISHIMA, M., BUSTO, R.: Mechanisms of cerebral vasodilation in hypoxia. J. appl. Physiol. **29**, 223–229 (1970a)

KOGURE, K., SCHEINBERG, P., REINMUTH, O.M., FUJISHIMA, M., BUSTO, R.: Regional cerebral blood flow in dogs local and remote effect of carbon dioxide. Arch. Neurol. (Chic.) **22**, 528–540 (1970c)

KONOLD, P., GEBERT, G., BRECHT, K.: The effect of potassium on the tone of isolated arteries. Pflügers Arch. ges. Physiol. **301**, 285–291 (1968)

KORNMÜLLER, A.E., PALME, F., STRUGHOLD, H.: Über Veränderungen der Hirnaktionsströme im akuten Sauerstoffmangel. Luftfahrtmed. **5**, 161–183 (1941)

KROGH, A.: Anatomie und Physiologie der Capillaren. Berlin: Springer 1924

KRUPP, P.: Zerebrale Durchblutung und elektrische Hirnaktivität. Basel-Stuttgart: Schwabe 1966

KRUPP, P., CARPI, A.: Die Beziehungen zwischen dem zerebrovasculären und elektrographischen Effekt der Hyperkapnie unter der Einwirkung von Barbituraten. Helv. physiol. pharmacol. Acta **22**, C78–C80 (1964)

KURIYAMA, H., OSA, T., ITO, Y., SUZUKI, H.: Excitation-contraction coupling mechanism in visceral smooth muscle. Advanc. Biophys. **8**, 115–190 (1976)

KUSCHINSKY, W., WAHL, M.: The functional significance of β-adrenergic and cholinergic receptors at pial arteries: A microapplication study. In: Cerebral circulation and metabolism (LANGFITT, T.W., MCHENRY, JR. L.C., REIVICH, M., WOLLMAN, H., eds). Berlin-Heidelberg-New York: Springer 1975a, pp. 470–472

KUSCHINSKY, W., WAHL, M.: Are alpha receptors involved in the adjustment of pial arterial resting tone? In: Blood flow and metabolism in the brain (HARPER, M., JENNETT, B., MILLER, D., ROWAN, J., eds). Edinburgh-London: Livingstone 1975b, pp. 2.3–2.9

KUSCHINSKY, W., WAHL, M.: In vivo evaluation of histamine receptors at pial arteries. In: Cerebral Function, Metabolism and Circulation (D.H. INGVAR, N.A. LASSEN, eds). Copenhagen: Munksgaard 1977, pp. 382–383

KUSCHINSKY, W., WAHL, M., BOSSE, O., THURAU, K.: The dependency of the pial arterial and arteriolar resistance on the perivascular H^+ and K^+ concentrations. Cerebral blood flow and intracranial pressure. Proc. 5th Int. Symp. Roma-Siena 1971, part I. Europ. Neurol. **6**, 92–95 (1971/72)

KUSCHINSKY, W., WAHL, M., BOSSE, O., THURAU, K.: Perivascular potassium and pH as determinants of local pial arterial diameters in cats. (A microapplication study). Circulat. Res. **31**, 240–247 (1972)

KUURNE, T., TROUPP, H., KASTE, M., VAPALAHTI, M.: Clinical and experimental intracranial pressure. Cerebral blood flow and intracranial pressure. Proc. 5th Int. Symp. Roma-Siena 1971, part II. Europ. Neurol. **8**, 188–191 (1972)

LANDAU, W.M., FREYGANG, W.H., ROWLAND, L.P., SOKOLOFF, L., KETY, S.S.: The local circulation of the living brain; values in the unanaesthetized and anaesthetized cat. Trans. Amer. neurol. Ass. **80**, 125–129 (1955)

LANGFITT, T.W., KASSELL, N.F., WEINSTEIN, J.D.: Cerebral blood flow with intracranial hypertension. Neurology (Minneap.) **15**, 761–773 (1965a)

LANGFITT, T.W., KUMAR, V.S. and MILLER, J.D.: Cerebral oedema caused by anoxia and changes in intracranial vascular pressures. In: Brain and Blood Flow, Ed.: R.W. ROSS RUSSELL, Pitman Medical and Scientific Publishing Co. Ltd. London, 386–392 1971

LANGFITT, T.W., MCHENRY, L.C., JR., REIVICH, M., WOLLMAN, H.: Cerebral circulation and metabolism. Berlin-Heidelberg-New York: Springer 1975

LANGFITT, T.W., WEINSTEIN, J.D., KASSELL, N.F.: Cerebral vasomotor paralysis produced by intracranial hypertension. Neurology (Minneap.) **15**, 622–641 (1965b)

LASSEN, N.A.: Cerebral blood flow and oxygen consumption in man. Physiol. Rev. **39**, 183–238 (1959)

LASSEN, N.A.: Assessment of tissue radiation dose in clinical use of radioactive inert gases, with examples of absorbed doses from $^{3}H_2$, ^{85}Kr and ^{133}Xe. Minerva nucl. **8**, 211–217 (1964)

LASSEN, N.A.: The luxury-perfusion syndrome and its possible relation to acute metabolic acidosis localized within the brain. Lancet **2**, 1113–1115 (1966)

LASSEN, N.A.: Brain extracellular pH: The main factor controlling cerebral blood flow. Scand. J. clin. Lab. Invest. **22**, 247–251 (1968a)

LASSEN, N.A.: On the regulation of cerebral blood flow in diseases of the brain with special regard to the "luxury perfusion syndrome" of brain tissue, i.e. a syndrome characterized by relative hyperemia or absolute hyperemia of the brain tissue. In: Progress in brain research. Vol. 30 (LUYENDIJK, W., ed). Amsterdam-London-New York: Elsevier 1968b, pp. 121–124

LASSEN, N.A., HØEDT-RASMUSSEN, K., SØRENSEN, S.C., SKINHØJ, E., CRONQVIST, S., BODFORSS, B., INGVAR, D.H.: Regional cerebral blood flow in man determined by krypton-85. Neurology (Minneap.) **13**, 719–727 (1963)

LASSEN, N.A., INGVAR, D.H.: The blood flow of the cerebral cortex determined by radioactive krypton-85. Experientia (Basel) **17**, 42–43 (1961)

LASSEN, N.A., INGVAR, D.H.: Die regionale Durchblutung des Gehirns und ihre Störungen. Verh. dtsch. Ges. Kreisl.-Forsch. **39**, 10–22 (1973)

LASSEN, N.A., MUNCK, O.: The cerebral blood flow in man determined by the use of radioactive krypton. Acta physiol. scand. **33**, 30–49 (1955)

LASSEN, N.A., MUNCK, O., TOTTEY, E.R.: Mental function and cerebral oxygen consumption in organic dementia. Arch. Neurol. Psychiat. (Chic.) **77**, 126–133 (1957)

LASSEN, N.A., PALVÖLGYI, R.: Cerebral steal during hypercapnia and the inverse reaction during hypocapnia observed by the ^{133}Xenon technique in man. Scand. J. clin. Lab. Invest. Suppl. 102 XIII D (1968)

LASSEN, N.A., PAULSON, O.B.: Partial cerebral vasoparalysis in patients with apoplexy: Dissociation between carbon dioxide responsiveness and autoregulation. In: Cerebral blood flow (BROCK, M., FIESCHI, C., INGVAR, D.H., LASSEN, N.A., SCHÜRMANN, K., eds). Berlin-Heidelberg-New York: Springer 1969, pp. 117–119

LAVRENTEVA, N.B., MCHEDLISHVILI, G.I., PLECHKOVA, E.K.: Distribution and activity of cholinesterase in nerve structures of the pial arteries: Histochemical investigation. Bull. exp. Biol. Med. **66**, 1282–1285 (1968)

LECHNER, H.: Impedanzmethoden. In: Der Hirnkreislauf. Stuttgart: Thieme 1972, S. 298–316

LECHNER, H., RODLER, H.: Eine neue Methode zur Registrierung intrakranieller Kreislaufveränderungen. Elektromedizin **6**, 75–77 (1961)

LECHNER, H., RODLER, H., GEYER, N.: Theorie der Entstehung der rheographischen Kurve. In: Rheoencephalographica (MARTIN, F., LECHNER, H., Hrsg.), S. 19–29. Wien: Wien. Med. Akademie 1965

LECHNER, H., RODLER, H., GEYER, N.: Die theoretischen Grundlagen der Rheographie und ihre praktischen Schlußfolgerungen. Elektromedizin **13**, 30–33 (1968)

LENNOX, W.G.: The cerebral circulation. XV. The effect of mental work. Arch. Neurol. Psychiat. (Chic.) **26**, 725–730 (1931)

LENNOX, W.G., GIBBS, E.L.: The blood flow in the brain and the leg of man and the changes induced by alterations of blood gases. J. clin. Invest. **11**, 1155–1177 (1932)

LEUSEN, I.: Regulation of cerebrospinal fluid composition with reference to breathing. Physiol. Rev. **52**, 1–56 (1972)

LEVER, J.D., SPRIGGS, T.L., GRAHAM, J.D.: A formol-fluorescence fine-structural and autoradiographic study of the adrenergic innervation of the vascular tree in the intact and sympathectomized pancreas of the cat. J. Anat. (Lond.) **103**, 15–34 (1968)

LEWIS, B.M., SOKOLOFF, S., WECHSLER, R.L., WENTZ, W.B., KETY, S.S.: A method for the continuous measurement of cerebral blood flow in man by means of radioactive krypton (Kr^{79}). J. clin. Invest. **39**, 707–716 (1960)

LEWIS, H.P., MCLAURIN, R.L.: Regional cerebral blood flow in increased intracranial pressure produced by increased cerebrospinal fluid volume, intracranial mass and cerebral edema. In: Intracranial pressure (BROCK, M., DIETZ, H., eds). Berlin-Heidelberg-New York: Springer 1972, pp. 160–164

LEYDEN, W.: Beiträge und Untersuchungen zur Physiologie und Pathologie des Gehirns. Virchows Arch. path. Anat. **37**, 519–559 (1866)

LIERSE, W.: Die Kapillardichte im Wirbeltiergehirn. Acta anat. (Basel) **54**, 1–31 (1963a)

LIERSE, W.: Die Kapillardichte im Rhinencephalon verschiedener Wirbeltiere und des Menschen. In: Progress in brain research. Vol. 3 (BARGMANN, W., SCHADE, P.J., Hrsg.), S. 230–236. Amsterdam-London-New York: Elsevier 1963b

LIERSE, W., HORSTMANN, E.: Quantitative anatomy of the cerebral vascular bed with especial emphasis on homogeneity and inhomogeneity in small parts of the gray and white matter. Acta neurol. scand. Suppl. 14, 15–19 (1965)

LINDEN, L.: The effect of stellate ganglion block on cerebral circulation in cerebrovascular accidents. Acta med. scand. **151**, Suppl. 301, 1–110 (1955)

LJUNGGREN, B., SIESJÖ, B.: Cerebral metabolic state during postischemic "recovery". Stroke **4**, 343 (1973)

LLUCH, S., GOMEZ, B., ALBORCH, E., MANRIQUE, M., URQUILLA, P.R.: Sympathetic control of cerebral blood flow in the unanesthetized goat. In: Cerebral circulation and metabolism (LANGFITT, T.W., MCHENRY, L.C., JR., REIVICH, M., WOLLMAN, H., eds). Berlin-Heidelberg-New York: Springer 1975, pp. 436–439

LUBSEN, N.: Experimental studies on the cerebral circulation of the unanaesthetized rabbit. I. Stimulation of the cervical sympathetic chain. Arch. néerl. Physiol. **25**, 287–305 (1940a)

LUBSEN, N.: Experimental studies on the cerebral circulation of the unanaesthetized rabbit. II. The action of adrenaline. Arch. néerl. Physiol. **25**, 306–322 (1940b)

LUDWIG, C.: In Lehrbuch der Physiologie des Menschen von Landois. Wien und Leipzig: Urban & Schwarzenberg 1885

LUDWIGS, N.: Über eine Modifikation der Methode nach GIBBS zur lokalisierten Durchblutungsmessung des Hirngewebes und die Gültigkeit der damit erhobenen Befunde. Pflügers Arch. ges. Physiol. **259**, 35–42 (1954)

LUDWIGS, N., SCHNEIDER, M.: Über den Einfluß des Halssympathicus auf die Gehirndurchblutung. Pflügers Arch. ges. Physiol. **259**, 43–55 (1954)

LÜBBERS, D.W.: The oxygen pressure field of the brain and its significance for the normal and critical oxygen supply of the brain. In: Oxygen transport in blood and tissue (LÜBBERS, D.W., LUFT, U.C., THEWS, G., WITZLEB, E., eds). Stuttgart: Thieme 1968, pp. 124–139

LÜBBERS, D.W.: Physiologie der Gehirndurchblutung. In: Der Hirnkreislauf (GÄNSHIRT, H., Hrsg.), S. 214–260. Stuttgart: Thieme 1972

LÜBBERS, D.W., INGVAR, D.H., BETZ, E., FABEL, H., SCHMAHL, F.: Sauerstoffverbrauch der Großhirnrinde in Schlaf- und Wachzustand beim Hund. Pflügers Arch. ges. Physiol. **281**, 58 (1964)

LÜBBERS, D.-W., LUFT, U.C., THEWS, G., WITZLEB, E. (Eds.): Oxygen Transport in Blood and Tissue. Thieme, Stuttgart 1968

LÜBBERS, D.W., STOSSECK, K.: Quantitative Bestimmung der lokalen Durchblutung durch elektrochemisch im Gewebe erzeugten Wasserstoff. Naturwissenschaften **57**, 311 (1970)

LÜLLMANN, H.: Calcium fluxes and calcium distribution in smooth muscle. In: Smooth muscle (BÜLBRING, E., BRADING, A.F., JONES, A.W., TOMITA, T., eds). London: Arnold 1970, pp. 151–165

LÜLLMANN, H., SIEGFRIED, A.: Über den Kalzium-Gehalt und den ^{45}Kalziumaustausch in Längsmuskulatur des Meerschweinchendünndarms. Pflügers Arch. ges. Physiol. **300**, 108–119 (1968)

LUYENDIJK, W.: Cerebral circulation. In: Progress in brain research. Vol. 30. Amsterdam-London-New York: Elsevier 1968

MACKENZIE, E.T., MCGEORGE, A.P., GRAHAM, D.I., FITCH, W., EDVINSSON, L., HARPER, A.M.: Breakthrough of cerebral autoregulation and the sympathetic nervous system. In: Cerebral Function, Metabolism and Circulation (D.H. INGVAR, N.A. LASSEN, eds). Copenhagen: Munksgaard 1977, pp. 48–49

MACKENZIE, E.T., YOUNG, A.R., STEWART, M., HARPER, A.M.: Effect of serotonin on cerebral function, metabolism and circulation. In: Cerebral Function, Metabolism and Circulation (D.H. INGVAR, N.A. LASSEN, eds), Copenhagen: Munksgaard 1977, pp. 76–77

MANGOLD, R., SOKOLOFF, L., CONNER, E., KLEINERMAN, J., THERMAN, P.O.G., KETY, S.S.: The effects of sleep and lack of sleep on the cerebral circulation and metabolism of normal young men. J. clin. Invest. **34**, 1092–1100 (1955)

MANN, L.I.: Effect of hypoxia on fetal cephalic blood flow, cephalic metabolism and the electroencephalogram. Exp. Neurol. **29**, 336–348 (1970)

MARTIN, F., KARBOWSKI, K., VANEY, P.: Rheoencephalographie. III. Etude de quelques paramètres, introduction à une analyse systematique des courbes rheoencephalographiques. Schweiz. Arch. Neurol. Psychiat. **93**, 14–25 (1964)

MATHEW, N.T., MEYER, J.S., HARTMANN, A.: Effect of α- and β-adrenergic blocking agents on regional cerebral blood flow and CO_2 responsiveness in patients with cerebrovascular disease. In: Cerebral circulation and metabolism (LANGFITT, T.W., MCHENRY, L.C., JR., REIVICH, M., WOLLMANN, H., eds). Berlin-Heidelberg-New York: Springer 1975, pp. 483–486

MCCALL, M.L., TAYLOR, H.W.: Effects of barbiturate sedation on the brain in toxaemia of pregnancy. J. Amer. med. Ass. **149**, 51–54 (1952)

MCDOWALL, D.G.: The effects of clinical concentrations of halothane on the blood flow and oxygen uptake of the cerebral cortex. Brit. J. Anaesth. **39**, 186–196 (1967)

MCDOWALL, D.G., HARPER, M.: The relationship between blood flow and extracellular pH of the cerebral cortex. In: Blood flow through organs and tissue (BAIN, W.H., HARPER, A.M., eds). Edinburgh-London: Livingstone 1968, pp. 261–271

MCHEDLISHVILI, G.I.: Functional behaviour of the vascular mechanisms of the brain: Its role in the regulation and in the disturbances of the cerebral circulation. Leningrad: Nauka 1968a

MCHEDLISHVILI, G.I.: Function of the vascular mechanisms in the brain. Their role in the regulation and pathology of cerebral circulation. Leningrad: Nauka 1968b

MCHEDLISHVILI, G.I.: Vascular mechanisms of the brain. Library of Congress, Catalog Card 70141241/ISBN/30306-10870-4 (1972). Consultant Bureau New York, A Division of Plenum Publ. Corp. New York 10011. A special research report/translated from Russian. Leningrad: Naukia Press 1968

MCHEDLISHVILI, G.I., NIKOLAISHVILI, L.S.: Zum venösen Mechanismus der funktionellen Dilatation der Piaarterien. Pflügers Arch. ges. Physiol. **296**, 14–20 (1967)

MCHEDLISHVILI, G.I., NIKOLAISHVILI, L.S.: Evidence of a cholinergic nervous mechanism mediating the autoregulatory dilatation of the cerebral blood vessels. Pflügers Arch. ges. Physiol. **315**, 27–37 (1970)

MCHENRY, L.C. JR., JAFFE, M.E., KENTON, E.J., COOPER, E.S., WEST, J.W., KAWAMURA, J., OSHIRO, T., GOLDBERG, H.I.: Vasodilator responsiveness-implications in cerebrovascular disease. In: Brain and blood flow (ROSS RUSSELL, R.W. ed). London: Pitman 1971, pp. 258–264

MCHENRY, L.C. JR., SLOCUM, H.C., HAYES, G.J.: The effects of hyperventilation on the cerebral circulation and metabolism. Trans. Amer. neurol. Ass. **89**, 223–225 (1964)

MCNAUGHTON, F.L.: The innervation of the intracranial blood vessels and dural sinuses. Proc. Ass. Res. nerv. ment. Dis. **18**, 178 (1938)

MEINIG, G., REULEN, H.J., HADJIDIMOS, A., SIEMON, C., BARTKO, D., SCHÜRMANN, K.: Induction of filtration edema by extreme reduction of cerebrovascular resistance associated with hypertension. In: Cerebral blood flow and intracranial pressure (FIESCHI, C. ed). Basel-München-Paris-London-New York-Sydney: Karger 1971/72, part II, pp. 97–103

MEINIG, G., REULEN, H.J., MAGAVLY, C., HASE, U., HEY, O.: Changes of cerebral hemodynamics and energy metabolism during increased CSF pressure and brain edema. In: Intracranial pressure (BROCK, M., DIETZ, H., eds). Berlin-Heidelberg-New York: Springer 1972, pp. 79–84

MELAMED, E., LARSEN, B.: Regional cerebral blood flow during voluntary conjugate eye movements in man. In: Cerebral Function, Metabolism and Circulation (D.H. INGVAR, N.A. LASSEN, eds). Copenhagen: Munksgaard 1977, pp. 530–531

MENDELOW, D.A., EIDELMAN, B.H., HATTINGH, J., KRAMER, B., MCCALDEN, T.A., SHIMELL, C., ROSENDORFF, C.: Autoregulation and cerebral metabolism after chemical sympathectomy in baboons. In: Cerebral Function, Metabolism and Circulation (D.H. INGVAR, N.A. LASSEN, eds). Copenhagen: Munksgaard 1977, pp. 52–53

MERCKER, H., SCHNEIDER, M.: Über Kapillarveränderungen des Gehirns bei Höhenanpassung. Pflügers Arch. ges. Physiol. **251**, 49–55 (1949)

METZGER, H.: Verteilung des O_2-Partialdruckes im Mikrobereich des Gehirngewebes. Polarographische Messung und mathematische Analyse. Habil.-Schrift Mainz 1972

MEYER, A.W.: Methode zum Auffinden von Hirntumoren bei Trepanation durch elektrische Widerstandsmessung. Zbl. Chir. **48**, 1824–1826 (1921)

MEYER, J.S.: Discussion remark in Cerebrovascular disease. Baltimore: Williams & Wilkins Comp. 1966, p. 214

MEYER, J.S., DENNY-BROWN, D.: The cerebral collateral circulation. I. Factors influencing collateral blood flow. Neurology (Minneap.) **7**, 447–458 (1957)

MEYER, J.S., GOTOH, F.: Metabolic and electroencephalographic effects of hyperventilation. Experimental study of brain oxygen and carbon-dioxide tension, pH, EEG, and blood flow during hyperventilation. Arch. Neurol. **3**, 539–552 (1960)

MEYER, J.S., GOTOH, F., FAVALE, E.: Cerebral metabolism during epileptic seizures in man. Electroenceph. clin. Neurophysiol. **21**, 10–22 (1966)

MEYER, J.S., KONDO, A., NOMURA, F., SAKAMOTO, K., TERAURA, T.: Cerebral hemodynamics and metabolism following brain trauma. Demonstration of luxury perfusion following brain-stem laceration. In: Cerebral blood flow. (BROCK, M., FIESCHI, C., INGVAR, D.H., LASSEN, N.A., SCHÜRMANN, K. eds). Berlin-Heidelberg-New York: Springer 1969a, pp. 199–201

MEYER, J.S., NOMURA, F., SAKAMOTO, K., KONDO, A.: Effect of stimulation of the brain-stem reticular formation on cerebral blood flow and oxygen consumption. Electroenceph. clin. Neurophysiol. **26**, 125–132 (1969b)

MEYER, J.S., TOYODA, M., SHINOHARA, Y., KITAMURA, A., RYN, T., WIEDERHOLT, J., GUIRAUD, B.: Regional cerebral blood flow (carotid perfusion) measured by clearance of hydrogen from cerebral venous blood. Scand. clin. Lab. Invest. Suppl. 102, XI: G (1968)

MEYER, M.W., KLASSEN, A.C.: Regional brain blood flow during sympathetic stimulation. In: Cerebral circulation and metabolism (LANGFITT, T.W., MCHENRY, JR., L.C., REIVICH, M., WOLLMAN, H., eds). Berlin-Heidelberg-New York: Springer 1975, pp. 459–461

MILLER, J.D., GARIBI, J., NORTH, J.B., TEASDALE, G.M.: False autoregulation after cold injury to the cerebral cortex. Stroke **4**, 332 (1973)

MILLER, J.D., STANEK, A.E., LANGFITT, T.W.: A comparison of autoregulation to changes in intracranial and arterial pressure in the same preparation. In: Cerebral blood flow and intracranial pressure. Europ. Neurol. **6**, 34–38 (1971/72)

MITCHELL, G., SCRIVEN, D.R.L., ROSENDORFF, C.: Adrenoceptors in intracerebral resistance vessels. Brit. J. Pharmacol. **54**, 11–15 (1975)

MIYAZAKI, M.: Effect of undesirable sound (noise) on cerebral circulation. Jap. Circulat. J. **35**, 931–936 (1972)

MOLNAR, L.: Sur le contrôle nerveux de la circulation

sanguine régionale des centres cerebraux. Budapest: Akadémiai Kiadó 1967

MOLNAR, L., SZANTO, J.: The effect of electrical stimulation of the vasomotor center on the cerebral blood flow. Quart. J. exp. Physiol. **49**, 184–193 (1964)

MONRO, A.: Observations on the structure and functions of the nervous system. Edinburgh: Creech 1783

MOSSO, A.: Über den Kreislauf des Blutes im menschlichen Gehirn. Leipzig: Vieth 1881

MRWA, U., RÜEGG, J.C.: Calcium activation of vascular contractile protein. In: Ionic Actions on Vascular Smooth Muscle (BETZ, E., ed). Berlin-Heidelberg-New York: Springer 1976, pp. 12–16

MÜLLER, U., ISSELHARD, W., HINZEN, D.H., GEPPERT, E.: Regionaler Energiestoffwechsel im Kaninchengehirn während kompletter Ischämie in Normothermie. Pflügers Arch. ges. Physiol. **320**, 168–180 (1970a)

MÜLLER, U., ISSELHARD, W., HINZEN, D.H., GEPPERT, E.: Elektrocorticogramm und regionaler Energiestoffwechsel des Kaninchengehirns in der postischämischen Erholung. Pflügers Arch. ges. Physiol. **320**, 181–194 (1970b)

MÜLLER-SCHAUENBURG, W.: Über einen Ansatz zur Trennung von Wärmeleitung und Wärmeabtransport durch das Blut – ein neues Verfahren zur quantitativen Messung der lokalen Gewebsdurchblutung. Med. Dissertation Tübingen 1972

MÜLLER-SCHAUENBURG, W., APFEL, H., BENZING, H., BETZ, E.: Quantitative measurement of local blood flow with heat clearance. Basic Res. Cardiol. **70**, 547–567 (1975)

MÜLLER-SCHAUENBURG, W., BETZ, E.: Gas and heat clearance comparison and use of heat transport for quantitative local blood flow measurements. In: Cerebral blood flow (BROCK, M. et al., eds). Berlin-Heidelberg-New York: Springer 1969, pp. 47–49

NAGAI, H., FURUSE, M., BANNO, K., IKEYAMA, A., MAEDA, S., KUCHIWAKI, H.: Some adjustment mechanism of brain metabolism during increased intracranial pressure. In: Intracranial pressure (BROCK, M., DIETZ, H., eds). Berlin-Heidelberg-New York: Springer 1972a, pp. 75–78

NAGAI, H., IKEYAMA, A., FURUSE, M., MAEDA, S., BANNO, K., HASUO, M., KUCHIWAKI, H.: Effect of increased intracranial pressure on cerebral hemodynamics. Cerebral blood flow and intracranial pressure. Proc. 5th Int. Symp. Roma-Siena 1971, part II. Europ. Neurol. **8**, 52–56 (1972b)

NELSON, E., RENNELS, M.: Electron microscopic studies on intracranial vascular nerves in the cat. Scand. J. clin. Lab. Invest. Suppl. 102 VI: A (1968)

NELSON, E., RENNELS, M.L., TAKAYANAGI, T.: Ultrastructural observations on the innervation of intracranial arteries. In: Brain and blood flow (ROSS RUSSELL, R.W., ed). London: Pitman 1971, pp. 248–253

NEUMANN, L., BETZ, E., BENZING, H.: Wirkung einer Unterbindung der Arteria cerebri media auf Durchblutung, Sauerstoffdruck und Säure-Basen-Haushalt in deren Versorgungsgebiet. Int. Z. angew. Physiol. **29**, 29–43 (1970)

NIELSEN, K.C., EDVINSSON, L., OWMAN, C.: Cholinergic innervation and vasomotor response of brain vessels. In: Cerebral circulation and metabolism. (LANGFITT, T.W., MCHENRY, L.C. JR., REIVICH, M., WOLLMAN, H., eds). Berlin-Heidelberg-New York: Springer 1975, pp. 473–475

NIELSEN, K.C., OWMAN, C.: Adrenergic innervation of pial arteries related to the circle of Willis in the cat (Fluorescent microscopy). Brain Res. **6**, 773–776 (1967)

NIELSEN, K.C., OWMAN, C.: Contractile response and amine receptor mechanisms in isolated middle cerebral artery of the cat. Brain Res. **27**, 33–42 (1971)

NOELL, W., SCHNEIDER, M.: Über die Durchblutung und die Sauerstoffversorgung des Gehirns im akuten Sauerstoffmangel. I. Mitteilung: Die Gehirndurchblutung. Pflügers Arch. ges. Physiol. **246**, 181–200 (1942a)

NOELL, W., SCHNEIDER, M.: Über die Durchblutung und die Sauerstoffversorgung des Gehirns im akuten Sauerstoffmangel. III. Mitteilung: Die arteriovenöse Sauerstoff- und Kohlensäuredifferenz. Pflügers Arch. ges. Physiol. **246**, 207–249 (1942b)

NOELL, W., SCHNEIDER, M.: Über die Durchblutung und die Sauerstoffversorgung des Gehirns im akuten Sauerstoffmangel. II. Mitteilung: Der Liquordruck. Pflügers Arch. ges. Physiol. **246**, 201–206 (1942c)

NOELL, W., SCHNEIDER, M.: Über die Durchblutung und die Sauerstoffversorgung des Gehirns. IV. Mitteilung: Die Rolle der Kohlensäure. Pflügers Arch. ges. Physiol. **247**, 514–527 (1944)

NORBERG, K., SIESJÖ, B.K.: CBF and oxidative metabolism in insulin induced hypoglycemic coma. In: Blood flow and metabolism in the brain (HARPER, A.M., JENNETT, W.B., MILLER, J.D., ROWAN, J.O., eds). Edinburgh-London: Churchill Livingstone 1975. pp. 9.33–9.34

NORCROSS, N.: Intracerebral blood flow: Experimental study. Arch. Neurol. Psychiat. (Chic.) **40**, 291–299 (1938)

NOTHNAGEL, H.: Die vasomotorischen Nerven der Gehirngefäße. Virchows Arch. path. Anat. **40**, 203–213 (1867)

NOVACK, P., KANDA, A., MILLS, L.C., KATZ, S., KATZ, R.: Effects of pentobarbital anesthesia upon cerebral blood flow and metabolism. In: 47th Ann. Meeting of the Federation of American Societies for Experimental Biology 1963. Fed. Proc. **22**, (2Pt1) 480 (1963)

NOVACK, P., SHENKIN, H.A., BORTIN, L., GOLUBOFF, B., SOFFE, A.M.: The effects of carbon dioxide inhalation upon the cerebral blood flow and cerebral oxygen consumption in vascular disease. J. clin. Invest. **32**, 696–772 (1953)

NOYONS, A.K.M., WESTENRIJK, N. v., JONGBLOED, J.: Recherches sur la régulation du débit circulatoire du cerveau. Arch. néerl. Physiol. **21**, 377–432 (1936)

NYLIN, G., BLÖMER, H., JONES, H., HEDLUND, S., RYLANDER, C.G.: Further studies on cerebral blood flow estimated with thorium-B-labelled erythrocytes. Brit. Heart J. **18**, 385–392 (1956)

NYLIN, G., HEDLUND, S., REGNSTRÖM, O.: Studies of the cerebral circulation with labelled erythrocytes in healthy man. Circulat. Res. **9**, 664–674 (1961a)

NYLIN, G., HEDLUND, S., REGNSTRÖM, O.: Cerebral circulation studied with labelled red cells in healthy males. Acta radiol. (Stockh.) **55**, 281–304 (1961b)

NYLIN, G., SILFVERSKIÖLD, B.P., LÖFSTEDT, S., REGNSTRÖM, O., HEDLUND, S.: Studies on cerebral blood flow in man, using radioactive-labelled erythrocytes. Brain **83**, 293–335 (1960)

OBERDÖRSTER, G., SAUM, R., BENNER, K.U., GEBERT, E., SOBOTKA, P., HIRSCH, H.: Die Erholung des Elektrokortikogramms nach kompletter Ischämie des Hundegehirns in Normothermie. Pflügers Arch. ges. Physiol. **307**, R 116 (1969)

OIKAWA, T., KANAYA, H., KIMOTO, S.: Regional cerebral blood flow during naming test in patients with speech disorders. In: Cerebral Function, Metabolism and Circulation (INGVAR, D.H., LASSEN, N.A., eds). Copenhagen: Munksgaard, 1977, pp. 536–537

OLDENDORF, W.H.: Clinical radioisotope studies of cerebral circulation time. In: Der Hirnkreislauf in Forschung und Klinik. Kongreßband d. II. Internat. Salzburger Symposions 1964, S. 204–212. Wien: Brüder Hollinek

OLDENDORF, W.H., KITANO, M.: Measurement of brain-circulation time by an intravenous radioisotope technique. J. nucl. Med. **5**, 377 (1964)

OLDENDORF, W.H., KITANO, M.: Isotope study of brain blood turnover in vascular disease. Arch. Neurol. (Chic.) **12**, 30–38 (1965)

OLESEN, J.: The influence of adrenaline, noradrenaline and angiotensin on the cerebral blood flow in man. In: Brain and blood flow (ROSS RUSSELL, R.W., ed). London: Pitman 1971, pp. 265–269

OLSSON, R.A., DAVIS, J.C., KHOURI, E.M., PATTERSON, R.E.: Evidence for an adenosine receptor on the surface of dog coronary myocytes. Circulation Res., **39**, 93–98 (1976)

OPITZ, E., PALME, F.: Darstellung der Höhenanpassung im Gebirge durch Sauerstoffmangel. II. u. III. Mitt. Pflügers Arch. ges. Physiol. **248**, 298–386 (1944)

OPITZ, E., SCHNEIDER, M.: Über die Sauerstoffversorgung des Gehirns und den Mechanismus von Mangelwirkungen. Ergebn. Physiol. **46**, 126–260 (1950)

OWMAN, C., FALCK, B., MCHEDLISHVILI, G.: Adrenergic structures of the pial arteries and their connections with the cerebral cortex. Byull. eksp. Biol. Med. **59**, 98–100 (1965)

PAGE, I.H.: Serotonin. Yearbook Med. Publ. Chicago 1968

PANNIER, J.L., LEUSEN, I.: Circulation to the brain of rats during acute and prolonged hypercapnia and hypocapnia. Stroke **4**, 326–327 (1973)

PATTERSON, J.L., JR., HEYMAN, A., BATTEY, L.L., FERGUSON, R.W.: Threshold of response of the cerebral vessels of man to increase in blood carbon dioxyde. J. clin. Invest. **34**, 1857–1864 (1955)

PAULSON, O.B.: Regional cerebral blood flow in middle cerebral artery occlusion. Scand. J. clin. Lab. Invest. Suppl. 102 pXVI: C (1968)

PAULSON, O.B.: Cerebral apoplexy (stroke): Pathogenesis, pathophysiology and therapy as illustrated by regional blood flow measurements in the brain. Stroke **2**, 327–360 (1971)

PAULSON, O.B., LASSEN, N.A., SKINHØJ, E.: Regional cerebral blood flow in apoplexy without arterial occlusion. Neurology (Minneap.) **20**, 125–138 (1970)

PEARCE, W.J., D'ALECY, L.G.: Normotensive hemorrhage and cerebral blood flow. In: Cerebral Function, Metabolism and Circulation (INGVAR, D.H., LASSEN, N.A., eds). Copenhagen: Munksgaard, 1977, pp. 44–45

PEERLESS, S.J., KENDALL, M.J.: The significance of the perivascular innervation of the brain. In: The Cerebral Vessel Wall (CERVOS-NAVARRO, J., BETZ, E., MATAKAS, F., WÜLLENWEBER, R., eds). New York: Raven Press 1976, pp. 175–182

PEIPER, U., WENDE, W.: Wirkung der extracellulären Wasserstoffionen-Konzentration auf die adrenerge Aktivierung des Gefäßmuskels. Pflügers Arch. ges. Physiol. **314**, 14–26 (1970)

PERL, W.: Heat and matter distribution in body tissues and the measurement of tissue blood flow by local clearance methods. J. theor. Biol. **2**, 201–235 (1962)

PICHLMAYR, J.: Das Verhalten der Hirndurchblutung bei Hunden unter verschiedenen Narkosearten. Z. Kreisl.-Forsch. **58**, 662–676 (1969)

PICKARD, J.D., MACKENZIE, E.T., DURITY, F., WELSH, F.A., LANGFITT, T.W., JENNETT, W.B., HARPER, A.M.: Effects of osmotic blood-brain barrier disruption on the responsiveness of the primate cerebral circulation. In: Blood flow and metabolism in the brain (HARPER, A.M., JENNETT, W.B., MILLER, J.D., ROWAN, J.O., eds). Edinburgh-London: Livingstone 1975, pp. 9.33–9.34

PICKERODT, V.: Die Wirkung von passiver Hyperventilation auf die Sauerstoffversorgung des Gehirns. Ärztl. Forsch. **25**, 57–67 (1971)

PIERCE, E.C., LAMBERTSEN, C.J., DEUTSCH, S., CHASE, P.E., LINDE, H.W., DRIPPS, R.D., PRICE, H.L.: Cerebral circulation and metabolism during thiopental anaesthesia and hyperventilation in man. J. clin. Invest. **41**, 1664–1671 (1962)

PLETCHKOVA, E.K., MCHEDLISHVILI, G.I., LAVRENTIEVA, N.B., NIKOLAISHVILI, L.S.: Evidence for a cholinergic mechanism responsible for the functional hyperemia in the cerebral cortex. In: Correlation of blood supply with metabolism and function. Proc. of an Intern. Symposion (MCHEDLISHvili, G.I., ed). Tbilisi: Georgian Academic Press Metsniereba 1969, pp. 172–184

Plum, F., Posner, J.B.: Blood and cerebrospinal fluid lactate during hyperventilation. Amer. J. Physiol. **212**, 864–870 (1967)

Polzer, K., Schuhfried, F.: Rheographische Untersuchungen am Schädel. Wien. Z. Nervenheilk. **3**, 295–299 (1950)

Posner, J.B., Plum, F., Zee, D.: Ventriculocisternal pH and cerebral blood flow. Arch. Neurol. (Chic.) **20**, 664–667 (1969)

Purves, M.J.: The effect of hypoxia, hypercapnia and hypotension upon carotid body blood flow and oxygen consumption in the cat. J. Physiol. **209**, 395–416 (1970)

Purves, M.J.: The physiology of the cerebral circulation. Cambridge: University Press 1972

Raichle, M.E., Posner, J.B., Plum, F.: Cerebral blood flow during and after hyperventilation. In: Brain and blood flow (Ross Russell, R.W., ed). London: Pitman 1971, pp. 223–228

Rapela, C.E., Buyniski, J.P.: Cerebral vascular responses to changes in the ionic osmolar composition of blood. In: Cerebral blood flow (Brock, M., Fieschi, C., Ingvar, D.H., Lassen, N.A., Schürmann, K., eds). Berlin-Heidelberg-New York: Springer 1969, pp. 106–110

Rapela, C.E., Green, H.D.: Autoregulation of canine cerebral blood flow. Circulat. Res. **15**, 205–212 (1964)

Rapoport, S.I.: Chronic effects of osmotic opening of the blood-brain barrier in the monkey. Science **176**, 1243–1245 (1972)

Rapoport, S.I.: Reversible opening of the blood-brain barrier by osmotic shrinkage of the cerebrovascular endothelium: Opening of the tight junctions as related to carotid arteriography. Small Vessel Angiography. St. Louis: Mosby 1973, pp. 137–151

Rapoport, S.I., Hori, M., Klatzo, I.: Reversible osmotic opening of the blood-brain barrier. Science **173**, 1026–1028 (1971)

Rapoport, S.I., Hori, M., Klatzo, I.: Testing of a hypothesis for osmotic opening of the blood-brain barrier. Amer. J. Physiol. **223**, 323–331 (1972)

Rapoport, S.I., Thompson, H.K.: Osmotic opening of the blood-brain barrier in the monkey, without associated neurological deficits. Science **180**, 971 (1973)

Rapoport, S.I., Thompson, H.K.: Effect of intravenous NH_4Cl and $NaHCO_3$ on the pH of the brain surface, as related to respiration and the blood-brain barrier. Exp. Neurol. **42**, 320–331 (1974)

Rapport, M.M., Green, A.A., Page, J.H.: Crystalline serotonin. Science **108**, 329–330 (1948)

Rees, J.E., Boulay, E.P.G.H. du, Bull, J.W.D., Marshall, J., Ross Russell, R.W., Symon, L.: Persistence of disturbance of regional cerebral blood flow after transient ischaemic attacks. In: Brain and blood flow (Ross Russell, R.W., ed). London: Pitman 1971, pp. 277–280

Reivich, M.: Zerebrale Autoradiographie. In: Der Hirnkreislauf (Gänshirt, H., Hrsg.), S. 331–341. Stuttgart: Thieme 1972

Reivich, M., Holling, H., Roberts, B., Toole, J.F.: Reversal of blood flow through the vertebral artery and its effect on cerebral circulation. New Engl. J. Med. **265**, 878–885 (1961)

Reivich, M., Jehle, J., Sokoloff, L., Kety, S.S.: Measurement of regional cerebral blood flow with C^{14}-antipyrine in awake cats. J. appl. Physiol. **27**, 269–300 (1969a)

Reivich, M., Kuhl, D., Wolf, A., Greenberg, J., Phelps, M., Ido, T., Casella, V., Fowler, J., Gallagher, B., Hoffman, E., Alavi, A., Sokoloff, L.: Measurement of local cerebral glucose metabolism in man with ^{18}F-2-Fluoro-2-Deoxy-D-Glucose. In: Cerebral Function, Metabolism and Circulation (Ingvar, D.H., Lassen, N.A., eds). Copenhagen: Munksgaard, 1977, pp. 190–191

Reivich, M., Marshall, W.J.S., Kassell, N.: Loss of autoregulation produced by cerebral trauma. In: Cerebral blood flow (Brock, M., Fieschi, C., Ingvar, D.H., Lassen, N.A., Schürmann, K., eds). Berlin-Heidelberg-New York: Springer 1969c, pp. 205–208

Reivich, M., Slater, R., Sano, N.: Further studies on exponential models of cerebral clearance curves. In: Cerebral blood flow (Brock, M., Fieschi, C., Ingvar, D.H., Lassen, N.A., Schürmann, K., eds). Berlin-Heidelberg-New York: Springer 1969b, pp. 8–10

Rich, M., Scheinberg, P., Belle, M.S.: Relationship between cerebrospinal fluid pressure changes and cerebral blood flow. Circulat. Res. **1**, 389–395 (1953)

Richter, H.: Collaterals between the external carotid artery and the vertebral artery in cases of thrombosis of the internal carotid artery. Acta radiol. (Stockh.) **40**, 108–112 (1953)

Ridge, J.W.: The distribution of cytochrome-oxidase activity in rabbit brain. Biochem. J. **102**, 612–617 (1967)

Ridley, H.: An experiment to discover the cause of the motion of the dura mater. Phil. Trans. B. **5**, 199–202 (1700)

Riegel, F., Jolly, F.: Über die Veränderungen der Piagefäße infolge von Reizung sensibler Nerven. Arch. path. Anat. **52**, 218–230 (1871)

Risberg, J., Ancri, D., Ingvar, D.H.: Correlation between cerebral blood volume and cerebral blood flow in the cat. Exp. Brain Res. **8**, 321–326 (1969b)

Risberg, J., Gustavsson, L., Ingvar, D.H.: Regional cerebral blood volume during paradoxical sleep. In: Cerebral blood flow (Brock, M., Fieschi, C., Ingvar, D.H., Lassen, N.A., Schürmann, K., eds). Berlin-Heidelberg-New York: Springer 1969a, pp. 101–103

Risberg, J., Ingvar, D.H.: Regional changes in cerebral blood volume during mental activity. Exp. Brain Res. **5**, 72–78 (1968)

RISBERG, J., INGVAR, D.H.: Increase of blood flow in cortical association areas during memorization and abstract thinking. In: Cerebral blood flow and intracranial pressure (FIESCHI, C., ed). Basel-München-Paris-London-New York-Sydney: Karger 1971/72. part I. Europ. Neurol. 6, 236–241

RISBERG, J., INGVAR, D.H.: Increase of regional cerebral blood volume during REM-sleep in man. 1st. Europ. Congr. Sleep Res. Basel: Karger 1973a, pp. 1–5

RISBERG, J., INGVAR, D.H.: Patterns of activation in the grey matter of the dominant hemisphere during memorization and reasoning. Studentlitteratur Lund, Schweden 1973b, pp. 1–47

RISBERG, J., INGVAR, D.H.: Multibolus technique for measuring the distribution of cerebral blood flow over short intervals in man. Circulat. Res. **31**, 889–898 (1973c)

ROACH, M.R.: The role of transmitters and sympathetic innervation in the control of cerebral blood flow. Specific sensitivity of cerebral vessels to pCO_2. In: Vascular smooth muscle (BETZ, E., ed). Berlin-Heidelberg-New York: Springer 1972, p. 130

ROBIN, E.D., WHALEY, R.D., CRUMP, C.H., BICKELMANN, A.C., TRAVIS, D.M.: Acid-base relations between spinal fluid and arterial blood with special reference to control of ventilation. J. appl. Physiol. **13**, 385–392 (1958)

ROBINSON, G.A., BUTCHER, R.W., SUTHERLAND, E.W.: Cyclic AMP. Ann. Rev. Biochem. **37**, 149–174 (1968)

RODLER, H.: A new way of rheoencephalography. Electroenceph. clin. Neurophysiol. **12**, 531 (1960)

ROLAND, P.E., LARSEN, B., SKINHØJ, E., LASSEN, N.A.: Regional cerebral blood flow increase due to treatment of somatosensory and auditive information in man. In: Cerebral Function, Metabolism and Circulation (INGVAR, D.H., LASSEN, N.A., eds). Copenhagen: Munskgaard, 1977, p. 540–541

ROLAND, P.E., SKINHØJ, E., LARSEN, B., LASSEN, N.A.: The role of different cortical areas in the organization of voluntary movements in man. Cerebral blood flow study. In: Cerebral Function, Metabolism and Circulation (INGVAR, D.H., LASSEN, N.A., eds). Copenhagen: Munksgaard, 1977, pp. 542–543

ROMANOV, V.A., GAEVYI, M.D.: Effect of stimulation of the tympanic nervous plexus on cerebral blood circulation and general arterial tension. Fiziol. Zh. (Mosk.) **57**, 697–703 (1971)

ROSENBLUM, W.I.: Can plasma skimming or inconstancy of regional hematocrit introduce errors in regional cerebral blood flow measurements or their interpretation. Stroke **3**, 248–254 (1972)

ROSENBLUM, W.I.: Some physiologic properties of nerves in the adventitia of cerebral blood vessels as revealed by fluorescence microscopy. In: The Cerebral Vessel Wall (CERVOS-NAVARRO, J., BETZ, E., MATAKAS, F., WÜLLENWEBER, R., eds). New York: Raven Press, 1976, pp. 183–189

ROSENDORFF, C., CRANSTON, W.I.: Application of the 133 Xe clearance method to the measurement of local blood flow in the conscious animal. In: Cerebral blood flow (BROCK, M., FIESCHI, C., INGVAR, D.H., LASSEN, N.A., SCHÜRMANN, K., eds). Berlin-Heidelberg-New York: Springer 1969, pp. 36–38

ROSOMOFF, H.C.: Adjuncts to neurosurgical anaesthesia. Brit. J. Anaesth. **37**, 246–261 (1965)

ROSS-RUSSELL, R.W.: Brain and blood flow. London: Pitman 1971

ROWAN, J.O., JOHNSTON, J.H., HARPER, A.M., JENNETT, W.B.: Perfusion pressure in intracranial hypertension. In: Intracranial pressure. Berlin-Heidelberg-New York: Springer 1972. pp. 165–170

ROY, C.S., SHERRINGTON, C.S.: On the regulation of the blood supply of the brain. J. Physiol. (Lond.) **11**, 85–108 (1890)

RÜEGG, J.C.: Smooth muscle tone. Physiol. Rev. **51**, 201–248 (1971)

RYDER, H.W., ESPEY, F.F., KIMBELL, F.D., PENKA, E.J., ROSENAUER, A., PODOLSKY, B., EVANS, J.P.: Modification of effect of cerebral blood flow on cerebrospinal fluid pressure by variation in craniospinal blood volume. Arch. Neurol. Psychiat. (Chic.) **68**, 170–174 (1952a)

RYDER, H.W., ESPEY, F.F., KIMBELL, F.D., PENKA, E.J., ROSENAUER, A., PODOLSKY, B., EVANS, J.P.: Influence of changes in cerebral blood flow on the cerebrospinal fluid pressure. Arch. Neurol. Psychiat. (Chic.) **68**, 165–169 (1952b)

RYZHOVA, N.M.: Control of local brain circulation by carbon dioxide. Fiziol. Zh. (Mosk.) **56**, 1020–1025 (1970)

SAGAWA, K., GUYTON, A.C.: Pressure-flow relationships in isolated canine cerebral circulation. Amer. J. Physiol. **200**, 711–714 (1961)

SCHAERTLIN, C.E.: Polarographische Messung der Sauerstoffspannung im Hirnblut bei Hypoxie. Helv. physiol. pharmacol. Acta **19**, 255–262 (1961)

SCHATZMANN, H.J.: Kalziumaufnahme und -abgabe am Darmmuskel des Meerschweinchens. Pflügers Arch. ges. Physiol. **274**, 295–310 (1961)

SCHEINBERG, P.: Simultaneous bilateral determinations of cerebral blood flow and arterial-cerebral venous oxygen and glucose differences. Proc. soc. exp. Biol. **74**, 575–578 (1950)

SCHEINBERG, P., BLACKBURN, J., RICH, M., SASLAW, S.: Effects of aging on cerebral circulation and metabolism. Arch. Neurol. Psychiat. (Chic.) **70**, 77–85 (1953)

SCHEINBERG, P., STEAD, E.A. JR.: The cerebral blood flow in normal male subjects as measured by the nitrous oxide technique. Normal values for blood flow, oxygen utilization, glucose utilization and peripheral resistance, with observations on the effect of tilting and anxiety. J. clin. Invest. **28**, 1163–1171 (1949)

SCHIEVE, J.F., WILSON, W.P.: The changes in cerebral vascular tone in experimental metabolic alkalosis and acidosis. J. clin. Invest. **31**, 658 (1952)

SCHIEVE, J.F., WILSON, W.P.: The changes in cerebral vascular resistance of man in experimental alcalosis and acidosis. J. clin. Invest. **32**, 33–38 (1953)

SCHINDLER, U.: Stoffwechsel-Untersuchungen am Cortex cerebri der Katze unter Hypercapnie. Dissertation Tübingen 1974

SCHINDLER, U., GÄRTNER, E., BETZ, E.: Energy-rich metabolites and EEG in hypoxia and in hypercapnia. In: Oxygen transport to tissue (BICHER, H.I., BRULEY, D.F., eds). New York: Plenum Publ. Corp. 1973, pp. 233–238

SCHMAHL, F.W., BETZ, E., DETTINGER, E., HOHORST, H.J.: Engergiestoffwechsel der Großhirnrinde und Elektroencephalogramm bei Sauerstoffmangel. Pflügers Arch. ges. Physiol. **292**, 46–59 (1966)

SCHMAHL, F.W., BETZ, E., TALKE, H.: Effects of transient carotid occlusion on the extramitochondrial redox system in the disturbed hemisphere. In: Cerebral blood flow and intracranial pressure. Proc. 5th Int. Symp. Roma-Siena 1971, part I. Europ. Neurol. **6**, 323–328 (1971/72)

SCHMAHL, F.W., BETZ, E., TALKE, H., HOHORST, H.J.: Energiereiche Phosphate und Metabolite des Energiestoffwechsels in der Großhirnrinde der Katze. Biochem. Z. **342**, 518–531 (1965)

SCHMIDT, C.F.: The intrinsic regulation of the circulation in the hypothalamus of the cat. Amer. J. Physiol. **110**, 137–152 (1934)

SCHMIDT, C.F.: The intrinsic regulation of the circulation in the parietal cortex of the cat. Amer. J. Physiol. **114**, 572–585 (1936)

SCHMIDT, C.F.: Der Kreislauf des Gehirns. Pflügers Arch. ges. Physiol. **251**, 571–584 (1949)

SCHMIDT, C.F.: The cerebral circulation in health and disease. Springfield, Ill.: Thomas 1950, p. 78

SCHMIDT, C.F.: Central nervous system circulation, fluid and barriers-introduction. In: Handbook of physiology. Bd. III (FIELD, J., ed). Washington: Amer. Physiol. Soc. 1961, pp. 1745–1750

SCHMIDT, C.F., HENDRIX, J.P.: The circulation of the brain and the spinal cord. Baltimore: Williams & Wilkins. Ass. Res. nerv. Dis. Proc. **18**, 229 (1938)

SCHMIDT, C.F., KETY, S.S., PENNES, H.H.: The gaseous metabolism of the brain of the monkey. Amer. J. Physiol. **143**, 33–52 (1945)

SCHMIDT, C.F., PIERSON, J.C.: The intrinsic regulation of the blood vessels of the medulla oblongata. Amer. J. Physiol. **108**, 241–263 (1934)

SCHMIDT-NIELSEN, K., PENNYCUIK, P.: Capillary density in mammals in relation to body size and oxygen consumption. Amer. J. Physiol. **200**, 746–750 (1961)

SCHNEIDER, M.: Durchblutung und Sauerstoffversorgung des Gehirns. Verh. dtsch. Ges. Kreisl.-Forsch. **19**, 3–25 (1953)

SCHNEIDER, M.: The metabolism of the brain in ischaemia and hypothermia. In: Metabolism of the nervous system (RICHTER, D., ed). London-New York-Paris-Los Angeles: Pergamon Press 1957, pp. 238–244

SCHNEIDER, M.: Über die Wiederbelebung nach Kreislaufunterbrechung. Thoraxchirurgie **6**, 95–106 (1958)

SCHNEIDER, M.: Zur Pathophysiologie des Gehirnkreislaufs. Acta neurochir. (Wien) Suppl. 7, 34–50 (1961)

SCHNEIDER, M.: Überlebens- und Wiederbelebungszeit von Gehirn, Herz, Leber, Niere nach Ischaemie und Anoxie. Forschungsber. d. Landes Nordrhein-Westfalen Köln-Opladen: Deutscher Verlag 1965

SCHRADER, J., NEES, S., GERLACH, E.: Evidence for a cell surface adenosine receptor on coronary myocytes and atrial muscle cells. Pflügers Arch., **369**, 251–257 (1977)

SCHÜLLER, M.: Über die Einwirkung einiger Arzneimittel auf die Gehirngefäße. Berl. klin. Wschr. Xi **294**, 305–307 (1874)

SCHULTZ, A.: Zur Lehre von der Blutbewegung im Innern des Schädels. St. Petersb. med. Zschr. **11**, 122–128 (1866)

SCHWARTZ, B., ZAREA, L.: Cerebral circulation in experimentally-induced cerebrovascular accidents (rabbit). Exp. Neurol. **23**, 474–484 (1969)

SCOTT, J.B., RUDKO, M., RADAWSKI, D., HADDY, F.J.: Role of osmolarity, K^+, H^+, Mg^{++}, and O_2 in local blood flow regulation. Amer. J. Physiol. **218**, 338–345 (1970)

SEM-JACOBSEN, C.W., STYRI, O.B., MOHN, E.: Simultaneous focal intracerebral blood flow measurements in man around 18 chronically implanted electrodes. In: Cerebral blood flow (BROCK, M., FIESCHI, C., INGVAR, D.H., LASSEN, N.A., SCHÜRMANN, K., eds). Berlin-Heidelberg-New York: Springer 1969, pp. 44–46

SENGUPTA, D., HARPER, A.M., JENNETT, W.B.: Cerebral blood flow in baboon following carotid ligation: Effects of hypoxia and hypotension. Stroke **5**, 330 (1973)

SEVERINGHAUS, J.W.: Cerebral blood flow in chronic hypoxia. Acta anaesth. scand. Suppl. **15**, 96 (1964)

SEVERINGHAUS, J.W.: Hypoxic respiratory drive and its loss during chronic hypoxia. Clin. Physiol. **2**, 57–79 (1972)

SEVERINGHAUS, J.W., CHIODI, H., EGER, E.I., BRANDSTATER, B., HORNBEIN, TH.: Cerebral blood flow in man at high altitude. Circulat. Res. **19**, 274–282 (1966)

SEVERINGHAUS, J.W., MITCHELL, R.A., RICHARDSON, B.W., SINGER, M.M.: Respiratory control at high altitude suggesting active transport regulation of CSF pH. J. appl. Physiol. **18**, 1155–1166 (1963)

SEYLAZ, J., AUBINEAU, P., EDVINSSON, L., MAMO, H., NIELSEN, K.C., OWMAN, C., SERCOMBE, R.: Regional differences in β-adrenergic effects on local cerebral blood flow and adrenergic innervation. In: Cerebral circulation and metabolism (LANGFITT, T.W., MCHENRY, L.C. JR., REIVICH, M., WOLLMAN, H., eds). Berlin-Heidelberg-New York: Springer 1975, pp. 454–458

SHACKELFORD, R.T., HEGEDUS, S.H.: Factors affecting

cerebral blood flow: Experimental review. Sympathectomy, hypothermia, CO_2-inhalation and papaverin. Ann. Surg. **163**, 771–777 (1966)

SHALIT, M.N., REINMUTH, O.M., SHIMOJYO, S., SCHEINBERG, P.: Carbon dioxide and cerebral circulatory control. III. The effects of brain stem lesions. Arch. Neurol. (Chic.) **17**, 342–353 (1967b)

SHALIT, M.N., REINMUTH, O.M., SHIMOJYO, S., SCHEINBERG, P.: A mechanism by which carbon dioxide influences cerebral circulation independent of a direct effect on vascular smooth muscle. In: Research on the cerebral circulation (MEYER, J.S., LECHNER, H., EICHHORN, O., eds). Springfield, Ill.: Thomas 1969, pp. 173–185

SHALIT, M.N., SHIMOJYO, S., REINMUTH, O.M.: Carbon dioxide and cerebral circulatory control. I. The extravascular effect. Arch. Neurol. (Chic.) **17**, 298–303 (1967a)

SHENKIN, H.A., CABIESES, F., NOORDT, G. VAN DEN, SAYERS, P., COPPERMAN, R.: The hemodynamic effect of unilateral carotid ligation on the cerebral circulation of man. J. Neurosurg. **8**, 38–45 (1951)

SHENKIN, H.A., HARMEL, M.H., KETY, S.S.: Dynamic anatomy of the cerebral circulation. Arch. Neurol. Psychiat. (Chic.) **60**, 240–252 (1948)

SHIMOJYO, S., REINMUTH, O.M., KOGURE, K., SCHEINBERG, P.: Cerebral blood flow and metabolism at different levels of hypoxia. Amer. Neurol. Ass. Jg. 1966, pp. 338–339

SHINOHARA, Y., SAKAI, F., ISHIHARA, T., KOBATAKE, K., NAKAHARA, K., GOTOH, F.: Nonparticipation of cholinergic mechanism in chemical control of cerebral vasomotor activity. In: Cerebral Function, Metabolism and Circulation (INGVAR, D.H., LASSEN, N.A., eds). Copenhagen: Munksgaard 1977, pp. 300–301

SIEGEL, G., JÄGER, R., NOLTE, J., BERTSCHE, O., ROEDEL, H., SCHRÖTER, R.: Ionic concentrations and membrane potential in cerebral and extracerebral arteries. In: Pathology of cerebral microcirculation (CERVOS-NAVARRO, J., ed). Berlin: Gruyter 1974b, pp. 96–120

SIEGEL, G., KOEPCHEN, H.P., ROEDEL, H.: Slow oscillations of transmembrane Na and K-fluxes in vascular smooth muscle. In: Vascular smooth muscle (BETZ, E., ed). Berlin-Heidelberg-New York: Springer 1972, pp. 1–6

SIEGEL, G., ROEDEL, H., JÄGER, R., BERTSCHE, O.: Relationship between membrane potential of vascular smooth muscle and external K^+ concentration. Pflügers Arch. ges. Physiol. **347**, R 14 (1974a)

SIESJÖ, B.K., NILSSON, L.: The influence of arterial hypoxemia upon labile phosphates and upon extracellular and intracellular lactate and pyruvate concentration in the rat brain. Scand. J. clin. Lab. Invest. **27**, 83–96 (1971)

SKINHØJ, E.: Regulation of cerebral blood flow as a single function of the interstitial pH in the brain. Acta neurol. scand. **42**, 604–607 (1966)

SKINHØJ, E.: The upper limit of autoregulation and the sympathetic system. In: Cerebral circulation and metabolism (LANGFITT, T.W., MCHENRY, L.C. JR., REIVICH, M., WOLLMAN, H., eds). Berlin-Heidelberg-New York: Springer 1975, pp. 487–488

SKINHØJ, E., PAULSON, O.B.: Carbon dioxide and cerebral circulatory control. Evidence of a nonfocal site of action of carbon dioxide on cerebral circulation [human]. Arch. Neurol. (Chic.) **20**, 249–252 (1969)

SÖDERBERG, U., WECKMANN, N.: Changes in cerebral blood supply caused by changes in the pressure drop along arteries to the brain of the cat. Experientia (Basel) **15**, 346–348 (1959)

SOKOLOFF, L.: The action of drugs in the cerebral circulation. Pharmacol. Rev. **11**, 1–85 (1959)

SOKOLOFF, L.: Local cerebral circulation at rest and during altered cerebral activity induced by anesthesia or visual stimulation. In: Regional chemistry, physiology and pharmacology of the nervous system (KETY, S.S., ELKES, J., eds). Oxford: Pergamon Press 1961, pp. 107–117

SOKOLOFF, L.: Control of cerebral blood flow: The effects of anesthetic agents. In: Uptake and distribution of anesthetic agents (PAPPER, E.M., ed). New York-Toronto-London: McGraw Hill Book Cie 1963, pp. 140–157

SOKOLOFF, L., GRAVE, G.D., JEHLE, J.W., KENNEDY, CH.: Postnatal development of the local cerebral blood flow in the dog. In: Cerebral blood flow and intracranial pressure (FIESCHI, D., ed). Basel-München-Paris-London-New York-Sydney: Karger 1971/72, part I, pp. 269–273

SOKOLOFF, L., MANGOLD, R., WECHSLER, R.L., KENNEDY, CH., KETY, S.S.: The effect of mental arithmetic on cerebral circulation and metabolism. J. clin. Invest. **34**, 1101–1108 (1955)

SOKOLOFF, L., REIVICH, M., PATLAK, C.S., PETTIGREW, K.D., DES ROSIERS, M.H., KENNEDY, CH.: The determination of local cerebral glucose consumption from the local uptake of (^{14}C) deoxyglucose. In: Blood flow and metabolism in the brain (HARPER, A.M., JENNETT, W.B., MILLER, J.D., ROWAN, J.O., eds). Edinburgh-London: Livingstone 1975, p. 15.9

SOMLYO, A.P., SOMLYO, A.V.: Vascular smooth muscle. I. Normal structure, pathology, biochemistry and biophysics. Pharmacol. Rev. **20**, 197–272 (1968b)

SOMLYO, A.P., SOMLYO, A.V.: Vascular smooth muscle. I. Pharmacology of normal and hypertensive vessels. Pharmacol. Rev. **22**, 250–353 (1970)

SOMLYO, A.V., SOMLYO, A.P.: Electromechanical and pharmacomechanical coupling in vascular smooth muscle. J. Pharmacol. exp. Ther. **159**, 129–145 (1968a)

SOMLYO, A.P., SOMLYO, A.V.: Ultrastructural aspects of activation and contraction of vascular smooth muscle. Fed. Proc. **35**, 1288–1293 (1976)

SPINA, A.: Experimentelle Untersuchungen über die Bildung des Liquor cerebrospinalis. Pflügers Arch. ges. Physiol. **76**, 204–218 (1898)

SPINA, A.: Über den Einfluß des hohen Blutdruckes auf die Neubildung der Zerebrospinal-Flüssigkeit. Pflügers Arch. ges. Physiol. **80**, 370–407 (1900)

STAVRAKY, G.W.: Response of cerebral blood vessels to electrical stimulation of the thalamus and hypothalamic regions. Arch. Neurol. Psychiat. (Chic.) **35**, 1002–1028 (1936)

STEWART, G.N.A.: A new method of measuring the velocity of the blood. J. Physiol. (Lond.) **11**, 15–18 (1890)

STÖHR, P.: Zur Innervation der Pia mater und des Plexus choroideus des Menschen. Anat. Anz. Erg.-H. 30, 54–63 (1921)

STONE, H.L., RAICHLE, M.E., HERNANDEZ, M.: Sympathetic innervation and carbon dioxide sensivity. In: Cerebral circulation and metabolism (LANGFITT, T.W., MCHENRY, L.C. JR., REIVICH, M., WOLLMAN, H., eds). Berlin-Heidelberg-New York: Springer 1975, pp. 428–430

STOSSECK, K., LÜBBERS, D.W., COTTIN, N.: Determination of local blood flow (microflow) by electrochemically generated hydrogen. Pflügers Arch. ges. Physiol. **348**, 225–238 (1974)

STROMBERG, D.D., FOX, J.R.: Pressures in the pial arterial microcirculation of the cat during changes in systemic arterial blood pressure. Circulat. Res. **31**, 229–239 (1972)

SUGANO, H., INANAGA, K.: Studies on the localized cerebral blood flow. Kyushu J. med. Sci. **12**, 9–13 (1961)

SUGAR, O., GERARD, R.W.: Anoxia and brain potentials. J. Neurophysiol. **1**, 558–572 (1938)

SUTHERLAND, E.W., ROBINSON, G.A., BUTCHER, R.W.: Some aspects of the biological role of adenosine 3′,5′-monophosphate (cyclic AMP). Circulation **37**, 279–306 (1968)

SUZUKI, H., TUKAHARA, Y.: Cerebral circulation during arousal reaction of EEG. Tohoku J. exp. Med. **84**, 316–328 (1965)

SVEINSDOTTIR, E., LASSEN, N.A.: Detector system for measuring regional cerebral blood flow. Stroke **4**, 365 (1973)

SVEINSDOTTIR, E., LASSEN, N.A. A 254-detector system for measuring regional cerebral blood flow. In: Cerebral circulation and metabolism (LANGFITT, W.T. et al., eds). Berlin-Heidelberg-New York: Springer 1975, pp. 415–417

SVEINSDOTTIR, E., LASSEN, N.A., RISBERG, J., INGVAR, D.H.: Regional cerebral blood flow measured by multiple probes: An oscilloscope and a digital computer system for rapid data processing. In: Cerebral blood flow (BROCK, M., FIESCHI, C., INGVAR, D.H., LASSEN, N.A., SCHÜRMANN, K., eds). Berlin-Heidelberg-New York: Springer 1969, p. 27–28

SVEINSDOTTIR, E., TORLÖF, P., RISBERG, J., INGVAR, D.H., LASSEN, N.A.: Monitoring regional cerebral blood flow in normal man with a computer-controlled 32-detector system. In: Cerebral blood flow and intracranial pressure (FIESCHI, C., ed). Basel-München-Paris-London-New York-Sydney: Karger 1971/72, part I, pp. 228–233

SYMON, L.: Observations on the leptomeningeal collateral circulation in dogs. J. Physiol. (Lond.) **154**, 1–14 (1960)

SYMON, L.: Studies of leptomeningeal collateral circulation in macacus rhesus. J. Physiol. (Lond.) **159**, 68–86 (1961)

SYMON, L.: A comperative study of middle cerebral pressure in dogs and macaques. J. Physiol. (Lond.) **191**, 449–465 (1967)

SYMON, L.: Experimental evidence for "intracerebral steal" following CO_2 inhalation. Scand. J. clin. Lab. Invest. 102 Suppl. 102–113 (1968)

SYMON, L.: The concept of intracerebral steal. Int. Anaesth. Clin. **7**, 597–615 (1969)

SYMON, L., ROSS RUSSELL, R.W.: The development of cerebral collateral circulation following occlusion of vessels in the neck. An experimental study in baboon. J. neurol. Sci. **13**, 197–208 (1971)

TAYLOR, H.W., MCCALL, M.L.: The cerebral effects of pentothal sodium in toxemias of pregnancy. J. Philad. gen. Hosp. **2**, 86–89 (1951)

THEWS, G.: Die Sauerstoffdiffusion im Gehirn. Ein Beitrag zur Frage der Sauerstoffversorgung der Organe. Pflügers Arch. ges. Physiol. **271**, 197–226 (1960)

THOMAS, H.: Licht- und elektronenmikroskopische Untersuchungen an den weichen Hirnhäuten und den Pacchionischen Granulationen des Menschen. Jb. Morph. Abt. 2: Z. mikroskop.-anat. Forsch. **75**, 269–327 (1966)

THORN, W., HEITMANN, R.: pH der Gehirnrinde vom Kaninchen in situ während perakuter, totaler Ischämie, reiner Anoxie und in der Erholung. Pflügers Arch. ges. Physiol. **258**, 501–510 (1954)

THORNER, M.W., LEWEY, F.H.: The effects of repeated anoxia on the brain. A histopathologic study. Amer. med. Ass. **115**, 1595–1600 (1940)

TISSEYRE, J.-P.: Débit sanguin métabolisme et vieillissement cérébral. (Sammlung Arbus-Bousser – textes receuillis). Selbstverlag der Laboratoires Dausse, Paris 1973

TODA, N.: The action of vasodilating drugs on isolated basilar, coronary and mesenteric arteries of the dog. J. Pharmacol. Exptl. Therap., **191**, 139–146 (1974)

TODA, N.: Responsiveness to potassium and calcium ions of isolated cerebral arteries. Amer. J. Physiol. **227**, 1206–1211 (1974)

TODA, N., FUJITA, Y.: Responsiveness of isolated cerebral and peripheral arteries to serotonin, norepinephrine, and transmural electrical stimulation. Circulat. Res. **33**, 98–104 (1973)

TODA, N., HAYASHI, S., FU, W.L.H., NAGASAKA, Y.: Serotonin antagonism in isolated canine cerebral arteries. Jap. J. Pharmacol. **26**, 57–63 (1976)

TOLANI, A.J., TALWAR, G.P.: Differential metabolism of various brain regions. Biochem. J. **88**, 357–362 (1963)

TRAYSTMAN, R.J., RAPELA, C.E.: Effect of sympathetic nerve stimulation on cerebral and cephalic blood flow. In: Cerebral circulation and metabolism (LANGFITT, T.W., MCHENRY, L.C., JR., REIVICH, M., WOLLMAN, H., eds). Berlin-Heidelberg-New York: Springer 1975, pp. 451–453

UEDA, H., HATANO, S., MOLDE, T., GONDAIRA, T.: Compartmental analysis of the human brain blood flow (discussion). Acta neurol. scand. Suppl. **14**, 90–91 (1965)

USINGER, W., PLESCHKA, K., ALBERS, C.: Der Einfluß der Vagotomie auf die Hirndurchblutung bei künstlich konstant gehaltenem Blutdruck. Pflügers Arch. ges. Physiol. **291**, 236–240 (1966)

VEALL, N., MALLETT, B.L.: The two-compartment model using Xe^{133} inhalation and external counting. Acta neurol. scand. Suppl. **14**, 83–84 (1965)

VESALIUS, A.: De humanis corporis fabrica. Liber VII, 1542. Nachdr. d. Ausg. 1542: Bruxelles: Impressions anastatique, Culture et Civilisation. Lebou 1964

VIERORDT, K.: Grundriß der Physiologie des Menschen. Tübingen: Laupp 1877

VLAHOV, V., ENZENROSS, H.G.: Einfluß der Ca^{++}-Ionen auf die Kontraktilität der glatten Muskulatur von Piagefäßen. Verh. dtsch. Ges. Kreisl.-Forsch. **39**, 129–132 (1973)

VYSHATINA, A.J.: Regional blood flow changes with electric stimulation of the reticular vasomotor formation of the medulla oblongata. Fiziol. Zh. (Mosk.) **56**, 733–741 (1970)

WAHL, M., DEETJEN, P., THURAU, K., INGVAR, D.H., LASSEN, N.A.: Micropuncture evaluation of the importance of perivascular pH for the arteriolar diameter on the brain surface. Pflügers Arch. ges. Physiol. **316**, 152–163 (1970)

WAHL, M., KUSCHINSKY, W.: The dilatory action of adenosine on pial arteries of cats and its inhibition by theophylline. Pflügers Arch. **362**, 55–59 (1976)

WAHL, M., KUSCHINSKY, W., BOSSE, O., NEISS, A.: Micropuncture evaluation of β-receptors in pial arteries of cats. Pflügers Arch. ges. Physiol. **348**, 293–303 (1974)

WAHL, M., KUSCHINSKY, W., BOSSE, O., OLESEN, J., LASSEN, N.A., INGVAR, D.H., MICHAELIS, J., THURAU, K.: Effect of l-norepinephrine on the diameter of pial arterioles and arteries in the cat. Circulat. Res. **31**, 248–256 (1972)

WAHL, M., KUSCHINSKY, W., BOSSE, O., THURAU, K.: Dependency of pial arterial and arteriolar diameter on perivascular osmolarity in the cat. Circulat. Res. **32**, 162–169 (1973)

WALLENFANG, TH., SCHUBERT, R., REULEN, H.J., SCHÜRMANN, K.: rCBF and regional energy metabolism in cold injury edema as affected by moderate and severe hypocapnia and hypercapnia. Stroke **4**, 332 (1973)

WALTZ, A.G., YAMAGUCHI, I., REGLI, F.: Cerebral vascular reactivity after sympathetic denervation. In: Brain and blood flow (ROSS RUSSELL, R.W., ed). London: Pitman 1971, pp. 178–181

WEBER, A.: Energized calcium transport and relaxing factors. Curr. Top. Bioenerget. **1**, 203–254 (1966)

WEBER, A., HERZ, R.: The binding of calcium to actomyosin systems in relation to their biological activity. J. biol. Chem. **238**, 599–605 (1963)

WEBER, A., MURRAY, J.M.: Molecular control mechanism in muscle contraction. Physiol. Rev. **53**, 612–673 (1973)

WECHSLER, R.L., DRIPPS, R.D., KETY, S.S.: Blood flow and oxygen consumption of the human brain during anesthesia produced by thiopenthal. Anesthesiology **12**, 308–314 (1951)

WEIDNER, A.: Energiestatus der Großhirnrinde der Katze während passiver Hyperventilation. Dissertation Marburg 1969

WEISS, CH., THIEMANN, V.: Oscillatory pressure induced changes of vascular resistance in autoregulation. Pflügers Arch. ges. Physiol. **343**, R 25 (1973)

WEISS, G.B., GOODMAN, F.R.: Effects of Ca^{++} on contraction, calcium distribution and movement in intestinal smooth muscle. J. Pharmacol. exp. Ther. **169**, 46–55 (1969)

WELCH, K.M.A., KNOWLES, L., SPIRA, P.: Local effect of prostaglandins on cat pial arteries. Europ. J. Pharmacol. **25**, 155–158 (1974)

WELLS, R.E., DENTON, R., MERRILL, E.W.: Measurement of viscosity of biologic fluid by cone plate viscometer. J. Lab. clin. Med. **57**, 646–656 (1961)

WENDE, W., PEIPER, U.: Wechselwirkung von Kalium und Noradrenalin auf die Spannungsentwicklung des isolierten Gefäßmuskels. Pflügers Arch. ges. Physiol. **320**, 133–141 (1970)

WEZLER, K., SINN, W.: Das Strömungsgesetz des Blutkreislaufs. Aulendorf: Cantor 1953

WILCKE, O.: Untersuchung der Hirndurchblutung mit radioaktiven Isotopen. In: Die zerebralen Durchblutungsstörungen des Erwachsenenalters (QUANDT, J., Hrsg.), S. 137–171. Stuttgart: Schattauer 1969

WILKINSON, I.M.S., BULL, J.W.D., DU BOULAY, G.H., MARSHALL, J., ROSS RUSSELL, R.W., SYMON, L.: The heterogeneity of blood flow throughout the normal cerebral hemisphere. In: Cerebral blood flow (BROCK, M., FIESCHI, C., INGVAR, D.H., LASSEN, N.A., SCHÜRMANN, K., eds). Berlin-Heidelberg-New York: Springer 1969, pp. 17–18

WILLIS, TH.W.: Cerebri anatome, cui accessit nervorum descriptio et usus. London 1664. Gesamtwerk: Venedig 1720

WODICK, R.: Möglichkeiten und Grenzen der Bestimmung der Blutversorgung mit Hilfe der lokalen Wasserstoffclearance. Habilitationsschrift Bochum 1973

WOLF, G.: Die Durchblutungsstörungen des Gehirns. Fortschr. Neurol. Psychiat. **27**, 487–548 (1959)

WOLFF, H.G.: The cerebral circulation. Physiol. Rev. **16**, 545–596 (1936)

Wolff, H.G., Forbes, H.S.: The cerebral circulation. V. Observations of the pial circulation during changes in intracranial pressure. Arch. Neurol. Psychiat. (Chic.) **20**, 1035–1047 (1928)

Wolff, H.G., Lennox, W.G.: Cerebral circulation. XII. The effect on pial vessels of variations in the O_2 and CO_2 content of the blood. Arch. Neurol. Psychiat. (Chic.) **23**, 1097–1120 (1930)

Wollman, H., Alexander, S.C., Cohen, P.J., Stephen, G.W., Zeiger, L.S.: Two-compartment analysis of the blood flow in the human brain. Acta neurol. scand. Suppl. **14**, 79–82 (1965)

Woodhall, B., Odom, G.L., Bloor, B.M., Golden, J.: Direct measurement of intravascular pressure in components of circle of Willis; contribution to surgery of congenital cerebral aneurysms and vascular anomalies of brain. Ann. Surg. **135**, 911–922 (1952)

Wüllenweber, R.: Messungen der Durchblutung des menschlichen Gehirns mit Thermosonden. Habilitationsschrift Bonn 1963

Wüllenweber, R.: Schwankungen der Hirndurchblutung unter physiologischen und pathophysiologischen Bedingungen. Acta neurochir. (Wien) **13**, 64–76 (1965a)

Wüllenweber, R.: Beobachtungen über den Einfluß der Atmung auf die lokale Hirndurchblutung des Menschen. Acta neurochir. (Wien) **13**, 506–516 (1965b)

Wüllenweber, R.: "Intracerebral steal" in man recorded by a heat clearance technique. Scand. J. clin. Lab. Invest. Suppl. 102, XIIIc (1968)

Wüllenweber, R., Gött, U., Szanto, J.: Beobachtungen zur Regulation der Hirndurchblutung. Acta neurochir. (Wien) **26**, 137–153 (1967)

Yamamoto, Y.L., Hodge, C.P., Phillips, K.P., Feindel, W.: Microflow patterns after experimental occlusion of middle cerebral artery demonstrated by fluorescein angiography and ^{133}Xenon clearance. In: Cerebral blood flow (Brock, M., Fieschi, C., Ingvar, D.H., Lassen, N.A., Schürmann, K., eds). Berlin-Heidelberg-New York: Springer 1969, pp. 123–126

Yamamoto, Y.L., Myles, T., Wolfe, L., Duszczyszyn, A., Hodge, C., Feindel, W.: Inhibition and reversal prostaglandin-induced cerebral vasospasm. In: Cerebral circulation and metabolism (Langfitt, T.W., McHenry, L.C., jr., Reivich, M., Wollman, H., eds). Berlin-Heidelberg-New York: Springer 1975, pp. 333–335

Zierler, K.L.: Equations for measuring blood flow by external monitoring of radioisotopes. Circulat. Res. **16**, 309–321 (1965)

Zupping, R.: Cerebral metabolism in patients with intracranial tumors. J. Neurosurg. **36**, 451–462 (1972)

Zwetnow, N.N.: Effects of increased cerebrospinal fluid pressure on the blood flow and on the energy metabolism of the brain. Acta physiol. scand. Suppl. **339**, 1–31 (1970)

Zwetnow, N.N., Kjällquist, A., Siesjö, B.K.: Cerebral blood flow during intracranial hypertension related to tissue hypoxia and to acidosis in cerebral extracellular fluids. In: Progress in brain research **30**, 87–92 (1968) (Luyendijk, W., ed). Amsterdam-London-New York: Elsevier 1968

Technik, Indikationen, Kontraindikationen und Komplikationen der zerebralen Angiographie

Von

M. NADJMI u. M. RATZKA

Mit 6 Abbildungen und 15 Tabellen

A. Einleitung

Die Erforschung der zerebralen Gefäße begann mit ihrer eingehenden anatomischen Beschreibung. Es folgten anatomische und physiologische Studien des Hirnkreislaufes unter Berücksichtigung meist experimenteller pathologischer Bedingungen und pharmakologischer Standpunkte (Tabelle 1). 1927 führte MONIZ die zerebrale Angiographie zur Darstellung der Hirngefäße in Röntgenbildern für klinisch diagnostische Zwecke ein und eröffnete mit den neuen diagnostischen Möglichkeiten auch einen neuen Weg der Hirnkreislaufforschung. Die seither weit verbreitete Angiogra-

Tabelle 1. Historische Methoden der Erforschung des Gehirnkreislaufs zusammengestellt nach Angaben von E. BETZ aus H. GÄNSHIRT (Hrsg.): Der Hirnkreislauf

Autor	Jahr	Veröffentlichung	Vorgehen
A. VESALIUS	1542	De humani corporis fabrica. Liber VII 1542	Anatomische Beschreibung der Hirngefäße
R.C. COLOMBO	1559	De re anatomica Libri XV. Venedig 1559 Deutsche Ausgabe Frankfurt 1609	Pulsationen des Gehirns sind mit denen des Herzens und der Arterien synchron. (Beobachtung durch Schädeldachfenster)
WILLIAM HARVEY	1628	Exercitio anatomica de motu cordis et sanguinis in animalibus Frankfurt/M 1628	Modernes Kreislaufkonzept. Beginn der experimentellen Kreislaufforschung
TH.W. WILLIS	1664	Cerebri anatome, cui accessit nervorum descriptio et usus. London 1664, Venedig 1720	Anatomische und physiologische Beobachtung der Hirngefäße
A. MONRO	1783	Observations of the structure and functions of the nervous System. Edinburg 1783 deutsch Leipzig 1887	Monro-Kellie – Doktrin: "the quantity of blood within the head must be the same, or nearly the same at all times."
G.K. KELLIE zu LEITH	1824	Reflections on the pathology of the brain. Trans. med. chir. Soc. Edinburg 1824 Beobachtungen durch Schädeldachfenster	
J.L. BRACHT	1830	Rech. exp. sur le syst. nerv. gangl. Paris 1830	Blutstauung im Gehirn nach Durchtrennung des Halssympatikus

Fortsetzung nächste Seite

Tabelle 1 (Fortsetzung)

Autor	Jahr	Veröffentlichung	Vorgehen
F.C. DONDERS	1850	Die Bewegung des Gehirns und die Gefäßfüllung der Pia mater auch bei geschlossenem unausdehnbarem Schädel unmittelbar beobachtet. Nederl. Lancet 1850 Abstracts in Schmidt Jb. ges. Med. 69 (1851) 16	Asphyxie und Erweiterung der zerebralen Gefäße.
A. SCHULTZ	1866	Zur Lehre von der Blutbewegung im Innern des Schädels. St. Petersb. Med. Z. 11 (1866) 122	Beobachtung der spontanen Weitenänderung der Piagefäße
H. NOTHNAGEL	1867	Die vasomotorischen Nerven der Gehirngefäße. Virchows Archiv path. Anat. 40 (1867) 203	Reaktion der Hirngefäße bei Schmerzreizen (am N. cruralis)
M. SCHÜLLER	1874	Über die Einwirkung einiger Arzneimittel auf die Hirngefäße. Berl. klin. Wschr. 11, 294; 305	Weite der Gehirngefäße unter Chloroformeinwirkung (bei Mensch und Tier)
G. GÄRTNER J. WAGNER	1887	Über den Hirnkreislauf. Wien. med. Wschr. (1887) 601–603; 640–642	Erhöhung der Gehirndurchströmung bei Anstieg des Aortendruckes
K. HÜRTHLE	1889	Untersuchungen über die Innervation der Gehirngefäße. Pflügers Arch. ges. Physiol. 44 (1889) 561	Messung des arterillen Blutdruckes im Circulus arteriosus cerebri
A. MYERSON R.D. HALLORAN H.L. HIRSCH	1927	Technic for obtaining blood from the internal jugular vein and internal carotid artery. Arch. Neurol. Psych. (Chic.) 17 (1927) 807	Karotis- und Jugularispunktion am Menschen
W. G. LENNOX	1932	The blood flow in the brain and the leg of man, and the changes induced by alterations of blood gases. J. clin. invest. 11 (1932) 1155	und Messung der arterio-venösen Sauerstoffdifferenz
E. MONIZ	1927	L'encéphalographie artérielle et son importance dans la localisation des tumeurs cérébrales. Rev. Neurol. 2 (1927) 72	Einführung der zerebralen Angiographie

phietechnik stellt die häufigste Untersuchung zum Nachweis von zerebralen Prozessen dar, sie hat nach allen Richtungen eine ungeahnte Entwicklung genommen und wird in ihrer Priorität erst seit wenigen Jahren durch die Computer-Tomographie abgelöst. Die Methode wurde in dem naturgemäß äußerst umfangreichen Schrifttum mehrfach unter verschiedenen Gesichtspunkten zusammenfassend dargestellt, so z.B. bei OLIVECRONA (1935), ELVIDGE (1937), GOULD et al. (1955), TÖNNIS und SCHIEFER (1959), DECKER (1960), KUHN (1960), KRAYENBÜHL und YASARGIL (1965), WEIBEL und FIELDS (1969), TAKAHASHI (1974), GÄNSHIRT et al. (1972), NEWTON und POTTS (1974), TAVERAS und WOOD (1976), HARWOOD-NASH und FITZ (1976) und vielen anderen.

Das Interesse an der ständigen Weiterentwicklung der Methode wird durch das reichhaltige Spektrum der Veröffentlichungen widergespiegelt. Die Vielfalt der Möglichkeiten, ein gestecktes Untersuchungsziel zu erreichen und zu neuen diagnostischen Gesichtspunkten zu kommen, wird ebenso dokumentiert wie eine teilweise extreme Verfeinerung neuer Methoden. Erste Ergebnisse von diagnostischem und teilweise therapeutischem Neuland werden zum Sammeln neuer Erfahrungsdimensionen gesichtet, festgehalten und immer wieder von physiologischen und anatomischen

Aspekten her überprüft. Diese Entwicklung setzt eine zunehmende apparative und personelle Spezialisierung voraus. Erst dann können auch schwierige und selten durchgeführte Untersuchungsmethoden im routinemäßigen Betrieb eine gleichmäßig gute Qualität der Ergebnisse garantieren. Die Aufrechterhaltung einer lebendigen Beziehung zu den klinischen Bereichen bleibt dabei für die Fruchtbarkeit jeder Arbeit entscheidend (RUGGIERO et al., 1973).

Ausblicke der weiteren Entwicklung ergeben sich in verschiedenen Richtungen. Wie bisher wird nach der weiteren Perfektionierung der Verfahrenstechniken zur Steigerung der Bildqualität und zur Senkung der Komplikationsquoten, besonders auf dem Sektor der spezialisierten Angiographie, gestrebt. Die breitere Einführung und Standardisierung der neuen Techniken, wie Serien-Schichtangiogramm, superselektive Angiographie, Angiographie zum therapeutischen Einsatz, Vergrößerungsangiographie, bis zum Vordringen in einen „mikroangiographischen Bereich" (DJINDJIAN, 1972) werden vorangetrieben.

B. Technik der zerebralen Angiographie

I. Ausstattung der angiographischen Arbeitsplätze

Zu einer voll funktionsfähigen Angiographieeinheit gehört heute eine Röntgenanlage, die simultan bzw. alternierend in zwei Bildebenen hohe Bildfrequenzen zuläßt und die mit einer elektronischen Bildverstärkeranlage ausgerüstet oder ausrüstbar ist, sowie ein Großbildwechsler, ebenfalls für hohe Bildfrequenzen in zwei Ebenen. Im allgemeinen wird bei Großbildwechslerbetrieb aber auch bei den schirmbildkinematographischen Verfahren die Aufnahmefrequenz rein mechanisch durch die Wechslerfrequenz oder die Bildgeschwindigkeit der Kameras begrenzt. Als Grundausstattung wird ein Großbildwechsler aus Gründen der Bildqualität vorzuziehen sein, und zwar in Form eines Folienwechslers, da sowohl die Gegenstromverfahren als auch die Katheterverfahren sowie die standardisierten Verfahren zur Bestimmung der Zirkulationszeit und Darstellung lokalisierter Durchblutungsstörungen höhere Bildfrequenzen erfordern (HUBER, 1972). Kassettenwechsler können nur noch für sehr beschränkte Fragestellungen eingesetzt werden.

Bei der Vergrößerungsangiographie wird auch bei der Benutzung von Hochleistungsdrehanodenröhren durch den sehr kleinen, zur scharfen Abbildung erforderlichen Fokus und die dadurch notwendige lange Belichtungszeit von etwa 0,5 s die Bildzahl pro Zeiteinheit begrenzt. Die Anfertigung simultaner bzw. alternierender Serien in zwei Ebenen während nur einer Kontrastmittelinjektion ist praktisch nicht durchführbar, da durch Streustrahlen in der jeweils anderen Bildebene die Bildqualität erheblich beeinträchtigt wird (WENDE et al., 1971; MISHKIN, 1974). Bei der Serienschichtangiographie, die als Simultan-Schichtung mit Kompositionskassetten durchgeführt wird, bestimmt die Dauer des Schichtvorganges, d.h. die Schichtgeschwindigkeit bei festgelegtem Schichtwinkel, die Anzahl der bei einem Injektionsvorgang möglichen Aufnahmephasen (NADJMI u. PÖSCHMANN, 1975). Die Auto-Angiotomographie (POOLE et al., 1974) bildet alle Phasen einer Angiographie in einer Schichtebene ab.

Zur Gegenstromangiographie sind wegen der großen Kontrastmittelmengen in bezug auf die Injektionszeit Überdruckinjektionseinrichtungen erforderlich (FARINAS, 1941; GOULD et al., 1955; MARSHALL u. LING, 1963; WAPPENSCHMIDT, 1966; WENDE u. TAENZER, 1965; NADJMI et al., 1968). Bei den selektiven Katheterverfahren und der Karotisangiographie wird der Einsatz einer automatischen Injektionseinrichtung (NEWTON u. POTTS, 1974; GREITZ, 1956; LODIN u. OTTANDER, 1967) aus Strahlenschutzgründen für den Arzt empfohlen; außerdem erlaubt eine automatische Injektionseinrichtung, mit Herzphasensteuerung über das EKG durch einen elektronischen Schwellenschalter zur Auslösung des Injektors in der Diastole, eine bessere Bildqualität mit weniger Kontrastmittel (HUBER, 1972; KLAUSBERGER u. VASS, 1966). Die Kathetermethoden erfordern den

Einsatz der Bildwandler-Fernsehkette, wobei zusätzliche Strahlenschutzeinrichtungen für Personal und Patienten vorhanden sein müssen. Der Patient wird durch eine Bleigummischürze (0,25 mm Pb) im Gonadenbereich und durch die Verwendung eines Bleigummivorhanges (0,5 mm Pb) in Höhe der Schultern, mit Halsausschnitt, geschützt. Die Dosisbestimmung während der Karotisangiographie (Wehmer, 1970) ergab 5 cm außerhalb und kaudal des Nutzstrahlenfeldes, bei korrekter Einblendung, eine Belastung von 16,5 Milliröntgen pro Aufnahme, in 60 cm Abstand von Feldmitte, hinter einer (0,25 mm Pb) Bleischürze, 0,05 Milliröntgen pro Aufnahme, ohne Bleischürze in 100 cm Abstand von Bildfeldmitte 0,5 Milliröntgen pro Aufnahme. Analoge Dosen gelten für das Personal. Durch den Bleigummivorhang reduziert sich die Strahlenbelastung auf die Injektionshand bei der Karotisangiographie um das 10- bis 20fache. Allein nach 240 Karotisangiographieserien zu 16 Aufnahmen, ohne Bleivorhang, würde die für ein Jahr höchstzulässige Röntgendosis bei beruflich Strahlenexponierten im Sinn der Strahlenschutzverordnung (60 rem an den Extremitäten und 5 rem Ganzkörperbelastung) erreicht (H. Betz in Gänshirt et al., 1972). Bei Durchführung der Untersuchung mit automatischer Injektion fällt die Belastung für das Personal völlig weg, da die Beatmung während des Ablaufs der Serie zur Gewährleistung verwacklungsfreier Aufnahmen kurz unterbrochen wird.

Zur Filmbearbeitung wurden allgemein automatische Entwicklungsmaschinen eingeführt. Der schnelle Auswurf der fertigen, trockenen Bilder nach 90 bis 180 s ermöglicht eine optimale Beurteilung noch während der Untersuchung, ohne die Entscheidungen über den weiteren Untersuchungsvorgang lange zu verzögern. In derselben Weise ist die photographische (Hacker u. Arburg, 1967), besser jedoch die elektronische Sofortsubtraktion (Decker u. Backmund, 1968) manchmal unentbehrlich, auch wenn für besondere Zwecke, aus Gründen der Bildqualität, anschließend noch weitere photographische Subtraktionen hergestellt werden sollen (Ziedses des Plantes, 1961).

II. Kontrastmittel

Nach Tierversuchen mit Wismutöl (Frank u. Alwens, 1910), Lipiodol (Sicard u. Forestier, 1923), Jodipin (Berberich u. Hirsch, 1923) konnten brauchbare Angiogramme am lebenden Menschen erst mit wasserlöslichen Halogenverbindungen erzielt werden. Strontiumbromid (Berberich u. Hirsch, 1923) und Natriumjodid (Dos Santos et al., 1929) erwiesen sich anfangs als zu different für die Gefäßwand und führten zu akuten Halogen-Intoxikationen mit Leber- und Nierenschädigungen. Für die ersten Versuche von zerebralen Angiographien wurden ebenfalls Brom- und Jodsalze (60–70%iges Strontiumbromid und 70%iges Lithiumbromid sowie 25%iges Natriumjodid; Moniz, 1927) verwendet. Moniz berichtete freimütig über die hohe Komplikationsrate mit 4 Todesfällen bei 150 Patienten, was möglicherweise, trotz größtem Interesse an der neuen Technik, die Verbreitung der Methode anfangs gehemmt haben mag. Mit der Einführung des Thorotrast 1931 durch Moniz und 1933 durch Löhr und Jacobi, einer 25%igen kolloidalen Lösung von Thoriumdioxyd mit einem alkalinisierenden Kohlehydratanteil schien das geeignete Kontrastmittel zur zerebralen Angiographie gefunden. Es bot bei sehr gutem Röntgenkontrast eine ausgezeichnete subjektive Verträglichkeit; auch objektive Nebenwirkungen wurden anfangs nicht beobachtet. Bald aber tauchten Verdachtsmomente auf über negative Langzeitwirkungen am retikuloendothelialen System (Held, 1932; Held u. Messe, 1932), konzerogene Wirkungen (Roussy et al., 1936) im Tierversuch bei Ratten mit sehr hohen Äquivalenzdosen (kurze Beobachtungszeit), über Retention von Thorotrast in den Hirngefäßen (Nordfield u. Russel, 1939), die in einem Fall die unmittelbare Todesursache darstellten (Eckström u. Lindgren, 1938). Später häuften sich die Mitteilungen über die Bildung von polymorphzelligen Sarkomen und über örtliche Thorotrastgranulome an der Injektionsstelle, z.B. bei 35 von 320 angiographierten Patienten (Bauer, 1949). Auch noch in den letzten Jahren werden Thorotrastome an der Injektionsstelle nach Angiographien beschrieben (Betz u. Matiar-Vahar, 1970); weiterhin finden sich Berichte über ausgedehnte Narbenbildungen der regionären Lymphbahnen (Wachsmuth, 1948), über ein Endothelsarkom der Leber (MacMahon et al., 1947) und Granulombildungen in den Glissonschen Scheiden der Leber.

Seit Ende der 40er Jahre verwendete man fast ausschließlich organische Jodsalze, anfangs aus der Diotrastgruppe (Diäthamolamin-, Diäthylamin-, Morpholin- oder Methylglucaminjodid), heute sind vorwiegend Diathrizoate und Jotalamate, insbesondere das reine Methyl-Glucaminsalz der Jotalaminsäure und Joxatalaminsäure in Gebrauch, in jüngster Zeit auch das Metrizamid. Je nach Art der Untersuchungsmethode werden von 3 bis zu 70 ml in einer Injektion verabreicht und bis zu 200 ml während einer Untersuchung, für besondere Verfahren sogar bis zu 500 ml (spinale Angiographie, Djindjian, 1972), wenn auch unter besonderen Schutzvorkehrungen zur Vermeidung von schweren Nebenwirkungen.

III. Vorbereitung zur Angiographie

Es gibt einige Veröffentlichungen über Arterienpunktionen ohne Anästhesie bei vernünftigen, gut mitarbeitenden Erwachsenen (Brenner u. Zaunbauer, 1966; Weickmann, 1969). In den meisten Fällen wird die Arterienpunktion zur zerebralen Angiographie, zumindest in lokaler Anästhesie, gelingen, selbst bei Kindern, die ausreichend sediert wurden (Nelhaus u. Chutorian, 1964). Es ist demnach in jedem Einzelfall die Entscheidung möglich, ob die Untersuchung in lokaler oder allgemeiner Anästhesie erfolgen soll. Die Diskussion über die Entscheidung ist vielfältig. Die überwiegende Anzahl der neueren Veröffentlichungen über angiographische Methoden zieht eine Durchführung der Untersuchung in Narkose vor, insbesondere wenn Komplikationen zu erwarten sind. Bei einer modernen, sachgemäß durchgeführten Narkose ergeben sich in der Tat einige Vorteile. Der Patient wird sowohl vor unter Umständen lang dauernden, subjektiv unangenehmen Prozeduren verschont; auch scheint es zu einer Herabsetzung der Komplikationsrate zu kommen; zumindest können eingetretene Komplikationen wesentlich besser beherrscht werden. Verhindert werden Schmerzreaktionen des Patienten, Komplikationen, die direkt oder indirekt von der vegetativen oder emotionellen Situation des Untersuchten abhängen, überschießende Vasoreaktionen usw. Durch die Arbeit am relaxierten Patienten wird manches einfacher und weniger traumatisch, begonnen schon bei der Arterienpunktion. Zur Beherrschung eingetretener Komplikationen besteht in der Intubationsnarkose die ideale Ausgangsposition, wenn es sich um schwere Kreislaufreaktionen, Atemstörungen, anaphyllaktische Reaktionen, also um Vorgänge handelt, die während der Narkose bemerkt werden können. Gegner der grundsätzlichen Narkoseanwendung weisen in neuesten Arbeiten darauf hin, daß sie bei Untersuchungen ohne Narkose teilweise bessere angiographische Ergebnisse erzielen und die Kreislaufbedingungen am wachen Patienten physiologischer studiert werden können (Ruggiero et al., 1973; Taveras u. Wood, 1976; grundsätzlich für Sedierung). Auch bei Untersuchungen in Notfällen, die früher sehr gerne ohne Narkose durchgeführt wurden, muß überlegt werden, ob nicht die Sicherheit des Verfahrens in Narkose, gerade bei bewußtseinsgetrübten, unruhigen oder komplikationsbedrohten Patienten (Aneurysma-Blutung), die evtl. Zeitersparnis aufwiegt, zumal viele dieser Patienten ohnehin erst grundversorgt werden müssen (Schock, Blutung, Atemwege, Multitraumatisierung) und die modernen Narkoseverfahren in derartigen Problemfällen nur ein geringes Risiko bedeuten (Tönnis u. Schiefer, 1959; Kazner et al., 1969; Schiefer, 1972; Walter et al., 1974).

Bei Vornahme einer Lokalanästhesie muß diese ausgiebig erfolgen; dennoch kann ein unangenehmes Druckgefühl im Augenblick der Gefäßpunktion nicht ganz vermieden werden. Darauf muß der Patient vorbereitet sein, damit es nicht zu einer Schreckreaktion mit Anspannung der Muskulatur im Punktionsbereich kommt.

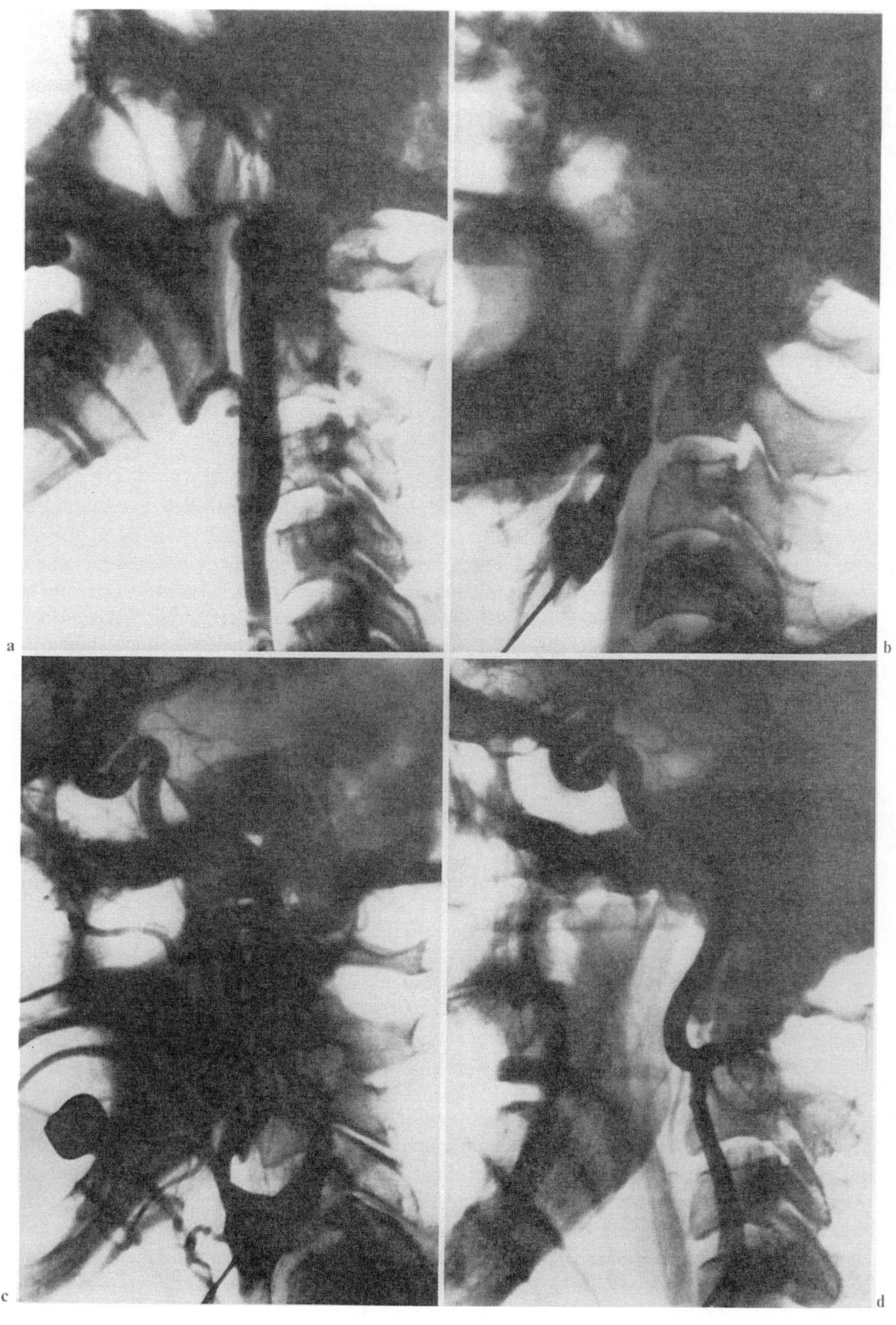

Abb. 1 a–d. Karotispunktion. Ideale tiefe Punktion der A. carotis communis (**a**), die Punktion im Bereich der Teilungsstelle ist nicht anzustreben (**b**, **c**). Punktion der A. carotis interna (**d**) mit leichtem Spasmus der Anfangsstrecke des Gefäßes

Die Lagerung erfolgt auf dem Rücken, Hebe- und Kippvorrichtungen (LYSHOLM-Tisch) ermöglichen passive Lageänderungen. Zur Karotispunktion ist eine Retroflexion des Halses erforderlich, die nach erfolgter Punktion wieder rückgängig gemacht werden muß, ohne daß abrupte Bewegungen des Patienten den Sitz der Kanülenspitze verändern. Dies erfolgt ebenfalls durch den Mechanismus des Tisches oder z.B. durch aufblasbare keilförmige Kissen unter den Schultern. Nackenrollen, die nach der Punktion herausgezogen werden müssen, stellen einen unvollkommenen Notbehelf dar.

Die Punktion und die Angiographie haben unter sterilen Kautelen zu erfolgen, Kathetermethoden setzen weitgehend die Beachtung der Asepsis wie im Operationssaal voraus. Eine gute Lagerung und Fixierung des Kopfes gelingt mit einem Formkeil aus Polyvinylschaum sowie mit einem Pflasterzug oder einer elastischen Binde. Das Halten des Kopfes durch eine dritte Person verbietet sich bei Berücksichtigung der Strahlenbelastbarkeit beruflich strahlenexponierter Personen und ist in allen Fällen entbehrlich. Zum reibungslosen und komplikationsfreien Ablauf der Untersuchung gehört, außer den entsprechenden räumlichen und technischen Voraussetzungen, eine gut eingespielte Arbeitsgruppe, die im Idealfall ohne Anweisungen jeden Handgriff beherrscht (BRENNER u. ZAUNBAUER, 1966).

IV. Die direkte Karotisangiographie

Die perkutane Punktion und Injektion der Arteria carotis communis am Hals ist ein einfaches, technisch wenig aufwendiges, schnell durchzuführendes Verfahren und wurde schon in den ersten Versuchen von MONIZ angestrebt, dann jedoch zugunsten der Freilegung wieder verlassen (zitiert nach SCHECHTER u. GUTIERREZ-MAHONAY, 1973). Eine Zeittafel der Entwicklung der Karotisangiographie gibt die Tabelle 2.

Tabelle 2. Direkte Karotis- und Vertebralisangiographie

Jahr	Autor	Methode
1927	MONIZ	Offene Punktion der Arteria carotis communis
1935	OLIVECRONA	Offene Punktion der Arteria vertebralis
1936	LOMAN und MYERSON	Perkutane Punktion der Arteria carotis communis
1937	BERCZELLER und KUGLER	Offene Punktion der Arteria vertebralis in Höhe des Atlasquerfortsatzes
1938	SJØQUIST	Offene Vertebralispunktion in Höhe der Eintrittsstelle in das Foramen des Proc. transv. des 6. HWK
1939	SCHALTENBRAND und WOLFF	Perkutane Karotisangiographie
1939	TURNBULL	Perkutane Karotisangiographie
1940	TAKAHASHI	Perkutane Vertebralisangiographie (im freien Anteil der Arterie vom Abgang bis zum Eintritt in die Foramina)
1942 1944 1945	KING ENGESET LOWMAN und DOFF	Direkte offene Vertebralispunktion Technik SJØQUIST
1946 1949 1950	FRØVIG SUGAR et al. LINDGREN	Perkutane Punktion der Arteria vertebralis im Verlauf zwischen den Foramina der HWK
1950	LINDGREN	Perkutane Vertebralispunktion in Höhe des Atlasquerfortsatzes

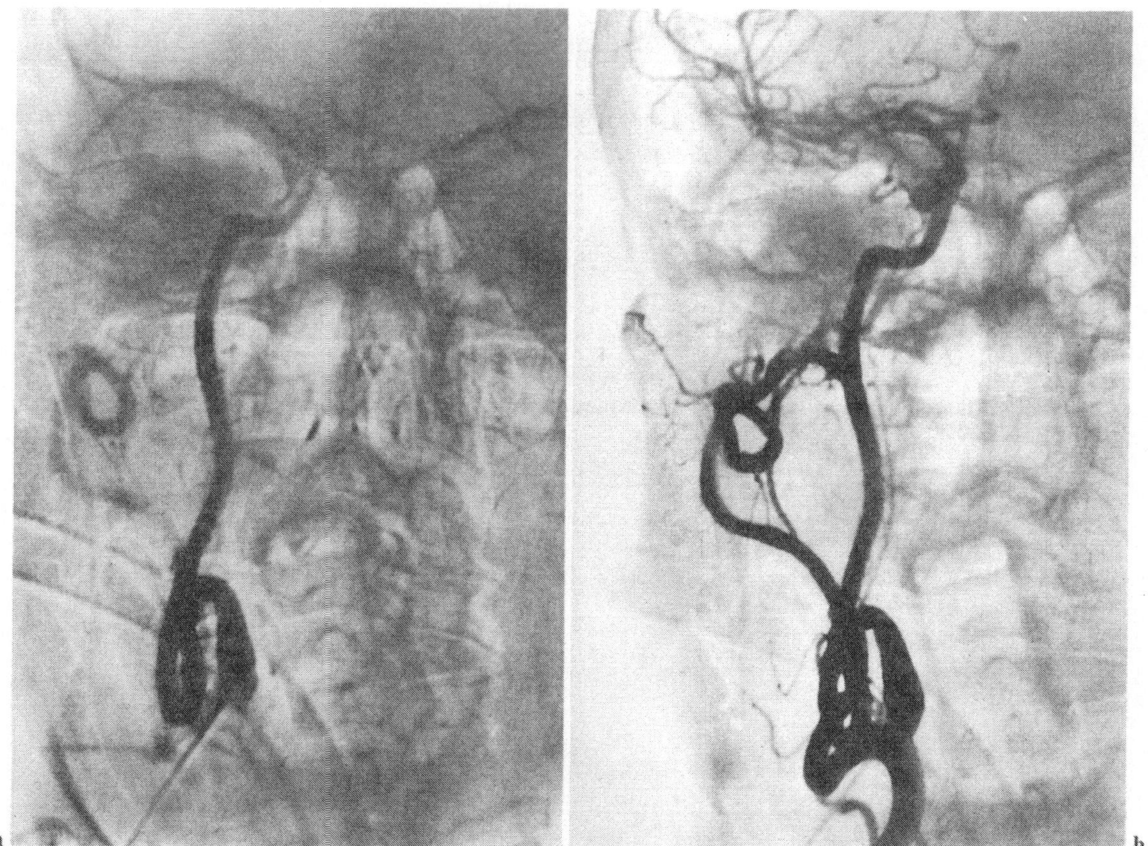

Abb. 2a u. b. Punktion der A. carotis interna bei tiefer Lage der Teilungsstelle und Schlingenbildung der A. carotis interna im proximalen Halsabschnitt

Medial des Musculus sternocleidomastoideus kann auf einer längeren Strecke die Pulsation der Arteria carotis, aber auch das Gefäß selbst und die Teilungsstelle getastet werden. Bei Retroflexionsstellung des Halses tritt das Gefäß in den Weichteilen noch mehr nach ventral, bei Überstrekkung beeinträchtigen die gestrafften Halsweichteile den Tastbefund wieder. Die Punktion ist im Bereich der Arteria carotis communis möglichst tief anzustreben und gelingt fast bei allen Patienten 3–4 cm proximal der Kommunisgabel. Der Einstich sollte nicht höher als etwa in Höhe des Schildknorpelunterrandes erfolgen. Bei sehr kräftigem Hals kann die Punktion erschwert sein, ebenso bei Tumoren am Hals, großen Hämatomen, Strumen, Verhärtungen nach Bestrahlung oder anderen Narben. In einem solchen Fall sollte in erster Linie daran gedacht werden, ein anderes Verfahren anzuwenden. Ist dies nicht möglich, wird hier nach Abdrängen des Hindernisses nach lateral, seltener nach medial, gelegentlich von lateral des Musculus sternocleidomastoideus noch eine Punktion möglich sein. Auf keinen Fall dürfen dabei aber unbekannte Risiken, wie Punktion durch nicht abgeklärte Tumoren, Tumorzellverschleppung, Punktion durch großzystische oder pulsierende Strumen, eingegangen werden. Die Punktion der Karotisgabel soll vermieden werden (TÖNNIS u. SCHIEFER, 1959; OLDENDORF, 1964). Es besteht die Gefahr der Reizung des Glomus caroticum und bei älteren Patienten der Ablösung thrombotischen Materials von arteriosklerotischen Plaques, da die Arteria carotis communis und Arteria carotis interna im Bereich der Teilungsstelle besonders häufig stenosierende Veränderungen tragen. OLDENDORF (1964) empfiehlt in diesen Fällen eher die Interna-Punktion, womit aber die korrekte Darstellung eben dieser stenosierenden Veränderungen nicht möglich ist. Die Interna-Punktion ist 1–3 cm oberhalb der

Karotisgabel möglich: Bei etwas mehr lateralwärts gerichteter Kanülenspitze wird die Arteria carotis interna, bei mehr medialwärts gerichteter Punktion die Arteria carotis externa erreicht. Die Einstichrichtung ist steiler, die Kanüle ist weniger gut im Gefäß zu fixieren. Vor der angiographischen Serie kann eine Testinjektion mit physiologischer Kochsalzlösung oder einem Farbstoff gemacht werden. Eine Verfärbung im Bereich der Glabella oder des Mundwinkels zeigen an, ob die Injektion in die A. carotis interna oder externa erfolgte. Besser ist die Gabe von etwas Kontrastmittel mit gleichzeitiger auf den Hals eingestellter Einzelaufnahme. Die Punktion im Bereich der Karotisgabel und das Vorschieben der Kanüle in die Arteria carotis interna oder externa werden bei älteren Patienten allgemein abgelehnt. Das Vorschieben in die Arteria carotis externa ist nach KRAYENBÜHL und YASARGIL (1965) in $^{2}/_{3}$ der Fälle technisch möglich, wenn der Kopf zur Gegenseite gedreht wird. Die hohe Internapunktion unmittelbar vor dem Eintritt des Gefäßes in die Schädelbasis (ECKER u. CHAMBERLAIN, 1947) wurde auf der Suche nach neuen sicheren Verfahren beschrieben, ebenso die Erleichterung der Punktion mit einer Hilfskanüle (GHERSI u. COSTALES, 1951), um ein Ausweichen der Arterie zu verhindern. Beide Techniken werden normalerweise nicht benötigt.

AARON et al. (1970) berichten über fünf verschiedene Methoden zur direkten Karotis externa-Punktion: „Methode de la Pitié", nach WICKBOM, 1948; LINDGREN, 1954; RUGGIERO, 1957; SALAMON, 1966 sowie die Katheterisierung der A. carotis externa aus der A. carotis communis (LIVERUD, 1958).

Zur Punktion werden kurzangeschliffene Kanülen von 0,8–1,6 mm Durchmesser verwandt. Es kann mit offener Kanüle punktiert werden oder mit eingeschliffenem (nicht überstehendem) spitzem Mandrin oder mit Trokar und spitzem Mandrin. Die Wahl der Kanüle bestimmt die Art des Vorgehens. Nur bei Punktion mit offener Kanüle kann in etwa einem Drittel der Fälle das sofortige pulsierende Ausströmen des Blutes während der Punktion (also ohne Verletzung der Gefäßhinterwand) beobachtet werden. In den verbleibenden Fällen und bei Punktion mit Trokar wird die Kanüle nach der Punktion durch vorsichtiges Zurückziehen in das Gefäßlumen gebracht und zeigt dann erst die kräftige arterielle Pulsation. Durch leichtes Vorschieben in das Gefäßlumen kann der Sitz der Kanüle etwas gesichert werden. Ein Vorschub von 5 mm reicht aus. Tritt beim Vorschieben ein Hindernis auf, muß sofort zurückgezogen werden, bis wieder kräftige Pulsationen zu sehen sind. Die Injektion hat dann zur Vermeidung von Intimaverletzungen besonders schonend zu erfolgen.

Wir verwenden Kanülen mit „Luer-Lok"-Ansatz zur festen Verbindung mit dem transparenten Ansatzschlauch und der Injektionsspritze. Das Material des Schlauches ist so fest, daß eine sichtbare Windkesselfunktion nicht mehr auftritt, aber noch so biegsam, daß bei Bewegungen am Spritzenende keine erheblichen Torsions- und Kippbewegungen an der Kanüle mehr auftreten. Dazu muß der Schlauch ausreichend lang sein. Während der Injektion liegt er in einem Bogen, so daß die Injektionsspritze etwa in einem Winkel von 90 Grad zur liegenden Kanüle gehalten wird, um einem Verschieben der Kanüle durch den Injektionsdruck vorzubeugen. Die Injektion sollte in etwa 2 s beendet sein, um stärkere Überlagerungen der Kreislaufphasen in den angiographischen Bildern zu vermeiden. Bei der Angiographie zur Kreislaufzeitbestimmung wird etwa ein Drittel des Kontrastmittels (3 ml) in wesentlich kürzerer Zeit in die Carotis interna injiziert (HUBER, 1972). Übermäßig schnelle Injektion großer Kontrastmittelmengen führt nicht zu kontrastreicheren Bildern. Durch die beanspruchte Windkesselfunktion der Gefäße und Abstrom von Kontrastmittel nach proximal können die Bilder sogar besonders flau sein; außerdem erhöht sich das Risiko eines Gefäßspasmus, und es kommt öfter zur Verlagerung der Kanüle während der Injektion (Gefahr der intra- oder paravasalen Injektion). Durch die Verwendung des transparenten Ansatzschlauches zwischen Injektionsspritze und Punktionskanüle werden paravasale Injektionen aber auch Mikroembolien, z.B. an den Netzhautgefäßen, am ehesten vermieden, die bei direktem Ansetzen der Spritze an die Punktionskanüle nach DECKER (1969) häufiger waren. Dabei ist die Strahlenexposition der Hände besonders hoch (s.o.).

V. Die direkte Vertebralisangiographie

Nach einer Periode fast ausschließlich operativer Angiographieverfahren wurden auch für die Vertebralisangiographie zwei perkutane Punktionsverfahren angegeben, die der Methode die weite Verbreitung sicherten (Tabelle 2). Die Punktion nach TAKAHASHI (1940) erfolgt im freien Anteil der Arteria vertebralis, unterhalb des Eintritts in das Foramen vertebrale des Querfortsatzes des sechsten Halswirbelkörpers. Die Methode ist weitgehend risikolos, aber technisch sehr schwierig. Selbst dem geübten Untersucher ist sie nur bei optimalen Verhältnissen, also bei langem schlankem Hals und kräftiger Vertebralarterie, möglich. Erst SUGAR (1949) und LINDGREN (1950) bzw. SJØGREN (1953) führten eine Methode ein, die – ähnlich wie die Karotispunktion – bei fast allen Patienten erfolgreich angewandt werden kann. Die Punktion ist schwieriger als die Punktion der Arteria carotis communis und setzt besondere Übung, Vorsicht und ein optimal eingespieltes Team voraus, führt dann allerdings zu sehr guten Ergebnissen (RUGGIERO et al., 1973). Nach Lagerung und Fixation des Kopfes, wie sie zur späteren Aufnahmeserie erforderlich sind, wird entweder lateral oder medial der Arteria carotis communis punktiert. Die mediale Punktion (SJØGREN, 1953) mit ihrem stark von medial nach lateral gerichteten Vorgehen soll die Gefahr der Verletzung des Duralsackes oder von Nervenwurzeln vermindern. Die Punktion soll in Richtung auf eine Lücke zwischen zwei Querfortsätzen vorsichtig, aber in einem Zug durchgeführt werden. Bei Knochenkontakt im Bereich eines Foramen intervertebrale kann vorsichtig zurückgezogen werden, um zu prüfen, ob die Punktion gelungen ist. Ist dies nicht der Fall, muß die Kanüle zurückgezogen und noch einmal punktiert werden. Mehrfache Korrektur der Nadelspitze durch tastendes Vorschieben der Nadel soll unbedingt vermieden werden, da dadurch die Zahl der Einstiche im Bereich des Gefäßes unkontrolliert vermehrt wird und die Verletzungsgefahr zunimmt. Bei Austritt von Liquor aus der Kanüle ist die Punktion in dieser Höhe, evtl.

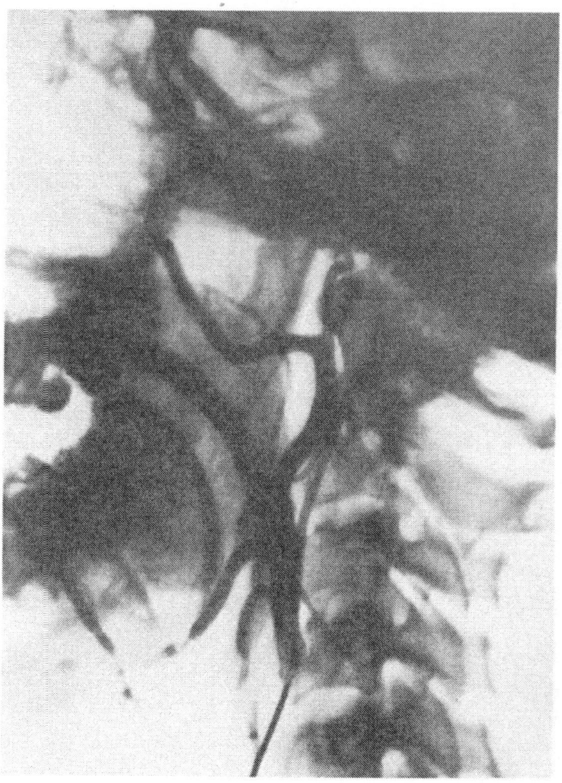

Abb. 3. Direkte Punktion der A. carotis externa, unmittelbar distal der Gabel der A. carotis communis

auf dieser Seite abzubrechen. Nach mehreren vergeblichen Versuchen soll ein anderer erfahrener Untersucher die Angiographie übernehmen. Die Punktion mit offener Kanüle wird von den meisten Untersuchern vorgezogen. Auch hier wird allgemein, jedoch nicht ausschließlich, die Narkoseuntersuchung bevorzugt. Verwendet werden Kanülen von 0,8–1,2 mm Durchmesser, die etwa 1–2 cm länger sind als für die Karotispunktion des jeweiligen Patienten erforderlich wäre. Bei geglückter Punktion kann man eine kräftige arterielle Pulsation des austretenden Blutes beobachten, und unter Umständen ist ein vorsichtiges Vorschieben der Kanüle um einige mm möglich, ohne daß die Pulsation nachläßt. Durch mehrfache Injektion von physiologischer Kochsalzlösung und anschließender Beobachtung des Blutrückstromes kann versucht werden, welche Injektionsgeschwindigkeit noch keinen Gefäßspasmus auslöst. Einzelaufnahmen mit wenig Kontrastmittel können über den Sitz der Kanüle Aufschluß geben.

Die erfolgreiche Injektion, ohne Extravasat oder Auslösung eines Gefäßspasmus, ist die eigentliche Schwierigkeit. Sie erfordert Erfahrung und Fingerspitzengefühl. Bei plötzlicher Erhöhung des Injektionswiderstandes ist ein Abbruch der Injektion erforderlich. Die Injektionsdauer ist etwas länger als bei der Karotisangiographie, die benötigte Kontrastmittelmenge kleiner (4–6 ml). Aufgrund der geschilderten Besonderheiten kommen automatische Injektoren nicht in Frage. Bei der großen Variationsbreite des Kalibers der Vertebralarterien gelingt gelegentlich die Punktion auf einer Seite nicht. Es muß dann die andere Seite untersucht werden. Da die linke Vertebralarterie, statistisch gesehen, meist kräftiger ist, empfiehlt sich der Beginn mit der linken Seite, wenn nicht ohnehin eine doppelseitige Untersuchung vorgesehen ist. Die von mehreren Autoren beschriebene Vertebralispunktion in Höhe des Atlasbogens (LINDGREN, 1956; MASLOWSKI, 1955; NAMIN, 1955) soll einen besseren Sitz der Kanüle gewährleisten. Die Methode hat sich jedoch nicht durchgesetzt, zumal die oft wesentliche Darstellung der Arteria vertebralis im Halsbereich damit nicht möglich ist.

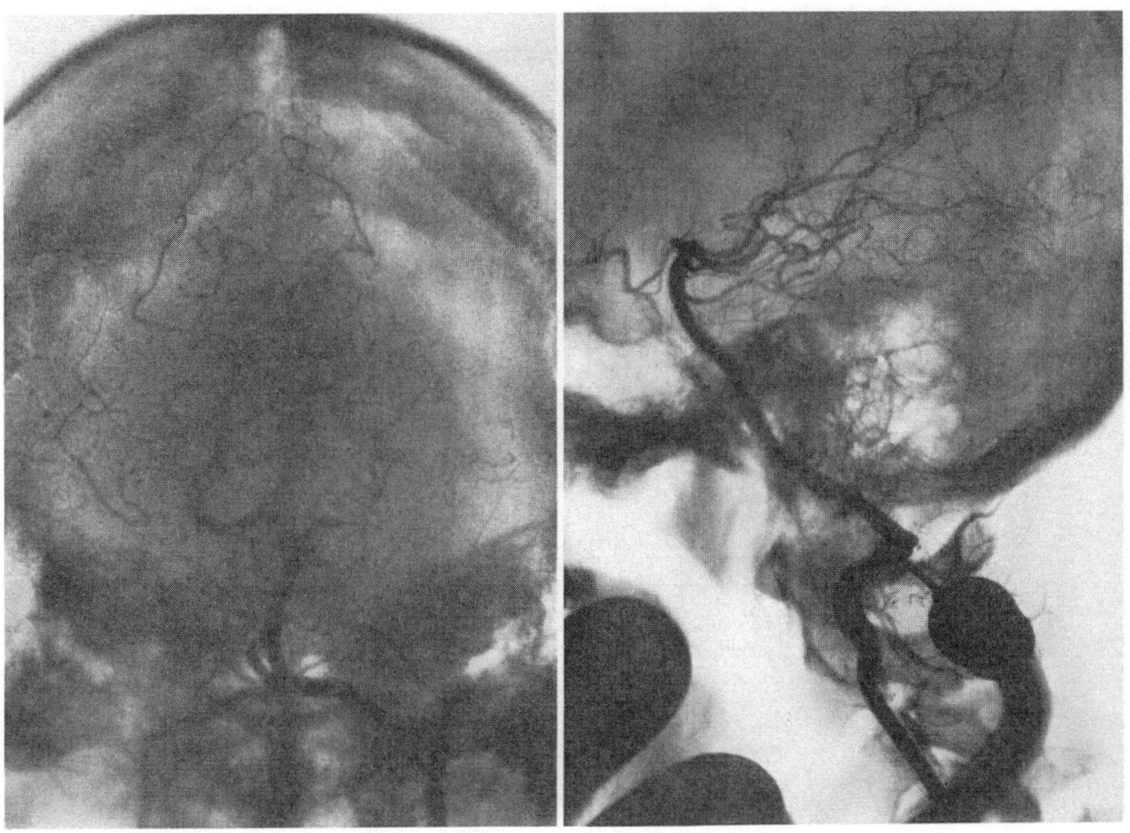

Abb. 4. Vertebralispunktion nach MASLOWSKI in Höhe des Sulcus vertebralis atlantis

Mit der oben beschriebenen Technik sind Aufnahmen in Spezialprojektion (nach TOWNE) durchaus möglich, wenn die Röhre im a–p Strahlengang entsprechend gekippt werden kann. Die Lagerung des Patienten oberhalb des Kassettenrandes zu dieser Projektion hat allerdings vor der Punktion zu erfolgen, da jegliche Umlagerung nach der Punktion zu vermeiden ist.

Gerade die Schwierigkeit des Verfahrens und seine besonderen Risiken hinsichtlich der Komplikationsrate (s.u.) haben der Entwicklung der indirekten Verfahren zur Darstellung des vertebrobasilären Gefäßsystems besonderen Auftrieb gegeben.

VI. Retrograde Punktionen und Gegenstromangiographie

Die Gegenstromangiographien entwickelten sich in Analogie zu den direkten Aortographieverfahren und von den ursprünglichen Versuchen her, die Arteria subclavia zur Darstellung des vertebrobasilären Kreislaufes zu punktieren (Tabelle 3). Ursprünglich wurde die Arteria subclavia operativ in unmittelbarer Nähe des Abganges der Arteria vertebralis aufgesucht, später wurde auch ein perkutanes Punktionsverfahren angegeben (SHIMIDZU, 1937). Zur Gegenstromangiographie ohne Verwendung von Kathetern eignen sich im Bereich der Neuroradiologie die Arteria cubitalis, die Arteria brachialis im Verlauf des Oberarms, die Arteria axillaris und die Arteria subclavia sowie die rechte Arteria carotis communis. Bei der direkten Punktion der Arteria subclavia in ihrer infraklavikulären Verlaufsstrecke kann die Injektion auch bei Erwachsenen noch manuell bewältigt werden. Die Bestrebungen, Pleurakomplikationen (Pneumothorax, Hämatothorax) zu vermeiden, führten konsequenterweise zur Punktion der Arteria brachialis. Bereits MONIZ diskutierte die Möglichkeit, ob die Füllung der hinteren Hirnarterien und des oberen Anteils der Arteria basilaris in einem seiner frühesten Angiogramme durch Abfluß von Kontrastmittel gegen den Strom der Arteria carotis communis und anterograde Füllung der rechten Vertebralarterie zustande gekommen war (zitiert nach SCHECHTER, 1972). Die Methode der retrograden perkutanen Karotispunktion rechts zur Darstellung der rechten Arteria vertebralis wurde von ELVIDGE (1938), ENGESET (1948) und ECKER (1951) beschrieben. Die A. carotis communis wurde distal der Freilegungs- und Punktionsstelle zur Injektion manuell komprimiert. ECKER

Tabelle 3. Retrograde Punktion und Gegenstromangiographie

1933	MONIZ	Offene Punktion der Arteria subclavia nahe der Abgangsstelle der Arteria vertebralis zur Vertebralisangiographie
1937	SHIMIDZU	Perkutane Subklaviapunktion zur Vertebralisdarstellung
1937	ELVIDGE	Offene retrograde Karotisinjektion rechts zur Darstellung der rechten Arteria vertebralis
1941 1945 1948	KRAYENBÜHL LIST POPPEN	Offene Subklaviapunktion Technik MONIZ
1948 1951	ENGESET ECKER	Perkutane retrograde Karotispunktion rechts zur Darstellung der rechten Arteria vertebralis
1955 1960	GOULD et al. KUHN	Offene retrograde Brachialisangiographie bei Kindern mit manueller Injektion und bei Erwachsenen mit manueller Injektion
1962 1963 1964 1965	SIGUEIRA et al. MARSHALL et al. WAPPENSCHMIDT WENDE und TAENZER	Perkutane retrograde Brachialisangiographie mit maschineller Injektion

(1951) injizierte in üblicher Richtung in die Arteria carotis communis; der Gegenstrom wurde ebenfalls durch Kompression der Arteria carotis communis distal der Punktionsstelle erzeugt.

Heute wird die Arteria brachialis meist im Bereich der Ellenbeuge aufgesucht, da hier die Punktion besonders einfach ist. Gelegentlich muß bei lokalen anatomischen Schwierigkeiten oder Fehlversuchen mit Hämatombildung die Verlaufsstrecke der Arteria brachialis am Oberarm gewählt werden. Punktiert wird mit Trokar und spitzem Mandrin durch die rückwärtige Gefäßwand, so daß erst beim Zurückziehen des offenen Trokars der arterielle, pulsierende Blutstrom sichtbar wird. Das Vorschieben der Kanüle gelingt meist einige cm weit. Auch hier darf dies nur ganz ohne Widerstand erfolgen, um Intimaverletzungen zu vermeiden. Nach einer vergeblichen Punktion mit Nachblutung sollte erst längere Zeit komprimiert werden, um ein größeres Hämatom zu vermeiden. Im Bereich der Arteria brachialis am Oberarm ist die Punktion etwas schwieriger, da das Gefäß schlechter gegen die Unterlage fixiert werden kann. Das Vorschieben des Trokars ist weniger weit möglich. Bei der Punktion ist besonders auf die Nervenverläufe zu achten. Bei geeigneter Lagerung des Arms (rechtwinklige Abduktion) ist die Punktion der Arteria axillaris meist gut möglich. Dieser Zugang wird für Katheterverfahren benutzt (Weibel u. Fields, 1969), jedoch ist bei gutem Kanülensitz auch eine Gegenstromangiographie möglich.

Die retrograde Brachialisangiographie gelingt bei den meisten Kindern. Die Methode läßt sich sicher ab dem 6. Lebensjahr einsetzen (Backmund, 1966, 1967). Nicht selten führt man sie schon bei Säuglingen erfolgreich durch. Bei sehr kleinen Kindern (bis zu 1–2 Jahren) wird unter Umständen eine manuelle Kontrastmittelinjektion vorgezogen. Sonst sind für die Gegenstromangiographie aus der Arteria cubitalis und der Arteria brachialis Überdruckinjektoren erforderlich, die das Kontrastmittel gegen den Blutstrom, über die Abgangsstelle der Arteria vertebralis hinaus oder bis in die Arteria anonyma (Truncus brachiocephalicus) gelangen lassen. In der darauffolgenden Diastole wird das Kontrastmittel, entsprechend dem physiologischen Blutstrom, in die großen Halsgefäße transportiert. Gelangt das Kontrastmittel bis zum Aortenbogen, kann es von rechts zur Darstellung beider Karotiden, seltener beider Vertebralarterien kommen; von links ist meist eine Mitdarstellung der linken Arteria carotis oder der Gefäße der Gegenseite nicht zu erwarten. Bei richtiger Technik kommt es nicht zu einer Überdruckinjektion in die Vertebral-Arterien oder in die rechte Arteria carotis communis, außer bei einem Verschluß oder bei einer hochgradigen Stenose der Arteria subclavia (subclavian steal-Syndrom), proximal des Abgangs der Arteria vertebralis. Die Injektoren sind seit Ende der 40er Jahre verbessert und die Bedienung vereinfacht worden. Bei den älteren druckgesteuerten Systemen wird eine Injektionsspritze in einen Injektorwagen gespannt, der beim Auslösen durch einströmende Druckluft vorgeschoben wird und so die Spritze entleert. Die Injektionsgeschwindigkeit wird durch den an einem Manometer einstellbaren Ausgangsdruck nach Erfahrungswerten gesteuert. Unabdingbare Sicherheitsvoraussetzung bei diesen Systemen ist, daß die Druckluft nicht direkt auf den Stempel der Injektionsspritze einwirken darf, damit bei Undichtigkeiten im System Luftembolien prinzipiell ausgeschlossen sind. Die neueren, volumengesteuerten Systeme bestehen meist aus einer großen Injektionsspritze als Kontrastmittelreservoir. Bei jeder Injektion kann die injizierte Kontrastmittelmenge, die Injektionsdauer oder die injizierte Kontrastmittelmenge pro Zeiteinheit („flow") und die Gesamtmenge direkt am Gerät eingestellt werden. Bei Erreichen eines festgelegten maximalen Injektionsdruckes schaltet das Gerät im Sinn einer automatischen Sicherung ab. Der Vorschub der Spritze erfolgt elektromotorisch über eine Schnecke. Auch bei diesem System werden sich sehr kurze Injektionszeiten (z.B. bei Tachykardie) wegen der Überdrucksicherung zur Ausnutzung nur einer Diastole zur Injektion nicht steuern lassen. Die bei der Injektion auftretenden Geschwindigkeiten des Kontrastmittels am Kanülenende sind in vergleichbaren Fällen bei beiden Systemen sicherlich dieselben. Eindeutige Prinzipvorteile bietet das neuere System, außer der sicheren und leichten Bedienung, vorwiegend bei der automatischen Karotisinjektion zur angiographischen Durchblutungsmessung, bei der durch einen über EKG herzphasengesteuerten Schwellenschalter sehr exakte Ergebnisse möglich sind. Häufiger Prinzipnachteil ist die Verwendung eines undurchsichtigen Spritzenzylinders (Metall), da die Sichtkontrolle des Kontrastmittels (Luftblasen) genommen ist. Die Kontrastmittelmenge pro Injektion der Gegenstromangiographien schwankt zwischen 25 und 50 ml. Nach den Füllungsbildern, die dabei erhalten werden, ist die Kontrastdichte der zerebralen Gefäße nicht größer als bei der direkten Injektion, da ein großer Anteil des Kontrastmittels andere Wege nimmt. TAVERAS und WOOD (1976) empfehlen zur retrograden Brachialisangiographie eine Injektions-Bolusmenge von 75 ml, wobei unter gewissen Umständen ein Teil des Injektionsgutes überschichtete physiol. Kochsalzlösung sein kann. Bei der rechtsseitigen Brachialisangiographie kommt in über 80% der Fälle über die Arteria anonyma (Truncus brachiocephalicus) die rechte Arteria carotis und das intrazerebrale Karotissystem mit zur Darstellung, in einem kleinen Prozentsatz die linke Arteria carotis, wenn der Abgang des Gefäßes in der Nähe des Abgangs der Arteria anonyma liegt oder die linke Arteria carotis communis mit von der (rechten) Arteria anonyma abgeht. Bei der gleichzeitigen Injektion in beide Brachialarterien mit zwei synchron geschalteten Injektoren oder einem Y-förmigen Schlauchverteilungsstück gelingt, außer einer sehr guten Darstellung der Verhältnisse der supraaortalen Gefäßabgänge, eine meist sehr kontrastkräftige Darstellung des vertebrobasilären Gefäßsystems, einschließlich einer guten Venenfüllung im Bereich der hinteren Schädelgrube. Es kann dabei auch häufiger die Darstellung des Abganges und des Anfangsstückes der Arteria spinalis anterior erwartet werden. Der Durchfluß durch den basalen Gefäßkranz kann durch eine manuelle Kompression der Arteria carotis communis am Hals der gleichen oder der Gegenseite gesteigert werden. Die Methode wird heute von den meisten Untersuchern in Intubationsnarkose durchgeführt. Ausnahmen werden nur bei primär bewußtseinsgestörten Patienten gemacht. Bei guter Einarbeitung gelingt es mit der Methode rasch, umfassend und ohne wesentliches Untersuchungsrisiko, die zerebralen Gefäße und vorgeschalteten großen supraaortalen Äste bis zum Abgang ausreichend darzustellen. Lediglich eine direkte linksseitige Karotisangiographie ist im gegebenen Fall zusätzlich erforderlich.

VII. Katheter-Angiographie

Als Vorläufer der Katheterangiographiemethoden kann die Aortographie angesehen werden, da von der direkten Aortographie, nach Punktion der Aorta im lumbalen Bereich, über die Katheteraorthographie von der Arteria femoralis, auch die Methoden der zerebralen Angiographie mit Kathetertechnik ableitbar sind (Tabelle 5 u. 6). Einen anderen Weg beschritt RADNER, der

Tabelle 4. Anhang Kathetertechnik

Gummikatheter	in der Pionierzeit der Katheterisierung von Venen: BLEICHRÖDER, 1912; FORSSMANN, 1929; KLEIN, 1930 und Arterien: FORSSMANN, 1931; ICHIKAWA, 1938; FARINAS, 1941; CHAVEZ, 1947
PVC-Katheter	(COURNARD-Katheter) COURNARD und RANGE (1941) (technisch) begrenzte Länge
PE-Katheter	seit 1948 Führungsdraht zur Röntgenkontrolle SELDINGER (1953) andere Möglichkeiten: Metallspitze, Kontrastfüllung
	Strahlendichte Katheter durch Einarbeitung von Schwermetallsalzen in die PE-Wand (z.B. Bleioxyd) ODMAN (1956)
	Vorgeformte Katheterspitzen in verschiedenen Formen gezielt bewegliche Katheterspitzen z.T. zur selektiven Angiographie ohne Führungsdraht
	Spezialkatheter zur intraarteriellen Therapie

Tabelle 5. Aortographie – Vorläufer der Kathetermethoden

1.	1929	Dos Santos	Punktion der Aorta abdominalis Weiterentwicklung zur „translumbalen Aortographie"
2.	1939	Robb und Steinberg	„intravenöse Aortographie"
3.	1948	Menesses Hoyes, Gomez Del Campo	Modifikation zur Darstellung der Aorta thoracalis. Verfahren wegen zu großer Komplikationsrisiken praktisch nicht angewandt
4.	1952	Wickbom	Direkte Punktion der Aorta ascendens, wegen Komplikationen bald verlassen
5.	1954	Smith	Aortographie durch perkutane Punktion des linken Ventrikels

Tabelle 6. Entwicklung der Kathetermethoden

1.	1941	Farinas	Femoralispunktion mit einem Trokar und Einführung eines Urethralkatheters (gab die Methode später wieder auf zugunsten direkter Kontrastmittelinjektion in den in der Arteria femoralis liegenden Trokar).
2.	1948	Radner	empfahl Einführung eines Katheters über eine Inzision über der rechten Arteria radialis (Arteria radialis mußte anschließend unterbunden werden. Gelegentlich gelang das Vorschieben wegen Gefäßspasmen oder anatomischer Besonderheiten nicht. Großkalibriger Katheter).
3.	1949	Jönsson	empfahl die retrograde Punktion der A. carotis communis (nach Freilegung) und Vorschieben des Trocars in den Aortenbogen. Wegen des Risikos der Aortenwandverletzung aufgegeben.
4.	1951	Pierce	perkutaner Femoraliskatheter durch das Lumen einer großkalibrigen Punktionskanüle. Methode damals sofort komplikationsärmer als Gefäßfreilegung. Größtes Risiko: noch zerebrale Komplikationen bei größeren Diotrast-Mengen.
5.	1953	Seldinger	Einführung der „Seldinger-Technik" Punktionsnadel und Katheter von gleichem Kaliber
6.	1956	Crawford	Retrograder Katheter durch die (freigelegte) Carotis communis zum Aortenbogen

Katheter-Methoden (Anhang Einsatzmöglichkeiten)

1. Thorakale Aortographie	durch unilateralen oder bilateralen infraklavikulären Subklavia-Katheter Brachialis- oder Axillaris-Katheter retrograden Katheter durch die Arteria carotis communis transfemoral
2. Darstellung des Truncus brachiocephalicus rechts	infraklavikulärer Subklavia-Katheter rechts Brachialis- oder Axillaris-Katheter rechts transfemoral
3. Darstellung des Abgangs der linken Arteria carotis	retrograder Katheder durch die linke Arteria carotis communis transfemoral
4. Selektive Darstellung der Karotiden oder Vertebral-Arterien	transfemoral; Brachialis- oder Axillaris-Katheter infraklavikulärer Subklavia-Katheter
5. Superselektive Methoden therapeutische Verfahren	transfemoral infraklavikulär

1947 bei Versuchen, die Koronararterien darzustellen, die Arteria radialis im distalen Drittel des Unterarms freilegte, einen Ureteren-Katheder vorschob und unter Schirmbildkontrolle die Tendenz des Katheters bemerkte, in die Vertebralarterie zu gleiten. Er beschrieb diese Methode zur Vertebralisangiographie. Das Verfahren wurde auch von HELMSWORTH et al. (1950) und anderen Autoren beschrieben. Die Fortschritte der Methodik waren anfangs eng an die Entwicklung in der Herstellung geeigneten Kathetermaterials geknüpft (Tabelle 4). Der Durchbruch kam mit der Beschreibung der SELDINGER-Technik 1953 und ihrer Einführung.

Die Katheterverfahren sind in mancher Beziehung aufwendiger. Sie erfordern erhöhten Zeitbedarf, größeren Personaleinsatz, Arbeiten unter aseptischen Bedingungen, wie im Operationssaal, Durchleuchtung mit erhöhter Strahlenbelastung auch für das Untersuchungspersonal, größere Vorsorgen wegen thrombembolischer Komplikationen. Auch bei den Katheterverfahren werden Extravasate, Gefäßwandverletzungen und subintimale Injektionen beobachtet. Bei Verlegung von Gefäßen durch zu große Katheter können ischämische Erscheinungen auftreten. Andererseits ist die Methode weitgehend universell und wird daher an vielen Instituten als Methode der Wahl eingesetzt. Schließlich sind die Verfahren im Bereich der selektiven und superselektiven Angiographien und anschließenden Techniken (z.B. Embolisierung) nicht zu umgehen. Im Idealfall wird von einer Arteria femoralis aus die Darstellung aller supraaortischen Gefäße, einschließlich des Aortenbogens, möglich sein. Bevorzugt wird die linke Arteria femoralis wegen des weniger geschlängelten Verlaufs der linken Arteria iliaca bis zur Aortenbifurkation (LINDGREN, 1956; NEWTON, 1963; HANAFEE, 1963). Die Femoralispunktion erfolgt in typischer Weise distal des Leistenbandes mit einem Trokar und spitzen Mandrin. Nach Zurückziehen des Mandrins wird der Trokar durch Vorschieben fixiert. Innerhalb der Kanüle kann nun ein flexibler, strahlendichter Führungsdraht eingebracht werden. Liegt dieser im Zielgebiet, wird die Kanüle über dem Draht entfernt und durch einen gleichkalibrigen Katheter ersetzt, der seinerseits in das Zielgebiet vorgeschoben werden kann. Nach Zurückziehen des Führungsdrahtes, bei verbleibendem Katheter, kann die Angiographie vorgenommen werden (SELDINGER-Prinzip). Durch die Verwendung verschieden starker Katheter und verschiedener vorgeformter Krümmungen an der Katheterspitze, die ihrerseits durch erneutes Einführen von elastischen Führungsdrähten, Zug, Drehung an Führungsdraht und Katheter in Lage und Form verändert werden können, lassen sich unter Schirmbildkontrolle die Katheterenden in die Abgänge der zu untersuchenden Gefäße einführen und selektive Angiographien der katheterisierten Gefäße vornehmen. Die Selektivität reicht bis zu kleinen Ästen der Arteria carotis externa (Arteria meningea media, Arteria pharyngea ascendens; DJINDJIAN, 1972), neuerdings auch distaler Abschnitte der Arteria carotis interna.

Manchmal gelingt die Angiographie nicht von einer Arteria femoralis aus; dann wird zunächst die Punktion und Katheterisierung der gegenseitigen Femoralarterie versucht. Bei Patienten ab dem 6. Dezennium ist die Katheterisierung von der Arteria femoralis aus in einem etwas größeren Prozentsatz technisch nicht durchführbar. Hierfür werden die dann erheblichen Schlängelungen der Arteria iliaca beider Seiten sowie Stenosen und arteriosklerotische Wandveränderungen verantwortlich gemacht. In diesen Fällen kann die Katheterisierung, entsprechend dem Wege der Gegenstromangiographie, von der Arteria brachialis oder der Arteria subclavia aus durchgeführt werden (ROY, 1965; WEIBEL u. FIELDS, 1969). Hierbei ist auf beiden Seiten eine selektive Darstellung der Vertebralarterie möglich, rechts auch die gemeinsame Darstellung der Arteria anonyma (Truncus brachiocephalicus). Die Darstellung der linken Arteria carotis ist unter Umständen etwas schwieriger. Gelegentlich, aber nur in Ausnahmefällen, kommt die retrograde Katheterisierung der Arteria carotis communis zur Darstellung des Aortenbogens bzw. des Karotisabgangs in Frage (BERK, 1960; VITEK, 1973). Die anterograde Katheterisierung der Arteria carotis zur selektiven Angiographie ist ebenfalls möglich (VITEK, 1973), bedeutet aber für den Untersucher ein größeres Strahlenrisiko und wird im allgemeinen nur bei technischen Schwierigkeiten oder Kontraindikation aller anderen Verfahren vorgenommen. Die Katheterisierung der direkt punktierten Arteria vertebralis (JAEGER, 1952) hat sich nicht eingeführt.

Die Injektion wird vorteilhafterweise ebenfalls mit automatischen Injektoren, gegebenenfalls mit über EKG herzphasengesteuertem Schwellenschalter vorgenommen (s.o.). Zur Kontrolle des Angiographieablaufs und der Vorbeugung von Komplikationen wurden Verfahrensregeln ausgearbeitet, deren Wirksamkeit und Vervollkommnung immer noch Gegenstand von Veröffentlichungen ist. Auch hier wird oft Allgemeinnarkose empfohlen. Für lange Untersuchungsabläufe können schonende, exzitationsfreie Verfahren angewendet werden. Eine kardio-vaskuläre Überwachung mit Monitoren empfiehlt sich. Die typischen Veränderungen während der Angiographie lassen sich gegen drohende Komplikationen abgrenzen. Eine EEG-Ableitung kann evtl. durchgeführt werden. Papaverin oder Lignocain-Injektionen können Spasmen im Arteriolenbereich vermindern. Die Messung der Ausscheidung läßt Schlüsse auf die Nierenfunktion zu. Temperaturmessungen an den Extremitäten können hinzukommen und vieles mehr. Antihistamine Substanzen und neuroleptische Substanzen mit einer Schutzwirkung gegen Katecholaminausschüttung und Hemmung der Formatio reticularis können bei Bedarf gegeben werden, ebenso Steroide, Diuretika oder Dextraninfusionen. Valium, auch intraarteriell appliziert (DOPPMAN et al., 1973), mag den depolarisierenden Effekt der Kontrastmittel an den Membranen der Motoneuronen verhindern. Durch Benetzung der Katheter mit Heparinlösungen (BJØRK, 1972) wird dem Auftreten von Thrombembolien vorgebeugt. Bei jeder bedrohlichen Situation kann die Untersuchung abgebrochen und unverzüglich reanimative Bemühungen eingesetzt werden (DJINDJIAN, 1972; WALLACE et al., 1972; DOUST u. REDMAN, 1972; PADOVANI et al., 1973; WALTER et al., 1974).

Die besten Möglichkeiten werden in einer neuroradiologischen Abteilung dann vorliegen, wenn alle Verfahren, je nach Bedarf und individuellen Gegebenheiten, mit der gleichen Perfektion abgewickelt werden können. Die prinzipielle Betonung eines Verfahrens in einer Abteilung ist meist nicht durch die Unbrauchbarkeit der anderen Methoden bedingt, sondern durch die besonderen diagnostischen Anforderungen in der Zusammenarbeit mit den Klinikern, der Größe des Durchgangs an Untersuchungen im Verhältnis zur Kapazität der Abteilung und ähnlichen, oft organisatorischen Gegebenheiten. Allerdings besteht weiterhin ein Trend zur immer höheren Spezialisierung der Methoden bis zu einem mikroangiographischen Bereich, wobei die reinen „Routineangiographien" durch andere Untersuchungsverfahren (Computer-Tomographie) an Bedeutung etwas zurückgedrängt werden.

C. Klinische Indikationen zur Angiographie

I. Allgemeines

Die Angiographie wird eingesetzt zur Abklärung lokalisierbarer Symptome des Schädels und Schädelinhalts (KRAYENBÜHL u. YASARGIL, 1965). Wenn möglich wird als weniger eingreifende, umfassend informierende Untersuchung die Computer-Tomographie (CT) nicht nur im Sinne einer Vorfelduntersuchung vorangestellt. Einige meist gefäßchirurgische Indikationen, die den asymptomatischen Patienten betreffen (WEIBEL u. FIELDS, 1969), insbesondere bei Annahme extrazerebraler Gefäßprozesse, sollten erst nach Durchführung einer Doppler-Sonographie der großen supraaortischen Äste der Angiographie zugeführt werden. Besondere Indikationen ergeben sich beim Kopfschmerz- bzw. Migränepatienten (RABE, 1971; JANZEN et al., 1972; Tabelle 7 u. 8). Man kann eine Unterscheidung treffen nach Indikationen, die ursprünglich die Darstellung einer tumorbedingten Raumforderung oder eines Tumors selbst bezwecken, und nach Indikationen, bei denen Gefäßveränderungen oder ihre Folgen gesucht werden. Ist die Diagnose klinisch eindeutig, kann die Angiographie nur dann indiziert werden, wenn die morphologische Darstellung

Tabelle 7. Indikationen zur Angiographie

1. Aneurysma
   Form und Lage
   zu- und abführende Gefäße, basale Gefäßspasmen, Kollateralen, Hämatom- und Ödembildung
2. arterio-venöses Aneurysma (Angiom)
   Abklärung der Zuflüsse von allen Seiten, postoperative Kontrolle
3. Gefäßstenosen oder -verschlüsse bei der Möglichkeit eines operativen Eingreifens
   Nachweis von Kollateralkreisläufen
   Circulus arteriosus cerebri, Externa-, Interna-Anastomose, direkte zerebrale End- zu-End-Anastomosen
4. zur Differentialdiagnose:
   Blutung – Thrombose – Embolie (Mikroangiom?)
   Venenthrombose (bzw. Hirndruck) bei maximaler Zirkulationsverzögerung
5. intrakranielle Verletzungen: epidurales, subdurales, intrazerebrales Hämatom
   Hirnödem
   traumatische arterio-venöse Fistel (Carotis interna – Sinus cavernosus)
6. intrakranielle raumfordernde Prozesse
   Lokalisation (supratentoriell, infratentoriell mit verschiedener Treffsicherheit)
   Artdiagnose
   Massenverschiebungen (Hernienbildung, Zysternenverquellung)
7. unilateraler Exophthalmus: retrobulbäre unilaterale Geschwülste u. Gefäßmißbildungen
8. Beurteilung des Operationserfolges und postoperativer Komplikationen

Tabelle 8. Klinische Indikationen zur Angiographie

1. bei dringendem klinischem Verdacht auf Tumor cerebri
2. bei intrakraniellen oder intrazerebralen Hämatomen, soweit eine chirurgische Intervention möglich ist
3. bei Hinweisen für diagnostisch unklare intrakranielle Druckerhöhung
   bei stenosierenden Gefäßerkrankungen
4. bei Patienten mit Verdacht auf Gefäßstenosen, soweit ein operatives Vorgehen vorgesehen ist
5. bei Patienten mit intermittierender Symptomatik
   a) bei Verdacht auf Steal-Syndrom oder unterschiedlichem Puls der oberen Extremitäten
   b) abgeschwächten oder fehlenden Pulsen einer Halsseite
   c) bei systolischem Geräusch hinter dem Kieferwinkel (Karotisgabel) oder der Supraklavikulärgrube (Subclavia), die nicht kardial bedingt sind
   d) durch Lageänderung des Kopfes oder Halses provozierbare Symptome von Karotisinsuffizienz oder vertebro-basilärer Insuffizienz
6. bei Schlaganfall mit zunehmender Symptomatik sofort, wenn Verdacht auf Stenosen oder Verschluß größerer Gefäße besteht und eine intrazerebrale Raumforderung auszuschließen ist
7. sonst bei Schlaganfällen erst bei Besserung der Symtomatik
8. bei kompletter Apoplexie zum Ausschluß einer massiven Hirnschwellung oder zur Indikationsstellung eines evtl. operativen Vorgehens
9. bei asymptomatischen Patienten mit Gefäßgeräuschen am Hals, wenn Eingriffe an anderen Gefäßen vorgesehen sind

des Befundes unumgänglich ist oder wenn sich zusätzliche Gesichtspunkte ergeben können. Sollten in keinem Fall mehr therapeutische Konsequenzen aus der Untersuchung möglich sein, sei es wegen der Art oder Schwere des Prozesses, dem Alter oder dem Allgemeinzustand des Patienten, sollte auf die Angiographie verzichtet werden. Abgesehen von Notfällen setzt die Angiographie die Ausschöpfung möglichst vieler anderer, einfacherer Untersuchungsmethoden voraus. In den letzten Jahren trat bei Sonderindikationen der Intensiv- und Transplantationsmedizin die Frage nach der angiographischen Darstellung des intravitalen Hirntodes wieder etwas mehr in den Vordergrund.

II. Intrakranielle Tumoren

Die Treffsicherheit der Methode ist bei supratentoriellen Prozessen etwa doppelt so hoch wie bei den infratentoriellen, obwohl auch bei diesen durch Verbesserung in der Durchführung und der Ausarbeitung der Angiogramme in den letzten Jahren noch erhebliche Fortschritte erzielt werden konnten (z.B. Huang u. Wolf, 1969, 1970). Einfache Verhältnisse liegen meist vor, wenn sich bei der Angiographie der Befund einer pathologischen Vaskularisation ergibt (Tumoranfärbung). Ist dies nicht der Fall, treten selbst im supratentoriellen Bereich gelegentlich Schwierigkeiten mit der genauen Lokalisation auf, die zusätzliche Maßnahmen erfordern, z.B. bei Verdacht auf Raumforderungen im Parietookzipital-Bereich und insbesondere bei mittellinien- oder basisnahen Tumoren. Je nach Art des Prozesses kommen als zusätzliche Untersuchungen noch eine Externadarstellung, Angiographien mit Kompression zur besseren Füllung des basalen Gefäßkranzes, Spezialprojektionen, Vergrößerungsangiographie oder Serienschichtangiographie in Frage. In manchen Fällen können selektive oder superselektive Verfahren zu besseren Ergebnissen führen.

Im Bereich der hinteren Schädelgrube erhalten die venösen Abflüsse ein besonderes Gewicht für die Beurteilung von Raumforderungen. Deswegen ist auf eine gute Füllung auch in den venösen Phasen besonders zu achten. Bei allen Prozessen, bei denen eine pathologische Gefäßanfärbung nicht sicher ist, kann vor der Fortsetzung der Maßnahmen eine Sofortsubtraktion über den weiteren Fortgang der Untersuchung entscheiden. Bei Darstellung einer pathologischen Vaskularisation können folgende Schlüsse gezogen werden: die Größe der „Anfärbung" erreicht vollständig oder nur teilweise das Ausmaß der Raumforderung; die pathologischen Gefäße lassen sich scharf oder nur unscharf gegen ihre Umgebung abgrenzen. Aus dem Aussehen und der Anordnung der pathologischen Gefäße können artdiagnostische Rückschlüsse und Aussagen über den Tumorkreislauf oder andere morphologische Details gezogen werden, ebenso auf die hämodynamischen Auswirkungen auf seine Nachbarschaft. Eine ausgedehnte „Anfärbung" bei nur geringer lokaler Raumforderung läßt Rückschlüsse auf den Malignitätsgrad zu: „raumersetzendes Tumorwachstum".

III. Extrakranielle raumfordernde Prozesse

In Frage kommen Tumoren oder Gefäßfehlbildungen, die sich an die Kreislaufgebiete der Arteria carotis externa und der Arteria vertebralis anschließen und im Bereich der Schädelbasis, am kraniozervikalen Übergang, im Bereich des Gesichtsschädels, der Orbitae und am Hals lokalisiert sind. Eine Sonderstellung nimmt der einseitige Exophthalmus ein. Direkte Tumoranfärbungen oder die Darstellung pathologischer Gefäße sind am wertvollsten. Die relativen Zeichen der Raumforderung durch Gefäßverlagerung sind wegen der größeren Variabilität der Gefäßverläufe nicht so sicher wie bei den intrakraniellen Tumoren. Selektive Verfahren führen in einigen Fällen zu besonders übersichtlichen Ergebnissen, der Vorteil der Gegenstromangiographie, besonders bei dieser Fragestellung, ist die Mitfüllung von Kreisläufen anderen Ursprungs (Truncus thyreocervicalis) und die Darstellung der Wechselwirkung dieser Kreisläufe in der Versorgung des pathologischen Prozesses, z.B. eine Mehrfachversorgung aus mehreren Arterienstämmen, Kollateral- und Umgehungskreisläufe.

IV. Intrakranielle oder intrazerebrale Hämatome

In der Regel ist eine Differenzierung zwischen intrazerebralen und extrazerebralen intrakraniellen Hämatomen aus dem charakteristischen Gefäßbild möglich. Schwierigkeiten in der Abgrenzung bestehen bei temporaler und parietookzipitaler Lokalisation, auch in der Abgrenzung gegenüber anderen Traumafolgen, insbesondere Hirntrümmerherden mit Begleitödem. Bei Darstellung meningealer Gefäße, die von der Kalotte abgedrängt werden, kann die Diagnose eines epiduralen Hämatoms erhärtet werden. Relativ selten scheinen Kontrastmittelextravasate zu sein. Wenn nicht, wie bei Traumen, der Mechanismus der Blutung klar ist, kann in Frühstadien die Blutungsursache nicht immer eindeutig bestimmt werden. Es finden sich nur indirekte Zeichen, etwa Gefäßkontrakturen bei Aneurysmen. Mikroangiome sind nur selten anfärbbar. Differentialdiagnostisch müssen Hirninfarkte und hypertonische Massenblutungen erwogen werden. Hierbei kann die CT-Untersuchung den entscheidenden differentialdiagnostischen Beitrag leisten.

V. Aneurysmen der Hirngefäße

Für therapeutische Entscheidungen ist die Darstellung von Form, Größe und Lage der Aneurysmen sowie die Beziehung zu den beteiligten Gefäßen nötig. Zur Darstellung der Prädilektionsorte, wie supraklinoidaler Carotis interna-Anteil, Ramus communicans anterior, Teilungsstelle der Arteria cerebri media, sind unter Umständen gesonderte Maßnahmen, wie Kompressionsangiogramme, anwendbar. Wegen des statistisch häufigen Auftretens multipler Aneurysmen ist eine 4-Gefäßangiographie, evtl. in 2 Sitzungen, erforderlich. Als besondere Projektionsverfahren werden halbschräge Aufnahmen, halbaxiale Aufnahmen und stereoskopische Angiographiebilder empfohlen (KRAYENBÜHL u. YASARGIL, 1972). Bleibt der Ausgangspunkt des Aneurysmas weiterhin unklar, können noch schichtangiographische Aufnahmen angeschlossen werden (RAMELLA, 1969; NADJMI et al., 1975). Das Verfahren kann auch zur besseren Darstellung großer, verzweigter oder teilweise thrombosierter Aneurysmen beitragen. Raumforderungen durch Blutungen nach Aneurysmaruptur, Gefäßspasmen oder Ausfall postaneurysmaler Arterienäste weisen auf das Ausmaß der Nebenreaktionen hin und tragen zu den therapeutischen Verhaltensrichtlinien bei. Wenn eine Frühdiagnostik unmittelbar nach Eintritt einer Subarachnoidalblutung nicht durch den klinischen Befund eines intrazerebralen Hämatoms erforderlich wird, soll die Angiographie innerhalb 3–10 Tagen nach der ersten Blutung stattfinden. Die Untersuchung soll wiederholt werden, wenn bei ausgeprägten Gefäßkontrakturen ein Aneurysmanachweis nicht gelingt, aber klinisch der dringende Verdacht auf ein Aneurysma weiterbesteht.

VI. Arteriovenöse Anastomosen und Angiome

Wir finden arteriovenöse Shuntbildungen häufig bei Tumoren, wo sie eine Besonderheit des pathologischen Kreislaufs darstellen. Ferner kommen die traumatischen Formen, insbesondere die traumatische Carotis-Sinus cavernosus-Fistel, zur Darstellung. Auch arterio-venöse Fisteln ungeklärter Genese ohne Angiomcharakter wurden beschrieben, z.B. bei EHRLICH et al. (1968) im Bereich der Arteria vertebralis. Die arteriovenösen Angiome nehmen eine Sonderstellung ein. Hier muß durch eine selektive Darstellung aller Gefäße im Sinn einer 4-Gefäß-Angiographie die hämodynamische Beziehung der Zu- und Abflüsse geklärt werden. Gleichzeitig kann im Serienangiogramm das Ausmaß des Shuntvolumens abgeschätzt werden. Auch hier empfehlen KRAYEN-

BÜHL u. YASARGIL (1965 u. 1972) stereoskopische Serienaufnahmen, NADJMI (1976) die Angiotomgraphie. Aus der Art der Anfärbung und der räumlichen Anordnung der pathologisch veränderten Gefäße kann das Ausmaß der Durchdringung von Hirngewebe, evtl. Anzeichen einer zusätzlichen intrazerebralen Blutung abgelesen werden. Die Indikation, das Vorgehen bei einer Operation oder überhaupt die Durchführbarkeit eines operativen Eingriffes lassen sich daraus ableiten.

VII. Schlaganfälle–intermittierende Symptomatik–Verdacht auf Gefäßstenosen

Beweisende angiographische Korrelate einer zerebrovaskulären Minderdurchblutung sind der Nachweis eines Gefäßverschlusses, eines Gefäßastverschlusses, von Stenosen und der Nachweis von Kollateralkreisläufen. Die Indikation zur Angiographie ist insbesondere gegeben, wenn durch ein chirurgisches Eingreifen eine entscheidende Verbesserung der klinischen Ausgangssituation erreicht werden kann.

Diese Fragestellung ist nicht ohne Angiographie zu klären; daher ergibt sich die unmittelbare Indikationsstellung meist aus anderen Kriterien.

1. Stenosierende Gefäßerkrankungen

Wichtig ist zunächst die Frage, ob und in welchem Ausmaße die großen supraaortischen Halsgefäße stenosiert sind, in zweiter Linie, inwieweit Gefäßwandveränderungen an anderen Gefäßen vorliegen, zumal am intrakraniellen Gefäßbaum. Bei einem geplanten operativen Eingriff, z.B. Endarteriektomie der Carotis communis oder interna, ist die Orientierung über die anderen großen Gefäßstämme, einschließlich der Abgangsverhältnisse, Möglichkeiten von Kollateralkreisläufen über den basalen Gefäßkranz und der Zustand der intrakraniellen Gefäße wesentlich. Liegt schon eine ausgeprägte Hemiparese vor, gelten andere Kriterien (s.u.).

2. Bei intermittierender Symptomatik

wird in allen Fällen zur Abklärung der Ursache eine Gefäßdarstellung erforderlich werden, insbesondere, wenn die Pulse einer Halsseite abgeschwächt oder aufgehoben sind, bei unterschiedlichem Puls oder Blutdruck der oberen Extremitäten oder bei Verdacht auf ein *Steal*-Syndrom. Das Gleiche gilt bei der Auskultation von systolischen Geräuschen hinter dem Kieferwinkel, entsprechend der Karotisgabel und über der Supraklavikulargrube, entsprechend der Arteria subclavia, die nicht kardial bedingt sind. Auch hier sollen Stenosen der supraaortischen Gefäßstämme aufgespürt werden. Eine operative Behandlung soll hier erfolgen, bevor irreversible zerebrale Kreislaufstörungen aufgetreten sind. Zu dieser Indikationsgruppe gehören Patienten, bei denen eine intermittierende Karotisinsuffizienz oder vertebrobasiläre Insuffizienz durch Lageänderung des Kopfes oder Halses provozierbar sind, sowie die Aumaurosis fugax.

3. Asymptomatische Patienten mit Gefäßgeräuschen am Hals, wenn Eingriffe an anderen Gefäßen vorgesehen sind

Durch die Angiographie sollen klinisch stumme Stenosen an den Halsgefäßen ausgeschlossen werden. Dadurch soll vermieden werden, daß ein geplanter gefäßchirurgischer Eingriff, z.B. eine Endarteriektomie an einer Extremität, durch einen zerebrovaskulären Insult kompliziert wird.

4. Schlaganfälle mit schnell progredienter Symptomatik

Bei Schlaganfällen mit schnell progredienter Symptomatik kann die Angiographie sofort indiziert sein, wenn Stenosen oder Verschlüsse der großen Gefäße vorliegen, um die 3- bis 6-Stundenfrist für eine mögliche Embolektomie einhalten zu können. Außerdem wird sich in diesen Fällen die Differentialdiagnose einer evtl. operablen intrazerebralen Raumforderung, wie Tumor, Tumorblutung, wachsendes Hämatom, stellen. Ist die 6-Stundenfrist schon längere Zeit verstrichen, wird bei unzweifelhaften Hirninfarkten vor einer geplanten Angiographie möglichst die Besserung der Symptomatik abgewartet.

5. Komplette Apoplexie

Beim kompletten Apoplex ist die Angiographie nur unter besonderen Voraussetzungen indiziert. Auch hier gilt die Frist, innerhalb derer versucht werden kann, einen Gefäßverschluß zu beheben, sowie die Möglichkeit des Ausschlusses einer operativ angehbaren Raumforderung oder des Ausschlusses einer massiven Hirnschwellung.

6. Migräne

Spezielle Anforderungen der Indikationsstellung gelten für Migränepatienten. Bei anamnestisch und klinisch unkomplizierter Migräne gilt die zerebrale Angiographie als nicht indiziert oder kontraindiziert, da einerseits faßbare pathologische Veränderungen im Angiogramm nicht erwartet werden können, andererseits die Patienten wegen ihrer Neigung zu Gefäßreaktionen (insbesondere Spasmen) als durch die Angiographie gefährdeter gelten (JANZEN, 1972); RABE (1971) fand bei typischem, unverwechselbarem Migränebild praktisch keine Überschneidungen mit den symptomatischen Migräneformen. Lediglich 5 von 340 Tumorpatienten hatten migräneähnliche Kopfschmerzen. Der migräneähnliche Kopfschmerztyp soll häufiger bei intermittierenden Liquorzirkulationsstörungen, ausgelöst am Aquädukt oder am vierten Ventrikel, als Symptom infratentorieller Tumoren auftreten (HEYCK, 1964; SCHÜRMANN u. ULBRICHT, 1966). Außer Anamnese und klinischer Symptomatik, die auf eine zerebrale Raumforderung hindeuten, galten zerebrale Krampfanfälle als wichtiges Differentialdiagnostikon, jedoch werden auch Beziehungen zwischen echter Migräne und Krampfanfällen diskutiert (BONHÖFFER, 1940; HEYCK, 1964).

PICHLER (1961) beschreibt als Ursachen symptomatisch bedingter Migränebeschwerden: präsklerotische Gefäßstörungen, Aneurysmen, Ventrikeltumoren, andere intrazerebrale Tumoren, Endangiitis obliterans, chronische Blei- und Nikotinvergiftung. BODECHTEL (1963) fügt insbesondere die zerebralen Angiome hinzu, wobei bei parietalem Sitz sensible Herdsymptome, bei okzipitalem Sitz typische Flimmerskotome (bis Hemianopsien) auftreten sollen. Beobachtungen hierzu finden sich schon bei MACKENZIE (1953) (12 von 50 Angiompatienten mit Migräneanamnese) und OLIVECRONA (1957) (4 von 107 Angiompatienten hatten Migräneanfälle). Die besondere Häufigkeit der Migräne bei den supraklinoidalen Aneurysmen der A. carotis interna, allerdings oft mit charakteristischer Begleitsymptomatik, führt zur symptomatischen Sonderform der „migraine ophthalmoplégique“. BAROLIN (1969) beschreibt eine posttraumatische Sonderform bei „Stauchungstraumen der Schädelwirbelsäuleneinheit“ und dadurch bedingt Irritation des Basilariszuflußgebiets, welche Parallelen zur (primär nicht traumatisch bedingten Sonderform) „Migraine cervical“ (bzw. Migraena cerebellaris (CHRAST) oder Basilarisarterienmigräne (BICKERSTAFF), beide zit. nach BAROLIN (1969), erkennen lassen.

Bleibende Schäden nach Migräneanfällen werden von CHARCOT (zit. nach INFELD), INFELD (1901), BONHÖFFER (1940), CONNOR (1962), BAROLIN (1969) beschrieben. Berichte über Todesfälle im Migräneanfall von BASSOE (1933), PETERS (1934), STÖRRING (1939), GUEST und WOLF (1964), HOLUB et al. (1965) weisen ebenfalls in die Richtung der Migräne mit morphologisch faßbaren zerebralen Ausfallmustern (ischämische und hämorrhagische Hirninfarkte).

Indikationen ergeben sich also bei erstmalig im Erwachsenenalter aufgetretener Migräne, bei negativer Familienanamnese oder bei ausgeprägter Begleitsymptomatik sowie den Formen komplizierter Migräne und Verdacht auf symptomatische Kopfschmerzformen. Es gelingt dabei gelegentlich, umschriebene intrazerebrale Gefäßspasmen nachzuweisen (NEWTON u. POTTS, 1974) was bei aller Diskussion um eine lokal gefäßabhängige (endzündliche?) Genese die Angiographie nur insofern rechtfertigt, als sich daraus therapeutische Konsequenzen ergeben können (antiphlogistische Behandlung oder Schlaganfalltherapie), obwohl die eigentliche Suche den Gefäßverschlüssen, Gefäßmißbildungen, Tumoren, Gefäßerkrankungen (Endangiitis obliterans, Moya-Moya), extrakraniellen Stenosen (Flimmerskotom/amaurosis fugax) usw. gilt.

Differentialdiagnostisch zusätzlich in Frage kommende Krankheitsbilder, wie der BING-Horton-Kopfschmerz (cluster-headache), evtl. die Arteriitis temporalis, sollten klinisch ausreichend abtrennbar sein und stellen keine Indikation zur Angiographie dar.

VIII. Intrazerebrale Drucksteigerung – dissoziierter Hirntod

Die Beobachtung des Kreislaufstillstands in den großen, zum Gehirn führenden Gefäßen bei irreversibler Hirndruckerhöhung oder intravitalem dissoziiertem Hirntod, wie sie z.B. bei GROS et al. (1959) mitgeteilt wird, bekommt eine neue Aktualität. Die Bedürfnisse der Intensivmedizin und der Transplantationsmedizin erfordern eine frühzeitige Diagnosestellung bei zerebralem Kreislaufstillstand. Durch eine gewisse Rechtsunsicherheit bei den Voraussetzungen zu dieser Indikation, deren Ursachen fast ausschließlich im außermedizinischen Bereich liegen, stellt sich die Frage nach einer besonders geeigneten, standardisierten Methode. Diese soll besonders einfach und schonend sein und jegliche Art von Artefakten ausschließen. Die doppelseitige Karotis- und Vertebralisangiographie wird, wie die selektiven Katheterdarstellungen der supraaortischen Gefäße, als zu aufwendig und in der Aussage zu unsicher beurteilt, da bei paravasalen Injektionen oder Gefäßspasmen Bilder wie beim extrazerebralen Kreislaufstillstand der großen Halsgefäße zustande kommen.

Weniger bedenklich erscheint die Gegenstromangiographie beider Brachialarterien und die Karotisangiographie links, wobei das Artefaktrisiko bei der direkten Karotispunktion links durch die drei im Gegenstromverfahren dargestellten großen Gefäßstämme praktisch ausgeglichen wird. Mehrere jüngste Arbeiten (GREITZ et al., 1973; KRÖSL u. SCHERZER (Hrsg.), 1973; BRADAC u. SIMON, 1974; BUSSE u. VOGELSANG, 1974) befassen sich eingehend und aufgrund eigener Untersuchungen mit diesem Thema. Als Methode der Wahl wird die Panarteriographie der großen Gefäße von einem großen Katheder im Aortenbogen aus empfohlen. Das Verfahren ist sehr einfach und wird als ausreichend sicher dargestellt. Während derselben Untersuchung kann eine Nierenarteriographie (Transplantationsmedizin) durch denselben Katheder angeschlossen werden. Als Nachteile werden eine relativ kontrastarme Gefäßdarstellung erwähnt. Auf den seitlichen Aufnahmen kommt noch hinzu die Überlagerung der Gefäßstämme beider Seiten. Die Aussagekraft steigt durch die Subtraktion dieser Angiogramme. GREITZ et al. (1973) empfehlen die Wiederholung der Untersuchung nach etwa 30 min.

Natürlich setzt die Indikationsstellung zu dieser Untersuchung die klinischen Zeichen des dissoziierten Hirntodes voraus: tiefes Koma mit Reaktionslosigkeit und fehlender Spontanatmung. Über 24 Std abgeleitetes O-Linien EEG. Das angiographische Bild allein ist nicht schlüssig, wie die Veröffentlichung von LEE et al. (1973) zeigt, wo ein „Stillstand"-Hirnarteriogramm durch einen Herzblock im Augenblick der Kontrastmittelinjektion möglicherweise als Folge einer Karotis-Sinus-Reaktion zustande kam. BUSSE u. VOGELSANG (1974) bestätigten die Anwendbarkeit der aortokranialen Panarteriographie auch bei Kindern und Kleinkindern. Lediglich im Säuglings- und Kleinkindesalter bis zu einem Jahr scheinen andere Kriterien des intravitalen Hirntodes zu gelten. MÜLLER (1973) nimmt an, daß der irreversible Funktionsverlust des Gehirns bei Neugeborenen und Säuglingen wegen der noch dehnbaren Schädel-Dura-Kapsel nicht mit letzter Sicherheit durch Angiographie nachgewiesen werden kann.

Ein Teil der **Einschränkungen zur Indikationsstellung** kann heute dadurch abgeklärt werden, daß vor der zerebralen Angiographie eine axiale computergesteuerte Tomographie des Schädels (CT) durchgeführt wird. Dies gilt vor allem bei unklaren Krankheitsbildern, desolaten Patienten sowie bei den (relativen) Kontraindikationen. Mit Hilfe des CT-Befundes kann die Situation genau eingeschätzt werden (Raumforderung, Hydrozephalus, Hirnödem, Infarktzonen, intrazerebrale Blutungen), und es ergeben sich entscheidende Hinweise für das weitere Vorgehen: Verzicht auf Angiographie, Art der Angiographie, Aufschub usw. Überhaupt kann für die CT gelten, daß die Indikation zur Angiographie die Ausschöpfung der anderen, weniger eingreifenden Untersuchungen voraussetzt, wenn immer die Möglichkeit dazu besteht.

Durch den vor der Angiographie erstellten CT-Befund ist es erstmalig möglich geworden, zerebrale Angiographiekomplikationen (Hirninfarkte) zu verifizieren (s.u.).

Bei nahezu allen aufgeführten Indikationen können viele wertvolle Vorinformationen gewonnen werden, die den Untersuchungsgang selbst erleichtern und optimieren lassen, wenn nicht die CT selbst schon das entscheidende Ergebnis erbracht hat. Selbst beim klinischen dissoziierten Hirntod (s.u.) aus unklarer Ursache ist noch vor Nachweis des zerebralen Kreislaufstillstandes eine Diagnose möglich. Bei der Indikationsgruppe der zerebrovaskulären Prozesse kann als weniger eingreifende Methode neben der CT die Doppler-Sonographie der zuführenden Gefäßstämme und extrakraniellen Kollateralen wertvoll sein.

IX. Therapeutische Eingriffe bei der Angiographie

Hier soll nur kurz hingewiesen werden auf die Embolisierungsverfahren mit Gelen, Baumwoll-, Plastik- und Metallkügelchen, die sich an die superselektiven Angiographien anschließen. Sie dienen im wesentlichen der Behandlung von ausgedehnten Gefäßgeschwülsten bzw. Angiomen (VLAHOVITCH u. FUENTES, 1976; LUESSENHOF et al., 1965; BOULOS et al., 1970; J. de Neuroradiologie 2 (1975): Sammelband therapeutische Embolisation, DJINDJIAN and MERLAND, 1978). Die Embolisierung von Tumoren, besonders meningealer Herkunft, vor der Operation, wurde ebenfalls versucht. Über die Verfahren ist schon reichlich Schrifttum vorhanden. Als weitere therapeutische Verfahren wurden die Stillung einer Aneurysmablutung oder Verschluß von Carotis-Sinus cavernosus-Fisteln durch Ballonkatheter mitgeteilt (WHOLEY et al., 1972; PICARD et al., 1974; SERBINENKO, 1974). Das Verfahren war ferner bei einer traumatisch bedingten unstillbaren Blutung aus Ästen der Arteria carotis externa anwendbar. Ebenso wird über Elektrokoagulationsverfahren durch selektive Katheterisierung berichtet (PHILLIPS, 1973). Es ist zu erwarten, daß sich die Anzahl der brauchbaren Verfahren vermehren und in die Angiographietechnik allgemein einführen läßt.

D. Kontraindikationen der zerebralen Angiographie

Absolute Kontraindikationen gibt es nicht.

Die relativen Kontraindikationen ergeben sich meist aus einer schwierigen klinischen Situation des Patienten, mit der Gefahr einer erheblichen Komplikationsrate durch Grunderkrankung oder Allgemeinzustand (Tabelle 9). Ist die Allgemeinstörung so erheblich, daß sich daraus ein weiteres therapeutisches Vorgehen verbietet, soll die Angiographie unterbleiben. Liegen lebensbedrohende Allgemeinstörungen, wie Diabetes mellitus, Niereninsuffizienz, eine erhebliche Blutdrucksenkung

Tabelle 9. Kontraindikationen

1. Schwere Allgemeinstörungen, die ein aktives Vorgehen bei dem zu erwartenden Krankheitsbild ausschließen.
2. Entgleister Diabetes mellitus, Niereninsuffizienz, Blutdrucksenkung, Blutverlust, Anämie, schwere Infekte, soweit die Angiographie bis nach Beseitigung der Störung aufschiebbar ist.
3. Bei Patienten mit zerebrovaskulären Erkrankungen, wenn
   a) ein schwerer Hypertonus besteht und keine Intubations-Narkose durchgeführt werden kann,
   b) ein Herzinfarkt erst kurz zurückliegt,
   c) häufig Krämpfe mit länger andauernder Bewußtlosigkeit auftreten,
   d) Anzeichen eines Hirnstamminfarkts vorliegen,
   e) eine Antikoagulation durchgeführt wurde (bei niedrigen Gerinnungswerten).

oder exzessive Blutdrucksteigerung, Blutverlust, schwere Anämie oder gefährliche Infekte, vor, sollte zuerst überlegt werden, ob nicht die Angiographie bis zur Beseitigung dieser Störungen aufschiebbar ist. So wird z.B. beim multitraumatisierten, bewußtlosen Patienten die Dringlichkeit zur Angiographie eher überschätzt, d.h. es darf nicht übersehen werden, daß Freilegung der Atemwege, Intubation, Schockbehandlung, Blutstillung, Fahndung nach inneren Verletzungen vordringlicher sein können, selbst wenn eindeutige zerebrale Herdsymptome oder Hinweise auf intrakranielle Drucksteigerung vorliegen.

Einen Aufschub verlangen schwere Gerinnungsstörungen oder eine Behandlung mit Heparin oder Dicumarol. Hyperkoagulopathien mit Neigung zu Thrombembolien können eine Kontraindikation darstellen. Ein doppelseitiger Verschluß beider Karotiden wird als Kontraindikation gegen eine Vertebralisangiographie angesehen. WEIBEL und FIELDS (1969) vertreten die Meinung, daß

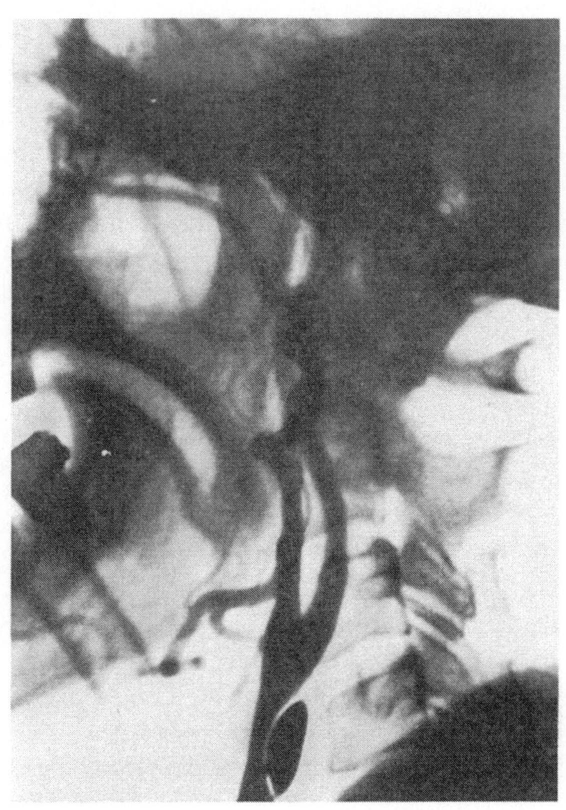

Abb. 5. Injektionskomplikationen. Kleines, manschettenförmiges Extravasat im Bereich der Punktionsstelle

bei Patienten mit zerebrovaskulären Erkrankungen nicht angiographiert werden soll, wenn ein schwerer Hypertonus besteht und keine Intubationsnarkose durchgeführt werden kann, wenn ein erwiesener Herzinfarkt erst kürzlich zurückliegt, häufig Krämpfe mit länger andauernder Bewußtlosigkeit auftreten oder Anzeichen eines Hirnstamminfarktes vorliegen. Die Kontraindikation ergibt sich bei diesen Fällen aus der erhöhten Komplikationsgefahr und fehlenden therapeutischen Konsequenzen aus dem Angiographieergebnis. Weitere Kontraindikationen ergeben sich zwanglos aus den denkbaren Komplikationen (s.u.), wenn aus irgendeinem Grund ein bestimmtes Komplikationsrisiko steigt.

E. Komplikationen der zerebralen Angiographie

Es hat sich grundsätzlich als schwierig erwiesen, Störungen, die nach zerebralen Angiographien auftreten, zuverlässig zu beurteilen. Bei schweren, plötzlich und während der Untersuchung auftretenden Zwischenfällen gelingt eine einwandfreie Zuordnung leicht. Die passageren, kleineren oder erst nach einem freien Intervall auftretenden Störungen erfordern ein vorher festgelegtes Konzept der Beobachtung, Befunderhebung und Dokumentation, da sonst ein erhebliches Maß an Unvollständigkeit und Zufälligkeit der Aussage zu erwarten ist. Auch können nur unter diesen Bedingungen die spontanen Schwankungen der Grunderkrankungen wiedererkannt und von den Komplikationen abgegrenzt werden. Der Wert der Einzelbeobachtung muß sich an der Aussage mehrerer möglichst großer prospektiver Studien kontinuierlicher Kollektive messen lassen. Mitteilungen, die alle diese Kriterien erfüllen, sind selten. Sicherheit besteht daher nur über die statistische Häufigkeit der schweren und letalen Komplikationen in Abhängigkeit zur Untersuchungsfrequenz, dem Alter der Probanden und der Grunderkrankung, während die Angaben über leichtere und passagere Komplikationen, auch hinsichtlich gemeinsamer Grunderkrankungen, erheblich streuen. Die schweren Komplikationen sind, obwohl häufig kasuistisch mitgeteilt, insgesamt so selten, daß die Verläufe nicht nur mitgeteilt werden, um etwa auf ihre Vermeidbarkeit hinzuweisen, sondern vorwiegend aus anderen Gründen, wie Beherrschung der Komplikation und klinischen evtl. operativen Verfahrensfragen. Die Vorstellungen über die Komplikationsmöglichkeiten stehen weitgehend fest, wenn sie auch noch laufend durch Randprobleme ergänzt werden. Hierbei tritt die Bedeutung der speziellen Kontrastmittelkomplikation in der Diskussion wieder hinter die Verfahrensfragen und das Problem um die Methode der Wahl zurück. Nach dem Stand der heutigen Erfahrung kann keines der gängigen Angiographieverfahren bei einwandfreier Abwicklung aus Gründen der Komplikationserwartung abgelehnt werden. Einzelne Vorbehalte, die die grundsätzliche Schädigungsmöglichkeit durch die eingreifende Untersuchungstechnik belegen, und zwar auch aufgrund pathologisch-anatomischer Untersuchungen, dürfen aber in ihrer Bedeutung nicht unterschätzt werden. Gerade sie tragen dazu bei, daß heute den vermeidbaren Störungen durch Punktion, Injektion und Kathetertechnik wieder die größte Beachtung geschenkt wird.

Die Schädigungsmöglichkeiten durch Punktion und Injektion gehen aus den Tabellen 10 u. 12 hervor. Es sind hier die verschiedensten Möglichkeiten nach großen Sammelstatistiken und Einzelveröffentlichungen aufgeführt, wie sie im bisherigen Schrifttum über Angiographie-Komplikationen mitgeteilt werden. Im Normalfall der Abteilungen mit großem angiographischen Durchgang ist von den Punktionsschäden am häufigsten die Durchstoßung der Gefäßrückwand, oft ja Teil der Methode, im Hinblick auf Komplikationen meist jedoch irrelevant. Kleinere Hämatome sind häufig, ohne daß Ausfälle mitgeteilt werden. Subjektive lokale Beschwerden durch Hämatome der Halsweichteile, der Arme (Brachialispunktion) und der Leistenbeugen und Oberschenkel (Femoralispunktion) sind häufig. Die übrigen Punktionsschäden sind selten und werden in der Litera-

Tabelle 10. Komplikationen bei der Punktion der Gefäße

1. Hämatom der Halsweichteile (meist harmlose Komplikation)	Kompression und Verlagerung der Trachea – Atemnot – begünstigt Auftreten von Pneumonien bei älteren Patienten flüchtige Rekurrenzparese Kompression der Jugularvenen (DUNSMORE) Absacken eines Hämatoms in das Mediastinum, besonders bei Kindern
2. Plexus- und Nervenschädigung (insgesamt seltene Komplikation)	Schädigung des Nervus recurrens und hypoglossus und vagus gelegentlich Reizung des Nervus sympathicus mit Pupillenerweiterung. Schädigung im Bereich des Plexus brachialis. Wurzelreizung mit Brachialis-Neuritis. Reizung des Glomus caroticum mit Kreislaufreaktionen. Schädigung des Nervus medianus und N. femoralis (je nach Punktion). (Nervenschädigungen sind häufiger bei der Vertebralis-Punktion als bei der Karotis-Punktion und den retrograden Verfahren.)
3. Fehlpunktionen	Punktion des Duralsackes (Vertebralis-Punktion) Mediastinalemphysem Punktion des Larynx oder Pharynx Punktion der Vena jugularis mit Luftembolie Pneumothorax und Hämatothorax bei Subklavia-Punktion (oder retrograder Karotis-Punktion)
4. Reaktionen am Ort der Punktion	Intramurale Hämatome, Dissoziation der Gefäßwände Skarifizierung der Gefäßhinterwand (RIMPAU) Aneurysma dissecans, Spätthrombose, Plaquebildung Zeichen lokaler zerebro-vaskulärer Insuffizienz Aneurysmabildung Thrombembolie (häufiger bei den Katheterverfahren) Arteriovenöse Fisteln (z.B. zwischen Arteria vertebralis und Plexus venosus vertebralis)
5. Gefäßkompression	Zu kräftige oder zu lange Kompression bei Punktionsversuchen oder nach der Angiographie.

Tabelle 11. Arteriovenöse Fisteln nach Gefäßpunktionen zur zerebralen Angiographie. Übersicht über die Literatur von 1956–1971 nach BERGQUIST et al. (1971)

Gesamtanzahl	24				
Auftreten des Gefäßgeräusches	sofort	bald (1–5 Tage)	Wochen	1–9 Jahre	unbekannt
	9	5	3	3	4
Heilungsquote	spontan 5		nach Operation (teilweise mehrfach) 11		

tur als Raritäten oder wegen besonderer therapeutischer Konsequenzen beschrieben (Tabellen 11 u. 13).

Das Hauptaugenmerk bei der Verhütung von Angiographie-Komplikationen gilt heute den Injektionsschäden, und zwar bei den direkten Punktionsverfahren insbesondere der intra- und paravasalen Injektion, bei den Katheter-Verfahren den lokalen Gefäßkomplikationen, wie arteriellen Thrombosen, Gefäßwand-Hämatomen und Nachblutungen, sowie den embolischen Ereignissen (Thromben, Plaques-Material, Fremdkörper). Von lokalen Komplikationen ist dabei die Arteria

Tabelle 12. Komplikationen durch den Injektionsvorgang

1. Intramurale Injektion	Einengung oder vorübergehender Verschluß des Gefäßlumens (ebenso auch bei paravasaler Injektion) Paresen, Aphasie, Hemianopsie, Bewußtseinsstörung, bulbäre Symptome
2. Intimaabhebung	durch Blutung oder Kontrastmitteldepots Plaquebildung, Thrombose, Aneurysma dissecans zentralnervöse Ausfälle
3. Embolien	Thrombembolien (häufiger bei Katheteruntersuchungen) von der Nadelspitze (bzw. Katheterspitze) oder aus dem Schlauch – Spritzen – und Verbindungssystem Luftembolien (Netzhautgefäße) Plättchen- und Cholesterinembolien (besonders Netzhautgefäße) (bei Mobilisierung von Material aus arteriosklerotischen Plaques) Baumwollfaserembolie (CHANSON) Mikro-Glaspartikel
4. Aneurysmaruptur	
5. Vasospasmen	
6. Intrathekale Injektion	bei Vertebralis-Punktion mit Reizerscheinungen und Verletzungen des Rückenmarks, Schädigung des Hirnstamms und basaler Hirnteile: Quadriplegien, Atemstörungen, Anopsie usw.

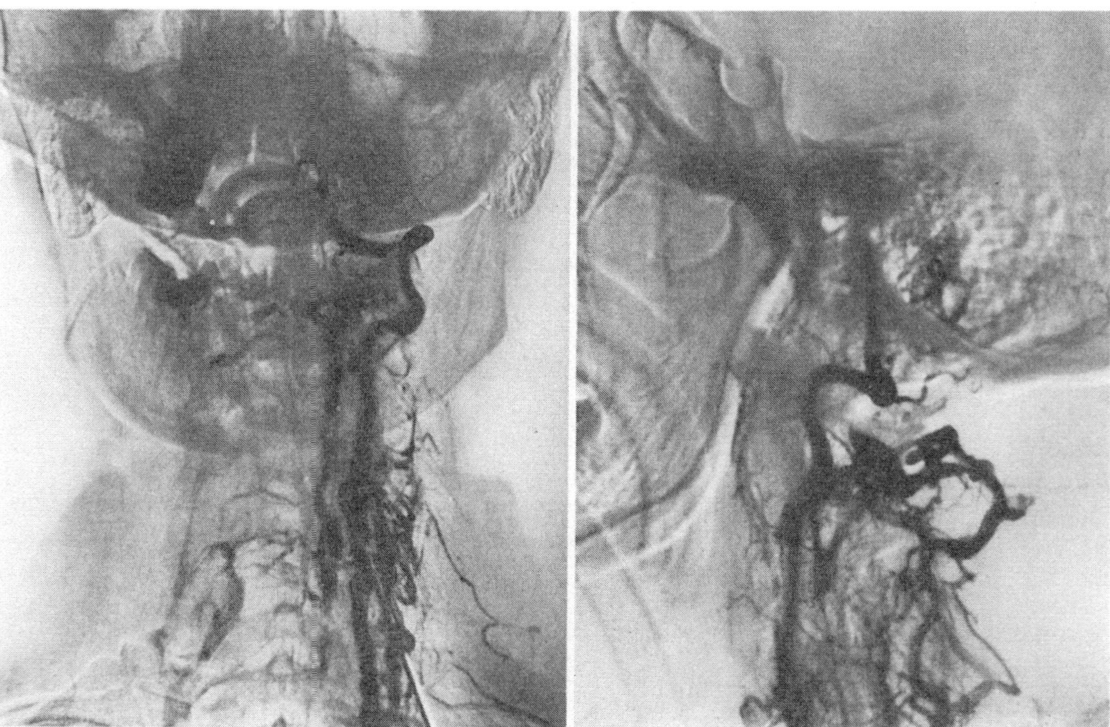

Abb. 6. Komplikation bei Vertebralispunktion: Die Kanüle durchstößt die Arterienwand, die Kanülenspitze liegt in der benachbarten Vene. Bei der Injektion kommt es zur gemeinsamen Darstellung der A. vertebralis und des vertebralen Venengeflechts. Keine Ausbildung einer av-Fistel (Beobachtungszeitraum 3 Jahre)

Tabelle 13. Aneurysmaruptur während zerebraler Angiographien
Literaturübersicht nach SHIRO WAGA et al. (1973)

Verteilung		n	Verfahren	n	Sitz d. Aneur.	n	Autoren	
Alter	23 J.	1	*Anaesth.*		*A. cer. med.*	3	BEAMER	1969
	31–40 J.	4	Lok.	6	*A. car. int.*		FERRARI	1969
	41–50 J.	4	Allg.	3	(Ram. com. post.)	5	GALLAGHER	1956
	51–60 J.	4	unbekannt	5	Ram. com. ant.	3	GOLDSTEIN	1967
	84 J.	1			Bifurkation	1	HOFF	1969
	♀	10	*Punktion*		Sonst.	2	JACKSON	1960
	♂	4	*direkt*	13	*A. basilaris*	1	JAMIESON	1954
			A. car. comm.	7			JENKINSON	1954
let. Ausgang		13	A. car. int.	5			LEHRER	1972
							MURPHY	1967
Gesamt		14	A. vertebr.	1			SAKAMOTO	1972
			indirekt				TRISKA	1962
			A. brachialis	1			VINES	1971
							WAGA	1973

brachialis häufiger betroffen als die Arteria femoralis. Auch hier besteht ein wesentlicher Bezug zur Grunderkrankung (s.u.).

Die Schäden durch das Kontrastmittel selbst sind im Normalfall die leichteren, passageren Komplikationen (Tabelle 14). Sie konnten durch die Entwicklung moderner Präparate stark zurückgedrängt werden.

Allgemeinen allergischen oder toxischen Wirkungen am Gesamtorganismus oder an Einzelorganen stehen spezielle zerebrale Reiz- und Ausfallerscheinungen gegenüber. Die allgemeinen Störungen lassen sich am besten aus den großen Statistiken über i.v. Pyelographien belegen. Die große Komplikationsrate bei PENDERGRASS et al. (1958) dokumentiert für den neuroradiologischen Bereich gleichzeitig die Vermeidbarkeit: i.v. Pyelogramme werden nicht in Narkose durchgeführt, es sind teilweise sehr große Kontrastmittelmengen angewandt worden. Über große Kontrastmittelzwischenfälle (anaphylaktischer Schock) wird in der modernen Angiographie-Literatur nicht mehr berichtet.

Gut erforscht sind die passageren Herz- und Kreislaufstörungen im Zusammenhang mit der Kontrastmittelinjektion (Tabelle 14). Eine EKG-Überwachung während des Eingriffs wurde schon mehrfach gefordert (DECKER, 1969; DJINDJIAN, 1972).

Unsicherer ist das Gebiet der funktionellen (zerebralen) Durchblutungsstörungen. Beim Menschen tritt im wesentlichen eine Gefäßdilatation, kein Spasmus, im Bereich der zerebralen Gefäße auf. Spasmen werden an den extrakraniellen Gefäßen, insbesonders nahe der Injektionsstelle, gefunden. Krankheitsbedingte Dauerspasmen (Subarachnoidalblutung) oder arteriosklerotisch verengte Gefäße verändern die lokale zerebrale Durchblutung entscheidend. Ihre Reaktion unter der Angiographie läßt sich im Einzelfall schwer voraussagen. Über Gefäßverlegungen durch Stase aggregierten Erythrozyten-Materials wird berichtet. Stillstand der Kontrastmittelsäule bei Injektionsschäden (s.o.) kann die zerebrale Zirkulation durch die längere Verweildauer des Kontrastmittels, besonders in einem gefäßgeschädigten Areal, entscheidend verschlechtern. Dies greift über zu den Befunden der zerebralen Reiz- und Ausfallserscheinungen, verursacht durch Schäden am Hirnparenchym selbst. Betroffen ist die Kapillarendothelmembran (Bluthirnschranke). Bei den heutigen Kontrastmitteln setzen größere Schädigungen eine komplexe Kausalitätskette voraus.

Besonders gefährdet sind Patienten mit erheblichen Gefäßprozessen, Hirndruck oder großen Schrankenstörungen (ausgedehnte Tumoren).

Die Häufigkeit der zerebralen Komplikationen (Tabelle 15) läßt den Schluß zu, daß sich seit der Einführung der modernen Kontrastmittel das Risiko der tödlichen Zwischenfälle und der

Tabelle 14. Kontrastmittelkomplikationen

1. Subjektives Hitzegefühl	bei intraarterieller Injektion	Chemorezeptoren
2. Herz- und Kreislaufstörungen	Absinken des Blutdruckes	Chemorezeptoren
	Verzögerung der Hirnzirkulation	Chemorezeptoren Viskosität Kreislaufwirkung
	Dilatation der kleinen Hirngefäße	Chemorezeptoren
	Verlegung kleiner oder arteriosklerotisch verengter Gefäße durch Erythrozyten	Viskosität Osmolarität
3. Zerebrale Reiz- und Ausfallserscheinungen		chemische Eigenschaften Osmolarität
a) direkte Toxizität	Veränderung der Bluthirnschranke (Gefäßpermeabilität) Intimaschwellung Ödem punktförmige Blutungen und Stase	in Abhängigkeit von Menge und Konzentration des Kontrastmittels Dauer der Kontrastmitteleinwirkung Intervalle zwischen der Kontrastmittelinjektion
		nachweisbar: pathologisch-anatomisch Evansblue Test Hirnszintigramm EEG
b) Verlängerung der Zirkulationsverlangsamung (siehe unter 2; Herz- und Kreislaufstörungen)	bei Hirndruck und zerebralen Gefäßprozessen	
4. Allgemeine Kontrastmittelwirkungen	Kopfschmerzen Schock (-fragmente) Haut- und Schleimhautkomplikationen Urtikaria Arzneimittelexanthem Rhinitis Konjunktivitis Glottisödem Asthma Lungenödem	Jodallergie Idiosynkrasie
	renale Symptome (tubuläre Insuffizienz)	allgemeine Toxizität

Zwischenfälle mit großen bleibenden Ausfällen nicht wesentlich verändert hat, wogegen die passageren Störungen weitgehend vermeidbar geworden sind. Auch hier liegen besondere Aspekte bei den Gefäßerkrankungen vor.

Eine etwas erhöhte Rate passagerer Komplikationen weisen alle Verfahren zur Vertebralisangiographie auf (YASARGIL, 1962; SCHIEFER, 1972). Davon werden den Kontrastmitteln im allgemeinen die passageren Amaurosen, Hemianopsien, visuellen Agnosien und Halluzinationen angelastet. In zweiter Linie kommen als Ursache die Gefäßverlegung (Katheter), zu große Kontrastmittelmengen oder Gefäßspasmen und paravasale Injektionen bei der direkten Punktion in Frage (MELARAGNO, 1972). Dem Katheterismus werden Komplikationen, wie Querschnitts-Syndrom durch Embolie der Spinalarterien oder in Form eines Spinalis anterior-Syndromes, angelastet (FLAMENT-DURAND, 1970; LYON, 1971). Lokale Traumatisierung, wie Verletzungen am Plexus brachialis

Tabelle 15. Häufigkeit zerebraler Komplikationen

1. Letale Zwischenfälle, älteres Schrifttum nach SCHIEFER (1959)

Thorotrast 1940–1954	5029	5	0,09%
Parabrodil (35–45%) 1951–1956	4868	9	0,1 %
Diodrast (35–50%) 1944–1955	6673	24	0,35%

2. Todesfälle, bleibende und vorübergehende Störungen nach WENDE in KAZNER et al. (1969), (Sammelstatistik)

	Angiogr.	+		bleibend		vorübergeh.	
Neurolog.-Neurochirurg. Krankengut	42395	47	0,11%	38	0,09%	502	1,19%
Zerebrale Gefäßerkrankg.	3073	58	1,9 %	73	2,4 %	63	2,1 %

oder an Nervenstämmen, kann der Brachialis- oder Axillarisangiographie folgen (DUBRICK et al., 1967). Bei sachgerechter Durchführung liegt die Komplikationsquote mit diesen Untersuchungen, wie ganz allgemein der Angiographien, nicht so hoch, daß eine Aufklärungspflicht über die im einzelnen möglichen Angiographierisiken bestehen würde (SCHIEFER, 1972). Von seiten der Grunderkrankung liegen besondere Verhältnisse bei den schweren stenosierenden Prozessen an extra- und intrakraniellen Gefäßen und bei den zerebralen Aneurysmen vor.

Das Alter selbst spielt, nach Ansicht der meisten Autoren, keine entscheidende Rolle, doch werden Herz-Kreislaufstörungen, schwere arteriosklerotische Veränderungen, diffuse Gefäßprozesse bei Hypertonie oder Diabetes mellitus meist erst in höheren Lebensaltern gefunden. So beobachteten PATTERSON et al. (1964) das Auftreten von bleibenden Ausfällen nach Angiographien nur bei Patienten ab dem 6. Lebensjahrzehnt, wobei jeweils ein Gefäßprozeß angenommen werden konnte. MCDOWELL et al. hatten 1959 über eine hohe Komplikationsrate im Alter, jedoch auch bei zerebralen Gefäßprozessen berichtet. Zusammenstellungen von SILVERSTEIN (1966) und WENDE (1969) dokumentieren die besondere Gefährdung der Gefäßkranken im Vergleich zu den Patienten des übrigen neurologischen und neurochirurgischen Krankengutes. Bei diesen zusammenfassenden Darstellungen weist SCHIEFER (1972) jedoch darauf hin, daß hier sehr unterschiedliche Kriterien bei der Annahme einer Komplikation zugrunde gelegt wurden. Besonders ungünstig liegt die Statistik für Schlaganfallpatienten, die im Koma angiographiert wurden, oder bei denen aus sonstigen Gründen eine schwere Störung des Allgemeinzustandes vorlag (MCDOWELL et al., 1959). Sie berichten von 11 Todesfällen nach 13 Angiographien an komatösen Patienten. In dem großen, fortlaufenden Krankengut von DECKER (1969) mit 24000 Angiographien hatten 7 der Patienten mit bleibenden oder letalen Komplikationen einen zerebralen Gefäßprozeß oder eine Karotisstenose im Halsbereich.

Die besonders hohe Komplikationsdichte dieses Krankengutes erklärt sich aus dem Zusammenwirken mehrerer Faktoren. Durch die Passage der beengten und vorgeschädigten Gefäße wird die zerebrale Durchblutung noch mehr verschlechtert, da gleichzeitig die Dauer der Kontrastmitteleinwirkung verlängert ist (RAUSCH et al., 1956; VOGELSANG, 1964). Die Gefährdung nimmt zu, sobald kleine Störungen des Untersuchungsablaufs, wie Gefäßwandschädigungen, Lumenverlegung von Gefäßen durch Katheter, Mikrothromben, Gefäßspasmen, hinzukommen oder Embolie von Plaque-Material (LINDNER et al., 1962) oder Herzrhythmusstörungen durch Karotis-Sinus-Reflexe, eine Bradykardie oder ein Blutdruckabfall auftreten, die sekundär zu einer schlechteren zerebralen Perfusion führen. Man ist deshalb übereingekommen, bei zerebralen Gefäßprozessen strengere Angiographieindikationen anzulegen (RÖTTGEN, 1952; TÖNNIS u. SCHIEFER, 1969; WEIBEL

u. FIELDS, 1969), wenn sich auch die Indikationsstellung durch die Möglichkeiten der operativen Eingriffe an den extrakraniellen Gefäßen erweitert haben (ZEITLER u. SCHOOP, 1979; HOWIESON, 1974).

Bei den Aneurysmen, die wegen einer ausgedehnten Subarachnoidalblutung angiographiert werden, besteht eine erhöhte Gefährdung durch die Engstellung der prä- oder postaneurysmatischen Gefäßstrecken und die Zirkulationsverlangsamung in diesem Bereich, die durch intrazerebrale Hämatome und Ödeme gesteigert werden kann. Über Verschlechterungen, unmittelbar nach einer Angiographie, im frischen Stadium einer Subarachnoidalblutung ist berichtet worden, aber bei den oft foudroyant verlaufenden Krankheitsbildern sind sie in der Beurteilung etwas unsicher. So berichtet bereits SCHIEFER 1959 über einen Todesfall unmittelbar vor Beginn der Angiographie. Eine Sammelstatistik der Aneurysma-Rupturen während einer Angiographie gibt Tabelle 13 wider, nach Literaturangaben von SHIRO WAGA et al. (1973). Diese Komplikation interessiert jedoch wegen des insgesamt nur sehr seltenen Auftretens vorwiegend im Hinblick auf den Verlauf und die Beherrschbarkeit der Störung. Die frühzeitige Angiographie ist wegen des Gipfels der Nachblutungsfrequenz in der ersten Woche nach der ersten Subarachnoidalblutung jedoch erforderlich. Die Auslösung einer Rezidivblutung als Komplikation, soweit sie der Untersuchung angelastet werden kann (PERRET u. NISHIOKA (1966) in einer großen Statistik von über 7000 Angiographien), zeigt eine wesentliche geringere Gefährdung als bei den schweren zerebralen Gefäßprozessen mit Allgemeinstörungen und Plegien, bei denen der Wert der Untersuchung sehr viel bestrittener ist. Die Gefährdung der Patienten steigt, bei Zugrundelegung dieser Arbeit, durch die im Frühstadium durchgeführte Angiographie vermutlich gar nicht an.

Bei zerebralen Raumforderungen größeren Ausmaßes, mit Zirkulationsverlangsamung, steigt die Gefährdung mit dem Ausmaß der Schädelinnendrucksteigerung an. Dennoch wird die Untersuchung in keinem Fall zu umgehen sein. Durch therapeutische Maßnahmen, die eine Verminderung des Hirndruckes zur Folge haben, lassen sich jedoch gleichzeitig die angiographischen Ergebnisse verbessern (GRANGE et al., 1967; HACKER u. ALONSO, 1969). Das Verfahren ist unterdessen weitgehend üblich.

Auch bei den frischen Schädelhirntraumen kann bei kunstgerechter Grundversorgung der Patienten und Durchführung in einer schonenden Narkose die Komplikationsrate im Vergleich zur bestehenden Gefährdung der Verletzten in Kauf genommen werden (TÖNNIS, 1959; SCHIEFER, 1972), wenn nicht zugunsten einer CT-Untersuchung auf die Angiographie verzichtet werden kann.

Das Literatur-Verzeichnis dieses Kapitels befindet sich am Schluß des nächsten Kapitels über „Normale Anatomie..." und gilt für beide Kapitel.

Normale Anatomie der zerebralen Arterien

Von

M. Nadjmi u. M. Ratzka

Mit 30 Abbildungen und 9 Tabellen

A. Einleitung

Die Kenntnis der normalen Anatomie der intrakraniellen Gefäße ist die unumgängliche Voraussetzung für die Beurteilung von Angiogrammen. Die angiographischen Techniken und ihre Entwicklung bis zum jetzigen Stand haben andererseits ganz wesentlich zur Erforschung der anatomischen Gefäßstrukturen, bis an die Grenzen des mikroskopischen Bereichs, beigetragen. Es haben sich hierzu sowohl selektive Techniken, unter Anwendung der direkten Vergrößerungstechnik, wie auch Verfeinerung der Injektionstechniken am anatomischen Präparat, teilweise in Verbindung mit feingeweblicher Präparation, bewährt. Deutliche Fortschritte konnten mit diesen Methoden auf dem Gebiete der Vaskularisationsterritorien kortikaler und subkortikaler Hirngefäßverzweigungen, den Aufzweigungen der Gefäße der hinteren Schädelgrube, des Hirnstammes und bei der Versorgung der Meningen der Schädelbasis noch in jüngster Zeit erzielt werden.

Aufgabe des vorliegenden Abschnittes sollte es sein, in relativ gedrängter Form einen Überblick über die normale Anatomie der intrakraniellen Arterien zu geben, zusammen mit einem Überblick der Originalien und Standardwerke über dieses Thema.

Die Einteilung des Kapitels folgt naturgemäß den anatomischen Gegebenheiten. Der Karotiskreislauf wird dem Vertebraliskreislauf vorangestellt. Um unnötige Wiederholungen zu vermeiden, andererseits aber zu einer geschlossenen Darstellung beizutragen, schien es praktisch, die Hirnstammgefäße sowohl des Karotiskreislaufes wie des vertebrobasilären Kreislaufes im Zusammenhang zum jeweiligen Abschnitt, ebenso eine Zusammenfassung der Kollateralkreisläufe, unter Einschluß des Circulus arteriosus Willisi, am Schluß des Kapitels einzufügen. Die primitiven karotidobasilären Verbindungen werden zusammen mit der A. basilaris erwähnt.

B. Karotiskreislauf

I. A. carotis communis

Die A. carotis communis entspringt rechts aus der A. anonyma (Truncus brachiocephalicus), links von der Höhe des Aortenbogens. Diese Anordnung soll in 64–70% der Fälle vorliegen, in 20–25% der Fälle entspringt die A. carotis communis der linken Seite, unmittelbar neben der A. anonyma oder geht aus der A. anonyma hervor; bei 4% der Fälle sollen die linke A. carotis communis, die linke A. vertebralis und die li. Arteria subclavia nebeneinander vom Aortenbogen abgehen, in weniger als 1% der Fälle entspringt die rechte A. carotis communis vom Aortenbogen. Die Angaben wurden von BOSNIAK (1964) aus einem großen anatomischen Untersuchungsgut (THOMSON, 1894; DE GARIS et al., 1933; WILLIAMS u. EDMONDS, 1935; LIECHTY et al., 1957; MARTIN et al., 1960; ROTH et al., 1961; BOSNIAK, 1964 zitiert nach KRAYENBÜHL u. YASARGIL, 1965) gewonnen. Andere Abgangsvarietäten zeigt das Schema von RAUBER-KOPSCH (1948), welches auch bei KRAYENBÜHL und YASARGIL (1957) abgebildet ist, jedoch ohne genaue Häufigkeitsangaben sowie HAUGHTON und ROSENBAUM (1974).

Die A. carotis communis zieht geradlinig mit gleichbleibendem Kaliber kranialwärts, wobei sie lateral der Trachea und des Larynx verläuft. In Höhe des Schildknorpeloberrandes kommt es zu einer kleinen, bogigen Erweiterung, zur spitzwinkligen oder U-förmigen Teilung in die beiden nahezu gleichstarken Äste: A. carotis externa und A. carotis interna. Der als leichte Gefäßerweiterung erkennbare Karotissinus (Sinus A. carotidis internae) setzt sich in die Carotis interna fort. Die Höhe der Karotisgabelung kann auf die Halswirbelkörper zwischen C 1/2 und C 6/7 projiziert sein; häufigster Sitz war C 4/5 mit 48,2%, es folgen C 3/4 mit 34,4%, C 5/6 mit über 13%, C 2/3 mit 3,7%; die beiden übrigen Höhen nur in Einzelfällen aus einem Untersuchungsgut von 658 Angiographien (KRAYENBÜHL u. YASARGIL, 1965).

II. A. carotis externa

Das sich zum Teil oberflächlich verzweigende Gefäß zur Versorgung des Gesichts und der Schädelwände war schon früh Objekt eingehender anatomischer Untersuchungen: VESALIUS (1543), HALLER (1757–1763), FARABEUF (1896), POIRIER (1896), LIVINI (1903), DESCOMPS (1912), HUARD und MONTAGNE (1931; zitiert nach AARON et al., 1970). Angiographische Studien wurden von Gruppen um SALAMON, DELMAS (nach AARON et al., 1970) sowie durch DJINDJIAN und Mitarbeiter (MERLAND, 1973), aber auch BELOU (1934), ORLANDINI (1951), VOENA und CARVALO (1959), LIE (1968) beigetragen, in den letzten Jahren durch die superselektive angiographische Technik und Anwendung von direkteren röntgenographischen Vergrößerungen erheblich verfeinert (SALAMON et al., 1974; MERLAND et al., 1975). Unter den Beschreibungen im extrakraniellen Bereich sei noch die Arbeit von LANZ und WACHSMUTH (1955) hervorgehoben. Weitere Untersuchungen befassen sich mit der Vaskularisation und dem Aufbau der Meningen teilweise vom feingeweblichen Standpunkt (LANG, 1971, 1973; hier auch eingehende weitere Literaturangaben).

Die A. carotis externa bei Kindern, oft im Kaliber etwas schwächer als die Carotis interna, beim Erwachsenen meist gleich stark, wird in 8 oder 9 Äste eingeteilt und stellt ein sehr differenziert verzweigtes Gefäßsystem mit ausgeprägter Kollateralenbildung dar. Die Art der Aufzweigung und damit Einteilung und Gruppierung der Hauptäste ist sehr variabel. Nach AARON et al. (1970) werden drei Hauptformationen, die etagenweise Aufteilung (division etagée) in 2 Typen, die Aufteilung mit gruppierten Gefäßabgängen (formes groupées) in 4 Haupttypen und die fächerförmige Aufteilung (formes en bouquet) unterschieden (Abb. 1).

Eine Übersicht über die Hauptäste und ihre Verzweigungen ergibt die Tabelle 1.

Die extrakraniellen Gefäße der A. carotis externa werden an anderer Stelle besprochen.

Versorgung der Schädelbasis

Die Innenseite der hinteren Schädelbasis wird von einer Gruppe lateraler und einer Gruppe medialer Gefäße versorgt.

Laterale Gefäße: Beteiligt sind der hintere Ast der A. meningica media oder die A. temporosquamosa, die einen subtentoriellen Ast unterschiedlicher Größe abgeben kann sowie der R. mastoideus meningeus der A. occipitalis externa, der durch ein hinter dem Mastoid gelegenes Foramen in die hintere Schädelgrube eintritt und ein Gebiet zwischen der A. meningica media im lateralen und der A. pharyngea ascendens im medialen Anteil versorgt.

Tabelle 1. Äste der Arteria carotis externa

A. thyroidea superior

A. laryngea superior
A. laryngea inferior
A. infrahyoidea
A. sternocleidomastoidea inferior
A. musc. infrahyoidei

A. lingualis

A. sublingualis
  R. mentalis
  R. maxillaris
  R. infrahyoideus
  R. hyoideus
A. profunda linguae
  Rr. linguales dorsales
A. dorsalis linguare

A. facialis

1. Segm.

A. palatina ascendens
  A. tonsillaris
  R. horizontalis (Gaumensegel)
  Rr. descendentes (Pharynx)
A. principalis glandulae submaxillaris
A. masseterica inferior
A. submentalis
  Rr. descendentes (gland. submax.)
  R. musc. infrahyoidei

2. Segm.

Aa. coronares superiores et inferiores
A. dorsalis nasi

A. pharyngea ascendens (A. pharyngomeningea)

R. anterior (pharyng. horizontalis)
R. medius (tympanicus ascendens)
R. posterior
  R. meningeus posterior

A. maxillaris interna

A. auricularis profunda
A. tympanica anterior
A. meningica media
R. meningicus accessorius
A. alveolaris mandibularis
A. masseterica
R. pterygoideus
A. temporalis profunda posterior
A. temporalis profunda anterior
A. buccalis
Aa. alveolares maxillares posteriores
Aa. alveolares maxillares anteriores
A. infraorbitalis
A. pterygopalatina
A. canalis pterygoidei
A. palatina descendens

A. occipitalis

1. Segm.

R. sternocleidomastoideus superior
A. cervicalis posterior

2. Segm.

Rr. ascendentes } zur Nacken-
Rr. descendentes } muskulatur
R. collateralis a. vertebr.

3. Segm.

R. internus
R. externus
Rr. meningei
  R. petromastoideus
R. posterior

A. auricularis posterior

R. auricularis
R. mastoideus

A. temporalis superficialis

Rr. parotidei
A. transversa faciei
A. masseterica superior (descendens)
A. temporalis profunda posterior
A. auricularis anterior
A. zygomatica orbitalis
R. anterior (frontalis)
R. posterior (temporoparietalis)

Die mediale Gefäßgruppe besteht aus dem Ramus meningicus posterior der A. pharyngea ascendens und dem R. meningicus der A. vertebralis. Die Gefäßgruppen haben vikariierende Versorgungsgebiete und weisen reichliche Anastomosen auf.

Versorgung der Meningen der Felsenbeinpyramiden und des Klivus

Die posterosuperiore Fläche der Pyramiden wird von den Rr. petrosi der A. meningica media versorgt, durch einen perforierenden R. meningicus der A. pharyngea ascendens, der durch das Foramen jugulare eintritt, einen R. meningicomastoideus der A. occipitalis externa und den R. temporosquamosus der A. meningica media im lateralen Anteil sowie durch die kavernösen Äste der A. carotis interna im medialen Anteil.

Die anterosuperiore Oberfläche der Felsenbeinpyramiden grenzt an die Versorgung der Regionen des Sinus cavernosus und der Keilbeine. Derzeit ist eine Differenzierung noch nicht möglich (Merland et al., 1975). Die meningeale Versorgung im Klivusbereich wird im oberen Anteil durch die im Kavernosusabschnitt der Carotis interna entspringenden meningealen Gefäße wie durch den Truncus meningo-hypophyseos versorgt, im unteren Anteil durch Äste der A. pharyngea ascendens, die sich nach medial und lateral auf den Klivus verteilen.

Bei der Vaskularisation der Meningen im Keilbeinbereich können eine laterale, eine mediale und eine Felsenbeinregion unterschieden werden. Im lateralen Bereich stammen die versorgenden Äste im basalen Abschnitt der Fossa temporalis von der A. meningica media. Der mediale Anteil, eine Region um Sella und Sinus cavernosus, bekommt Zuflüsse aus der A. carotis interna, durch die Rr. capsulares und Rr. meningei sowie von der A. carotis externa, einerseits aus der A. meningica accessoria, die aus der A. maxillaris interna oder der A. meningica media abgehen kann und durch das Foramen rotundum zieht, andererseits durch das Keilbeinsegment der A. meningica media, von dem ein Ast zum kleinen Keilbeinflügel und zur Region des Sinus cavernosus abgegeben wird. Im Bereich der Fissura orbitalis superior können noch mediale Äste der A. ophthalmica an der Versorgung teilnehmen.

Die Versorgung der Meningen der vorderen Schädelgrube wird im lateralen Anteil und im Bereich der Orbitadächer durch die frontobasalen Äste der A. meningica media übernommen, im medialen Anteil durch die A. ethmoidalis anterior, welche auch einen Ast zur Falx abgibt und anschließend nach dorsal durch die A. ethmoidalis posterior (beide aus der A. ophthalmica). Letztere nimmt, zusammen mit Ästen der Kavernosus-Region, an der Versorgung des Keilbeins teil.

Die differenzierte Darstellung der Versorgungsbezirke der Meningen im Bereich der Schädelbasis ist im wesentlichen erst durch die äußerst verfeinerte superselektive Injektionstechnik der einzelnen Äste der A. carotis externa möglich geworden (MERLAND et al., 1975, DJINDJIAN u. MERLAND, 1978).

Die A. meningea media ist das stärkste die Dura versorgende Gefäß, gelegentlich auch der stärkste Ast der A. maxillaris interna. Sie tritt, zusammen mit dem Ramus meningeus des Nervus mandibularis, durch das Foramen spinosum in das Endokranium ein und teilt sich in wechselnder Höhe meist in 2, gelegentlich in 3 Äste. Beide verlaufen an der Oberfläche der Dura und folgen den Gefäßfurchen der Tabula interna des Schädeldaches. Der vordere Ast zieht zur vorderen Schädelgrube, zu den Orbitae und bis zu den Nasenhöhlen, während der hintere Ast einen sphenoparietalen Verlauf aufweist. Die Versorgung umfaßt die Dura mater der Großhirnhemisphären, die Schädelknochen und mit perforierenden Ästen teilweise äußere Weichteile des Schädels. Die Versorgung der Dura der hinteren Schädelgrube und des Tentoriums ist komplex und stark wechselnd. Zuflüsse werden von den Ästen der A. carotis interna aus dem Kavernosus-Abschnitt, der A. pharyngea ascendens im Klivusbereich und meningealen Ästen der A. vertebralis, der A. occipitalis interna sowie zum Teil feinsten Ästchen der Kleinhirnarterien abgegeben.

Das Kollateralennetz der Äste der A. carotis externa bildet im Bereich der Vaskularisation des Gesichts, des Schädels und der Meningen, insbesondere im Bereich der Endverzweigungen, reichliche Möglichkeiten zu Kompensation- und Umgehungskreisläufen bei lokalen Prozessen. Die Möglichkeit der Kollateralverbindungen zu anderen Kreisläufen, insbesondere der A. carotis interna und der A. vertebralis, sind in einem eigenen Kapital über Kollateralkreisläufe dargestellt (s.u.). Es handelt sich meist um präformierte Anastomosen, die – insbesondere bei pathologischen Kreislaufverhältnissen – wirksam werden.

III. A. carotis interna

1. Stamm

Die A. carotis interna verläuft geradlinig kranialwärts zur Apertura externa des Karotiskanals der Schädelbasis, in den Halsweichteilen, ebenfalls ohne Äste abzugeben und dadurch mit gleichbleibendem Lumen. Dieses Segment weist im Kindesalter eine physiologische Schlängelung auf,

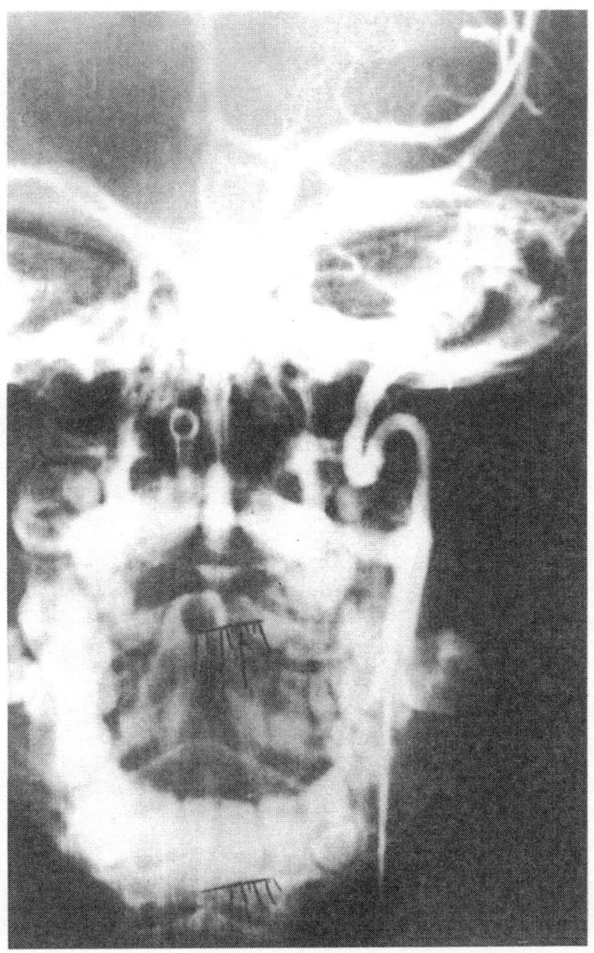

Abb. 1. Schleifenbildung der A. carotis interna im Halsbereich; im Kleinkindesalter physiologisch

die im höheren Alter durch Elongation des Gefäßes erneut auftreten kann. Vor dem Eintritt in den Karotiskanal wird eine nach medialwärts konvexe Biegung unterschiedlichen Ausmaßes ausgeführt. Der Verlauf innerhalb des Canalis caroticus folgt den knöchernen Strukturen. Die angiographische Darstellung dieses Segmentes zeigt die Form des knöchernen Kanals, der einen geraden, schräg nach medial und aufwärts gerichteten oder bogigen Verlauf nehmen kann. Der Kanal endet in der Gegend der Pyramidenspitze. Die A. carotis interna wendet sich nun medial- und rostralwärts zur Lateralfläche des Keilbeinkörpers. In dieser Höhe beginnt die Einteilung nach Fischer (1938) in 5 Segmente:
C5 Ganglionabschnitt,
C4 horizontaler, nach vorne ziehender Abschnitt,
C3 Verbindungsstück, Siphonknie,
C2 horizontaler, nach dorsal gerichteter Abschnitt,
C1 Endabschnitt.
Die Segmente C2 bis C5 werden seit Moniz (1940) als Karotissiphon zusammengefaßt.

Im ganglionären Segment ist die Arterie zuerst durch eine dünne knöcherne Lamelle oder ein bindegewebiges Septum vom Mittelteil des darauf liegenden Ganglion Gasseri getrennt, steigt dann fast senkrecht in einer Furche an der Lateralfläche des Keilbeinkörpers (Sulcus caroticus), an der medialen Seite des Ganglion trigeminale Gasseri, an dessen frontalem Pol nach oben.

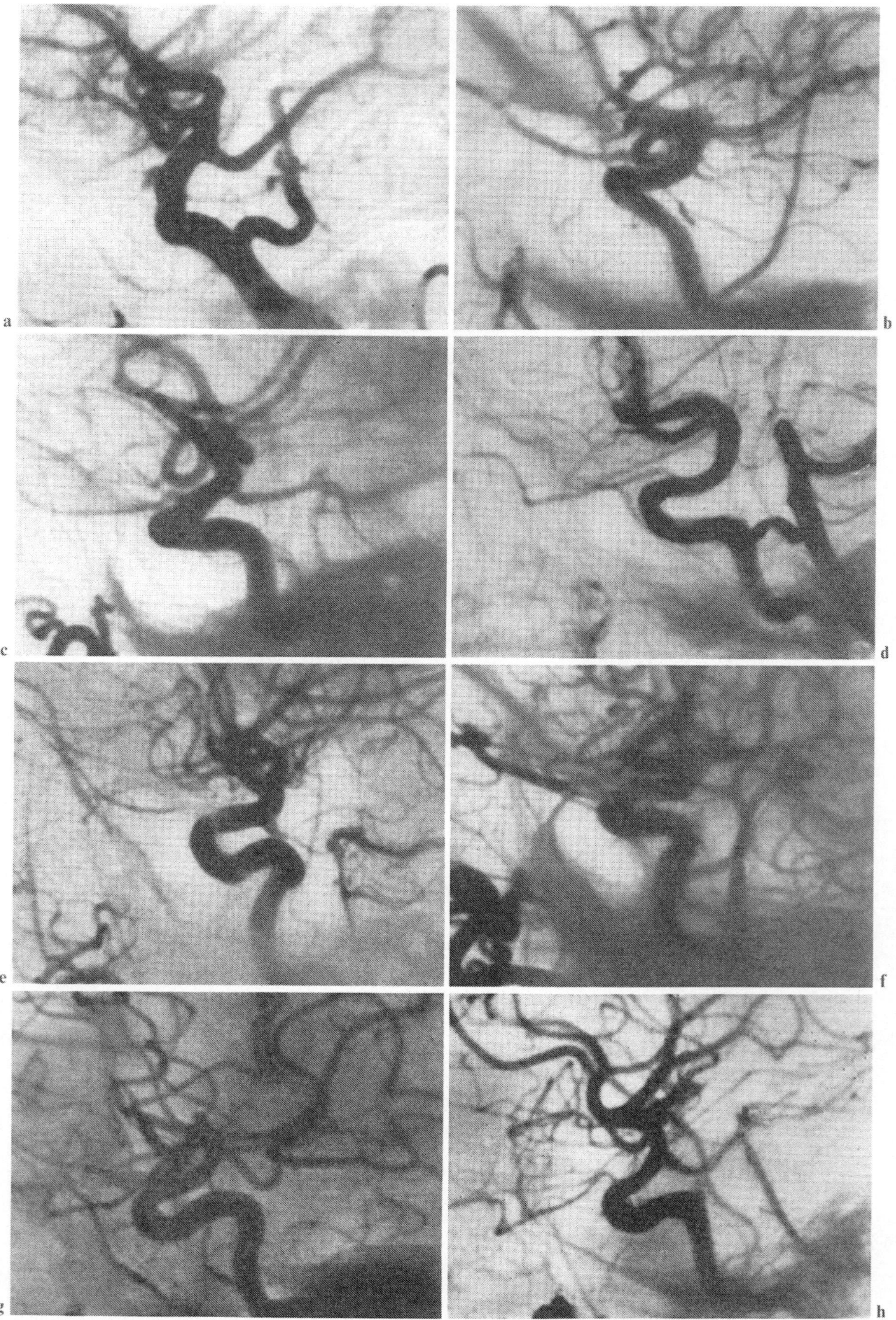
a
b
c
d
e
f
g
h

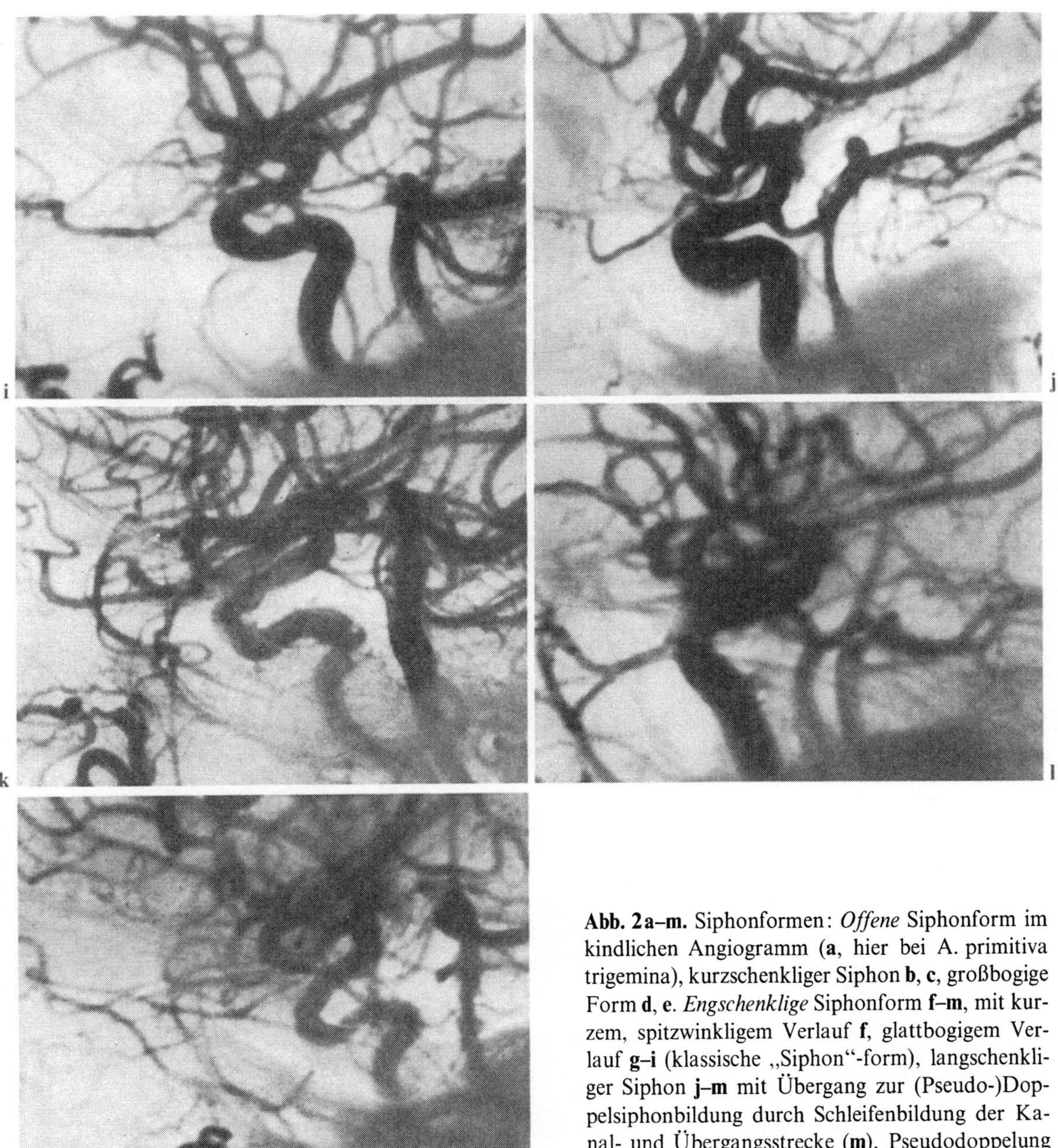

Abb. 2a–m. Siphonformen: *Offene* Siphonform im kindlichen Angiogramm (**a**, hier bei A. primitiva trigemina), kurzschenkliger Siphon **b**, **c**, großbogige Form **d**, **e**. *Engschenklige* Siphonform **f–m**, mit kurzem, spitzwinkligem Verlauf **f**, glattbogigem Verlauf **g–i** (klassische „Siphon"-form), langschenkliger Siphon **j–m** mit Übergang zur (Pseudo-)Doppelsiphonbildung durch Schleifenbildung der Kanal- und Übergangsstrecke (**m**), Pseudodoppelung durch engbogigen Verlauf der Anfangsstrecke der A. cerebri media im seitlichen Strahlengang **e, k, j**

Hier befindet sie sich bereits im Sinus cavernosus, wo sie nach einer weiteren Biegung rostralwärts zur Basis des Processus clinoideus anterior zieht, wo das Karotisknie C3 eine meist engschenklige rostralwärts konvexe Biegung beschreibt. In diesem Segment erfolgt der Durchtritt durch die Dura, mit okzipitalwärts gerichtetem Verlauf am medialen Rand des Processus clinoideus anterior im Abschnitt C2, der zusammen mit dem C1 (End-) Abschnitt zisternal und supraklinoidal angeordnet ist, in relativ gestrecktem Verlauf bis zur Bifurkation der A. carotis interna.

Im Bereich des Sinus cavernosus ist die A. carotis interna durch je eine Dura-Duplikatur an ihrem Eintritt und am Übergang zum zisternalen Abschnitt sowie durch das bindegewebige Trabekelwerk des venösen Blutleiters noch weitgehend fixiert. Der obere, zisternal gelegene Siphonschenkel und der Endabschnitt liegen relativ frei beweglich im Subarachnoidalraum und bieten zur Beurteilung von intrakraniellen Raumforderungen besonders wertvolle Hinweise. Kanal- und

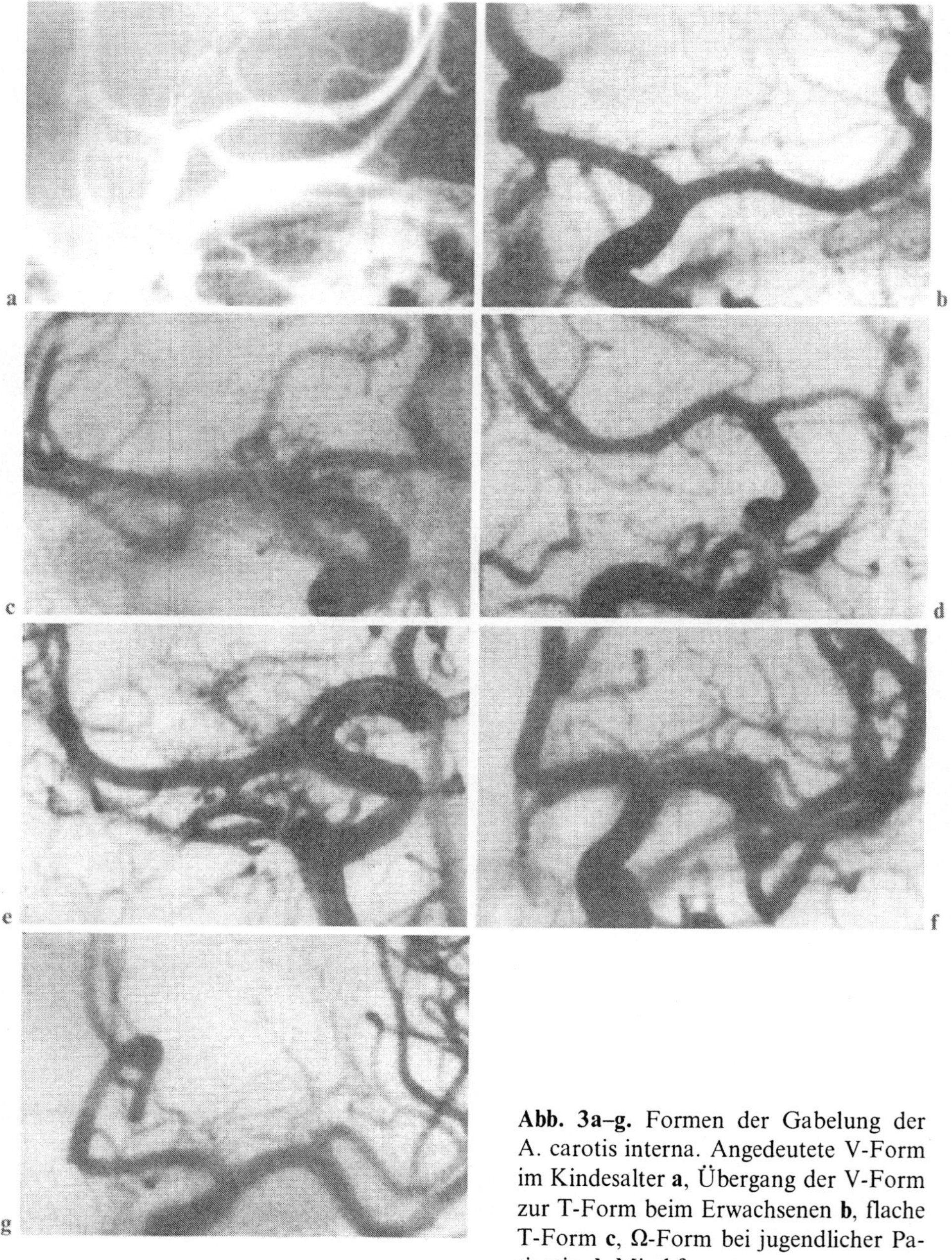

Abb. 3a–g. Formen der Gabelung der A. carotis interna. Angedeutete V-Form im Kindesalter **a**, Übergang der V-Form zur T-Form beim Erwachsenen **b**, flache T-Form **c**, Ω-Form bei jugendlicher Patientin **d**, Mischformen **e–g**

Kavernosusabschnitt stellen im funktionellen Sinn eine „Übergangsstrecke" des Gefäßsystems vom extrakraniellen zum intrakraniellen Typ dar, was sich im wesentlichen im Wandbau zeigt. Die Muskelfasern und elastischen Elemente der Tunica media vermindern sich auf etwa $^1/_4$ der extrakraniellen Schichtdicke; auch die Tunica externa und adventitia werden dünner, die Lamina elastica interna dicker (LANG, 1965; VIEHWEGER u. JENSEN, 1968; ZÜLCH, 1971). Die Einsparungen an Wandmaterial sind möglich, da die Arterien innerhalb der Schädelhöhle entweder von Liquor oder von venösem Blut (Sinus cavernosus) umgeben sind und der Flüssigkeitsdruck einen Teil der Stützfunktionen der Gefäßwand übernimmt (LANG, 1965).

Insbesondere mit dem Siphonabschnitt beschäftigen sich einige sehr eingehende Arbeiten (RUEDINGER, 1888; FUCHS, 1924; DÖRFLER, 1935; POLI u. ZUCHA, 1940; SPATZ, 1943; FALK, 1952; H. FISCHER, 1954; PLATZER, 1956 und 1957; TEUFEL, 1964; MOISSL, 1972). Die Arbeiten befassen sich mit der genauen anatomischen Analyse, teilweise unter Einbeziehung embryologischer und vergleichend anatomischer Gesichtspunkte sowie mit funktionellen Gesichtspunkten des Karotissiphons als arterieller Übergangsstrecke, strömungsdynamischen Problemen und – damit im Zusammenhang – mit ätiopathogenetischen Untersuchungen des Siphons als Prädilektionsort arteriosklerotischer Veränderungen.

Varianten im zervikalen Bereich betreffen vorwiegend den Verlauf, der nach MONIZ und LIMA (1943), KRAYENBÜHL und YASARGIL (1965), WEIBEL und FIELDS (1965), RAIMONDI (1972), HAUGHTON und ROSENBAUM (1974), DILENGE und HÉON (1974), HARWOOD-NASH und FITZ (1966) in starker Abhängigkeit vom Lebensalter, durch Krümmungen und Schleifenbildung, gekennzeichnet sein kann. So finden KRAYENBÜHL und YASARGIL im Kollektiv der bis zu 20jährigen einen geradlinigen Verlauf bei 86,4%, bei den über 50jährigen nur noch in 34%. HUEBNER (1967) vertritt die Ansicht, daß die A. carotis interna bei dorsalem Abgang der A. carotis communis vorwiegend gestreckt, bei lateralerem Ursprung mehr oder weniger bogig verläuft. Dadurch werden weitgehend die Nachbarschaftsbeziehungen des Gefäßes im Zervikalbereich bestimmt. Die gestrecktere Arterie liegt in der Tiefe der Halsweichteile nicht unmittelbar der Pharynxwand an, während eine starke gewundene A. carotis interna in direkte Beziehung zur Seiten- oder Hinterwand des Schlundes oder der Gaumentonsille treten kann (CAIRNEY, 1924; STREIT, 1932; RICKENBACHER, 1972). Bei KRAYENBÜHL und YASARGIL (1965) werden die Verlaufsvarianten im extrakraniellen Abschnitt, im Karotiskanal und im Bereich des Siphons in einem eigenen größeren Untersuchungsgebiet und nach Angaben von MONIZ et al. (1933), LAZORTHES (1961) und DILENGE (1962) eingehend statistisch dargestellt. Es werden bis zu 7 verschiedene Siphon-Formvarianten unterschieden, die zum Teil zu pathologischen, insbesondere elongierten Gefäßformen überleiten und andererseits gegen pathologische Veränderungen durch Raumforderungen (bei gestrecktem Verlauf) differentialdiagnostisch abgegrenzt werden müssen. Dabei werden die angiographischen Variationen des Siphon- und Carotis interna-Anteils im a-p Bild der Angiogramme (KRAYENBÜHL u. YASARGIL, 1965) berücksichtigt. Mit der Frage des Abstandes des Karotissiphons von der Mittellinie befaßt sich eine topometrische Untersuchung von NADJMI (1967).

Äste der A. carotis interna

In der extrakraniellen Verlaufsstrecke werden von der A. carotis interna in der Regel keine Äste abgegeben. Die Äste der intrakraniellen Verlaufsstrecke können als extradurale, durale und intradurale Äste unterschieden werden.

2. Extradurale Äste

Die extraduralen Äste sind von sehr kleinem Kaliber und können angiographisch nicht abgegrenzt werden. Sie ziehen innerhalb des Canalis caroticus zur Paukenhöhle (Ramus carotidotympanicus). Ein weiterer Ast ist die A. canalis pterygoidei.

3. Äste des Kavernosus-Abschnittes

Im Sinus cavernosus wird eine größere Anzahl von Gefäßen abgegeben, die – besonders unter pathologischen Bedingungen – angiographisch sichtbar werden (McCONNEL, 1953; BERNASCONI u. CASSINARI, 1956; FRUGIONI et al., 1960; DE LA TORRE u. NETZKY, 1960; CORTES et al., 1964; KRAMER u. NEWTON, 1965). Eine schematische Einteilung geben SCHNÜRER und STATTIN (1963) sowie PARKINSON (1964), wogegen McCONNEL (1953) vorwiegend die hypophysären Äste der Aa. capsulares hervorhebt. PARKINSON unterscheidet drei Hauptstämme,

den Truncus meningo-hypophyseus,
die A. sinus cavernosi inferior und
die Aa. capsulares.

Der erste Ast ist der Truncus meningo-hypophyseus. Er entspringt der Konvexität der dritten Biegung (Curvatura cavernosa posterior) am Beginn des unteren Siphonschenkels, genau unterhalb der Eintrittstelle des N. oculomotorius. Parkinson fand den Truncus in allen 200 Präparaten (Parkinson, 1964, 1965). Der Stamm soll bei den meisten Individuen nahezu das gleiche Kaliber wie die A. ophthalmica haben. Er verzweigt sich unmittelbar nach dem Abgang in einen tentoriellen Ast, welcher zu den Meningen des Klivus zieht, und in die A. hypophysea inferior. Beide Äste sollen auch in den lateralen Angiogrammen sichtbar sein (Schnürer u. Stattin, 1963).

Der tentorielle Ast des Truncus meningo-hypophyseus zieht nach dorsal und lateral und gibt noch innerhalb des Sinus cavernosus Zweige zum N. oculomotorius und N. trochlearis sowie zum Dach des Sinus cavernosus ab. Er anastomosiert mit den meningealen Ästen der A. ophthalmica sowie meningealen Ästen der A. pharyngea ascendens (Wallace et al., 1967; Djindjian et al., 1968). Er versorgt Teile des Tentoriums und der Falx cerebri und kommuniziert mit dem gleichnamigen Gefäß der Gegenseite. Ähnlich wie andere Duragefäße soll er an einem geschlängelten Verlauf erkennbar sein. Bei einer Länge von über 40 mm soll dies als Hinweis für einen pathologischen Befund gelten, die normale Länge soll zwischen 5 und 35 mm schwanken (Schnürer u. Stattin, 1963). Der zu den Meningen des Klivus ziehende Ast durchquert den hinteren unteren und medialen Abschnitt des Sinus cavernosus (Wallace et al., 1967), verzweigt sich auf dem Dorsum sellae und dem Klivus, anastomosiert mit dem Ast der Gegenseite und sendet einen Zweig zum Nervus abducens. Außerdem besteht eine Kollateralverbindung zur A. meningea posterior und anderen meningealen Ästen der A. vertebralis.

Die A. hypophysea inferior versorgt die Neurohypophyse und die Dura des Sellabodens. Die angiographische Darstellung gelingt, wenn der Karotissiphon das Dorsum sellae nicht verdeckt (Hacker, 1970).

Die A. sinus cavernosi inferior, als zweiter Ast, fand sich in 80% der Präparate Parkinsons (1964). Sie soll etwa 5 mm distal des Truncus meningo-hypophyseus von der lateralen Seite des infraklinoidalen Siphonschenkels entspringen und den Sinus cavernosus und die unteren, angrenzenden Hirnhäute versorgen. Endverzweigungen ziehen zum Ganglion Gasseri. Kollateralverbindungen mit der A. meningica media im Bereich des Foramen spinosum durch das Foramen rotundum und andere kleine Foramina dieser Gegend sowie mit meningealen Ästen der A. ophthalmica werden beschrieben (Margolis u. Newton, 1969).

Etwas weiter distal entspringen die beiden Aa. capsulares (McConnel, 1953), die bei 50% der Untersuchten gefunden wurde. Die untere Kapselarterie geht von der unteren medialen Seite der A. carotis interna ab, läuft medianwärts zur unteren Umhüllung des Hypophysenvorderlappens, anastomosiert mit der A. hypophysea inferior und biegt, wie diese Zweige, zum Sellaboden ab. Die vordere Kapselarterie entspringt an der medialen Seite der A. carotis interna kurz vor dem Durchtritt durch das Diaphragma sellae, zieht ebenfalls medianwärts zum vorderen Rand des Selladaches und anastomosiert mit dem Ast der Gegenseite.

4. Intradurale Äste der A. carotis interna

Außer der A. hypophysea superior (Ferner u. Kautzky, 1959) und mehreren feinen Ästchen, die zusammen mit anderen kleinen Arterien aus der A. cerebri posterior und dem Ramus communicans posterior als „untere Gefäßgruppe" an der Versorgung des Chiasma opticum teilhaben (Bergland u. Ray, 1969), – die entsprechende „obere Gefäßgruppe" besteht aus kleinen Ästen der A. cerebri anterior – handelt es sich vorwiegend um die A. ophthalmica, die A. communicans posterior und die A. choroidea anterior. In diesem Bereich befinden sich auch einige entwicklungsgeschichtliche Besonderheiten, die beim erwachsenen Menschen als Anomalie anzusehen sind, (A. primitiva trigemina, Rete mirabilis, s.u.).

Die A. ophthalmica

Ihr Abgang erfolgt unmittelbar nach dem Durchbruch der A. carotis interna durch das Diaphragma sellae im zisternalen Segment und der Konvexität des Siphonknies, und zwar meist an der medialen Seite des Gefäßes (DECKER, 1955; LENZI, 1955). Sie tritt mit dem N. opticus, an dessen lateraler oder medio-basaler Seite liegend, durch den Canalis opticus des Os sphenoidale in die Orbita, zieht unter leichten Windungen um den N. opticus zur medialen Orbitawand, zur Mitte des nasalen Augenwinkels, wo die Aufteilung in die divergierenden Endäste, die A. supratrochlearis und A. dorsalis nasi, erfolgt. Während ihres schraubenförmigen Verlaufs um den N. opticus gibt sie zahlreiche Äste ab, die in eine okuläre und eine orbitale Gruppe eingeteilt werden. Häufige Anastomosen der orbitalen Gruppe zu Ästen der A. carotis externa bestehen zwischen den Aa. musculares mit der A. infraorbitalis, den Aa. ethmoidales anterior und posterior mit Rami meningici, den Aa. palpebrales superior und inferior mit Ästen der A. temporalis superficialis und A. infraorbitalis der Aa. frontales media und lateralis mit Ästen der A. temporalis superficialis, der A. dorsalis nasi mit der A. angularis, der A. lacrimalis mit der A. meningica media (KRAYENBÜHL u. YASARGIL, 1965; NEWTON u. POTTS, 1974). Diese Anastomosen erscheinen, insbesondere bei Tumoren im Bereich der Orbitae, der vorderen Schädelbasis, der vorderen Schädelgrube sowie bei Verschluß der A. carotis interna im Angiogramm dilatiert. Die übrigen Aufzweigungen der A. ophthalmica kommen, insbesondere in den seitlichen angiographischen Bildern, sehr gut zur Abbildung, vor allem wenn auf die Darstellbarkeit dieses Gefäßbereichs besondere Rücksicht genommen wird (Wahl von Belichtungswerten für den Gesichtsschädel, Subtraktion der Angiogramme, Vergrößerungstechnik). In den übrigen Übersichtsangiogrammen soll sie bei 75 bis 98% der Fälle nachweisbar sein (CURRY u. CULBRETH, 1951; TARTARINI u. GUIGNI, 1955; TÖNNIS u. SCHIEFER, 1959; DECKER, 1955; DILENGE et al., 1961; DALY u. POTTS, 1963; WHEELER u. BAKER, 1964; KRAYENBÜHL u. YASARGIL, 1965), geringfügig häufiger bei Punktion der A. carotis interna. Der Aderhautplexus des Auges wird nach DALY und POTTS (1963) in 37%, nach WHEELER und BAKER (1964) in 54% und nach KRAYENBÜHL und YASARGIL (1965) in 51% dargestellt (zitiert nach KRAYENBÜHL u. YASARGIL, 1965). Man kann in den seitlichen Angiogrammen den parallel unter dem Planum sphenoidale leicht aszendierenden Verlauf von meist 1–1,5 cm Länge, das Ansteigen zum Orbitadach und den bogigen Verlauf oberhalb des Bulbus gut differenzieren, die äußeren Gefäßanteile die Aa. palpebrales frontales und dorsales nasi sollen in unter 5% der Angiogramme nachweisbar sein (KRAYENBÜHL u. YASARGIL, 1965). In der üblichen a-p Projektion wird der Anfangsabschnitt der A. ophthalmica durch die A. carotis interna oder die frontobasalen Gefäße verdeckt. KRAYENBÜHL und YASARGIL konnten die A. ophthalmica in 32% der Fälle gut abgrenzen. Bei Orbita-Projektion und leichter Drehung des Kopfes zur Seite soll das Gefäß in der Angiographie immer gut abgegrenzt werden können.

A. communicans posterior

Sie entspringt am Ende des oberen Siphonschenkels an der Grenze zwischen dem C2- und C1-Segment, zieht innerhalb der basalen Zisterne über den Rand des Diaphragma sellae zwischen der Sella und dem Tuber cinereum okzipitalwärts in Richtung des freien Tentoriumrandes und ist dem N. oculomotorius an dessen Medialseite unmittelbar benachbart. Das Gefäß schließt den hinteren Bogen des Circulus arteriosus cerebri und verbindet das Karotissystem mit dem vertebro-basilären Gefäßsystem. Auf seinem kurzen Verlauf werden funktionell wichtige Arteriolen zum Chiasma, dem N. oculomotorius und zum Hirnstamm abgegeben. Die Variationen betreffen vor allem Kaliber und Verlauf und demonstrieren den Endstand der embryonalen Individualentwicklung einer sehr variantenreichen Gefäßverbindung. Das Kaliber kann von mehreren Millimetern, wobei die Arterie im Lumen stärker sein kann als die A. cerebri posterior, bis zur hochgradigen Hypoplasie schwanken. Meist nimmt das Kaliber des Gefäßes in der embryonalen Entwicklung und noch im Kindesalter allmählich ab, so daß ein starkes Kaliber bei Erwachsenen wesentlich seltener als bei Feten oder Säuglingen gefunden wird (DE VRIESE, 1905; PADGET, 1945).

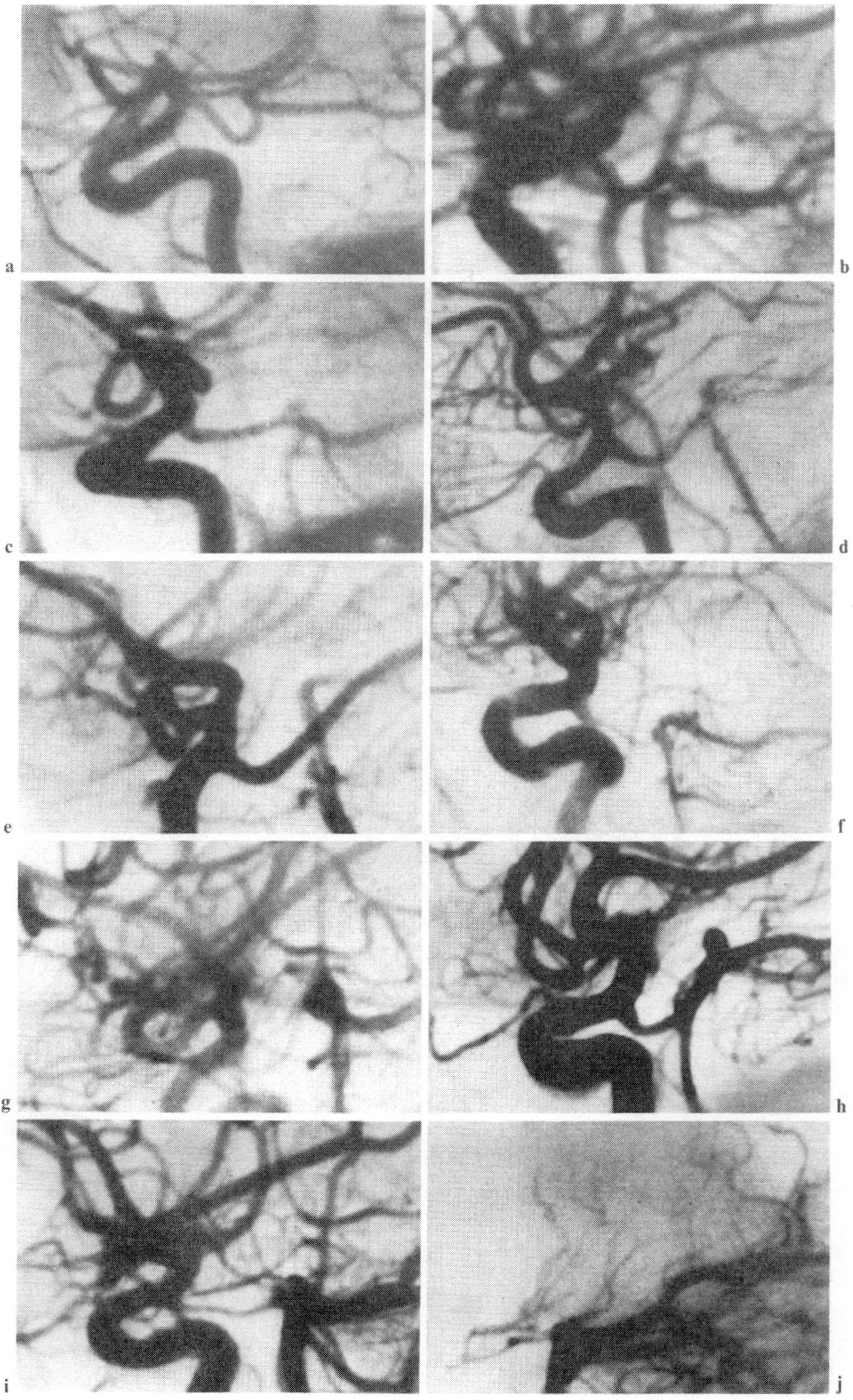
a
b
c
d
e
f
g
h
i
j

Die Arterie soll in 3–11% der Fälle einseitig, in 0,3–1,5% der Fälle doppelseitig fehlen. Sie war häufig Objekt eingehender anatomischer Untersuchungen (WINDLE, 1888; STOPFORD, 1916; FETTERMAN u. MORAN, 1941; PADGET, 1954; MITTERWALLNER, 1955; KRAYENBÜHL u. YASARGIL, 1957; WELLS, 1960; HASSLER u. SALTZMAN, 1963). Angiographisch kann das Gefäß in den seitlichen Projektionen gut, in den a-p Projektionen nur bei halbaxialem Strahlengang dargestellt werden. Die Füllung gelingt sowohl im Karotisangiogramm, besonders bei Interna-Punktion, als auch im Vertebralisangiogramm, hier häufiger bei Kompression einer A. carotis interna (SALTZMAN, 1963).

Die Darstellung ist bei Kindern häufiger. Der Abgang kann sich trichterförmig ektatisch darstellen und die Form eines Infundibulums bilden (SALTZMAN, 1959). Diese Veränderung ist im höheren Alter häufiger (HASSLER u. SALTZMAN, 1963; KRAYENBÜHL u. YASARGIL, 1965; WOLLSCHLAEGER u. WOLLSCHLAEGER, 1974). Der Verlauf kann gestreckt, nach kranial oder kaudal konkav ansteigen oder gewellt bzw. geknickt sein.

Weitere Angaben finden sich bei der Besprechung der A. cerebri posterior. Die Äste der A. communicans anterior werden im Kapitel über die subkortikalen Gefäße der Äste der A. carotis interna beschrieben, ebenso die A. choroidea anterior, die als letzter Ast der A. carotis interna wenige Millimeter oder unmittelbar distal der A. communicans posterior im supraklinoidalen Abschnitt entspringt.

IV. A. cerebri anterior

1. Verlauf

Die A. cerebri anterior ist der mediale Ast der Carotis interna-Gabel. Sie geht vom supraklinoidalen Abschnitt der A. carotis interna, etwa in Höhe des Processus clinoideus anterior, ab. Eingehende Untersuchungen beschäftigten sich schon frühzeitig, aber auch bis in die jüngste Zeit mit ihrem Verhalten in normalen und pathologischen anatomischen Präparaten, im Angiogramm sowie mit den kortikalen und subkortikalen Versorgungsarealen. Als wesentliche Autoren können genannt werden: HEUBNER (1872), WINDLE (1888), CAVATORTI (1904), BLACKBURN (1907), BEEVOR (1908), AYER und AITKEN (1909), SHELLSHEAR (1920), FOIX und HILLEMAND (1925), CRITCHLEY (1930), E. FISCHER (1938), ALEXANDER (1942), WORINGER und GERNEZ (1948), CURRY und CULBRETH (1951), LINDGREN (1954), LAZORTHES et al. (1955–1961), MITTERWALLNER (1955), KAPLAN (1956, 1973, 1975), ANDERSON (1958, 1963), TÖNNIS und SCHIEFER (1959), OSTROWSKI et al. (1960), DILENGE und CONSTANS (1963), WESTBERG (1963, 1964, 1966), WILSON (1963), KRAYENBÜHL und YASARGIL (1965), KAPLAN und FORD (1966), LAZORTHES und SALAMON (1971), FARNARIER (1972), PERCHERON (1973), LIN und KRICHEFF (1974), MARINO (1974), WADDINGTON (1974), GEORGE et al. (1975), LAZORTHES et al. (1975), RING (1975) und SALAMON et al. (1975). Weiterhin praktikabel ist die Einteilung der A. cerebri anterior in 5 Abschnitte nach FISCHER (1938; A1 bis A5) im einzelnen: Pars praecommunicalis (A1), gegenüber der Pars postcommunicalis (A2 bis A5): Pars ascendens (A2 bis A3), Pars horizontalis dorsalis (A4 bis A5). Im Bereich der Pars praecommunicalis werden subkortikale, im Bereich der Pars postcommunicalis kortikale Äste abgegeben. Eine eigene Stellung nimmt die A. communicans anterior ein.

◀ **Abb. 4a–j.** Formen der A. communicans posterior. Direkter Abgang der A. cerebri posterior von der A. carotis interna **a–c**, **e** (fehlende Pars basilaris der A. communicans posterior). Kräftige A. communicans posterior mit Anschluß an die Basilarisgabel **d**, **f**, **h**. Infundibuläre Erweiterung des Abganges von der A. carotis interna **d**, **h**, **i**. Je nach Siphon, flache Verlaufsform **a**, **b**, **c**, **i**, **j** oder ausgeprägt basalwärts konvexbogiger Verlauf **g**, **h**, selbst bei fehlender Pars basilaris **e**. Filiforme Darstellung **j**, dennoch gute Füllung der von der A. communicans posterior abgehenden Rr. thalamoperforatae

2. Pars praecommunicalis (A1)

Gleichbedeutend werden die Ausdrücke Pars circularis, Pars horizontalis oder Pars chiasmatis gebraucht. Die Pars praecommunicalis ist das mediale Stück der T-förmigen Carotis interna-Gabel bis zum Abgang der A. communicans anterior. Sie verläuft oberhalb des Processus clinoideus anterior nach medial und rostralwärts gerichtet zwischen dem Chiasma opticum und dem Trigonum olfactorium, entlang der Stria olfactoria medialis, bis unmittelbar an die Lamina terminalis, wo die A. communicans anterior abgeht (KRAYENBÜHL u. YASARGIL, 1965). Im Angiogramm kann der Verlauf des Gefäßabschnitts horizontal, aufsteigend oder absteigend sein, entsprechend einer T-, V- oder Pilzform der Internagabel. Ausgeprägte Pilzform leitet zu den Gefäßprozessen (Elongation und Schlängelung) über.

Die mäßig ausgeprägten Verlaufsvarianten zeigen eine gewisse Altersabhängigkeit (KRAYENBÜHL u. YASARGIL, 1965). Kaliber-Seitendifferenzen sind häufig. Hypoplasie einer Pars praecommunicalis wird selten (WINDLE (1888) 1%, KRAYENBÜHL u. YASARGIL (1965) 4%, BLACKBURN (1907) 8%, CAVATORTI (1904) 11%, MITTERWALLNER (1955) 15%) beobachtet. Die Aplasie wird noch seltener gefunden (0,3 bis 1,3%; CURRY u. CULBRETH, 1951; MITTERWALLNER, 1955; TÖNNIS u. SCHIEFER, 1959; KRAYENBÜHL u. YASARGIL, 1965). Bei fehlender oder nur sehr schmächtig angelegter Pars praecommunicalis kann im Karotisangiogramm der gleichen Seite die Füllung der A. cerebri anterior vollständig ausbleiben. Im kontralateralen Karotisangiogramm stellen sich dann meist beide vorderen Hirnarterien dar. Sehr seltene Varianten sind die Verdoppelung oder Inselbildung der A. cerebri anterior, die von BUSSE (1921) und MITTERWALLNER (1955) beschrieben wurden. Die Fusion der beiden vorderen Hirnarterien, anstelle einer A. communicans anterior oder über eine längere Strecke als gemeinsamer A. cerebri anterior-Stamm (WINDLE, 1888; MONIZ, 1940; CURRY u. CULBRETH, 1951), wird eher den Normvarianten des Anfangsteils der Pars postcommunicalis zuzurechnen sein. Im Angiogramm ist der Verlauf der Pars praecommunicalis im a-p Strahlengang ein wichtiger Indikator für die frontobasalen und suprasellären topographischen Verhältnisse. Im seitlichen Strahlengang wird der Gefäßabschnitt, außer bei erheblichen Verlagerungen oder Schleifenbildungen, im wesentlichen orthograd getroffen. Ausgeprägte Schleifen sind, gegenüber säckchenförmigen Aneurysmen, oft nur durch Spezialaufnahmen (Schrägserie, stereoskopische Aufnahmen, Angiotomographie) zu differenzieren.

Selten geht aus der A. praecommunicalis eine A. frontalis inferior bzw. fronto-orbitalis medialis als gemischter, dienzephaler und kortikaler Ast ab. Im übrigen nehmen nur die Aa. perforantes (A. centralis brevis bzw. diencephalica und A. centralis longa bzw. A. recurrens HEUBNER, 1872) ihren Ursprung in diesem Segment. Sie werden an anderer Stelle im Zusammenhang besprochen.

3. Pars postcommunicalis (A2 bis A5)

Die ersten beiden Abschnitte (A2 und A3) bilden die Pars ascendens der A. cerebri anterior. Die Segmente beider Seiten liegen paramedian, unmittelbar nebeneinander, in der Cisterna corporis callosi, mit Kontakt zur medianen Hemisphärenfläche, nur wenige Millimeter von der Lamina terminalis entfernt.

Der ventral-konvexe Bogen (A2) umschließt die Regio par-olfactoria und geht in Höhe des Rostrum corporis callosi in einen dorsalkonvexen Bogen über. Als Grenze beider Segmente wird der Scheitelpunkt des dorsal-konvexen Bogens mit dem Abgang der A. frontopolaris angenommen, wogegen die A. frontobasalis im Verlauf der A2-Strecke nach fronto-basal und lateral zieht. Die Variabilität dieses Gefäßabschnitts in der angiographischen Darstellung ist relativ groß. In den a-p Projektionen kann ein wellenförmiges Ausschwingen um die Mittellinie um 2–10 mm (KRAYENBÜHL u. YASARGIL, 1965), besonders der A2-Strecke, beobachtet werden. In den seitlichen Bildern ist die oben beschriebene zweifache Biegung großen Schwankungen unterworfen. Die „physiologische Konkavität", also der dorsalkonvexe Bogen von A2 und A3, kann

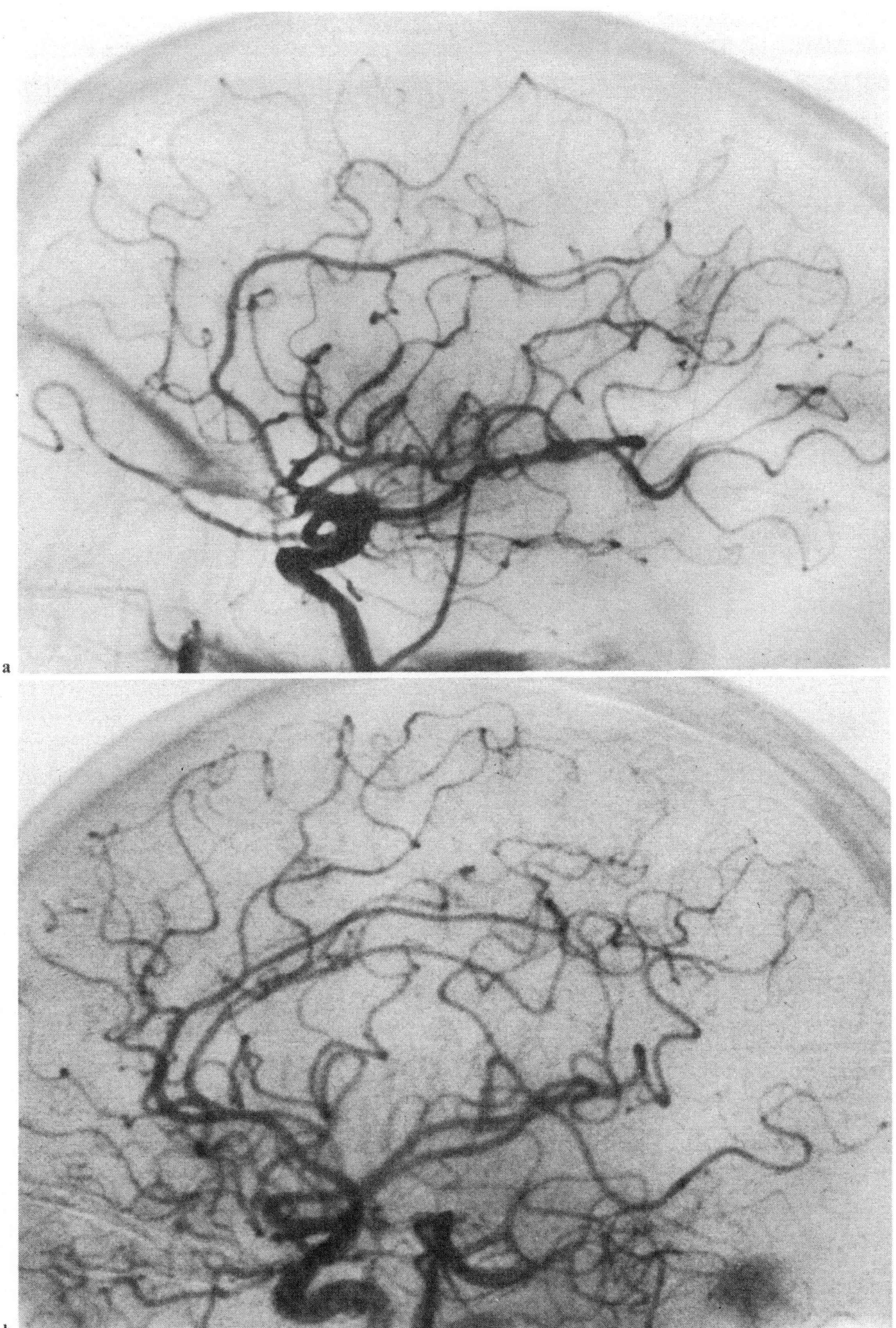

Abb. 5a u. b (Legende s. nächste Seite)

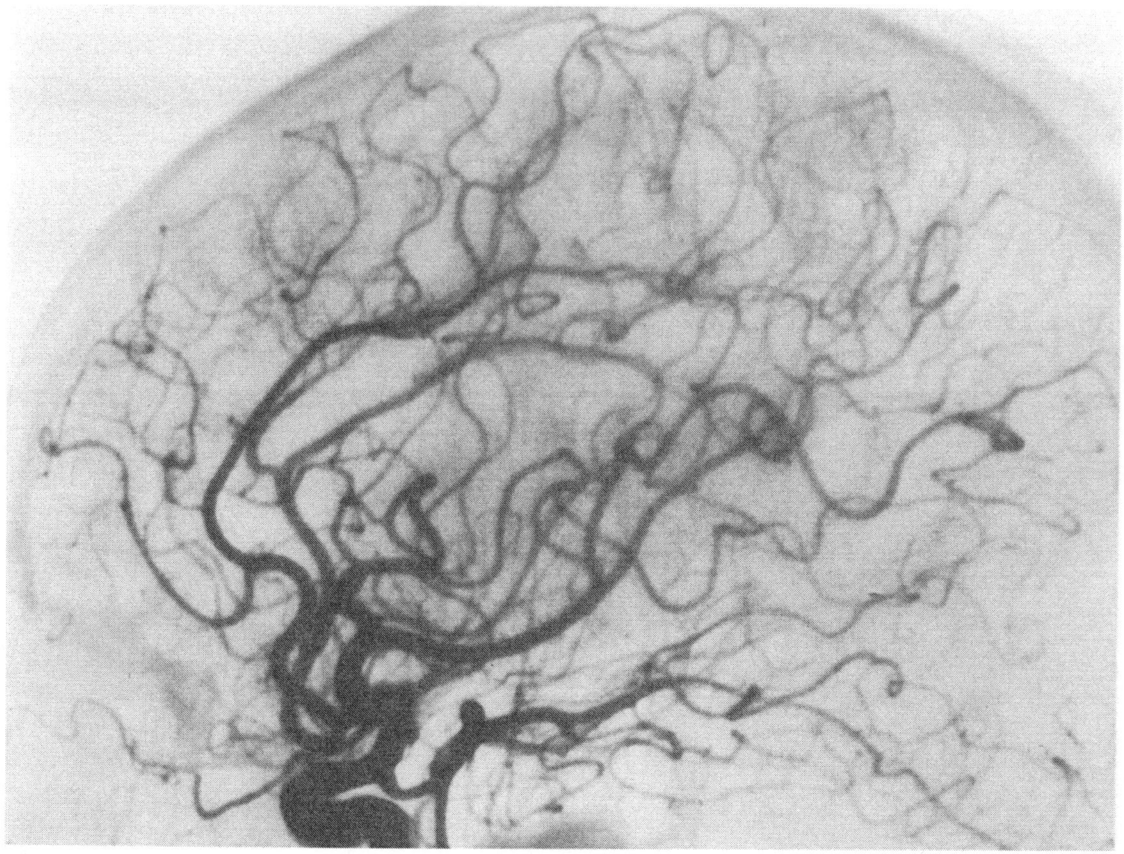

Abb. 5a–c. Verlauf und Aufteilung der A. cerebri anterior. Gefäßbild bei Dolichozephalie **a**, bei normozephaler Schädelkonfiguration **b** und bei Turrizephalie **c**. Stark unterschiedlicher Verlauf der A. cerebri anterior beider Seiten bei Schädelasymmetrie **c** und unterschiedliche Höhe der Aufteilung

völlig fehlen (BONNAL u. LEGRE (1958) in 35%). Gelegentlich kann ein völlig gestreckter, fast geradliniger Verlauf dieser Segmente mit wimpelartigen Abgängen der kortikalen Äste (KRAYENBÜHL u. YASARGIL, 1965 in 0,2%), unabhängig von der Altersverteilung, beobachtet werden. Bei sehr starker Ausprägung des dorsalkonvexen Bogens kann, besonders bei Kindern, die Abgrenzung gegen eine fronto-basale Raumforderung notwendig werden. Bei LINDGREN (1954) wird die Pars horizontalis als A. cerebri anterior, die Pars ascendens bereits als A. pericallosa bezeichnet, was sich jedoch nicht allgemein eingeführt hat.

Pars horizontalis dorsalis (A4 bis A5)

Nachdem meist noch im A3-Segment ein zweiter ventralkonvexer Bogen um das Balkenknie beschrieben wird, liegt die A. cerebri anterior im Bereich des A4- und A5-Segments, der Oberseite des Balkens im Sulcus corporis callosi, im Verlauf bis an das Splenium eng an. Die Abschnitte werden nach FISCHER (1938) in das frontale Segment A4 und das parietale Segment A5, durch eine Frontalebene durch den Scheitelpunkt der Kranznaht, unterteilt. Nach Abgang der A. callosum marginalis aus dem Bereich des Balkenknies wird der Hauptstamm des Gefäßes im allgemeinen als A. pericallosa bezeichnet. Im A5-Segment wird schließlich die A. frontalis posterior oder A. parietalis interna (der A. cerebri anterior) abgegeben. In beiden Segmenten werden kleinere horizontale Äste nach lateral zur Balkenoberseite und vertikale Äste zum Gyrus cinguli abgegeben, die in den a-p Projektionen der Angiogramme den Sulcus longitudinalis corporis collosi in Form eines Schnurrbarts sichtbar erscheinen lassen (HUANG u. WOLF, 1964 in 17% der Fälle).

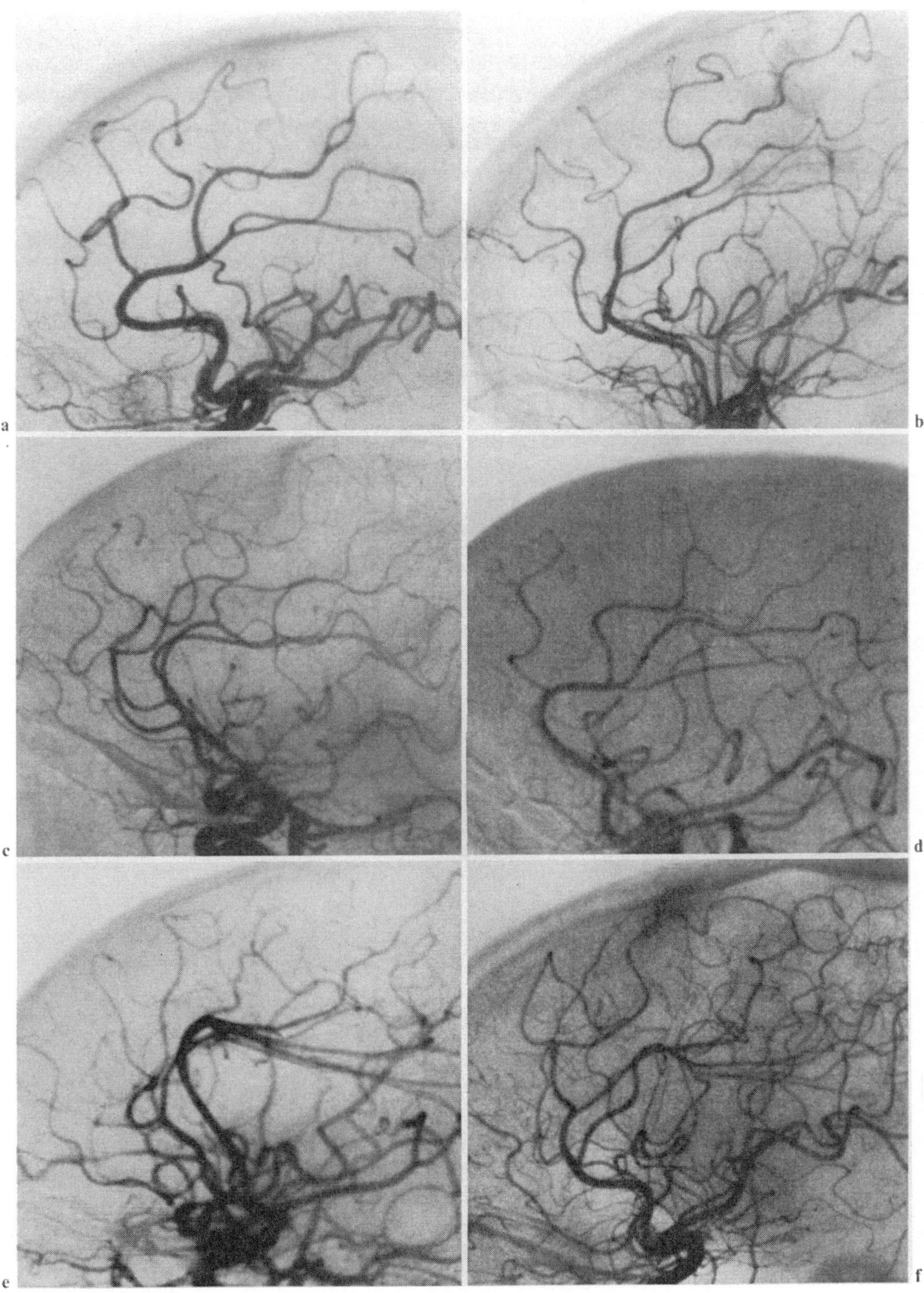

Abb. 6a–f. Verlauf und Aufteilung der A. cerebri anterior. Ausgeprägter Stamm der A. cerebri anterior mit tangential abgehenden kaliberschwächeren Ästen. Kräftige A. calloso-marginalis, die das Kaliber der A. pericallosa übersteigt **a**, frühe Aufteilung in A. pericallosa und A. calloso-marginalis **b**, nahezu symmetrisch auf beiden Seiten **c**, Trifurkation des Anteriorstammes **d**, ungeteilter Anteriorstamm **e** bis zur fächerförmigen Aufteilung und deszendierender Perikallosaverlauf (keine Raumforderung), weniger ausgeprägt, jedoch auch mit fächerförmiger Teilung der A. pericallosa **f**

Die A. calloso-marginalis im Anfangsabschnitt und die A. pericallosa haben enge Beziehungen zur Falx cerebri, deren Variationen vorwiegend durch die A. pericallosa angiographisch dokumentiert werden (Abstand über dem Balkenknie durchschnittlich 10 mm, über dem Splenium corporis callosi 1–3 mm). In den a-p Projektionen der Angiogramme sollen in 18% der Fälle (KRAYENBÜHL u. YASARGIL, 1965) bzw. in 25% der Fälle (DILENGE, 1962) durch Anastomosen der A. pericallosa und calloso-marginalis, unter der Falx zur Mittellinie die parietalen Äste der Gegenseite zur Darstellung kommen. Die Variationen dieser Segmente sind natürlich in den seitlichen angiographischen Bildern deutlicher. Sie umfassen Abgangsvarianten, wie die frühe oder späte Aufteilung in die A. calloso marginalis und A. pericallosa, bei früher Aufteilung dementsprechend Abgang der A. frontopolaris oder auch frontobasalis von der A. calloso marginalis usw, Verlaufsvarianten mit ventralkonvexen Schleifen, zeltförmigem Ansteigen oder steilem Abstieg der A. pericallosa oder frühzeitige Aufteilung der kortikalen Äste im hinteren Balkenbereich. Die Variationen sind bei KRAYENBÜHL und YASARGIL (1965) im einzelnen in ihrer Häufigkeit beschrieben und schematisch dargestellt.

4. Kortikale Äste

Die kortikalen Äste der A. cerebri anterior lassen sich nach KRAYENBÜHL und YASARGIL (1965) einteilen in

A. frontobasalis (synonym A. frontoorbitalis, A. frontalis (medialis) inferior),
A. frontopolaris (synonym A. frontalis anterior (interna)),
A. calloso-marginalis (synonym A. frontalis medialis) mit Aufteilung in die A. praefrontalis (A. frontalis medialis interna) und A. cingularis (A. frontalis posterior interna),
A. pericallosa,
A. frontalis posterior (synonym A. parietalis interna oder A. parietalis posterior) mit Aufteilung in die A. praecentralis, A. praecunea und A. parietooccipitalis (medialis).

Französische Autorengruppen, z.B. um SALAMON (MOSCOW et al., 1974; RAYBAUD et al., 1975) bevorzugen die Einteilung in

A. orbitofrontalis,
A. frontopolaris,
A. frontalis interna anterior,
A. frontalis interna media,
A. frontalis interna posterior,
A. paracentralis,
A. parietalis interna superior,
A. parietalis interna inferior.

Im A2-Segment entspringt die A. frontobasalis von der A. cerebri anterior. Sie kann jedoch auch von der A. frontopolaris oder der A. calloso-marginalis abgegeben werden. Sie verläuft parallel zum Bulbus olfactorius, nahe der basalen Mantelkante, nach rostralwärts und versorgt die mediobasale („orbitale") Fläche des Stirnhirns. Die A. frontopolaris zieht nach schräg oben und rostralwärts um die Mantelkante des Stirnpoles, wo die Endverzweigungen, wie auch bei den nachfolgenden kortikalen Gefäßen, die Hirnkonvexität etwa ein bis zwei Querfinger breit umgreifen.

Die A. calloso-marginalis kann, nach Abgang im Bereich des Balkenknies, parallel zur A. pericallosa bzw. zum Hauptstamm im Sulcus cinguli verlaufen. Ihre Endäste biegen noch vor der Balkenmitte kranialwärts und versorgen die mediale Fläche des Stirnhirns bis zum oberen Anteil des Gyrus centralis.

Die A. frontalis posterior, im A4- oder A5-Segment entspringend, zieht nach dorsal und schräg aufwärts zu den dorsalen Stirnhirn- und vorderen Parietalhirnanteilen, vor allem zum Bereich des Gyrus praecentralis und Anteilen des Praecuneus. In der Fissura parieto-occipitalis werden häufig Anastomosen mit den kortikalen Endästen der A. cerebri posterior gefunden.

Die kortikalen Endäste selbst weisen, relativ unabhängig von den häufigen Variationen der Hauptäste, was den Verlauf, die Aufteilung, mögliche Duplikationen, Triplikationen einzelner Gefäße betrifft (BAPTISTA, 1963), eine weitgehende Formenkonstanz auf. In den seitlichen angiographischen Bildern können sie immer identifiziert werden (RAYBAUD et al., 1975).

A. communicans anterior

Die vordere Verbindung im Circulus arteriosus cerebri (Willisi), mit einer Länge von 0,1–3 mm die kürzeste zerebrale Arterie (KRAYENBÜHL u. YASARGIL, 1965), weist eine besonders große Formvariation auf, die von DE ALMEIDA (1931) eingehend untersucht wurde. Er unterscheidet 20 verschiedene Ausprägungsformen als Endzustände einer individuellen embryonalen Entwicklung. Eine Schematisierung in Hauptgruppen ist nach einzelnen Merkmalen, wie doppelte Anlage, Winkelbildung in V- oder Y-Form, netzförmige Ausbildung, dünne, langgezogene Gefäßanlage, kurze weitlumige Verbindung usw., vorgenommen worden. MITTERWALLNER (1955) findet bei 360 Präparaten in 0,3% der Fälle keine A. communicans anterior. Angiographisch wird das Gefäß im allgemeinen nicht dargestellt. Es läßt sich wegen seines kurzen Verlaufes oft nur schwer abgrenzen. Meist sind es technische Faktoren, wie Überdruck bei der Injektion, besondere Strömungsverhältnisse während der Gefäßdarstellung, veränderte Druckgradienten durch Gefäßkompression oder Gefäßverschlüsse oder ein hypoplastisches präkommunikales Anteriorsegment der Gegenseite, die durch eine Füllung beider Aa. cerebri anteriores bei der Angiographie das Vorhandensein der A. communicans anterior dokumentieren. Oft ist die Darstellung zum Nachweis oder Ausschluß eines säckchenförmigen Aneurysmas erforderlich, da die Arterie einen der hauptsächlichen Ursprungsorte dieser Anomalien darstellt. In den a-p Aufnahmen ist, durch Kopflagerung bzw. Änderung der Projektionsrichtung, die Darstellung aus verschiedenen Blickwinkeln möglich, während das Gefäß in den seitlichen Aufnahmen orthograd projiziert wird. Die Arterie kann, je nach Verlauf der Gabel der Arteria carotis interna, schon vor der Höhe des Processus clinoideus anterior, bis zur Mitte des Planum sphenoidale liegen. Auch der Abstand von der Frontobasis kann zwischen einigen Millimetern und 3 cm schwanken (KRAYENBÜHL u. YASARGIL, 1965). Eine fehlende Darstellung bei Karotisangiographie beider Seiten, mit jeweiliger Kompression der Carotis interna der Gegenseite, kann die Vermutung einer Hypoplasie oder fehlenden Anlage des Gefäßes unterstützen, beweist sie jedoch nicht, da sie viel häufiger z.B. bei sackförmigen Aneurysma- oder anderen pathologischen Befunden (6 bis 8,2% nach KRAYENBÜHL u. YASARGIL (1965), 7,1% nach SEDZIMIR (1959) auftritt, als eine Aplasie zu erwarten ist (unter 1%).

5. Äste der A. communicans anterior

Die A. communicans anterior gibt mehrere sehr feine Aa. perforantes zum Diencephalon ab, außerdem gelegentlich eine A. cerebralis anterior media (synonym A. corporis callosi superior oder A. mediana corporis callosi), die nach DE VRIESE (1907) auch in der menschlichen Embryonalentwicklung regelmäßig, zumindest passager, angelegt ist und einer unpaaren, vorderen Hirnarterie der Säugetiere entsprechen soll. WINDLE (1888) beschrieb sie in bis zu 4,5% der Fälle seiner anatomischen Präparate. Bei den anderen Autoren (BLACKBURN, 1907; ADACHI, 1929; DE ALMEIDA, 1931; MITTERWALLNER, 1955) wurde das Gefäß in bis zu 10% der Fälle beobachtet. LAZORTHES (1961) fand es in einem relativ kleinen Beobachtungsgut von 35 Sektionen sogar in 20%. Er unterscheidet langes, mittellanges oder kurzes Gefäß und bringt die persistierende Anlage mit der Hypoplasie oder Aplasie einer A. cerebri anterior in Verbindung. Die angiographische Darstellung des Gefäßes ist schwierig. Abbildungen finden sich bei CURRY und CULBRETH (1951) sowie bei KRAYENBÜHL und YASARGIL (1965). Sichere Angaben über die Häufigkeit dieser Arterie in den Angiogrammen sind wegen der relativ seltenen Beobachtung wohl noch nicht möglich.

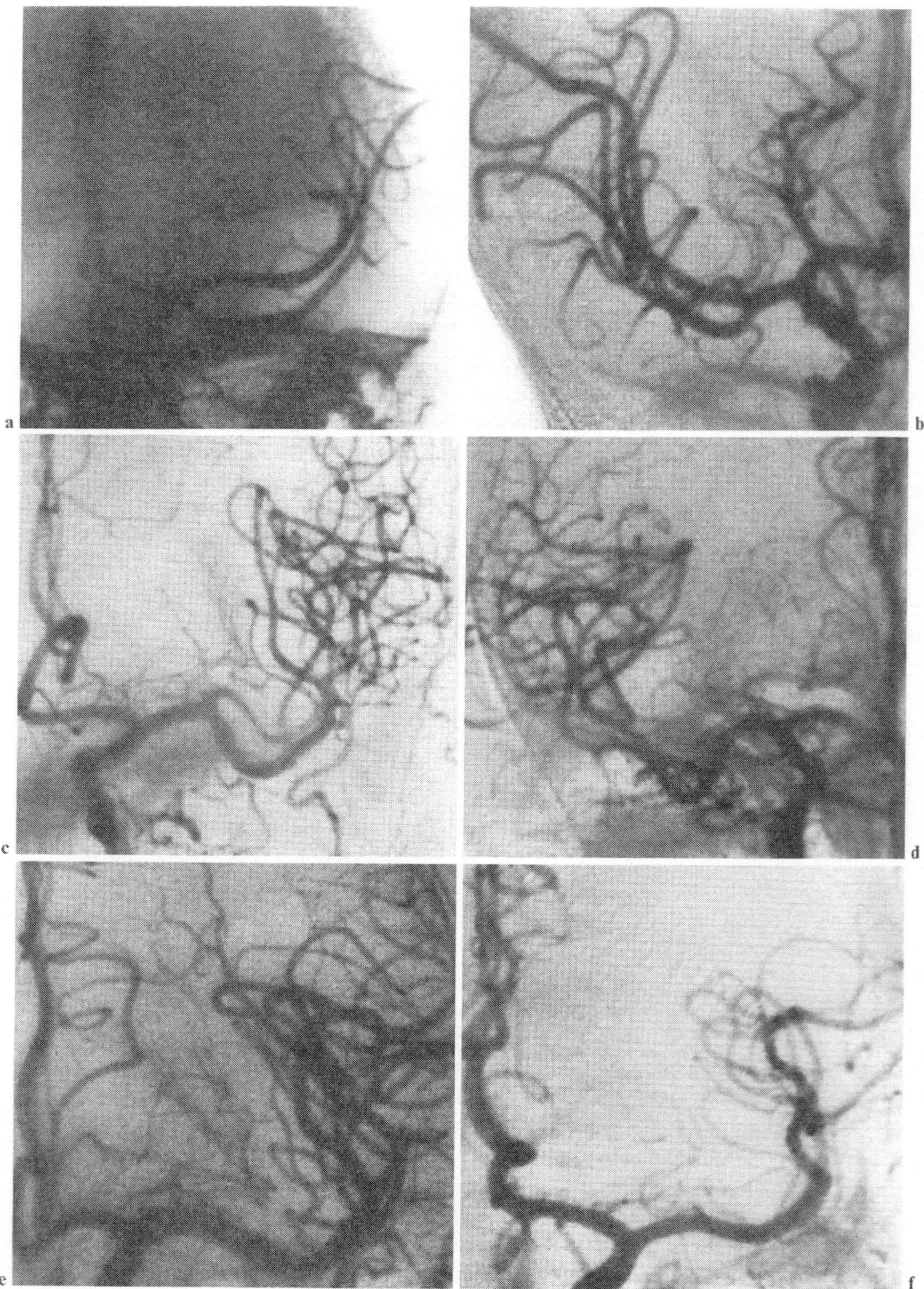

Abb. 7a–g. Aufteilung der A. cerebri media. Sehr frühe Bifurkation **a**, **b**, Bifurkation, Trifurkation im mittleren Keilbeinabschnitt **c**, **d**, späte Mediateilung am Übergang zur Inselschwelle **e**, **f**, ungleicher Teilungstyp im Karotisangiogramm beider Seiten **g**

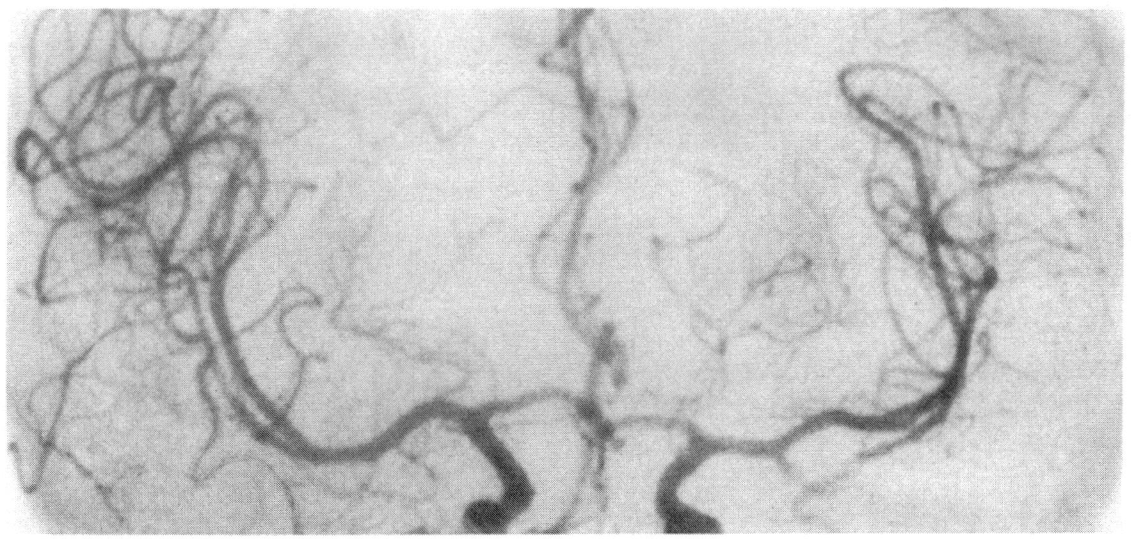

Fig. 7g

V. A. cerebri media

1. Stamm

Die A. cerebri media, als stärkster Ast der A. carotis interna, wird als ihre direkte Fortsetzung angesehen. Die Einteilung erfolgt üblicherweise in 5 Abschnitte (M1 bis M5, analog zur Einteilung der Segmente der A. cerebri anterior bei FISCHER, 1938). Die Abschnitte werden auch als Pars sphenoidalis (Keilbeinabschnitt), Pars insularis (Inselabschnitt), Pars opercularis und Pars terminalis (Endaufzweigungen) bezeichnet. Diese Unterscheidung ist sowohl nach anatomischen wie angiographischen Kriterien möglich. Die Äste können in kortikale und zentrale Arterien (zu den Basalganglien) eingeteilt werden.

2. Pars sphenoidalis

Die Pars sphenoidalis (M1) ist der Verlauf des Gefäßes vom Abgang horizontal auf dem Keilbeinflügel nach lateral und etwas nach dorsalwärts gerichtet bis zur Inselgrenze. Je nach der individuellen Gefäßentwicklung, in Anpassung an die Schädelform und durch sekundäre Veränderungen (arteriosklerotische Elongation) kann der Bogen der sphenoidalen Verlaufsstrecke sehr unterschiedliche Formen aufweisen; mitbestimmt durch die Mediateilungsstelle, die die Form einer Bifurkation oder Trifurkation haben kann und deren Lage zwischen Abgang der A. cerebri media und dem Inselgebiet sehr variabel ist, einschließlich asymmetrischer Verhältnisse beider Aa. cerebri mediae bei *einem* Individuum (statistische Angaben über Formvarianten bei KRAYENBÜHL u. YASARGIL, 1965). Eine frühe Teilung (Pseudobifurkation) kann durch den Abgang der A. orbito-frontalis der A. cerebri media vorgetäuscht werden. Die durchschnittliche Länge dieses Segments beträgt, nach HERMAN et al. (1963) und JAIN (1964), 14 bis 16 mm (5–30 mm). Außer der A. orbito-frontalis, die nach KRAYENBÜHL und YASARGIL (1965) in 6% der Fälle nachzuweisen ist, gehen in diesem Segment nur zentrale Äste zum Hirnstamm ab, die an anderer Stelle gemeinsam behandelt werden. Bei stark medialem Abgang kann die A. fronto-orbitalis in a-p Projektion einen ähnlichen Verlauf wie die A. ophthalmica aufweisen. Bis etwa zur Pubertät verläuft die A. cerebri media schon im Keilbeinabschnitt mehr oder weniger stark nach lateral ansteigend.

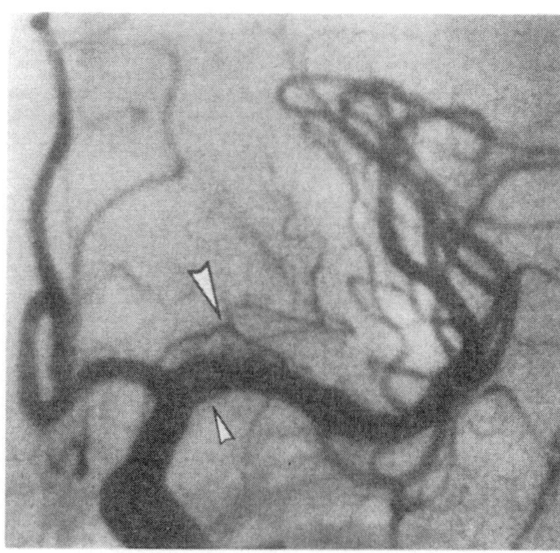

Abb. 8. Fenestration der A. cerebri media im Keilbeinabschnitt. ▷ Kräftige Darstellung der A. choroidea anterior in ap Projektion. Seltene, klinisch nicht relevante Variante, die gegen Schleifenbildung bei frühzeitiger Teilung des Mediastammes abzugrenzen ist.

In etwa 3% fand sich bei autoptischen Untersuchungen von Crompton (1962) und Jain (1964) eine A. cerebri media accessoria, als von der A. cerebri anterior oder von der A. carotis interna nach lateralwärts zur Sylvischen Furche ziehender Ast zur Versorgung der fronto-laterobasalen Hirnabschnitte. In 2 Fällen entstammten diesem Gefäß Aa. perforantes zum Hirnstamm. Eine angiographische Abgrenzung gelang wegen des nahezu kongruenten Verlaufs zum Stamm der A. cerebri media nicht.

3. Pars insularis (M2)

Am Übergang von der Pars sphenoidalis zur Pars insularis teilt sich die A. cerebri media meist in 2, seltener in 3 Hauptäste (9:1; Jain, 1964), die zunächst eine kurze Strecke horizontal verlaufen, um am Limen insulae rechtwinklig nach oben abzuknicken. Die anschließende schlingenförmige Anordnung des Inselgefäßfächers ist entwicklungsgeschichtlich bedingt durch das Einsinken der Inselregion, ab etwa der 4. Fetalwoche, und das Vorschieben des frontalen, parietalen und temporalen Operculums, um deren Ränder geschlungen die kortikalen Endäste der A. cerebri media radiär in einem Kreissegment von 270 Grad, ausstrahlend an der Hirnoberfläche, erscheinen (Villiger u. Ludwig, 1946; Ranson u. Clark, 1948; Ferner u. Kautzky, 1959). Die Aa. insulares (Inselschlingen oder Sylvische Gefäßgruppe) zeigen in Form und Anordnung gewisse Variationen, sind jedoch insgesamt von einer solchen Beständigkeit, daß sie im einzelnen identifiziert werden können (de Almeida, 1931; Dilenge, 1962; Ring, 1963, 1974; Krayenbühl u. Yasargil, 1965; Ring u. Waddington, 1967). Zur besseren Abgrenzung der Varianten der Sylvischen Gefäße von pathologischen Befunden, insbesondere Raumforderungen und Gefäßastverschlüssen, wurden zahlreiche Hilfskonstruktionen mit Linien, Meßfiguren und Schablonen angegeben. Das Knie der A. cerebri media, also die Umschlagstelle zum Inselabschnitt, soll in a-p Projektionen der Angiogramme durchschnittlich etwa 3 cm Abstand zur temporalen Kalotte aufweisen (Chase u. Taveras, 1963). Die arterielle Achse von Moniz (1940) bildet mit einer Geraden durch die Protuberantia occipitalis interna und das Zentrum der Sella einen Winkel zwischen 36 und 49 Grad (Woringer u. Gernez, 1948; Hodes et al., 1953; Ring, 1962). Die Gerade durch das Os incisivum zum Syphonknie in der seitlichen Projektion (Syphon-Inzisivum-Linie, Krayenbühl u. Richter, 1952) wird in ihrer Richtung durch die Sylvische Gefäßgruppe fortgesetzt. Die Klino-Parietal-

Linie nach CHASE und TAVERAS (1963) zwischen dem vorderen Klinoidfortsatz und dem Punkt an der Lamina interna der Kalotte, 2 cm oberhalb der Lambdanaht, wird durch die Sylvischen Gefäße, bei Erwachsenen maximal um 10 mm, bei Kindern maximal um 15 mm, überragt. Das Sylvische Dreieck wird durch die Schlingenreihen der Inselgefäße bestimmt, wobei die oberen Schlingenköpfe der Richtung des Sulcus insularis superior, die tiefere Reihe der Richtung des Sulcus Sylvii entsprechen (SCHLESINGER, 1953; TAVERAS u. WOOD, 1964; 1976; WOLLSCHLAEGER u. WOLLSCHLAEGER, 1964; VLAHOVITCH, 1964). Der am weitesten medial gelegene Schlingenkopf soll nach CHASE und TAVERAS (1963) von der parietotemporalen Kalotte maximal 4,3 cm entfernt sein („angiographic sylvian point“). RAYBAUD et al. (1975) geben durchsichtige Schablonen für die Lokalisation der kortikalen Äste der vorderen und mittleren Hirnarterie an. Weitere topometrische Untersuchungen zur Lage der Mediaäste und der Hirnwindungen finden sich bei MICHOTEY et al. (1975), RING (1975) und WADDINGTON (1975), wogegen SALAMON et al. (1975) die Lokalisation der Fissuren und Sulci des Gehirns nach den Gefäßverläufen orientieren.

4. Pars opercularis (M3)

Es werden damit die Gefäßabschnitte bezeichnet, in welchen sich die Mediaäste mit Verlaufsrichtung nach frontal, parietal, parietookzipital und temporal um die Ränder der Opercula schlingen, wobei im frontalen und parietalen Bereich Schleifenbildungen zustande kommen, im temporalen Bereich meist eine flache lateralwärts gerichtete Biegung. In parietookzipitaler Richtung setzen die Aa. gyri angulares weitgehend geradlinig den Mediaverlauf fort. In der angiographischen a-p Projektion entsprechen die frontalen und parietalen operkulären Äste den aufsteigenden „Kandelaberarterien“; die absteigenden Äste der Sylvischen Gruppe ziehen zum Temporalbereich.

5. Kortikale Äste

Im operkulären Bereich ist die Aufteilung in die Endäste mit kortikalem Verlauf schon weitgehend vollständig. Sie versorgen die Großhirnhemisphären an der Oberfläche. Die Grenzen zu den Versorgungsgebieten der A. cerebri anterior und A. cerebri posterior sind relativ konstant. Es werden folgende Äste unterschieden:

A. orbitofrontalis (synonym: A. frontobasilis lateralis, A. frontalis inferior lateralis)
A. praecentralis (A. praerolandica)
A. centralis (A. rolandica)
A. parietalis anterior
A. parietalis posterior
A. gyri angularis (A. pli curbe)
A. temporalis anterior und media
A. temporalis posterior

Hinzu kommen fast regelmäßig eine A. praefrontalis, eine A. temporo-occipitalis und eine A. temporo-polaris (RAYBAUD et al., 1975), die, wie schon oben erwähnt, von den letzteren Autoren durch eine an knöcherne Fixpunkte des Schädels angelegte durchsichtige Schablone, insbesondere zum Nachweis der Mediaastverschlüsse, bestimmt werden können.

Die Versorgungsgebiete der einzelnen Mediaäste zeigt Tabelle 2. In den angiographischen Bildern kommt es zu vielfältigen Überlagerungen der Mediaäste untereinander sowie mit anderen kortikalen Gefäßen aus der A. cerebri anterior und der A. cerebri posterior. In den a-p Aufnahmen zeigen die temporalen Äste einen horizontalen oder leicht laterobasalwärts gerichteten Verlauf. Die A. gyri angularis liegt lateral der parietalen Kandelabergefäße in einer fast horizontalen lateralkonvexen Biegung. Die terminalen Verzweigungen der A. gyri angularis und der A. parietalis posterior verlaufen tangential, entlang der Tabula interna kranialwärts, bis nahe an die Mittellinie,

Tabelle 2. Versorgungsareale der kortikalen Äste der A. cerebri media zusammengestellt nach Angaben von KRAYENBÜHL und YASARGIL (1965) und RAYBAUD et al. (1975)

	(nach KRAYENBÜHL u. YASARGIL, 1965)	(nach RAYBAUD et al., 1975)
A. orbitofrontalis	G. frontalis med., frontobasale laterale Abschnitte, Pars triangularis des G. frontalis inferior	lateraler Anteil des orbitalen Abschnittes des Frontallappens
A. praefrontalis		Pars opercularis des G. frontalis med. Pars triangularis front., G. frontalis sup., Pars orbitalis inf. (kaudaler Anteil)
A. praecentralis	Operculum des G. frontalis inferior, G. praecentralis außer Mantelkante	hinterster Anteil des G. frontalis inferior, unteres Drittel oder untere Hälfte des G. praecentralis, vorderer Anteil des zentralen Operculum und Ränder des Sulcus praecentralis
A. centralis	G. centralis, Lobulus parietalis superior	(gewöhnlich 2 Arterien) mittleres Drittel des G. praecentralis, G. centralis, Gebiete in der Tiefe des Sulcus praecentralis, unterer Anteil des G. postcentralis
A. parietalis anterior	hinteres Ende des G. frontalis medius, G. centralis	mittlerer Anteil des G. postcentralis (nur A. parietalis anterior) die ersten beiden G. parietales, ein Teil des G. supramarginalis (gemeinsam)
A. parietalis posterior	Lobulus parietalis inferior	
A. gyri angularis	G. angularis, G. marginalis	Teil des G. supramarginalis, größter Teil des G. angularis
A. temporo-occipitalis		unterer Teil des G. angularis, hinterer Anteil des G. temporalis superior, laterale Fläche des Okzipitallappens
A. temporalis anterior	G. temporalis superior und medius	G. temporalis medius und superior (gemeinsam). Die einzelnen Territorien variieren, meist ist ein Gefäß dominant
A. temporalis media	(vorn und Mitte)	
A. temporalis posterior	G. temporalis superior, medius und inferior (hinten)	
A. temporopolaris		Temporalpol. Beitrag zur Vaskularisation des Uncus zusammen mit Ästen der A. cerebri posterior

wo es zu Überlagerungen mit den Endverzweigungen der A. pericallosa und A. marginalis kommt. Gleichzeitig projiziert sich in diese Region die allerdings stark geschlängelte A. meningica media (Ramus posterior) und A. occipitalis externa. In den lateralen Projektionen ziehen die A. temporalis anterior und A. temporalis media weitgehend in Richtung der Gefäßachse nach dorsal und überlagern die Anfangsstrecke der A. gyri angularis. Die A. temporalis posterior steigt nach kaudal S-förmig ab und kann sich mit dem Anfangsabschnitt der A. cerebri posterior überlagern. Sie soll gelegentlich als Ast der A. gyri angularis oder A. parietalis posterior entspringen. Kranial von ihr, in fast paralleler Richtung, kann die A. temporo-occipitalis verlaufen. Vor der A. temporalis anterior mit steilem, basalwärts gerichtetem Verlauf ist die A. temporopolaris abgrenzbar. Die A. praecentralis und A. centralis enden vor der Mantelkante. Die parietalen Arterien überlagern sich, besonders bei steilem absteigendem Verlauf der A. pericallosa, mit Ästen der vorderen Hirnarterie zu einer besonders gefäßreichen Zone, deren mediale und laterale überlagernde Anteile jedoch bei speziellen Techniken (Angiotomographie, stereoskopische Aufnahmen) gut differenziert werden können. Wie schon erwähnt, ist das Muster der terminalen Mediaäste sehr konstant. Feine Kollateralen können in den Grenzgebieten der Vaskularisation, zwischen A. cerebri anterior, A. cerebri media und A. cerebri posterior, auch physiologischerweise nachgewiesen werden. Das Fehlen der A. cerebri media oder einzelner ihrer stärkeren Äste aufgrund anatomischer Varianten oder Anomalien wird in der Literatur nicht beschrieben.

VI. Subkortikale Gefäße der Äste der A. carotis interna

1. Allgemeines

Den kortikalen Verzweigungen der A. carotis interna können subkortikale Vaskularisationsterritorien im weitesten Sinn gegenübergestellt werden. Wenn man von den schon erwähnten Ästen der A. pericallosa, der A. cerebri anterior und der A. corporis callosi dorsalis der A. cerebri posterior (A. pericallosa posterior) zum Balken absieht, handelt es sich im wesentlichen um die vorderen Anteile der arteriellen Versorgung des Hirnstammes und der Endhirnkerne und Endhirnbahnen (LEEDS, 1974). Die Einteilung in mediane, mediolaterale, laterale und posteriore Gefäßgruppen gelingt nur bis zum Mesenzephalon. Im Übergangsbereich, zwischen Mesenzephalon und Dienzephalon, beginnen die hier zu besprechenden Gefäße. Es handelt sich um Äste, die die vorderen Anteile des Mesenzephalon durchziehen, Endverzweigungen zur Versorgung des Gebietes abgeben und ihren Verlauf zum Dienzephalon fortsetzen. Sie stammen aus der A. cerebri posterior, den Aa. choroideae posteriores, der A. communicans posterior und der A. choroidea anterior. Soweit sie von der Versorgung durch die A. cerebri posterior abhängen, werden sie dort (s.u.) eingehend besprochen.

2. Äste der A. communicans posterior

Äste der A. communicans posterior sind die Aa. thalamoperforatae anteriores, mehrere kräftige, ähnlich den Aa. perforantes der A. cerebri posterior verlaufende Äste, die nach GEORGE et al. (1975) in ein interpedunkuläres, paraventrikuläres (hypothalamisches) und ein thalamisches Segment eingeteilt werden. Sie können auch als Aa. diencephalicae inferiores bezeichnet werden (LANG, 1965) und versorgen das Gebiet zwischen Hypophysenstiel und Corpora mammilaria bis zum Foramen Monroi und der Adhaesio interthalamica nach dorsal. Sie weisen ein Kaliber von 0,2–0,8 mm auf und sind insbesondere in den Vertebralisangiogrammen, eventuell nach Kompression der gleichseitigen A. carotis interna, nachweisbar (GEORGE et al., 1975). Das Segmentum interpedunculare kann sehr klein sein oder in Angiographien scheinbar fehlen. Je proximaler die Arterien von der A. communicans posterior abgehen, desto spitzer ist der Winkel im Anfangsteil zur A. communicans posterior und desto länger die Verlaufsstrecke der Gefäße im Segmentum interpedunculare. Die Äste ziehen nach dorsal zum Tractus opticus und treten in enger Beziehung zur lateralen Wand des 3. Ventrikels in den Hypothalamus. Die Schleife um den Tractus opticus kann in den Angiogrammen durch ihre deutliche frontalwärts gerichtete Konkavität identifiziert werden. Sie bezeichnet die Übergangszone zwischen dem Segmentum interpedunculare und dem Segmentum paraventriculare.

Das paraventrikuläre Segment hat im seitlichen Strahlengang der Angiogramme, im Gegensatz zum mesenzephalen Segment der hinteren thalamoperforierenden Arterien, einen wellenförmigen Verlauf, der jedoch gelegentlich fehlen kann (GEORGE et al., 1975). Im a-p Strahlengang liegen sie von der lateralen Wand des 3. Ventrikels im Abstand von 2–5 mm nach lateral entfernt, aber immer medial der inneren Kapsel. In Höhe der Massa intermedia wird mit etwa 1 mm der geringste Abstand erreicht. Hier biegen die Äste scharf nach lateral zum Thalamus ab und bilden das thalamische Segment als dichtes Büschel feiner Endäste zur Versorgung des ventralen und paraventrikulären Kerns des Thalamus.

3. A. choroidea anterior

Die A. choroidea anterior bildet mit Ästen der Aa. choroideae posteriores die Gruppe der oberen dienzephalen Arterien. Sie entspringt zwischen dem Abgang der A. communicans posterior und der Bifurkation der A. carotis interna, nur wenig von beiden entfernt. Gelegentlich ist der Abgang auf der Bifurkationsstelle gegen die A. cerebri media hin verschoben. Der Abgang von der A. cerebri media im Anfangsabschnitt soll in fast 12% der Fälle (CARPENTER et al., 1955) erfolgen, nach MITTERWALLNER (1955) und SJÖGREN (1956) in etwa 2,5% der Fälle. Abgang von der A. communicans posterior wird von CARPENTER et al. (1955) in 6,7%, von HROMADA (1957) in 1,9%, von SJÖGREN (1956) in 3,8%, von MORELLO und COOPER (1953) in über 8% von MITTERWALLNER (1955) jedoch nur in 0,3% ihrer Fälle beobachtet. Eingehende Beschreibungen aus anatomischer, klinisch-pathogenetischer, angiographischer Sicht stammen von CURRY und CULBRETH (1952), HOFF und OSLER (1952), COOPER (1953), CARPENTER et al. (1955), LENZI (1955), MITTERWALLNER (1955), MORELLO und COOPER (1955), MOUNIER-KUHN et al. (1955), JEFFERSON und SHELDON (1956), SJÖGREN (1956), HROMADA (1957), PERTUISET et al. (1962), OTOMO (1965) und GOLDBERG (1974).

Die Arterie zieht okzipitalwärts, verläuft längs des medialen Randes, an der Unterseite des Tractus opticus, bis zum vorderen Pol des Corpus geniculatum laterale divergierend. Hier angekommen, dringt ein Ast der Arterie durch die Fissura choroidea in den Plexus choroideus im Bereich der Spitze des Unterhorns ein. Weitere Äste versorgen den Hypocampus bis in die Gegend des Globus, in Höhe des Abganges der Hinterhörner der Seitenventrikel, wo etwa die Versorgungsgrenze des Gefäßes verläuft und Anastomosen zu den Aa. choroideae posteriores bestehen. Im Anfangsabschnitt abgegebene Ästchen versorgen den Anfangsteil des Tractus opticus; weitere feine Äste ziehen durch die Substantia perforata anterior zum hinteren Schenkel der Capsula interna im basalen Anteil zum Anfangsteil der Sehstrahlung zum medialen Anteil der Spitze des Globus pallidus, dem Schwanz des Nucleus caudatus, dem Nucleus hypothalamicus, ventrolateralen Teilen des Thalamus sowie rostralen Anteilen von Substantia nigra, Nucleus ruber, Ansa lenticularis, Nucleus amygdalae, Tuber cinereum und Corpus mamillare (KRAYENBÜHL u. YASARGIL, 1965). In den Angiogrammen kann sie häufig abgegrenzt werden. Die Angaben schwanken von 75% (MONIZ, 1940) bis 96% (DILENGE, 1962), wobei die Abgrenzung im seitlichen Strahlengang noch häufiger als im a-p Strahlengang gelingt (KRAYENBÜHL u. YASARGIL, 1965). Das Gefäß weist in den Angiogrammen sowohl im seitlichen wie im a-p Strahlengang einen charakteristischen Verlauf auf, der zu der Diagnose auch kleinerer Raumforderungen im Bereich des oberen Hirnstammes sowie durch ihre Lage am Tentoriumrand bei Raumforderungen in der hinteren Schädelgrube und bei Massenverlagerungen herangezogen werden kann. Der Verlauf im seitlichen Angiogramm ist zunächst einige mm weit kaudalwärts gerichtet, dann wird ein flacher, kaudalwärts konvexer Bogen von 1–1,5 cm Länge beschrieben. Nach einem fast horizontal bzw. parallel zu den Felsenbeinen gerichteten Verlauf von etwa 2 cm wird schließlich ein großer frontalwärts konkaver Bogen beschrieben. In den a-p Projektionen wird das Gefäß durch die feinen lentikulostriären Gefäße überlagert, von denen es sich lediglich durch den geradlinig nach lateral ansteigenden Verlauf abhebt.

4. Äste der A. communicans anterior und der A. cerebri anterior

Der Anschluß der Vaskularisation in rostraler Richtung wird durch die Rami striati aus der A. cerebri anterior und der A. cerebri media hergestellt, die den Globus pallidus versorgen und zum Telenzephalon weiterziehen, sowie durch die Aa. diencephalicae inferiores anteriores aus der A. cerebri anterior und der A. communicans anterior: mehrere, bis zu 0,6 oder 1,0 mm weite Äste zur Pars impar ventriculi telencephali, mit den angrenzenden hypothalamischen Gebieten und der Lamina terminalis (MURPHY, 1954; OSTROWSKI et al., 1960; LAZORTHES, 1961; LEEDS, 1974). Sie werden auch als A. centralis brevis (diencephalica) bezeichnet; eine mediale und eine laterale werden unterschieden. Die laterale Gruppe mit Abgang im Bereich des proximalen Abschnittes des präkommunikalen Segmentes der A. cerebri anterior besteht aus 8–12 Gefäßen, die von der dorsalen Zirkumferenz der A. cerebri anterior meist gruppenweise entspringen und dorsalwärts ziehend die Substantia perforata durchsetzen. Die mediale Gruppe, meist 4–10 Arterien, entspringt vom distalen Abschnitt des präkommunikalen Segments der A. cerebri anterior und von der A. communicans anterior und zieht ebenfalls nach dorsal. Das Versorgungsgebiet beider Gefäßgruppen umfaßt rostrale Anteile von Nucleus paraventricularis, Nucleus dorsomedianus, Nucleus praeopticus, Nucleus supraopticus, Nucleus tuberis, rostrale Anteile des Infundibulums, die Commissura anterior und das Genu corporis callosi. Die Grenze des Versorgungsbereichs stellt etwa die Gegend des Foramen Monroi dar.

A. centralis longa (Synonym: Aa. striatae anteriores et mediales, A. recurrens HEUBNER). Das Gefäß wurde 1872 von HEUBNER erstmalig beschrieben. Es entspringt im distalen Abschnitt des präkommunikalen Segments, meist unmittelbar vor Abgang der A. communicans anterior. CRITCHLEY (1930) fand es in seinem Sektionsgut in 80% der Fälle mit typischem Verlauf, PADGET (1944) beschreibt das Gefäß als regelmäßig, wenn auch mit Variationen hinsichtlich Kaliber und Verlauf. LAZORTHES (1961) fand es in allen seinen Präparaten. WESTBERG (1963) konnte das Gefäß in einem Fall nicht unter den anderen perforierenden Ästen abgrenzen, in einem Fall war es doppelt angelegt. Die Arterie zieht in einem relativ engen Bogen lateralwärts bis etwa zur Höhe der Karotisgabel und tritt dann, dorsalwärts ansteigend, durch den medialen Teil der Substantia perforata. Ihr Versorgungsgebiet kann den Bulbus olfactorius, unter Umständen mit angrenzenden Hirnrindenarealen, umschließen, vor allem jedoch den vorderen Schenkel der inneren Kapsel, die rostralen und medialen Anteile von Putamen, Pallidum und Caput nuclei caudati. Angiographisch kann die Arterie in den a-p Projektionen nachgewiesen werden. Der Anfangsabschnitt kann durch das präkommunikale Segment der A. cerebri anterior verdeckt sein. In den lateralen Bereichen und im seitlichen Strahlengang ist das Gefäß gegen die zentralen Äste der A. cerebri media nicht abgrenzbar.

5. Äste der A. cerebri media

Die zentralen Äste der A. cerebri media lassen sich in eine innere, mittlere und äußere Gruppe aufteilen, die in Anzahl und Kaliber etwas variieren. Am Abgang wird der Gefäßfächer häufig mit einem Kamm verglichen.

Die innere Gruppe entspringt in der Nähe der Gabel der A. carotis interna von der A. cerebri media. Es handelt sich meist um 1 bis 2 feine Ästchen. Die in der Mitte gelegene Hauptgruppe entspringt dem Stamm der A. cerebri media und setzt sich aus 5 bis 8 Ästen unterschiedlichen Kalibers zusammen, wobei die stärksten Äste meist lateral angeordnet sind. Diese Gefäßgruppe findet sich praktisch im gesamten Untersuchungsgut konstant.

Die äußere Gruppe entspringt in der Nähe der Teilungsstelle der A. cerebri media oder von einem der Hauptäste, bevorzugt dem oberen. Meist handelt es sich um 2 oder 3 mittelkräftige Arteriolen. Die Gesamtzahl der zentralen Arterien der A. cerebri media soll zwischen 6 und 12 Gefäßen variieren, bei einem Mittelwert von 8 (LAZORTHES et al., 1975). Sämtliche Gefäße ziehen nach ihrem Abgang nach dorsal, wobei sie zur Mitte hin konvergieren, und zwar am stärksten die Gefäße der äußeren Gruppe. Sie ziehen durch die Substantia perforata nach oben, die hierbei gebildete, leicht nach lateral konkave Kurve von engem Radius markiert den Sitz

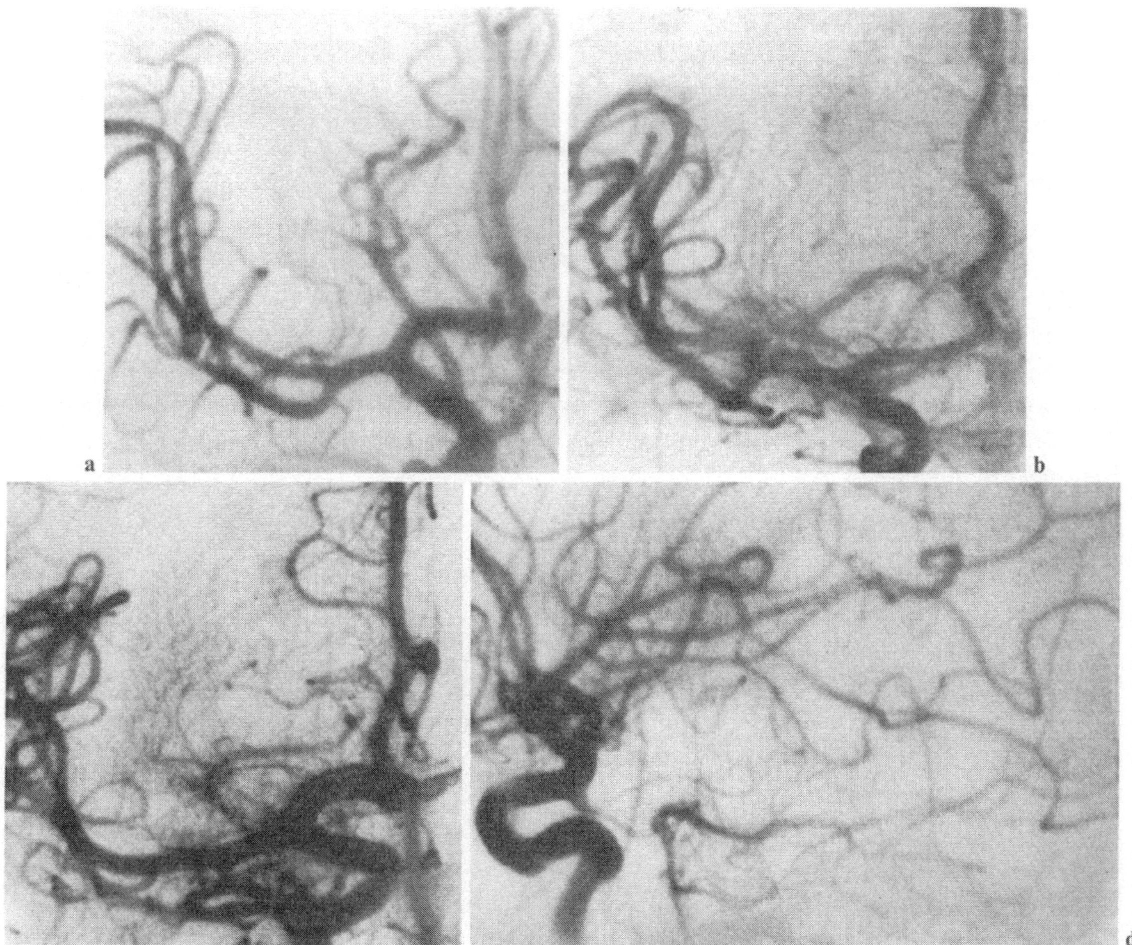

Abb. 9a–d. Darstellung der striolentikulären Gefäße der A. cerebri anterior und A. cerebri media im a-p Strahlengang **a**, **b** als zarte Äste, als bürstenartige präkapilläre Gefäßgruppe **c** und der A. choroidea anterior **b** a-p und seitlich

der Substantia perforata anterior. Vor diesem Punkt verlaufen die zentralen Äste im wesentlichen in einer Ebene (LAZORTHES et al., 1975). Innerhalb des Gehirns fächern sich die Arterien in anterio-posteriorer und transversaler Richtung auf, um zu ihren Versorgungsgebieten zu gelangen. Hier unterscheidet LAZORTHES (1965) eine vordere von einer hinteren Gruppe. Die vordere Gruppe soll den rostralen Anteil des Putamen und den äußeren Anteil des Globus pallidus versorgen, zum vorderen Schenkel der inneren Kapsel ziehen, um schließlich im Kopf und im vorderen Anteil des Körpers des Nucleus caudatus ihre Endverzweigungen zu bilden.

Die hintere Gruppe, etwas medial und unterhalb der ersteren lokalisiert, läuft nach dorsal zum mittleren Anteil des Nucleus lenticularis. Es handelt sich also beim Versorgungsgebiet der zentralen Äste der A. cerebri media um telenzephale subkortikale Kerngebiete und Bahnen, was von LAZORTHES et al. (1956), LAZORTHES et al. (1960), KAPLAN und FORD (1966) und PERCHERON (1973) bestätigt wird. Diese teilen die zentralen Versorgungsareale des Telenzephalon, wie oben beschrieben, auf die A. choroidea anterior, die A. recurrens HEUBNER und die zentralen Äste der A. cerebri media auf, denen der größte Anteil zukommt. Variationen und vikariierende Versorgung sind häufig. Im vorderen Anteil stehen die zentralen Äste der A. cerebri media bei der Abgrenzung der Versorgungsareale in Wechselbeziehung mit der A. recurrens HEUBNER, in den dorsalen Anteilen mit der A. choroidea anterior.

C. Das vertebro-basiläre Gefäßsystem

Frühe grundlegende Untersuchungen über das vertebrobasiläre Gefäßsystem veröffentlichten DURET 1874, TESTUT 1900, STOPFORD 1916, FOIX und HILLEMAND 1925, SHELLSHEAR 1927 und ADACHI 1928. Vergleichende Untersuchungen von klinischen Befunden, Angiogrammen, Leichenangiogrammen und pathologisch-anatomischen Präparaten führten (im Gegensatz zur Karotisangiographie im supratentoriellen Bereich) zu unterschiedlichen Beurteilungen der Wertigkeit von Angiogrammen für die Darstellung pathologischer Veränderungen, insbesondere von Raumforderungen im Bereich des vertebro-basilären Gefäßsystems (LAZORTES et al., 1950; LINDGREN, 1950; DECKER, 1951; COLUMELLA, 1952; SJÖGREN, 1953; RUGGIERO und CONSTANS, 1954; HAUGE, 1954). Eine genauere Standardisierung der normalen und pathologischen Verhältnisse des vertebrobasilären Kreislaufs war erforderlich. Hierzu führten vor allem die Arbeiten von KRAYENBÜHL und YASARGIL (1957), LAZORTHES (1961), BAKER (1961), WOLF et al. (1962), GREITZ und SJÖGREN (1963), LOEB und MEYER (1965), STEPHENS und STILWELL (1969) sowie HUANG und WOLF (1969).

I. Arteria Vertebralis

Die Arteria vertebralis wird allgemein in 4 Verlaufsstrecken (3 extrakranielle und 1 intrakranielle) eingeteilt. Sie entspringt als erster und oft stärkster Ast medial des Musculus scalenus anterior aus dem kranialwärts konvexen Teil des Bogens der A. subclavia. Die Abgangsstelle liegt links etwas weiter proximal als rechts. Ein Abgang von Aortenbogen zwischen den Ursprungsstellen der linken A. subclavia und der linken A. carotis communis ist ebenfalls möglich. Weitere Abgangsvarianten sind der Ursprung aus der A. carotis communis oder A. carotis interna (3–4‰ nach LINDGREN, 1950), mit Verlauf nur durch wenige Foramina intervertebralia oder direktes Eintreten in das Foramen occipitale magnum (HYRTL, 1887; CHANAMIRJAN, 1929; TIWISINA, 1957). Hierher gehört die seltene Variante der sog. A. primitiva hypoglossica (BATUJEFF, 1889; OERTEL, 1922; LINDGREN, 1950; TAKEUCHI u. YOSHIOKA, 1963). Noch seltener sollen andere Abgangsvarianten, z.B. von der A. thyroidea (inferior), vorkommen (KRAYENBÜHL u. YASARGIL, 1957; TÖNNIS u. SCHIEFER, 1959). Das kurze, prävertebrale Anfangsstück, die *1. Strecke*, verläuft links annähernd senkrecht, rechts etwas schräg nach medial und dorsal in der Tiefe der Halsweichteile vor dem Musculus scalenus ant. nach kranial, kreuzt die anderen Halsgefäße und links den Ductus thoracicus. Es bestehen enge Beziehungen zum Plexus vertebralis des Halssympathikus. Der Gefäßabgang wird teilweise durch das Ganglion stellatum umfaßt. Kurz vor dem Eintritt in das Foramen costotransversarium des 6. HWK liegt dem Gefäß häufig das kleine Ganglion vertebrale benachbart. Die Begleitvene liegt etwas lateral und vor der Arterie. Schleifen- und Knickbildungen dieser Gefäßstrecke werden beobachtet (WEIBEL u. FIELDS, 1969), gehören aber meist zu pathologischen (arteriosklerotischen) Veränderungen. Nach Eintritt in das Foramen costotransversarium des 6., seltener des 5. Halswirbelkörpers (in Ausnahmefällen des 2. bis 4. oder 7. Halbswirbelkörpers: TESTUT, 1921; ADACHI, 1928; auch Verläufe völlig außerhalb der Querlöcher wurden beobachtet: WACKENHEIM u. BABIN, 1969), beginnt der vertebrale Teil, im funktionellen Sinn eine „Übergangsstrecke“ (RICKENBACHER, 1972) als *2. Strecke.* Das Gefäß steigt durch die Querfortsatzlöcher nahezu senkrecht nach oben und kreuzt im Foramen die an den Zwischenwirbellöchern austretenden zervikalen Nervenwurzeln. Begleitet wird es von der V. vertebralis, dem Plexus venosus vertebralis und dem N. vertebralis. Diese Verlaufsstrecke ist gekennzeichnet durch enge Beziehungen zu den benachbarten knöchernen Strukturen, insbesondere der Unkovertebral-Region, was sich besonders bei starken Bewegungsausschlägen der Halswirbelsäule oder bei knöchernen Umbauveränderungen der Unkovertebral-Region auswirkt. Dadurch wie durch arteriosklerotische Elongation des Gefäßes, können stärkere Kurven- und Windungsbildungen auftreten (HARZER u. TÖNDURY, 1966). Über die strömungsphysiologische Bedeu-

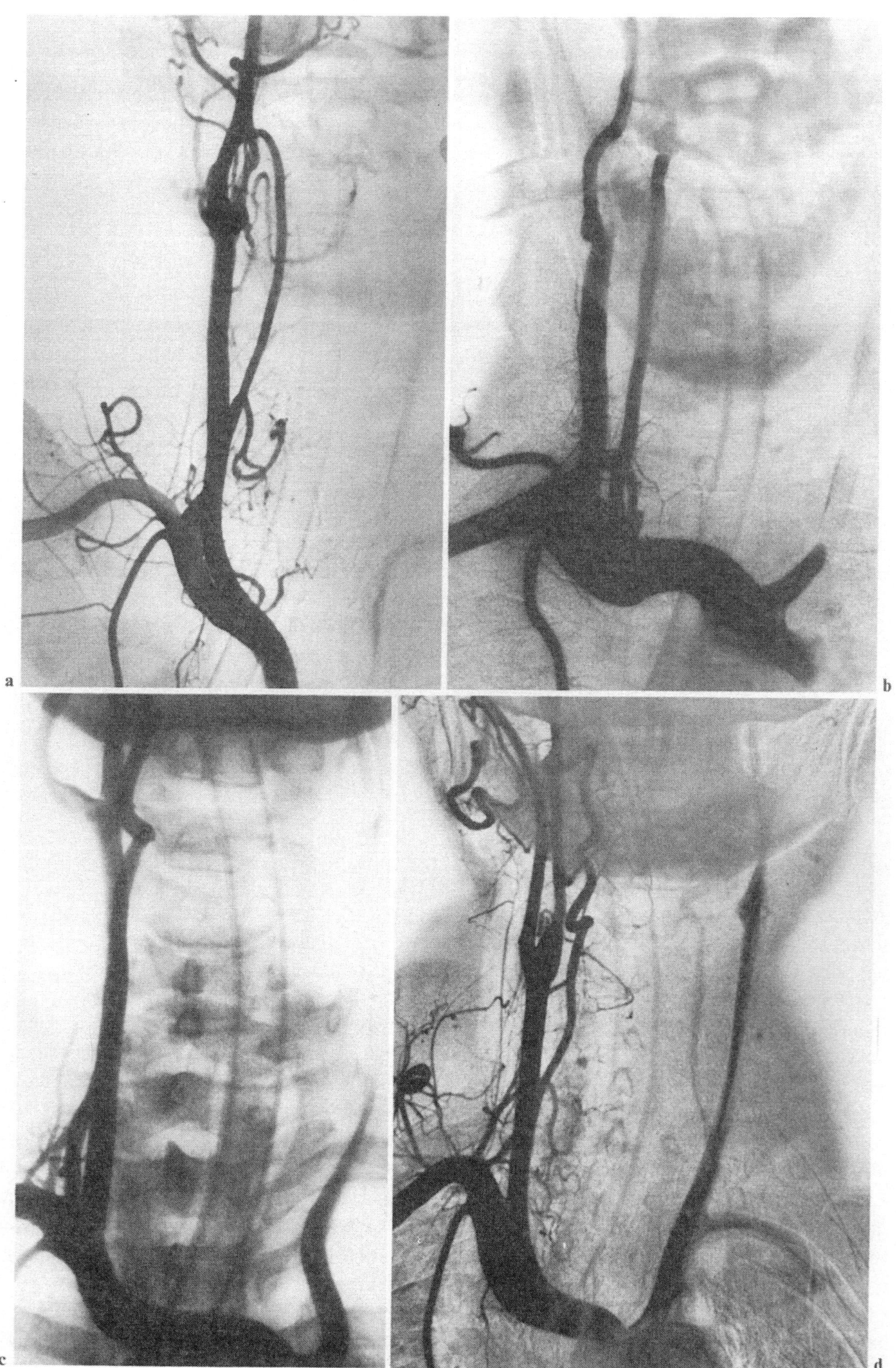

Abb. 10a–d (Legende s. Seite 358)

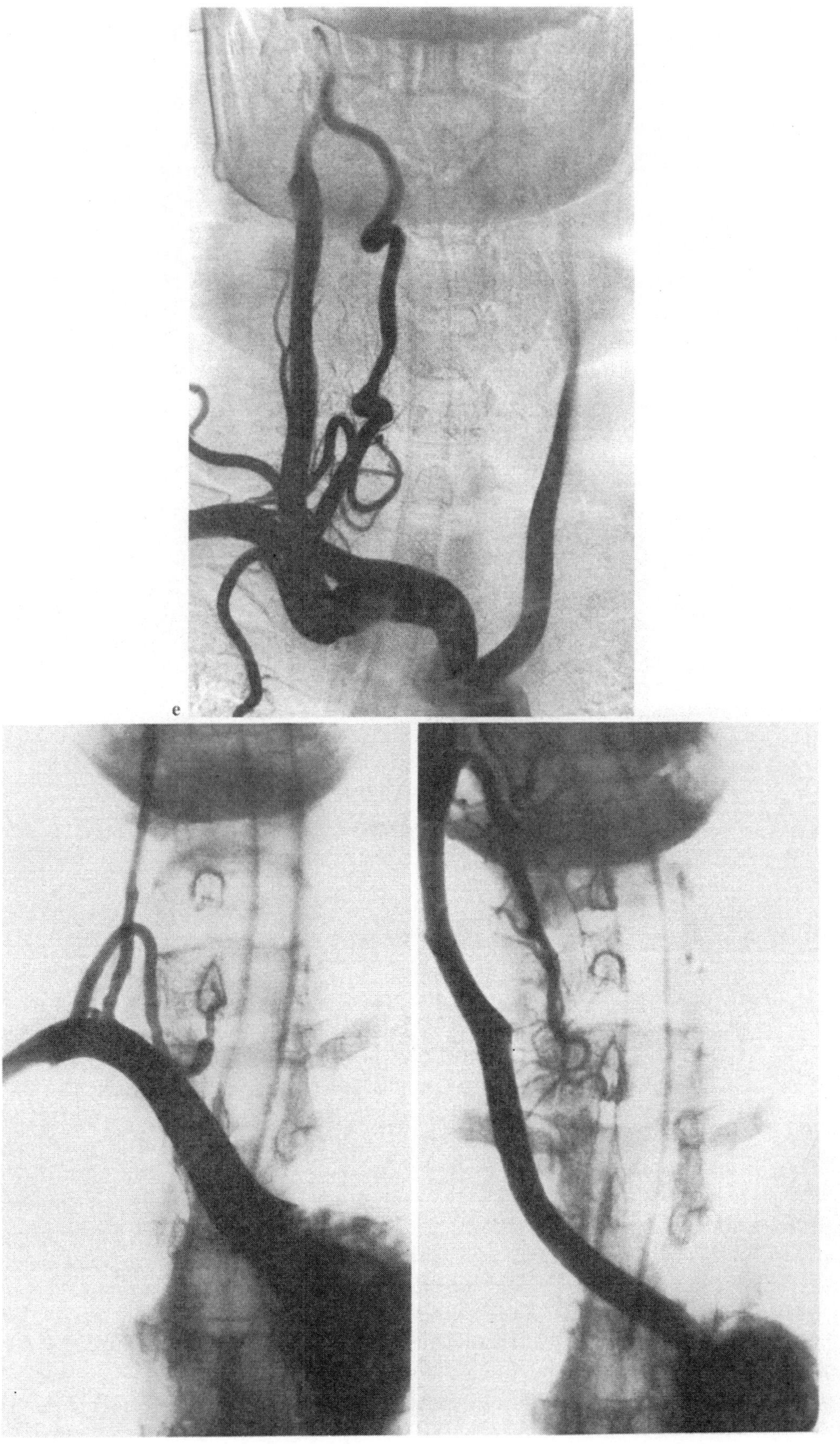

Abb. 10e u. f

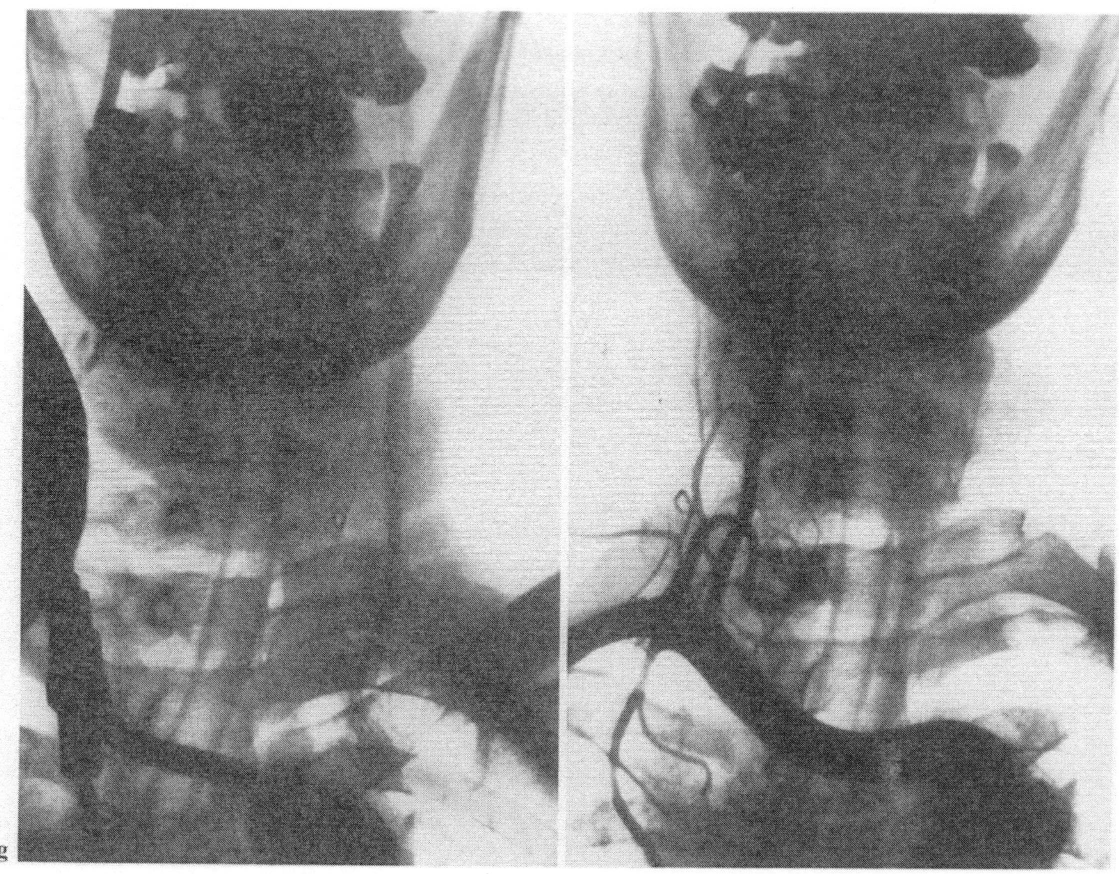

Abb. 10a–g. A. anonyma (Truncus brachiocephalicus). Klassische Form **a**. Häufigste Variante: Abgang der linken A. carotis communis von der A. anonyma oder gemeinsam mit der A. anonyma **b–e**. Abgang der rechten A. carotis communis von der Aorta **f, g** sogar proximal der A. anonyma **g**

tung der durch Knochen eingeschlossenen Verlaufsstrecken (2 und 3) sowie ihre Krümmungen wurden vielfältige Untersuchungen angestellt (RÜDINGER, 1888; GEGENBAUER, 1899; de KLEYN u. NIEUWENHUYSE, 1927; de KLEYN u. VERSTEEGH, 1933; TATLOW-BAMMER, 1957; KUNERT, 1957; TIWISINA, 1957; WEIBEL u. FIELDS, 1969). Die *3. Strecke* mit den Reserveschlingen für die Kopfbewegungen beginnt nach Durchtritt durch das Foramen costotransversarium des Axis. Das Gefäß wendet sich nach dorsal und lateral (1. Krümmung), durchtritt nach einem lateralwärts konvexen Bogen (2. Krümmung) das Querloch des Atlas, biegt rechtwinklig nach dorsal (3. Krümmung) und beschreibt einen lateralkonvexen Bogen um die Massa lateralis atlantis, um auf dem hinteren Atlasbogen im Sulcus a. vertebralis, der gelegentlich zu einem Foramen ausgebildet sein kann (KIMMERLE, 1930; KRAYENBÜHL u. YASARGIL, 1957), nahezu horizontal nach medial und dorsal zu ziehen. Zwischen Atlas und Okziput verläuft die A. vertebralis im „subokzipitalen Dreieck", umgeben vom Sinus atlanto-occipitalis (ZOLNAI, 1964). Nach einer weiteren (4.) Krümmung nach ventral und kranial wird die Membrana atlanto-occipitalis posterior und die Dura im Bereich der Austrittsstelle des 1. Zervikalnerven durchbohrt, und das Gefäß tritt in die *4. Strecke* mit intrakraniellem Verlaufsanteil. Die Arterie verläuft auf dem Klivus konvergierend mit der gegenseitigen, bis zur Vereinigungsstelle, mit Ausbildung der A. basilaris. In dieser subarachnoidalen, nicht mehr an die Knochenstrukturen gebundenen Strecke, hat das Gefäß bei gestrecktem Verlauf Beziehungen zum N. hypoglossus und zur Radix spinalis des N. accessorius, bei stark geschlängeltem Verlauf auch zu den Nerven der Vagusgruppe (RICKENBACHER, 1964; KERBER et al., 1972).

Takahashi (1974) rechnet das 4. Segment vom Verlauf im Sulcus a. vertebralis an. Wackenheim (1974) unterscheidet 5 Segmente, wobei das 4. ebenfalls nach Durchtritt durch das Foramen costotransversarium des Atlas, das 5. nach Durchtritt durch die Dura beginnt (intrakranielles Segment), entsprechend dem subokzipitalen und intrakraniellen Abschnitt nach Rickenbacher (1964).

Die A. vertebralis gibt in ihren ersten drei Verlaufsstrecken kleinere Muskeläste ab, darunter einen etwas kräftigeren im Bereich des Sulcus a. vertebralis (des Atlas). Diese Muskeläste versorgen nicht nur die Nackenmuskulatur, sondern geben auch Rami spinales (radikuläre und radikulomedulläre Arterien für die Medulla im zervikalen Bereich) und Rami meningei zum Wirbelkanal ab, die sowohl mit den segmentären spinalen und muskulären Ästen der A. occipitalis (A. carotis externa), des Truncus thyreocervicalis und Truncus costocervicalis wie den longitudinalen spinalen Arterien (A. spinalis anterior, Aa. spinales posteriores) reiche Anastomosen bilden. Die A. meningica anterior der A. vertebralis entspringt am Übergang vom 2. zum 3. Segment, unmittelbar vor der 1. Krümmung in Axishöhe. Sie tritt in den Spinalkanal ein, verläuft nach kranial und medial an seiner Vorderfläche und versorgt die Dura des Foramen occipitale magnum. Nach Newton (1968) wird sie in 48% der Angiogramme nachgewiesen. Die A. meningica posterior der A. vertebralis (in 35% der Angiogramme nachweisbar: Newton, 1968) entspringt in der extrakraniellen Verlaufsstrecke zwischen Atlasbogen und Foramen occipitale magnum, verläuft nach kranial und medial zum Hinterrand des Foramen, tritt in die hintere Schädelgrube ein, verläuft mittelliniennah in der Falx cerebelli, wo sie sich in einen medialen Ast, der bis zur Falx cerebri reichen kann, und einen lateralen Ast für die Versorgung der medialen und kaudalen Anteile der Dura der hinteren Schädelgrube aufteilt. Der mediale Ast darf im Angiogramm nicht mit dem Vermienast der A. cerebelli inferior posterior (s.u.) verwechselt werden. Im intrakraniellen Segment gibt die A. vertebralis, sogleich nach dem Duradurchtritt, die A. spinalis posterior ab, die lateral um die Medulla läuft und ventral und lateral der dorsalen Wurzeln kaudalwärts zieht. Sie bildet, ergänzt von den segmentalen Rami spinales, eine lange dorsale Anastomosenkette; auch eine Vereinigung mit der A. spinalis posterior der Gegenseite zu einem unpaaren Gefäß wurde beschrieben (Krayenbühl u. Yasargil, 1972). Das Gefäß ist bei Anwendung der Subtraktionstechnik in bis zu 4% der Angiogramme nachweisbar (Schechter u. Zinngiesser, 1964). In unterschiedlicher Höhe geht in diesem Segment in der Regel auch die A. cerebelli inferior posterior ab (s.u.). Die A. spinalis anterior, die Schechter und Zinngiesser (1964) in bis zu 50% der Fälle angiographisch fanden, entspringt dem der Mittellinie zugewandten Kreisbogen der A. vertebralis, vereinigt sich in unterschiedlicher Höhe mit dem gegenüberliegenden Gefäßstamm meist zu einem median vor der Fissura mediana anterior verlaufenden, unpaaren Gefäß und versorgt die ventralen medianen und paramedianen Anteile der Medulla. Sie bildet mit den segmentalen Spinalarterien eine ventrale Anastomosenkette. Hinzu kommen noch einige perforierende Äste, die die Medulla oblongata und den unteren Brückenabschnitt mit versorgen.

Beide Vertebralisstämme können im Kaliber stark differieren, wobei Kaliberunterschiede geringen Ausmaßes aber auch Kaliberverhältnisse bis 1:12 vorkommen. Der Weitenunterschied beider Gefäße stellt die häufigste Variation dar. Das völlige Fehlen einer Vertebralarterie wurde sogar in großen Kollektiven (Mitterwallner, 1955; Busch, 1966) nicht festgestellt. Im Kollektiv von Busch (1966; 1000 Gehirne) zeigten sich bei 15% der Gefäßpaare Kaliberunterschiede von mehr als 1:2 (1:3 bis 1:8, 1 Fall 1:12). Bei einem Drittel aller Präparate bestanden signifikante Seitendifferenzen. Statistisch gesehen ist die linke Vertebralarterie etwas häufiger das weitere Gefäß, wobei die Prozentangaben leicht streuen (Duret, 1874; Testut, 1900; Longo, 1905; Blackburn, 1907; Stopford, 1925; Morel u. Wildi, 1953; Mitterwallner, 1955; Neimanis, 1956; Krayenbühl u. Yasargil, 1957; Taveras und Wood, 1964; Busch, 1966; Voigt et al., 1972; Newton u. Mani, 1974). In weitem Abstand folgen als Varianten die verschiedenen Spielarten von mangelnder Vereinigung oder Verdoppelung bzw. Fenestration der Endstrecke. Beide Anomalien gehen auf Störungen in der embryonalen Entwicklung bei der Ausbildung der A. basilaris zurück. Nach Padget (1948) werden etwa am 28. Tag in der Hinterhirnregion bilaterale

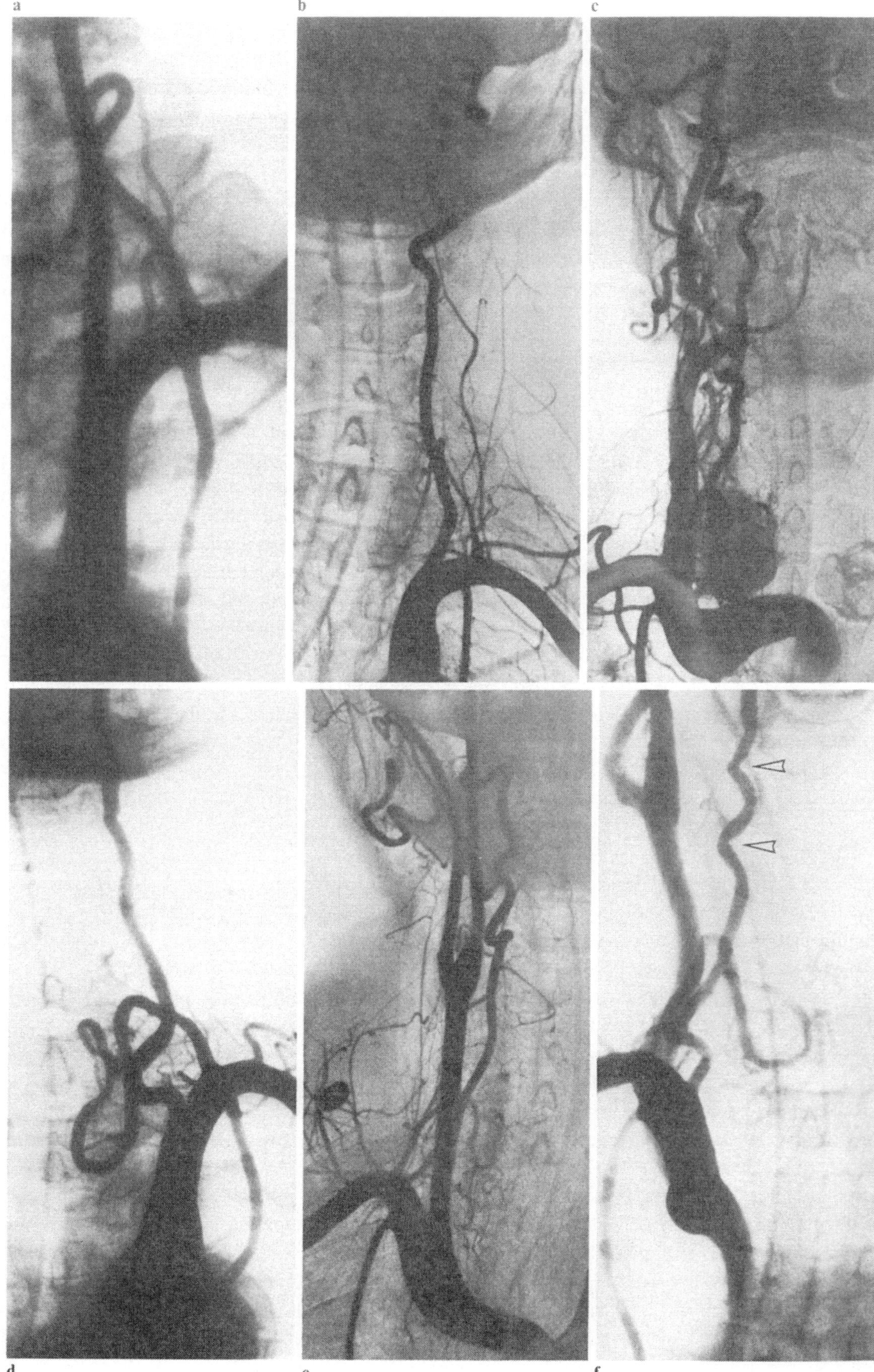
a
b
c
d
e
f

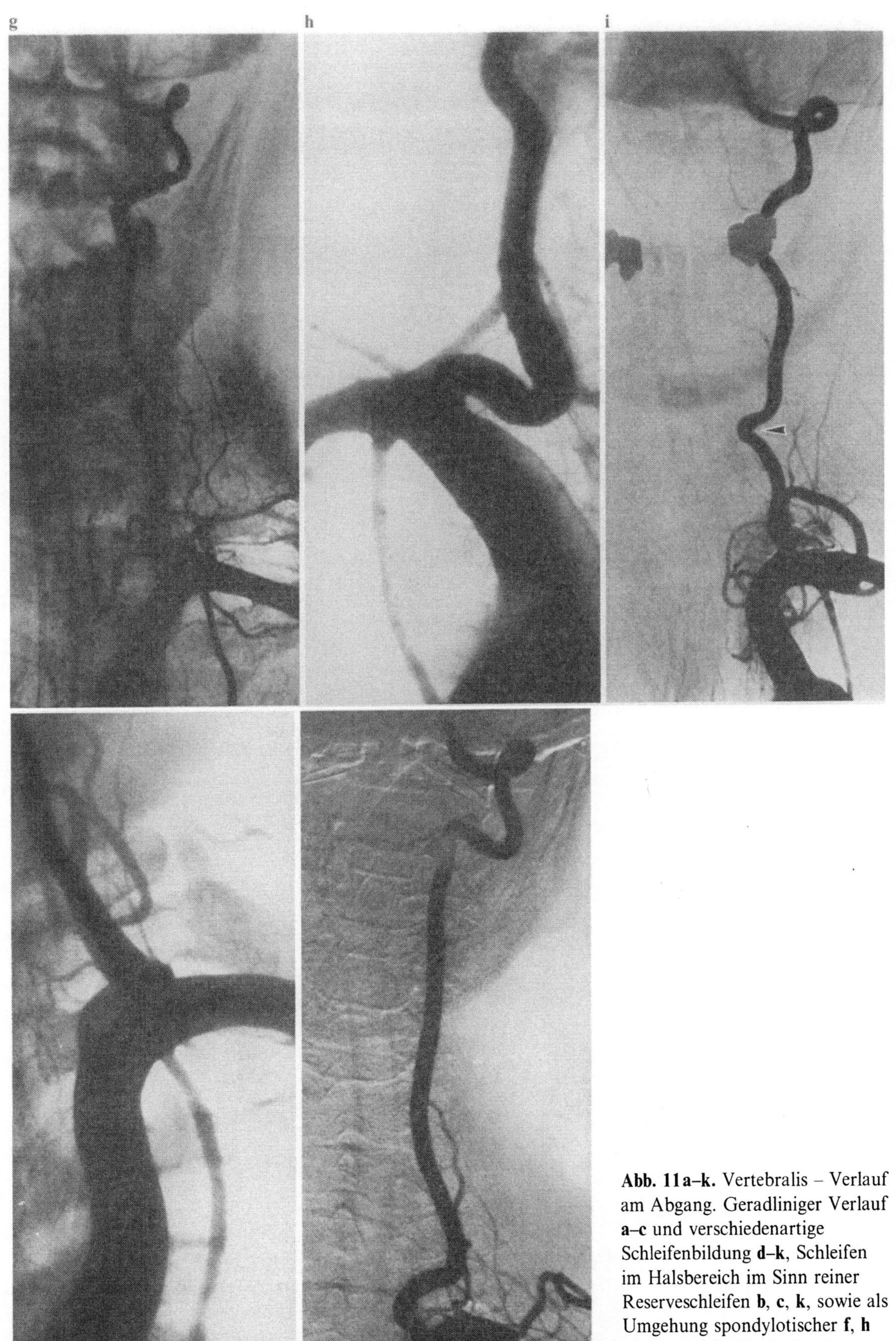

Abb. 11a–k. Vertebralis – Verlauf am Abgang. Geradliniger Verlauf **a–c** und verschiedenartige Schleifenbildung **d–k**, Schleifen im Halsbereich im Sinn reiner Reserveschleifen **b**, **c**, **k**, sowie als Umgehung spondylotischer **f**, **h** und spondylarthrotischer **i** Zacken deutbar

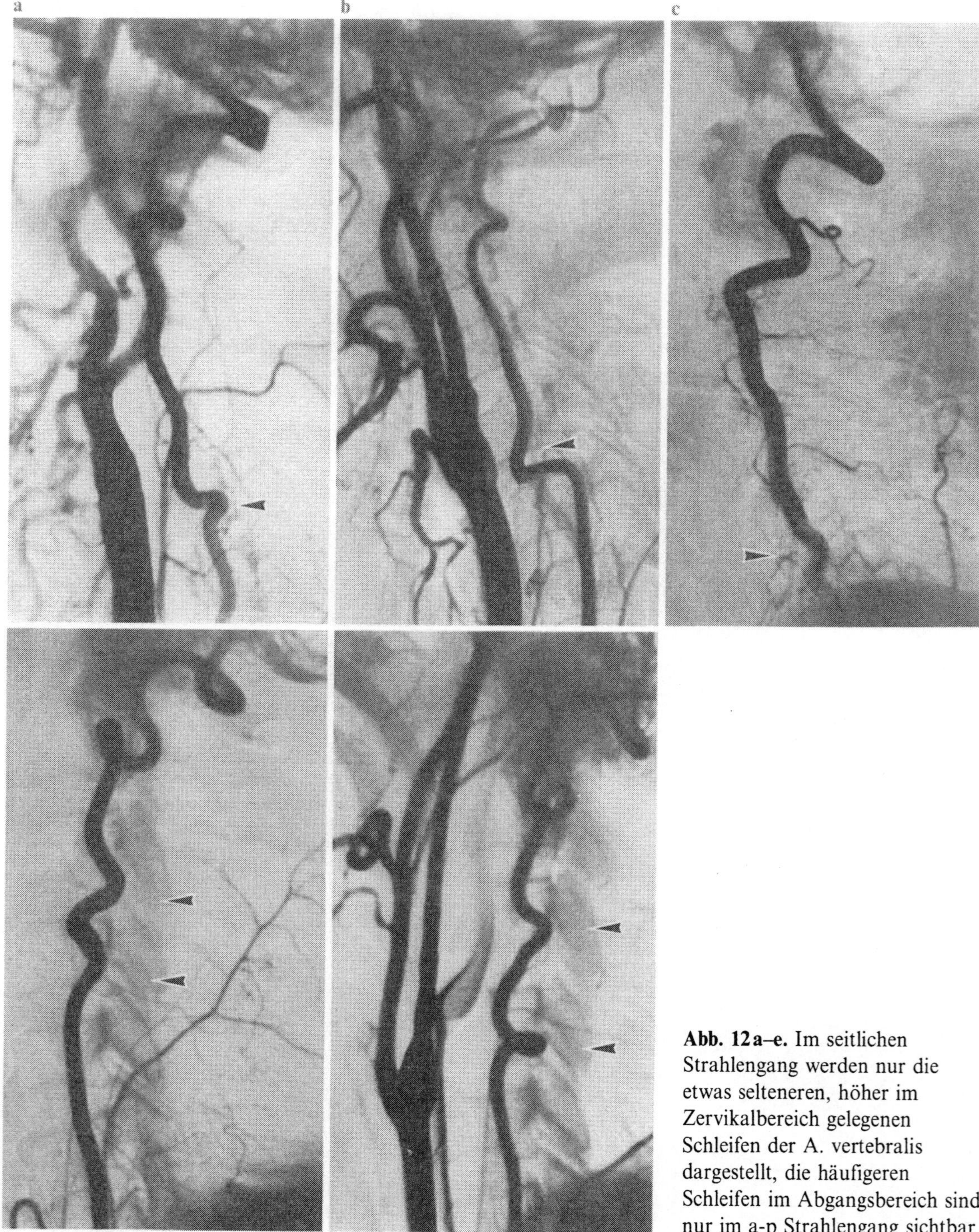

Abb. 12a–e. Im seitlichen Strahlengang werden nur die etwas selteneren, höher im Zervikalbereich gelegenen Schleifen der A. vertebralis dargestellt, die häufigeren Schleifen im Abgangsbereich sind nur im a-p Strahlengang sichtbar

longitudinale Neuralarterien sichtbar, die lateral mit den primitiven Hinterhirnplexus in Verbindung stehen. Ihr Hauptzufluß stammt aus der A. primitiva otica und hypoglossica. Die A. basilaris entsteht durch Verschmelzung der Neuralarterien. Eine Fenestration der A. vertebralis, immer in der atlanto-okzipitalen Übergangsstrecke, bedeutet das Persistieren eines lateralen Kanals, der parallel zu den Neuralarterien verläuft. Die Beobachtungen über die Vertebralisfenestration sind zahlreich. Sie findet sich in 0,25–6% des Beobachtungsgutes bei Hirnsektionen (KADYI,

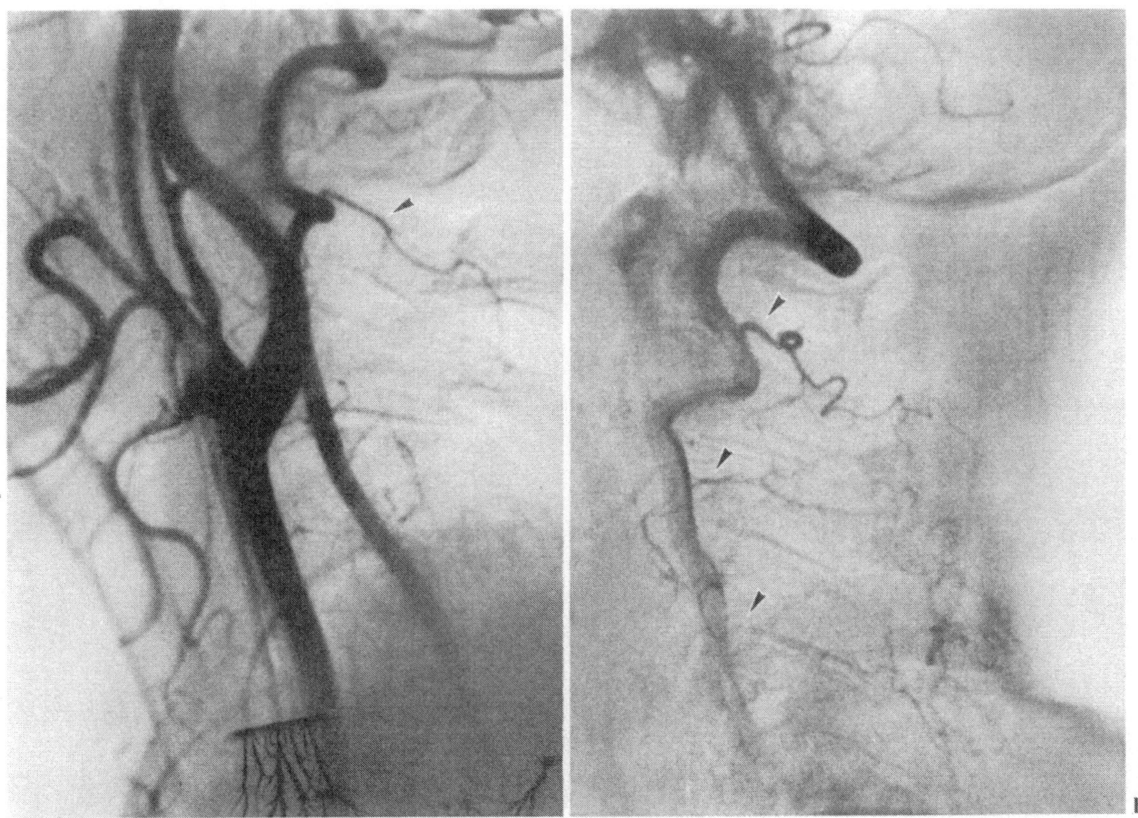

Abb. 13a u. b. Segmentale Äste der A. vertebralis (►) in Höhe der Atlasschleife (**a**) und im gesamten Zervikalbereich mit Anastomosenbildung (**b**)

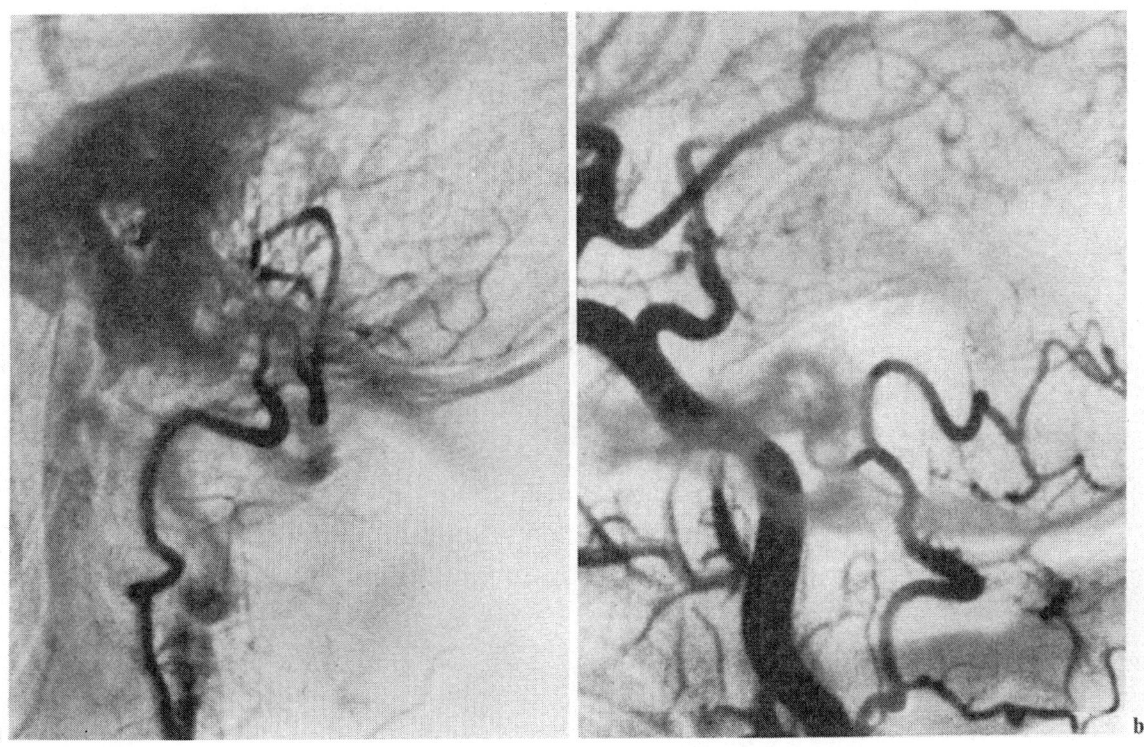

Abb. 14a u. b. Hypoplastisches Endstück der A. vertebralis, die in der A. cerebelli inferior posterior endet (**a**) bzw. noch eine schmale Verbindung zur A. basilaris aufweist (**b**) (gleichzeitig besteht eine A. trigemina primitiva)

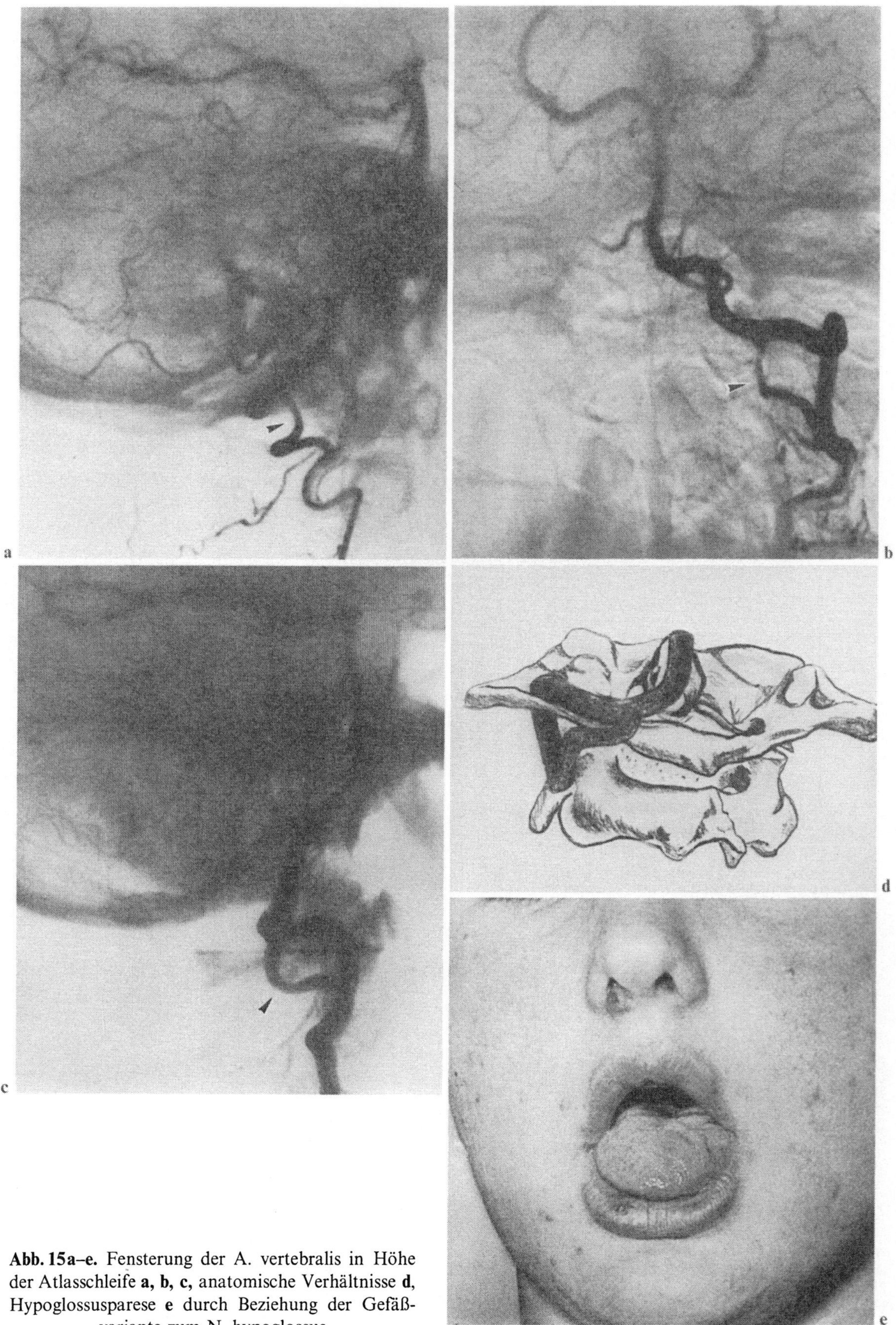

Abb. 15a–e. Fensterung der A. vertebralis in Höhe der Atlasschleife **a, b, c,** anatomische Verhältnisse **d,** Hypoglossusparese **e** durch Beziehung der Gefäßvariante zum N. hypoglossus

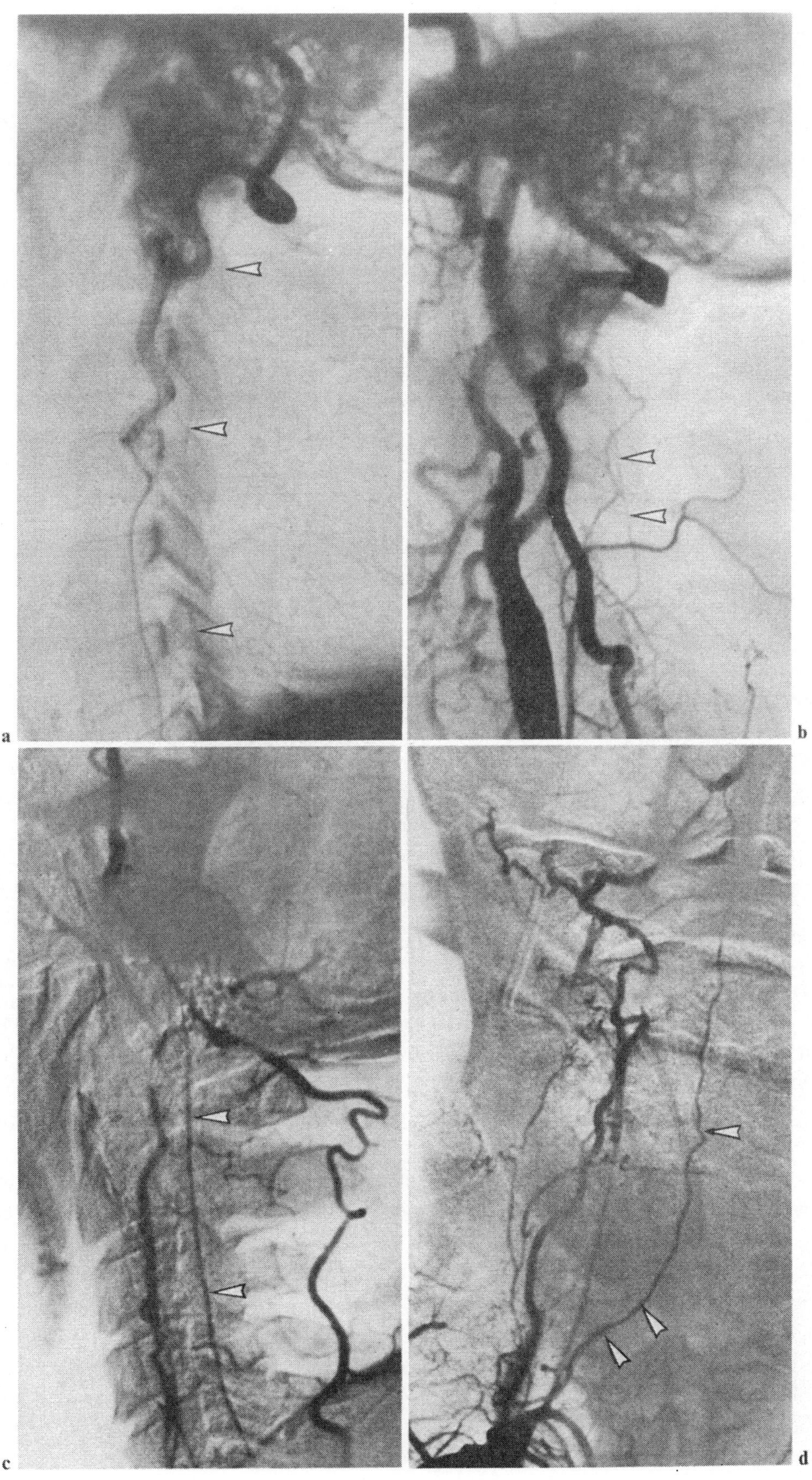

Abb. 16a–d. Darstellung der A. spinalis anterior bei regelrechten Kreislaufverhältnissen **a**, **b**, starke Kaliberzunahme im Rahmen kollateraler Kreisläufe bei Vertebralisverschluß **c**, **d**

1866; OGLE, 1895; STOPFORD, 1916; ANSAROFF, 1925; ADACHI, 1928; SCHMEIDEL, 1936; MITTERWALLNER, 1955; KRAYENBÜHL u. YASARGIL, 1957; THOMAS et al., 1959; BUSCH, 1966; WOLLSCHLÄGER et al., 1967). Angiographischer Nachweis der Vertebralisfensterung wird ab 1968 beschrieben (NADJMI u. SCHWIND, 1968; HANDA et al., 1968; MIZUKAMI et al., 1968; MAKI et al., 1969; KOWADA et al., 1970; TAKAHASHI et al., 1970; SHIMIZU et al., 1972; KAWAMOTO et al., 1972; KOWADA et al., 1973; TEAL et al., 1973; SCHMIDT u. PFINGST, 1973). Die fehlende Vereinigung der Vertebralarterien zur A. basilaris findet sich als Hemmungsmißbildung (fehlende Verschmelzung der primitiven Neuralarterien), wobei die A. basilaris verdoppelt ist oder eine Fensterung aufweist (s.u.) oder bei Hypoplasie einer der Vertebralarterien. Dabei kann noch eine rudimentäre Verbindung oder eine weitere entwicklungsgeschichtlich begründete Variante (A. primitiva hypoglossica persistens) vergesellschaftet sein (BATUJEFF, 1889; BLACKBURN, 1907; CAVATORTI, 1907; BERRY u. ANDERSON, 1909; HIRKO, 1919; OERTEL, 1922; LINDGREN, 1950; MCMINN, 1953).

II. Arteria cerebelli inferior posterior

Die A. cerebelli inferior posterior läßt sich bei den (direkten und indirekten) Vertebralisangiographien in 88 bis 96% der Fälle darstellen (LINDGREN, 1950; KRAYENBÜHL u. YASARGIL, 1957, 1965, 1972; GREITZ u. SJÖGREN, 1963; FIEGEL u. NADJMI, 1971; VOIGT et al., 1972). Bei der anatomischen Präparation fehlt das Gefäß in 2–21% der Fälle (ADACHI, 1928; LANDOLT, 1949; MITTERWALLNER, 1955; LANG u. KOLLMANNSBERGER, 1961; MÜLLER, 1975). Dabei stammt der niedrigste Wert von 2% bei MITTERWALLNER (1955) aus dem größten Untersuchungsgut, der höchste Wert von 21% bei ADACHI (1928) kommt daher, daß Gefäße, die nicht aus der A. vertebralis entspringen, außer Acht gelassen wurden. Das Gefäß fehlt rechts doppelt so häufig wie links (VOIGT et al., 1972). In einzelnen Fällen ist es doppelt angelegt (MITTERWALLNER, 1955; MÜLLER, 1975). Kaliberunterschiede beider Seiten sind nicht ausgeprägt.

1. Verlauf

Die *A. cerebelli inferior posterior* geht in der Regel in mittlerer Höhe des 4. (intrakraniellen) Abschnittes der A. vertebralis ab. KRAYENBÜHL und YASARGIL (1957) fanden den Abgang des Gefäßes in diesem Bereich in 69% der Fälle, 3 bis 10 mm oberhalb der Ebene des Foramen occipitale magnum, in 9% in Höhe des Atlasbogens und in 12% der Fälle höher, im Bereich der Vereinigungsstelle der Vertebralarterien. Die Variationsbreite des Gefäßabganges reichte bei anatomischen Präparaten von 6–36 mm Abstand zur Vereinigungsstelle, mit einer Häufung bei 12–21 mm (LANG u. KOLLMANNSBERGER, 1961), in einem kleineren Kollektiv, bei MÜLLER (1975), von 12 mm oberhalb bis 24 mm unterhalb der Spitze des Vereinigungswinkels der Vertebralarterien. Die Arterie soll in 82,3% der Fälle von der A. vertebralis, in 5,2% von der A. basilaris entspringen und in 6,5% der Fälle fehlen (VOIGT et al., 1972). Dabei geht das Gefäß in 2,6% der Fälle rechts, in 1,7% der Fälle links und in 0,8% der Fälle beidseits von der A. basilaris ab. Auch bei KRAYENBÜHL und YASARGIL (1957) wird in 5,2% der Fälle der Abgang von der A. basilaris angegeben, bei MITTERWALLNER (1955) in 0,5% der Fälle. Diese Autorin findet in 0,5% der Fälle eine doppelte Anlage des Gefäßes. Der besonders tiefe Abgang der A. cerebelli inferior posterior im Bereich des 3. (extraduralen) Abschnittes der A. vertebralis wird bei LANDOLT (1949), bei KRAYENBÜHL und YASARGIL (1957), bei MEGRET (1972) und RICKENBACHER 1964 zitiert von TÖNDURY (1970) beschrieben. Die Ursache liegt in entwicklungsgeschichtlichen Varianten (HOCHSTETTER, 1891; STREETER, 1918; PADGET, 1948; SCHMEIDEL, 1933). Über das Auslaufen der hypoplastischen A. vertebralis in der A. cerebelli inferior posterior, ohne oder mit nur rudimentärer Verbindung zur A. basilaris, wird ebenfalls berichtet, und zwar übereinstimmend in 0,2%

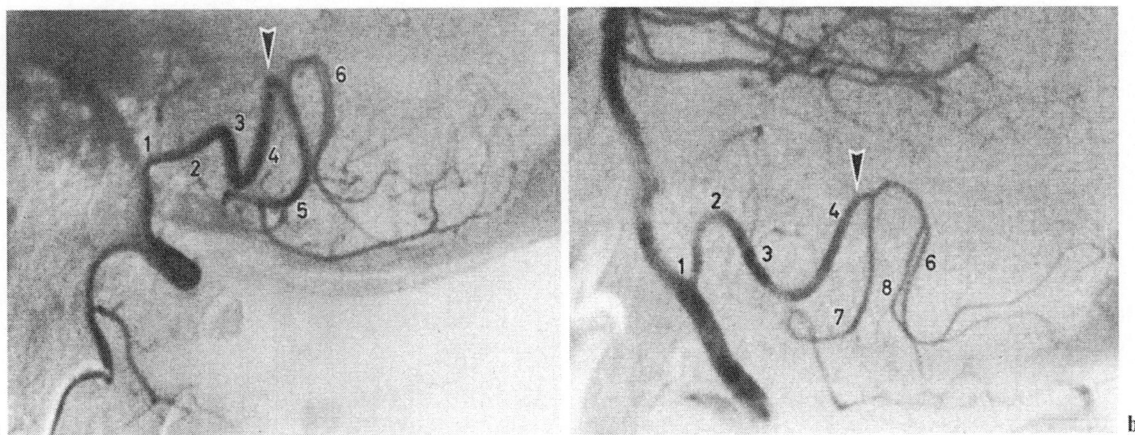

Abb. 17a u. b. A. cerebelli inferior posterior, klassische Verlaufsform und Aufteilung **a** u. **b**: Segmentum medullare anterius (*1*) Segmentum medullare laterale (*2*) Segmentum medullare posterius (*3*) Segmentum supratonsillare (*4*) Ramus tonsillohemisphaericus (*5*) **a** Segmentum vermiculare (*6*) Ramus tonsillaris (*7*) **b**, Ramus hemisphaericus (*8*) **b**, Choroidaler Punkt

der Fälle von MITTERWALLNER (1955) und BUSCH (1966), ebenso bei KRAYENBÜHL und YASARGIL (1972), auf beiden Seiten als Rarität bei CAVATORTI (1907), außerdem bei OERTEL (1922) und McCULLOUGH (1962). In angiographischen Arbeiten erscheint diese Verlaufsform statistisch häufiger, so bei FIEGEL und NADJMI (1971) in 2,5% der Fälle, bei TAKAHASHI (1974) in bis zu 4% der Fälle.

Bei TSCHERNYSCHEFF und GRIGOROWSKI (1929) wurde als Hauptmerkmal des Gefäßverlaufs die Aufteilung in einen medialen und lateralen Zweig angegeben. Die Beschreibung eines „klassischen" Verlaufs der A. cerebelli inferior anterior mit einer kaudalen und kranialen Schleife geben COLUMELLA (1952) und HAUGE (1954). Nach KRAYENBÜHL und YASARGIL (1957) soll das Gefäß in 99% der Fälle im Angiogramm den typischen S-förmigen Verlauf in antero-posteriorer Richtung oberhalb des Foramen occipitale magnum aufweisen. Als markante Punkte wurden immer die Spitze der kaudalen und kranialen Schleife angesehen, gleichzeitig wurde auf den natürlichen Variantenreichtum dieser Formation hingewiesen. Diese ursprüngliche Einteilung:

Stamm – kaudale Schleife – kraniale Schleife
- Ventrikeläste
- Vermienast
- Hemisph.-Ast

findet sich auch bei GREITZ und SJÖGREN (1963), wo auf die besondere Bedeutung des Arcus chorioideus (s.u.) als Orientierungspunkt eingegangen wird. KRAYENBÜHL und YASARGIL (1965) unterscheiden:

Pars cisternalis –	Pars medullaris –	Arcus chorioideus –	Aufteilung
(Stamm)	(kaudale Schleife)	(Endabschnitt der kraniellen Schleife)	

Dieselbe Einteilung braucht MEGRET (1972) mit anderer Benennung:

Segment initial (preamygdalien)
Segment intermédière (amygdalien)
Segment terminal.

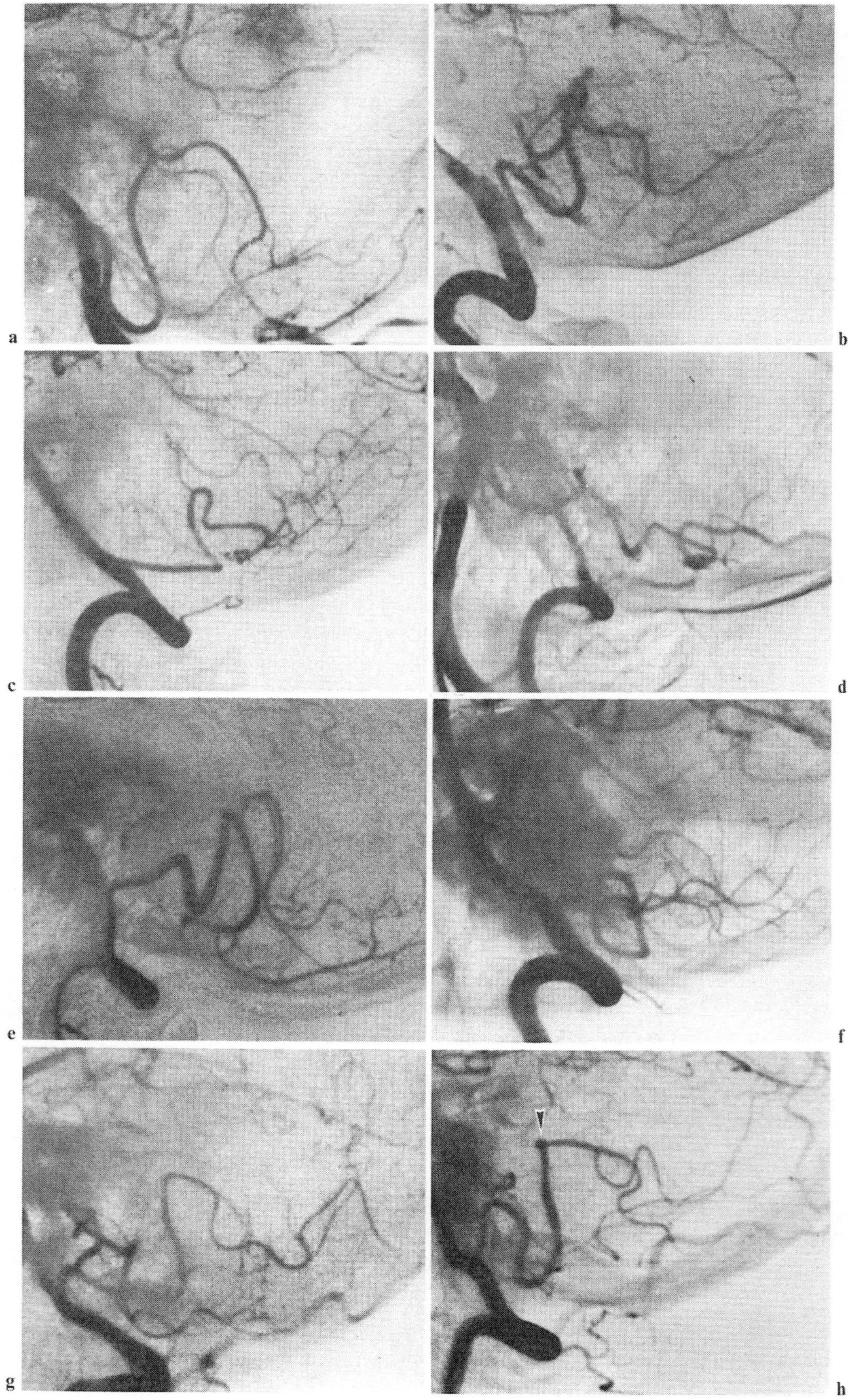

Abb. 18a–h

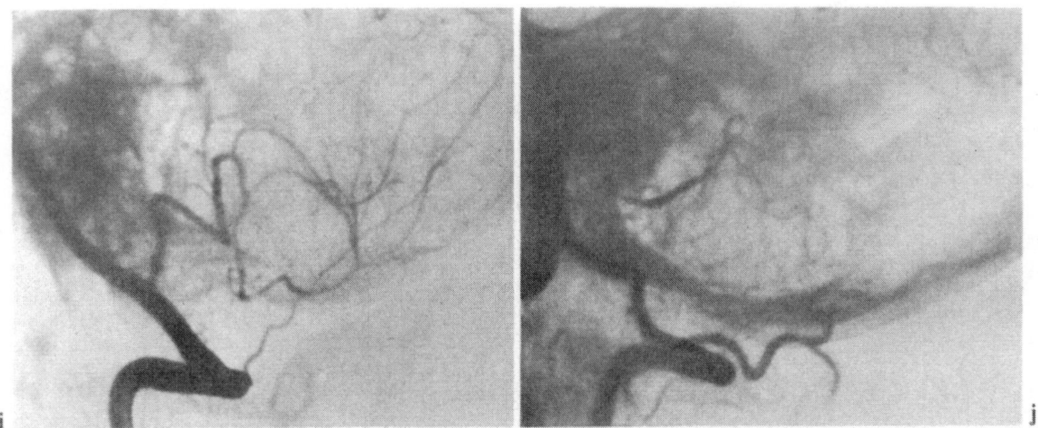

Abb. 18a–j. Verlaufsformen der A. cerebelli inferior posterior bei mittlerer Abgangshöhe. 1. absteigendes zisternales Segment bzw. Anfangsstück **a**, **b**, mit unmittelbarem Übergang in eine kaudale Schleife **a**, Doppelschleifenbildung des Segmentum medullare laterale **b**. 2. weitgehend gestreckter Verlauf des Anfangsstücks mit völlig gestrecktem Verlauf des Segmentum tonsillare laterale **c**, sehr flachbogige Schleifen **d**, gestrecktes Segmentum medullare laterale und Übergang in normal weite Schleifen **e**, rundbogige Schleifenbildung **f**. 3. ansteigendes Anfangsstück. Frühzeitige Aufteilung in Vermien- und Tonsillohemisphärenast **g**, rechtwinklige Richtungsänderung und Aufteilung am choroidalen Punkt ► **h**, kleinbogiger Verlauf **i** bzw. fast verstrichene Schleifen **j**

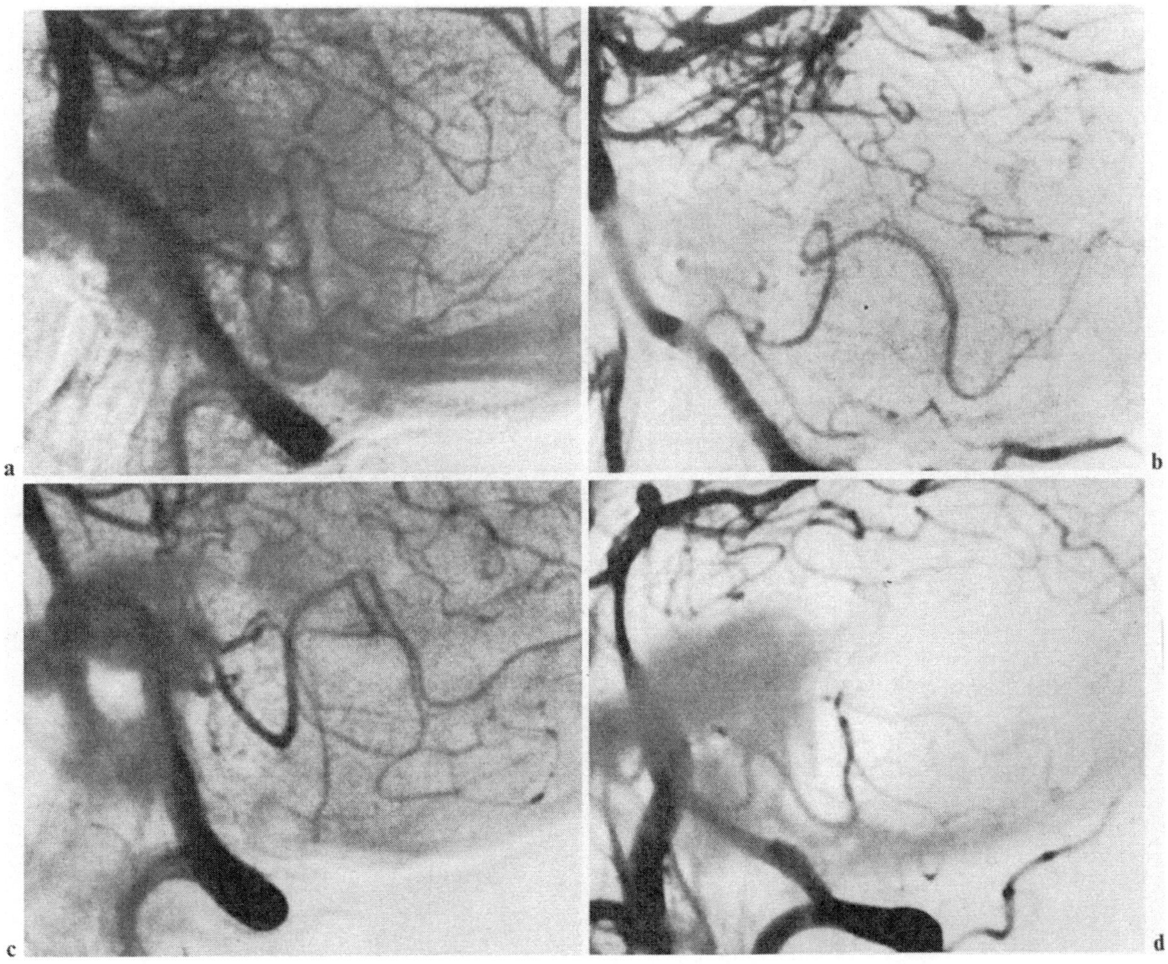

a
b
c
d

Abb. 19a–d. A. cerebelli inferior posterior mit hohem Abgang (in der Nähe der Vereinigung der Vertebralarterien) mit gestrecktem Verlauf des Segmentum medullare anterius und laterale **a**, mit flachbogigem Verlauf der kaudalen Schleife **b**, engschenkligem Verlauf der kaudalen Schleife bei elongierter Vertebralisendstrecke **c** mit gut ausgeprägter kranialer und kaudaler Schleife **d** (bei Turrizephalie)

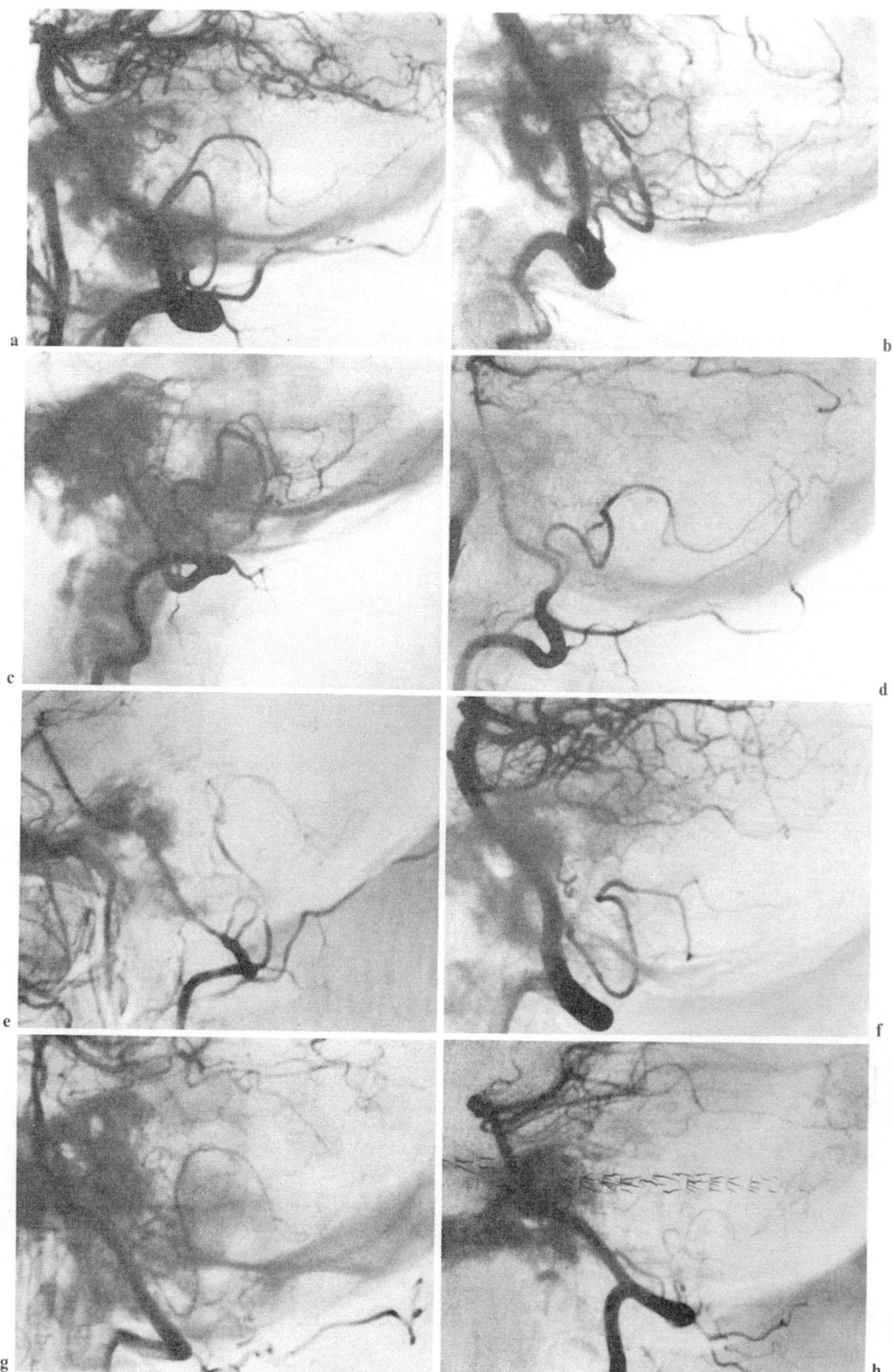

Abb. 20a–h

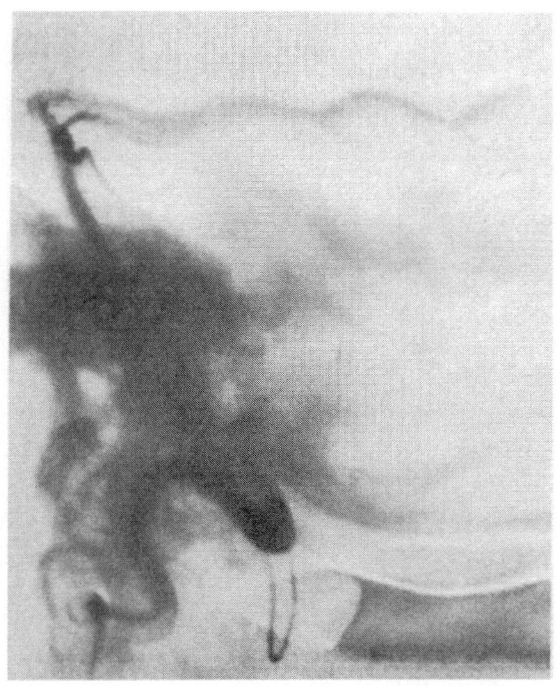

Abb. 21. Tiefliegende Tonsillenschleife bei Arnold-Chiari-Syndrom

Die Einteilung in Segmente nach WOLF et al. (1962) in:

1. Segment (Pars cisternalis und absteigender Schenkel der kaudalen Schleife)
2. Segment (aufsteigender Schenkel der kaudalen Schleife und aufsteigender Schenkel der kranialen Schleife)
3. Segment (absteigender Schenkel der kranialen Schleife, meist schon Ramus tonsillo-hemisphericus)

benennt als Segmente die mehr oder weniger geradlinigen Elemente zwischen den markanten Schleifenscheiteln. Diese Einteilung wurde von HUANG und WOLF (1966) in 6 Segmente weiter differenziert und in dieser Form von TAKAHASHI (1974) übernommen:

1) Segmentum medullare anterius	zisternales Segment (GREITZ)
2) Segmentum meduallare laterale	absteigender Schenkel der kaudalen Schleife
3) Segmentum medullare posterius	aufsteigender Schenkel der kaudalen Schleife
4) Segmentum supratonsillare	Arcus choroideus (GREITZ)
5) Segmentum retrotonsillare superius	absteigender Schenkel der kranialen Schleife
6) Segmentum vermiculare	Vermienast.

In dieser „klassischen“ Verlaufsform (Abb. 17), mit Ursprung der A. cerebelli inferior posterior im mittleren Bereich des 4. Abschnitts der A. vertebralis, zieht das *Segmentum medullare anterius*, vorwiegend dorsalwärts und etwas kaudalwärts gerichtet, um den Vorderrand der Medulla oblongata. Die Höhe des Abganges von der A. vertebralis bestimmt dabei entscheidend die Verlaufsrichtung und Konfiguration der ersten beiden Segmente. Das Gefäß zieht durch die Wurzelbündel des N. hypoglossus zu den Wurzeln des N. glossopharyngeus und N. vagus und liegt meist auf Niveau der Olive der Medulla an (KRAYENBÜHL u. YASARGIL, 1965). In a-p Projektion kann der Anfangsabschnitt ebenfalls in Abhängigkeit von der Höhe des Abgangs medial oder lateral der A. vertebralis erscheinen (WOLF et al., 1962).

◀ **Abb. 20a–h.** A. cerebelli inferior posterior mit tiefem Abgang (Ebene des Foramen occipitale magnum und darunter). Ansteigender Verlauf der Angangsstrecke **a–d** mit ausgiebiger **a**, **b** und flacher Schleifenbildung **c**, **d**. Absteigender Verlauf der Anfangsstrecke **e–h** mit ausgiebiger Schleifenbildung **e–g**. Nahezu gestreckter Verlauf **h**. Der letzte Befund leitet zu den Verlaufsanomalien über (Arnold-Chiari-Syndrom)

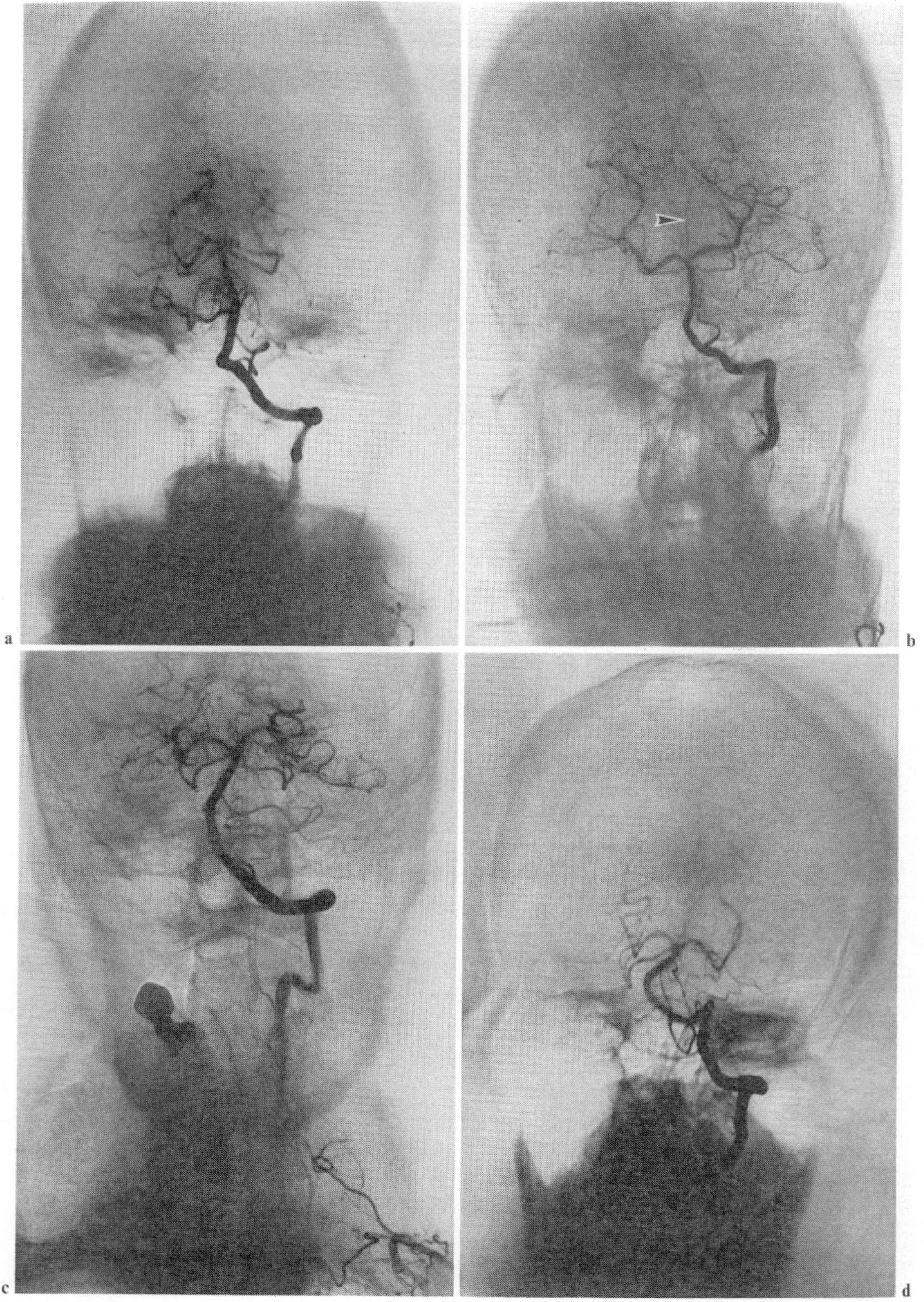

Abb. 22a–e. Darstellung der A. cerebelli inferior posterior im a-p Strahlengang. Verlauf der medullären Schleife, je nach Höhe des Abganges, lateral **a–c** oder medial **d–e**, mittelständiger Verlauf des Vermienates **b**, **d**

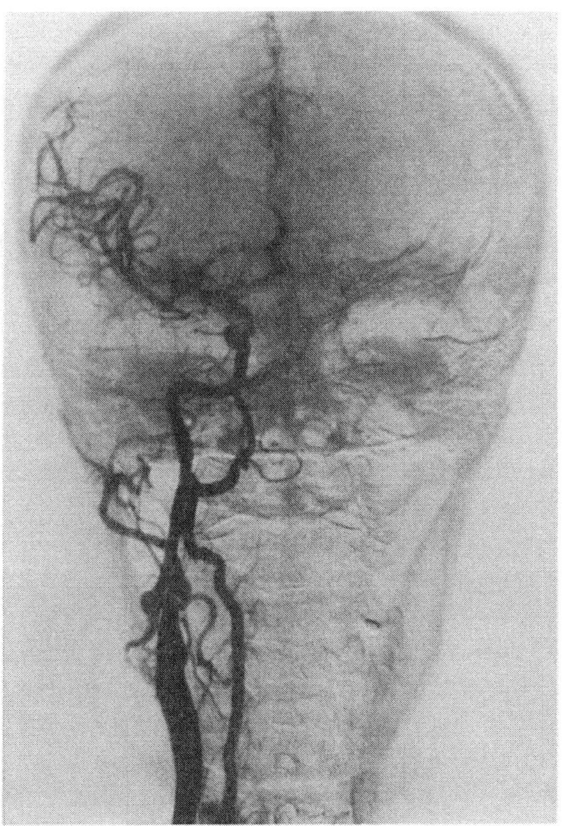

Abb. 22e

Das *Segmentum medullare laterale* setzt den nach dorsal gerichteten Verlauf zum unteren Anteil der Tonsillenvorderfläche fort. Das Segment kreuzt die laterale Tonsillenfläche. In 10% der Fälle verläuft es dorsal und kaudal der Tonsille (MARGOLIS u. NEWTON, 1974; MÜLLER, 1975). Diese häufige Variante, mit tiefem Wendepunkt der kaudalen Schleife – teilweise weit unterhalb der Ebene des Foramen occipitale magnum – soll bei der Arnold-Chiari-Mißbildung häufiger vorkommen. Der Verlauf im Zervikalkanal bildet dann die Form einer Haarnadel (GREITZ u. SJÖGREN, 1963), während die Schleife bei der Tonsillenherniation eher weit ist (WOLF et al., 1962). In a-p Projektion entspricht die laterale Ausdehnung des Segments der lateralen Kontur der Medulla oblongata.

Das *Segmentum medullare posterius* wendet sich zunächst bogenförmig zum Obex fossae rhomboideae, wo einzelne feine Ästchen in das retrooliväre Gebiet abgegeben werden und kleinere Anastomosen zu Ästen der A. cerebelli inferior anterior zu finden sind, dann aufwärts in der Rinne zwischen Rautengrube und Kleinhirn, an der Hinterfläche der Medulla bzw. der Kleinhirnschenkel, und beschreibt einen engen Bogen zur Kleinhirnunterfläche. Als Ast dieses Segments kann der Ramus tonsillo-hemisphericus abgehen, der an der Tonsillenvorderfläche zum unteren Tonsillenpol zieht und sich mit einem lateralen Ast an der Versorgung des unteren Anteils der Kleinhirnhemisphären beteiligt. Die ersten drei Segmente bilden die kaudale (medulläre) Schleife).

Das *Segmentum supratonsillare* (Spitze der kranialen Schleife, Arcus choroideus) verläuft medial oder kranial des oberen Tonsillenpoles. Der Beginn des Segments liegt dem Velum medullare inferius unmittelbar an und markiert den „choroidalen Punkt", d.h. die Stelle, an der ein oder mehrere Äste zum Plexus choroideus des 4. Ventrikels abgegeben werden (WOLF et al., 1962; GREITZ u. SJÖGREN, 1963). Der Punkt befindet sich auf einer Meßlinie, etwa an der Markierung des vorderen Drittels der Verbindungsstrecke, zwischen dem Vorderrand des Foramen occipitale magnum und Torcular (TAKAHASHI et al., 1973). Andere Meßpunkte auf der TWININGschen Linie bzw. der „Auditory line" (WOLF et al., 1962) sowie auf der Verbindungslinie der Protuberantia occipitalis interna und der Spitze der Basilarisgabel (MEGRET, 1972; WACKENHEIM, 1974) werden angegeben. Dies ist möglich, weil die Spitze der kranialen Schleife weniger Variationen aufzuweisen scheint als die der kaudalen. Sie wird bestimmt durch die Anheftstelle des Velum medullare im Bereich des Nodulus. Nur wenn eine Lücke zwischen dem Velum und dem Nodulus besteht, kann in einigen Fällen die Schleife bis auf die Höhe des Fastigiums des 4. Ventrikels aufsteigen. Bei der Form des Segmentes bestimmt dies, ob eine enge oder weite Schleife entsteht (WOLF et al., 1962). Im absteigenden Anteil des Segments können Anastomosenäste aus der A. cerebelli inferior anterior aufgenommen werden, ferner Rami tonsillares zur medialen Tonsillenfläche und zum Nodulus, die sich – ebenso wie die Äste zum Plexus – besonders bei pathologischen Kreislaufsituationen oder Tumoren in diesem Bereich deutlich zeigen (TAKAHASHI et al., 1973). Auch die Aufteilung des Stammes in mediale (Vermien-) und laterale (Hemisphären-)Äste kann in diesem Abschnitt oder aber im nächsten Segment erfolgen.

Das *Segmentum retrotonsillare superius* verläuft nach dorsal und kaudal an der hinteren Tonsillenfläche im Sulcus retrotonsillaris. Auf dieser Verlaufsstrecke, bis zum unteren lateralen Tonsillenrand, kann sich das Gefäß in einen oft sehr unterschiedlich starken, medialen oder lateralen Ast aufteilen. Der mediale oder Vermien-Ast stellt bei kräftiger Ausbildung das letzte Segment dar. Der laterale Ast (Hemisphärenast) kann auch als Ramus tonsillo-hemisphericus ausgebildet sein und gibt dann, außer den Ästen zu den lateralen Anteilen des Lobulus biventer, Lobulus gracilis, Lobulus semilunaris inferior und Lobus semilunaris superior, Äste ab, die von der Hinterfläche der Tonsille nach vorn und lateral verlaufen. Weitere Ausgangspunkte von Hemisphärenästen sind, in der Reihenfolge der Häufigkeit, das Segmentum medullare laterale, das Segmentum supratonsillare, das Segmentum medullare posterius, selten auch das Segmentum medullare anterius (WOLF et al., 1962; KRAYENBÜHL u. YASARGIL, 1957, 1965; HUANG u. WOLF, 1969; TAKAHASHI, 1973). Im Angiogramm sind die Hemisphärenäste im seitlichen Bild, etwa 1 bis 1,5 cm oberhalb und parallel zur Okzipitalschuppe aufsteigend, fast immer sichtbar (KRAYENBÜHL u. YASARGIL, 1957), können aber auch kalottennah und durch den Knochen verdeckt verlaufen. In a-p Projektion ist der Ramus tonsillohemisphericus oft nur schwer abgrenzbar, so daß die kraniale Schleife unvollständig erscheint.

Das *Segmentum vermiculare* richtet sich nach dorsal und apikal und umgibt bogenförmig den Unterwurm. Ein stärkerer Ast ist der Ramus suprapyramidalis. Im Verlauf im Sulcus paramedianus (valleculae) werden multiple Ästchen zum Unterwurm der Aa. vermis caudales sowie an die medialen Anteile des Lobulus biventer, Lobulus gracilis, Lobulus semilunaris inferior und Lobulus semilunaris superior abgegeben. Oft sollen reichlich Anastomosen zur Gegenseite und zu Ästen der A. cerebelli superior bestehen. Im Angiogramm sind die Vermienäste im seitlichen Bild nicht immer zu sehen. Sie bilden eine nach unten, im hinteren Anteil nach hinten konvexe (hintere oder 3.) Schleife um die Copula pyramidis. Der Verlauf im a-p Bild ist lateralwärts konvex, im Gegensatz zur medialwärts konvex verlaufenden kranialen Schleife, bei der der medial konvexe Bogen der medialen Ausbuchtung der Tonsille in die Vallecula entspricht (WOLF et al., 1962). Beide Schleifen formen das allerdings stark projektionsabhängige Bild des S-förmigen Verlaufs in der a-p Projektion. Der Verlauf des Vermienastes ist in beiden Strahlenrichtungen sehr konstant, besonders der a-p Verlauf in der Mittellinie, bzw. wenige Millimeter paramedian. Bei der Beurteilung von Verlagerungen ist auch hier der gleichzeitige Nachweis deformierter Gefäßstrecken entscheidend.

2. Verlaufsvarianten

Die Verlaufsvarianten der A. cerebelli inferior posterior sind so zahlreich, daß WACKENHEIM (1974) resignierend feststellt, man könne bei jedem Autor (COLUMELLA, 1952; HAUGE, 1954;

RUGGIERO, 1954; GREITZ u. SJÖGREN, 1963) etwas anderes lesen. Hauptprinzip der Variationen ist die gegenseitige Ergänzung der Stromgebiete der Kleinhirnarterien bei entwicklungsgeschichtlich bedingten Abgangs- und Verlaufsvarianten. Dies ergibt sich schon im „Normalfall" aus der Vielzahl der oben beschriebenen Kollateralen, die sich noch vermehren ließen. So beschreibt z.B. ATKINSON (1949) in seiner Arbeit über die A. cerebelli inferior anterior konstante Anastomosen von Ästen dieses Gefäßes zu den Wurzeln des VII. bis X. Hirnnerven mit Endästen der A. cerebelli inferior posterior. LAZORTHES et al. (1950) nennen 3 Typen des Verlaufs der A. cerebelli inferior posterior nach der Versorgung:

Typ 1: (normal) sichert die Versorgung des Vermis und der Unterseite der gleichseitigen Kleinhirnhemisphäre,
Typ 2: (extensiv) es besteht ein Kollateralkreislauf zur Kleinhirnhemisphäre der Gegenseite,
Typ 3: (regressiv) die Arterie versorgt die lateralen und rostralen Abschnitte der Hemisphäre, der Rest wird von der Gegenseite vaskularisiert.

GREITZ (1956) orientiert seine Einteilung in 3 Typen am Gefäßverlauf:

Typ 1: entspricht dem oben beschriebenen klassischen Verlauf. Bei Abgang des Gefäßes von der A. vertebralis erreicht der zisternale Abschnitt den unteren Tonsillenpol und geht in die kaudale Schleife über.
Typ 2: Bei Abgang von der A. vertebralis steigt der zisternale Abschnitt an, die kaudale Schleife fehlt, das Gefäß erreicht zuerst den oberen Tonsillenpol.
Typ 3: Bei Abgang von der A. basilaris verläuft der zisternale Abschnitt nahezu horizontal und erreicht den oberen Tonsillenpol.

HUANG und WOLF (1969) geben 6 häufigere Varianten (A bis F) an, dabei fehlt in 3 Fällen eine ausgeprägte kaudale Schleife, in 2 Fällen eine deutliche kraniale Schleife, 1 Fall zeigt die Ausbildung der Segmente 4 bis 6 (Segmentum supratonsillare) durch die A. cerebelli inferior anterior. Von TAKAHASHI (1974) wird diese Einteilung übernommen und zusätzlich eine Aufgliederung der Häufigkeit von 10 Abgangsvarianten in seinem Beobachtungsgut erstellt (TAKAHASHI et al., 1968, Abb. 17–20).

Bei der Hypoplasie dere A. cerebelli inferior posterior kann das Gefäß durch den medialen Ast der A. cerebelli inferior anterior oder sogar durch einen Ast der A. cerebelli superior ersetzt werden. Auch der Verlauf der einzelnen Segmente ist sehr variationsreich. Die extremen Verläufe der kaudalen und kranialen Schleife wurden bereits erwähnt. Sowohl bei aufgehobener wie bei besonders tiefer kaudaler Schleife, aber auch bei fehlender kranialer Schleife (Typ B, C und F der Einteilung nach HUANG u. WOLF, 1969) kann, statt des Segmentum medullare laterale, ein Segmentum medullare mediale entstehen. MARGOLIS und NEWTON (1972) wiesen darauf hin, daß der Arcus choroideus bis zu 10 mm unterhalb des Velum medullare inferius des 4. Ventrikels verlaufen kann, nach WACKENHEIM (1974) z.B. auch bei der Arnold Chiari-Mißbildung. Die Erkenntnis über die relative „Unzuverlässigkeit" des Gefäßverlaufes zur Beurteilung von Raumforderungen der hinteren Schädelgrube hat die Einsicht gefördert, die differenzierten kleineren, „sicheren" Kriterien (Verlauf des Vermienastes, der Hemisphärenäste und Lage des Punktum choroideum) dem relativ unsicheren „Eindruck" über den Gesamtverlauf des Gefäßes überzuordnen. Die schon erwähnten Meßpunkte für den chorioidalen Punkt verlieren, nach Beobachtungen von MARGOLIS und NEWTON (1972), nicht völlig ihre Bedeutung. Nach WOLF et al. (1962) befindet sich der chorioidale Punkt selten tiefer als 1 mm unterhalb der „auditory line", das ist eine Parallele zur TWININGschen Linie durch den Unterrand des Meatus acusticus internus. Die anteroposteriore Lage des Punktes als Lot auf die TWININGsche Linie, d.h. die Verbindungslinie zwischen dem Tuberculum sellae und der Protuberantia occipitalis interna, soll sich ebenfalls in einem engen Rahmen bewegen und zwischen den Markierungspunkten in 52 und 60% der Streckenlänge, vom Tuberculum sellae aus gemessen, zu finden sein. Nach MEGRET (1972) und WACKENHEIM (1974) schneidet das Mittellot auf die Verbindungslinie zwischen der Protuberantia occipitalis interna und der Spitze der Basilarisgabel die A. cerebelli inferior posterior im chorioidalen Punkt.

III. Arteria basilaris

1. Verlauf

Die A. basilaris hat einen einfachen, relativ konstanten Verlauf. Sie wird durch die Vereinigung der Vertebralarterien, etwa in Höhe des Sulcus pontomedullaris, gebildet und verläuft meist ohne wesentliche Kaliberabnahme (BUSCH, 1966) in einer flachen, medianen Grube der Ponsvorderfläche zum Klivus nach rostral (TAKAHASHI, 1974). Nach Abgabe ihrer Äste teilt sie sich in der Cisterna interpeduncularis, unmittelbar nach Durchtritt zwischen den beiden Nn. abducentes, in die Aa. cerebri posteriores. Äste sind die Aa. cerebelli superiores, Aa. cerebelli inferiores anteriores, in einzelnen Fällen auch Aa. auditivae internae bzw. cerebelli mediae. Die pontinen Äste können in 2 Gruppen eingeteilt werden, die medialen und transversalen pontinen Arterien. Die zahlreichen kleinen medianen Ponsäste ziehen nach kaudal und dringen senkrecht in den Pons ein. Die transversalen pontinen Äste entspringen von der postero-lateralen Fläche der A. basilaris und verlaufen nach lateral und dorsal um den Pons. In Anzahl und Kaliber sind sie variabel. Sie geben in ihrem Verlauf perforierende Äste ab. Diese pontinen Äste sind in den Angiogrammen in den lateralen Projektionen nur schwach, in den halbaxialen Projektionen nur selten zu sehen. GABRIELSON und AMUNDSEN (1969) konnten sie allerdings, bei Anwendung besonderer Sorgfalt, in 84% in den lateralen und in 41% in den a-p Projektionen nachweisen. Zahlreiche der früheren Arbeiten über die A. basilaris beschäftigen sich besonders mit Länge, Kaliber und Verlauf des Gefäßes, besonders anhand anatomischer Präparate, teilweise in Beziehung zu Körpergröße, Alter, Geschlecht, arteriosklerotischen Veränderungen sowie im Hinblick auf Anomalien und pathologische Veränderungen (LONGO, 1905; CAVATORTI, 1907; RENDALL, 1909; BERRY u. ANDERSON, 1909; DAVY, 1916; STOPFORD, 1916; ADACHI, 1928; MITTERWALLNER, 1955; KRAYENBÜHL u. YASARGIL, 1957; LANG u. KOLLMANNSBERGER, 1961; BUSCH, 1966; HAVERLING, 1974). Eine eingehende Standardisierung der Verlaufsvarianten, unter Einschluß der Literaturangaben, versuchten VOIGT et al. (1972). Hervorgehoben werden Verlaufsvarianten in Kollektiven von gefäßgesunden Erwachsenen, erwachsenen Patienten mit arteriosklerotischen Veränderungen und Kindern. Die Besonderheiten des Basilarisverlaufs im kindlichen Angiogramm, unter Berücksichtigung der Arbeiten von SCHIEFER und VETTER (1957), TAVERAS und POSER (1959), PARAICZ und SZESNASY (1959), RAIMONDI und WHITE (1967), LA TORRE et al. (1969), DECKER und BACKMUND (1970), BRADAC und SIMON (1971), HARWOOD-NASH u. FITZ (1976) sind: auffallend weiter Klivus-Basilarisabstand, relativ große Basilaris-Gesamtlänge und höchster Überstand der A. basilaris über den Apex des Dorsum sellae (auch im Vergleich zu den Untersuchungskollektiven mit arteriosklerotisch elongierten Gefäßen). Die Veränderungen sind bis zum 3. Lebensjahr ausgeprägt und erst gegen das 10. Lebensjahr ausgeglichen. Sie erklären sich aus den sich wechselseitig beeinflussenden Größen und Wachstumsbeziehungen zwischen Hirnstamm und Schädelbasisstrukturen. Dabei nimmt das Gefäß bei Kindern einen überwiegend geradlinigen Verlauf in der Sagittalebene mit der geringsten Seitenabweichung vergleichbarer Kollektive, trotz relativ großer Gesamtlänge des Gefäßes (PARAICZ u. SZENASY, 1959; DECKER u. BACKMUND, 1970; VOIGT et al., 1972). Im Kollektiv der Gefäßgesunden beginnt der Grenzbereich der „Basilarisanpressung" bei einem Abstand von 2 mm vom Klivus, der „Basilarisabdrängung" bei 12 bis 13 mm Klivusabstand. Der Abstand der A. basilaris vom Apex des Dorsum sellae in antero-posteriorer Richtung beträgt im Mittel 7,2 mm (2–13 mm), im Einklang mit den Ergebnissen von KRAYENBÜHL und YASARGIL (1957).

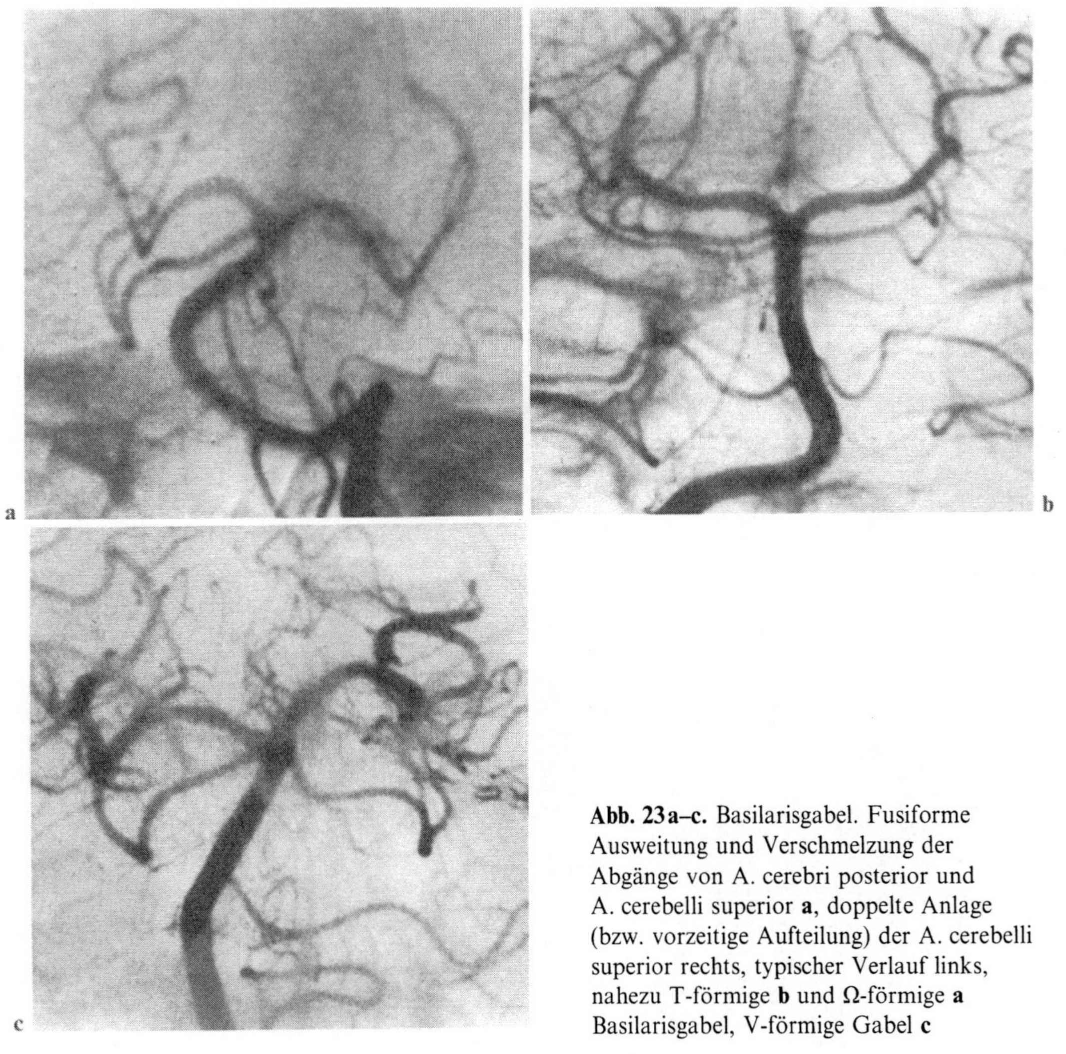

Abb. 23a–c. Basilarisgabel. Fusiforme Ausweitung und Verschmelzung der Abgänge von A. cerebri posterior und A. cerebelli superior **a**, doppelte Anlage (bzw. vorzeitige Aufteilung) der A. cerebelli superior rechts, typischer Verlauf links, nahezu T-förmige **b** und Ω-förmige **a** Basilarisgabel, V-förmige Gabel **c**

Dies ist bei der Beurteilung einer eventuellen Dorsalwärtsverlagerung der Basilarisgabel zu berücksichtigen, die für verschiedene Krankheitsbilder angegeben wird: retrosellärer Tumor (YASARGIL, 1962), dilatierter, nach kaudal herniierter 3. Ventrikel, z.B. bei Aquäduktstenose (SCATCLIFF et al., 1965; SCHECHTER u. ZINNGIESSER, 1967; LA TORRE et al., 1969). Der hier angegebene Grenzwert von 9 mm ist vermutlich zu eng gefaßt. Die Seitenabweichung aus der Medianen betrug bei den Gefäßgesunden bis zu 11 mm nach rechts und 8 mm nach links bei einem gestreckten geradlinigen Verlauf in 67% der Fälle (MITTERWALLNER (1955) 82%, BUSCH (1966) 84%). Diese Angabe schwankt jedoch, je nach Zusammensetzung des Kollektivs, am stärksten (CAVATORTI (1907) 16%, ADACHI (1928) 25%. BOERI und PASERINI (1964) 25%). Der Basilarisüberstand über den Apex des Dorsum sellae betrug im Mittel 2 mm, korrespondierend mit den Ergebnissen von KRAYENBÜHL und YASARGIL (1957) und BOERI und PASERINI (1964), die einen Überstand in 30% der untersuchten Fälle fanden. Das Kollektiv der Patienten mit arteriosklerotisch veränderten Gefäßen wies eine um 10 mm (25%) gesteigerte Gesamtlänge des Gefäßes auf. Der Maximalwert für den Basilarisüberstand war verdoppelt (15 mm) bei 3 $^{1}/_{2}$fachem Mittelwert. Extreme Werte bestanden bei der Seitenabweichung, die deutlich über denen der Vergleichsgruppe mit infratentoriellen Raumforderungen lagen. Der Klivus-Basilarisabstand war nicht signifikant verändert. Häufig ergibt sich durch den starken Basilarishochstand das Symptom der Eindellung des Bodens des 3. Ventrikels, beschrieben von COLUMELLA (1952), SJÖGREN (1953), GREITZ und LÖF-

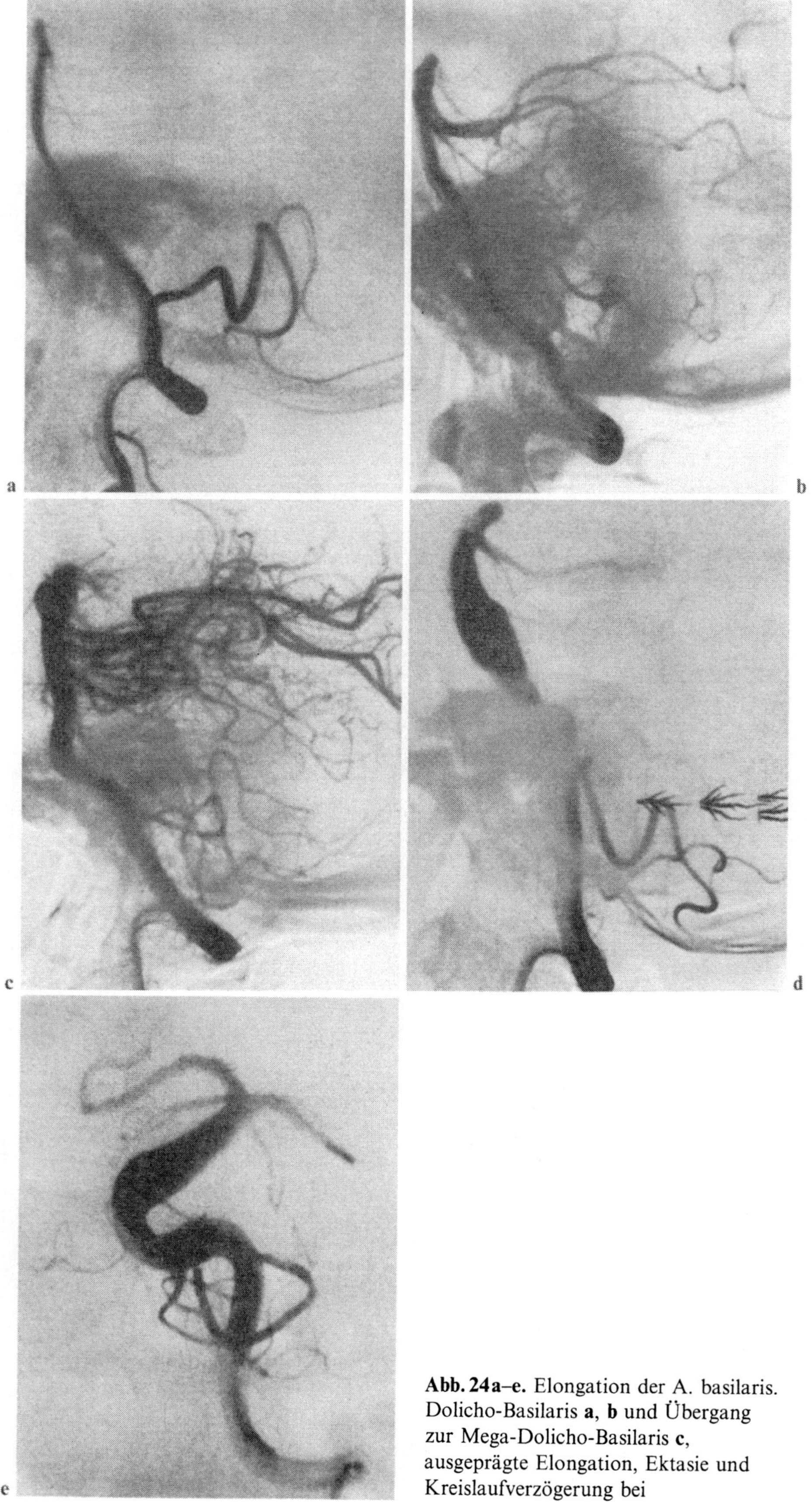

Abb. 24a–e. Elongation der A. basilaris. Dolicho-Basilaris **a**, **b** und Übergang zur Mega-Dolicho-Basilaris **c**, ausgeprägte Elongation, Ektasie und Kreislaufverzögerung bei Mega-Dolicho-Basilaris **d**, **e**

STEDT (1954), RUGGIERO und CONSTANS (1954), KRAYENBÜHL und YASARGIL (1957), TATELMAN (1958), BOERI und PASSERINI (1964), DETTORI et al. (1966). Entsprechend der Trias: Elongation, Schlängelung, Ektasie, findet man in dieser Gruppe durchschnittlich höhere Werte für das Gefäßkaliber.

2. Varianten

Ausgeprägte Normvarianten weisen die Form und Höhe der Vereinigungsstelle sowie der Basilarisgabel auf. Sie sind durch Länge und Verlauf des Gefäßes bedingt. Die „typische" Vereinigungsstelle am kaudalen Brückenrand fanden CAVARTORTI (1907) in 49%, STOPFORD (1916) in 48%, KRAYENBÜHL und YASARGIL (1957) in 66%, BUSCH (1966) in 50%. Der Verlauf der Vertebralarterien vor der Vereinigung kann gestreckt, einseitig gestreckt oder beidseits gewunden sein, was – auch im Zusammenhang mit den Kaliberunterschieden der Vertebralarterien – die Variabilität des Vereinigungswinkels und die Höhe der Vereinigung maßgeblich beeinflussen soll (RICKENBACHER, 1964; BUSCH, 1966; VOIGT et al., 1972). Bei starker Elongation und Schlängelung wurde als Anomalie sogar ein Überkreuzen der Vertebralarterien vor der Vereinigung beschrieben (BUSCH, 1966).

Die Basilarisgabel kann W- oder V-Form aufweisen, je nachdem, ob die A. basilaris weiter oder weniger weit in die Cisterna interpeduncularis nach kranial reicht. Bei relativ flachem Verlauf wird eine Omega- oder Schlingenform (LINDGREN, 1950) oder eine T-Form (LINDGREN, 1950; BUSCH, 1966; FIEGEL u. NADJMI, 1972) beschrieben.

Zu den Anomalien sind in erster Linie Fälle zu zählen, bei denen die Vereinigung der Vertebralarterien partiell oder total ausbleibt. Der geringste Verschmelzungsdefekt ist ein nur innerhalb des Gefäßes sichtbares, meist nur einige Millimeter langes Septum, welches sich auf der Gefäßoberfläche nur durch eine diskrete ventrale und dorsale Furche bemerkbar macht (BLACKBURN, 1907; DAVY, 1916; BUSCH, 1966). Totale Verdopplung der A. basilaris wird bei RIBES-CHAUSSIER (1928) und CAVATORTI (1908) beschrieben.

Eine relativ häufige weitere Ausprägungsform (bis zu 2% im anatomischen Untersuchungsgut) ist die Ausbildung von Fenstern bzw. Ösen, meist im proximalen Anteil der A. basilaris. Möglichkeiten der Ausprägungsform nach Literaturangaben und einigen eigenen Beobachtungen finden sich bei KRAYENBÜHL und YASARGIL (1957). In Einzelfällen bleibt die Verschmelzung der Vertebralarterien völlig aus (LONGO, 1905; BLACKBURN, 1907; DAVY, 1916; STOPFORD, 1916; ADACHI, 1928; MITTERWALLNER, 1955; KRAYENBÜHL u. YASARGIL, 1957; BUSCH, 1966; MÜLLER, 1975).

3. Karotidobasilare Verbindungen

Ebenfalls als Anomalie sind die persistierenden primitiven Arterien aufzufassen, welche in Form von karotido-basilären oder karotido-vertebralen Anastomosen verlaufen. Die häufigste dieser Verbindungen, die entwicklungsgeschichtlich Kollateralen vom Karotissystem zu den basalen longitudinalen Neuralarterien entspricht, und die sich im Regelfall bis auf die A. communicans posterior zurückbilden, ist die A. primitiva trigemina. Sie entspringt in der Regel vom Kavernosus-Abschnitt der A. carotis interna, zieht durch den Sinus cavernosus nach dorsal, tritt medial vom 1. Trigeminusast und lateral des N. oculomotorius aus dem Sinus aus, verläuft dann nach medial und verbindet sich mit der A. basilaris in deren mittlerem Abschnitt vor dem Klivus. Nach der Erstbeschreibung am erwachsenen Menschen durch QUAIN 1844 beschäftigten sich zahlreiche Veröffentlichungen im anatomischen Bereich mit dem Gefäß (TÜNGEL, 1860; DURET, 1874; TARENIETZKI, 1880; FLESCH, 1882; HOCHSTÄTTER, 1885; DECKER, 1886; SMITH, 1909; OERTEL, 1922; KOTRNETZ, 1931; ÖKRÖS, 1934; HASENJÄGER, 1937; HULTQUIST, 1941; SUNDERLAND, 1941; HARRISON u. LUTRELL, 1950). Der angiographische Nachweis gelang zuerst SUTTON (1950). Es folgten zahlreiche Veröffentlichungen (FRUGIONI, 1952; PHILLIPIDES et al., 1952; HARRISON

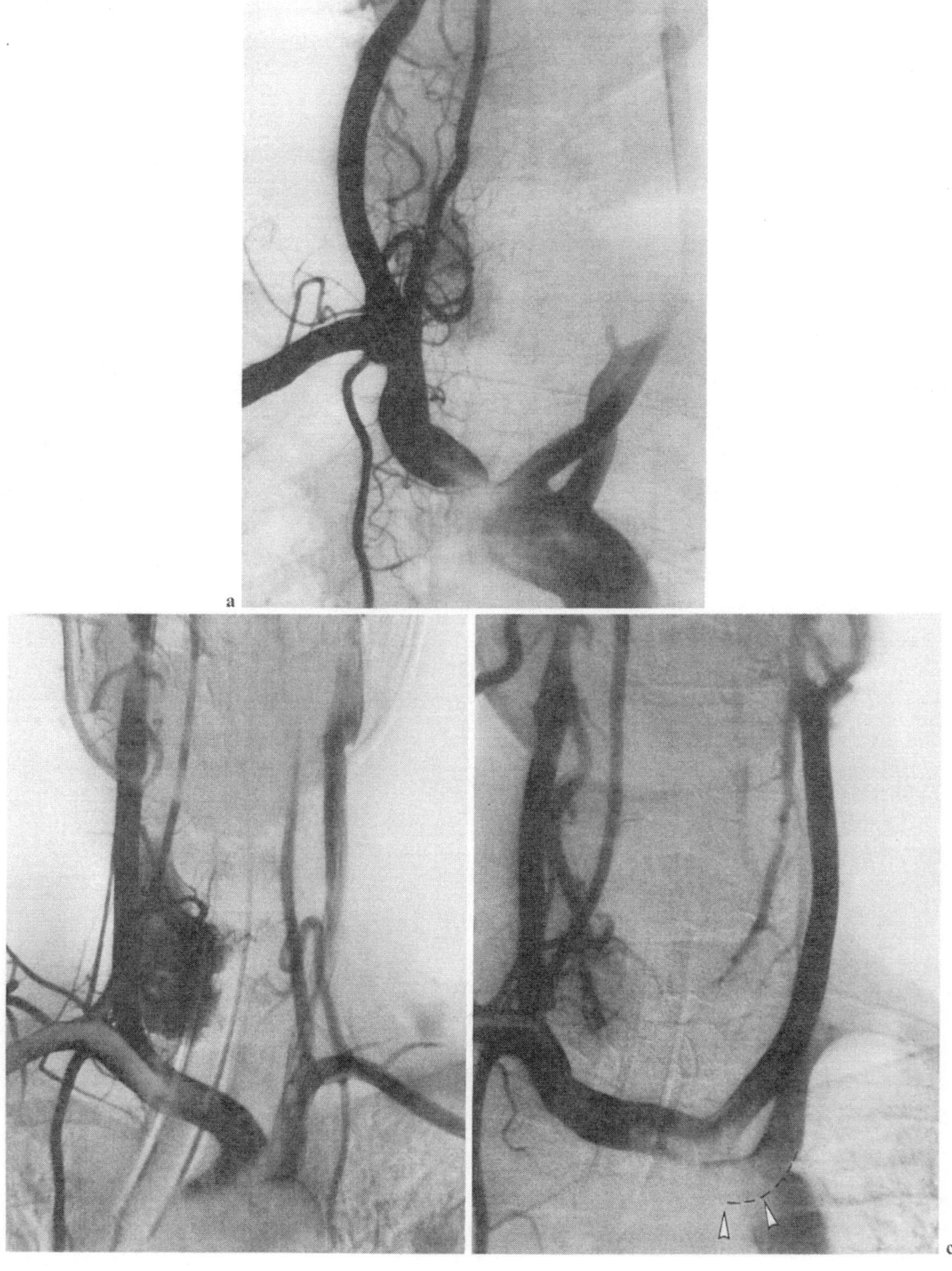

Abb. 25a–c. Seltene Darstellung des kompletten Aortenbogens mit allen supraaortalen Ästen im rechtsseitigen retrograden Brachialisangiogramm **a**, **b** sowie mit dextroponierter linker Arteria subclavia **c**

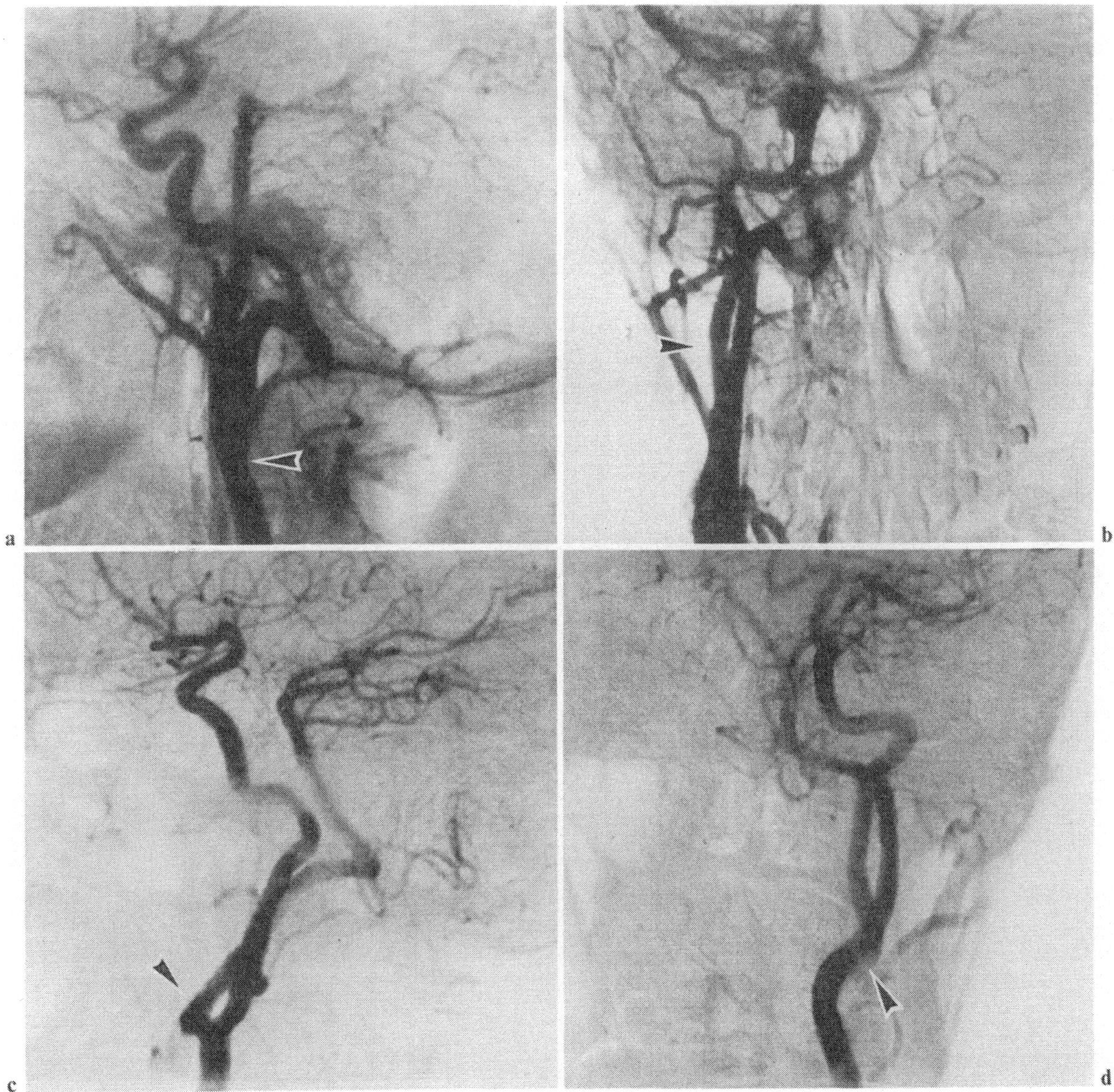

Abb. 26a–d. A. hypoglossica primitiva (2 Fälle). Abgang einer sehr kaliberkräftigen linksseitigen Vertebralarterie in Höhe des Atlas aus der Arteria carotis interna (im ap und seitlichen Strahlengang)

u. LUTRELL, 1953; SICCURO u. BAGGIORE, 1953; KLOSS, 1953; MONTRIEUL, 1956; STENVERS et al., 1953; GESSINI u. FRUGIONI, 1954; LINDGREN, 1954; MURTAGH et al., 1955; POBLETE u. ANSENJO, 1955; SCHÄRER, 1955; BREA, 1956; GROS et al., 1956; TÖNNIS et al., 1957; KRAYENBÜHL u. YASARGIL, 1957; SCHIEFER u. WALTER, 1958; SALTZMANN, 1959; NADJMI, 1961; CAMPBELL u. DYKEN, 1961; HUBER, 1961; WISE u. PALUBINSKAS, 1964; LEMAHIEV et al., 1967; DICKMANN et al., 1967; FIELDS, 1968; SUTTON, 1971). 150 Fälle der Weltliteratur wurden in der Sammelarbeit von LIE (1968) zusammengefaßt. Die Arbeiten befassen sich mit der eingehenden Verlaufsbeschreibung im Angiogramm, der Korrelation zu klinischen Krankheitsbildern, insbesondere der Subarachnoidalblutung, zur Kombination der Anomalien mit anderen entwicklungsgeschichtlich bedingten Gefäßmißbildungen, artero-venösen Angiomen, der Kombination mit Aneurysmen und der hämodynamischen Bedeutung der Anastomose, insbesondere bei hochgradigen stenosierenden Gefäßprozessen oder anlagebedingt hypoplastischen Gefäßen (LIE, 1968) und im Sinn von *Steal*-Syndromen bei sonst unveränderten zerebralen Kreisläufen (CAMPBELL u. DYKEN, 1961; HUBER, 1961).

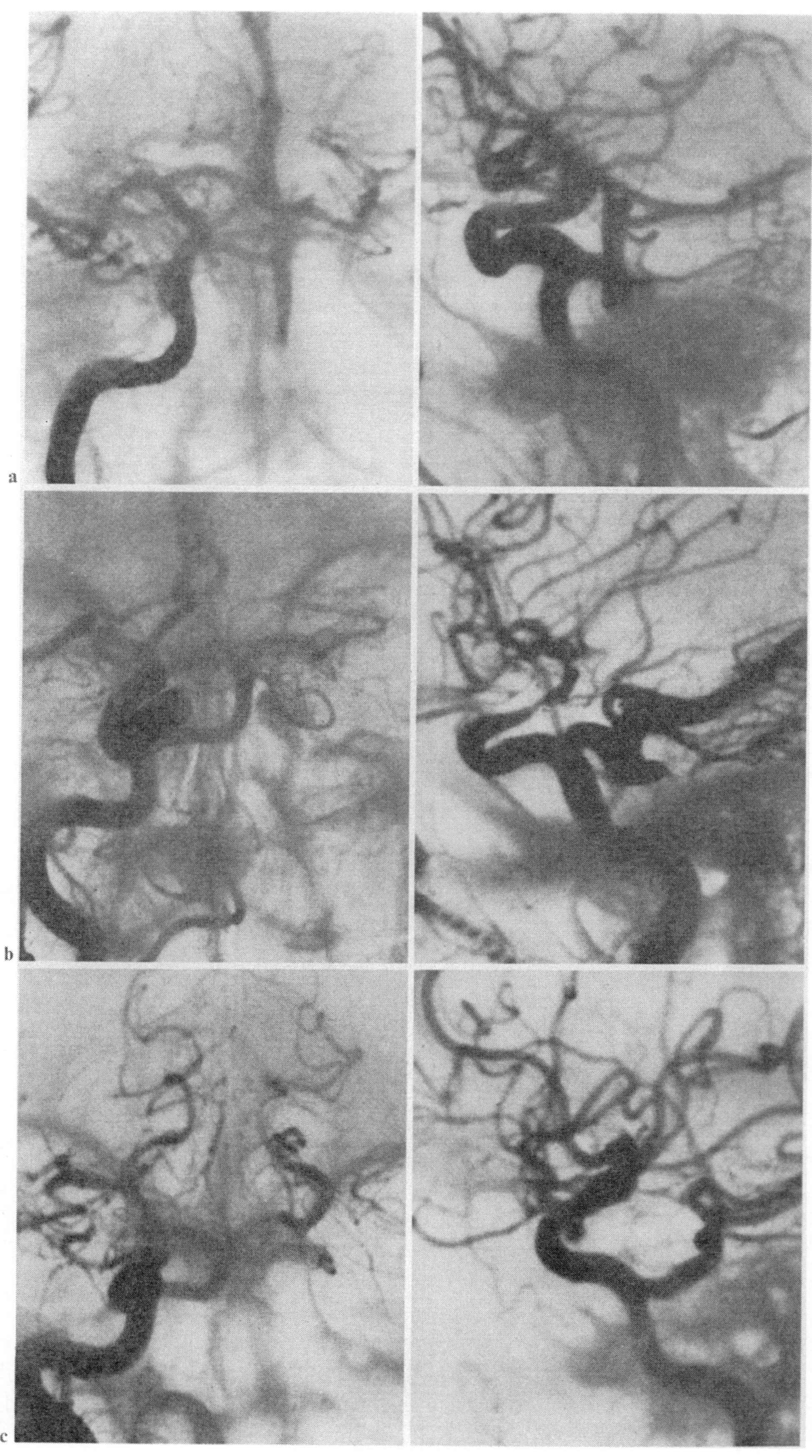

Abb. 27a–f. Formen der A. trigemina primitiva. Kräftiger Gefäßstamm mit gleichem Kaliber wie die A. carotis interna **a** oder nur geringfügig kleinerem Gefäßquerschnitt **b**, **c**. S-förmig geschwungene Formen **a**, **b**, **d**, **e**,

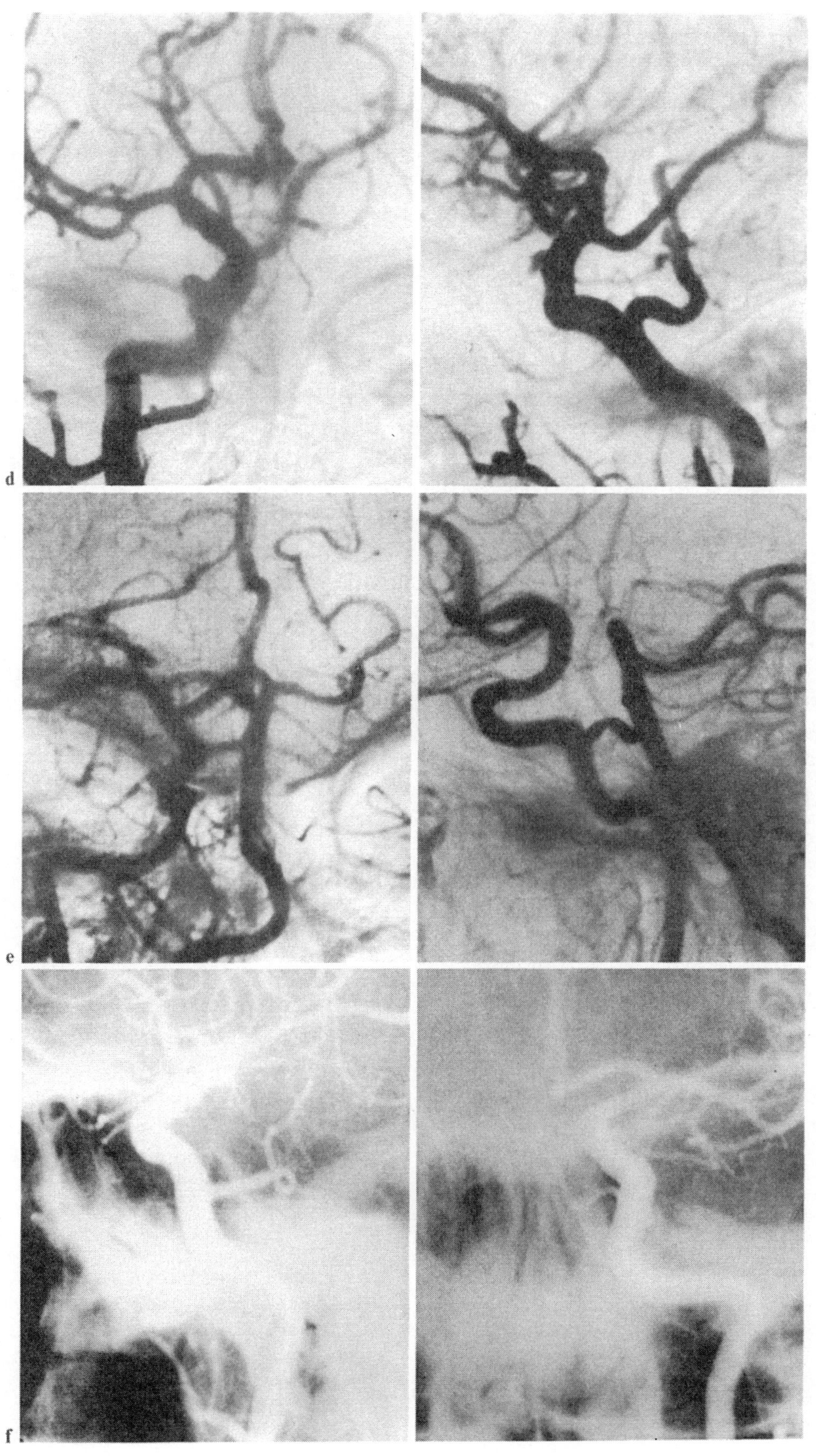

ausgeprägt basalwärts konvexbogiger Verlauf **c**, gestreckte Verlaufsform **f**, kleine Anastomosenkaliber **e**, **f**, unterschiedliche Höhe der Einmündung in die A. basilaris, sehr hohe **c**, **f**, sehr tiefe Einmündung **d**

Die Frage, ob es sich bei den Aneurysmen des Kavernosusabschnitts der A. carotis interna um rudimentäre Anlagen der A. primitiva trigemina handelt, wird diskutiert (PADGET, 1948; TIWISINA, 1964).

Topographisch die nächstliegende karotido-basiläre Anastomose ist die A. primitiva acustica (otica), die jedoch im Untersuchungsgut weitaus am seltensten erscheint. Sie zieht, gemeinsam mit dem 7. und 8. Hirnnerven, durch den Meatus acusticus internus. Die anatomische Beschreibung findet sich bei ALTMANN (1947). LIE (1968) berichtet über drei angiographisch nachgewiesene Fälle. Etwas häufiger wird die A. primitiva hypoglossica gefunden. Sie entspringt aus der A. carotis interna, etwa in Höhe des 1. bis 3. Halswirbels, verläuft durch den Kanal des N. hypoglossus, um die A. basilaris oder die A. vertebralis zu erreichen. Anatomische Beschreibungen stammen von BATUJEFF (1889), OERTEL (1922), MORRIS und MOFFAT (1956). Angiographische Arbeiten stammen von DALLE ORE (1954), LINDGREN (1950), BEGG (1961), GERLACH et al. (1962), BRUETMANN und FIELDS (1963), GILMARTIN (1963), PERRYMANN et al. (1963), SCOTT (1963), UDVARHELI und LAI (1963), JACKSON (1964), EADIE et al. (1964), SUTHERLAND und DONALDSON (1972), GOMBI et al. (1973), HUBER und RIVOIR (1974), WIEDNER und SCHREYER (1976). Eine Übersicht über 20 in der Literatur veröffentlichte Fälle, einschließlich der eigenen, gibt SUTTON (1971). Ebenfalls eine seltene Anomalie eines aus der Embryonalzeit persistierenden Gefäßes stellt die „erste zervikale (inter-) segmentale Arterie" (SUTTON, 1971) bzw. persistierende proatlantale Arterie (LIE, 1968) dar, die von der A. carotis interna (auch A. carotis externa, LIE, 1975) in Höhe des Atlas oder Axis abgeht und sich mit der horizontalen Strecke der A. vertebralis auf dem Atlasbogen verbindet. Die erste Beobachtung stammt von GOTTSCHAU (1885). Angiographisch wurden 5 Fälle beschrieben (LUCARELLI u. DE FERRARI, 1960; SAMRA et al., 1968; FLYNN, 1968; CONFORTI et al., 1966; HUTCHINSON u. MILLER, 1970; LIE, 1975). Eine relativ seltene Anomalie der A. basilaris ist die sog. Mega-Dolicho-Basilaris (TIWISINA, 1964; BOERI u. PASERINI, 1964; DETTORI et al., 1966), die jedoch, wegen der korrelierten klinischen Symptomatik bei noch unklarer Genese, zu den pathologischen Veränderungen des Gefäßes überleitet.

IV. A. cerebri posterior

1. Verlauf

Die A. cerebri posterior geht ursprünglich aus der A. carotis interna ab (Pars carotica), die Verbindung zur A. basilaris (Pars basilaris) wird erst später angelegt bzw. wirksam. Morphologisch bildet sie beim Erwachsenen in der Regel den Endast der A. basilaris. Sie stellt also ein Zwischenglied zwischen dem Karotiskreislauf und dem vertebrobasilären Gefäßsystem dar. Hieraus sich ergebende Varianten sind der einseitige und doppelseitige Abgang des Gefäßes von der A. carotis interna, das entsprechende Verhalten der Aa. communicantes posteriores und die Form des

Tabelle 3. Darstellbarkeit der A. cerebri posterior im Karotisangiogramm (nach KRAYENBÜHL u. YASARGIL, 1965)

ELVIDGE	1938	14%	TÖNNIS-PIA	1952	36%
FERNANDEZ et al.	1939	32%	SCARCELLA	1952	29%
MONIZ	1940	20%	TARDINI et al.	1955	26,8%
LIST et al.	1945	15%	SCHIEFER-VETTER	1957	37,3%
ENGESET	1948	23,5%	RABIOTTI-SAGINARO	1958	18%
WICKBOM	1948	20–25%	DECKER-HIPP	1958	15–20%
GREEN-ARANA	1948	34%	DILENGE	1962	40%
CURRY-CULBRETH	1951	33%	KRAYENBÜHL-YASARGIL	1964	35,7%
KRAYENBÜHL-RICHTER	1952	15–20%			

Anfangsstückes der hinteren Hirnarterien, in Beziehung zur Ausbildung der A. basilaris (s.o.) (WINDEL, 1888; DE VRIESE, 1905; FAWCETT u. BLACHFORD, 1905; STOPFORD, 1925; PADGET, 1945; SUNDERLAND, 1948; MITTERWALLNER, 1955; KRAYENBÜHL u. YASARGIL, 1957; HOYT et al., 1974). Hypoplasie oder Atresie der Pars basilaris entsprächen einem Karotisabgang, Rückbildung der Pars carotica einem Basilarisabgang. Dazwischen liegen die Übergangsmöglichkeiten, repräsentiert z.B. durch wechselnde Angaben über die Darstellbarkeit im Karotisangiogramm zwischen 14 und 40% (Tab. 3).

2. Aufteilung und kortikale Äste

Insgesamt ist der Verlauf der A. cerebri posterior konstant. Die von ihr abhängigen Gefäße kann man, nach dem Versorgungsbereich, in kortikale Gefäße (zum Okzipital- und Temporalbereich) sowie dienzephale und mesenzephale Äste einteilen, letztere werden durch weitere Hirnstammäste vorwiegend aus dem Bereich des Circulus arteriosus cerebri (WILLIS) ergänzt (s.u.). Der Verlauf des Gefäßes gliedert sich in 4 bis 5 topographisch definierte Abschnitte:

Segmentum interpedunculare	Pars praecommunicalis (P1)	
Segmentum crurale		
Segmentum cisternae ambientis Segmentum cisternae quadrigeminae	Pars postcommunicalis (P2)	Pars circularis (basilaris)
Kortikale Äste	Pars corticalis (P3–P4) (KRAYENBÜHL u. YASARGIL, 1965)	

(WACKENHEIM u. BRAUN, 1970; MARGIOLIS et al., 1971; TAKAHASHI, 1974)

Die vier kortikalen Äste sind die
A. occipitotemporalis anterior (anterior temporal artery)
A. occipitotemporalis posterior (posterior temporal artery)
A. parietooccipitalis
A. calcarina
(WACKENHEIM u. BRAUN, 1970; MARGIOLIS et al., 1971) bzw.:
A. occipitalis lateralis (A. temporooccipitalis) P3
A. occipitalis medialis (A. occipitalis interna) P4.

Dabei entspricht die A. parietooccipitalis in dieser Einteilung einer Endaufzweigung der A. occipitalis medialis bzw. einer späten Aufteilung des Hauptstammes (siehe auch unten; KRAYENBÜHL und YASARGIL, 1965).

Die dienzephalen und mesenzephalen Arterien können folgendermaßen eingeteilt werden:

Aa. thalamoperforatae posteriores
Aa. colliculi quadrigemini et corporis geniculati
Aa. choroideae posteriores medialis et laterales
Aa. pericallosae posteriores
Circulus arteriosus pericallosus (WACKENHEIM u. BRAUN, 1970);
nach KRAYENBÜHL und YASARGIL (1965) in:
Aa. paramedianae (Aa. interpedunculares und Aa. intercrurales perforantes)
Aa. thalamicae (mediales et laterales)
Aa. quadrigeminae
A. choroidea posterior media
Aa. choroideae posteriores laterales (anterior / superior)
A. corporis callosi dorsalis.

Nach SCHLESINGER (1976), in Übereinstimmung mit FOIX u. HILLEMAND (1925), in Aa. paramedianae und Aa. circumferentiae mit eingehender Aufgliederung (s.u.).

Verlauf. Das Segmentum interpedunculare ist das kurze (0,5–1 cm lange) Anfangsstück der A. cerebri posterior bis zum Abgang der A. communicans posterior. Es ist ventro-lateralwärts gerichtet und erscheint so in den halbaxialen a-p Projektionen des Angiogrammes. In den lateralen Bildern projiziert es sich in der Regel orthograd und ist gar nicht zu sehen („Basilarisknopf"). Hier gehen zentrale Äste zum Hirnstamm ab (s.u.). Im Segmentum crurale wird die anterolaterale Fläche des Hirnschenkels umlaufen. In der Cisterna ambiens geht die Arterie in das Segmentum cisternae ambientis über. Sie liegt zwischen Mittelhirn und Gyrus hippocampus dem Hirnschenkel an, in unmittelbarer Nähe der V. basilaris und wird durch den N. occulomotorius, weiter kaudal durch den N. trochlearis von der A. cerebelli superior getrennt. Die ersten drei Segmente formen das charakteristische V, W, Omega oder T der Basilarisgabel (peduncular fork; RADNER, 1951). Im proximalen Anteil des Segmentum cisternae ambientis oder bereits im Segmentum crurale kann als einzelner Stamm oder mit mehreren Ästen die A. occipito-temporalis anterior abgehen (die gelegentlich aus der A. occipitotemporalis posterior entspringt). Diese Arterie verläuft rostralwärts und lateralwärts unter dem Gyrus hippocampi und versorgt den vordern Anteil der Unterfläche des Temporallappens. Ihre Äste erscheinen im Vertebralisangiogramm im seitlichen Bild vor der A. basilaris in der mittleren Schädelgrube. Etwa in der Mitte des einen kranialwärts konkaven Bogen beschreibenden Segmentes entspringt gewöhnlich die A. occipito-temporalis posterior, die gelegentlich einen Ast zur vorderen Temporalregion abgibt und entlang dem Gyrus hippocampi zum Gyrus lingualis verläuft. Zahlreiche kleine Äste entspringen an der Unterseite des Temporallappens und angrenzenden Okzipitallappens. Die distalen Verzweigungen können mit Ästen der A. calcarina im hinteren Drittel der Fissura calcarina anastomosieren. Eine mittlere A. occipitotemporalis kommt inkonstant vor (GALLOWAY u. GREITZ, 1960). Der Arterienstamm nähert sich wieder der Mittellinie und erreicht in der Cisterna quadrigemina den geringsten Abstand zum Gefäß der Gegenseite (WACKENHEIM u. BRAUN, 1970: 1–3 cm, gemessen am freien Tentoriumrand, wo sie auch bindegewebig fixiert ist; FERNER u. KAUTZKY, 1959) im Segmentum cisternae quadrigeminae. Hier erreicht der Hauptstamm, bzw. nach Spaltung der lateralen Äste (P3), die A. occipitalis medialis (P4) als Fortsetzung des Hauptstammes die Fissura longitudinalis superior und endet an der Innenfläche des Occipitallappens.

Die A. parieto-occipitalis im Sinn von WACKENHEIM und BRAUN (1970), MARGOLIS et al. (1971), TAKAHASHI (1974), A. occipitalis medialis (KRAYENBÜHL u. YASARGIL, 1965) stellt die direkte Verlängerung des Segmentum cisternae quadrigeminae der A. cerebri posterior dar. MARGOLIS et al. (1971, 1974) finden den Abgang häufiger im Segmentum cisternae ambientis oder zusammen mit der A. calcarina durch Bifurkation des Stammes der A. cerebri posterior im proximalen Drittel der Fissura calcarina. Der Unterschied in der Nomenklatur (s.o.) trägt zu dieser Auffassung bei. Nahe der Zeltspitze werden Äste A. corporis callosi dorsalis, A. parietooccipitalis (im Sinn von KRAYENBÜHL u. YASARGIL, 1965) zum Isthmus gyri fornicati, dem Splenium, dem Pulvinar thalami, den Vierhügeln, zur Epiphyse und zur Rinde des Cuneus und des Gyrus lingualis abgegeben. Der Hauptstamm der A. parieto-occipitalis trifft auf den dorsal des Balken gelegenen Anteils des Gyrus cinguli, teilt sich in mehrere kortikale Äste zur Medialfläche des Parietookzipitallappens. Andere größere Äste ziehen zum Praecuneus und tief in die Fissura parieto-occipitalis.

Die A. calcarina entsteht gewöhnlich bei der Bifurkation des Stammes der A. cerebri posterior im rostralen Drittel des Sulcus calcarinus. Am Ursprung liegt sie unmittelbar neben dem parieto-occipitalen Ast, beschreibt aber gleich eine scharfe Biegung tief in die Fissura calcarina. Das Gefäß kann in 60% der Fälle mit zwei Stämmen abgehen: Abgang von der A. parietooccipitalis in 16% oder der A. temporalis posterior in 6% der Fälle werden beschrieben (MARGOLIS et al., 1971). Die Blutversorgung der Sehrinde durch zusätzliche Gefäße aus der A. parietooccipitalis, der A. temporalis posterior oder beiden lag in 50% der Fälle vor. Dabei betonen POLYAK (1957) und SMITH and RICHARDSEN (1966), daß sich die A. calcarina nicht exklusiv auf die Versorgung der primären Sehrinde beschränken muß (SHELLSHEAR, 1927; ABBIE, 1938). Angiographisch erscheint die A. occipitotemporalis posterior in der lateralen Projektion kaudal der A. calcarina und A. parieto-occipitalis und wird durch die A. cerebelli superior überlagert. In der halbaxialen a-p Projektion dehnt sie sich vom Ursprung lateralwärts, anschließend dorsalwärts aus. Die A. parieto-occipitalis ist in der lateralen Projektion der oberste kortikale Ast. In der halbaxialen Projektion erscheint der proximale Anteil von den kortikalen Ästen am weitesten medial, während die distalen Verzweigungen sich lateral der A. calcarina erstrecken. Die A. calcarina kann man in den seitlichen angiographischen Bildern leicht an ihrem gestreckten Verlauf zwischen den parieto-occipitalen Ästen, die kranial liegen, und den kaudalwärts gelegenen hinteren okzipito-temporalen Ästen identifizieren. Im frontalen Bild projiziert sich das Anfangsstück lateral der parieto-okzipitalen und medial der okzipito-temporalen Äste. Die Aufzweigungen werden von den okzipito-lateralen Ästen überlagert, können jedoch durch Vergleich einer klassischen mit einer halbaxialen a-p Projektion differenziert werden.

3. Die dienzephalen und mesenzephalen Äste

Eine umfassende Darstellung der arteriellen Versorgung des Hirnstammes aus anatomischer Sicht gibt SCHLESINGER 1976. Seine Klassifizierung, die den kleinsten Verästelungen der Gefäße folgt, ist anatomisch topographisch orientiert und die Nomenklatur sehr detailliert auf die versorgten anatomischen Strukturen des Hirnstammes bezogen.

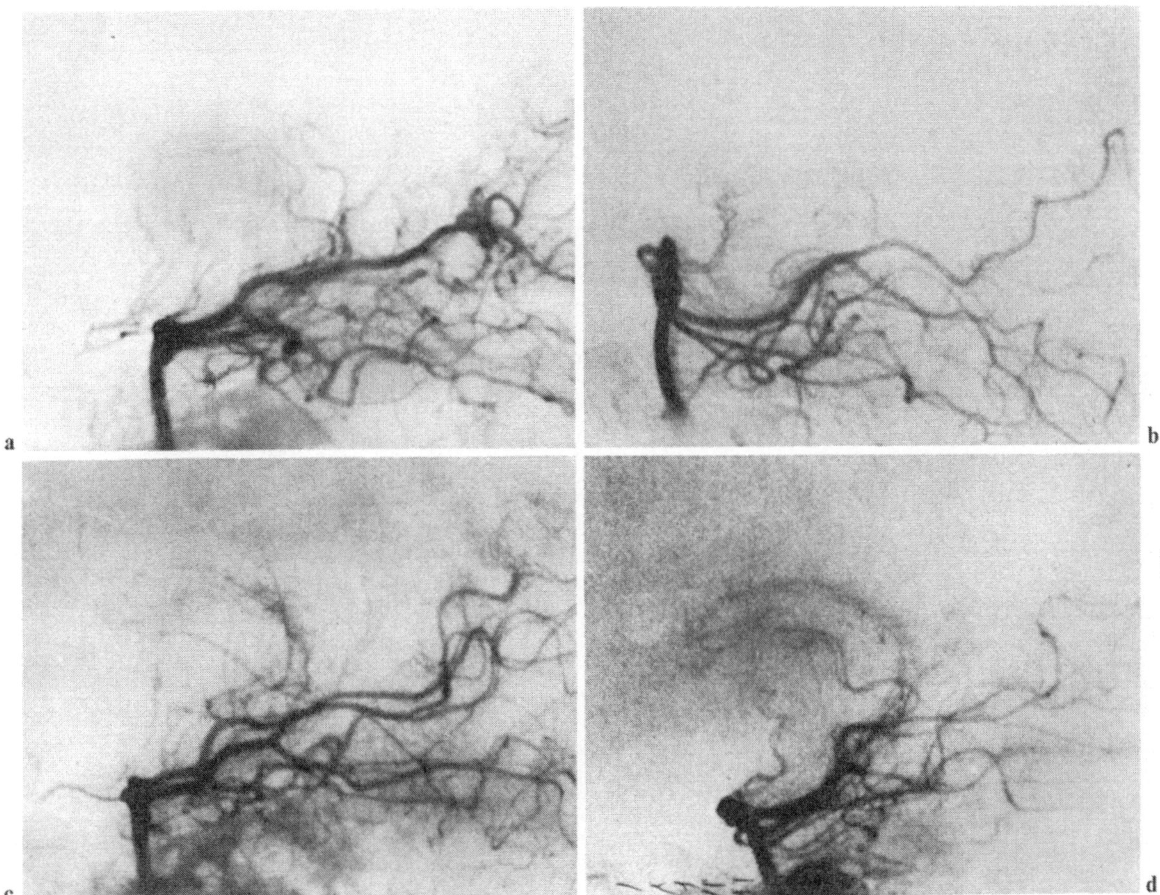

Abb. 28a–d. Darstellung der A. thalamoperforatae im seitlichen Strahlengang und der Aa. Choroideae posteriores **a**, **b**, Abgang perforierender Gefäße von der A. communicans posterior und der A. cerebri posterior, kräftige Darstellung der hinteren Choroidalarterien **a–d** und Plexusfärbung **a**, **c**, **d**

Tabelle 4. Aufteilung der dienzephalen und mesenzephalen Äste der A. cerebri posterior (zusammengestellt nach Angaben von SCHLESINGER, 1976)

Aa. Paramedianae				
Arteria tubero-thalamica	Rr. hypothalamici			Nucl. ventralis anterior (anteromedialer Anteil)
	R. medialis			Lamina zwischen Nucl. anterior u. Nucl. lateralis
				Nucl. dorsomedialis (rostraler Anteil)
				Nucl. parataenialis
	R. lateralis			Nucl. ventralis anterior (Thalami)
Arteriae mammillares	Aa. paramammillares lat.			laterale Fläche des Corpus mamillare
	Aa. paramammillares med.			mediale Fläche des Corpus mammillare
	Aa. intramammillares			
Arteria interpe-duncularis profunda	R. posterior			Nucl. ruber (oberer Anteil) mit Kapsel
	Rr. hypothalamici posteriores			Nucl. parafascicularis
				Centrum medianum
	R. anterior			Radiatio rubrothalamica
	(A. subthalamo-thalamica)			Forel ś Feld
				kraniale Fläche der Kapsel des Nucl. ruber
				Nucl. ventro-postero-lateralis (mittlerer Anteil)
Aa. circumferentiales				
Arteria chorioidea medialis („orale" und „kaudale" Variante)	R. medialis			Plexus chorioideus des III. Ventrikels
	R. lateralis	R. centralis	R. med.	Nucl. dorsomedialis (lateraler Anteil)
				Nucl. dorsomedialis (Zentrum)
				Nucleus anterior (Cauda)
			R. lat.	Nucl. dorsomedialis (hinterer Anteil)
				Nucl. dorsolateralis (nach cranial angrenzender Anteil)
		Rr. subependym.		Nucl. parataenialis (kaudaler Anteil)
				Nucl. paraventricularis (kaudaler Anteil)
Arteria chorioidea posterio-lateralis	R. lateralis	suprathalamischer Anteil des Pl. chorioid.		Plexus chorioideus des Seitenventrikels (Temporalhorn)
	R. medialis			Plexus chorioideus des Seitenventrikels (hinterer Anteil)
	Rr. parenchymatosi			Nucl. pulvinaris thalami (oberer Anteil)
				Nucl. caudatus (hintere Fläche der Cauda)
				angrenzender hinterer Schenkel der Capsula interna
				oberer und mittlerer Anteil des Nucl. externus thal.
Arteriae geniculo-thalamicae	Aa. geniculothalamicae laterales			hinterer Schenkel der Capsula interna
				Zona incerta bis Nucleus ventro-postero-lateralis
	Aa. geniculothalamicae mediales			hinterer Pol des Nucl. dorsomedialis
				Nucl. parafascicularis
				Zentrum medianum
arteriae intergeni-culothalam.	Aa. intergeniculo-thalamicae		ant.	Untere $^{2}/_{3}$ des Nucl. lateralis thalami
			post.	obere Anteile des Nucl. externus thalami
			med.	ausgedehnte Verzweigung in der postero-ventralen Kerngruppe.
	Aa. basigeniculatae ant. laterales			Ganglion geniculatum
	(Aa. genicul. propr.)			Sehstrahlung
	(Aa. intrageniculatae med.)			kurze diffuse Aufzweigungen

Tabelle 4. (Fortsetzung)

arteria pulvinaris inferior	R. medialis R. lateralis	dorsale Fläche der Nucl. pulvinaris medialis, ventro-postero-medialis, ventro-postero-lateralis Nucl. pulvinares inf. et lateralis
arteria praetectalis		Brachium quadrigem. superior, Pars dorsalis hinterer Pol des Nucl. habenulae
arteria cingulo-thalamica	(3–5 Äste)	Nucleus anterior thalami Nucl. ventralis anterior thalami Nucl. dorsomedialis (rostraler Anteil) Nucl. paratаenialis et paraventricularis
arteria splenio-thalamica	R. medialis R. lateralis	Nucl. parataenialis et paraventricularis Nucl. dorsomedialis (dorsaler Anteil) und angrenzende Abschnitte des Nucl. externus.

Die Einteilung unterscheidet zuerst die extraparenchymalen von den intraparenchymalen Arterien, wobei die intraparenchymalen Gefäße die terminalen Aufzweigungen der extraparenchymalen oder subarachnoidalen Stämme darstellen. Das zweite Einteilungsprinzip stammt von Foix und Hillemand (1925) und unterscheidet die paramedianen von den zirkumferentialen Gefäßen.

Die Gegenüberstellung der Einteilung der Hirnstammgefäße ergibt die Tabelle 4, die schematisch die Einteilung der von der A. cerebri posterior abhängigen Hirnstammgefäße bis zu den Endverzweigungen nach Schlesinger (1976) zeigt. Die Ergebnisse wurden aus Injektionspräparaten, subtiler Präparation und mikroskopischer Untersuchung gewonnen. Sie stellen repräsentative Beispiele der Gefäßversorgung dar. Die detaillierte Beschreibung des Gefäßverlaufes wurde in der Tabelle weggelassen.

Diese hochdifferenzierte Darstellungsweise ist beim heutigen Stand der Untersuchungstechnik für die Angiographie am Lebenden nicht anwendbar. Hierzu reicht die Einteilung nach Wackenheim und Braun (1970; Tabelle 5), die unter Einschluß der Arbeiten vorwiegend von Rouviere (1940), Namin (1955), Columella (1956), Lazorthes et al. (1956–1961), Löfgren (1958), Thevenot (1959), Pernkopf (1960), Galloway und Greitz (1960), Potts und Taveras (1963), Westberg (1966), Djindjian und Bories (1967), Ruggiero (1967), Isfort (1967), Wackenheim et al. (1968) erstellt wurde.

Die *Aa. thalamo-perforatae posteriores* entspringen vom Segmentum interpedunculare der A. cerebri posterior, zum Teil vom Endabschnitt der A. basilaris. Es handelt sich um 2 bis 6 relativ kaliberschwache Gefäße, die durch die Fossa interpeduncularis nach kranial und dorsal verlaufen. Sie können im a-p Bild nur schlecht, im lateralen angiographischen Bild leichter abgegrenzt werden. Der zisternale Abschnitt verläuft kranial- und ventralwärts und tritt in das Parenchym ein, indem er eine sanfte, basalwärts gerichtete Kurve beschreibt. Der parenchymale Abschnitt verläuft geradeaus kranialwärts und gegen die Mittellinie zu. Wackenheim und Braun (1970) unterscheiden 5 verschiedene radioanatomische Typen mit unterschiedlichem Abgang und zisternalem Verlauf. Einige ähnlich verlaufende Gefäße mit Ursprung aus der A. communicans posterior werden als Aa. thalamo-perforatae anteriores bezeichnet.

Aa. colliculi quadrigemini und Aa. corporis geniculati. Sie entspringen vom Segmentum cisternae ambientis oder vom Segmentum cisternae quadrigemini der A. cerebri posterior und versorgen die Vierhügelregion und die Corpora geniculata. Man kann sie nur selten in den Angiogrammen erkennen, und zwar nur im seitlichen Strahlengang, wenn sowohl die Aa. thalamo-perforatae posteriores, als auch die Aa. choroideae posteriores gut dargestellt sind. Wackenheim und Braun

Tabelle 5. Mesenzephale und dienzephale Äste der Arteria cerebri posterior (zusammengestellt nach Angaben von WACKENHEIM u. BRAUN, 1970; KRAYENBÜHL u. YASARGIL, 1965; SCHLESINGER, 1976)

WACKENHEIM und BRAUN (1970)	KRAYENBÜHL und YASARGIL (1965)	SCHLESINGER (1976)
Aa. thalamoperforatae	Aa. paramedianae	Aa. paramedianae
	Aa. interpedunculares	A. tuberothalamica
Aa. colliculi quadrigemini	Aa. intercrurales perforantes	A. mammillaris
Aa. corporis geniculati		Aa. interpedunculares prof.
A. chorioidea posterior medialis	Aa. thalamicae mediales laterales	A. interpedunculares sup.
		A. perforans N. oculomotorii
Aa. chorioideae posteriores laterales		A. circumflexa N. oculomotorii
	A. quadrigemina	Aa. mesencephali laterales
A. pericallosa posterior		Aa. circumferentiae
(Circulus arteriosus pericallosus)	A. choroidea posterior media	A. choroidea posterior medialis
		Aa. choroideae posteriores laterales
	Aa. choroideae posteriores laterales	Aa. geniculothalamicae
		Aa. intergeniculothalamicae
	A. corporis callosi	A. pulvinaris inferioris
		Aa. basigeniculatae laterales
		Aa. basigeniculatae mediales
		A. protectalis
		A. cingulothalamica
		A. spleniothalamica

(1970) unterscheiden einen Typ mit kräftigem Abgang und Aufteilung im zisternalen Abschnitt vom Typ mit direktem Abgang von zwei Ästen (20%) von der A. cerebri posterior.

Aa. choroideae posteriores. Es handelt sich um sehr kaliberkräftige, für die Versorgung des Mesenzephalon besonders bedeutende Gefäße, die in ihrem Muster eine große Vielfalt aufweisen. Nach wie vor werden zwei klassische Gruppen, nämlich die medialen und lateralen hinteren Choroidalarterien, unterschieden. Die A. choroidea posterior media entspringt im Segmentum interpedunculare oder im Segmentum crurale der A. cerebri posterior. Sie läuft in der Cisterna ambiens parallel zur hinteren Hirnarterie, um den Hirnstamm zur Vierhügel-Zisterne. Hier steigt sie kranial- und rostralwärts lateral der Epiphyse und bildet den Umriß einer „3". Schließlich verläuft sie in die Gegend des Foramen Monroi im Velum interpositum, neben der V. cerebri interna. Auf dieser Verlaufsstrecke versorgt sie den Plexus choroideus des 3. Ventrikels. Bei guter Aufnahmetechnik kann man die A. choroidea posterior media auch in der a-p Projektion nachweisen. In den seitlichen Projektionen wird das den Hirnstamm umschlingende Segment durch die A. cerebri posterior überlagert. Das anschließende Segment bis zur Vierhügelzisterne, welches die „3" bildet, ist in den Angiogrammen gut abgrenzbar. Es wird regelmäßig in der Gegend der Pinealis, vor der A. choroidea posterior lateralis, gefunden. In manchen Angiogrammen kann man noch die Aufteilung in 2 Äste finden. Die übliche „3" findet sich nach WACKENHEIM und BRAUN (1970) in 40% der Fälle, in weiteren 40% findet sich ein etwas uncharakteristischer gewellter Verlauf. Die restlichen Verläufe zeigen einen weiten Bogen, in dem die untere, dorsalwärts konvexe Krümmung sehr kurz ist und im teilweise durch die A. cerebri posterior überlagerten Gebiet liegt.

Aa. choroideae posteriores laterales. Es handelt sich um zwei bis sechs Arterien auf jeder Seite. Sie nehmen ihren Ursprung vom Segmentum crurale oder dem Segmentum cisternae ambientis der A. cerebri posterior, ziehen sofort in die Fissura choroidea und versorgen den Plexus choroideus des Seitenventrikels. Ein vorderer Ast versorgt den Plexus im vorderen Anteil des Temporalhorns zusammen mit der A. choroidea anterior. Hintere Äste ziehen durch die Fissura choroidea über den Thalamus zum Plexus im Trigonumbereich und zur Tela choroidea auf dem Thalamus. Angiographisch ist ein Nachweis in den a-p Projektionen praktisch nicht möglich. Auf den seitlichen Bildern beschreiben die Arterien einen großen, rostralwärts konvexen Bogen oberhalb des Pulvinar thalami. Teilweise überlagern sie sich mit Ästen der A. choroidea posterior media. Mit der A. choroidea anterior wird ein oft kräftig angefärbtes Kollateralennetz gebildet.

Die *A. pericallosa posterior* entspringt gewöhnlich aus der A. parieto-occipitalis der A. cerebri posterior in der Cisterna quadrigemina. Sie verläuft in einer flachen Kurve nach dorsal und kranialwärts um den hinteren unteren Balkenrand, tritt in die Cisterna pericallosa ein und zieht rostralwärts über den Balken, wo sie ein reiches Kollateralennetz mit der A. pericallosa (anterior) bildet. Sie kann sich bis zum Gyrus cinguli ausdehnen und dann den Sulcus calloso- marginalis versorgen. Angiographisch konnte das Gefäß von Wackenheim und Braun (1970) nur in den seitlichen Projektionen identifiziert werden. Die sichere Abgrenzung von der A. choroidea posterior lateralis ist nötig, da beide ähnlich verlaufen. Bei gut dargestellter A. choroidea posterior lateralis verläuft der Bogen der A. pericallosa posterior etwa 1 cm weiter dorsal. Ein zu großer Abstand kann einem pathologischem Befund entsprechen (Galloway et al., 1964).

V. A. cerebelli superior

In der embryonalen Entwicklung wird das Mesenzephalon schon bei 7–10 mm Embryolänge von einem kräftigen Ast der A. basilaris versorgt, welcher als A. cerebelli superior sichtbar wird (Rickenbacher, 1974), während die A. cerebelli inferior anterior und die A. cerebelli inferior posterior einem Arteriengeflecht im Bereich des Myelenzephalon entstammen und erst von 20–40 mm Embryolänge an erkennbar werden. Die Entstehung aus einem Geflecht erklärt den im endgültigen Zustand variablen Ursprung und Verlauf der vorderen und hinteren A. cerebelli inferior, im Gegensatz zur relativen Konstanz der A. cerebelli superior (Stopford, 1916). Aus phylogenetischer Sicht kommt Critchley (Chritchley u. Schuster, 1933) zum Schluß, daß sich die A. cerebelli superior aus der A. cerebelli alpha und beta der niederen Wirbeltiere ableitet, was die regelmäßige Aufteilung in 2 Primäräste und die häufigste Variante, nämlich doppelten Abgang von der A. basilaris, erklären soll. Der Abstand des Ursprungs von der Basilarisgabel liegt bei 1–4 mm (Lang u. Kollmannsberger, 1961; Müller, 1975). Blackburn (1907) fand eine Verdoppelung in 4% der Fälle, in weiteren 4% der Fälle eine sofortige Aufteilung der Arterie nach dem Abgang in zwei Äste, Stopford (1916) in 28% und Adachi (1928) in 36% der Fälle, Mitterwallner (1955) in 21%, Krayenbühl und Yasargil (1957) in nur 2,5% der Fälle eine direkte Verdoppelung. Hinzu kommen noch 3% bei einem zusätzlichen Ast aus der A. cerebri posterior und über 20% mit Teilung unmittelbar nach Abgang der A. cerebelli superior. Critchley (Critchley u. Schuster, 1933) unterscheidet, als seltene Anomalie, den Abgang der A. cerebellaris superior vom Anfangsteil der A. cerebri posterior bei Fällen mit fehlender A. cerebelli superior, deren Versorgungsgebiet teilweise von verschiedenen Verzweigungen der A. cerebri posterior übernommen werden kann. Eine doppelte Anlage werde oft dadurch hervorgerufen, daß die A. marginalis direkt aus der A. basilaris, statt aus der A. cerebelli superior entspringe. Das Versorgungsgebiet umfaßt nach Critchley und Schuster (1933) in Brücke und Mittelhirn den überwiegenden Anteil der Brückenhaube, den größten Teil des Nucleus ruber, die Substantia nigra, die oberen zwei Drittel des Brachium conjunctivum, einen Teil der lateralen Schleife und das Wurzelgebiet des Nervus trigeminus, im Bereich des Kleinhirns im wesentlichen die obere Kleinhirnfläche bis an den Hemisphärenrand, den Oberwurm sowie, durch subkortikale Äste, das Mark, Nucleus dentatus, Nucleus emboliformis und Nucleus globosus. Im Verlauf des Gefäßstammes können, in Übereinstimmung mit Mani und Newton (1968), drei Segmente unterschieden werden: das Segmentum cisternae interpeduncularis-cruralis, das Segmentum cisternae ambientis und das Segmentum cisternae quadrigeminae; an Ästen: der marginale Ast (A. marginalis cerebelli), Hemisphärenäste und der Oberwurmast (A. vermicularis superior).

Nach dem Abgang von der A. basilaris verläuft die A. cerebelli superior zunächst parallel zur A. cerebri posterior in der Cisterna interpeduncularis-cruralis, entsprechend der Ausdehnung der Crura cerebri nach lateral. Zwischen diesem Abschnitt und dem entsprechenden Segment der A. cerebri posterior findet sich der Nervus oculomotorius. Das Segmentum cisternae ambientis ist durch das Tentorium cerebelli von der A. cerebri posterior sowie von der V. basilaris (ROSENTHAL) getrennt und geht in das Segmentum cisternae quadrigeminae über. Im vorderen Abschnitt des Segmentum cisternae ambientis, bereits am Rande der Hirnschenkel, kann die Aufteilung in zwei Äste erfolgen, die entlang dem Nervus trochlearis eng nebeneinander herlaufen. Unmittelbar lateral der Vierhügel ändern die Äste ihre Richtung und wenden sich kaudal- und lateralwärts. Die A. marginalis cerebelli verläuft stärker lateral und erreicht die obere Begrenzung des Kleinhirnbrückenwinkels. Im Fall einer doppelt angelegten A. cerebelli superior entspricht der untere Ast der A. marginalis cerebelli, der obere Ast dem Segmentum cisternae ambientis. Der laterale Ast beschreibt dann eine haarnadelförmige Kurve und erreicht den vorderen Rand des Kleinhirns, wo er Äste an die Seitenteile des Lobulus quadrangularis abgibt und einen Ast zur Versorgung des Lobulus semilunaris superior. Das mediale Hauptgefäß zieht bis zur Oberfläche des Kleinhirns und endet in 2 oder 3 Gefäßbündeln, am weitesten medial liegend die A. vermicularis superior (MANI u. NEWTON, 1968; HOFFMANN et al., 1974) bzw. „Aa. vermis craniales" (KRAYENBÜHL u. YASARGIL, 1957), zur Versorgung der oberen Wurmanteile. Feinere Äste gehen in die Fissuren des Kleinhirnwurmes ab, als erster die A. cerebellaris praecentralis. Etwas weiter lateral finden sich noch mehrere Hemisphärenäste. Zwischen den Vierhügeln und der oberen Inzisur haben CRITCHLEY und SCHUSTER (1933) ein Netzwerk feiner Anastomosen als „Plexus pedunculi" beschrieben. Einige Äste sollen rostralwärts ziehen und sich mit kleinen, rückläufigen Ästen der A. cerebri posterior vereinigen. Kleine Äste aus dem mesenzephalozerebellären Teil des Gefäßes erlauben die Darstellung des oberen Anteils des Daches des 4. Ventrikels (HUANG et al., 1968). Man kann zweierlei zarte Äste unterscheiden. Medial liegen sie zwischen der Lingula und dem Lobulus centralis. Etwas weiter lateral finden sich stärkere Äste, die zwischen den oberen Kleinhirnschenkeln und dem Lobulus centralis liegen. Die letzteren können weiter zum Nucleus dentatus ziehen (LAZORTHES et al. (im Druck), MARINI DE ARANJO, 1975; beide zitiert nach SCIALFA et al., 1975). Der Nachweis dieser Gefäße gelingt bei Vergrößerungstechnik und Subtraktion häufig im seitlichen und gelegentlich im a-p Strahlengang. In den seitlichen Projektionen der Angiogramme beschreibt die A. cerebelli superior zunächst einen nach kranial konvexen Bogen im Verlauf des Segmentum cisternae interpeduncularis-cruralis, steigt dann nach oben zum Tentoriumrand auf, um sich im Bereich des Segmentum cisternae ambientis in die Äste aufzuteilen, die okzipitalwärts stark absteigend verlaufen. Dadurch wird die typische Zeltform im seitlichen Strahlengang erzielt. In den a-p Aufnahmen verlaufen die Aa. cerebelli superiores weitgehend parallel zu den Aa. cerebri posteriores, werden streckenweise von diesen überdeckt und beschreiben durch ihren halbkreisförmigen Verlauf um den Pons, wie die Aa. cerebri posteriores, eine W-, V- oder Omegaform.

VI. A. cerebelli inferior anterior

Die A. cerebelli inferior anterior entspringt relativ konstant im proximalen Abschnitt der A. basilaris, in unmittelbarer Nähe der Vereinigungsstelle der Vertebralarterien (KRAYENBÜHL u. YASARGIL, 1957), statistisch gesehen, in 9–14 mm nach LANG und KOLLMANNSBERGER (1961), in 9–15 mm nach MÜLLER (1975) von der Vereinigungsstelle, mit einer Häufung bei 9–10 mm. Fehlende Anlage wird im Kollektiv von MITTERWALLNER (1955) in 1,1% der Fälle angegeben, eine doppelte Anlage in bis zu 6% (MITTERWALLNER, 1955; LANG u. KOLLMANNSBERGER, 1961; GERALD et al., 1973; SCIALFA et al., 1975). Andere Autoren nennen bei doppelter Anlage das weiter rostral gelegene

Gefäß A. cerebelli media (KRAYENBÜHL u. YASARGIL, 1957), A. cerebello-labyrinthi (SMALTINO et al., 1971; CAILLE et al., 1974; VOGELSANG, 1974), oder es wird bei entsprechendem Verlauf ein direkter Abgang der A. labyrinthi (auditiva interna) von der A. basilaris angenommen.

Grundlegende anatomische und radioanatomische Beschreibungen gaben TSCHERNISCHEFF und GRIGOROWSKY (1929), SUNDERLAND (1945), ATKINSON (1949), BASSET (1952), TAKAHASHI et al. (1968 u. 1974). Die ursprüngliche Beschreibung GRIGOROWSKYS betreffend Aufteilung in einen medialen und lateralen Ast wurde vorwiegend aufgrund der a-p Projektion der Angiogramme folgendermaßen ergänzt: Der Stamm der A. cerebelli inferior anterior zieht etwas nach kaudal und lateral, zur Furche zwischen Pons und Medulla oblongata, gibt eine Anzahl feiner Äste zum Pons und zu den Oliven ab und kreuzt den Kleinhirnbrückenwinkel. Hier verläuft die Arterie in Kontakt entweder mit den ventralen oder dorsalen Flächen der Wurzeln des N. facialis, N. intermedius und N. acusticus und kann die A. auditiva interna abgeben, die in den Meatus acusticus internus zieht, sowie gelegentlich eine A. fossae bulbi lateralis (Artère de la fossette laterale du bulbe (FOIX u. HILLMAND, 1925), die jedoch auch von der A. basilaris oder A. vertebralis abgegeben werden kann). Im Kleinhirnbrückenwinkel teilt sie sich in 2 Hauptäste (TAKAHASHI, 1968), bzw. 4 bis 5 Endäste (KRAYENBÜHL u. YASARGIL, 1957). Ein Hauptast verläuft lateralwärts zu Tegmentum und Flocculus sowie in der Fissura horizontalis zwischen dem Lobulus semilunaris superior und inferior cerebelli und gibt reichlich Kollateralen zu Ästen der A. cerebelli superior und A. cerebelli inferior posterior ab. Der mediale Ast verläuft abwärts zum Lobulus biventer, ebenfalls mit reichlich Kollateralen zur A. cerebelli inferior posterior. Die Verlaufsstrecke des Gefäßes kann in 3 größere Abschnitte eingeteilt werden: pontines Segment, vom Ursprung aus der A. basilaris bis zur lateralen Ponsfläche im Kleinhirnbrückenwinkel, flokkuläres Segment, im Verlauf um den Flocculus (1 bis 2 Schleifen), bis zum Eintritt in die Fissura horizontalis (s.o.) und die Äste, die wiederum in Rr. superficiales und Rr. fissurales gruppiert werden können (MÜLLER, 1975). Beim Versuch, einen „typischen" Gefäßverlauf herauszuarbeiten, mit welchem die zahlreichen Varianten verglichen werden können, kommen NAIDICH und KRICHEFF (1975) zu einer hochdetaillierten Beschreibung, insbesondere nach der Analyse brauchbarer lateraler Projektionen in etwas verfeinerter Technik, wogegen die früheren Veröffentlichungen meist auf die Unmöglichkeit der Analyse der seitlichen angiographischen Bilder, wegen ihrer Überlagerung mit den Felsenbeinmassiven, hinwiesen (Tabelle 6).

Tabelle 6. Typischer Verlauf der A. cerebelli inferior anterior (zusammengestellt nach Angaben von SCIALFA et al., 1975)

	kaudale Schleife		„M"-Segment		oder	einfache Meatus-Schleife
			Meatusschleife			
		arteria rostrolateralis	Bracchiumschleife			Bracchium-Segment
			supraflokkuläres Segment			
			aufsteigende Arterie			
			absteigende Arterie			
arteria cerebelli inferior anterior				retroflokkuläres Segment		
				untere Äste zum Lob. semilunaris		
				untere Äste zum Lob. biventer		
				Biventer-Segment		
				aufsteigender Hemisphärenast		
				Kollateralen zur A. cerebelli inferior posterior		
		arteria caudomedialis	kaudale Schleife			
			laterale Schleife			
			Biventer-Segment			

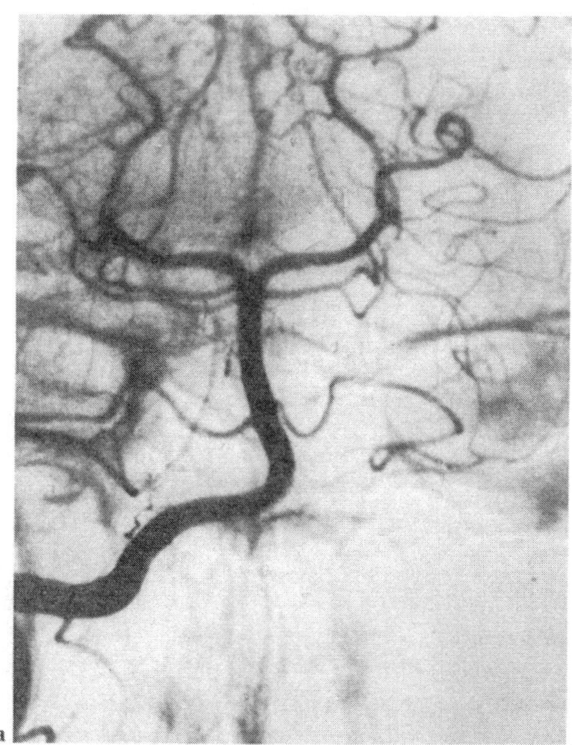

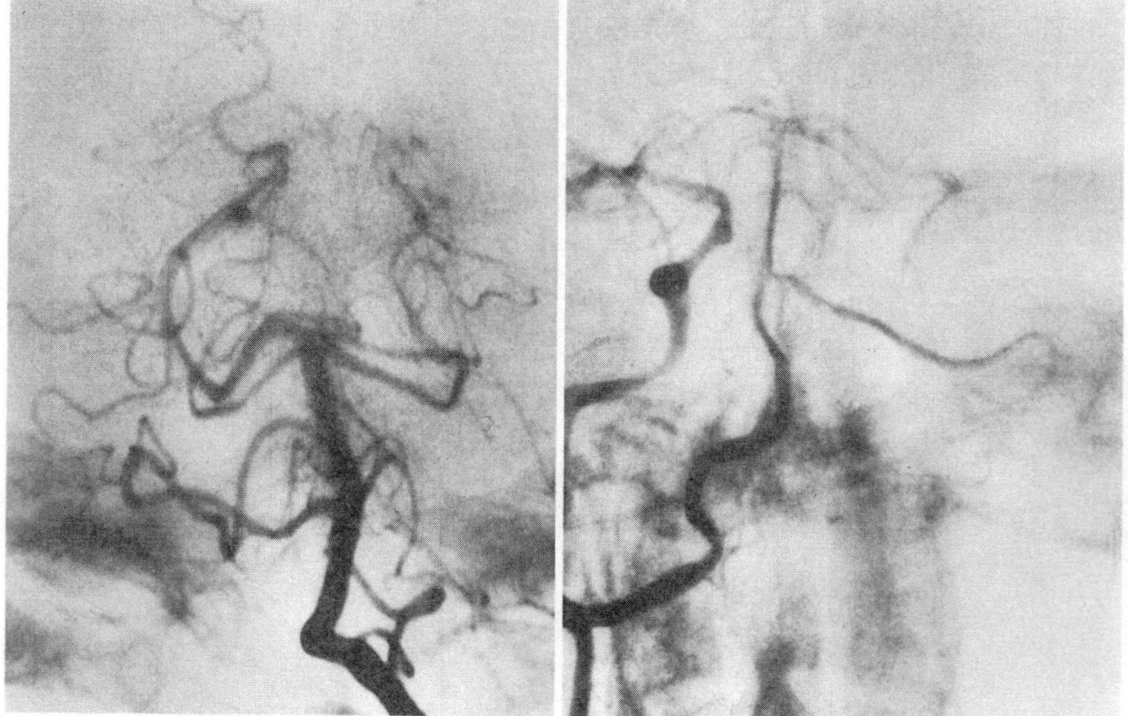

Abb. 29a–e. A. cerebelli inferior anterior (AICA). Beidseits klassischer symmetrischer Verlauf **a** bei fehlender ▶ A. cerebelli inferior posterior (links), sehr kräftige AICA **b** (rechts), ektatische AICA links (long type) **c**, kräftige AICA **d** (rechts) (long type) bei normaler Ausprägung links, kräftige AICA **e** und A. cerebelli inferior posterior auf einer Seite bei stark ausschwingendem Verlauf der elongierten A. basilaris

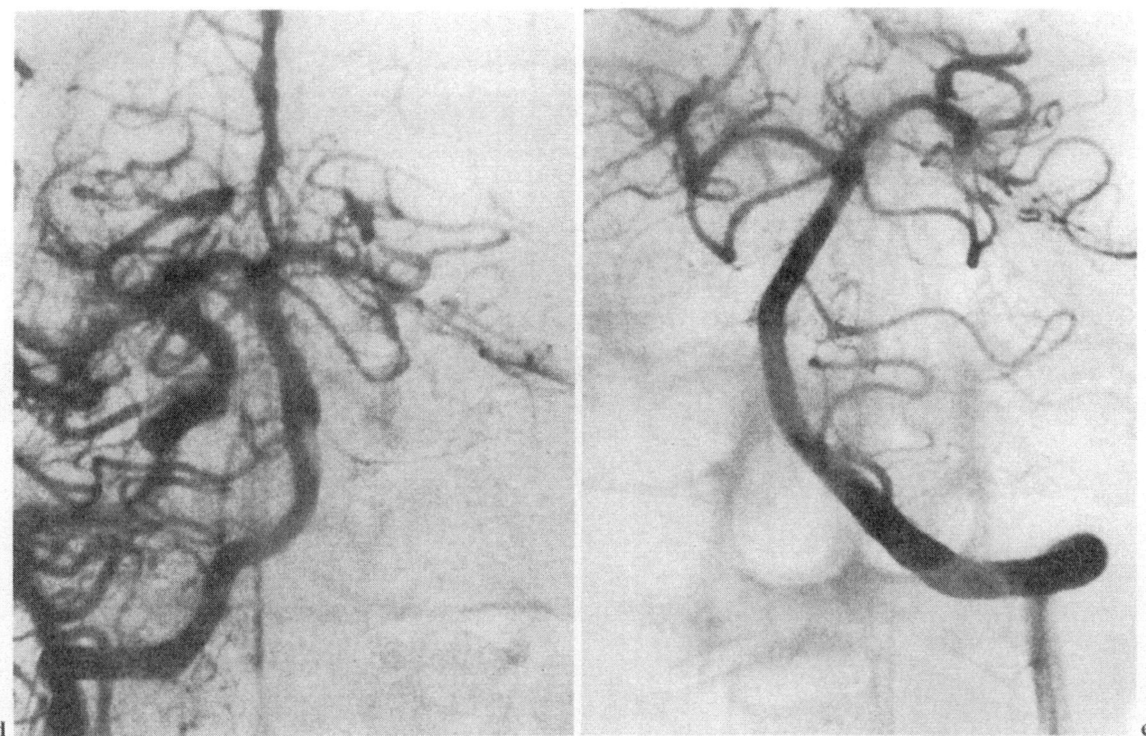

Abb. 29d u. e

Die Beschreibung der Verlaufsvarianten kann nach verschiedenen Gesichtspunkten erfolgen. SCIALFA et al. (1975) unterscheiden 3 Typen des Gefäßverlaufs, gleichzeitig Vaskularisationstypen im Sinn der (entwicklungsgeschichtlichen) Gefäßanlage:

(1) *Short type:* (41%) kurzes kaliberschwaches Gefäß, Aufteilung in Höhe des N. acusticus und des Flocculus mit feinen Ästen zum Pons und zu kranialen Anteilen der Medulla (STOPFORD, 1916; FOIX u. HILLEMAND, 1925; ATKINSON, 1949), gelegentlich mit Zuflüssen zur lateralen Portion des Plexus choroideus. Wenn bedeutende Äste zu den Hirnnerven VII und VIII vorliegen, wurde dieser Gefäßtyp oft A. auditiva interna bzw. A. cerebelli labyrinthi genannt (siehe auch GERALD et al., 1973). SCIALFA et al. (1975) ziehen für diese Äste die Bezeichnung „branches to the acoustico-facial bundle“ vor.

(2) *Intermediate type:* (34%) mit etwas stärkerem Kaliber und antero-lateraler Verlaufsrichtung zum Kleinhirnbrückenwinkel und zur antero-lateralen Fläche des Kleinhirns (Sulcus horizontalis; s.o.).

(3) *Long type:* (25%) großkalibrige Gefäße, die das Versorgungsgebiet der oben beschriebenen Typen überdecken und sich dann auf die Kleinhirnunterfläche fortsetzen, wo ein ausgedehntes Versorgungsareal bestehen kann.

MÜLLER (1975) unterscheidet vier Verlaufstypen (I bis IV), die sich den Typen nach SCIALFI et al. (1975) etwa folgendermaßen zuordnen lassen: Typ I (53%) entspricht dem „short type“, die Typen II (16%) und III (25%) etwa dem „intermediate type“, Typ IV (6%), bzw. noch Anteile des Typ III, dem „long type“. Eine Sonderform dieses Zwischentyps beschreiben auch SCIALFA et al. (1975): Zwei Gefäße, eines vom „intermediate type“, eines vom „long type“, gehen auf einer Seite aus einem gemeinsamen Stamm hervor. SCIALFA et al. (1975) heben zudem hervor, daß das Kaliber der A. cerebelli inferior anterior nicht unbedingt umgekehrt proportional dem der A. cerebelli inferior posterior zu sein braucht. Ebenso wie Kombinationen der verschiedenen Typen auf beiden und auf einer Seite (Doppelanlage) erscheinen, können auch eine A. cerebelli inferior anterior vom „long type“ und eine kräftig ausgebildete A. cerebelli inferior posterior zusammen auf einer Seite angelegt sein.

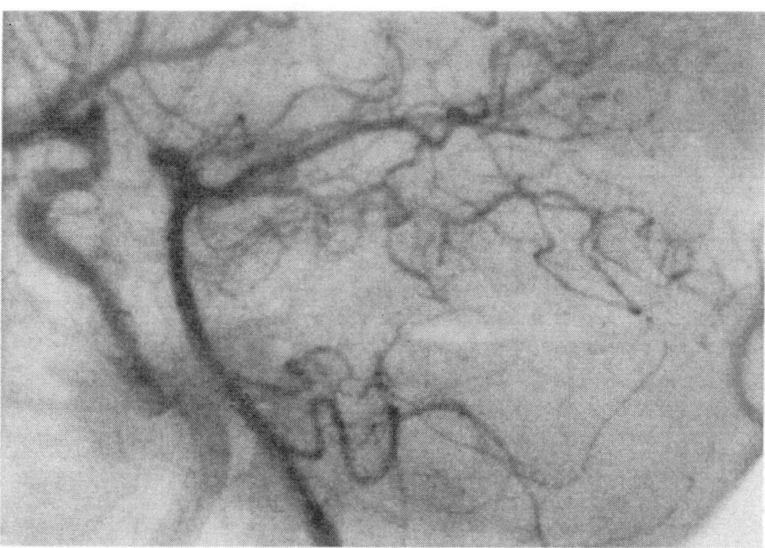

Abb. 30. Optimale Darstellung der Gefäße der hinteren Schädelgrube insbesondere der A. cerebelli inferior anterior im seitlichen Strahlengang durch modifizierte Technik: Die kV-Zahl wird auf 85–95 angehoben, der mAs-Wert entsprechend gesenkt. Die bessere Durchstrahlung der Felsenbeinpyramiden verhindert den Auslöscheffekt bei der Subtraktion

Eingehende Beschreibungen der A. auditiva interna (A. labyrinthi) geben SMALTINO et al. (1971), CAILLE et al. (1974) und WENDE et al. (1975). An einem großen Kollektiv von 238 untersuchten Gefäßen wird von WENDE et al. (1974) und WENDE und NAKAYAMA (1975) die Variabilität des Abganges (45,4% von der A. cerebelli inferior anterior, 24,4% von der A. cerebelli superior, 16% von der A. basilaris, 5,4% von der A. cerebelli inferior posterior) und insbesondere die Bildung des Gefäßes aus zwei Stämmen in 8,8% (6,7% aus der A. cerebelli superior und A. cerebelli inferior anterior, 1,3% aus der A. cerebelli superior und A. cerebelli inferior anterior, 1,3% aus der A. cerebelli superior und A. cerebelli inferior posterior, 0,8% aus der A. basilaris und der A. cerebelli superior) hervorgehoben. Die Anwendung besonderer Techniken zur Darstellung des Gefäßes, wie Röntgenvergrößerungstechnik, Subtraktion, evtl. Angio-Tomographie, wird in den verschiedenen Arbeiten besprochen (SMALTINO et al., 1971; WENDE et al., 1971, 1974; VOGELSANG, 1974; WENDE u. NAKAYAMA, 1975).

D. Kollateralkreisläufe

I. Allgemeines

Den klassischen kollateralen Kreislauf bildet der bereits 1664 von TH. WILLIS beschriebene basale Hirngefäßkranz. Die übrigen zerebralen Gefäße sollten in funktionellem Sinn „Endarterien" sein (COHNHEIM, 1872). Diese Theorie wurde bereits durch vielfältige anatomische Untersuchungen der nachfolgenden Jahre sowie in jüngerer Zeit durch die Darstellbarkeit zahlreicher Kollateralen im Angiogramm fast aller Hirnareale widerlegt (HEUBNER, 1872; DURET, 1874; FAY, 1925; PFEIFER, 1930; COBB, 1931; HILLER, 1936; CAMPBELL et al., 1938; WOLFF, 1938; BÖLÖNI, 1951, VAN DEN EEKEN u. ADAMS 1953; RICHTER, 1953; LIN, 1955; FROWEIN, 1956; KRAYENBÜHL u. YASARGIL, 1957; 1958, 1964, 1965; MOUNT u. TAVERAS, 1957; GILLILAN, 1959; TÖNNIS u. SCHIEFER, 1959; VAN DEN BERGH 1961; BERRY, 1961; HARRISON u. HEARN, 1961; KAPLAN, 1961; MEYER u. GOTOH,

1961; MEYER et al., 1962; PITTS, 1962; FARIS et al., 1963; KAMEYAMA u. OKINAKA, 1963; KRAYENBÜHL, 1963; BOSNIAK, 1964; NEWTON u. WYLIE, 1964; TAVERAS u. WOOD, 1964; WOLLSCHLAEGER u. WOLLSCHLAEGER, 1964; BURROWS u. LASCELLES 1965; FIELDS et al., 1965; WEIDNER et al., 1965; HAWKINS, 1966; HUBER, 1966; ELMOHAMED et al., 1967; SINDERMANN, 1967; ROBERT, 1969; WEIBEL u. FIELDS, 1969; DORNDORFF u. GÄNSHIRT, 1972; HUBER, 1972; KRAYENBÜHL u. YASARGIL, 1972; RICKENBACHER, 1972).

Die angiographischen Arbeiten befassen sich zum Teil mit den kollateralen Kreisläufen bei zerebralen Gefäßverschlüssen, da verschiedene kollaterale Verbindungen überhaupt nur oder aber besser bei pathologischen Kreislaufverhältnissen zur Darstellung kommen.

II. Circulus arteriosus cerebri

Der Circulus arteriosus cerebri (WILLISI) trägt als weitgehend konstant und kaliberkräftig ausgeprägte Kollateralverbindung zwischen beiden Aa. cerebri anteriores einerseits und den Karotiden und der A. basilaris, auch unter normalen Bedingungen zur reibungslos seitengleichen Blutversorgung in den supratentoriellen und Stammhirnversorgungsarealen bei. Er umgibt an der Hirnbasis das Chiasma, die Lamina terminalis, das Infundibulum, das Tuberculum cinereum, die Hypophyse, die Corpora mammillaria, die Substantia perforata und einen Teil der Crura cerebri. Die Häufigkeit der symmetrischen Ausbildung des basalen Gefäßkranzes wird in der Literatur sehr unterschiedlich beurteilt. ADACHI und HASEBE (1928) 73%, ALPERS et al. (1959) 52,5%, GODINOV (1929) 43%, DORNDORF u. GÄNSHIRT (1972) 40%. HODES et al. (1953) geben einen sehr niedrigen Wert von 18% an, ebenso FAWCETT u. BLACHFORD (1905) 11%. In der Mitte liegen die Angaben um 25% von RIGGS (1937), KLEISS (1941), MOREL und WILDI (1953), KRAYENBÜHL u. YASARGIL (1957), DECKER und HIPP (1958), WOLLSCHLÄGER u. WOLLSCHLÄGER (1974). Die Abweichungen ergeben sich zum Teil aus den Beurteilungskriterien. So werden Kaliberunterschiede bei ALPERS et al. (1959) zwischen symmetrischen Teilen des Circulus arteriosus cerebri als nicht abnorm angesehen, wenn das kleinere Gefäß einen Außendurchmesser von mehr als 1 mm hatte. ALPERS et al. (1959); ALPERS und BERRY (1963) beschreiben als Varianten bzw. Anomalien: fehlendes Gefäß, strangförmige oder fadendünne Gefäße, zusätzliche Gefäße, abnormen Gefäßabgang, Fusion der A. cerebri anterior und multiple Anomalien. Die seltenste Variante sind fehlende Gefäße (0,6%). RIGGS (HODES et al., 1953) findet in ihrem Untersuchungsgut von „1647 Autopsien und tausenden anschließenden Untersuchungen" immer ein feines Ästchen, was die scheinbare Lücke zwischen den Gefäßen überbrückt, ebenso MOREL und WILDI (1953) bei einem Untersuchungsgut von 763 Präparaten. Fusion der Aa. cerebri anteriores ist in 1,7% der Fälle zu finden (fehlende A. communicans anterior), vergleichbare Angaben bei DE VRIESE (1904) 1,8%, KLEISS (1942) 1%. Multiple Anomalien (Kombinationen der oben genannten; Aneurysmen waren ausgeschlossen) waren in 13,4% der Fälle angelegt, abnormer Abgang (meist „embryonale" Abgangsform der A. cerebri posterior von der A. carotis interna) in 14,6%, zusätzliche Gefäße, ausschließlich im vorderen Kreis, die A. cerebri anterior und A. communicans anterior betreffend 18,9%, strangförmige Gefäße schließlich in 27,4% der Fälle mit 4- bis 5-fachem Überwiegen des hinteren Gefäßkranzes. Anomalien im Bereich des hinteren Gefäßkranzes sind auch nach PADGET (1945) bei Zusammenfassung von mehr als 1000 Literaturfällen häufiger. Sie unterscheidet hier 4 Grundmöglichkeiten: eine Übergangsform, eine „primitive", schwache und eine unvollständige Anlage. KRAYENBÜHL und YASARGIL (1957) schließen sich diesem Schema an und berichten über eine ähnliche statistische Verteilung. Doppelt so häufig sollen Anomalien am Circulus arteriosus cerebri auftreten, wenn gleichzeitig sackförmige Aneurysmen vorhanden sind (BUSSE, 1921; DANDY, 1928; FORBUS, 1930; SLANY, 1938; PADGET, 1944; MANGHI et al., 1957). KRAYENBÜHL und YASARGIL (1957) heben die Übereinstimmung der Ergebnisse bei näherer Betrachtung des systematischen Vorgehens der einzelnen Autoren, die große Formkonstanz des basalen Hirnkranzes und die Seltenheit ausgefallener Variationen hervor, die in ihrer Wertigkeit nicht überschätzt werden sollen. Die funktionelle Bedeutung des Circulus arteriosus cerebri liegt mehr im potentiellen Wert (ROGERS, 1947) bei pathologischen Kreislaufbedingungen, da unter normalen Verhältnissen eine Passage des Bluts von einer in die gegenüberliegende Seite des Circulus nicht zu erwarten ist (TÖNNIS u. SCHIEFER, 1959; GRYSPEERDT, 1963).

Tabelle 7. Möglichkeiten von Kollateralen der Äste der A. vertebralis (nach WEIBEL u. FIELDS, 1969)

	ipsilateral	kontralateral
Rr. spinales	A. spinalis anterior A. spinalis posterior A. cervicalis ascendens (Tr. thyreocervicalis) A. cervicalis profonda (Tr. costocervicalis)	
Rr. musculares	A. occipitalis (A. carotis externa) A. cervicalis ascendens A. cervicalis profunda	
R. meningeus		R. meningeus
A. spinalis posterior	A. spinalis anterior Rr. spinales	A. spinalis posterior
A. spinalis anterior	A. spinalis posterior Rr. spinales	
Aa. medullares		
A. cerebelli inferior posterior	A. cerebelli inferior anterior (A. basilaris) A. cerebelli superior (A. basilaris)	

Tabelle 8. Kollaterale Kreisläufe (zusammengestellt nach Angaben von DORNDORF u. GÄNSHIRT, 1972)

I. Carotis-Vertebralis-Verbindungen
   1. Okzipitalis-Anastomose
   2. A. communicans posterior
   3. Choroidea-Anastomose
   4. Balkenanastomose
   5. Leptomeningeale Verbindungen

II. Querverbindungen zwischen gleichnamigen Hirnarterien

III. Vertikale gleichseitige Kollateralen proximal des Circulus arteriosus cerebri
   1. Aorta-Subclavia-Kollateralen
   2. A. subclavia-, A. carotis externa-, A. carotis interna-Kollateralen
   3. A. subclavia-, A. carotis externa-, A. vertebralis-Kollateralen
   4. A. carotis externa-, A. carotis-interna-Kollateralen
   5. Circulus arteriosus cerebri (WILLISI)

IV. Leptomeningeales Anastomosennetz

III. Andere Kollateralkreisläufe

Der Circulus arteriosus cerebri ist die einzige Kollaterale, die sich unter physiologischen Bedingungen, allenfalls unter Zuhilfenahme eines Kunstgriffes (Kompression der ipsi- oder kontralateralen A. carotis interna oder A. vertebralis bei der Karotis- oder Vertebralis-Angiographie: SALZMANN, 1959; GRYSPEERD, 1963), mit einiger Konstanz angiographisch darstellen läßt. Er gehört mit dem leptomeningealen Anastomosennetz zu den sofort verfügbaren Kollateralen (SIMON et al., 1962; HANDA et al., 1965), ebenso die persistierenden primitiven Kollateralverbindungen, wie die A. primitiva trigemina, A. primitiva acustica und A. primitiva hypoglossica, die zervikalen intersegmentalen Arterien (s.u.) sowie sehr selten etwa Verbindungen zwischen A. carotis externa und A. carotis interna, wie die A. stapedia und das Rete mirabile (ASK-UPMARK, 1935; DANIEL

Tabelle 9. Kollaterale Kreisläufe (zusammengestellt nach Angaben von KRAYENBÜHL u. YASARGIL, 1965)

I. Circulus arteriosus extracranialis

Verbindungen zwischen Ästen der A. carotis externa untereinander und zur Gegenseite

II. Circulus arteriosus duralis

Verbindungen zwischen Ästen der A. meningea media und Ästen anderer meningealer Gefäße sowie mit Ästen der A. carotis externa und A. carotis interna

III. Circulus arteriosus cerebralis basilaris (WILLISI)

IV. Circulus arteriosus interhemisphaericus und intrahemisphaericus corticalis und subcorticalis

1. Verbindungen der A. frontopolaris, A. callosomarginalis und A. pericallosa untereinander und mit den verschiedenen Ästen der A. cerebri media
2. Verbindungen der Äste der A. cerebri media untereinander und mit der A. cerebri posterior
3. Verbindungen der A. pericallosa, A. corporis callosi dorsalis und der A. parietooccipitalis
4. Verbindungen der A. pericallosa und A. callosomarginalis zu Ästen der Gegenseite
5. Verbindungen zwischen A. choroidea anterior und Aa. choroid. post.
6. Verbindungen zwischen den Gefäßsystemen (präkapillär) kortikaler und subkortikaler Strukturen

V. Circulus arteriosus cerebellaris

1. Verbindungen zwischen Ästen der A. cerebelli inferior posterior, A. cerebelli inferior anterior und A. cerebelli superior untereinander und über die Mittellinie
2. Verbindungen zwischen Ästen der A. cerebelli superior und der A. cerebri posterior

VI. Circulus arteriosus transcranialis

1. Verbindungen zwischen Ästen der A. ophthalmica und den Aa. frontales und Aa. nasales sowie Ästen der A. carotis interna
2. Verbindungen zwischen Ästen der A. ophthalmica mit Ästen der A. meningea media und der A. ethmoidalis
3. Verbindungen des Ramus meningeus der A. vertebralis und Ästen der A. occipitalis externa

VII. Circulus arteriosus spinalis

Verbindungen zwischen Ästen der A. spinalis anterior und der A. spinalis posterior zur Gegenseite und zu spinalen Ästen der A. vertebralis und anderen segmentalen spinalen Arterien

VIII. Circulus arteriosus vertebrocervicalis

Verbindungen zwischen Muskelästen der A. vertebralis und Muskelästen der A. carotis externa und der A. subclavia

IX. Circulus arteriosus primitivus

A. primitiva trigemina
A. primitiva auditiva (otica)
A. primitiva hypoglossica

et al., 1953; MOUNT u. TAVERAS, 1957; SOLNITZKI, 1960; WEIDNER et al., 1965; HAWKINS 1966; MINAGI u. NEWTON, 1966; HAWKINS u. SCOTT, 1967; TEAL et al., 1973). Die Unterscheidung in sofort und mit Latenz verfügbare Kollateralen führt zur Vorstellung, daß vorgebildete, aber nicht gängige Gefäßanlagen eröffnet werden müssen, da die Funktion der sog. ständig verfügbaren Anastomosenverbindungen, Strömungsumkehr, Bildung von Umgehungskreisläufen usw. im wesentlichen nur vom Druckgradienten bzw. dessen Änderungen abhängt. Einen Überblick über die vorwiegend bei Gefäßprozessen wirksamen Kollateralen gibt Tabelle 7 und 8. Die Darstellung der Kollateralverbindungen im normalen Angiogramm wird bei KRAYENBÜHL und YASARGIL (1965) detailliert statistisch belegt und die Ursachen für das Zustandekommen dieser Phänomene erläutert (Tabelle 9).

Literatur

AARON, C., DOYON, D., FISCHGOLD, H., METZGER, J., RICHARD, J.: Artériographie de la carotide externe – étude anatomo-radiologique et clinique. Paris: Masson et Cie. 1970

ABBIE, A.A.: Blood supply of visual pathways. Med. J. Austr. **2**, 199–202 (1938)

ADACHI, B.: Das Arteriensystem der Japaner, Bd. I. Kaiserl. Universität Kyoto, 1928

ALAJOUANINE, TH., CASTAIGNE, P., LHERMITTE, FR., GAUTHIER, J.C.: Les anastomoses des artères cérébrales: leur rôle de suppléance. Sem. Hôp. Paris **35**, 1133–1143 (1954)

ALEXANDER, L.: The vascular supply of the strio-pallidum. Res. nerv. Dis. **21**, 77–132 (1942)

ALMEIDA, F. DE: Note sur les collatérales de l'artère communicante cérébrale antérieure. Arch. Anat. Antrop. Lisboa **13**, 551–556 (1931)

ALPERS, B.J., BERRY, R.C.: Circle of Willis in cerebral vascular disorders. The anatomical structure. Arch. Neurol. (Chic.) **8**, 398–402 (1963)

ALPERS, B.J., BERRY, R.C., PADDISON, R.M.: Anatomical studies of the circle of Willis in normal brain. Arch. Neurol. Psychiat. (Chic.) **81**, 409–418 (1959)

ALTMANN, F.: Anomalies of the internal carotid artery and its branches; their embryological and comparative anatomical significance. Report of a new case of persistent stapedial artery in man. Laryngoskope (St. Louis) **57**, 313 (1947)

ANDERSON, K.N.: A study of the anatomical variations in the basilar arterial system, with special reference to altered hemodynamics following unilateral ligation of a vertebral artery. Medical Thesis, University of Washington, School of Medicine, 1958

ANDERSON, K.N.: Angiographic localization of small intracerebral hematomas. Acta radiol. **1**, 173–182 (1963)

ANSAROFF, N.: Bull. Inst. rech. biol. Univ. Perm **3**, 248 (1925)

ASK-UPMARK, E.: Carotid sinus and cerebral circulation. Anatomical, experimental and clinical investigation, including some observations on rete mirabile caroticum. Acta psychiat. neurol., Suppl. **6**, 1–374 (1935)

ATKINSON, W.J.: The anterior inferior cerebellar artery – its variations, pontine distribution and significance in the surgery of cerebello-pontine angle tumors. J. Neurol. Neurosurg. Psychiat. **12**, 137–151 (1949)

AYER, J.F., AITKEN, H.F.: A report on the circulation of the basal ganglia. Boston med. surg. J. **160**, Suppl. 18 (1909)

BACKMUND, H.: Neuroradiologie bei Säuglingen und Kleinkindern. Radiologe **11**, 449–453 (1966)

BACKMUND, H.: Zerebrale Kontrastmitteluntersuchungen im Säuglings- und Kleinkindesalter. Fortschr. Med. **23** 1020–1021 (1067)

BAKER, A.B.: The medullary blood supply and the lateral medullary syndrome. Neurology (Minneap.) **11** (10), 852–861 (1961)

BAPTISTA, A.G.: II. Studies on the arteries of the brain. Neurology (Minneap.) **13**, 825–835 (1963)

BAROLIN, G.S.: Migräne und Trauma. Wien. Z. Nervenheilk. **27**, 45–76 (1969)

BASSETT, D.L.: A stereoscopic atlas of human anatomy. Sect. I: The central nervous system. Portland: Sawyer's Inc. 1952

BASSOE, P.: Migraine. J. Amer. med. Ass. **101**, 599–605 (1933)

BATUJEFF, N.: Eine seltene Arterienanomalie (Ursprung der A. basilaris aus der A. carotis interna). Anat. Anz. **4**, 282–285 (1889)

BAUER, K.H.: Thorotrastschäden und Thorotrastomgefahr. Chirurg **13**, 387–389 (1949)

BEAUVIEUX, RISTICH-GOELMINO: De la vascularisation du centre cortical de la macula. Arch. Opthal. (Paris) **43**, 5–20 (1926)

BECKER, H.M.: Steal-Effekt: Natürliches Prinzip der Kollateralisation arterieller Verschlüsse. Med. Klin. **64**, 882–887 (1969)

BEEVOR, C.E.: The cerebral arterial supply. Brain **30**, 403–425 (1908)

BEGG, A.C.: Radiographic demonstration of the „hypoglossal artery". A rare type of persistent anomalous carotid basilar anastomosis. Clin. Radiol. **12**, 187–189 (1961)

Belou, P.: Revision anatomica del sistema arterial. Buenos Aires 1934

Berberich, J., Hirsch, S.: Die röntgenographische Darstellung der Arterien und Venen am Lebenden. Münch. klin. Wschr. **2**, 2226–2228 (1923)

Berczeller, A., Kugler, H.: Freilegung der Arteria vertebralis am Sulcus atlantis. Beitrag zur Arteriographie des Stromgebietes der Arteria vertebralis-basilaris. Langenbecks Arch. klin. Chir. **190**, 810–815 (1937)

Bergh, R. van den: De subcorticale Angioarchitectur van het menselijk telencephalon. Bruxelles: Arscia Nietgava 1961

Bergland, R., Ray, B.S.: The arterial supply of the human optic chiasm. J. Neurosurg. **31**, 327–334 (1969)

Bergquist, E., Bergström, K., Hugosson, R., Jorulf, H.: Complicated arteriovenous fistula after vertebral angiography. Neuroradiology **2**, 170–175 (1971)

Berk, M.E.: Combined carotid-vertebral angiography a method of vertebral angiography. Brit. J. Radiol. **33**, 780–783 (1960)

Bernasconi, V.: Abnormal origin of the middle meningeal artery from the opthalmic artery. Neurochirurgica **8**, (3) 81–85 (1965)

Bernasconi, V., Cassinari, V.: Un segno carotidografico tipico di meningioma del tentorio. Chirurgia (Milan) **11**, 586–588 (1956)

Bernsmeier, A., in Bodechtel, G.: Differentialdiagnose neurologischer Krankheitsbilder. Stuttgart: Thieme 1963

Berry, R.G.: Discussion of „Collateral circulation of the brain". Neurology (Minneap.) **11**, 20–22 (1961)

Berry, R.J.A., Anderson, J.H.: A case of nonunion of the vertebrals with consequent abnormal origin of the basilaris. Anat. Anz. **35**, 54–65 (1909–1910)

Betz, H., Matiarvahar, H.: Bulbäre Syndrome bei zervikalen Thorotrastomen. Nervenarzt **41**, 226 (1970)

Bjørk, L.: Heparin coating of catheters against thromboembolism in percutaneous catheterization for angiography. Acta radiol. (Diagn.) **12**, 576 (1972)

Blackburn, J.W.: Anomalies of the encephalic arteries among the insane: A study of arteries at the base of the encephalon in two hundred and twenty consecutive cases of mental disease, with special reference to anomalies of the circle of Willis. J. comp. Neurol. Psychol. **17**, 493–509 (1907)

Bleichröder, F.: Intra-arterielle Therapie. Klin. Wschr. **49**, 1503 (1912)

Bodechtel, G.: Differentialdiagnose neurologischer Krankheitsbilder. Stuttgart: Thieme 1963

Boeckem, Fr.K.: Komplikationen bei Femoralis-, Vertebralis- und Brachialgegenstromarteriographie. Nervenarzt **41**, 566 (1970)

Bölöni, F.: Etude sur la vascularisation du lobe frontal au point de vue phylogénétique. Acta anat. (Basel) **12**, 110–134 (1951)

Boeri, R., Passerini, A.: The megadolichobasilar anomaly. J. Neurol. Sci. **1**, 475–484 (1964)

Bonhöffer, K.: Dauerausfallserscheinungen bei Migräne. Dtsch. med. Wschr. 521–523 (1940)

Bonnal, J., Legre, J.: L'angiographie cérébrale. Paris: Masson et Cie. 1958

Bosniak, M.A.: An analysis of some anatomic-roentgenologic aspects of the brachiocephalic vessels. Amer. J. Roentgenol. **91**, 1222–1231 (1964)

Bosniak, M.A.: Cervical arterial pathways associated with brachio-cephalic occlusive disease. Amer. J. Roentgenol. **91**, 1232–1244 (1964)

Boulos, R., Kricheff, I., Chase, N.: Value of cerebral angiography in the embolization treatment of cerebral arteriovenous malformations. Radiology **97**, 65–70 (1970)

Bradac, G.B., Simon, R.S.: Pneumencephalographic studies of the development of the brain stem and skull base in childhood. Neuroradiology **2**, 111–114 (1971)

Bradac, G.B., Simon, R.S.: Angiography in brain death. Neuroradiology **7**, 25–28 (1974)

Brea, G.B.: Sulla persistensa della anastomosi carotido basilare. Sist. nerv. **8**, 17–23 (1956)

Brenner, H., Zaunbauer, W.: Einfluß technischer Faktoren auf Verlauf und Komplikationen bei cerebraler Angiographie. Hrsg. K.E. Loose. Stuttgart: Thieme 1966

Bruetman, M.E., Fields, W.S.: Persistent hypoglossal artery. Arch. Neurol. Psychiat. (Chic.) **8**, 269–372 (1963)

Burrows, E.H., Lascelles, R.G.: The contribution of radiology to the diagnosis and prognosis of occlusions of the middle cerebral artery and its branches. Brit. J. Radiol. **38**, 481–493 (1965)

Busch, W.: Beitrag zur Morphologie der A. basilaris (Untersuchungsergebnisse an 1000 Gehirnen). Arch. Psychiat. Nervenkr. **208**, 326–344 (1966)

Busse, O.: Aneurysmen und Bildungsfehler der A. communicans anterior. Virchows Arch. path. Anat. **229**, 178 (1921)

Busse, O., Vogelsang, H.: Transfemorale cerebrale Panarteriographie zur Bestimmung des Hirntodes. Fortschr. Röntgenstr. **121**, 5, 630–634 (1974)

Caillé, J.M., Pinon, J., Boussens, J.: Anatomic radiological study of the cerebello-labyrinthine arterial system. Fortschr. Hals-Nas.-Ohrenheilk. **21**, 47–60 (1974)

Cairney, J.: Tortuosity of the cervical segment of the internal carotid artery. J. Anat. (Lond.) **59**, 87–96 (1924)

Campbell, A., Alexander, L., Putnam, T.J.: Vascular pattern in various lesions of the human central nerves system. Arch. Neurol. Psychiat. (Chic.) **39**, 1150–1202 (1938)

Campbell, R.L., Dyken, M.L.: Four cases of carotid basilar anastomoses associated with central nervous system dysfunction. Neurol. Neurosurg. Psychiat., N.S. **24**, 250–253 (1961)

Carpenter, M.B., Noback, C.R., Moss, M.L.: The

anterior choroidal artery: The origin, course, distribution and variations. Arch. Neurol. Psychiat. (Chic.) **71**, 714–722 (1955)

CAVATORTI, P.: Di una rara variazione delle arterie della base dell' encefalo nell' uomo. Monit. zool. ital. **18**, 294–297 (1907)

CAVATORTI, P.: Il tipo normale e le variazione delle arterie della base dell' encefalo nell' uomo. Monit. zool. ital. **19**, 248 (1908)

CHANAMIRJAN, A.: Variation der Wirbelarterien. Anat. Anz. **68**, 163 (1929)

CHANSON, J.L., LANDERS, J.W., SWANSON, E.E.: Cotton fibre embolism. A frequent complication of cerebral angiography. Neurology (Minneap.) **13**, 558 (1963)

CHARCOT: Zit. nach INFELD, 1901

CHASE, N.E., TAVERAS, J.M.: Temporal tumors studied by serial angiography – A review of 150 cases. Acta radiol. **58**, 225–238 (1963)

CHAVEZ, I., DORBECKER, N., CELIS, A.: Direct intracardiac angiocardiography, its diagnostic value. Amer. Heart J. **33**, 560 (1947)

COBB, ST.: The cerebral circulation. The question of „endarteries of the brain and the mechanism of infarction". Arch. Neurol. Psychiat. (Chic.) **25**, 273–280 (1931)

COHNHEIM, J.: Untersuchungen über die embolischen Prozesse. Berlin: August Hirschwald 1872

COLUMELLA, F.: L'angiografia dell'arteria vertebrale e il suo valone diagnostico. Chirurgica (Pavia) **7**, 185–194 (1952)

COLUMELLA, F., PAPO, T.: Vertebral angiography in supratentorial expansive processes. Acta radiol. **46**, 178 (1956)

CONFORTI, P., ARMENSE, B., GALLIGIONI, F.: Anomalous carotid-vertebral anastomosis: primitive cervical segmental artery. Neurochirurgica (Stuttg.) **9**, 99 (1966)

CONNOR, C.R.: Complicated migraine. Lancet **1962**, 1072–1074

COOPER, J.S.: Ligation of anterior choroidal artery for involontary movements. Parkinsonism. Psychiat. Quart. **27**, 317–319 (1953)

CORTES, O., CHASE, N.E., LEEDS, N.: Vizualization of tentorial branches of internal carotid artery in intracranial lesions others than meningiomas. Radiology **82**, 1024–1028 (1964)

COURNAND, A., RANGE, H.A.: Catheterization of right auricle in man. Proc. Soc. exp. Biol. (N.Y.) **46**, 452 (1941)

CRAWFORD, P., MOLNAR, W., KLASSEN, K.P.: Transcarotid aortography. J. thorac. Surg. **32**, 46–52 (1956)

CRITCHLEY, M.: The anterior cerebral artery and its syndrome. Brain **53**, 120–165 (1930)

CRITCHLEY, M., SCHUSTER, P.: Beiträge zur Anatomie und Pathologie der Arteria cerebellaris superior. Z. ges. Neurol. Psychiat. **144**, 681–741 (1933)

CROMPTON, M.P.: The pathology of ruptured middle cerebral aneurysms. Lancet **1962 II**, 421–425

CURRY, R.W., CULBRETH, G.G.: The normal cerebral angiogram. Amer. J. Roentgenol. **65**, 345–373 (1951)

DALLE, ORE: Zit. nach T.A. LIE, Congenital anomalies of the carotid arteries. Amsterdam: Excerpta Medica Foundation 1968

DALY, R., POTTS, G.: Demonstration of the ophthalmic artery and the choroid plexus of the eye by carotid angiography. Neurology (Minneap.) **13**, 120–122 (1963)

DANDY, W.E.: Arteriovenous aneurysm of brain. Arch. Surg. **17**, 190–243 (1928)

DANIEL, P.M., DAWES, J.D.K., PRICHARD, M.L.: Studies of the carotid rete and its associated arteries. Phil. Trans. B **237**, 173–208 (1953)

DAVY: Zit. nach J.S.B. STOPFORD. The arteries of the pons and medulla oblongata. J. Anat. Phys. **50**, 131 (1916)

DECKER, F.: Über eine seltene Varietät der Arterien der Hirnbasis. S.-B. phys.-med. Ges. Würzb. **38** (1886)

DECKER, K.: Technik und diagnostische Möglichkeiten der perkutanen Vertebralis-Angiographie. Acta neurochir. (Wien) **2**, 74–80 (1951)

DECKER, K.: Die Arteria ophthalmica im Katorisangiogramm. Fortschr. Röntgenstr. **82**, 667–673 (1955)

DECKER, K.: Klinische Neuroradiologie. Stuttgart: Thieme 1960

DECKER, K.: Komplikationen bei Angiographien der Hirngefäße – eine Übersicht nach 24000 Untersuchungen. Zbl. Neurochir. **30**, 299–302 (1969)

DECKER, K., BACKMUND, H.: Angiographie des Hirnkreislaufes. Stuttgart: Thieme 1968

DECKER, K., BACKMUND, H.: Pädiatrische Neuroradiologie. Stuttgart: G. Thieme 1970

DECKER, K., HIPP, E.: Der basale Gefäßkranz; Morphologie und Angiographie. Anat. Anz. **105**, 100 (1958)

DETTORI, P., CRISTI, G., DALBUONO, S.: Anomalia megadoligobasilare. Studio clinicoradiologico di 8 casi. Radiol. med. (Torino) **52**, 1259–1273 (1966)

DICKMANN, G.H., PARDAL, C., AMEZUA, J.L., ZAMBONI: Persistencia de la arteria trigeminal. 7 cases. Acta neurochir. (Wien) **17**, 205–216 (1967)

DILENGE, D.: L'angiographie de l'artère carotide interne. Paris: Masson et Cie. 1962

DILENGE, D., CONSTANS, J.P.: Semiologie angiographique de l'artère cérébrale antérieure. Acta radiol. **1**, 248–256 (1963)

DILENGE, D., FISCHGOLD, H., DAVID, M.: L'artère ophthalmique. Aspects angiographiques. Neurochir. **7**, 249–257 (1961)

DILENGE, D., HÉON, M.: The internal carotid artery. In: NEWTON and POTTS, Radiology of the skull and brain II, 2, St. Louis: Mosby 1974

DISTELMAIER, P., WAPPENSCHMIDT, J.: Eine atypische Bildung des Endabschnittes der A. vertebralis und der Arteriae cerebellares inferiores posteriores. Fortschr. Röntgenstr. **124**, 253–256 (1976)

DJINDJIAN, R.: The future for angiography in Neuroradiology. Neuroradiology **3** 175–176 (1972)

DJINDJIAN, R., BORIES, J.: Principes généraux du diagnostic des processes expansifs intra-crânieux par l'angiographie vertebrale. In: Diagnostico neuroradiologico (Solé ILENAS et WACKENHEIM), TORAY, ed., vol. 1, pp. 343–352. Barcelona 1967

DJINDJIAN, R., COPHIGNON, J., COMOY, J., HOUART, R., REY, J.: Polymorphisme neuro-radiologique des fistules carotido-caverneuses. Neurochir. **14**, 881–890 (1968)

DJINDJIAN, R., MERLAND, J.J.: Super-Selective Arteriography of the External Carotid Artery. Springer Verlag, Berlin-Heidelberg-New York 1978

DÖRFLER, J.: Ein Beitrag zur Frage der Lokalisation der Arteriosklerose der Hirngefäße mit besonderer Berücksichtigung der Arteria carotis interna. Arch. Psychiat. Nervenkr. **103**, 180–190 (1935)

DOPPMAN, J.L., ALBERTSON, K., RAMSEY, R., SALTZ, S.L.: Intra-arterial Valium: Its safety and effectiveness. Radiology **106**, 335 (1973)

DORNDORF, W., GÄNSHIRT, H.: Die Klinik der arteriellen zerebralen Gefäßverschlüsse. In: GÄNSHIRT, H., Der Hirnkreislauf. Stuttgart: Thieme 1972

DOS SANTOS, R., LAMAS, A., PEREIRA CALDAS, J.: L'artériographie des membres de l'aorte et ses branches abdominales. Bull. Soc. Chirurgie Paris **55**, 587–601 (1929)

DOUST, B.D., REDMAN, H.C.: The myth of 1 ml/kg in angiography. A study to determinate the relationship of contrast medium dosage to complications. Radiology **104**, 557 (1972)

DOYON, D., MARKOVITZ, P., AARON, C., SIMON, J., RICHARD, J., GASQUET, U., PAUGAM, P.: Etude radioanatomique de la carotide externe. J. Radiol. Electrol. **48**, (5), 301–307 (1967)

DUBRICK, S., MASLAND, W., MISHKIN, M.: Brachial plexus injury following axillary artery puncture. Radiology **88**, 271–273 (1967)

DUNSMORE, R., SCOVILLE, W.B., WHITCOMB, B.B.: Complications of angiography. J. Neurosurg. **8**, 110–118 (1951)

DUQUESNEL, J., POUILLAUDE, J.-M., FROMENT, J.-C., PAPILLON, D.: De la présence de fragments de verre dans les opacifants vasculaires. J. Radiol. Electrol. **54**, 297 (1973)

DURET, H.: Recherches anatomiques sur la circulation de l'encéphale. Arch. Physiol. **1**, 316 (1874)

EADIE, M.J., JAMIESON, K.G., LENNON, E.A.: Persisting carotid-basilar anastomosis (18 personal cases) J. neurol. Sci. **1**, 501–511 (1964)

ECKER, A.: The normal cerebral angiogram. 190pp. Springfield: Charles C. Thomas 1951

ECKER, A., CHAMBERLAIN, R.H.: An additional approach to the internal carotid artery for cerebral angiography. J. Neurosurg. **4**, 444–450 (1947)

EECKEN, H.M. VAN DER, ADAMS, R.D.: The anatomy and functional significance of the meningeal arterial anastomoses of the human brain. J. Neuropath. **12**, 132–157 (1953)

EHRLICH, F.E., CAREY, L., KITRINOS, N.P.: Congenital arteriovenous fistula between the vertebral artery and vertebral vein. Case Report J. Neurosurg. **29**, 629 (1968)

EKSTRÖM, G., LINDGREN, A.G.H.: Gehirnschädigungen nach cerebraler Angiographie mit Thorotrast. Zbl. Neurochir. **3**, 227–248 (1938)

ELMOHAMED, A., HEMPEL, K.J., KAEMPFER, W.: Über Anastomosen zwischen linker und rechter A. meningica media, sowie deren Verhalten zum Sinus sagittalis superior. Tag. Dtsch. Neuropath. u. Neuroanat. Düsseldorf, 1967

ELVIDGE, A.R.: The cerebral vessels studied by angiography. Ass. Res. nerv. Dis. **1**, 110–149 (1937)

ELVIDGE, A.: The cerebral vessels studied by angiography. J. neuro. ment. Dis. **18**, 110–149 (1938)

ENGESET, A.: Cerebral angiography with perabrodil (carotis angiography). Acta radiol., Suppl. **56**, 207 (1944)

ENGESET, A.: About the angiographic visualization of the posterior cerebral artery, especially by intracarotid injection of contrast. Acta radiol. **30**, 152–162 (1948)

FALK, P.: Pathophysiologische Studie über die Carotis interna im Carotiskanal. Zur Pulsation der Carotis interna im Carotiskanal. Arch. Ohr.-, Nas.- u. Kehlk.-Heilk. **160**, 77–92 (1952)

FARINAS, P.L.: New technique for arteriographic examination of abdominal aorta and its branches. Amer. J. Roentgenol. **46**, 641–645 (1941)

FARIS, A.A., POSER, CH.M., WILMORE, W., AGNEW, C.H.: Radiologic visualisation of neck vessels in healthy men. Neurology (Minneap.) **13**, 386–396 (1963)

FARNARIER, PH.: L'artère cérébrale antérieure. Thèse Médicine, Marseille: 1972

FAWCETT, E., BLACHFORD, J.V.: The circle of Willis: An examination of 700 specimen. J. Anat. Physiol. **40**, 63–70 (1905–1906)

FAY, T.: The cerebral vasculature. Preliminary report of study by means of roentgen ray. J. Amer. med. Ass. **84**, 1727–1730 (1925)

FERNANDEZ, BARAHONA, ALVES, ABEL: A angiografia cerebral nos oligofrenicos. Arch. Med. leg. Lisboa **8**, (1939)

FERNER, H., KAUTZKY, R.: Angewandte Anatomie des Gehirns und seiner Hüllen. Handbuch der Neurochirurgie (OLIVECRONA-TÖNNIS), Grundlagen, Bd. I, 1, S. 2–89. Berlin-Göttingen-Heidelberg: Springer 1959

FETTERMAN, G.H., MORAN, T.J.: Anomalies of circle of Willis in relation to cerebral softening. Arch. Path. **32**, 251–257 (1941)

FIEGEL, A., NADJMI, M.: Variationen der Arterien und ihre topometrischen Verhältnisse im retrograden Brachialisangiogramm. Röntgen-Bl. **24** (2), 73–90 (1971)

FIELDS, W.S.: The significance of persistent trigeminal artery. Radiology **91**, 1096–1101 (1968)

FIELDS, W.S., BRUETMAN, M.E., WEIBEL, J.: Collateral

circulation of the brain. Monogr. Surg. Sci. **2**, 183–259 (1965)
FISCHER, E.: Die Lageabweichung der vorderen Hirnarterie im Gefäßbild. Zbl. Neurochir. **3**, 300–313 (1938)
FISCHER, H.: Verlauf und Form der Hirnarterien und ihre funktionelle Bedeutung. Anat. Anz. Erg. Bd. **100**, 355–361 (1954)
FLAMENT-DURAND, J.: Etude Anatomoclinique d'un Cas de Paraplegie survenue après une Aortographie Abdominale. Acta neurol. belg. **70**, 523 (1970)
FLESCH: Zit. nach OERTEL, Über die Persistenz embryonaler Verbindungen zwischen der A. carotis interna und der A. vertebralis und ihre Bedeutung für den Circulus arteriosus Willis. Anat. Anz. **55**, Erg.-Bd. 281 (1922)
FLYNN, R.A.: External carotid origin of the dominant vertebral artery, case report. J. Neurosurg. **29**, 300–301 (1968)
FOIX, CH., HILLEMAND, P.: Note sur la disposition générale des artères de l'axe encephalique. C.R. Soc. Biol. (Paris) **92**, 31–33 (1925)
FOIX, CH., HILLEMAND, P.: Les artères de l'axe encephalique jusqu'au diencephale inclusivement. Rev. neurol. **2**, 705–739 (1925)
FORBUS, W.D.: On origin of miliary aneurysm of superficial cerebral arteries. Bull. Johns Hopk. Hosp. **47**, 239–285 (1930)
FORSSMAN, W.: Die Sondierung des rechten Herzens. Klin. Wschr. **2**, 2085 (1929)
FORSSMAN, W.: Über Kontrastdarstellung der Höhlen des lebenden rechten Herzens und der Lungenschlagader. Münch. med. Wschr. **78**, 481 (1931)
FRANK, O., ALWENS, W.: Kreislaufstudien am Röntgenschirm. Münch. med. Wschr. **57**, 950 (1910)
FRØVIG, A.G.: Dobbeltsidig obliterasjon av arteriae carotides communes. Nord. Med. **29**, 611 (1946)
FROWEIN, R.: Angiographische Befunde bei cerebralen Gefäßerkrankungen und ihre Beziehung zu den klinischen Syndromen. Acta radiol. **46**, 381–389 (1956)
FROWEIN, R.: Ergebnisse der funktionellen Angiographie bei cerebralen Gefäßprozessen und ihre Beziehung zu den hirnpathologischen Syndromen. Habilitationsschrift Frankfurt/Main, 1956
FRUGIONI, C.: Persistenza dell'anastomosi carotidobasilare Chirurgia **7**, 327–334 (1952)
FRUGIONI, P., NORI, A., GALLIGIONI, F., GIAMUSSO, V.: Particular angiographic sign in meningiomas of the tentorium: Artery of Bernasconi and Cassinary. Neurochirurgica **2**, 142–152 (1960)
FUCHS, E.: Krümmungen der A. carotis interna im Canalis caroticus und Sinus cavernosus. Anat. Anz. **59**, 279–286 (1924)
GABRIELSEN, T.O., AMUNDSEN, P.: The pontine arteries in vertebral angiography. Amer. J. Roentgenol. **106**, 296–302 (1969)
GÄNSHIRT, H. (Hrsg.): Der Hirnkreislauf. Physiologie, Pathologie, Klinik. Stuttgart: Thieme 1972
GALLOWAY, J.R., GREITZ, T.: The medial and lateral choroid arteries. An anatomic and roentgenographic study. Acta radiol. **53**, 353–366 (1960)
GALLOWAY, J.R., GREITZ, T., SJÖGREN, S.E.: Vertebral angiography in the diagnosis of ventricular dilatation. Acta radiol. (Diagn.) **2**, 321–333 (1964)
GARIS, G.F. DE, BLACK, I.H., RIEMENSCHNEIDER, E.A.: Pattern of aortic arch in American white and negro stocks, with comparative notes on certain other mammals. J. Anat. (Lond.) **67**, 599–619 (1933)
GEGENBAUER, C.: Lehrbuch der Anatomie des Menschen, 7. Aufl. Leipzig: Wilh. Engelmann 1899
GEORGE, A.E., SALAMON, G., KRICHEFF, I.I.: Angiography of the thalamoperforating arteries with special emphasis on arteriography of the third ventricle. Advances in cerebral angiography. Berlin-Heidelberg-New York: Springer 1975
GERALD, B., WOLPERT, S.M., HAIMOVICI, H.: Amer. J. Roentgenol. **118**, 617 (1973)
GERLACH, J., JENSEN, H.P., SPULER, H., VIEHWEGER, G.: Traumatic carotido-cavernous fistula combined with persisting primitive hypoglossal artery. J. Neurosurg. **20**, 885–887 (1963)
GERLACH, J., SPULER, H., VIEHWEGER, G.: Die Persistenz der A. primitiva hypoglossica. Arch. Psychiat. Nervenheilk. **203**, 164 (1962)
GESSINI, L., FRUGIONI, P.: Considerazioni sulla persistenza della amastomosi carotido basilare. Riv. Neurol. **24**, 338–348 (1954)
GHERSI, J.A., COSTALES, A.M.: La angiographia cerebral. Intentos para asegurar la punción carotidea percutánea. Técnica de las dos agujas. Sémana méd. **3017**, 870–871 (1951)
GILLIAN, L.A.: Significant superficial anastomoses in the arterial blood supply to the human brain. J. comp. Neurol. **113**, 55–74 (1959)
GILMARTIN, D.: Hypoglossal artery associated with internal carotid stenosis. Brit. J. Radiol. **36**, 849 (1963)
GODINOV, V.M.: The arterial system of the brain. Amer. J. physic. Anthropol. **13**, 359–388 (1929)
GOLDBERG, H.J.: The anterior chorioidal artery. In NEWTON and POTTS, Radiology of the skull and brain II, 2, St. Louis: Mosby 1974
GOMBI, R., KELEMEN, J., KARSAI, K., LUDANI, ZS.: Arteria hypoglossica primitiva persistens. Magy. Radiol. **25**, 215 (1973)
GOTTSCHAU, M.: Zwei seltene Varietäten der Stämme des Aortenbogens. Arch. Anat. Entwickl.-Gesch. (Lpz.) **245** (1885)
GOULD, P.L., PEYTON, W.T., FRENCH, L.A.: Vertebral angiography by retrograde injection of the brachial artery. J. Neurosurg. **12**, 369–374 (1955)
GRANGE, R.A., HAWKINS, T.D., SAMUEL, J.R.: The influence of arterial carbon dioxide tension on the angiographic appearance of intracranial tumors. Vortrag 8. Symposium Neuroradiologicum 1967. Acta radiol. **9**, 292 (1969)
GREEN, J.R., ARANA, R.: Cerebral angiography: Clinical evaluation based on 107 cases. Amer. J. Roentgenol. **59**, 617–650 (1948)

GREITZ, T.: A radiologic study of the brain circulation by rapid serial angiography of the carotid artery. Acta radiol., Suppl. 140 (1956)

GREITZ, T., GORDON, E., KOLMODIN, G., WIDEN, L.: Aortocranial and carotid angiography in determination of brain death. Neuroradiology **5**, 13–19 (1973)

GREITZ, T., LÖFSTEDT, S.: The relationship between the third ventricle and the basilary artery. Acta radiol. **42**, 85–100 (1959)

GREITZ, T., SJÖGREN, S.E.: The posterior inferior cerebellar artery. Acta radiol. **58**, 284–297 (1963)

GROS, CH., MINVIELLE, J., VLAHOVITCH, B.: Anastomoses artérielles intracraniennes, étude artériographique et clinique. Neuro-chirurgie **2**, 281–302 (1956)

GROS, C., VLAHOVITCH, B., ROILGEN, A.: Images angiographiques d'arrêt, circulation encephalique total dans les souffrances aigues du tronc cerebral. Neuro-chirurgie **5**, 113 (1959)

GRYSPEERD, G.L.: Angiographic studies of the blood flow in the circle of Willis. Acta radiol. **1**, 298–313 (1963)

GUEST, I.A., WOLF, A.L.: Fatal infarction of brain in migraine. Brit. med. J. 225–226 (1964)

HACKER, H.: Gefäßdiagnostik bei Tumoren der Selaregion. Radiologe **10**, 445–449 (1970)

HACKER, H., ALONSO, A.: Karotisangiographie nach Entwässerung – bessere Darstellung von Hirntumoren. Neurochirurgia (Stuttg.) **12**, 187 (1969)

HACKER, H., ARBURG, C.: Schnellverfahren für die Subtraktion in der täglichen Routine. Fortschr. Röntgenstr. **107**, 803–806 (1967)

HANAFEE, W.: Axillary artery approach to carotid, vertebral, abdominal aorta, and coronary angiography. Radiology **81**, 559–567 (1963)

HANDA, H., HANDA, J., KOYAMA, T.: Agenesis of the corpus callosum associated with multiple developmental anomalies of the cerebral arteries. Brain and Nerve (Tokyo) **20**, 317–326 (1968)

HANDA, J., MEYER, J.S., HUBER, P., YOSHIDA, K.: Time course of development of cerebral circulation. J. vascular Dis. **2**, 271 (1965)

HARRISON, C.R., HEARN, J.B.: A new aspect of collateral circulation in occlusion of internal carotid artery. J. Neurosurg. **18**, 542–545 (1961)

HARRISON, C., LUTRELL, C.: Persistent carotid basilar anastomosis. J. Neurosurg. **10**, 205–215 (1953)

HARWOOD-NASH, D.C., FITZ, CH.R.: Neuroradiology in infants and children. St. Louis: Mosby 1976

HARZER, K., TÖNDURY, G.: Zum Verhalten der A. vertebralis in der alternden Halswirbelsäule. Fortschr. Röntgenstr. **104**, 687–699 (1966)

HASEBE, K.: Arterien der Hirnbasis. In: ADACHI, B., Das Arteriensystem der Japaner, Bd. I, S. 111–134. Kaiserl. Universität Kyoto 1928

HASENJÄGER, TH.: Ein Beitrag zu den Abnormitäten des Circulus Willis. Zbl. Neurochir. **1**, 34 (1937)

HASSLER, O., SALTZMAN, G.T.: Angiographic and histologic changes in infundibular widening of the posterior communicating artery. Acta radiol. **1**, 321–327 (1963)

HAUGE, T.: Catheter vertebral angiography. Acta radiol., Suppl. **109** (1954)

HAUGHTON, V.M., ROSENBAUM, A.E.: The normal and anomalous aortic arch and brachiocephalic arteries. In: NEWTON and POTTS, Radiology of the skull and brain II, 2, St. Louis: Mosby 1974

HAVERLING, M.: The tortous basilary artery. Acta radiol. **15**, 241–249 (1974)

HAWKINS, D.T.: The collateral anastomoses in cerebrovascular occlusion. Clin. Radiol. **17**, 203–219 (1966)

HAWKINS, T.D., SCOTT, W.C.: Bilateral rete carotidis in man. Clin. Radiol. **18**, 163–165 (1967)

HELD, A.: Thorotrast und Infektion. Zur Frage der Blockierung des reticuloendothelialen Systems. Fortschr.-Röntgenstr. **45**, 330 (1932)

HELD, A., MEESE: Die Leberzirrhose im Röntgenbild nach Thorotrast. Fortschr. Röntgenstr. **45**, 451 (1932)

HELMSWORTH, J.A., GUIRE, J.M.C., FELSON, B.: Amer. J. Roentgenol. **64**, 196 (1950)

HERMANN, L.H., OSTROWSKI, A.Z., GURDJAN, E.S.: Perforating branches of the middle cerebral artery. Arch. Neurol. (Chic.) **8**, 32–35 (1963)

HEUBNER, O.: Zur Topographie der Ernährungsgebiete der einzelnen Hirnarterien. Zbl. med. Wiss. **10**, 817 (1872)

HEYCK, H.: Der Kopfschmerz. Stuttgart: Thieme 1964

HILLER, F.: Die Zirkulationsstörungen des Rückenmarks und Gehirns. Im Handbuch der Neurologie von BUMKE und FOERSTER, Bd. 11. Berlin: Springer 1936

HIRKÔ, G.: Zwei Fälle von Arterienvarietäten. Tokyo-Igakkwai-Zasski **23**, 280 (1919)

HOCHSTETTER, F.: Über 2 Fälle einer seltenen Varietät der A. carotis interna. Arch. Anat. Physiol., 396–400 (1885)

HOCHSTETTER, F.: Entwicklungsgeschichte des Gefäßsystems. Ergebn. Anat. Entwickl.-Gesch. **1**, 696 (1891)

HODES, PH.J., CAMROY, F., RIGGS, H.E., BLY, P.: Cerebral angiography: Fundamental in anatomy and physiology. Amer. J. Roentgenol. **70**, 61–82 (1953)

HOFF, H., OSLER, G.: Neurologie auf Grundlagen der Physiologie. Dtsch. med. Wschr. **77**, 33–36 (1952)

HOFFMANN, H.B., MARGOLIS, M.TH., NEWTON, TH.H.: The superior cerebellar artery. Normal gross and radiographic anatomy. In: NEWTON and POTTS, Radiology of the skull and brain II, 2. St. Louis: Mosby 1974

HOLUB, V., CHRAST, B., SAXL, O.: Tödlicher Ausgang eines kindlichen Migräneanfalles. Kinderärztl. Prax. **33**, 539 (1965)

HOWIESON, J.: Complications of cerebral angiography. In: NEWTON and POTTS (eds.), Radiology of the skull and brain, Vol. 2, Book 1, p. 1034. St. Louis: Mosby 1974

HOYT, W.F., NEWTON, TH.H., MARGOLIS, M.TH.: The posterior cerebral artery. Embryology and development anomalies. In: NEWTON and POTTS, Radiology of the skull and brain II, 2. St. Louis: Mosby 1974

HROMADA, J.: Anatomische Bemerkungen über die A. choroidea anterior in Bezug auf die Cooper'sche Operation bei der Behandlung des Parkinsonismus. Zbl. Neurochir. **17**, 209–217 (1957)

HUANG, Y.P., WOLF, B.S.: Angiographic features of the pericallosal cistern. Radiology **82**, 14–23 (1964)

HUANG, Y.P., WOLF, B.S.: Angiographic features of fourth ventricle tumors with special reference to the posterior inferior cerebellar artery. Amer. J. Roentgenol. **107**, 543–564 (1969)

HUANG, Y.P., WOLF, B.S.: Differential diagnosis of fourth ventricle tumors from brain stem tumors in angiography. Neuroradiology **1**, 4–79 (1970)

HUANG, Y.P., WOLF, B.S., ANTIN, S.P., OKUDERA, T., KIM, I.H.: Angiographic features of aquaeductal stenosis. Amer. J. Roentgenol. **104**, 90–108 (1968)

HUBER, P.: Die A. trigemina primitiva. Betrachtungen zur klinischen Bedeutung der carotido-basilären Anastomose. Dtsch. Z. Nervenheilk. **181**, 612–633 (1961)

HUBER, P.: Die prognostische Bedeutung des angiographisch sichtbaren Kollateralkreislaufes bei Verschlüssen der A. cerebri media. Fortschr. Röntgenstr. **104**, 82–89 (1966)

HUBER, P.: Angiographische Funktionsdiagnostik des Hirnkreislaufs. In: GÄNSHIRT, H., Der Hirnkreislauf. Stuttgart: Thieme 1972

HUBER, P., RIVOIR, R.: Aneurysm on a persistent left hypoglossal artery. Neuroradiology **6**, 277 (1974)

HUEBNER, H.J.: Zum Verlauf der A. carotis interna im Bereich des Halses. Anat. Anz. **121**, 489–496 (1967)

HULTQUIST, G.T.: Zur Kenntnis der Morphologie und funktionellen Bedeutung der Anomalien der basalen Hirnarterien. Z. Neurol. **173**, 468 (1941)

HUTCHINSON, N.A., MILLER, J.D.R.: Persistent proatlantal artery. J. Neurol. Neurosurg. Psychiat. **33**, 524 (1970)

HYRTL: Lehrbuch der Anatomie des Menschen. Wien 1887

INFELD, M.: Zur Kenntnis der bleibenden Folgen des Migräneanfalls. Wien. klin. Wschr. **14**, 673–675 (1901)

ISFORT, A.: Spontane Hirnblutungen, Vol. 1. Berlin: Schering A.G. 1967

ITO, J., MAEDA, H., INOUE, K., ONISHI, Y.: Fenestration of the middle cerebral artery. Neuroradiology **13**, 37–39 (1977)

JACKSON, F.E.: Syncope associated with persistent hypoglossal artery. J. Neurosurg. **21**, 139–141 (1964)

JAEGER, R.: Surg. Clin. N. Amer. **32**, 1565 (1952)

JAIN, K.K.: Some observations on the anatomy of the middle cerebral artery. Canad. Surg. **7**, 134–139 (1964)

JANZEN, R.: Postangiographische Spätreaktionen der Hirngefäße bei Migräne-Kranken. Beitrag zum Pathomechanismus des Migräneanfalles. Z. Neurol. **201**, 24 (1972)

JEFFERSON, A., SHELDON, P.: Transtentorial herniation of the brain as revealed by the displacement of arteries. Acta radiol. **46**, 480–498 (1956)

JÖNSSON, G.: Thoracic aortography by means of cannula inserted percutaneously into common carotid artery. Acta radiol. **31**, 376–386 (1949)

KADYI, H.: Über die Blutgefäße des menschlichen Rückenmarkes. Anat. Anz. **1**, (1866)

KAMEYAMA, M., OKINAKA, S.: Collateral circulation of the brain. With special reference to arteriosclerosis of the major cervical and cerebral arteries. Neurology (Minneap.) **13**, 279–286 (1963)

KAPLAN, H.A.: Arteries of the brain: An anatomic study. Acta radiol. **46**, 364–370 (1956)

KAPLAN, H.A.: Collateral circulation of the brain. Neurology (Minneap.) **11**, 9–15 (1961)

KAPLAN, H.A.: The blood vessels of the brain in 3 D. stereo publications. Brooklyn, New York 1 1973

KAPLAN, H.A.: The anatomy of the perforating arteries of the basal ganglia. Advances in cerebral angiography. Berlin-Heidelberg-New York: Springer 1975

KAPLAN, H.A., FORD, D.H.: The brain vascular system. Amsterdam: Elsevier Publ. Comp. 1966

KAWAMOTO, K., TANAKA, M., MIKI, M., SOMEDA, K.: Fenestration of the vertebobasilar system. Brain Nerve (Tokyo) **24**, 811–815 (1972)

KAZNER, E., KUBICKI, ST., KUNZE, ST., SCHIEFER, W., WENDE, S.: Die Bedeutung der klinischen Zusatzuntersuchungen für die Differentialdiagnose zerebrale Massenblutung – Hirninfarkt. Fortschr. Neurol. Psychiat. **37**, 225–250 (1969)

KERBER, C.W., MARGOLIS, M.T., NEWTON, TH.H.: Tortous vertebrobasilar system: A cause of cranial nerve signs. Neuroradiology **4**, 74–77 (1972)

KIMMERLE, A.: Mitteilungen über einen eigenartigen Befund am Atlas. Röntgenpraxis **2**, 479 (1930)

KING, A.B.: Demonstration of the basilar artery and its branches with thorotrast. Bull. Johns Hopk. Hosp. **70**, 81–89 (1942)

KLAUSBERGER, E.M., VASS, K.: Die Wirkung eines Medikaments auf die zerebrale Durchblutung im herzphasengesteuerten Angiokinematogramm. Wien. klin. Wschr. **78**, 113–117 (1966)

KLEIN, O.: Zur Bestimmung des zirkulatorischen Minutenvolumens beim Menschen nach Fickschem Prinzip. Münch. med. Wschr. **77**, 131 (1930)

KLEISS, E.: Die verschiedenen Formen des Circulus arteriosus cerebralis Willisi. (Eine statistische Untersuchung von 325 menschlichen Gehirnen.) Anat. Anz. **92**, 216–230 (1941/1942)

KLEYN, A. DE, NIEWEHUYSE: Schwindelanfälle und Nystagmus bei einer bestimmten Stellung des Kopfes. Acta oto-laryng. (Stockh.) **11** (1927)

KLEYN, A. DE, VERSTEIGH, C.: Über verschiedene Formen von Menières Syndromen. Dtsch. Z. Nervenheilk. **132**, 157 (1933)

KLOSS, K.: Persistierende Carotis-Basilaris-Anastomose als Ursache einer Subarachnoidalblutung. Zbl. Neurochir. **13**, 166–171 (1953)

KOTRNETZ, H.: Über eine für die Chirurgie der Hypophyse wichtige Gefäßvarietät. Langenbecks Arch. klin. Chir. **168**, 111 (1931)

KOWADA, M., YAMAGUCHI, K., TAKAHASHI, H.: A case of two fenestrations of the left vertebral artery. Brain Nerve (Tokyo) **22**, 469–472 (1970)

KOWADA, M., YAMAGUCHI, K., TAKAHASHI, H.: Fenestration of the vertebral artery with a review of 23 cases in Japan. Radiology **103**, 343–346 (1972)

KRAMER, R., NEWTON, TH.H.: Tentorial branches of the internal carotid artery. Amer. J. Roentgenol. **95**, 826–830 (1965)

KRAYENBÜHL, H.: Das Hirnaneurysma. Schweiz. Arch. Neurol. Psychiat. **47**, 155 (1941)

KRAYENBÜHL, H.: Die Bedeutung des zerebralen Kollateralkreislaufes bei organischen Hirnleiden für deren neurochirurgische Behandlung. Schweiz. med. Wschr. **93**, 111–119 (1963)

KRAYENBÜHL, H., RICHTER, H.R.: Die zerebrale Angiographie. Stuttgart: Thieme 1952

KRAYENBÜHL, H., YASARGIL, M.G.: Die vaskulären Erkrankungen im Gebiet der A. vertebralis und A. basilaris, S. 1–170. Stuttgart: Thieme 1957

KRAYENBÜHL, H., YASARGIL, M.G.: Der cerebrale collaterale Kreislauf im angiographischen Bild. Acta neurochir. (Wien) **6**, 30–80 (1958)

KRAYENBÜHL, H., YASARGIL, M.G.: Verschluß der A. cerebralis media. Ergebnisse der klinischen und katamnestischen Untersuchungen. Schweiz. Arch. Neurol. Neurochir. Psychiat. **94**, 287–304 (1964)

KRAYENBÜHL, H., YASARGIL, M.G.: Die zerebrale Angiographie, 2. Aufl. Stuttgart: Thieme 1965

KRAYENBÜHL, H., YASARGIL, M.G.: Angiographie der Hirngefäße. In: Lehrbuch der Röntgendiagnostik, hrsg. von H.R. SCHINZ, W.E. BAENSCH, W. FROMMHOLD, R. GLAUNER, E. VEHLINGEN, J. WELLAUER, Bd. I. Stuttgart: Thieme 1965

KRAYENBÜHL, H., YASARGIL, M.G.: Das normale Hirngefäßbild im angiographischen Bild. Aus: Der Hirnkreislauf, Hrsg. GÄNSHIRT, S. 161–200. Stuttgart: Thieme 1972

KRÖSL, W., SCHERZER, E.: Die Bestimmung des Todeszeitpunktes. Wien: Mandrich 1973

KUHN, R.A.: Brachial cerebral angiography. J. Neurosurg. **17**, 955–971 (1960)

KUHNERT, W.: Pathologische Veränderungen an der A. vertebralis und ihre Bedeutung für die cerebrale Durchblutung. Dtsch. Arch. klin. Med. **204**, 375–392 (1957)

LANDOLT, F.: Zur Topographie der Kleinhirnarterien: Abnorme Verlaufsformen der A. cerebellaris inferior posterior. Schweiz. Arch. Neurol. Psychiat. **64**, 329–337 (1949)

LANG, J.: Mikroskopische Anatomie der Arterien. Angiologica **2**, 225–284 (1965)

LANG, J.: Zur Vaskularisation der Dura mater cerebri I. Z. Anat. Entwickl.-Gesch. **135**, 20–34 (1971)

LANG, J.: Zur Vaskularisation der Dura mater cerebri II. Z. Anat. Entwickl.-Gesch. **141**, 223–236 (1973)

LANG, J., KOLLMANNSBERGER, A.: Beitrag zur Anatomie der Kleinhirnarterien. Morph. Jb. **102**, 170–179 (1961)

LANZ, T. VON, WACHSMUTH, W.: Praktische Anatomie, Hals. Berlin-Göttingen-Heidelberg: Springer 1955

LAZORTHES, G.: Vascularisation et circulation cérébrales, Vol. 1. Paris: Masson 1961

LAZORTHES, G., BASTIDE, G., ROULLEAU, J., AMARAL-GOMES, F.: Les artères du thalamus. Verh. 1. Europ. Anat. Anz. **109**, 828–831 (1960–1961)

LAZORTHES, G., GOUAZE, A., SALAMON, G.: Vascularisation cérébrales. Paris: Masson (in press) Zit. nach: SCIALFA, G., BANK, W., MEGRET, M., CORBAZ, J.M. The posterior fossa arteries. In: Advances in cerebral angiography. Berlin-Heidelberg-New York: Springer 1975

LAZORTHES, G., POULHES, J., ESPAGNO, J.: Les artères du cervelet. C. R. Ass. Anat. 279–288 (1950)

LAZORTHES, G., POULHES, J., GAUBERT, J.: Les artères et les territoires vasculaires de l'hypothalamus. Applications neurochirurgicales. Presse méd. **64**, 1701–1703 (1956)

LAZORTHES, G., SALAMON, G.: The arteries of the thalamus. An anatomical and radiological study. J. Neurosurg. **34**, 23–26 (1971)

LAZORTHES, G., SALAMON, G., GOUAZE, A., ZADEH, J.: The central arteries of the brain. – Classification and territories of vascular supply. In: Advances in cerebral angiography. Berlin-Heidelberg-New York: Springer 1975

LEE, K.F., SHU-REN LIN, LEE, J.J.: A stillstand cerebral arteriogram secondary to heart block. A case report with discussion of mechanism. Neuroradiology **5**, 233–236 (1973)

LEEDS, N.E.: The striate arteries and the artery of HEUBNER. In: NEWTON and POTTS, Radiology of the skull and brain II, 2. St. Louis: Mosby 1974

LELLI, G.F.: Compartamento dell'arteria auditiva interna e dei suoi rami labirintici nell'uomo. Z. Anat. Entwickl.-Gesch. **110**, 48 (1939)

LEMANHIEV, S.F., CALLIAOW, L., PATTYN, G.: Les anastomoses carotido-basilaires primitives. J. belge Radiol. **50**, 337–348 (1967)

LENZI, M.: Sulla semiologica angiografica dell'arteria coroidea anteriore. Radiol. chir. (Basel) **24**, 202–210 (1955)

LIE, T.A.: Congenital anomalies of the carotid arteries. Excerpta med. (Amst.) 1968

LIE, T.A.: Classification regarding the nomenclature of the „so-called" segmental and presegmental arteries (with special reference to the proatlantal intersegmental artery and its variants). In: Advances in cerebral angiography, pp. 310–314. Berlin-Heidelberg-New York: Springer 1975

LIECHTY, J.D., SHIELDS, T.W., ANSON, B.J.: Variations pertaining to aortic arches and their branches with comments on surgically important types. Quart. Bull. Northw. Univ. Med. Sch. **31**, 136–143 (1957)

LIN, J.P., KRICHEFF, I.I.: The normal anterior cerebral artery complex. In: NEWTON and POTTS, Radiology of the skull and brain II, 2. St. Louis: Mosby 1974

LIN, P.M., SCOTT, M.: Collateral circulation of the external carotid artery and the internal carotid artery through the ophthalmic artery. Radiology **65**, 755–761 (1955)

LINDGREN, E.: Some aspects on the technique of tumors in the posterior fossa. Acta radiol. **34**, 331 (1950)

LINDGREN, E.: Röntgenologie einschließlich Kontrastmethoden. In: Handbuch der Neurochirurgie, Bd. 2. Berlin-Göttingen-Heidelberg: Springer 1954

LINDGREN, E.: Another method of vertebral angiography. Acta radiol. **46**, 257–261 (1956)

LINDNER, D.W., HARDY, W.G., THOMAS, L.M., GURDJIAN, E.S.: Angiographic complications in patients with cerebro-vascular disease. J. Neurosurg. **19**, 179–185 (1962)

LIST, C.F., BURGE, C.H., HODGES, F.J.: Intracranial angiography. Radiology **45**, 1–14 (1945)

LIVERUD, K.: Techniques in percutaneous carotid and vertebral angiography with polyetylene catheters. J. Oslo Cy. Hosp. **8**, 220–242 (1958)

LIVINI, F.: Arteria carotis externa. Arch. ital. Anat. Embriol. **2**, 653–741 (1903)

LODIN, H., OTTANDER, H.G.: The circulation through the anterior communicating cerebral artery on automatic contrast injection. Clin. Radiol. **18**, 268–271 (1967)

LOEB, C., MEYER, J.S.: Strokes due to vertebro-basilar disease. Springfield: Ch. Thomas 1965

LÖFGREN, F.O.: Vertebral angiography in the diagnosis of tumors in the pineal region. Acta radiol. **60**, 108–124 (1958)

LÖHR, W., JACOBI, W.: Die kombinierte Enzephaloarteriographie Fortschr. auf dem Gebiet der Röntgenstr. und Nuklearmedizin Erg. Bd. 44. Leipzig: Thieme 1933

LOMAN, J., MYERSON, A.: Visualization of the cerebral vessels by direct injection of thorium dioxide (Thorotrast). Amer. J. Roentgenol. **35**, 188–193 (1936)

LONGO, L.: Le anomalie del poligono di Willis nell-'uomo studiate comparativamente in alcuni mammiferi et nuelli. Anat. Anz. **27**, 170–200 (1905)

LOWMAN, R.M., DOFF, S.D.: Arteriography for the demonstration of intracranial aneurysms. Amer. J. Roentgenol. **53**, 341–347, 1945

LUCARELLI, S., FERRARI, U. DE: Studio clinico-radiologico di un caso di origine anomalla (dall'a carotide externa) dell'arteria vertebrale sinistra. Radiol. med. (Torino) **64**, 963 (1960)

LUESSENHOP, A.J., KACHMANN, R., SHEVLIN, W., FERRERO, A.A.: Clinical evaluation of artificial embolization in the management of large cerebral malformations. J. Neurosurg. **23**, 400–412 (1965)

LYON, L.W.: Transfemoral vertebral angiography as a cause of an anterior spinal artery syndrome. Case report. J. Neurosurg. **35**, 328 (1971)

MACMAHON, H.E., MURPHY, A.S., BATES, M.J.: Endothelial cell Sarkoma of liver following Thorotrast injections. Amer. J. Path. **23**, 585–681 (1947)

MACKENZIE, I.: The clinical presentation of the cerebral angioma. A review of 50 cases. Brain **76**, 184–219 (1953)

MAKI, Y., WATANABE, M., NAKATA, Y., ONO, Y., SHIRAI, S.: Angiographic demonstration of the vertebral artery. Clin. Neurol. Rinsha shinkeigaku **9**, 199–204 (1969)

MANGHI, E., SANGINARIO, M., ROSELLI, R., BOERI, F.: Variazioni anatomiche e emodinamiche nella porzione anteriore del poligono di Willis. – Studio angiografico in diverse condizioni cliniche. Riv. Neuropsichiat. **3**, 356–368 (1957)

MANI, R.L., NEWTON, TH.H., GLICKMAN, M.G.: The superior cerebellar artery: An anatomic roentgenographic correlation. Radiology **91**, 1102–1108 (1968)

MANI, R.L., NEWTON, TH.H., GLICKMAN, M.G.: The superior cerebellar artery: Arteriographic changes in the diagnosis of posterior fossa lesions. Radiology **92**, 1281–1287 (1969)

MARGOLIS, M.TH., NEWTON, TH.H.: The posterior inferior cerebellar artery. In: NEWTON and POTTS, Radiology of the skull and brain II, 2. St. Louis: Mosby 1974

MARGOLIS, M.TH., NEWTON, TH.H.: Collateral pathways between the cavernous portion of the internal carotid and external carotid arteries. Radiology **93**, 834–835 (1969)

MARGOLIS, M.TH., NEWTON, TH.H.: Borderlands of the normal and abnormal posterior inferior cerebellar artery. Acta radiol. **13**, 163–176 (1972)

MARGOLIS, M.TH., NEWTON, TH.H., HOYT, W.F.: Cortical branches of the posterior cerebral artery. Anatomic-radiologic correlation. Neuroradiology **2**, 127–135 (1971)

MARGOLIS, M.TH., NEWTON, TH.H., HOYT, W.F.: The posterior cerebral artery. Gross and roentgenographic anatomy. In: NEWTON and POTTS, Radiology of the skull and brain II, 2. St. Louis: Mosby 1974

MARINI DE ARANJO, M.: Zit. nach G. LAZORTHES, A. GOUAZE, G. SALAMON, Vascularisation et circulation cérébrales. Paris: Masson et Cie. (1975)

MARINI DE ARANJO, M.: Zit. nach SCIALFA, G., W. BANK, M. MEGRET, J.M. COBBAZ, The posterior fossa arteries in advances in cerebral angiography. Berlin-Heidelberg-New York: Springer 1975

MARINO, R.J.: Estudo esperimental anatomo-radiologico e esteriotaxico do territorio vascular cortical da arteria cerebral anterior. Tese de Docencia. Sao Paulo, 1974

MARSHALL, T.R., LING, J.T.: Direct percutaneous non-catheter left and right brachial angiography (left panarteriography – right cerebral angiography). Radiology **80**, 258–260 (1963)

MARTIN, M.J., WHISNANT, J.P., SAYRE, G.P.: Occlusive vascular disease in extracranial cerebral circulation. Arch. Neurol. (Chic.) **3**, 530–538 (1960)

MASLOWSKI, H.A.: Vertebral angiography: Percutaneous lateral atlanto-occipital method. Brit. J. Surg. **43** 1–8 (1955)

McConnel, E.M.: Arterial blood supply of human hypophysis cerebri. Anat. Rec. **115**, 175–203 (1953)

McCoullough, A.W.: Some anomalies of the cerebral arterial circle (of Willis) and related vessels. Anat. Rec. **142**, 537–543 (1962)

McDowell, F.H., Schick, R.W., Frederick, W., Dunbar, H.S.: An arteriographic study of cerebrovascular disease. Arch. Neurol. (Chic.) **1**, 435–442 (1959)

McMinn, R.M.H.: A case of nonunion of the vertebral arteries. Anat. Rec. **116**, 283 (1953)

Megret, M.: Repérage des artères chorioidennes de l'artère cérébelleuse postéro-inferieure. Strasbourg 1972

Melaragno, R.: Lateral syndrome of the medulla oblongata (Wallenberg's syndrome) as a complication of a vertebral angiography. A case report. Arch. Neuro-psiquiat. (S.Paulo) **30**, 78 (1972)

Meneses Hoyes, J., Gomez del Campo, C.: Angiography of thoracic aorta and coronary vessels, with direct injection of opaque solution into aorta. Radiology **50**, 211–213 (1948)

Merland, J.J.: Arteriographie superselective des branches de la carotide externe. Thesis J.J. Merland, Paris: VI, 1973

Merland, J.J., Djindjian, R., Bories, J.: Superselective arteriography of the branches of the external carotid artery. Recent findings concerning the exo- und endrocranial base of the skull. In: Advances in cerebral angiography. Berlin-Heidelberg-New York: Springer 1975

Meyer, J.S., Gotoh, F.: Interaction of cerebral hemodynamics and metabolism. Neurology (Minneap.) **11**, 45–65 (1961)

Meyer, J.S., Gotoh, F., Tazaki, Y., Hamaguchi, K., Ishikawa, S., Nouailhat, F., Symon, L.: Regional cerebral blood flow and metabolism in vivo. Arch. Neurol. (Chic.) **7**, 560–581 (1962)

Michotey, P., Moscow, N.P., Salamon, G.: Anatomy of the cortical branches of the middle cerebral artery. In: Newton and Potts, Radiology of the skull and brain II, 2. St. Louis: Mosby 1974

Minagi, H., Newton, Th.H.: Carotid rete mirabile in man. Radiology **86**, 100–102 (1966)

Mishkin, M.M.: Direct serial magnification angiography. In: Newton and Potts, Radiology of the skull and brain I. St. Louis: Mosby 1974

Mitterwallner, F. v.: Variationsstatistische Untersuchungen an den basalen Hirngefäßen. Acta anat. (Basel) **24**, 51–88 (1955)

Mizukami, M., Mine, T., Tomita, T.: Window formation of vertebral artery (vertebral diastemato artery); and the association with cerebral aneurysm and/or arteriovenous malformation. Brain Nerve (Tokyo) **20**, 1271–1276 (1968)

Moissl, G.: Über die vaskulär bedingten pathologischen Veränderungen des Karitissiphons im zerebralen Angiogramm. Inaug.-Dissertation, Würzburg, 1972

Moniz, E.: L'encephalographie arterielle, son importance dans la localisation des tumeurs cerebrales. Rev. neurol. **2**, 72 (1927)

Moniz, E.: Die zerebrale Arteriographie und Phlebographie. Ergänzungsband zum „Handbuch der Neurologie" II. Berlin: Springer 1940

Moniz, E., Lima, P.A., Caldas, P.: A filmogem da circulaçao cerebral. A medicina contemporanca, No 3. Zit. nach: Krayenbühl, H., und Yasargil, M.G. Die cerebrale Angiographie. Stuttgart: Thieme 1965

Moniz, E., Pinto, A., Alvez, A.: Artériographie du cervelet et des autres organes de la fosse postérieure. Bull. Acad. Med. Paris **109**, 758–760 (1933)

Montrieul, B., zitiert nach Gros, Ch., Minvielle, J., Vlakowitch, B.: Anastomose artérielle intracranieune, étude artériographique et clinique. Neurochir. **2**, **3**, 281 (1956)

Morel, F., Wildi, E.: Examen anatomique du polygone du Willis et de ses anomalies. Etude statistique. V. Int. Neurol. Kongress Lissabon, 1953. Zbl. Neurochir. **13**, 174–175 (1953)

Morello, A., Cooper, I.S.: Arteriographic anatomy of the anterior choroidal artery. Amer. J. Roentgenol. **73**, 748–751 (1955)

Morris, E.D., Moffat, D.B.: Abnormal origin of the basilary artery. Anat. Rec. **125**, 701–705 (1956)

Moscow, N.P., Michotey, P., Salamon, G.: Anatomy of the cortical branches of the anterior cerebral artery. In: Newton and Potts, Radiology of the skull and brain II, 2. St. Louis: Mosby 1974

Mounier-Kuhn, A., Bouchet, A., Costaz, G.: Contribution à l'etude anatomique radiologique et chirurgicale de l'artère choroidenne antérieure. Neurochirurgie **1**, 345–370 (1955)

Mount, L.A., Taveras, J.M.: Arteriographic demonstration of the collateral circulation of the cerebral hemispheres. amer. med. Ass. Arch. Neurol. Psychiat. **78**, 235–253 (1957)

Müller, D.: Zur Frage des sogenannten Hirntodes bei Neugeborenen und im frühen Kindesalter. In: Krösel, W., Scherzer, E. (eds.), Die Bestimmung des Todeszeitpunktes. Wien: Mandrich 1973

Müller, J.: Über Lage und Ursprungszonen der Kleinhirnarterien und deren Quellgefäße. Inaug.-Dissertation, Würzburg, 1975

Murphy, J.P.: Cerebrovascular disease. The Year Book Medical Publishers Inc. Chicago: 1954

Murtagh, F., Stauffer, H.M., Harley, R.D.: A case of persistent carotid-basilar anastomosis associated with aneurysm of the homolateral middle cerebral artery manifested by oculomotory palsy. J. Neurosurg. **12**, 46 (1955)

Nadjmi, M.: Über die A.primitiva trigemina im Carotis- und Vertebralisangiogramm. Dtsch. Z. Nervenheilk. **182**, 231–237 (1961)

Nadjmi, M.: Zerebrale Gefäße im Angiotomogramm. Stuttgart: Thieme 1977

Nadjmi, M., Braun, H., Cavallini, L., Nippert, M.: Hämodynamische und physikalische Aspekte der retrograden Brachialisangiographie. Dtsch. Z. Nervenheilk. **194**, 328–343 (1968)

Nadjmi, M., Pöschmann, A.: Über ein Gerät zur Serien-Angio-Tomographie. Fortschr. Röntgenstr. **123**, 4, 299–301 (1975)

NADJMI, M., SCHWIND, F.: In: G. SCHALTENBRAND, Spezielle neurologische Untersuchungsmethoden. Stuttgart: Thieme 1968

NAIDICH, T.P., KRICHEFF, J.J.: The anterior inferior cerebellar artery in profile anatomic-radiographic correlation in the lateral projection. In: Advances in cerebral angiography. Berlin-Heidelberg-New York: Springer 1975

NAMIN, D.: Percutaneous vertebral angiography. J. Neurosurg. **11**, 442–457 (1954)

NAMIN, P.: L'angiographie vertebrale. Paris: Doin et Cie. 1955

NEIMANIS, G.: Über Kaliberschwankungen und Verlaufsanomalien des intrakraniellen Abschnittes der A. vertebralis. Z. Path. **67**, 461 (1956)

NELHAUS, G., CHUTORIAN, A.: Narcosis for neuroradiologic procedures in children. Arch. Neurol. (Chic.) **10**, 485–496 (1964)

NEWTON, T.H.: The axillary artery approach to arteriography of the aorta and its branches. Amer. J. Roentgenol. **89**, 275–283 (1963)

NEWTON, TH.H., GOODING, C.A.: Catheter techniques in pediatric cerebral angiography. Amer. J. Roentgenol. **104**, 63–65 (1968)

NEWTON, TH.H., KERBER, CH.W.: Techniques of catheter cerebral angiographies. In: NEWTON and POTTS, Radiology of the skull and brain I. St. Louis: Mosby 1974

NEWTON, TH.H., KRAMER, R.A., MANI, J.R.: Catheter technique in vertebral arteriography. Radiology **87**, 691–695 (1966)

NEWTON, TH.H., MANI, R.L.: The vertebral artery. In: NEWTON and POTTS, Radiology of the skull and brain II, 2. St. Louis: Mosby 1974

NEWTON, TH.H., POTTS, D.G. (eds.): Radiology of the skull and brain, Vol. 2, Book 1. St. Louis: Mosby 1974

NEWTON, TH.H., WYLIE, E.J.: Collateral circulation associated with occlusion of the proximal subclavian and innominate arteries. Amer. J. Roentgenol. **91**, 394–405 (1964)

NIELSEN, K.A., OWMAN, C.: Adrenergic innervation of pial arteries related to the circle of Willis in the cat. Brain Res. **6**, 773–776 (1967)

NORTHFIELD, D.W.C., RUSSEL, D.S.: The fate of thorium dioxide (thorotrast) in cerebral angiography. Lancet **1937/I**, 377–381

ODMAN, P.: Thoracic aortography by means of a radiopaque polythelene catheter inserted percutaneously. Acta radiol. **45**, 117–124 (1956)

ÖKRÖS, A.: Abnormitäten des Circulus arteriosus Willisi in Beziehung zur angiographischen Untersuchung des Gehirns. Magy. orv. Arch. **35** (1934)

OERTEL, O.: Über die Persistenz embryonaler Verbindungen zwischen der A. carotis interna und der A. vertebralis und ihre Bedeutung für den Circulus arteriosus Willisi. Anat. Anz. **55**, Erg.-Band 281 (1922)

OGLE, J.W.: Note on a nerve piercing the walls of an artery. J. Anat. (Lond.) **29**, (1895)

OLDENDORF, W.H.: Technical factors related to the complications of carotid angiography. Bull. Los Angeles neurol. Soc. **29**, 163–176 (1964)

OLIVECRONA, H.: Bericht über arteriographische Darstellung der Arteria vertebralis. Tagg. Brit. Neuro. Surg. 1935. Zbl. Chir. **32**, 1904 (1935)

OLIVECRONA, H.: Das arteriovenöse Aneurysma der Karotis- und Vertebralisgebiete. Dtsch. Z. Nervenheilk. 1957

ORLANDINI, I.: Il sistema arterioso della testa et del collo. Bologna: Capelli 1951

OSTROWSKI, A., WEBER, J.E., GURDJIAN, E.S.: The proximal anterior cerebral artery; an anatomic study. Arch. Neurol. (Chic.) **3**, 661–664 (1960)

OTOMO, E.: The anterior chorioidal artery. Arch. Neurol. (Chic.) **13**, 656 (1965)

PADGET, D.H.: The circle of Willis: Its embryology and anatomy. In: DANDY, W.E., Intracranial arterial aneurysms. New York: Comstock Publ. Co. 1945

PADGET, D.H.: The development of cranial arteries in the human embryo. Contributions to embryology. Carneg. Inst. Washington **212**, 205–262 (1948)

PADGET, D.H.: Designation of the embryonic intersegmental arteries in reference to the vertebral artery and vertebral stem. Anat. Rec. **119**, 349 (1954)

PADOVANI, J., KASBARIAN, M., FAURE, F., LEYNAUD, D.: Prévention des accidents de l'angiographie par cathétérisme artériel. Notre statistique. J. Radiol. Électrol. **54**, 113 (1973)

PARAICZ, E., SZESNAZY, E.: Über die Carotisangiographie im Kindesalter. Acta neurochir. (Wien) **7**, 350–363 (1959)

PARKINSON, D.: Collateral circulation of cavernous carotid artery. Anatomy. Canad. J. Surg. **7**, 251–268 (1964)

PARKINSON, D.: A surgical approach to the cavernous portion of the carotid artery. Anatomical studies and case report. J. Neurosurg. **23**, 474–483 (1965)

PATTERSON, R.H., GOODELL, H., DUNNING, H.S.: Complications of carotid arteriography. Arch. Neurol. (Chic.) **10**, 513–520 (1964)

PENDERGRASS, H.P., TONDEREAU, R.L., PENDERGRASS, E.P., RITCHIE, D.J., HILDRETH, F.A., ASKOVITZ, S.I.: Reactions associated with i.v. urography. Historical and statistical review. Radiology **71**, 1–12 (1958)

PERRET, G.H., NISHIOKA, H.: Cerebral angiography. An analysis of the diagnostic value and complications of carotid and vertebral angiography in 5484 patients. J. Neurosurg. **25**, 98–114 (1966)

PERCHERON, S.: The anatomy of the arterial supply of the human thalamus and its use for the interpretation of the thalamic vascular pathology. Exc. Neurol. **205**, 1–13 (1973)

PERNKOPF, E.: Topographische Anatomie des Menschen, Bd. 1. Berlin-Göttingen-Heidelberg: Urban & Schwarzenberg 1960

PERTUISET, B., ARON, D., DILENGE, D., MAZALTON,

A.: Les syndromes de l'artère choriodiénne antérieure. Rev. neurol. **106**, 286 (1962)

PERYMAN, G.R., GRAY, G.H., BRUST, R.W., CONLON, P.C.: Interesting aspects of cerebral angiography with emphasis on some unusual congenital variations. Amer. J. Roentgenol. **89**, 372–384 (1963)

PETERS, R.: Tödliche Gehirnblutung bei menstrueller Migräne. Beitr. path. Anat. **93**, 209–218 (1934)

PFEIFER, R.A.: Grundlegende Untersuchungen für die Angioarchitektonik des menschlichen Gehirns. Berlin: Springer 1930

PHILIPIDES, D., MONTRIEUL, B., DE HAYNIN, G., HERRENSCHMIDT, M.: Anéurysme de l'artère basilaire identifié par l'arteriographie. Presse Med. **58**, 1227 (1952)

PHILLIPS, J.F.: Electrocoagulation transcatheter of blood vessels. Invest. Radiol. **8**, 295 (1973)

PICARD, I., LEPOIRE, J., MONTAUT, J., HEPNER, J., ROLAND, J., GUYONNAUD, J.C., JACOBS, F., ANDRE, J.M.: Endarterial occlusion of carotid cavernous fistulas using a balloon tipped catheter. Neuroradiology **8**, 5–10 (1974)

PICHLER, E.: Der Kopfschmerz. Im Almanach für Neurologie und Psychiatrie. München: Lehmann 1961

PIERCE, E.C.: Percutaneous femoral artery catheterization in man with special reference to aortography. Surg. Gynec. Obstet. **93**, 56–74 (1951)

PITTS, F.W.: Variations of collateral circulation in internal carotid occlusion. Neurology (Minneap.) **12**, 467–471 (1962)

PLATZER, W.: Der Carotissyphon und seine anatomische Grundlage. Fortschr. Röntgenstr. **84**, 200–206 (1956)

PLATZER, W.: Die Variabilität der Arteria carotis interna im Sinus cavernosus in Beziehung zur Variabilität der Schädelbasis. Morph. Jb. **98**, 225–243 (1957)

POBLETE, R., ASENJO, A.: Anastomosis carotidobasilar par persistencia de la arteria trigeminal primitiva. Neurocirugia (Chile) **11**, 1–5 (1955)

POIRIER, P., NICOLAS, A.: Traité d'anatomie humaine (Angélogie), II, 2, pp. 669–691. Paris: Masson et Cie. 1896

POLI, D., ZUCHA, J.: Beiträge zur Kenntnis der Anomalien und der Erkrankungen der A. carotis interna. Zbl. Neur. **5**, 209 (1940)

POLYAK, S.L.: The vertebral visual system, pp. 609–615. Chicago: Univ. Chicago Press 1957

POOLE, G.J., POTTS, D.G., NEWTON, TH.H.: Angiotomography. In: NEWTON and POTTS, Radiology of the skull and brain I. St. Louis: Mosby 1974

POTTS, D.G., TAVERAS, J.M.: Differential diagnosis of space occupying lesions in the region of the thalamus by cerebral angiography. Acta radiol. **1**, 373–384 (1963)

QUAIN, R.: The anatomy of the arteries of the human body. London: Taylor and Walton 1844

RABE, W.: Die Indikation zu neuroradiologischen Untersuchungen bei Migräne. Fortschr. Neurol. Psychiat. **39**, 401 (1971)

RABIOTTO, A., SAGNINARIO, M.: La visualisazzione dell'arteria cerebrale posteriore nell' angiografia carotidea. Ann. Radiol. diagn. (Bologna) **30**, 18–32 (1957)

RADNER, S.: Intracranial angiography via the vertebral artery. Acta radiol. **28**, 838–842 (1947)

RADNER, S.: Thoracal aortography by catheterization from radial artery: preliminary report of a new technique. Acta radiol. **29**, 178–180 (1948)

RADNER, S.: Vertebral angiography by catheterization. A new method employed in 221 cases. Acta radiol., Suppl. **87** (1951)

RAIMONDI, A.J.: Pediatric neuroradiology. Philadelphia: Saunders 1972

RAIMONDI, A.J., WHITE, H.: Cerebral angiography in the newborn and infant: General principles. Ann. Radiol. **10**, 147–164 (1967)

RAMELLA, G.: Angio-Tomography for the Study of Endocranial Aneurysms. Acta neurochir. (Wien) **21**, 285 (1969)

RANSON, S.W., CLARK, S.L: Anatomy of the nervous system. Philadelphia: W.B. Saunders Co. 1948

RAUBER-KOPSCH, F.: Lehrbuch der Anatomie des Menschen, Bd. II. Leipzig: Thieme 1948

RAUSCH, FJ., SCHIEFER, W., STRUCK, G.: Über den Wert der zerebralen Angiographie für die Diagnose arteriosklerotischer Gefäßprozesse. Fortschr. Neurol. Psychiat. **24**, 512–520 (1956)

RAYBAUD, CH., MICHOTEY, P., BANK, W., FARNARIER, PH.: Angiographic-anatomic study of the vascular territories of the cerebral convolutions. Advances in cerebral angiography. Berlin-Heidelberg-New York: Springer 1975

RENDALL: Zit. nach BERRY, R.J.A., J.H. ANDERSON, A case of nonunion of the vertebrales with consequent abnormal origin of the basilaris. Anat. Anz. **35**, 515 (1909)

RIBES-CHAUSSIER: Zit. nach ADACHI, B., Das Arteriensystem der Japaner, Bd. I. Kaiserl. Universität Kyoto, 1928

RICHTER, H.R.: Collaterals between the external carotid artery and the vertebral artery in cases of thrombosis of the internal carotid artery. Acta radiol. **40**, 108–112 (1953)

RICKENBACHER, J.: Der suboccipitale und intracranielle Abschnitt der Arteria vertebralis. Z. Anat. Entwickl.-Gesch. **124**, 171–178 (1964)

RICKENBACHER, J.: Normale und pathologische Anatomie des Hirngefäßsystems. In: GÄNSHIRT, Der Hirnkreislauf. Stuttgart: Thieme 1972

RIGGS, H.E.: Anomalies of circle of Willis. Trans. Philadelphia Neurol. Soc., Dez. 1937

RIGGS, H.E., GRIFFITHS, J.Q.: Anomalies of the circle of Willis in persons with nervous and mental disorders. Arch. Neurol. Psychiat. (Chic.) **39**, 1353–1356 (1938)

RIMPAU, A.: Zur Morphologie der Carotispunktion. Virchows Arch. path. Anat. **330**, 156–171 (1957)

RIMPAU, A., SEILS, H.: Pathologisch-anatomische Befunde an der Punktionsstelle bei der Hirnarteriographie und Betrachtungen zur Punktionstechnik. Fortschr. Röntgenstr. **87**, 191–199 (1957)

RING, B.A.: Middle cerebral artery; anatomical and radiographic study. Acta radiol. **57**, 289–300 (1962)

RING, B.A.: Angiographic recognition of occlusions of isolated branches of the middle cerebral artery. Amer. J. Roentgenol. **89**, 391 (1963)

RING, B.A.: Normal middle cerebral artery. In: NEWTON and POTTS, Radiology of the skull and brain II, 2. St. Louis: Mosby 1974

RING, B.A.: The cerebral cortical arteries. In: Advances in cerebral angiography. Berlin-Heidelberg-New York: Springer 1975

RING, B.A., WADDINGTON, M.M.: Angiographic identification of the motor strip. J. Neurosurg. **26**, 249–254 (1967)

ROBB, G.P., STEINBERG, I.: Visualization of chambers of the heart, the pulmonary circulation and the great blood vessels in man; a practical method. Amer. J. Roentgenol. **41**, 1–17 (1939)

ROBERT, F.: Der Einfluß des Kontrastmittels auf den Kollateralkreislauf beim Verschluß der A. cerebri media. Radiol. clin. Biol. (Basel) **38**, 357–371 (1969)

RÖTTGEN, P.: Die Röntgendiagnostik zerebraler Durchblutungsstörungen. Nauheimer Fortbildungslehrgänge **18**, 26–38 (1952)

ROGERS, L.: The function of the circulus of Willis. Brain **70**, 171–178 (1947)

ROTH, G., BAUMGARTNER, J., MORSIER, G. DE: Artériographique vertébrale par voie sousclavière et aortographie. Psychiatr. Neurol. Neurochir. (Amst.) **64**, 202–213 (1961)

ROUSSY, G., OBERLING, C.H., GUERIN, M.: Über Sarkomerzeugung durch kolloidales Thoriumdioxyd bei der Ratte. Strahlentherapie **56**, 160 (1936)

ROUVIERE, H.: Anatomie humaine descriptive et topographie. Paris: Masson et Cie., édit. 1940

ROY, P.: Amer. J. Roentgenol. **94**, 1 (1965)

RUEDINGER, J.: Über die Hirnschlagadern und ihre Einschließung in Knochenkanälen. Arch. Anat. Entwickl.-Gesch. 97–108 (1888)

RUGGIERO, G., CONSTANS, T.P.: L'artériographie vertébrale. Rev. neurol. **90**, 1–13 (1954)

RUGGIERO, G., JAY, M.: Une technique pour l'artériographie de la carotide externe. Acta radiol. **50**, 452–459 (1958)

RUGGIERO, G., SCIALFA, G., CRISTI, G.: The value of direct percutaneous puncture technique in vertebral angiography. Neuroradiology **6**, 104–109 (1973)

RUGGIERO, R.: Technique Neuroradiologique. Paris: Masson 1957

SALAMON, G.: Technique de ponction percutanée de l'artère carotide externe. Ann. Radiol. **9**, 11–12, 855–856 (1966)

SALAMON, G., FAURE, J., RAYBAUD, C., GRISOLI, F.: Normal external carotid artery. In: NEWTON and POTTS, Radiology of the skull and brain II. St. Louis: Mosby 1974

SALAMON, G., GUERINEL, G., DEMARD, F.: Etude radio-anatomique de l'artère carotide externe. Ann. Radiol. **11**, 3–4, 199–215 (1968)

SALAMON, G., RAYBAUD, CH., MICHOTEY, P., FARNARIER, PH.: Anatomic and radiographic study of the fissures and sulci of the brain. Advances in cerebral angiography. Berlin-Heidelberg-New York: Springer 1975

SALTZMAN, G.F.: Persistent primitive trigeminal artery studied by cerebral angiography. Acta radiol. **51**, 329–336 (1959)

SALTZMAN, G.F.: Angiographic demonstration of the posterior communicating and posterior cerebral arteries. Acta radiol. **52**, 1–20 (1959)

SALTZMAN, G.F.: Circulation through the anterior communicating artery studied by carotid angiography. Acta radiol. **52**, 194–208 (1959)

SALTZMAN, G.F.: Circulation through the posterior communicating artery in different tests. Acta radiol. Diagnosis **1**, 313–298 (1963)

SAMRA, K.A., SCONVILLE, W.B., YAGHNAI, M.: Anastomosis of carotid and basilar arteries. Persistent primitive trigeminal artery and hypoglossal artery. Report of two cases. J. Neurosurg. **30**, 622–625 (1969)

SCATCLIFF, J.H., MISHKIN, M.M., HYDE, I.: Vertebral angiography: an evaluation of methods. Radiology **85**, 14–22 (1965)

SCARCELLA, A.: Studio arteriografico della cerebrale posteriore visualizzata athraverso la carotide interna. Arch. Neurochir. (Firenze). Ref. Zbl. Neurochir. **12**, 307 (1952)

SCHAERER, J.P.: A case of carotid-basilar anastomosis with multiple associated cerebrovascular anomalies. J. Neurosurg. **12**, 62–65 (1955)

SCHECHTER, M., GUTIERREZ-MAHONEY, G.G.: The evolution of vertebral angiography. Neuroradiology **5**, 157–164 (1973)

SCHECHTER, M., ZINNGIESSER, L.H.: The anterior spinal artery. VII. Symposium Neuroradiologicum, New York, 1964

SCHIEFER, W.: In: GÄNSHIRT, Der Hirnkreislauf. Stuttgart: Thieme 1972

SCHIEFER, W., VETTER, K.: Das cerebrale Angiogramm in den verschiedenen Altersstufen. Zbl. Neurochir. **17**, 218–232 (1957)

SCHIEFER, W., WALTER, W.: Die Persistenz embryonaler Gefäße als Ursache von Blutungen des Hirns und seiner Häute. Acta neurochir. (Wien) **7**, 7 (1959)

SCHLESINGER, B.: The insulo-opercular arteries of the brain, with special reference to angiography of striothalamic tumors. Amer. J. Roentgenol. **70**, 555–563 (1953)

SCHLESINGER, B.: The upper brain stem in the human. – Its nuclear configuration and vascular supply. Berlin-Heidelberg-New York: Springer 1976

SCHMEIDEL, G.: Die Entwicklung der A. vertebralis beim Menschen. Gegenbauers morph. Jb. **71**, 315–435 (1933)

SCHMEIDEL, G.: Über merkwürdige Varietäten des intracraniellen Teiles der A. vertebralis des erwachsenen Menschen. Gegenbauers morph. Jb. **77**, 110–123 (1936)

SCHMIDT, H., PFINGST, E.: Zur Doppelung der Arteria vertebralis. Fortschr. Röntgenstr. **118**, 636–640 (1973)

SCHNÜRER, L., STATTIN, S.: Vascular supply of intracranial dura from internal carotid artery with special reference to its angiographic significance. Acta radiol. (Diagn.) **1**, 441–450 (1963)

SCHÜRMANN, K., ULBRICHT, W.: Differentialdiagnose des Kopfschmerzes Fortschr. Med. **84**, 104–105 (1966)

SCHÜRMANN, K., ULBRICHT, W.: Kopf- und Gesichtsschmerz bei intrakraniellen Erkrankungen I u. II. Fortschr. Med. **84**, 93–99, 132–139 (1966)

SCIALFA, G., BANK, W., MEGRET, M., CORBAZ, J.M.: The posterior fossa arteries. (1) The morphology and variation of the anterior inferior cerebellar artery. (2) The angiographic localization of the fourth ventricle. In: Advances in cerebral angiography. Berlin-Heidelberg-New York: Springer 1975

SCOTT, H.S.: Carotid basilar anastomosis. Persistent hypoglossal artery. Brit. J. Radiol. **36**, 847 (1963)

SEDZIMIR, C.B.: An angiographic test of collateral circulation through the anterior segment of the circle of Willis. J. Neurol. Neurosurg. Psychiat. **22**, 64–68 (1959)

SELDINGER, S.L.: Catheter replacement of the needle in percutaneous arteriography. Acta radiol. **39**, 368–376 (1953)

SERBINENKO, F.A.: Balloon catheterization and occlusion of major cerebral vessels. J. Neurosurg. **41**, 125–145 (1974)

SHELLSHEAR, J.L.: The basal arteries of the fore-brain and their functional significance. J. Anat. (Lond.) **55**, 27–35 (1920)

SHELLSHEAR, J.L.: A contribution to the knowledge of the arterial supply of the cerebral cortex in man. Brain **50**, 236–253 (1927)

SHIMIDZU, K.: Beiträge zur Arteriographie des Gehirns – eine einfache percutane Methode. Langenbecks Arch. klin. Chir. **188**, 295–316 (1937)

SHIMIZU, Y., IMAI, T., RAI, M., HIDA, K.: Two cases with fenestration of the vertebral artery. Brain Nerve (Tokyo) **24**, 1185–1189 (1972)

SHIRO WAGA, AKINDRI KONDO, KOZO MORITAKE, HAJIME HANDA: Rupture of intercranial aneurysma during angiography. Neuroradiology **5**, 169 (1973)

SICARD, J.A., FORESTIER, G.: Injections intravasculaires d'huile jodée sous contrôle radiologique. C. R. Soc. Biol. (Paris) **88**, 1200–1202 (1923)

SICCURO, A., BAGGIORE, P.: Le tronc anastomotique carotide-basilare. V. Int. Neurol. Kongress, Lissabon, 1959

SIGUEIRA, E.B., KARRAS, B.G., CANNON, A.G., BUCY, P.C.: Percutaneous brachial cerebral angiography. J. Neurosurg. **19**, 1050–1057 (1962)

SILVERSTEIN, A.: Arteriography of stroke. Arch. Neurol. (Chic.) **15**, 206 (1966)

SIMON, M., RABINOW, K., HORENSTEIN, S.: Proximal subclavian artery occlusion and reversed vertebral blood flow to the arm. Clin. Radiol. **13**, 201 (1962)

SINDERMANN, F.: Krankheitsbild und Kollateralkreislauf bei einseitigem und doppelseitigem Carotisverschluß. J. Neurol. Sci. **5**, 9–25 (1967)

SJÖGREN, S.E.: Percutaneous vertebral angiography. Acta radiol. **40**, 113–123 (1953)

SJÖGREN, S.E.: The anterior chorioidal artery. Acta radiol. **46**, 143 (1956)

SJOQUIST, O.: Arteriographische Darstellung der Gefäße der hinteren Schädelgrube. Chirurg **10**, 377–380 (1938)

SLANY, A.: Anomalien des circulus arteriosus Willisi und ihre Beziehung zur Aneurysmenbildung an der Hirnbasis. Virchows Arch. path. Anat. **301**, 62 (1938)

SMALTINO, F., BERNINI, F., ELEFANTE, R.: Normal and pathological findings of angiographic examination of the internal auditory artery. Neuroradiology **2**, 216–222 (1971)

SMITH, G.E.: Note on a anomalous anastomosis between the internal carotid and basilar arteries. J. Anat. Physiol. (Lond.) **43**, 310–312 (1909)

SMITH, C.G., RICHARDSON, W.F.: The course and distribution of the arteries supplying the visual (striate) cortex. Amer. J. Ophthal. **61**, 1391–1396 (1966)

SMITH, P.W., WILSON, C.W., CREGG, H.A., KLASSEN, K.P.: Cardioangiographie. J. thorac. Surg. **28**, 273 (1954)

SOLNITZKY, O.: Collateral circulation in cerebral vascular insufficiency. Georgetwon med. Bull. **14**, 19–31 (1960)

SPATZ, H.: Anomalien und Erkrankungen der Carotis interna. Zbl. ges. Neurol. Psychiat. **103**, 38–40 (1943)

STENVERS, H.W., BANNENBERG, P.M., LENSHÖCK, CH.: Anastomosis carotido-basilaire persistante. Rev. Neurol. **6**, 575 (1953)

STEPHENS, R.B., STILWELL, D.L.: Arteries and veins of the human brain. Springfield: Ch. Thomas 1969

STÖRRING, G.E.: Über Apoplexien im relativ jugendlichen Alter. Z. ges. Neurol. Psychiat. **167**, 405–409 (1939)

STOPFORD, J.S.B.: The arteries of the pons and medulla oblongata. (I) J. Anat. Physiol. (Lond.) **50**, 132–164 (1916). (II) J. Anat. Physiol. (Lond.) **50**, 225–280 (1916). (III) J. Anat. Physiol. (Lond.) **51**, 250–277 (1917)

STREETER, G.L.: The developmental alterations in the vascular system of the brain of the human embryo. Contr. Embryol. Carneg. Instn Washington **8**, 5–35 (1918)

STREIT, H.: Beiderseitige Schleifenbildung der Carotis interna in der Höhe der Gaumenmandeln. Zbl. Hals-, Nas.- u. Ohrenheilk. **30**, 351–352 (1932)

SUGAR, O., HOLDEN, L.B., POWELL, C.P.: Vertebral angiography. Amer. J. Roentgenol. **61**, 166–182 (1949)

SUNDERLAND, S.: An anomalous anastomosis between the internal carotid and basilar arteries. Aust. N.Z. J. Surg. **11**, 140–142 (1941)

SUNDERLAND, S.: The arterial relations of the internal meatus. Brain **68**, 23–27 (1945)

SUTHERLAND, G.R., DONALDSON, A.A.: Persistent hypoglossal artery complicated by internal carotid artery stenosis. Clin. Radiol. **23**, 222 (1972)

SUTTON, D.: The vertebro-basilary system and its vascular lesions. Clin. Radiol. **22**, 271–287 (1971)

SYMON, L., ISHAKAWA, S., MEYER, J.S.: Cerebral arterial pressure changes and development of leptomeningeal collateral circulation. Neurology (Minneap.) **13**, 237 (1963)

TAKAHASHI, K.: Perkutane Punktion der Vertebralis am Hals. Arch. Psychiat. Nervenkr. **111**, 373–379 (1940)

TAKAHASHI, M.: Atlas of vertebral angiography. Berlin: Urban & Schwarzenberg; Tokyo: Igaku Shoin Ltd. 1974

TAKAHASHI, M.: The anterior inferior cerebellar artery. In: Radiology of the skull and brain, Vol. 2, Book 2, pp. 1796–1808. St.Louis: C.V. Mosby 1974

TAKAHASHI, M., KAWANAMI, H., WATANABE, N., MATSUOKA, S.: Fenestration of the extracranial vertebral artery. Radiology **96**, 359–360 (1970)

TAKAHASHI, M., OKUDERA, T., TANAKA, M., KITAMURA, K., YONEMASU, Y.: Angiographic diagnosis of cerebellar medulloblastomas: Evaluation with pre- and postoperative vertebral angiographies. Amer. J. Roentgenol. **118**, 622–632 (1973)

TAKAHASHI, M., WILSON, G., HANAFEE, W.: The anterior inferior cerebellar artery: Its radiographic anatomy and significance in the diagnosis of extra axial tumors of the posterior fossa. Radiology **90**, 281–287 (1968)

TAKEUCHI, K., YOSHIOKA, M.: Über die A.primitiva hypoglossica. Med. Klin. **25**, 1032 (1963)

TALAIRACH, J., SZIKLA, G.: Atlas d'anatomie stéréotaxique du télencéphale. Vol. 1. Paris: Masson et Cie. 1967

TARENIECKY (1880): Zit. nach: OERTEL, O., Über die Persistenz embryonaler Verbindungen zwischen der A.carotis interna und der A.vertebralis und ihre Bedeutung für den Circulus arteriosus Willisi. Anat. Anz. **55**, Erg.-Band 281 (1922)

TARTARINI, E., GUIGNI, L.: Studio arteriografico del sifone carotideo in condizioni normali e pathologiche. Sist. nerv. **3**, 3–31 (1951)

TATELMAN, L.: The angiographic evaluation of cerebral atherosclerosis. Radiology **70**, 801–807 (1958)

TATLOW, W.F.T., BAMMER, H.G.: Syndrome of vertebral artery compression. Neurology (Minneap.) **7**, 331 (1957)

TAVERAS, J.M., POSER, C.N.: Roentgenological aspects of cerebral angiography in children. Amer. J. Roentgenol. **82**, 371–385 (1959)

TAVERAS, J.M., WOOD, E.H.: Diagnostic neuroradiology, Vol. 2. Baltimore: Williams and Wilkins 1976

TEAL, J.S., RUMBAUGH, C.L., BERGERON, R.T., SEGALL, H.D.: Anomalies of the middle cerebral artery, duplication and early bifurcation. Amer. J. Roentgenol. **118**, 567–575 (1973)

TEAL, J.S., RUMBAUGH, C.L., BERGERON, R.T., SEGALL, H.D.: Angiographic demonstration of fenestration of the intradural intracranial arteries. Radiology **106**, 123–126 (1973)

TEAL, J.S., RUMBAUGH, C.L., BERGERON, R.T., SEGALL, H.D.: Congenital absence of the internal carotid artery associated with cerebral hemiatrophy, absence of external carotid artery and persistence of the stapedial artery. Amer. J. Roentgenol. **118**, 534 (1973)

TESTUT, L.: Traité d'anatomie humaine II Angiologie système nerveux central. Vol. 5. Paris: Doin 1905

TESTUT, L.: Traité d'anatomie humaine, 7. Aufl., Bd. II, Paris: Doin 1921

TEUFEL, J.: Einbau der A. carotis interna in den Canalis caroticus unter Berücksichtigung des transbasalen Venenabflusses. Morph. J. **106**, 178–274 (1964)

THEVENOT, C.: Les artères du system nerveux central. Vol. 1. Paris: Vigot Frères 1954

THOMAS, G.T., ANDERSON, K.N., HAIN, R.F., MERENDINO, K.A.: The significance of abnormalous vertebro-basilar artery communications in operations of the heart and great vessels; an illustrative case with review of the literature. Surgery **46**, 747–757 (1959)

THOMSON, A.: Third annual report of commitee of collective investigation of anatomical society of Great Britain and Ireland. J. Anat. Physiol. (Lond.) **27**, 183–194 (1894)

TIWISINA, TH.: Funktionale und organische Durchblutungsschäden der Vertebralis-Basilaris-Strombahn. Hippokrates (Stuttg.) **28**, 202–205 (1957)

TIWISINA, TH.: Die Vertebralisangiographie. Theoretische und klinische Medizin in Einzelausgaben, Bd. 18. Heidelberg: Dr. Alfred Hüthig 1964

TÖNDURY, G.: Angewandte und topographische Anatomie, 4. Aufl. Stuttgart: Thieme 1970

TÖNNIS, W.: Inwieweit ist die Kontrastmitteldiagnostik bei frischen Kopfverletzungen notwendig bzw. berechtigt? Hefte Unfallheilk. **60**, 99–107 (1959)

TÖNNIS, W., PIA, H.W.: Die Geschwülste der mittleren Schädelgrube im Arteriogramm. Zbl. Neurochir. **12**, 145–165 (1952)

TÖNNIS, W., SCHIEFER, W.: Zirkulationsstörungen des Gehirns im Serienangiogramm. Berlin-Göttingen-Heidelberg: Springer 1959

TÖNNIS, W., SCHIEFER, W.: Zirkulationsstörungen des Gehirns im Serienangiogramm. Berlin-Heidelberg-New York: Springer 1969

TÖNNIS, W., SCHIEFER, W., WALTER, W.: Zur Differentialdiagnose intracranieller Blutungen. Dtsch. Z. Nervenheilk. **176**, 666–692 (1957)

TORRE, E. DE LA, NETZKY, M.G.: Study of persistent primitive maxillary artery in human fetus: Some homologies of craniel arteries in man and dog. Amer. J. Anat. **106**, 185–195 (1960)

TORRE, E. DE LA, OCCHIPIUTTI, E., POLLICITA, A.: Backward displacement of the upper part of the basilar artery in infantile hydrocephalus. Acta radiol., N.S. **8**, 385–392 (1969)

TSCHERNISCHEFF, A., GRIGOROWSKY, I.: Über die arterielle Versorgung des Kleinhirnes. Arch. Psychiat. Nervenkr. **85**, 483–540 (1929)

TÜNGEL (1860): Zit. nach OERTEL, O., Über die Persistenz embryonaler Verbindungen zwischen der A.carotis interna und der A.vertebralis und ihre

Bedeutung für den Circulus arteriosus Willisi. Anat. Anz. **55**, Erg.-Bd. 281 (1922)

TURNBULL, F.: Cerebral angiography by direct injection of the common carotid artery. Amer. J. Roentgenol. **41**, 166–172 (1939)

UDVARHELY, G.B., LAI, M.: Subarachnoid hemorrhage due to rupture of an aneurysm on a persistent left hypoglossal artery. Brit. J. Radiol. **36**, 843 (1963)

VIEHWEGER, G., JENSEN, H.P.: Obliterierende cerebrale Gefäßerkrankungen im Kindesalter. Deutscher Röntgenkongreß 1967, Teil A, 183–185 (1968)

VILLIGER, E., LUDWIG, E.: Gehirn und Rückenmark, 14. Aufl. Basel: Benno Schwabe 1946

VITEK, J.J.: Femorocerebral angiography: Analysis of 2000 consecutive examinations, special emphasis of carotid arteries catheterization in older patients. Amer. J. Roentgenol. **118**, 633 (1973)

VLAHOVITCH, B., FUENTES, J.M.: Embolization of cerebral angiomas by catheterization of cortical arteries. Neuroradiology **11**, 243–245 (1976)

VLAHOVITCH, B., GROS, C., ABID-YAZDI, I.J., FERNANDEZ-SERRAT, A.: Repérage du sillon insulaire supérieure dans l'angiographie carotidienne de profil. Neuro-chirurgie **10**, 91–99 (1964)

VOENO, G., CAVALO, A.: Studio angiografico del sistemo carotideo nelle neoplasie cervico-faciali. Arch. Ital. **70**, Suppl. **6**, 1017–1080 (1959)

VOGELSANG, H.: Die Bestimmung der Durchflußgeschwindigkeit im Carotisangiogramm und deren diagnostische Bedeutung bei cerebralen Gefäßerkrankungen. Nervenarzt **35**, 31–34 (1964)

VOGELSANG, H.: Angiographische Studie zur Darstellbarkeit von Arterien im Meatus acusticus internus. (A. cerebelli labyrinthi und A. auditiva int.) Radiologe **14**, 548–550 (1974)

VOIGT, K., BRANDT, TH., SAUER, M.: Röntgenanatomische Variationsstatistik zur topographischen Beziehung zwischen A. basilaris und Schädelbasisstrukturen. Neuroradiologische Untersuchungen an Vertebralis- und Brachialisangiographien. Arch. Psychiat. Nervenkr. **215**, 376–395 (1972)

VRIESE, B. DE: Sur les artères de la base du cerveau. Verh. anat. Ges. **18**, 88–99 (1904)

VRIESE, B. DE: Sur la signification morphologique des artères cerebrales. Arch. Biol. (Liège) **21**, 357–457 (1905)

WACHSMUTH, W.: Untersuchung über die gewebsschädigende Wirkung von Thorotrast. Chirurg **19**, 390 (1948)

WACKENHEIM, A.: Roentgendiagnosis of the cervicooccipital region. Berlin-Heidelberg-New York: Springer 1974

WACKENHEIM, A., BABIN, E.: Excursion extratransversaire de l'artère vertébrale. Presse med. **77**, 1213–1214 (1969)

WACKENHEIM, A., BRAUN, J.P.: Angiography of the mesencephalon. Berlin-Heidelberg-New York: Springer 1970

WACKENHEIM, A., BRAUN, J.P., BRADAC, G.B.: Angiographie der Tumoren des Mittelhirns und seiner Nachbarschaft. Radiologe **8**, 354–363 (1968)

WADDINGTON, M.M.: Atlas of cerebral angiography. Boston: Little Brown & Co. 1974

WALLACE, S., GOLDBERG, H.I., LEEDS, N.E., MISHKIN, M.M.: The cavernous branches of the internal carotid artery. Amer. J. Roentgenol. **101**, 34–46 (1967)

WALLACE, S., MEDELLIN, H., JINGH, D. DE, GIACTURCO, C.: Systemic heparenisation for angiography. Amer. J. Roentgenol. **116**, 204 (1972)

WALTER, L., SMITH, A.L., LARSON, C.PH.: Anesthesia for neuroradiologic procedures. In: NEWTON and POTTS, Radiology of the skull and brain I. St. Louis: Mosby 1974

WAPPENSCHMIDT, J.: Anwendung und Leistungsbreite der linksseitigen Brachialisarteriographie in der neurologischen Diagnostik. Fortschr. Röntgenstr. **104**, 540–546 (1966)

WAPPENSCHMIDT, J.: Die Gegenstromarteriographie, Methode, Indikation und Leistungsbreite in der Diagnostik neurogener Krankheitsbilder. Habilitationsschrift Bonn 1969

WEHMER, H.: Strahlendosismessungen bei Funktionsuntersuchungen. Diss. Heidelberg 1970

WEIBEL, J., FIELDS, W.S.: Atlas of arteriography in occlusive cerebrovascular disease. Stuttgart: Thieme 1969

WEICKMANN, F.: Grundlagen der angiographischen Diagnostik zerebraler Gefäßprozesse. In: Die zerebralen Durchblutungsstörungen des Erwachsenenalters, hrsg. von J. QUANDT. Stuttgart: Schattauer 1969

WEIDNER, W., HANAFEE, W., MARKHAM, CH.H.: Intracranial collateral circulation via leptomeningeal and rete mirabile anastomoses. Neurology (Minneap.) **15**, 39–48 (1965)

WELLS, CH. W.: The cerebral circulation. The clinical significance of current concepts. Arch. Neurol. (Chic.) **3**, 319–331 (1960)

WENDE, S., NAKAYAMA, N.: Anatomical variations of the internal auditory artery. In: Advances in cerebral angiography. Berlin-Heidelberg-New York: Springer 1975

WENDE, S., NAKAYAMA, N., SCHWERDTFEGER, P.: Internal auditory artery (embryology, anatomy, angiography, pathology). J. Neurol. **210**, 21–31 (1975)

WENDE, S., SCHINDLER, K., MORITZ, G.: Der diagnostische Wert der angiographischen Vergrößerungstechnik mit Feinstfokusröhren in 2 Ebenen. Radiologe **11**, 471 (1971)

WENDE, S., TAENZER, V.: Technik und Wert der perkutanen Brachialis-Zerebralangiographie. Fortschr. Röntgenstr. **103**, 143–150 (1965)

WENDE, S., ZIELER, E., NAKAYAMA, N.: Cerebral magnification angiography. Berlin-Heidelberg-New York: Springer 1974

WESTBERG, G.: The recurrent artery of HEUBNER and the arteries of the central ganglia. Acta radiol. **1**, 949–954 (1963)

Westberg, G.: The arteries of the cerebral ganglia. VII. Symposium Neuroradiologicum, New York, p. 32, 1964

Westberg, G.: Arteries of the basal ganglia. Acta radiol. (Diagn.) **5**, 581–596 (1966)

Wheeler, G.E., Baker, H.L., Jr.: The ophthalmic artery complex in angiographic diagnosis. Radiology **83**, 26–35 (1964)

Wholey, M., Kessler, L., Boehnke, M.: A percutaneous ballon catheter technique for the treatment of intercranial aneurysma). Acta radiol. (Diagn.) **13**, 286 (1972)

Wickbom, I.: Angiography of the carotid artery. Acta radiol., Suppl. **72** (1948)

Wickbom, I.: Thoracic aortography after direct puncture of the aorta from the jugulum. Acta radiol. **38**, 343 (1952)

Wiedner, F., Schreyer, H.: Seltene Anomalien cerebraler Gefäße (einseitige Aplasie der A. carotis interna. Persistenz der A. hypoglossica). Fortschr. Röntgenstr. **124**, 3, 245–249 (1976)

Williams, G.D., Edmonds, H.W.: Variations in arrangement of branches arising from aortic arch in American whites and negroes. Anat. Rec. **62**, 139–146 (1935)

Willis, Thomas: Cerebri anatomia nervorumque descriptis et usus. London 1664

Wilson Mc. Clure: The anatomical foundation of neuroradiology of the brain. London: J.A. Churchill Ltd. 1963

Windle, B.C.A.: On the arteries forming the circle of Willis. J. Anat. Physiol. (Lond.) **22**, 289–293 (1888)

Wise, B.L., Palubinskas, A.J.: Persistent trigeminal artery (carotid-basilar anastomosis). J. Neurosurg. **21**, 199–206 (1964)

Wolf, B.S., Newman, Ch.M., Khilnani, M.T.: The posterior inferior cerebellar artery on vertebral angiography. Amer. J. Roentgenol. **87**, 322–337 (1962)

Wolff, H., Schaltenbrand, G.: Die perkutane Angiographie der Hirngefäße. Zbl. Neurochir. **4**, 233–241 (1939)

Wolff, H.: Cerebral blood vessels – anatomical principles. Proc. Res. nerv. ment. Dis. **18**, 29–68 (1938)

Wollschlaeger, P.B., Wollschlaeger, G.: Arterial anastomoses of the human brain (a radiographic-anatomical study). VII. Symposium Neuroradiologicum, New York, 1964

Wollschlaeger, P.B., Wollschlaeger, G.: The ACA/ICA and MCA/ICA ratio. VII. Symposium Neuroradiologicum, New York, p. 36, 1964

Wollschlaeger, G., Wollschlaeger, P.B., Lukas, F.V., Lopez, V.F.: Experience and result with postmortem cerebral angiography performed as routine procedure of the autopsy. Amer. J. Roentgenol. **101**, 68–87 (1967)

Woringer, E., Gernez, A.: L'artériogramme cérébral. Essai de définition des frontières de l'artériogramme carotidien normal et de ses variations. Presse méd. **73**, 881–882 (1948)

Yasargil, M.G.: Die Vertebralisangiographie. Ihre Bedeutung für die Diagnose der Tumoren. Acta neurochir., Suppl. **9**, 1–108 (1962)

Zeitler, E., Schoop, W.: Der Wandel der Indikation zur Angiographie bei der arteriellen Verschlußkrankheit. Fortschr. Röntgenstr. **112**, 291 (1970)

Ziedses des Plantes, B.G.: Subtraktion. Stuttgart: Thieme 1961

Zolnai, B.: Die zwischen der A. vertebralis und zerebralen Venen bestehende Verbindung am atlanto-occipitalen Abschnitt beim Menschen. Anat. Anz. **114**, 400–407 (1964)

Zülch, K.J.: Gibt es einen Spasmus der Hirngefäße? Radiologe **11**, 429–435 (1971)

Angiographic Diagnosis of Supratentorial Space-Occupying Processes

By

Hans Henrik Jacobsen

With 75 Figures

Until a few years ago the neuroradiologist had at his disposal the use of pneumoencephalography, ventriculography with its different modifications, and angiography when he wanted to (1) establish the existence or absence of an intracranial space-occupying lesion, (2) to determine its location, and (3) to make an attempt to determine its nature.

In every neuroradiologic department there would be many cases in which two or all of these methods had to be used on the same patient, often combined with gamma-scanning and/or with ultra-sound examinations. Therefore the attempts to localize a space-occupying lesion as exactly as possible have forced many authors into a meticulous research of the angiologic normal anatomy, including the many variations, combined with studies of the pathologic anatomy, not only concerning the dislocations of the cerebral vessels, but also the architecture of the cerebral and meningeal arteries and veins. In this way several intracranial vessels, so far unknown to the anatomists, were found and named. Quite naturally a certain disruption of the nomenclature could not be avoided, but the broad international communication between neuroradiologists has already created more uniformity in this matter. Our knowledge of the cerebral and meningeal vessels is now much more comprehensive and exact than 20 years ago.

During the last years it has been said that this great normal and pathoanatomic work has been more or less wasted, because most of this topographic and "histologic" diagnostic work could have been left to computer-assisted tomography.

In the departments which own one of these machines it must be confessed that – especially when dealing, as in this chapter, with supratentorial expanding processes – the number of cerebral angiographies and pneumoencephalographies have obviously decreased, as at the same time topographic and histologic diagnosis have both become safer. But, on the other hand, there still are areas inside the skull where the CT-scanner cannot be used. The classic cerebro-angiographic methods will still be of value in the exact elucidation of vascular malformations and in such cases where a planned operation makes it necessary to visualize the vessels supplying and draining a tumor. To this might be added that the CT-scanners are still so expensive that not every neuroradiologic department will be able to make use of this magnificent invention for a number of years.

A. The Topographic Diagnosis (Herniations)

From the inner side of the skull wall dura sends its processes into the skull cavity: falx cerebri, tentorium cerebelli, falx cerebelli, and diaphragma sellae. They divide the cavity into more communicating compartments, caudally communicating with the spinal canal through the foramen magnum. The dural septa are strong; being built up of fibrous connective tissue; only strong forces can dislocate them; the only movable part is the low and weak anterior portion of the falx cerebri, which can be moved from side to side. The brain tissue is soft, and even a hard tumor inside or outside the brain will hardly per se be able to dislocate the falx or tentorium; the hemisphere involved first has to utilize the capacity of its surrounding subarachnoid space; when no more of this is left, it must penetrate into other compartments. The separating walls are the dural septa but to them must be added the sharp ridge between the anterior and the middle fossa, which is known by radiologists as the sphenoid ridge. The medial part of this is the posterior edge of the lesser wing of the sphenoid bone, laterally continuing in a strong bony ridge up to the pterion. If a tumor creates a lack of space in the anterior fossa, part of the frontal lobe may make its way over this ridge down into the anterior part of the middle fossa. Such dislocations of the brain substance, which may be found far from the expanding lesion itself, are called herniations. We speak about herniations from side to side under the falx, herniations in descending or ascending direction through the tentorial notch and descending or ascending sphenoid-ridge herniations. These different types will be discussed in the following pages, but it must be borne in mind that a tumor, cyst, or hematoma may cause a dislocation of the arteries and veins lying in close proximity without causing any herniation. Thus the herniation is a kind of a remote effect, while the tumor itself can cause local displacements. An expanding lesion may be found without herniation, but the opposite phenomenon is never seen. If a very large expanding lesion in one hemisphere is found without herniation from side to side, one should be prepared to find a similar lesion in the opposite hemisphere creating an equilibrium.

The herniations were first described by pathologists who saw the sharp indentations in the cerebellar tonsils when these were pressed down into the foramen magnum; similar sharp grooves were seen in the uncus and the parahippocampal gyrus when one or both hemispheres were pressed down into the tentorial notch. Similar, but much more shallow grooves may be found in normal brains, especially when the tentorial incisure is large enough to permit the inferior medial part of the temporal lobe to occupy some of the space between the brain stem and the tentorial edge.

The severity and duration of herniations differ. In severe cases the squeezing of the brain substance against the sharp edge may have the effect of obstructing the veins and/or arteries, and in this way infarctions may follow the herniation.

In cases with a previously known tumor in one hemisphere and contralateral paresis, an ipsilateral paresis may occur; one explanation may be that the peduncle of the opposite side is pressed against the tentorial edge because the brain stem is pushed away by the herniated part of the temporal lobe; (another explanation naturally may be another tumor or the well-known phenomenon that a glioma has penetrated the corpus callosum and has grown out in the contralateral hemisphere).

The literature on herniations is abundant. Among the more extensive recent descriptions concerning the vascular disturbances characterizing the different types of herniations TAVERAS and WOOD (1964), KRAYENBÜHL and YAŞARGIL (1965), and NEWTON and POTTS (1974) should be mentioned. These works give such exact descriptions of the vascular disturbances corresponding to each type and sub-type of herniations that it is possible for the descriptions and tables to be used as an exact diagnostic clue. It should be remembered, however, that, in addition to each of these descriptions, the local vascular changes caused by the expanding lesion itself must be considered. Furthermore, the reader of these extensive and excellent descriptions must make clear to himself that they will never be sufficient to a radiologist, who does not have a great routine in the evaluation of angiograms, but to the neuroradiologic expert they are an extremely valuable aid. "Herniations are of course not the primary object of cerebral angiography" said AZAMBUJA et al., (1956b), and with these words they stated that many space-occupying lesions have their own vascular changes: hypo- or avascular zones, hypervascular regions, perhaps pathologic vessels, and that some tumors have a characteristic vascular architecture. In such cases the topographic diagnosis is made *eo ipso* and, furthermore, in some cases we have obtained information about the nature of the lesion. This shows that the distinction between topographic and "histologic" diagnosis is vague.

I. Subfalcine Herniation

This midline dislocation was said by TAVERAS and WOOD (1964) to be the most common among the supratentorial herniations. The vessels indicating the midline shift are the anterior cerebral artery with its branches and the deep veins. The mode of dislocation provides information about the site of the expanding lesion. It is obvious that the posterior third of the pericallosal artery must remain on its own side to which it is fixed by the posterior part of the falx, which in turn is fixed to the ridge of the roof of tentorium. Likewise, the posterior part of the vein of Galen is fixed to the anterior point of the same ridge – the point called "le carrefour falco-tentoriel" by the French. So even if we have to deal with great dislocations of the anterior cerebral artery, its posterior portion will always return to the midline, and this return will often take place in a sudden bend, which TAVERAS and WOOD (1964) called a step (Figs. 21c and 39). This step may also be seen in cases with a slight dislocation, but it is never seen if, by accident, an oblique view should be the result of the intended frontal projection. A frontal mass will displace the artery in a smooth arc, and this arc does not necessarily end in a step (Figs. 23a and 28a). The anterior part of the pericallosal artery is situated at a lower level than the lower edge of the falx, but farther behind where its normal position is higher than the edge of the falx it will be forced back to the midline, unless the herniation is so violent that the cingulate gyrus follows the herniated hemisphere under the falcine edge; in that case the profile view will show the callosomarginal artery lying at a lower level than the pericallosal. The more moderate herniation will show the callosomarginal artery sticking to the midline, looking like a rein trying to keep the more dislocated pericallosal artery *in situ* (the callosomarginal sign; Fig. 14a and b, and 21c). The dislocation of the deep veins in these frontal masses will depend on the size of the expanding lesion.

A mass lying a little more posteriorly, that is to say still in the frontal lobe but behind the origin of the pericallosal artery will create a different picture: now the pericallosal artery is dislocated so that the greater part of it is parallel to the midline with a step anteriorly and posteriorly – "the square shift" of TAVERAS and WOOD (1964) (Fig. 21c). Here we may also find an anterior displacement of the Sylvian point.

The parieto-occipital masses will cause what is called the posterior subfalcine herniation. Here the anterior part of the pericallosal artery is located in the midline but the direction of the artery will be backward, laterally till suddenly the artery returns to the midline with a sharp bend (Fig. 28a); this herniation will further show a dislocation of the deep veins, especially of the posterior two-thirds of the internal cerebral vein and the anterior part of the vein of Galen, the posterior portion of which cannot leave the midline as it is fixed to the beginning of the straight sinus (Fig. 29a). The more profoundly situated masses will give a still greater dislocation of the deep veins. In slight, posterior herniations the displacement of the veins will be more pronounced than the arterial dislocation.

In lesions extending through the whole length of a hemisphere the whole length of the pericallosal artery will be displaced, possibly followed by the callosomarginal artery. If the herniation is not too big, the picture will bear some resemblance to the square shift, but the steps on leaving and returning to the midline may be more blunt (Fig. 14a). Just as the callosomarginal sign may indicate a downward displacement of the cingulate gyrus, this capsize may manifest itself in the frontal view if the small vessels, which are often visible in the pericallosal cisterns, are tilted. This picture corresponds to the tilting of the pericallosal cisterns seen in pneumoencephalography (Fig. 31a).

Finally it should be noted that a cerebral hemiatrophy – traumatic or congenital – may cause a midline shift without the presence of any expanding lesion.

II. Tentorial Herniation

The ascending and descending transtentorial herniations were through described by AZAMBUJA et al. (1956a and b). In an autoptic material they found descending herniation in 80% of 79 supratentorial tumors. The first patho-anatomic description of this kind of herniation was given by MEYER (1920), who was also the first author to demonstrate that the vessels might be squeezed between the herniated brain substance and the sharp edge of the tentorium with infarction as the result.

A distinction between different subtypes is necessary: the herniation will be bilateral in cases where it is caused by a midline tumor (tumors of the corpus callosum, tumors within the third ventricle, bilateral meningiomas of the falx, etc.) or symmetric, bilateral expanding lesions. The grade of the herniation among other factors will depend on the width of the tentorial notch, which should have no relation to the width of the skull (PLAUT, 1963). This herniation is not as common as the unilateral ones. It will cause a downward dislocation of the brain stem and may be of the central parts of the cerebellum; angiographically it will·present itself with a backward and downward dislocation of the upper part of the basilar artery; likewise, it will show displacement of the deep cerebral veins in the same direction: the vein of Galen and the upper part of the basal vein.

The unilateral descending transtentorial herniation, i.e., the unilateral temporal-lobe herniation, was analysed by AZAMBUJA et al. in 1956. The authors distinguished between anterior, posterior, and complete herniations and observed that the anterior is often followed by the posterior resulting in complete herniation. The vessels that should be evaluated especially are the anterior choroidal artery, the posterior communicating and posterior cerebral arteries, the basilar artery, and the deep cerebral veins. In the anterior herniations part of the uncus gyri hippocampi is pressed down in the antero-lateral part of the tentorial notch, where by the mesencephalon is dislocated to the opposite side and may undergo a rotation. Normally the anterior choroidal artery starts its course in a medially convex arc, surrounding the uncus, but in an anterior herniation the artery will be dislocated further medially, and the arc will be widened (Fig. 25a). Here one must be aware that an expanding lesion in the uncus itself may cause a similar widening of the arterial bow, but it does not necessarily produce a dislocation toward the midline. At the same time the lateral view will show a stretching of the artery, particularly in its cisternal part; it may be dislocated downward or more rarely upward, depending on whether the portion of the temporal lobe over or below the choroid fissure is herniated. The displacement of the posterior communicating and posterior cerebral arteries may be very difficult to evaluate in the anterior herniations; one might expect a downward dislocation, and this may also be the case, but the natural course of the posterior communicating artery descends to different degrees, so the change should be considerable before it is reliable. The more posteriorly the herniation is located, the more likely a steep descending course will indicate a true herniation. At the same time the posterior communicating and posterior cerebral arteries will be pressed medially in the frontal view (Fig. 1a and b, and 33a). Some other vessels in the ambient cistern, e.g., the posterior portion of the basal vein will also be pushed medially when the herniation reaches the posterior part of the tentorial incisure. In the case of a great herniation through a narrow incisure it may be seen that the posterior cerebral artery, following its way from its pathologically depressed origin below the herniation to its normal site on the medial, inferior surface of the

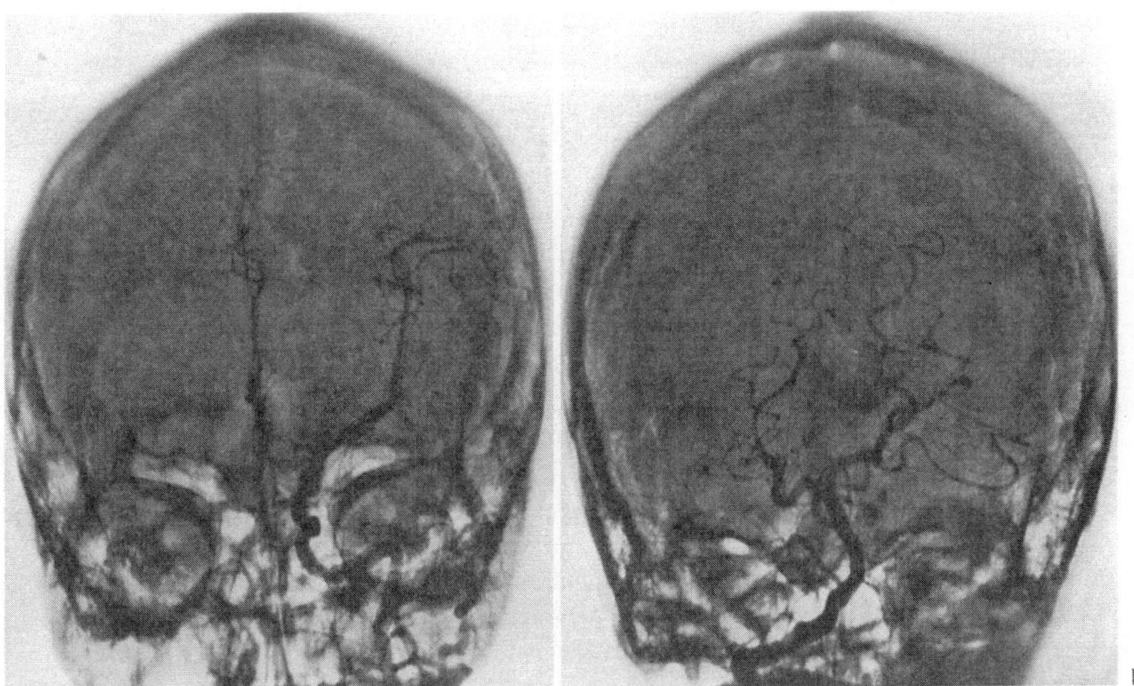

Fig. 1a and b. Aneurysma sacculatum a. carotidis int. sin. Hematoma intracerebrale lobi temporalis sin. Man, 51 years. Elevation and medial dislocation of middle cerebral artery; more moderate dislocation of anterior choroidal artery. Left posterior cerebral and superior cerebellar arteries are pressed medially, indicating a middle and posterior tentorial herniation (corresponds with depression in side-views). Filling of bilocular aneurysm via posterior communicating artery is seen in Fig. 1b. Operation: intracerebral hematoma extending through temporal lobe

occipital lobe will be squeezed in passing the tentorial edge; then the frontal view will show a short but distinct stenosis (HOYT, 1960).

It should be mentioned here that the dislocated posterior communicating or posterior cerebral artery – or the herniated brain substance – may press the oculomotor nerve against the petroclinoid ligament (JOHNSON and YATES, 1956a and b). The same authors offered an explanation of the multiple hermorrhages that are often seen at autopsy after severe tentorial herniations: when the mesencephalon is stretched and pushed downward, the many delicate arterial branches from the basilar artery may rupture inside the brain stem. Under the same circumstances the compressed brain stem may cause a narrowing or an occlusion of the aqueduct. It has been mentioned that the contralateral peduncle of the mesencephalon may be pressed against the tentorial edge causing ipsilateral motor disturbances.

Before we end the discussion of the tentorial herniations we must add that combinations of tentorial and other herniations can be found, e.g., tentorial and subfalcine (Fig. 25a and b) or tentorial and foramen magnum-herniations, but it also must be mentioned that a tentorial herniation may take the opposite direction:

The ascending tentorial herniation will be caused by expanding lesions in the posterior fossa, not only tumors or leptomeningeal cysts but also malformations such as that of Arnold-Chiari or Dandy-Walker (NEWTON and POTTS, 1974). The brain stem and the adjacent parts of the cerebellum will be pushed up through the tentorial notch followed by the stretched superior cerebellar arteries. The basilar artery will be pushed forward against the clivus and the posterior cerebral arteries will be stretched in their anterior portions and spread from each other. The vein of Galen is elevated and so is the posterior portion of the basal vein. As shown by HUANG et al. (1966) the precentral cerebellar vein is elevated, and under the same circumstances HARA et al. (1966) demonstrated an upward, forward dislocation of the thalamoperforating arteries.

III. Sphenoid-Ridge Herniation

CRONQVIST (1965) examined 45 patients with frontal expansive lesions and descending herniation over the sphenoid ridge. In 24 cases he found dorsal dislocation and compression of the carotid siphon; in 17 cases he found the lateral part of the middle cerebral artery displaced backward. In 10 cases the anterior portion of the middle cerebral artery was elevated, in 12 cases the same arterial portion was depressed. This difference is surprising, but can be explained: just behind the sphenoid ridge is found the anterior part of the Sylvian fossa; this is large in its antero-medial part, and here the first portion of the artery is less intimately connected to the surface of the brain, so the herniating part of the frontal lobe may find its way over (especially medially) or below the artery (especially the lateral herniations). The temporal horn with its lower position will always be depressed. WELCH and CRAIGMILE (1963) in similar cases found kinking of the supraclinoid part of the siphon over the optic nerve or the lateral edge of the chiasm; STØVRING (1968) found kinking over the dorsum sellae, over the anterior clinoid process, and over the clino-tentorial ligament. There is no doubt his statements are correct but some of his pictures have a certain resemblance to arteriosclerotic plaques, so one should take this differential diagnosis into consideration in less pronounced cases. Similar observations were made by HEISKANEN (1964). The evaluation of a dislocation of the anterior portion of the basal vein may be difficult because of the great variability at the beginning of this vein (WOLF and HUANG, 1966).

A corresponding herniation may be found near the midline if the gyrus rectus is herniated over the sphenoid limbus and the anterior part of the sellar diaphragm down into the pituitary fossa. TAVERAS and WOOD (1964) have seen two cases at autopsy, but revising the angiograms they did not find the posterior displacement of the anterior cerebral arteries nor the lateral dislocation of the siphons, which might have been expected.

An ascending herniation over the sphenoid ridge is known. It was mentioned by NEWTON and POTTS (1974). A temporal mass should press temporal-lobe substance over the ridge up into the anterior fossa between the sphenoid ridge and the middle cerebral artery. This artery, together with the anterior choroid artery, should be elevated (Fig. 24a).

IV. Other Herniations

Herniations through congenital, traumatic, or surgical defects in the skull may be found, the latter often being connected with recurrence of an operated tumor. Brain vessels may be found outside an occipital postoperative bony defect, but this does not necessarily indicate a new or recurring space-occupying lesion.

The very important herniations through the foramen magnum will be discussed in Encyclopedia of Medical Radiology, Vol. XIV/1B, p. 99ff.

B. The More Exact Localization of the Space-Occupying Lesions

While herniations may be regarded as the remote effects of an expanding lesion, giving rough information about the site of the process inside one or another of the dural compartments, there will be numerous local signs giving more exact indications of the location. However, the significance of the herniations should not be underestimated as they per se may indicate a disastrous development. TAVERAS and WOOD (1964) and KRAYENBÜHL and YAŞARGIL (1965) give very exact classifications of the regions inside and outside the encephalon – with a detailed account of the stretchings and displacements of arteries and veins, each of which indicating the location and the size of the space-occupying lesions. Each of the two pairs of authors have their own mode of classification, which in a survey might be cooperated, and both pairs of authors agree that it may be impossible to detect or localize every space-occupying lesion via the angiographic route.

In an attempt to avoid the sharp separation of the different regions, which all the same is difficult to maintain in practice, we want to start with a description of the dislocations caused by the *suprasellar expanding lesions*. They may be pituitary tumors penetrating the sellar diaphragm, craniopharyngiomas, meningiomas of the tuberculum sellae, epidermoid tumors, optic gliomas, and chordomas. Each of these processes can stay in the midline, they can tilt forward or backward or to a greater or lesser extent to one side, or their growth can be stronger on one side than on the other.

It has been discussed whether pneumoencephalography or angiography was to be preferred in this site of tumors; CHASE and TAVERAS (1961) stated that the most reliable diagnosis was obtained with encephalography, whereas angiography had the advantage that aneurysms could be excluded and a pathologic vasculation of a tumor could be seen. POWELL et al. (1974) used magnification combined with subtraction, and thereby obtained the same advantages as CHASE and TAVERAS, but additionally they were able to identify the meningo-pituitary branches from the internal carotid in all of their 41 pituitary adenomas and the capsular arteries in 36 of the 41 cases. In the frontal projection they preferred the central beam tilted 5° caudally instead of the usual 25°.

A tumor extending forward or straight upward will stretch the siphon and elevate the first (horizontal) portion of the anterior cerebral artery (Fig. 2) – as a rule on both sides – so that these two arteries ascend on their way toward the midline. This evaluation may be difficult because a slight ascent is normal in many individuals; but if this ascent is accompanied by a stretching in a caudally concave arc or semicircle the course is pathologic. A tumor extending laterally from the pituitary fossa will press the cavernous part of the carotid siphon laterally.

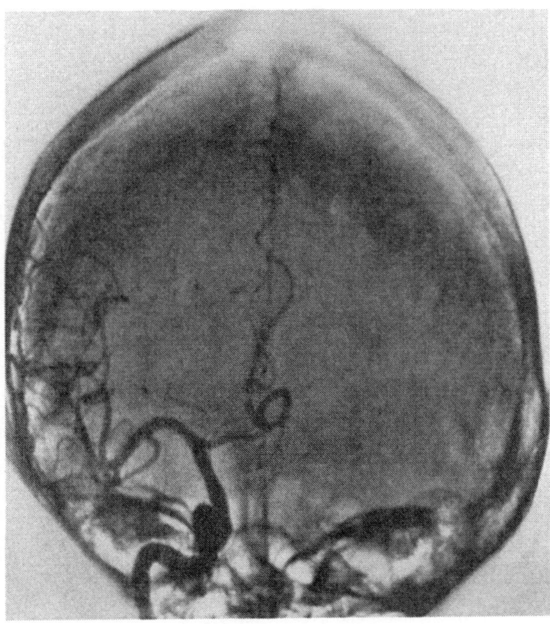

Fig. 2. Suprasellar chromophobe adenoma. Woman, 47 years. Bitemporal hemianopia. Right carotid: stretching of siphon, elevation of transverse portion of anterior cerebral artery (and of beginning of basilar vein). Operation: chiasm was dislocated upward and backward by a cystic tumor. Histology: chromophobe adenoma

The very large tumors impressing the floor of the third ventricle may reach the foramen of Monro elevating and squeezing the angulus venosus and elevating the internal cerebral vein, stretching the septal veins. The tumors directed backward may not change the siphon nor the anterior cerebral arteries (BULL, 1973), but they may elevate the internal cerebral vein and the vein of Galen, and growing into the interpeduncular cistern may squeeze the posterior communicating arteries from each other; in such cases the vertebral angiography will show a backward dislocation of the upper part of the basilar artery, a stretching and posterior displacement of the thalamoperforating arteries (KRAMER et al., 1973), an elevation of the medial posterior choroidal arteries and a backward dislocation of the anterior pontomesencephalic vein.

CHASE and TAVERAS (1963) and later TAVERAS and WOOD (1964) discussed the *parasellar tumors*, which may be intradural or extradural. The intradural tumors represent the same lesions as mentioned under the suprasellar processes growing laterally, whereas the extradural parasellar expanding lesions to some extent differ from the suprasellar masses. However, they found extradural parasellar meningiomas extending to the sphenoid sinus and to the nasopharynx, and some pituitary adenomas may make their way laterally, undermining the cavernous sinus. More commonly this location of expanding lesions is represented by carcinomas from the mucous membrane in the sphenoid sinus or from the nasopharynx. To this we may add some cases of juvenile angiofibromas extending from the nasopharynx, one of them destroying the surroundings of the foramen lacerum on its way up into the parasellar region (SIEMSSEN et al., 1967 – see also THIBAUT, 1963). The parasellar tumors may displace the pre- and/or cavernous portion of the carotid siphon, the direction of the dislocation depends to the greatest extent on the mass.

Anterior to the sellar region is the *subfrontal region*. The most important masses occurring in this region are the meningiomas arising from the planum sphenoidale, the medial portion of the lesser wing or from the olfactory groove. From the same location of tumors KRAYENBÜHL and YAŞARGIL (1965) counted the gliomas of the basal part of the frontal lobe. It will be clear that the anteriorly extending suprasellar space-occupying lesions will give the same dislocation of the vessels as the posteriorly situated midline tumors in the subfrontal region, namely: the ascending portion of the anterior cerebral arteries will be pushed upward, backward, and stretched in a downward anteriorly concave bow; if the mass is lateral to the midline the arteries will be forced to the opposite side. It should be noted that the concave arc may appear as a normal finding, in pathologic cases, however, the arteries will be stretched and followed by other signs of vascular dislocation: the upper part of the carotid siphon is pushed backward and downward, the septal vein is lifted and often stretched, the internal cerebral vein may be elevated and pushed backward with increased curvature. As most of the extracerebral masses in this region are meningiomas, there will be a difference in the picture of the extra- and intracerebral masses. An enlarged ophtalmic artery with visible branches to the tumor indicates a meningioma. Often subtraction will turn out to be necessary in this distinction.

The lesions of the optic chiasm region, cystic arachnoiditis, or gliomas, especially the spongioblastomas have nothing characteristic to show in angiography. The spongioblastomas often show osseous changes – the J-shaped sella, and possibly one or both foramina optica become enlarged. Likewise the tumors in the hypothalamic region – most commonly gliomas – will present themselves like posterior suprasellar expanding lesions. In some cases it is easier to distinguish these lesions from the real suprasellar space-occupying lesions orginating from the pituitary fossa by using encephalography (cf. Figs. 44a and b).

Ascending to the *fronto-polar region* it will be found that space-occupying lesions may be extracerebral – as hematomas or meningiomas – or intracerebral as the different kinds of gliomas: the ascending portion of the pericallosal artery will be dislocated backward and, if the mass is not located in the midline, to one side. Here it should be remembered that the anterior part of the falx is low and relatively soft, so in our opinion this midline shift does not necessarily mean a true herniation. The behavior of the frontopolar artery will be different: it may build

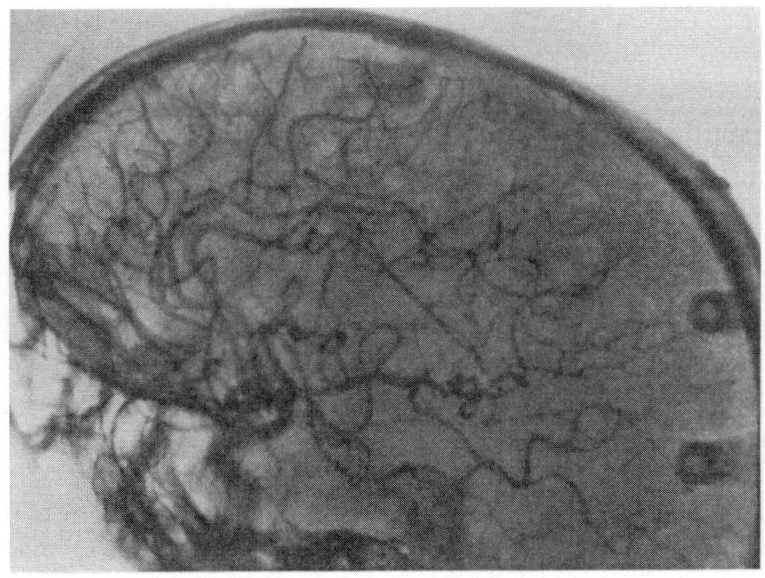

Fig. 3. Normal variant of anterior cerebral artery

a marginal vessel surrounding a noninfiltrating tumor. The great tumors in this region will influence the septal vein, that may be stretched, and the internal cerebral vein again may show an increased curvature; in extracerebral hematomas, as usual, the cerebral vessels will not reach the inner table of the skull.

Penetrating deeper into the *anterior portion of the frontal lobe* we will find similar changes; especially in the lower anterior portion of the frontal lobe a mass will influence the lenticulostriate arteries as established by ANDERSEN (1958, 1963), they may be stretched and/or dislocated medially or laterally, depending on the site of the mass (Fig. 32a and b).

Following the midline upward and backward to the sulcus centralis we will face the *parasagittal frontal masses* which again may be intracerebral or extracerebral; they may cause a depression and flattening of the supracallosal portion of the pericallosal artery, but here a warning is necessary because in normal cases one may find a sudden reduction in the lumen of this artery and an apparent depression of its posterior half (Fig. 3). The first time we saw this picture we misinterpreted it, and only a normal pneumoencephalography, a normal gamma-scan, and intense clinical observation saved our patient from a fruitless operation. In this region a shift from the midline, often with the afore-mentioned "step", indicates a subfalcine herniation. Other displacements may be found, e.g. depression of the septal vein and the internal cerebral vein.

The expanding lesions on the *supracallosal medial surface of the frontal lobe* may be extracerebral as the meningiomas of the falx or intracerebral as the wellknown gliomas of the gyrus cinguli. Meningiomas of the falx, beyond a depression of the branches of the anterior cerebral artery, may cause a dislocation to the same side as the site of the tumor; the glioma of the cingulate gyrus may separate the callosomarginal from the pericallosal artery. Furthermore, it may invade the corpus callosum and extend into the opposite hemisphere, forming what is called a butterfly glioma (cf. Fig. 7a and b). This possibility has to be taken in consideration if a great tumor near the midline (for instance evaluated by its pathologic vascular architecture) gives no shift of the midline vessels.

The space-occupying processes related to the *convexity of the frontal lobe* represent so many different kinds of extra- and intracerebral lesions that an enumeration would seem meaningless. It should just be mentioned that abscesses of the brain are often found in the region of the middle cerebral artery and its branches. From the upper portion of the convexity a mass will produce a depression of the upper margin of the Sylvian triangle, a spreading and stretching of the opercular arteries, a depression of the Sylvian group of arteries; in the lower-situated masses the same branches will be pushed medially, and if the mass continues backward into the parietal lobe, the Sylvian point may be displaced downward, medially, and forward. The deep veins are generally shifted across the midline. In the anteriorly situated masses in this group the lenticulostriate arteries are dislocated medially.

The lesions located in the *medullary substance in the same region* between the cortex and the lateral wall of the lateral ventricle will give a similar displacement of the vessels and further, and this is especially true for gliomas, one will see the medullary veins are larger and more distinct than in normal cases (HUANG and WOLF, 1964; HOOSHMAND et al., 1974). The same will be the case in space-occupying lesions in the *deeper portion of the parietal lobe.*

Continuing backward behind the Rolandic sulcus we come to the *convexity of the parietal lobe*. Here, as in the previously mentioned regions may be found intra- and extracerebral expanding lesions of different kinds. Among the extracerebral lesions the extracerebral hematomas and hygromas should be mentioned; here, as over the corresponding frontal convexity region, arachnoid cysts and meningiomas may also be found (Fig. 42a and b). One will find dislocation of the Sylvian point in an anterior direction (Fig. 11a); a medial dislocation will be met in the more superficially lying tumors; the peripheral, dorsal branches of the middle cerebral artery will be spread from each other and are often stretched, but one must note the great variability in the course of the pial arteries in this region. The total Sylvian group of arteries may be pressed forward (Fig. 4), and the single vessels of it will be twisted. In this region one will also find the posterior cerebral artery dislocated downward and medially. While the deep veins – the internal cerebral and the vein of Galen – are almost constantly dislocated to the opposite side we often find the anterior cerebral artery remaining in the midline, if not, we may find a slight dislocation posteriorly, ending in a steep step.

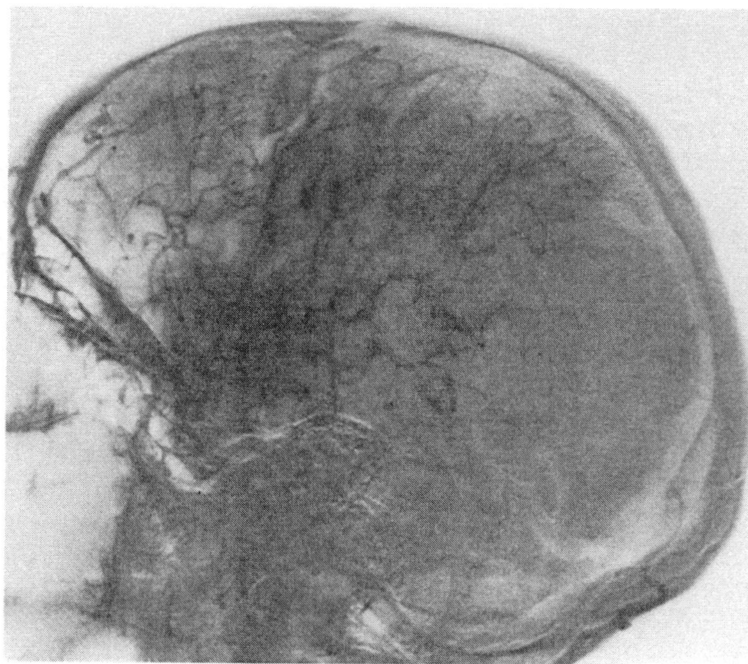

Fig. 4. Hematoma epidurale traumaticum. Man, 45 years. Frontal and oblique views were typical of a posteriorly situated epidural hematoma. This profile view in a late arterial phase shows forward dislocation of peripheral branches of middle and posterior cerebral arteries

The upper part of the parietal convexity is the *parietal parasaggittal region.* The same different kinds of space-occupying lesions are met. Three facts should be noted: (1) a certain distance between the inner table of the skull and the superior sagittal sinus, seen in the profile view, is not indicative of an epidural hematoma, because in some individuals this sinus has its normal place an inch or so down in the falx, but if in the frontal view one finds the sinus together with its veins from the convexities (the superior superficial veins) at a correponding distance from the inner table with an avascular zone in between, the diagnosis of an epidural hematoma is certain (Fig. 11b), (2) as mentioned earlier, there is a great variability in the peripheral distribution of the branches of the middle cerebral artery, so the decision whether there is or is not a little spreading and stretching of these vessels is very difficult, (3) furthermore, as also mentioned previously, the posterior portion of the pericallosal artery may seem to be depressed where it is lying over the posterior part of the corpus callosum.

The vascular dislocations characteristic for this region are: a depression of the pericallosal artery which usually remains in the midline; if, however, a larger tumor is located in the transitional region between frontal and parietal lobes, a depression of the corpus callosum and a herniation of the cingulate gyrus may be found with the angiographic displacements discussed under the subfalcine herniations. The Sylvian point will be depressed, and the same is the case with the internal cerebral vein which will also be flattened. A meningioma arising from the junction between the falx and the superior sagittal sinus may involve and more or less occlude the sinus; this diagnostic problem is solved in oblique frontal views giving a sufficient survey of the sinus in all its length.

Related to the *medial surface of the parietal lobe* extra- and intracerebral lesions may again be found. Among the first are the meningiomas of the falx (there is no sharp border-line between this region and the medial surface of the frontal lobe). We have observed a wedge-shaped meningioma squeezing in from above between the falx and the brain surface and an angiographically similar subdural hematoma which did not continue over the convexity (JACOBSEN, 1955). In both cases the peripheral branches of the anterior cerebral artery were displaced from the midline. These branches may surround a meningioma or a glioma, but in the gliomatous tumor they usually will not be dislocated from the midline. The pericallosal artery may be depressed, and as a token of a subfalcine herniation it may be displaced to the opposite side, with a sharp step back to the midline. Involving the gyrus cinguli intracerebral masses will separate the callosomarginal from the pericallosal artery. The deep veins may be depressed and dislocated to the opposite side in the case of a herniation.

Lesions in the *region of the occipital lobe* will behave different by depending on their location: lateral, inferior, medial, posterior. The infero-medial border of the occipital lobe with its close relation to the edge of the tentorial notch may be pushed upward and laterally by an ascending tentorial herniation with an elevation and lateral displacement of the posterior branches of the posterior cerebral artery. A tentorial meningioma will give different displacements: if it is located near the "carrefour falco-tentoriel," the displacement will correspond to that of the ascending tentorial herniation; spreading more over the cerebral surface of the tentorium it will elevate the posterior branches of the middle cerebral artery and the Sylvian point. It should be observed that a tentorial meningioma will cause an enlargement of the tentorial artery from the carotid siphon (Fig. 20a and b). It is difficult to establish more general trends, especially in the intracerebral masses in this region; here as in some of the upper parietal convexity masses a pneumoencephalogram may be helpful, if not necessary.

Masses in or immediately about the *Sylvian fissure* most often are meningiomas from the Pterion. They may intrude into the fissure separating its lips and pushing the branches of the middle cerebral artery in a medial direction. Like the few gliomas seen in this region, the meningiomas may split and stretch the branches of the middle cerebral artery so they are situated as vessels surrounding the tumor.

Caudal to the Sylvian fissure the *temporal lobe* extends from the facies cerebralis of the major wing of the sphenoid bone backward to the occipital lobe, into which it passes without any natural border-line. On account of its length it is necessary to distinguish between the anterior, middle, and posterior temporal region, even if there are not border-lines. Extra- and intracerebral lesions may be found. Among the extracerebral lesions, the sub- or epidural hematomas should be mentioned, which especially in the anterior portion of the region are difficult to distinguish from other space-occupying lesions; they will show an elevation of the transversal portion of the middle cerebral artery, an upward, medial dislocation and a straightening of its bow, and possibly a shift of the anterior part of the anterior cerebral artery; the anterior part of the Sylvian vessels will be elevated depending on the size and the extension backward of the process. The anterior choroidal artery may be stretched and pushed medially (Fig. 25a and b). But this picture, which provides nothing but the location of the lesion, may be changed completely by the aid of the angiotomography in the frontal plane; with this procedure Glickman et al. (1973) disclosed 17 subtemporal among 115 subdural hematomas, demonstrating an avascular zone below the temporal lobe; they found the anterior temporal branch of the middle cerebral artery less reliable.

A little farther posteriorly it may be impossible to distinguish the parasellar lesions from the temporal; it is known that for instance a chromophobe pituitary adenoma or a chordoma may extend so far laterally that they give the picture of a subtemporal expanding lesion. The farther backward we follow this region, the more the intracerebral processes (e.g., gliomas) will dominate the picture, which is to say that the horizontal portion and the bow of the middle cerebral artery may keep their normal position while the elevation of the Sylvian branches will grow more emphasized; here we also find an elevation and medial dislocation of the basal vein (Fig. 24a and b), possibly a medial dislocation of the anterior choroid artery and a shift of the deep veins. In the middle and posterior temporal region we may find a sign indicating an intracerebral versus an extracerebral subtemporal lesion, as for instance a meningioma. The latter will elevate the temporal lobe and its vessels *in toto*, whereas the intracerebral lesions will expand the temporal lobe and only elevate the main branches of the middle cerebral artery; hereby the arterial branches descending on the lateral surface will keep their site but they will be stretched in their descending course, draping over the temporal lobe. This sign was called "the draping sign" (Fig. 5) by Taveras and Wood (1964), who added that it should be used cautiously because it can be seen in extracerebral lesions in the medial part of the middle fossa, elevating electively the medial part of the temporal lobe; however, in that case one will also find a sharp elevation of the anterior choroidal artery. Before leaving this region it should be added that the angiogram may be influenced by upward herniations through the tentorial notch and from meningiomas of the tentorium, among these are the so-called saddle-tumors extruding from the tentorial edge and extending into the posterior as well as into the middle fossa; naturally such lesions will be able to dislocate the posterior cerebral artery medially and possibly upward. Finally, we should mention the rarely seen neurinomas of the trigeminal nerve or ganglion.

Having discussed the vascular displacements of the more superficially located space-occupying lesions, we will now examine the more profound processes.

The expanding lesions in the *thalamus* will give a different picture depending on which portion of the ganglion is affected. This is well understood regarding the fact that the upper part of the thalamus is on a higher level than the stria terminalis that covers the thalamostriate vein; this vein therefore may be depressed or elevated; and together with the movable part of the vein of Galen and the internal cerebral vein it will be pushed across the midline. In contrast to this the anterior cerebral artery will remain in the midline, but the great branches of the middle cerebral artery, and with them the Sylvian point, may be dislocated laterally. The anterior choroidal artery may be enlarged and may together with the posterior choroidal artery, especially

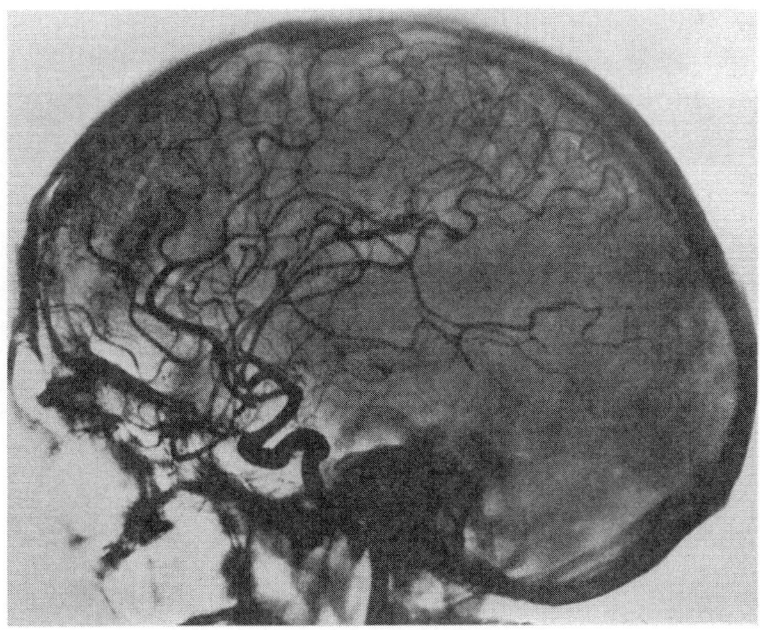

Fig. 5. The "draping sign" in a temporal spaceoccupying process

the lateral branch, describe a straightened and widened bow (GALLOWAY and GREITZ, 1960).

This angiographic picture will be altered if a thalamic tumor extends into the frontal lobe; in which case a depression and lateral dislocation of the lenticulostriate arteries will occur, or if it extends laterally into the temporal lobe or downward into the brain stem.

Most tumors in the *pineal region* are true pinealomas originating from the pineal body. Others may occur as tentorial meningiomas, gliomas, or metastases from the quadrigeminal plate. For the establishment of these tumors most authors consider ventriculography to be the most safe method (TOD et al., 1974). In spite of this, the pinealomas will show certain vascular signs: as pointed out by LÖFGREN (1958) and described more exactly by GALLOWAY and GREITZ (1960) the arc of the medial posterior choroidal artery will be expanded. Furthermore, an elevation of the vein of Galen together with a stretching of the internal cerebral vein may be seen. In the cases where a tumor in this region occludes the aditus ad aquaeductum we will meet the usual signs of a ventricular dilatation: expanding of the normal bow of the pericallosal arteries, a lateral displacement of the Sylvian vessels, a depression of the lenticulostriate arteries, and the sign, which was regarded by TAVERAS and WOOD (1964) as the most reliable: the lateral displacement of the thalamostriate veins, thereby causing a widening of the angle between these veins and the internal cerebral veins in the frontal view.

It has been discussed whether the true pinealomas should be regarded as intra- or extraventricular tumors; from our point of view this discussion is without great interest inasmuch as the tumor originates from the posterior wall of the third ventricle from which it often projects into the posterior part of the ventricle wiping out the contour of the suprapineal and pineal recesses. More frequently, perhaps, it will expand backward and downward over the quadrigeminal plate into or below the posterior part of the tentorial incisure.

The *intraventricular masses* are easier to detect by ventriculography than by angiography (Fig. 6a and b). If for some reason angiography is the first neuroradiologic examination, we run the risk that it may be completely negative, or just show the signs of hydrocephalus which often accompanies intraventricular tumors. Blush of the tumor may be seen.

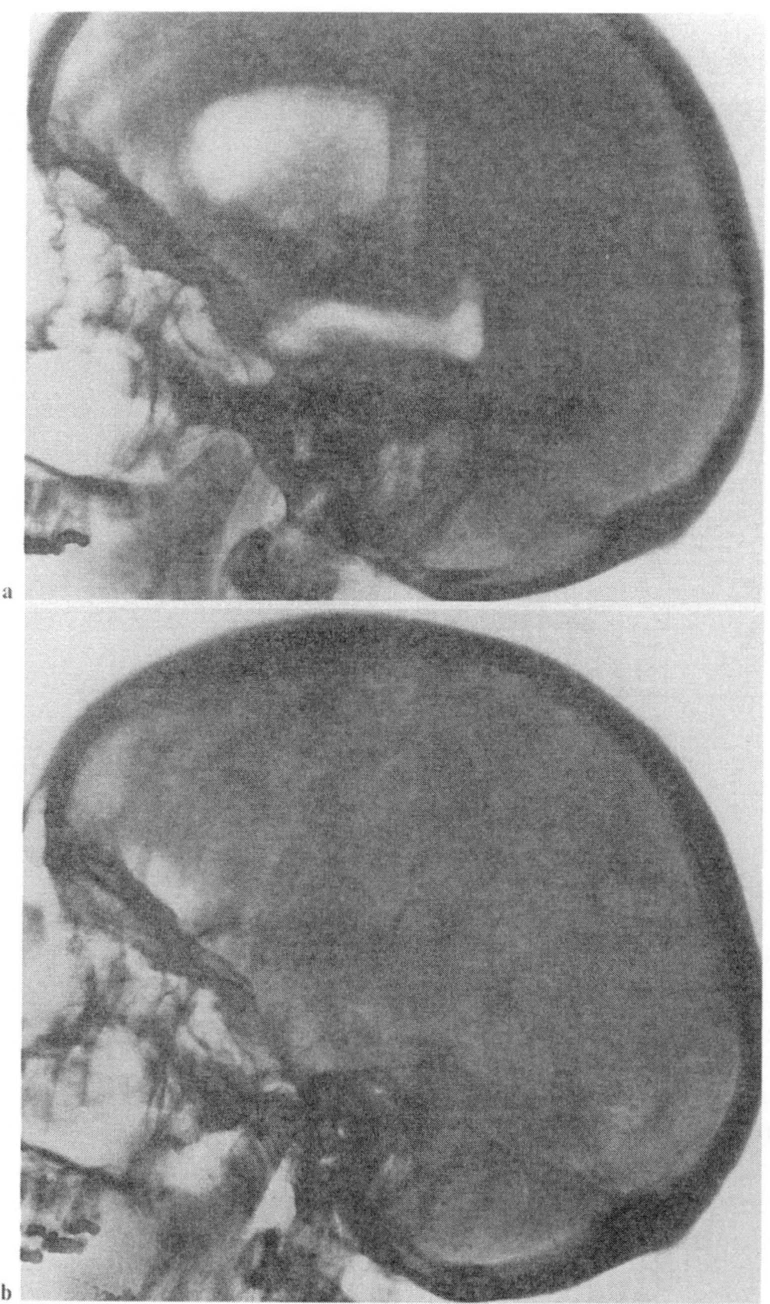

Fig. 6a and b. Astrocytoma in third ventricle. Woman, 45 years. Amenorrhea, increasing headache, uncharacteristic visual disturbances. Encephalography: mass growing up in third ventricle to the foramen of Monro. Right carotid: posterior dislocation of angulus venosus with stretching of septal vein. Operation: Tumor supposed to originate from optic chiasm. Histology: astrocytoma isomorphicum

Expanding lesion of the *corpus callosum* will most frequently be gliomas (OSBORN and POOLE, 1975). Just like the pinealomas and the intraventricular masses, they are easier to detect by pneumography – in this case encephalography sooner than ventriculography. But certain angiographic signs may be of interest. Depending on the location – anterior, intermediate, or posterior – a more or less local elevation of the pericallosal artery may be seen; in the venous phase one may see an enlarged distance between the inferior sagittal sinus and the depressed

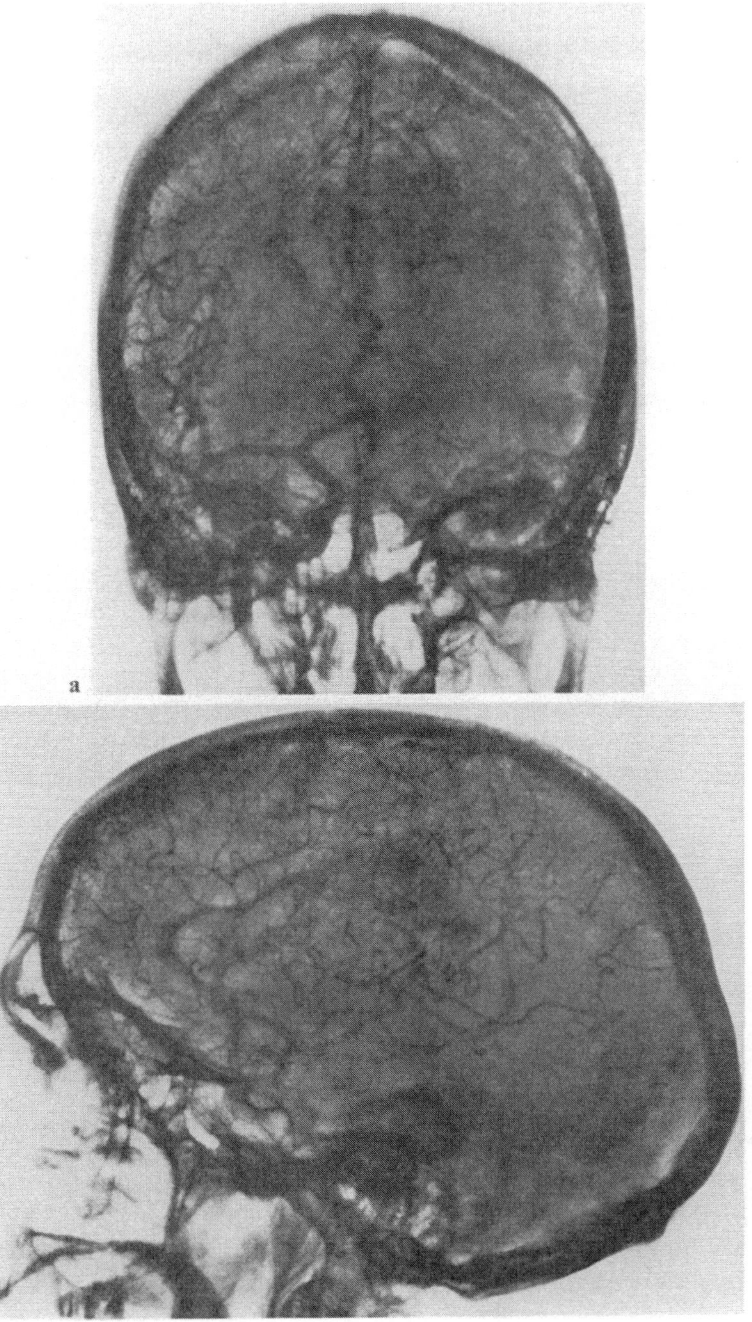

Fig. 7a and b. Glioblastoma corporis callosi. Man, 55 years. Short anamnesis. Symmetrical tumor vessels, some running in a certain order, others not. Calibration irregular. Elevation of posterior portion of pericallosal artery (depression of the internal cerebral vein). Diagnosis: malignant glioma extending from corpus callosum into both hemispheres. No operation, no autopsy

internal cerebral vein. Pathologic vessels may occur in cases of malignant gliomas, and it should be remembered that the corpus callosum, in addition to its natural function as a large collection of commissural tracts, may serve as a bridge for a glioblastoma which originating in one hemisphere, penetrating the corpus callosum, may infiltrate the other hemisphere forming a so-called butterfly glioma (Figs. 7a and b and 8).

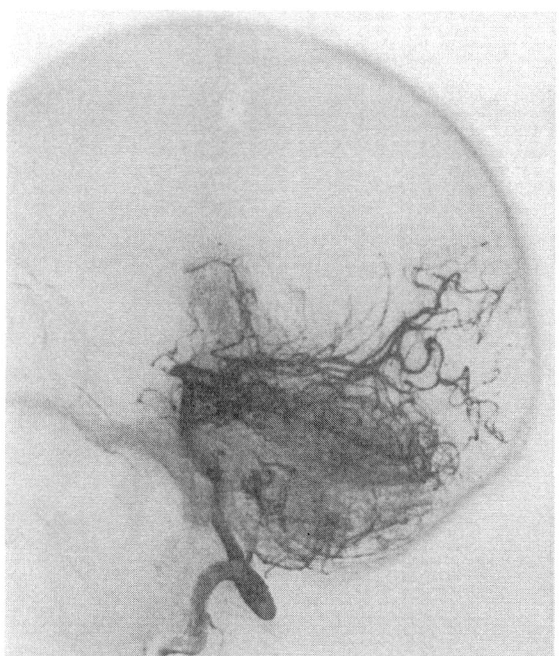

Fig. 8. Astrocytoma corporis callosi. Woman, 34 years. Distension and backward dislocation of posterior pericallosal arteries; medial posterior choroidal arteries are pushed forward. Operation disclosed, corresponding to this, a tumor in splenium of corpus callosum. Histology: astrocytoma polymorphicum

C. The Vascular Architecture of the Different Space-Occupying Processes

The space-occupying lesions to be discussed are the following:

1. hematomas and hygromas,
2. empyemas,
3. non-neoplastic cysts,
4. neoplastic tumors,
5. abscesses,
6. edema,
7. granulomas,
8. parasites.

As for example intracerebral hematomas and many neoplastic tumors will be conjoined by edema, and neoplastic tumors may start clinically with bleeding, it will be seen that there are no distinct border-lines between some of the different headings of this scheme. These different lesions with regard to their angiographic behavior: displacements, changes in the vascular architecture, and possible changes in the blood flow will be discussed in the following.

I. Hematomas

Most hematomas, intra- as well as extracerebral, are traumatic. Others may occur spontaneously as for instance those caused by diseases of the blood (Fig. 9), defects in the coagulating mechanism as anticoagulating therapy, hypovitaminosis, vascular diseases as malformations, or severe arteriosclerosis. In infants and children as well as adult patients we will find cases without any trauma in the anamnesis (Fig. 10); in some of them it may be true that no trauma has occurred, in others we may suppose a slight trauma as an eliciting factor where some of the diseases just mentioned are present.

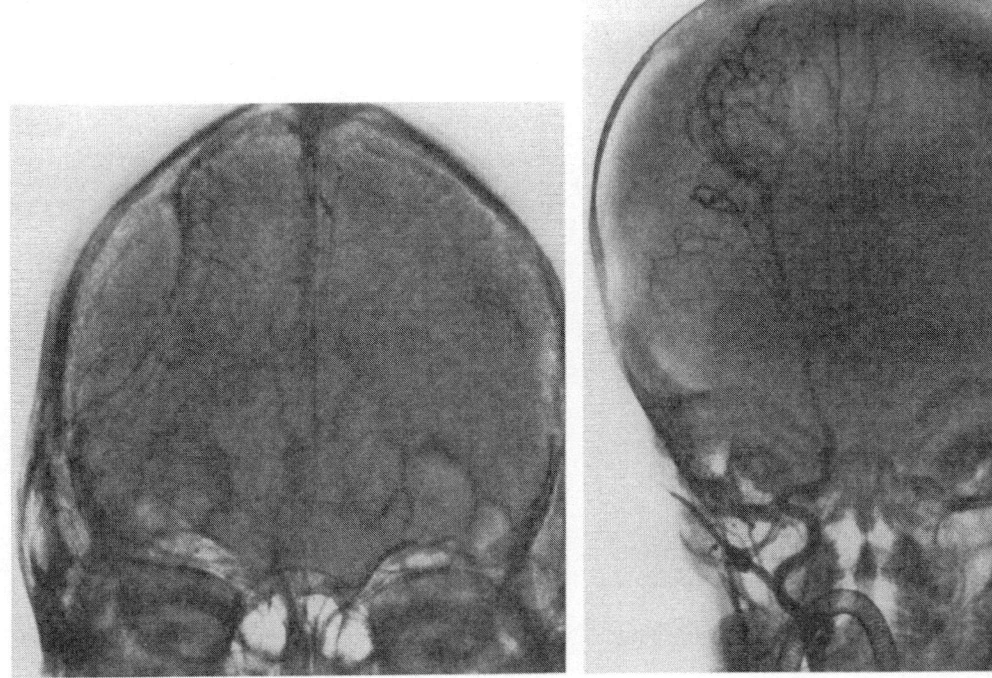

Fig. 9 Fig. 10

Fig. 9. Hematoma subdurale. Man. 69 years. 9 months previously a myeloid leukemia was diagnosed; he developed a hemorrhagic diathesis. During the last two weeks he had a slight but increasing hemiparesis. This frontal view shows a typical biconvex avascular zone. The midline shift was so moderate that we suspected a similar process on the opposite side, but after evacuation nothing further was done

Fig. 10. Hematoma subdurale chronicum non traumaticum, cystis arachnoidealis. Girl $8^1/_2$ years. Born with bilateral aniridia, buphtalmos dx. Increasing periphery of the skull. Right carotid: stretching of siphon, that continues in a vertical middle cerebral artery. Up to 3-cm broad avascular zone between theca and brain. No shift of midline vessels. Two operations disclosed a chronic subdural hematoma on both sides, a right-sided arachnoid cyst, partial aplasia of right frontal lobe, and total aplasia of right temporal lobe

Traumatic hematomas are discussed in Chapt. 1, p. 75ff. and part B (XIV 1/B), p. 1ff. As the angiographic picture is the same for traumatic and nontraumatic hematomas, we only want to emphasize a few facts here: if in a frontal view we find the superior sagittal sinus together with the superior superficial veins separated from the inside of the theca by an avascular zone, it is clear that an epidural hematoma is the diagnosis (Fig. 11a and b), but if in a side-view we find the same sinus placed 1–2 cm below the internal table of the theca it does not necessarily mean an epidural hematoma, for in some cases this sinus has found its natural location between the two strata of the falx at this lower level.

Most authors agree that if the middle meningeal artery is placed at a certain distance medial to the internal lamina of the temporal squama building a medially convex bow, it demonstrates the presence of a temporal epidural hematoma (CRONQUIST and KÖHLER, 1963) but as shown by MCGRATH and SONDERHEIMER (1973) this is not always true. The subtemporal epidural hematomas may be very difficult to distinguish from the dilaceration of the temporal lobe; for this purpose GLICKMAN et al. (1973) recommended and demonstrated the submento-vertical projection, which they performed without appreciable extension of the neck. It should be possible to make the same differential diagnosis with frontal multisectional angiotomography.

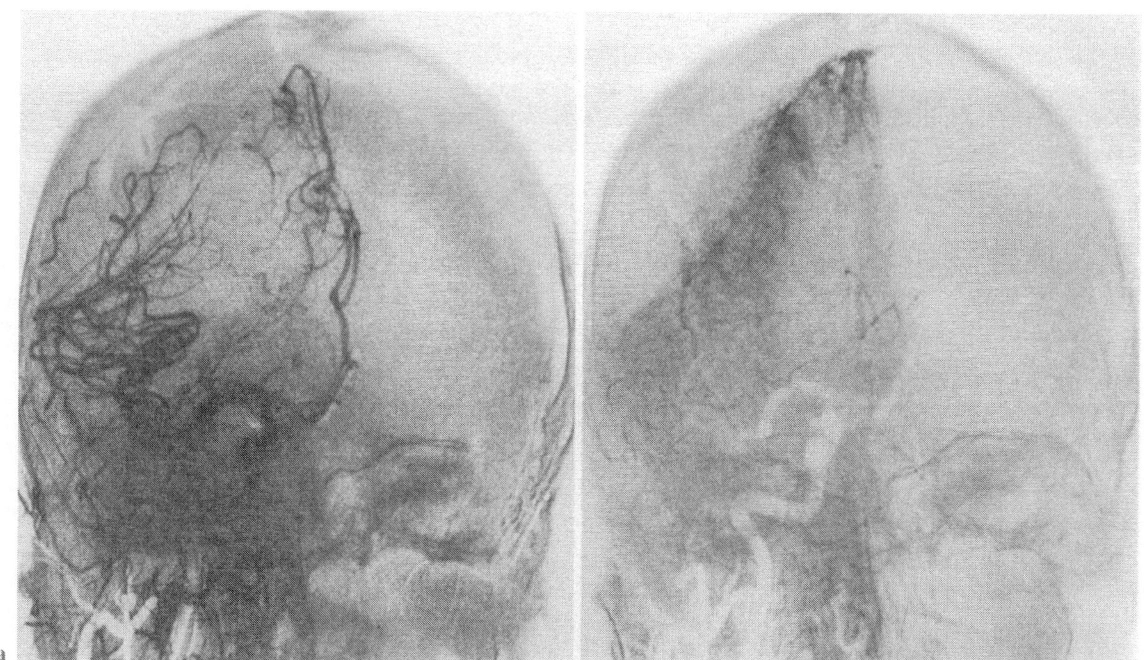

Fig. 11a and b. Hematoma epidurale traumaticum. Man, 53 years. Traffic accident. Surface of brain, superficial veins, and superior sagittal sinus are depressed by an avascular zone. Note compression of veins in surface of compressed right hemisphere. Sylvian point is dislocated anteriorly

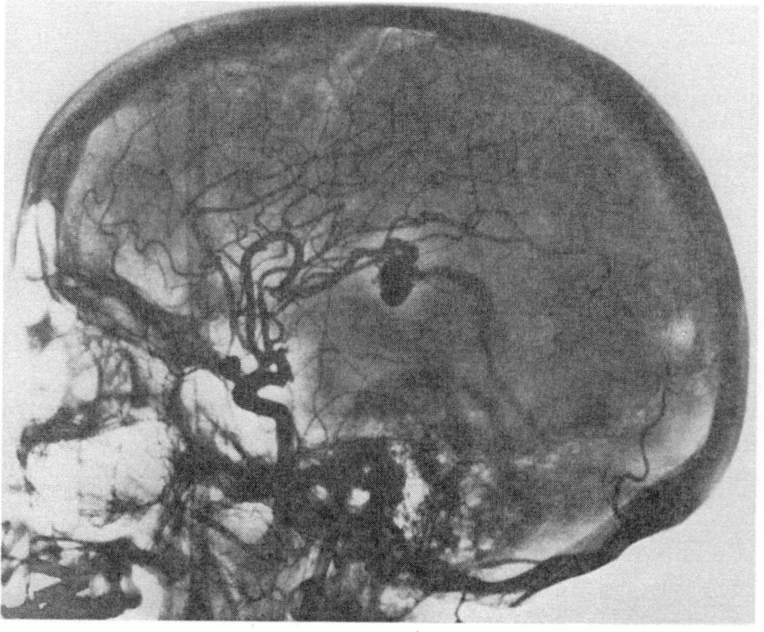

Fig. 12. Angioma arteriovenosum. Hematoma intracerebrale. Woman, 47 years. Enlarged branch of Sylvian group supplies a well-demarcated a–v angioma. Total Sylvian group is elevated by an intracerebral temporal hematoma. Furthermore, a saccular aneurysm was seen in trifurcation on middle cerebral artery in frontal and oblique views

With regard to intracerebral hematomas (Figs. 12–14) it should be mentioned that, whether they are traumatic or not, they will be accompanied by a considerable edema during the first days, so the vascular displacement will exaggerate the size of the hematoma itself; but the edema will decrease very early and soon the absorption of the hematoma will set in, so the

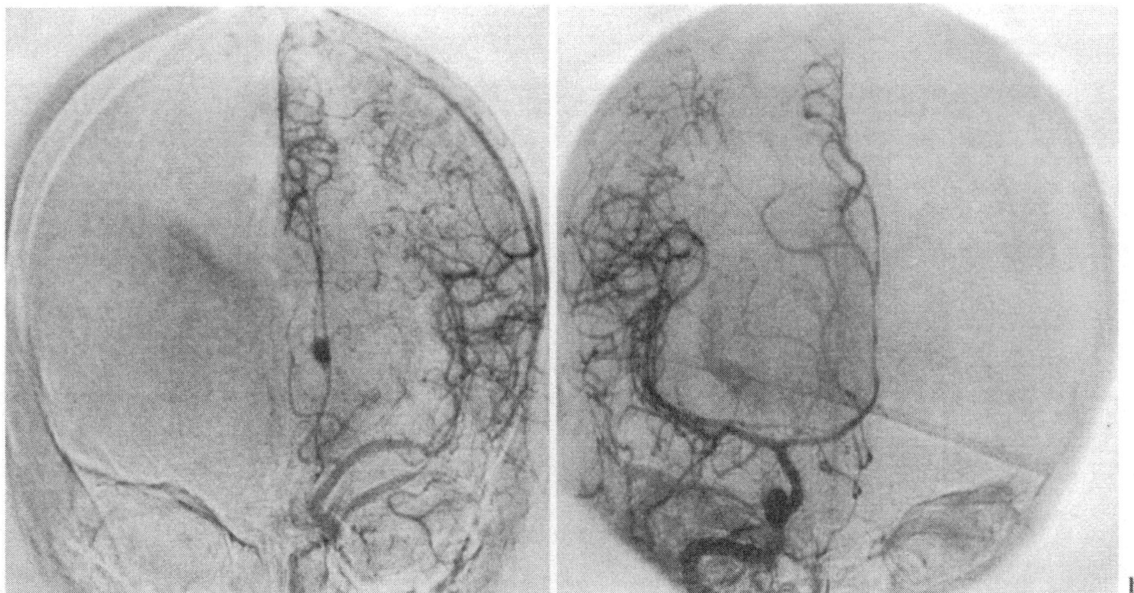

Fig. 13a and b. Aneurysma sacculatum a. pericallosae *sin.* hematoma intracerebrale lobi frontalis bilateralis inprimis *dx.* Woman, 50 years. Saccular aneurysm on left pericallosal artery. Dislocation to the left of both pericallosal arteries. Spastic arteries. Operation disclosed an intracerebral hematoma extending across midline

surgeon may allow himself to assume an expectative attitude. We have been able to follow this development in several cases with the CT-scanner, enabling us to avoid repeated angiographic examinations. It must be added that the CT-scanner depicts the difference between edema and hematoma very clearly.

The hygromas have been considered to be the final result of a subdural hematoma that has not been resorbed, and this is probably true for the greater part. In the angiogram it cannot be distinguished from a subdural hematoma. In some cases, however, the fluid content has been found to be identical with that of the cerebrospinal fluid, so TAVERAS and WOOD (1964), in agreement with NEWTON and POTTS (1974), presumed that a tear of the arachnoid membrane may cause the fluid to flow out into the subdural space. It must be admitted that this mechanism does not seem quite clear, but a kind of a meningeal cyst could occur in this way.

II. Empyemas

It might seem peculiar to make a distinction between the empyemas and brain abscesses, but from an angiographic point of view we have found it most practical. We are aware that an extracerebral accumulation of pus may be found simultaneously with an intracerebral accumulation, i.e., the true abscess. The etiologic factors are almost the same, although the penetrating injury plays a bigger role in the occurrence of the empyema. The reason why we wish to discuss the empyemas here is that the angiographic picture may be exactly the same as that of the subdural hematoma. We have seen collections of pus in layers several centimeters deep, but more often they must be measured in millimeters, (and in such cases we will meet the same differential diagnostic difficulties as in the thin subdural hematomas – without taking the clinical information into account – that a thin avascular extracerebral zone may show an extracerebral accumulation as well as a cortical atrophy). In some cases two factors may separate the picture of an empyema from that of a subdural hematoma: (1) the edema of the brain caused by the infection may cause a greater shift of the midline in empyemas than in subdural hematomas,

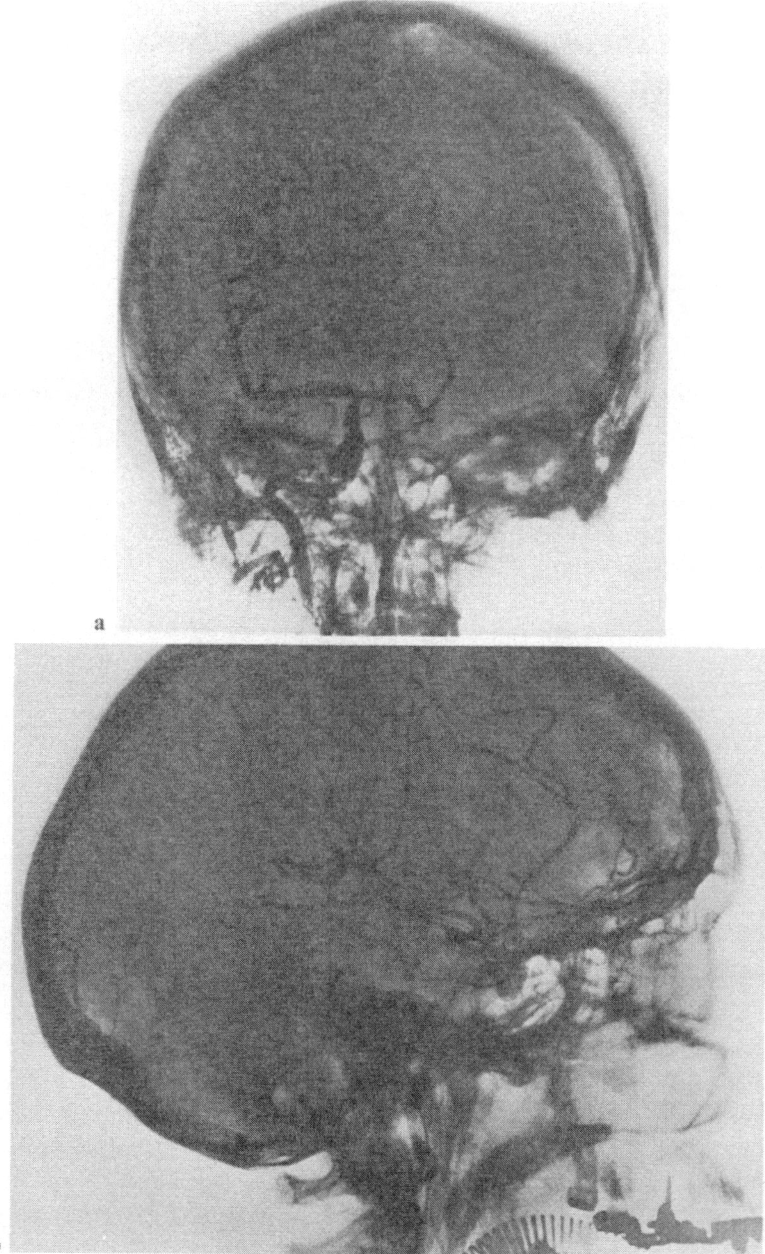

Fig. 14a and b. Intracerebral frontal hematoma. Woman, 57 years. The shift of anterior cerebral artery is largest anteriorly; posteriorly it returns to midline without a step. Branches of Sylvian arteries pressed backward. Operation: intracerebral hematoma in right frontal lobe (125 ml)

(2) the vessels of the surface of the brain may change their caliber in empyemas as shown by GREITZ (1964) in three cases of tuberculous meningitis. LEEDS et al. (1971) had three patients with meningitis purulenta and narrow arteries. SEGALL et al. (1973) stated: "acute meningitis in children may be associated with vasoconstriction of blood vessels at the base of the brain and also at the periphery. Areas of vasodilatation may coexist."

Furthermore, there may be some difference in the appearance of the avascular zone in extracerebral hematomas and empyemas as shown by FERRIS et al. (1964): they found the inner limitation more irregular in empyemas than in hematomas and a vascular pooling in the wall of the empyema collection.

Just as the subdural hematomas in rare cases (Jacobsen, 1955) may occur between the falx and the medial surface of one hemisphere, a case of an interhemispheric empyema has been described by Vesin and Bohutora (1972). Epidural empyemas are known, Handel et al. (1974) published a report on four cases. Angiographically they found an avascular biconvex zone, and they emphasized that the downward displacement of the superior sagittal sinus caused by the avascular mass, has the same significance as in the epidural hematomas, namely that the accumulation is extradural.

III. Non-neoplastic Cysts

As the aim of this chapter is to discuss the space-occupying lesions, porencephalic cysts will not be dealt with here. The colloidal cysts of the third ventricle are regarded by most authors as tumors (Zülch, 1975). The cysts of the septum pellucidum, the Verga cysts, and the more important subarachnoidal or arachnoidal cysts remain to be discussed. The two cysts or cavities first mentioned should be regarded as anatomic variations, although it must be admitted that the cavum (or cystis) septi pellucidi often occurs together with other malformations, such as agenesis of the corpus callosum. This cyst is located between the two normal membranes constituting the septum pellucidum. The cavum of Verga is situated more posteriorly and is only seen if the fornix after having contacted the inferior surface of the corpus callosum looses this contact anteriorly to the splenium. Both of them may or may not communicate with the ventricles or with the subarachnoid space; the septal cyst is pushed in between the medial walls of the anterior portion of the pars centralis of the lateral ventricles; it is visualized in pneumoencephalography and to our knowledge neither the septal cyst nor the cavum Vergae play any role in the angiographic picture.

Subarachnoid cysts may be seen over the convexities, in the chiasmatic region, in the posterior fossa, in the paracollicular region, and rarely between the hemispheres (Newton and Potts, 1974). Very often the pneumographic picture in children will show an accumulation of air in the velum interpositum. This has been described as a cyst but in our opinion this is not correct.

Starkman et al. (1958) objected to the term subarachnoid cysts because in the many cases in which these cysts communicate with the subarachnoid space, they are not true cysts; and if they do not communicate they are not subarachnoid but arachnoid cysts because their internal membrane is a sheet of arachnoidea. Their etiology is obscure, some are supposed to be a kind of congenital malformation, often combined with other malformations, such as an agenesis of the temporal operculum, and they may be found in infants (Fig. 10); Dee et al. (1974) found an arachnoid cyst in a neonate; in other cases they are assumed to have a traumatic or inflammatory origin; the theories of Taveras and Wood (1964) and Newton and Potts (1974) about some types of hygromas, quoted on p. 435, should be mentioned here. They may be found incidentally in necropsies from "normal" old people, but in children they may act as real expanding lesions causing increased intracranial pressure or, especially when located in the posterior fossa or in the tentorial incisure, hydrocephalus.

In some cases, again especially in children, the skull picture may be characteristic with elevation of the lesser wing of the sphenoid bone, anterior dislocation of the major wing, and thinning and bulging of the squama of the temporal bone. When communicating with the subarachnoid space they quite naturally are shown better by pneumoencephalography than by arteriography (Baumgarten and Kemperdick, 1973), but the cysts over the convexity may also be established by angiography: an avascular zone inside the theca, a straightening of the carotid siphon, an elevation of the horizontal portion of the middle cerebral artery and possibly a medial dislocation of the basal vein; there is usually little or no shift of the anterior cerebral artery (Robinson, 1964).

The cysts in the pituitary-chiasmatic region may seemingly have their origin *in loco*, while others ascend from the pituitary fossa; cystic expansions of Rathke's pouch are found among the latter; the craniopharyngiomas may be mentioned here, but they must be regarded as true tumors. The cysts in this region may ascend to the level of the foramen of Monro (PATRIQUIN, 1973), and cause hypothalamic disturbances. Such large cysts will push the basilar artery and the thalamoperforating arteries backward and elevate the internal cerebral vein.

IV. Neoplastic Tumors

A multitude of different tumors may be found inside the skull but it would be meaningless to systematically deal with all of them; therefore we have chosen to discuss the tumors giving a more or less characteristic angiographic picture, emphasizing the differential diagnostic problems. ZÜLCH (1975) gave an excellent survey of the anatomy and pathophysiology of the different intracranial tumors, their preferred location, age, and sex.

The tumors will act angiographically by their space-occupying function, their vascular architecture, their influence on the local or more general changes of the blood flow, and finally by their remote effects, such as herniation or blocking of the flow of the cerebrospinal fluid. The space-occupying influence is independent of the grade of malignancy, and the grade of malignancy says little about the prognosis in so far as a histologically benign tumor placed at a surgically disadvantageous site may be deleterious in a short time. A large and highly malignant glioblastoma may demand very little space on account of its infiltrating growth, whereas a large benign meningioma is space-occupying with massive vascular dislocation. With regard to the vascular architecture it can generally be said that that of malignant gliomas will amost always differ from that of meningiomas. The blood flow again will be different in gliomas, meningiomas, and metastatic tumors. The remote effect of herniations and the influence on the herniated blood vessels or on the pathways of the cerebrospinal fluid has been discussed; to this we should add that an effect on the cerebrospinal flow may be caused not only by the "Massenverschiebung" but also by the compression of the foramina of Monro or the aditus ad aquaeductum by tumors in the intimate neighborhood of these channels.

Meningiomas. In the many cases studied by ZÜLCH (1975), these tumors were the most common among the intracranial neoplastic lesions: 16%. They are benign, slow growing, capsulated, often highly vasculated tumors; with the exception of the relatively rare intraventricular meningiomas they are extracerebral tumors, which do not invade the cerebral parenchyma. They have their origin in the meninges.

WICKBOM in NEWTON and POTTS (1974) and others believe that meningiomas originate in the dura; other authors maintain they come from the arachnoid membrane (ROSENCRANTZ and STATTIN, 1972); in both cases it is difficult to explain how they can appear intraventricularly. TAVERAS and WOOD are of the opinion that they originate from arachnoid cells, included in the dura; the same opinion was held by TRAUB (1961). They may affect the underlying bone in different ways; most frequently forming a hyperostosis on the inside of the skull (and this in its turn may reaffect the tumor forming an umbo in its base (ZÜLCH, 1975); in other cases it may invade the bone forming an irregular compound of osteolytic and osteoplastic spots; growing through the theca the meningioma may appear as a prominence outside, sometimes with spicula. In ZÜLCH's opinion (1975) the invasion of the bone may be taken as a sign of malignancy; this does not correspond with our experience nor with that of TRAUB (loc. cit.) who is aware that a sarcomatous meningioma is apt to destroy the bone, but who holds the opinion that an impression or infiltration of the bone does not necessarily mean a malignant meningioma.

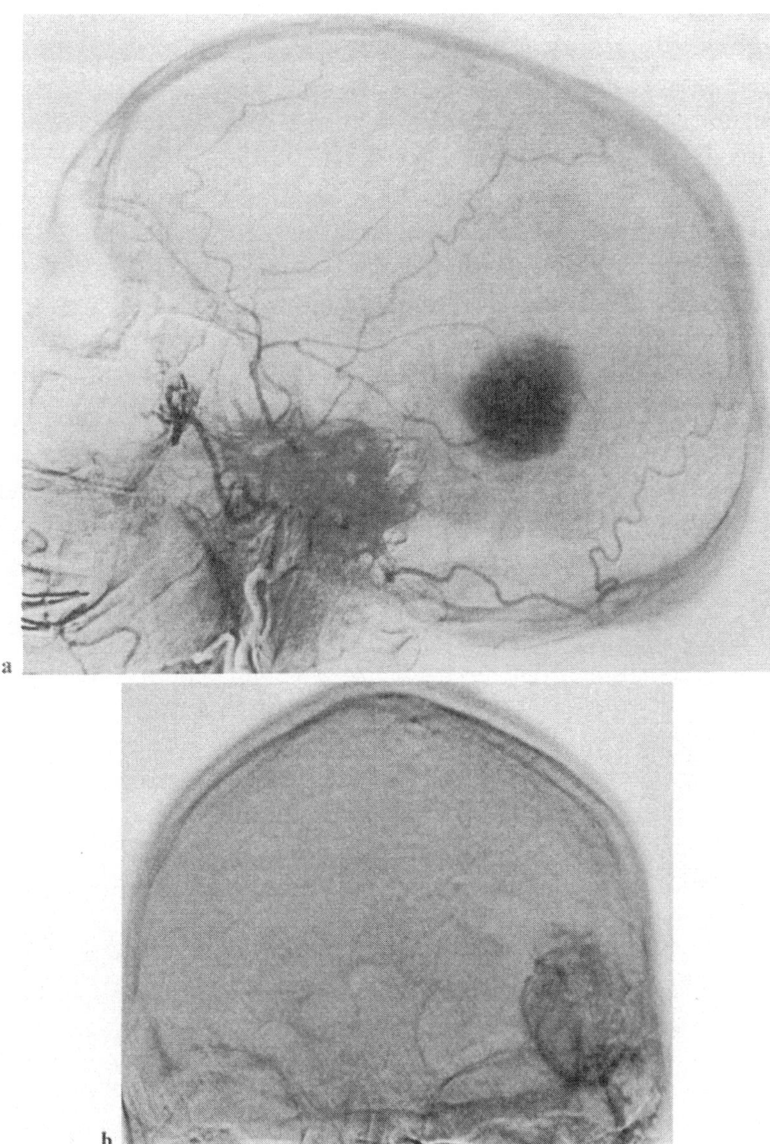

Fig. 15a and b. Meningioma. Woman, 56 years. General epileptic seizure one month earlier. Left external carotid: sharply delineated, round 3-cm large tumor, mainly supplied from meningeal arteries (pictures taken during injection in common carotid are not shown). Operation: tumor was easily enucleated. Histology: meningeoma oligomitoticum

The size of the tumor varies from a pin head to a man's fist; they are usually solitary, but more than one hundred have been counted in one patient (ZÜLCH, 1975). Several small tumors are often found incidentally at necropsy. Two or three meningiomas may be found together with neurinomas in patients with Recklinghausen's neurofibromatosis. A meningioma coincident with a malignant glioma has been observed. SACKETT and his coworkers (1974) collected 52 cases to which they added two cases of their own. The meningiomas may occur in the facial bones: KENDALL (1973) had 5 cases with operated meningiomas; 4–18 years after the operation he found osseous changes in the zygoma and the maxilla, which were found to be nonmalignant meningiomas. This picture may be very like the changes caused by fibrous dysplasia. JACOBSEN and VRAA-JENSEN (1949) showed a picture of this bone disease spreading from the orbital roof out into the zygoma. They found a central radiolucency which they felt would not be found in the osseous changes of a meningioma. ROSENCRANTZ and STATTIN (1972) found meningiomas penetrating the normal foramina and fissures like dumb-bell tumors – some of them invading orbita. In our own department, we recently demonstrated an orbital tumor by CT-scanning; there was no tumor to be found in the cranial cavity; the histologic diagnosis was meningioma. Moreover, we have examined a man who had been operated upon 9 and 10 years previously for a meningioma in his left middle fossa. When he came to us he had a stenosis of his left external acoustic meatus. A tomographic examination disclosed a pillowy mass protruding from the roof which showed a slight bony destruction. Microscopy showed meningioma with no signs of malignancy.

Most meningiomas receive their arterial supply from branches of the external carotid artery, especially from the middle meningeal artery (Fig. 15a and b). An enlargement of this artery may manifest itself in an enlargement of the foramen spinosum (LINDBLOM, 1936). Among meningeal vessels derived from the internal carotid should be mentioned the ethmoid branches from the opthalmic artery, small meningeal arteries from the top of the carotid siphon and the tentorial artery, originating from the subarachnoid portion of the carotid siphon and taking its course backward near the free edge of the tentorium (Figs. 16a and b, 20a) (BERNASCONI and CASSINARI, 1956). However, large meningiomas invading the pia, but not the brain, may receive pial arteries in their periphery.

The usual picture of a meningioma is that of a well-defined space-occupying lesion, surrounded by the arciform arteries separated from each other by the tumor. In rare cases the tumor appears to be only slightly vasculated (Figs. 17a and b, 20a and b), in most cases it is hypervasculated, partly with pathologic vessels spreading funnel-shaped from the base of the tumor or appearing in more irregular windings (Fig. 16a and b) and partly with a homogeneous stain, appearing in the late arterial phase but persisting for many seconds into the middle or late venous phase (Figs. 18a and b, 19a and b). The stain in the glioblastomas, when it occurs, appears earlier than in the meningiomas; and although the pathologic vessels of the meningiomas may appear irregular and twisted, they never show the irregularity of their lumen so characteristic of the malignant gliomas in which the irregularity in course and caliber caused WICKBOM (1953) to speak of "a bizzare pattern" (cf. Figs. 16a and b with 36). Furthermore, arterio-venous fistulas are rare in meningiomas but characteristic in glioblastomas; however, as shown by STATTIN (1966) and KIEFFER et al. (1973) such anastomoses may occur (Fig. 19a). STATTIN (1966) recommended subtraction for their visualization.

Meningiomas may be found in children (MERTEN et al., 1974), but they occur mainly between 45 and 60 years of age (ZÜLCH, 1975).

The most common location is in the parasagittal region, i.e., along the superior sagittal sinus, in the angle between the falx, the sinus, and the dura of the convexity, i.e., in the region where we find the greatest number of granulationes arachnoideales (Figs. 16a and b, 19a and b). Here they may assume the size of a tangerine; greater anteriorly and posteriorly, somewhat smaller in the middle third, because in this region, near to the motor cortex they will elicit symptoms even when only small in size. In this location they may invade and possibly occlude the superior sagittal sinus; this is especially the case in bilateral tumors. The origin of the tumor may be placed farther inferiorly in the falx, these meningiomas may also be bilateral. Other meningiomas are placed far from the falx over the convexity of the brain. They may be flat in the form of the so-called meningiomas "en plaque". If such a tumor is supplied exclusively from the external carotid branches it may appear very similar to an extracerebral hematoma if angiography is performed by injection in the internal carotid. The angioblastic meningiomas are often located over the convexity (Fig. 16a and b); they show a very rapid flow; for this reason they have been regarded as malignant tumors, but this is not necessarily the case (KIEFFER et al., 1973), surgically they may be difficult to handle (TELENIUS, 1966). The meningiomas of the olfactory groove, or of the cribriform plate of the ethmoid bone elsewhere

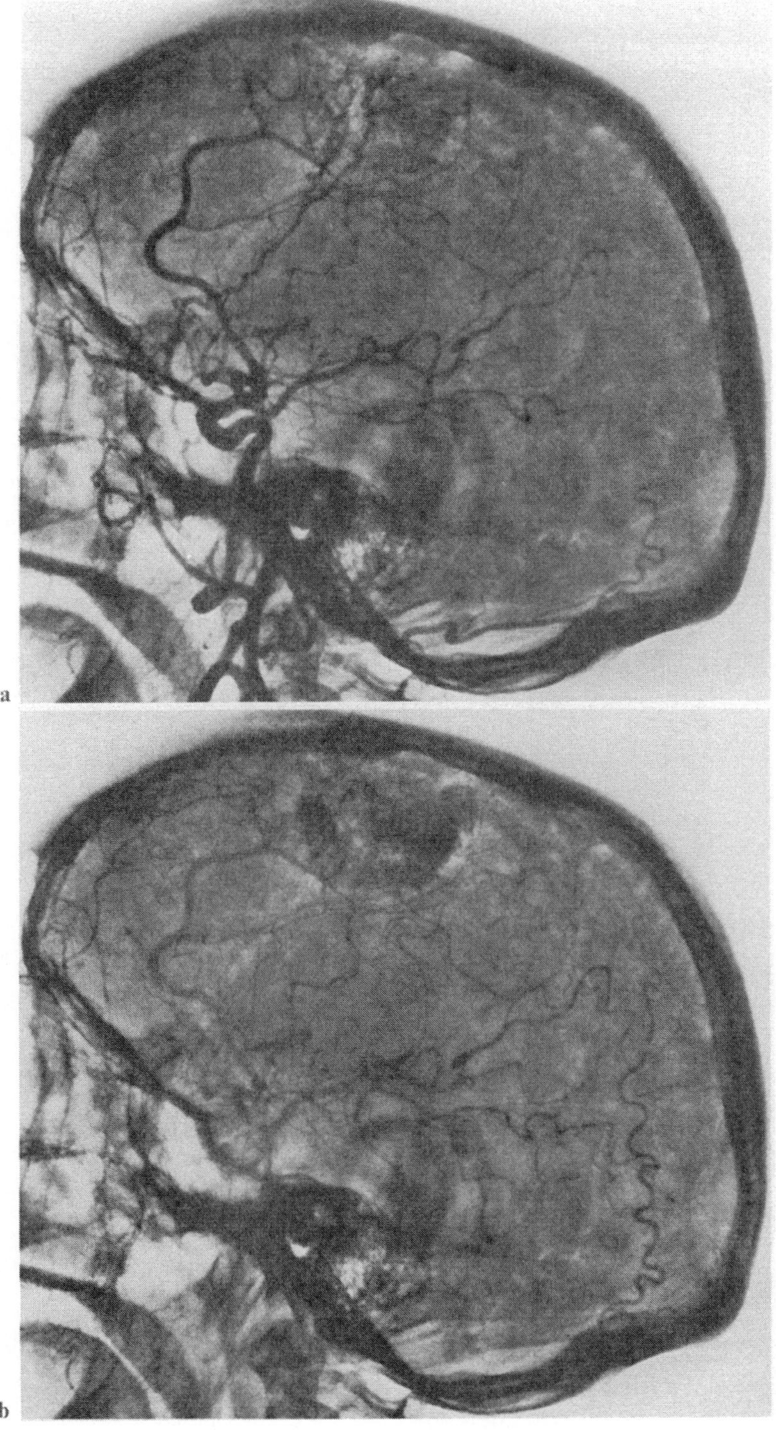

Fig. 16a and b. Meningioma. Woman, 59 years. Slight symptoms for many years. Left common carotid: a wide anterior cerebral and a wide and tortuous anterior branch of middle meningeal artery supply a $4^1/_2$-cm large, sharply delineated parasagittal tumor, in the late arterial phase. Fig. 16b shows almost homogeneous stain without shunt. Operation and histology: meningeoma oligomitoticum

may grow very large; it is difficult to distinguish them from the tumors of the sphenoid planum. Both types may show hyperostotic bone changes but in some respects they differ from the sphenoid-ridge meningiomas. To detect a stain in these highly vasculated regions subtraction may be valuable (GREGORIUS and BENTSON, 1975). Continuing posteriorly we meet the presellar

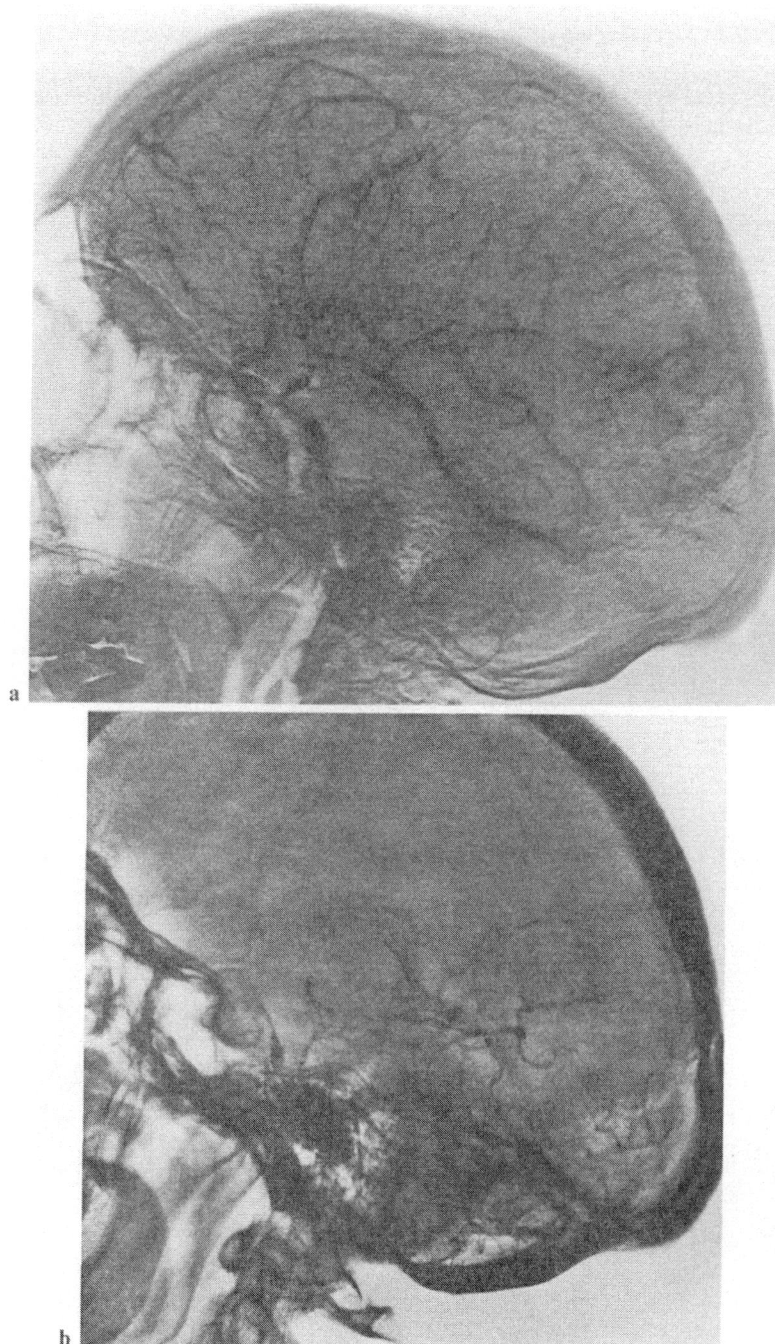

Fig. 17a and b. Meningioma falcis cerebri. Man, 43 years. Vague symptoms for 16 years. Right-sided hemianopia and loss of memory for 6 months. Left carotid and vertebral angiography: $4 \times 4 \times 4$ cm big tumor close to midline. Scanty, irregular tumor vessels without diffuse stain. Cranially a curved marginal vein. Operation and histology: meningeoma falcis (typus transitionalis)

meningiomas. In my own department we missed five of them before we had the possibility of using the subtraction technique and tomography in combination with pneumoencephalography. The surgeons operated upon the patients because the visual disturbances indicated a tumor in this region. The meningiomas here may compress the pituitary gland and invade the sphenoid sinus. From this location the tumor may also follow the sheath of the optic nerve and extend

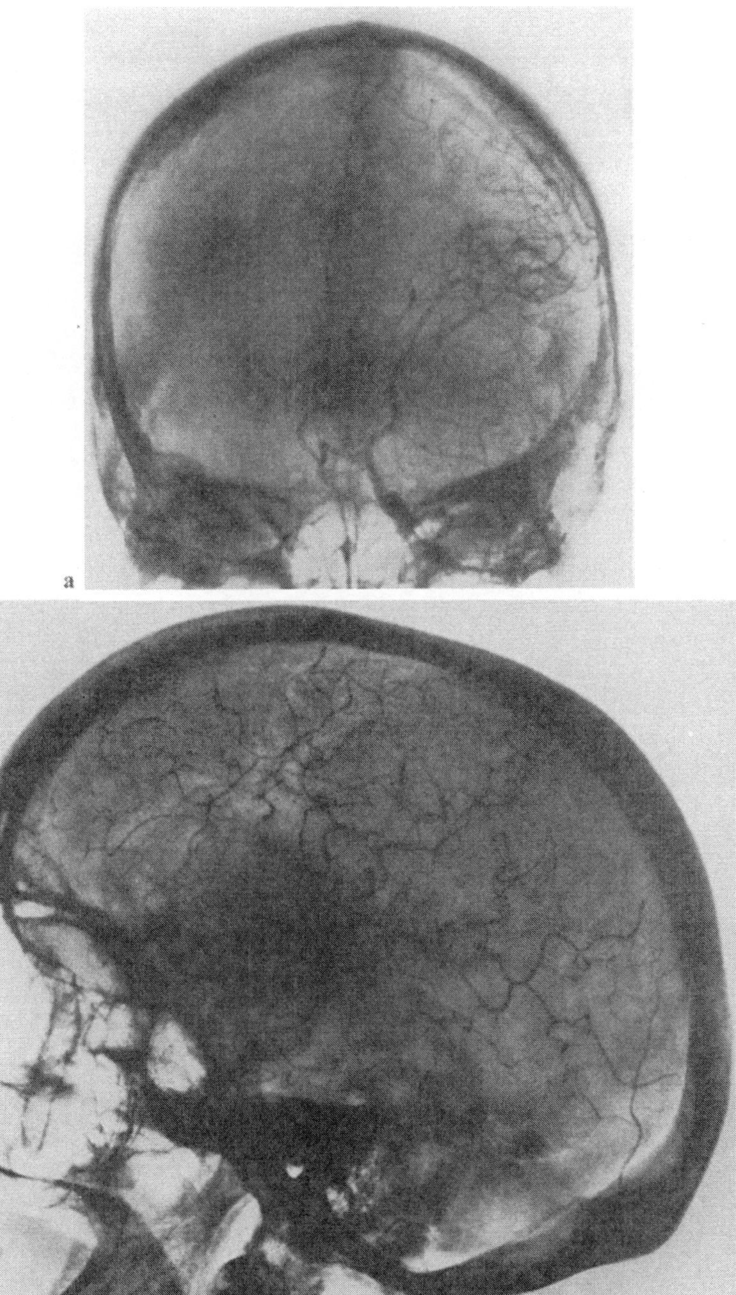

Fig. 18a and b. Meningioma (sphenoid ridge). Woman, 58 years. Left common carotid: 6 × 6 × 6 cm big tumor with diffuse stain, mainly sharply delineated (Fig. 18a shows an earlier arterial phase than Fig. 18b). Basis on left sphenoid ridge. (Top of siphon tilted backward: descending sphenoid ridge herniation not shown.) Operation: meningioma with its base on lateral sphenoid ridge; vascular supply from meningeal vessels and from middle cerebral artery. Histology: meningeoma oligomitoticum

into the orbit. From the sphenoid ridge, medial and lateral meningiomas may take different directions; extending posteriorly they can even reach the posterior fossa. En route they can squeeze vessels and nerves. The smaller tumors of this region may appear as tumors en plaque. From the roof of the cavum of Meckel meningiomas may spread out into the middle fossa. The tentorial meningiomas may be found on the upper or lower surface or both (Fig. 20a

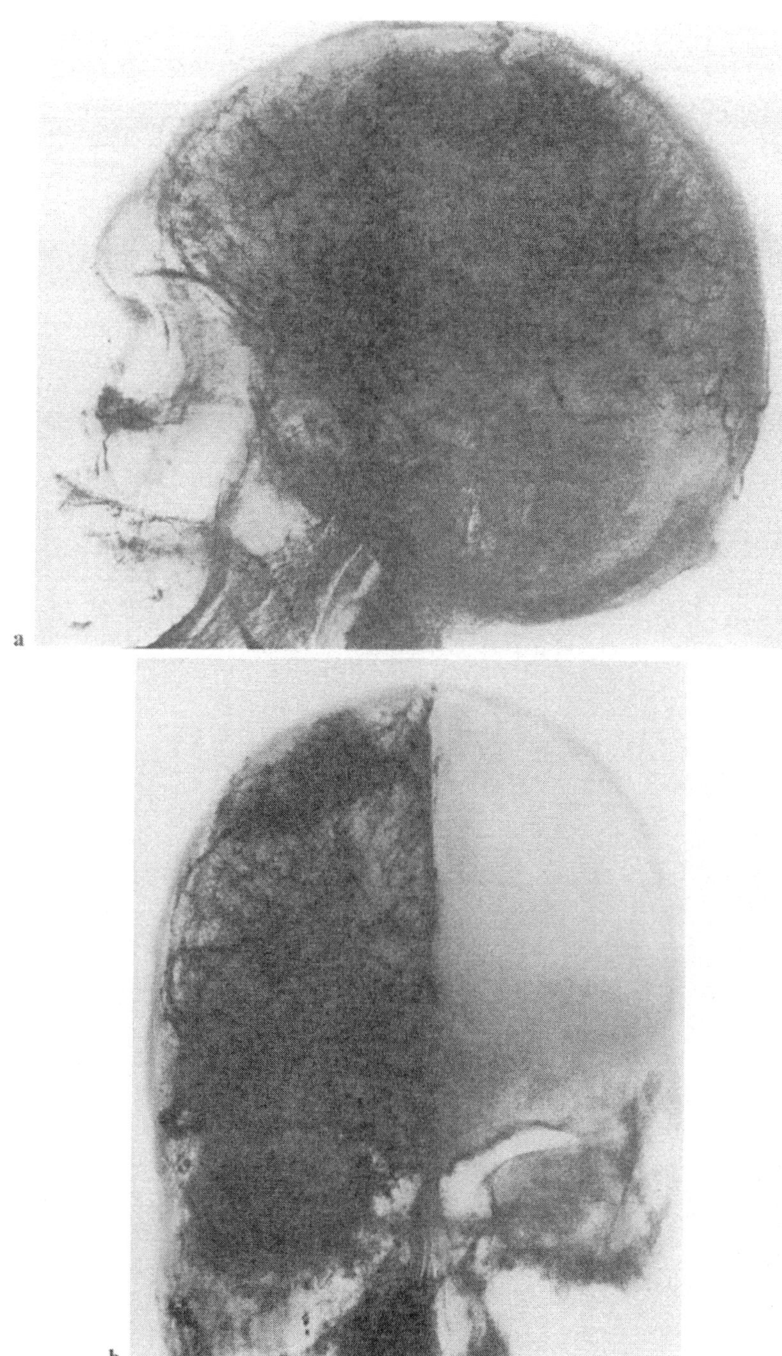

Fig. 19a and b. Meningioma parasagittale. Man, 66 years. Focal seizures for several years. Right common carotid: in late arterial phase diffuse stain in a parasagittal meningioma, sharply delineated. Early filling of one or two superficial veins. Operation: meningioma invading superior sagittal sinus. Histology: meningeoma

and b). Lying near the tentorial edge they may press the brain stem with the consequenses discussed earlier in this chapter. Tentorial meningiomas obtain their main blood supply from the tentorial artery.

Finally, among the supratentorial meningiomas the intraventricular meningiomas should be mentioned. In the lateral ventricles they can obtain a very large size, especially in the trigonum;

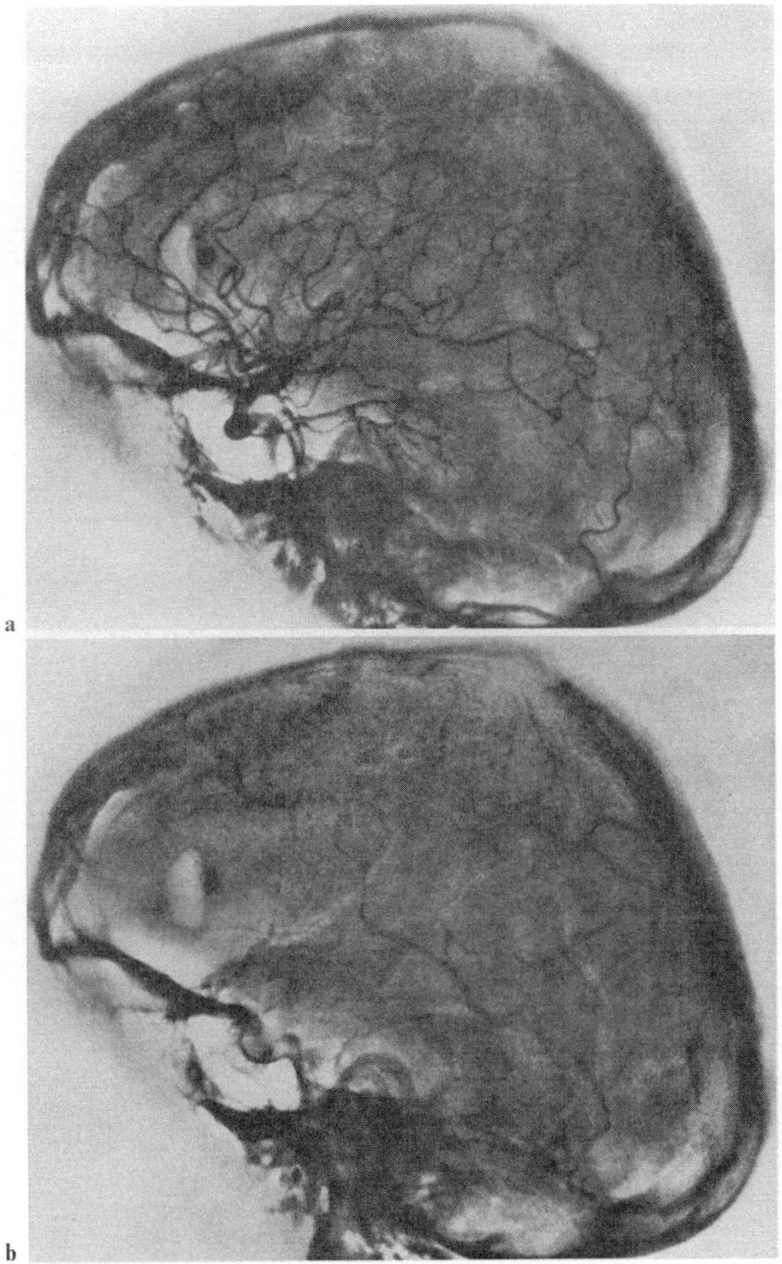

Fig. 20a and b. Meningioma tentorii sin. Woman, 48 years. A hypertrophic tentorial artery (not to be confused with a horizontal branch of the middle meningeal artery, located $^1/_2$ cm higher) supplies vasculated tumor which in later phases appears well delineated. Vessels are not as irregular as in malignant gliomas. Operation: a meningioma originating from medial portion of tentorium extending into middle fossa, posterior fossa, and tentorial notch. Histology: fibroblastic meningioma

they originate from the choroid plexus, they are supplied by the anterior and posterior choroid arteries (FALK, 1955), and they often calcify. All meningiomas may calcify but it is our impression that the calcification is not as common as once assumed, for instance among 29 presellar meningiomas GREGORIUS and BENTSON (loc.cit.) found only two with visible calcification. From the velum interpositum a meningioma may go down into the third ventricle.

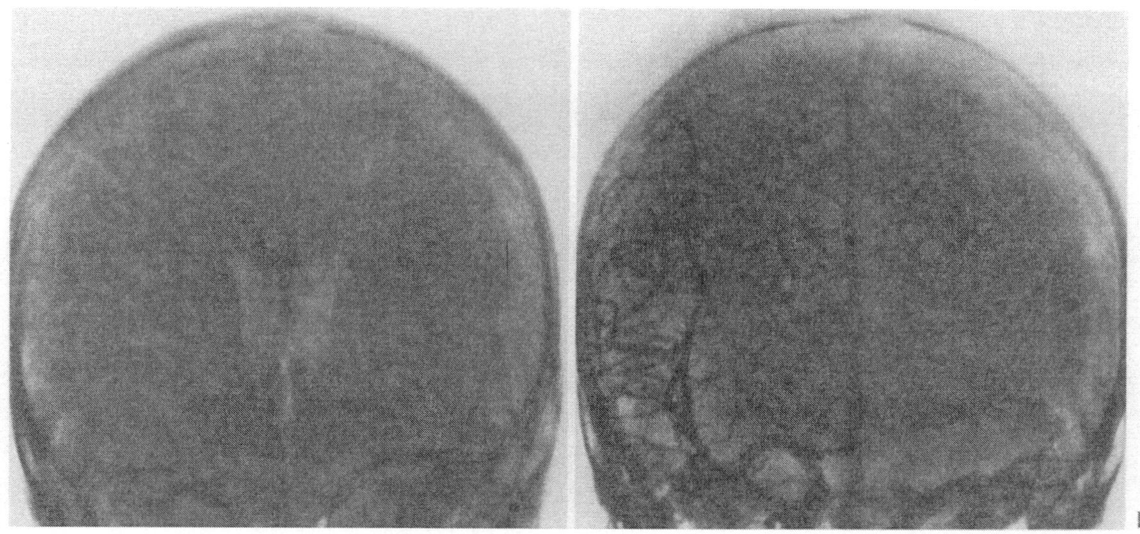

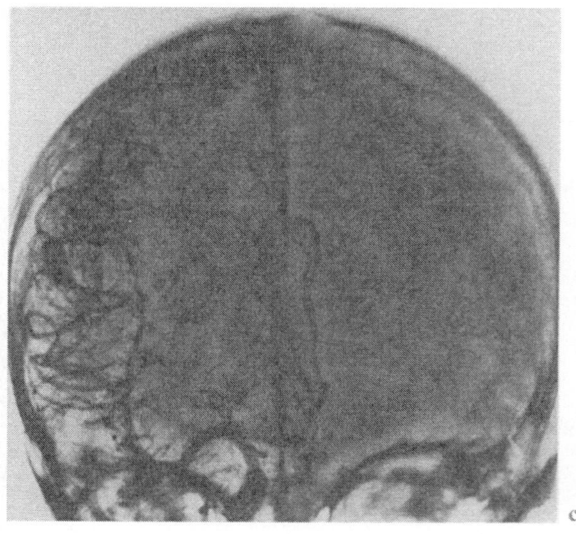

Fig. 21a–c. Rapidly growing glioblastoma. Man, 59 years. For one year slowly increasing left hemiplegia. January 1974: right carotid angiography was negative. A slight indentation of right anterior horn was noted on PEG. May 1974: violent extension of malignant vessels with a–v shunt. Square shift of pericallosal artery with sharp step and calloso-marginal sign. (In another patient we saw a similar development in three weeks, but the films could not be reproduced.)

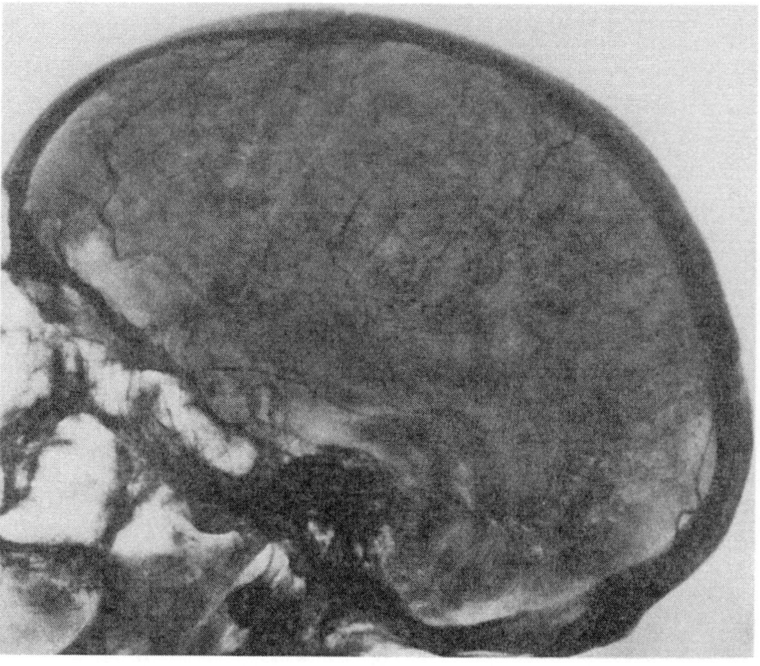

Fig. 22

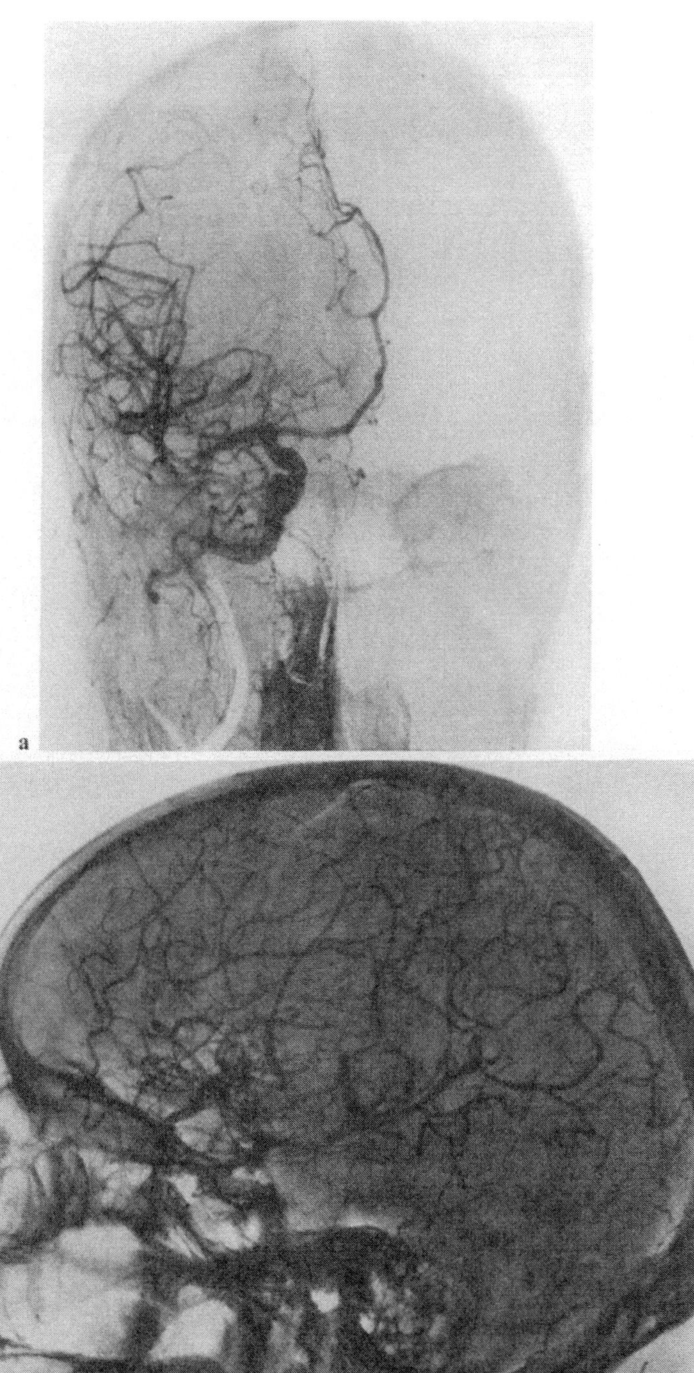

Fig. 23a and b. Glioblastoma multiforme. Woman, 72 years. Irregularly calibrated vessels and a–v shunts. Lenticulostriate arteries take part in supply of tumor; they are depressed and pushed medially. Pericallosal artery dislocated in a bow without step

---

◀ **Fig. 22.** Glioblastoma multiforme resembling an abscess. Man, 61 years. Right carotid: this tumor, showing an avascular center, might have some resemblance to an abscess, but vessels in highly vasculated periphery are so irregular in course, size, and caliber that malignancy is unquestionable. Histologic diagnosis: glioblastoma multiforme

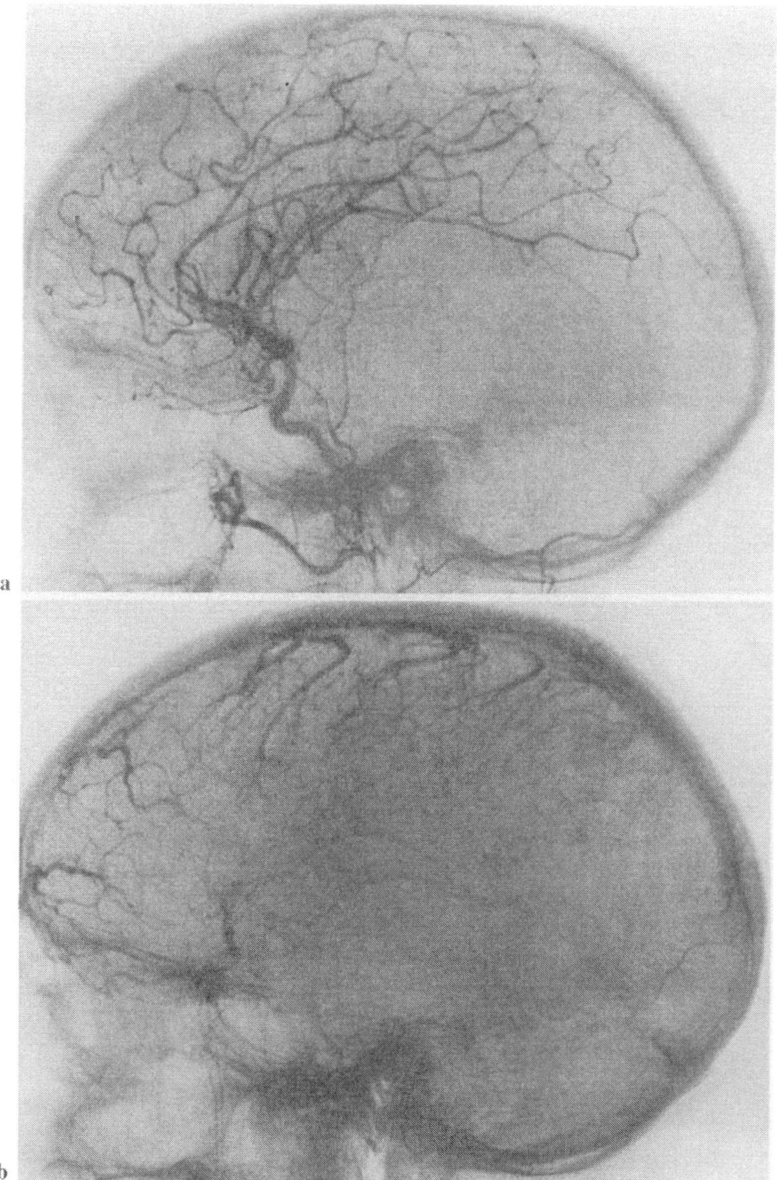

Fig. 24a and b. Glioblastoma of left temporal lobe. Boy, 11 years. Arciform elevation and compression of Sylvian group of arteries; steep elevation of anterior choroidal artery (which in frontal view was pressed to midline). Elevation of basal vein, posterior $^{3}/_{4}$ of which makes a downward concave bow. Beginning of this veins is elevated separately. Thus, pictures show an expanding lesion in middle and posterior portion of temporal lobe with an ascending herniation over sphenoid ridge. No tumor vessels. Operation and histology: glioblastoma multiforme

Glioblastomas. Most authors consider glioblastomas as the second most common intracranial tumors; in ZÜLCH'S cases (1975) they totalled 12.2%. The preferred age group is between 45 and 65 years of age – similar to the meningiomas. The male sex is preferred in contrast to the meningiomas. Belonging to the great group of gliomas, i.e., tumors originating from the supporting tissue – the glia – of the central nervous system, these tumors are principally quite different from the meningiomas. They are intracerebral, and as the lowest differentiated of the group of gliomas, the glioblastomas are highly malignant. Most meningiomas are slowly growing tumors; the patients may have a very long anamnesis. The malignant glioma (glioblastoma

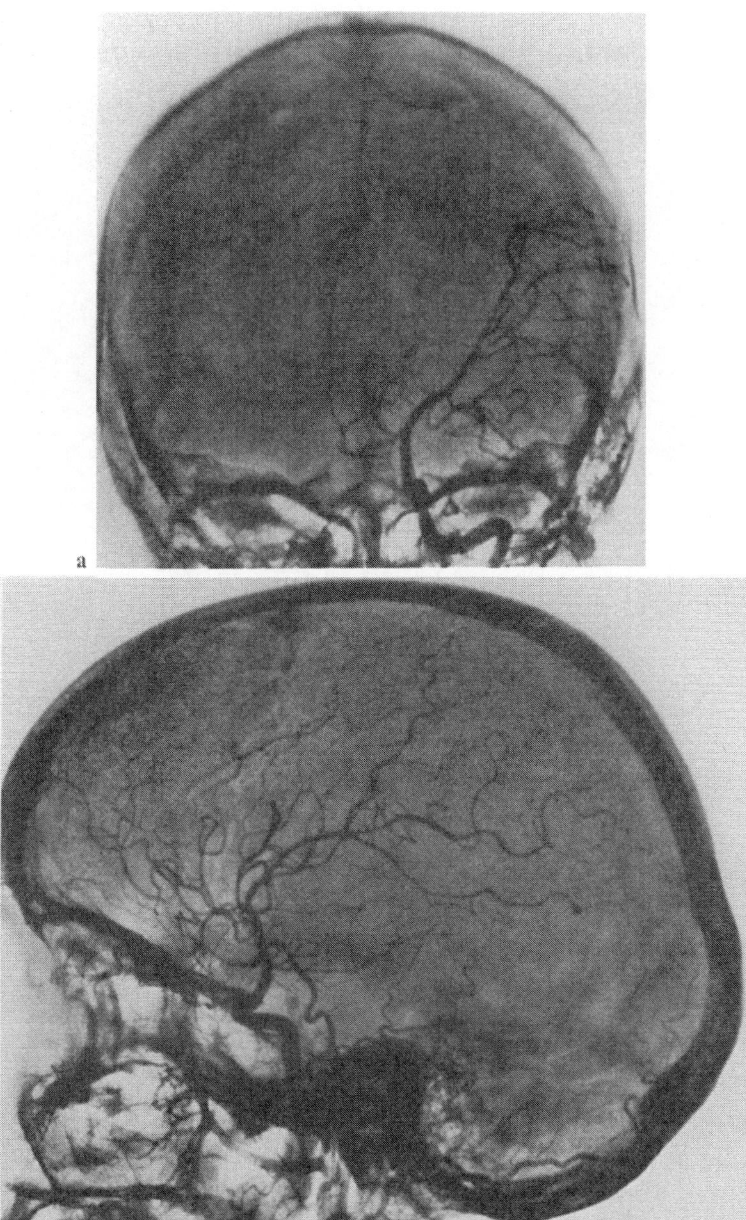

Fig. 25a and b. Glioblastoma multiforme. Woman, 54 years. Upper part of siphon is raised – continuing in the straightened and elevated middle cerebral artery. Anterior and middle portions of anterior cerebral artery dislocated to the right; anterior choroidal artery pushed almost to midline and slightly depressed: combination of subfalcine and anterior tentorial herniation. No tumor vessels. Operation and histology: glioblastoma in left temporal lobe

multiforme) may develop its symptoms and signs and its angiographic changes in few weeks (Fig. 21a–c) (KRAYENBÜHL and YASARGIL, 1965; JACOBSEN and OLIVARIUS, 1966; CRONQVIST, 1967; LIN and SIEW, 1971).

Angiographically they may present themselves in different manners: as observed by ZÜLCH (1975) they may be: well circumscribed (Fig. 22) or they may extend more diffusely (Fig. 37a and b) in the parenchyma; they may appear highly vasculated, which is characteristic, or they may be almost avascular (Figs. 23–25). They may be found everywhere in the cerebrum, sometimes in the brain stem, but they almost never occur in cerebellum. As they are growing infiltratively

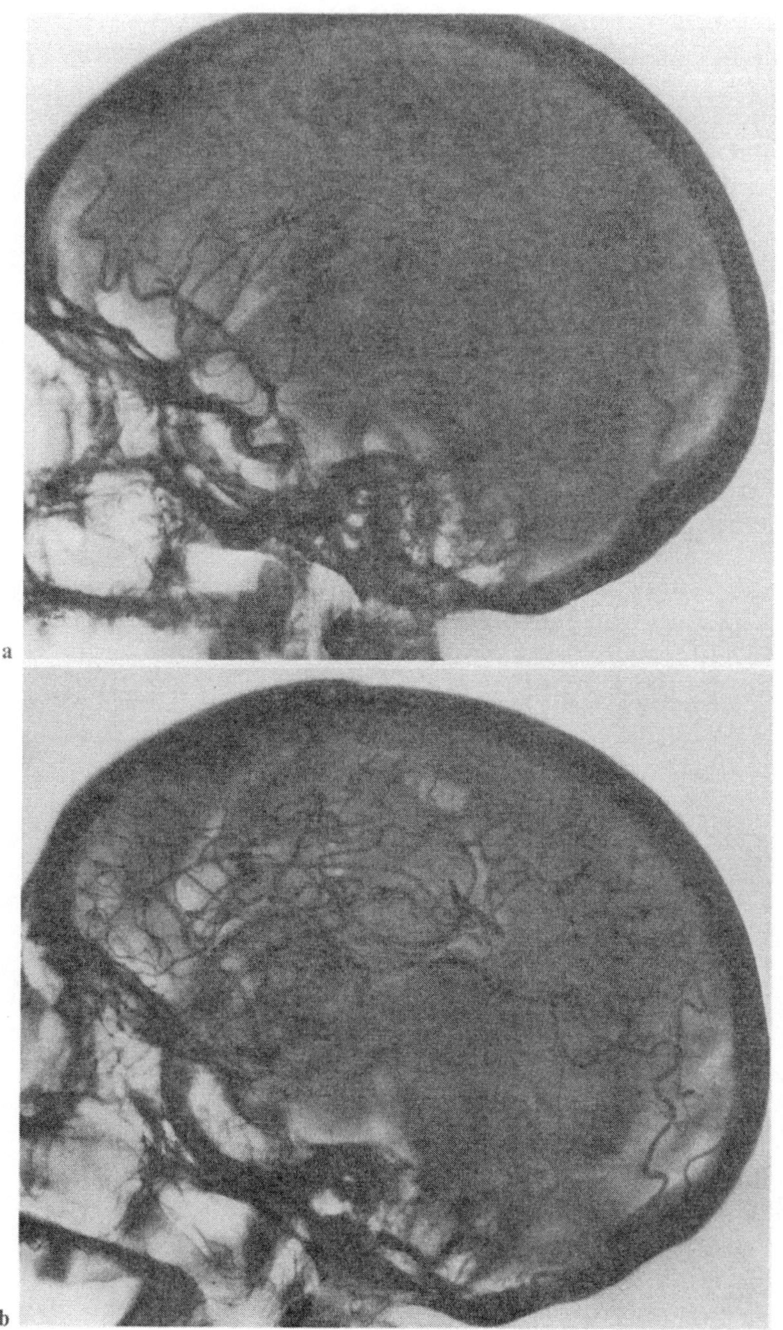

Fig. 26a and b. Malignant recurrence. Woman, 50 years. In Sept. 1974 she was operated upon after a right-sided carotid angiography showed a temporal space-occupying lesion without tumor vessels. Operation was not radical (**a**). In March 1975 there were symptoms and signs of recurrence: the angiography then (**b**) showed a ball of most irregularly calibrated malignant vessels. No reoperation, no autopsy

more than they are space-occupying one can meet even great glioblastomas only causing a moderate shift of the midline vessels (Fig. 29a), but the lack of shift may also be caused by the fact that the glioblastoma has invaded the corpus callosum, crossed the midline, and spread out into the opposite hemisphere in the form of a butterfly glioma (Fig. 7a and b).

We know little about the history of development, it is generally supposed that the glioblastoma may develop from more benign forms of gliomas; we do know, however, that in many cases

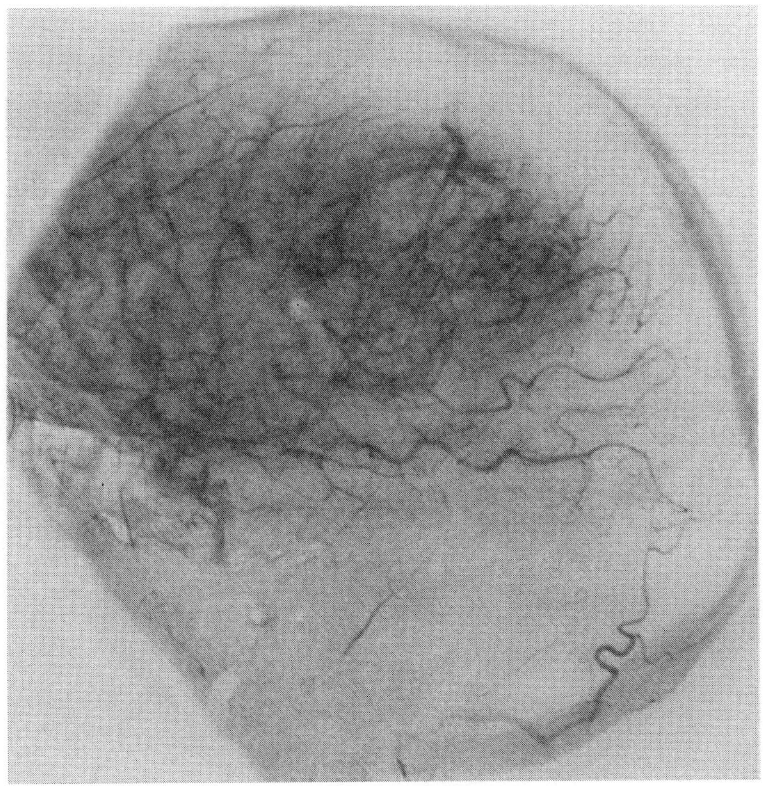

Fig. 27. Glioblastoma. Man, 49 years. Transferred from another hospital for operation if possible. Right carotid: vasculated tumor, 8 cm long, deep in right hemisphere. Hypovascular center (necrosis). Early filling of superficial and deep veins. Structure and size were certified by CAT-scanning, as was the unsharp limitation. Surgeons desisted from operation because of malignant character, size, and site of tumor

of recurrence of an operated benign glioma, the tumor has "degenerated" into the malignant form (Fig. 26a and b).

As mentioned by KRAYENBÜHL and YAŞARGIL (1965) three different forms of vascular architecture may be seen: (1) The angiomatous group is characterized by its abundance of vessels, irregular in course and caliber, often fed by enlarged cerebral arteries and drained by great veins to the deep cerebral veins. In some cases it may be impossible, in the radiogram, to distinguish this tumor from an arterio-venous angioma (Fig. 38b and c). (2) A group with diffuse stain similar to the stain of the meningiomas but as a rule without the sharp border of the meningioma. The stain seen with a magnifying glass or examined by the magnification technique will consist in coarser vessels than seen in the stain of meningiomas. The stain of the meningiomas appears late in the arterial phase and persists in most of the venous phase; the stain of the glioblastomas appears earlier in the arterial phase, almost simultaneously with the first appearance of the first observed draining veins, and the stain disappears very quickly. However, AZAR-KIA et al. (1974) reported four cases of delayed stain in glioblastomas.

These two groups may be represented in the same tumor. (3) In the third group no tumor vessels are visible; this form manifests itself by one or more early filled veins; if they do not show a dislocation of the surrounding vessels they can be mistaken for an arterio-venous malformation or the "luxurious flow" characterizing certain vascular lesions, e.g., infarcts. We can meet glioblastomas with an avascular or hypovascular center surrounded by a more or less dense ring of pathologic vessels; the avascular center is a necrotic, cystic, or hemorrhagic portion (Figs. 27, 28a and b) of the tumor, and the picture may have some likeness to an abscess (Fig. 22).

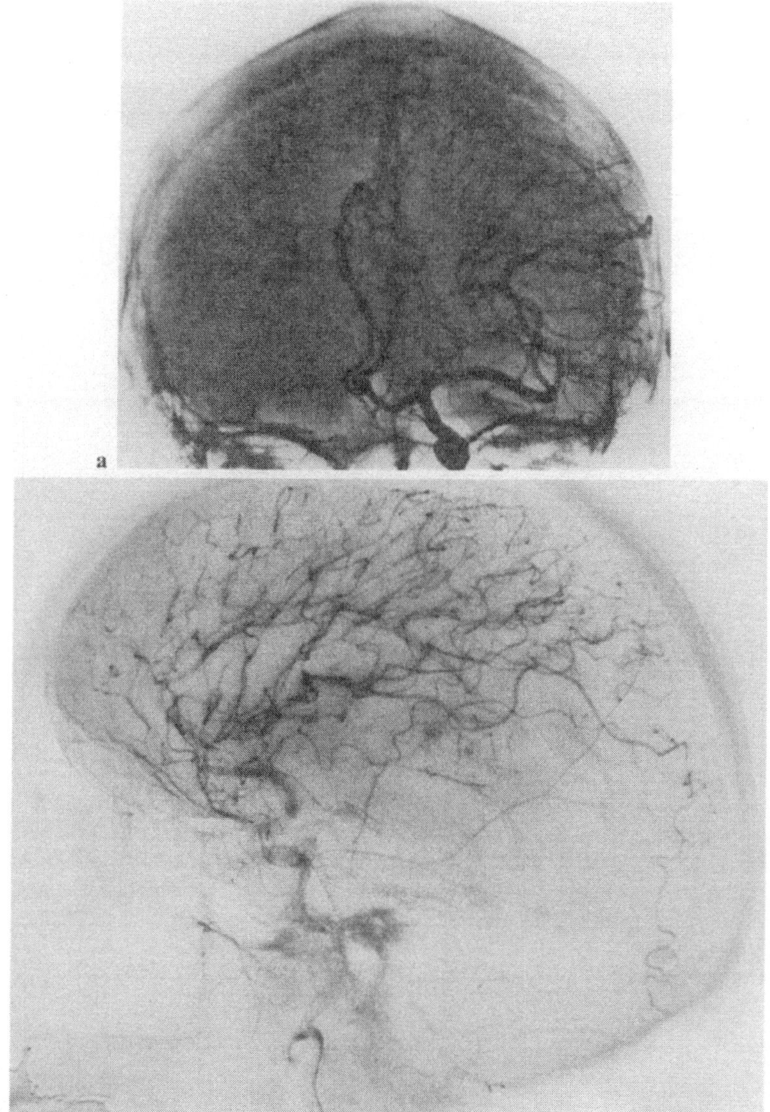

Fig. 28a and b. Glioblastoma multiforme, hematoma intracerebrale. Woman, 63 years. Anamnesis very short. Shift of pericallosal artery increasing posteriorly, ending in a step. Middle cerebral artery elevated and dislocated medially with stretching of its lateral branches. Slight occurrence of pathologic vessels in posterior portion of temporal lobe. Operation: hematoma (30 ml); behind this suspect tissue. Histology: glioblastoma multiforme

In a few cases we have seen a bundle of irregularly calibrated arteries converging in a straight or slightly twisted course from the parietal theca to the deep veins – almost in a cone; the filling of the deep veins appears in an early arterial phase (Figs. 29a and b). If the glioblastoma penetrates the cortex of one hemisphere it may infiltrate the dura and in this way take some of its arterial supply from the meningeal arteries. The most common vascular architecture (the first and second group of KRAYENBÜHL and YAŞARGIL, 1965) is almost the same for the glioblastomas and the metastatic tumors; often the metastases are better demarcated, and a multiplicity of tumors will speak in favor of metastases. It will be understood that in some cases the diagnosis is so safe that a superfluous operation may be omitted, but in most cases the diagnosis cannot be made with absolute certainty (cf. Fig. 39).

The more benign tumors of the neuroepithelium. The gangliocytoma (ganglioglioma, neuroblastoma, neuroastrocytoma – ZÜLCH, 1975) amounts to 0.4%, a slowly growing, benign tumor composed

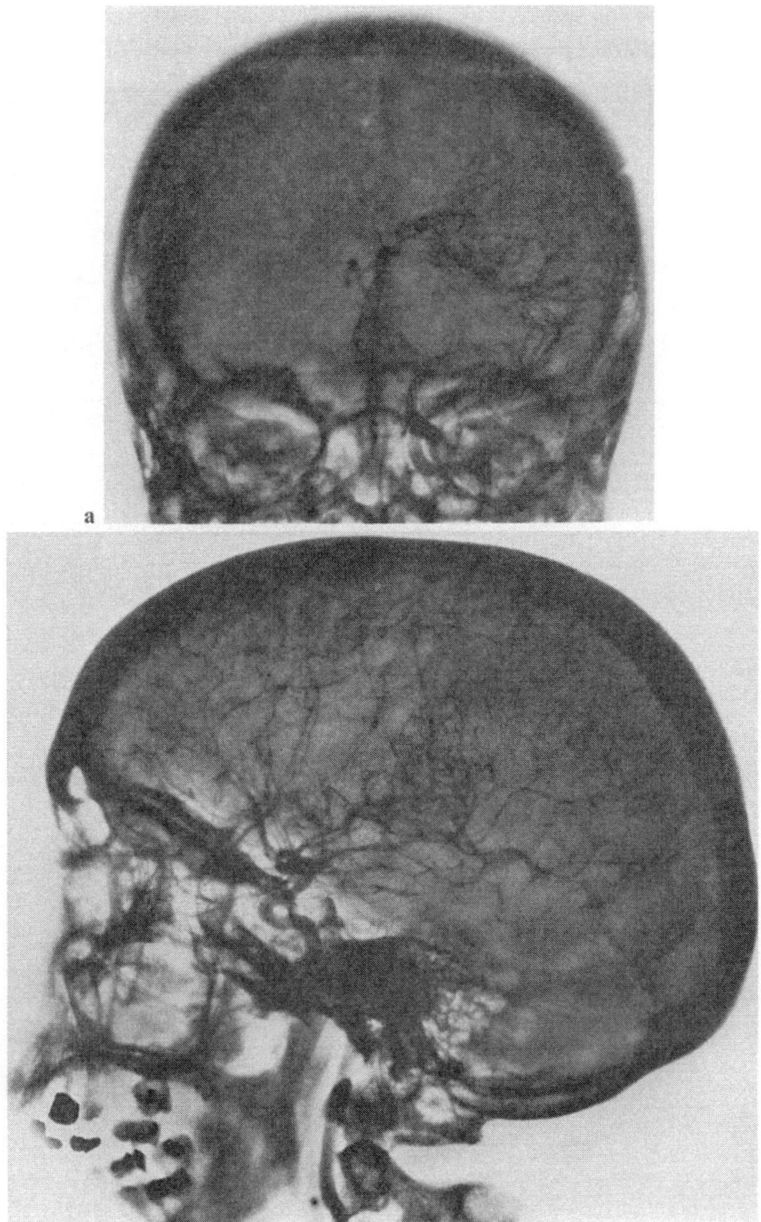

Fig. 29a and b. Glioblastoma multiforme. Woman, 35 years. Very short anamnesis. Wedge-shaped, irregularly calibrated collection of arteries converging to deep veins, shunting in an early arterial phase. Moderate shift of deep veins; posterior portion of vein of Galen remains in midline. Operation and histology: ut supra

of ganglion cells and astrocytes. It usually occurs within the three first decades of life (KATZ et al., 1972), is generally located in the temporal lobe, where it may form large cysts. Their vascularization is poor, calcification may be found. In rare cases they may dedifferentiate and assume the malignity of the glioblastoma. TAVERAS and WOOD (1964) stated that "they are thought to be related to the polar spongioblastomas." They should have no characteristic angiographic features.

The *ependymomas* (4.3% according to ZÜLCH, 1975) may occur inside the ventricles or as extraventricular tumors, most often they are seen originating from the ependyma of one lateral ventricle extending out into the hemisphere. They usually occur in the first two decades of life; this tumor forms the prevalent supratentorial glioma of this age-group. There is one danger connected to the operation upon it: as its surface is tufted, the tufts may loosen and metastasize inside the cerebrospinal fluid space. Most of the tumors are partially cystic, they may calcify, but less frequently than the astrocytomas and oligodendrogliomas. NEWTON and POTTS (1974) found some hypervascularization in children. Beyond this no angiographic characteristics are mentioned.

In the same connection ZÜLCH (1975) mentioned the *colloid cysts* or *ependymal cysts*. According to BATNITZKY et al. (1974) it forms 0.5% of all "brain tumors"; it may be found in all age-groups and is said by the same authors to be *the* tumor of the third ventricle. It is said (ZÜLCH, 1975; TAVERAS and WOOD, 1964) to originate from the paraphysis, the cystic anlage from which the telencephalon is developed, i.e., this epithelial tumor has its stalk or its base connected to the choroid plexus in the upper, anterior wall of the foramen of Monro. Although its size is as a rule limited to 2 cm, it will be understood that this tumor may occlude one or both foramina of Monro, intermittently or constantly. The diagnosis is safer by ventriculography than by arteriography, but certain angiographic signs should be mentioned. POTTS and TAVERAS (1963) in two cases found elevation of the anterior portion, depression of the posterior portion of the internal cerebral vein, the anterior portion making a sharp curve, concave downward. In the frontal view the thalamostriate vein describes a medial downward concave curve in contrast to the tumors of septum pellucidum which will depress the anterior portion of the internal cerebral vein. The change in course of the thalamostriate vein is not found in any of the 25 cases of BATNITZKY et al. (1974). These authors agree that pathologic vessels or tumor strain are never seen (whereas the intraventricular meningiomas and the plexus-papillomas will show stain). Calcification is never seen.

The *plexus-papilloma* is a highly vascularized benign tumor originating from the choroid plexus. ZÜLCH (1975) stated its occurrence as 0.6% of intracranial tumors; the figure according to TAVERAS and WOOD (1964) is a little lower. The preferred age group according to ZÜLCH is between 25 and 35 years, however, TAVERAS and WOOD found the highest number of cases were in the first decade of life. In the lateral ventricle the tumor appears in the trigonum region, and from there it may penetrate into the brain substance, though always with a clear-cut demarcation without infiltration. In this region the tumor may be highly calcified. Although this location is the most common in children, calcification is rare at this age. In adults it is more commonly found in the fourth ventricle. A close histologic relationship to "normal" ependymoma and transitional forms may be found. Big cysts may be connected to the tumor and it is often accompanied by a communicating hydrocephalus, especially in children; the explanation of this may be an excessive production of cerebrospinal fluid from the highly enlarged fluid-producing surface. In the third and lateral ventricles the tumor is fed by the posterior and anterior choroid arteries. In the arterial phase one will see many small tortuous vessels, in the venous phase an almost homogeneous stain (NEWTON and POTTS, 1974). Early appearance of draining veins is described (KRAYENBÜHL and YAŞARGIL, 1965), and malignancy is seen (BANNA, 1971). Spontaneous and postoperative metastases occur.

Among the ependymoma-like tumors ZÜLCH (1975) mentions those *accompanying the tuberous sclerosis*. They are found close to the lateral ventricle; they are more or less cystic, often calcified, and may obtain the size of a tangerine. NEWTON and POTTS (1974) and FITZ et al. (1974) also mentioned more malignant tumors in this connection. KRAYENBÜHL and YAŞARGIL found many thin, slightly twisted neoplastic vessels in the late arterial phase together with malformations of the veins and dural sinuses. HILAL et al. (1971) found small arterial occlusions in children, but these observations must be taken as belonging more to the disease per se rather than to the accompanying tumors.

The *astrocytoma* in the material of ZÜLCH (1975) represented 6.6% of intracranial tumors. The age-group between 35 and 45 years is preferred, but it is also found in children. There are different subtypes: the tumor may be firm, circumscribed, solid – almost cartilagineous

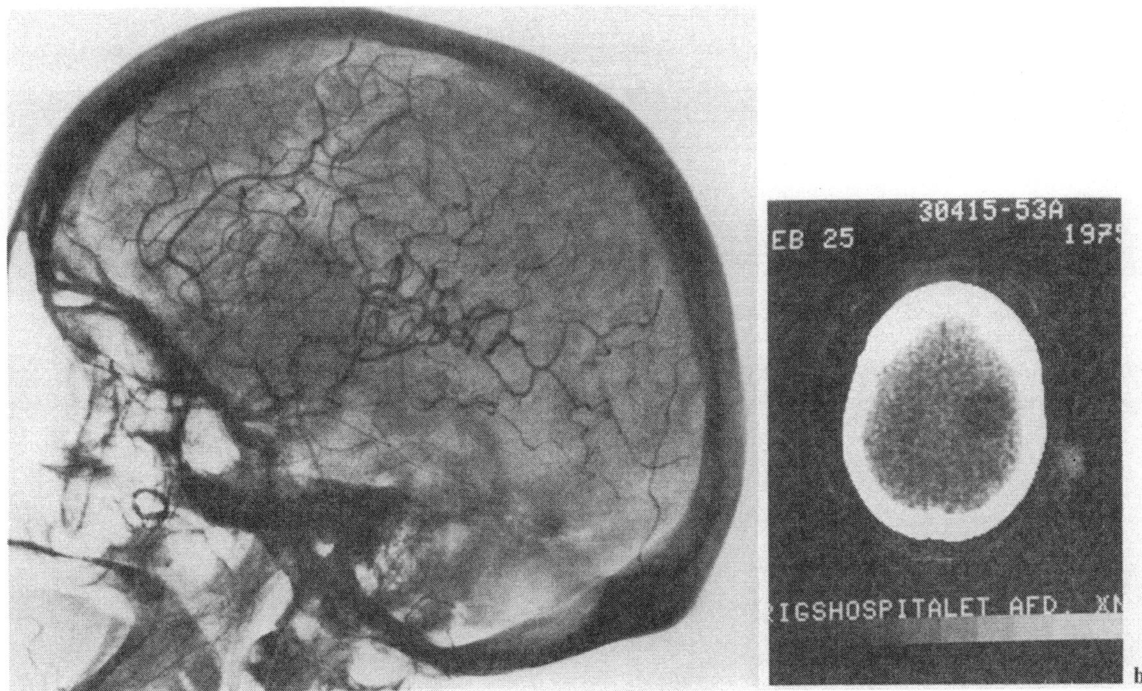

Fig. 30a and b. Astrocytoma. Man, 26 years. Repeated focal seizures starting in left arm for 2 years. EEG, gamma-scanning, encephalography, and two angiographies in right carotid were all negative. To demonstrate the negative result of neuroradiologic examination it would be necessary to show 83 reproductions which is not possible. CAT-scan shows what we called a cyst in upper part of right hemisphere. Operation: a cystic tumor – size of a ping-pong ball was enucleated. Histology: astrocytoma isomorphicum

– or more soft, tough, without definite borders; others are soft, but not tough, more like edema. These subgroups may be found mixed in one tumor. The growth is partially expanding, partially infiltrating. An astrocytoma may break through the cortex like a mushroom, thus causing spreading and distension of the cortical arteries and veins. Very often they are cystic; the tumor may appear as one large cyst with a small solid tumor somewhere in its wall. Calcification is rare. They are most frequently found in the hemisphere, especially in its frontal portion. They may originate from the thalamus, the brain stem, and the spinal cord (Figs. 6a and b, 30–33). Their cerebellar occurrence should not be forgotten, but in ZÜLCH'S (1975) specification the cerebellar astrocytomas are counted as spongioblastomas. From one hemisphere the tumor may invade the corpus callosum and infiltrate the septum pellucidum and/or the opposite hemisphere.

From a pathologic point of view this tumor may be called benign or semibenign, but only in rare cases can the surgeon be sure that removal has been complete; and in 10% of the tumor preparations removed, foci will be found with the malignant character of the glioblastoma.

The angiographic appearance will vary. The expanding force has been mentioned if the tumor penetrates the cortex. If a thalamic astrocytoma extends into the Sylvian fissure, and if it shows some grade of vascularization, the picture can be very difficult to distinguish from an intrasylvian meningioma (TAVERAS and WOOD, 1964); in this connection we should also mention GVOZDANOVIĆ'S study (1955) in the superficial veins in cases of intracranial expanding lesions. The vascular architecture may vary, at any rate these tumors are less vasculated than the glioblastomas; sometimes no tumor vessels are to be seen, in other cases such vessels may appear. The number and also the degree of twisting being variable. Some authors consider the appearance of pathologic vessels as a sign of malignancy; we should be satisfied with the statement that this evaluation

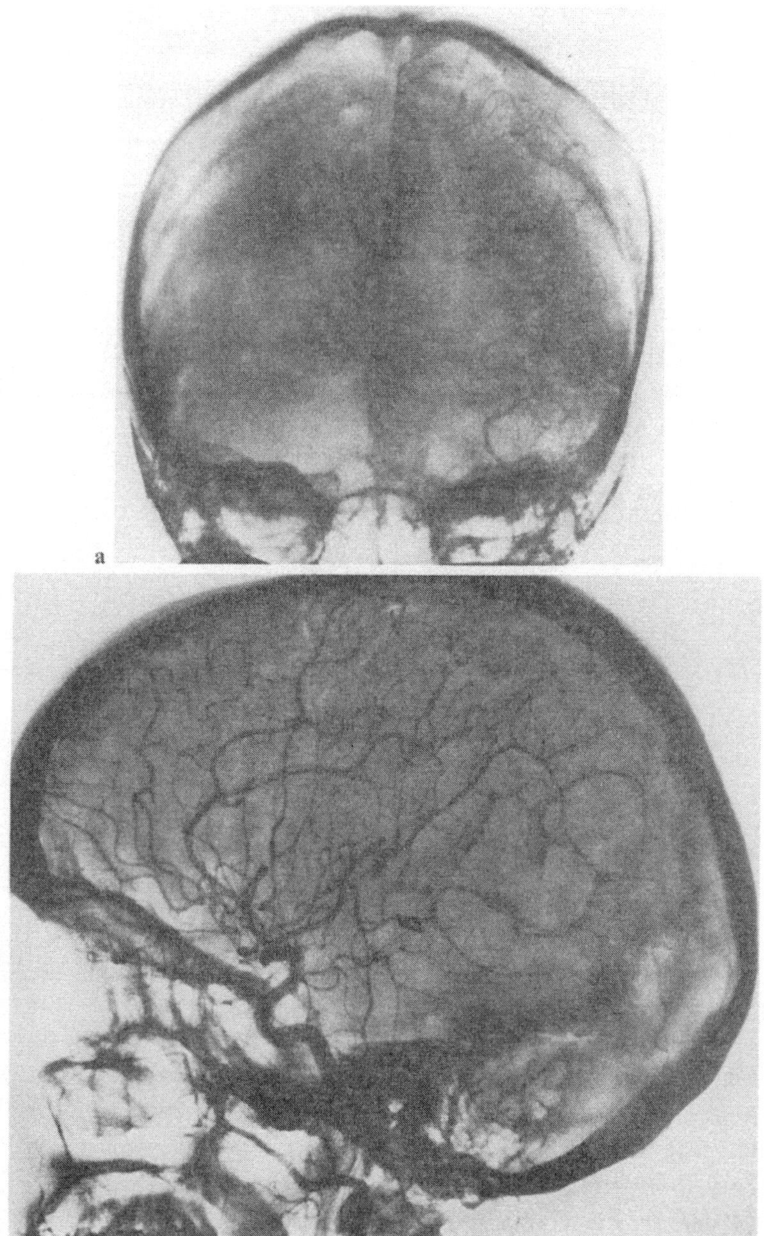

Fig. 31a and b. Astrocytoma, with calcifications. Woman, 37 years. 1-cm shift to the right of midline-vessels; Fig. **a** shows a slight but significant tilting of small vessels in right and left sulcus cinguli. Posteriorly the peripheral branches of middle cerebral artery are stretched and spread about the calcifications. No tumor vessels were found. Operation, histology: ut supra

is difficult if not impossible. In benign astrocytomas arterio-venous fistula are practically never seen (KRAYENBÜHL and YAŞARGIL, 1965).

Oligodendrogliomas represent 9.6% of intracranial tumors (ZÜLCH, 1975). The age-group between 30 and 55 years is most commonly affected. They may be seen in children, and then as a rule located to the thalamus. In adults they may occur everywhere in the hemisphere, more frequently in their anterior parts, and more frequently located in the cortex than in the white matter. They may expand the cortex, and they may break through the cortex and adhere to

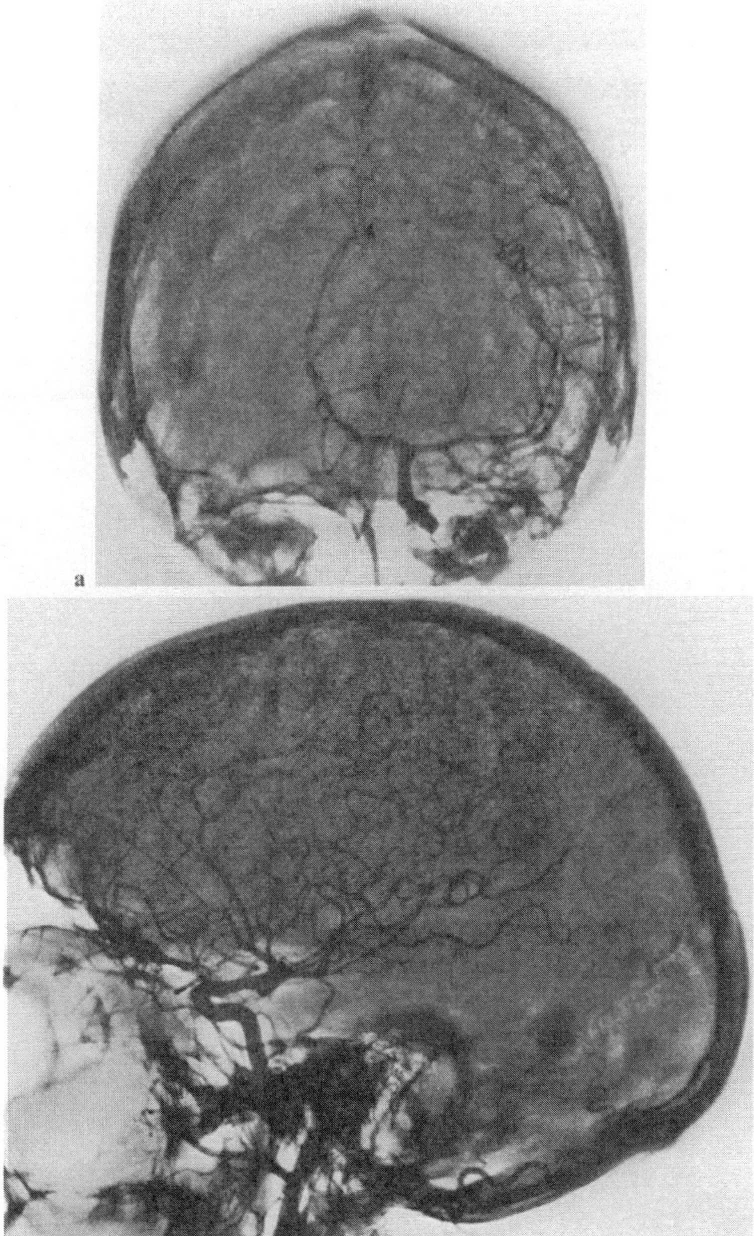

Fig. 32a and b. Astrocytoma. Man, 56 years. $2^1/_2$-cm arciform dislocation of anterior and middle portion of anterior cerebral artery (only slight deviation of deep veins). Top of the siphon pushed backward (same with angulus venosus). Sylvian and lenticulostriate arteries dislocated laterally and slightly depressed. No tumor vessels. Diagnosis: great frontal space-occupying process. Operation: soft, grayish-red bleeding tumor expanding diffusely in left hemisphere. Histology: astrocytoma polymorphicum

the dura without infiltration. From the relatively rare parasagittal location they may invade the corpus callosum. Their growth is slow, and they often calcify. KALAN and BURROWS (1962) examined the frequency of calcification in the different types of gliomas and found radiologically visible calcification in this type of glioma in 46.7%, in ependymomas in 14.6%, in astrocytomas of all grades of Kernohan – that is including glioblastomas – in 6.3%, and in medulloblastomas in 1%. The tumor is called semibenign, but ZÜLCH (1975) stated that the polymorphous and highly vasculated type should be called semimalignant.

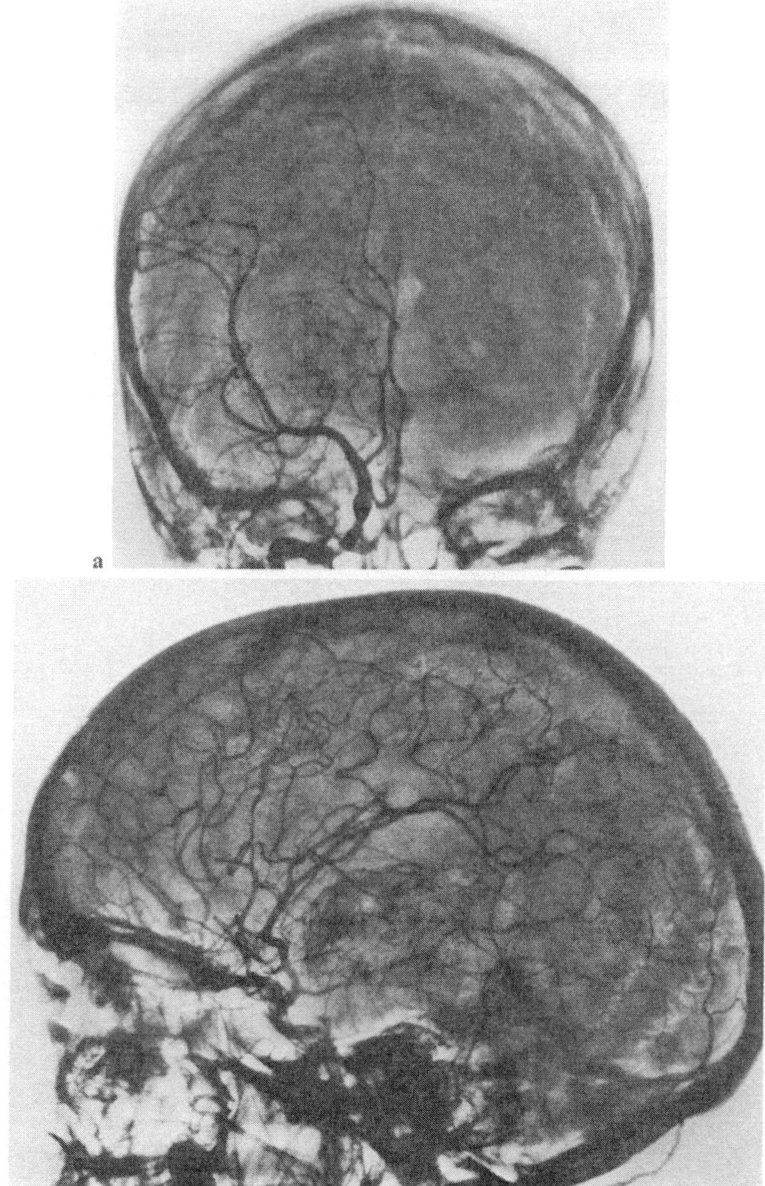

Fig. 33 a and b. Astrocytoma. Girl, 15 years. Highly vascularized tumor in region of basal ganglia – supplied by middle and posterior cerebral arteries. Course of middle cerebral artery and stretching of its lateral branches indicates that an avascular portion of tumor – or maybe an edema – extends to operculum. Posterior cerebral artery is dislocated medially; its anterior portion downward: anterior tentorial herniation. Operation and histology: subtotal removal, astrocytoma isomorphicum

The difference in vascularization may explain these different conceptions: generally ZÜLCH (1975) describes this tumor as rather vascular with an abundance of smaller vessels, whereas KRAYENBÜHL and YAŞARGIL (1965) stated that as a rule they found no tumor vascularization, but sometimes a homogeneous rather diffuse stain; and NEWTON and POTTS (1974) said that they may give a slight stain.

Metastases inside the fluid space may be seen spontaneously and after surgery. In cases of recurrence we have seen a vascularization like that of a glioblastoma, and it was mentioned by TAVERAS and WOOD (1964) that as well as astrocytomas, oligodendrogliomas may undergo malignant metaplasia at any time during their development.

The *spongioblastoma polare* was described by ZÜLCH (1975) and other authors including the cerebellar astrocytomas; this is the reason why his figure of percentual occurrence amounts to 6. This tumor is most frequently found in the age-group between 10 and 25 years. The most common supratentorial location is the optic nerves. The tumor may go through the optic foramen as a dumb-bell tumor, as a rule enlarging the foramen. Parenthetically it may be ponted out that whereas in earlier days we diagnosed optic gliomas by means of angiography and orbitography with a positive contrast media, we now exclusively use the computer-assisted tomograph, which delineates the optic nerve with great accuracy.

The intracranial spongioblastoma in most cases is accompanied by a cyst, and often a very large one. The tumor grows expansively, but in spite of the macroscopically clear cleavage there is some infiltration from the periphery. It may grow through the terminal lamina and fill the third ventricle. The most common supratentorial angiographic finding is that of a slight stain in a small tumor of the wall, and the dislocation and spreading of the greater vessels caused by the cyst.

Medulloblastomas amount to 4.2% of intracranial tumors; they occur mainly in children between 7 and 12 years of age and almost exclusively in the posterior fossa, from which metastases may move in cranial as well as in caudal direction. In their monograph, KRAYENBÜHL and YAŞARGIL (1965) reproduced the pictures of two supratentorial cases showing a diffuse, faint, homogeneous staning. It was not stated whether these two tumors occurred primarily in the cerebrum or if they might be supposed to be metastatic implants from the posterior fossa.

In ZÜLCH's material (1975) *metastases* represent 7.1% of intracranial tumors. They may occur in any part of the brain, and they also may be seen in the dura, in which they may be implanted or be firmly adherent. In the cerebrum they are usually located subcortically; they are rarely seen in the basal ganglia (TREVISAN and DETTORI, 1972). Most of them are sharply delineated and round (ZACHRISSON, 1963) (Figs. 34a and b, 35); their size rarely exceeds that of a hen's egg, but those found near to the central sulcus are small, because they will give symptoms in an early phase of their development (ETHELBERG and VAERNET, 1953). Like the glioblastomas they are often surrounded by a large edema, an observation that has been clearly confirmed by the use of the CT-scanner. In ZACHRISSON's material (1963), 124 patients, i.e., 10% showed multiple ocurrence, although only one hemisphere was examined; this multiplicity is regarded as characteristic of this type of tumor. As stated by NEWTON and POTTS (1974) this differential diagnosis versus other tumors is not reliable in all cases: meningiomas may be multiple and glioblastomas may show separate hypervasculated areas (Figs. 36–40).

The vascular architecture is highly varyiable. WICKBOM (1953) found pathologic vessels in 19 out of 38 verified metastases. TREVISAN and DETTORI (1972) performed 75 angiographies (carotis/vertebralis) in 62 patients with verified metastases; only 29 of these showed pathologic vascularization (cf. Fig. 39). A clear classification of the neoplastic vascularization is given by ZACHRISSON (1963): the metastases may appear (1) with a homogeneous stain like meningiomas (Fig. 34a and b), (2) show an avascular center surrounded by a highly vascularized periphery (Fig. 35), (3) contain large, irregular vessels, often with arterio-venous shunts, (4) show a network of delicate tortuous vessels. To this should be added that the pathologic vessels are often seen at the end of one single artery because the metastases are of embolic nature (NEWTON and POTTS, 1974). The possible avascular center represents a central necrosis, and small cysts may occur in the tumor. In contrast to the glioblastomas, the metastases are usually drained to the superficial veins. Naturally the brain metastases will obtain their arterial supply from the internal carotid or/and the vertebral-basilar arteries, but some participation from the external carotid has been described. KLAUSENBERGER (1972) reported a patient with subtotal occlusion of the right carotid siphon; a highly vasculated tumor in the right occipital lobe was supplied by branches of the right occipital artery; it also had some small branches from the right posterior cerebral artery; the histologic diagnosis was carcinoma.

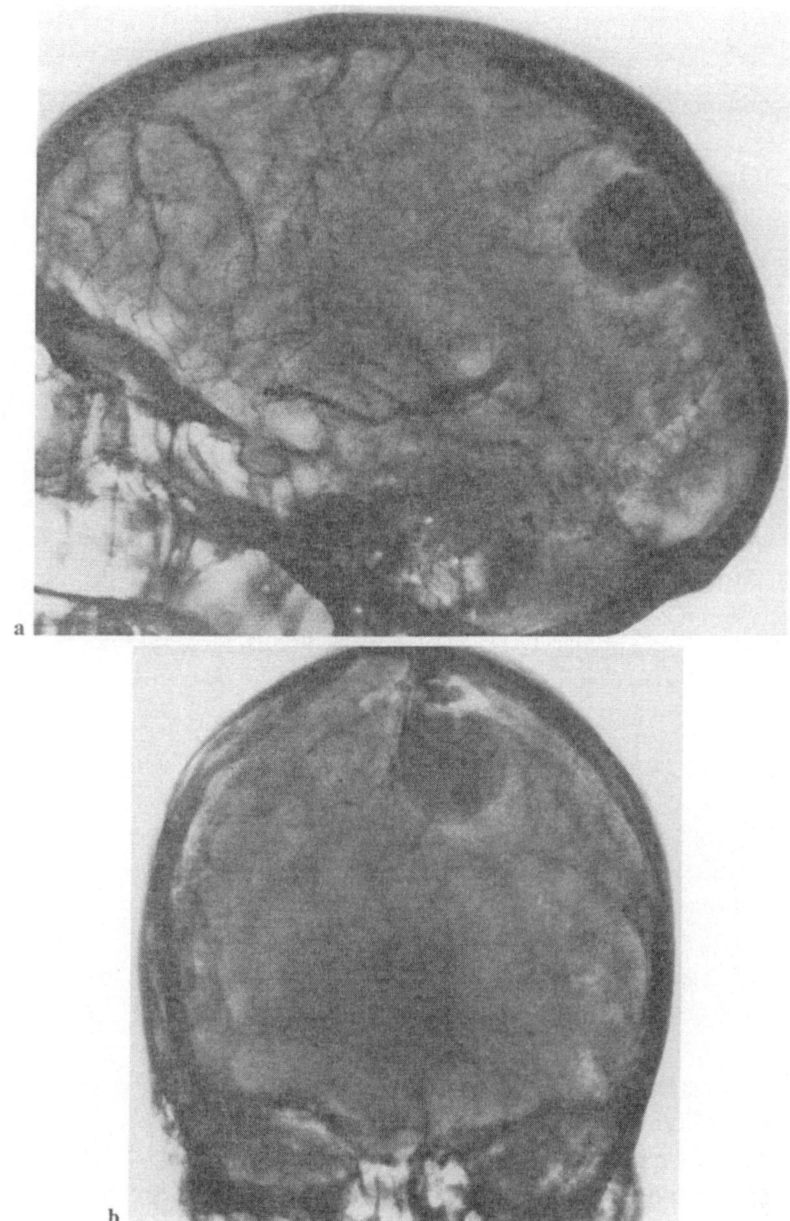

Fig. 34a and b. Metastasis from rhabdomyosarcoma. Woman, 18 years. Operated upon 3 years previously for a rhabdomyosarcoma originating in right quadriceps muscle. Postoperative roentgen treatment. Now visual disturbances for a few months. Left carotid: in the upper, medial portion of the occipital lobe a $3^1/_2$ cm large round, sharply delineated highly vascularized tumor with almost homogeneous stain, supplied from peripheral branches of anterior and middle cerebral arteries. Operation: tumor was well delineated "looking like a typical metastasis." Histology: rhabdomyosarcoma

From what has been said it is obvious that differential diagnosis may be difficult and in some cases impossible. First of all – in our opinion – one should not cultivate what in the older German literature has been called "Die voraussetzungslose Radiologie"; one must always know the case reports before planning and performing a neuroradiologic examination. But still several cases will be left, in which no primary tumor is known. Some metastases look like meningiomas, yet the stain of the metastases usually appears and disappears in earlier phases

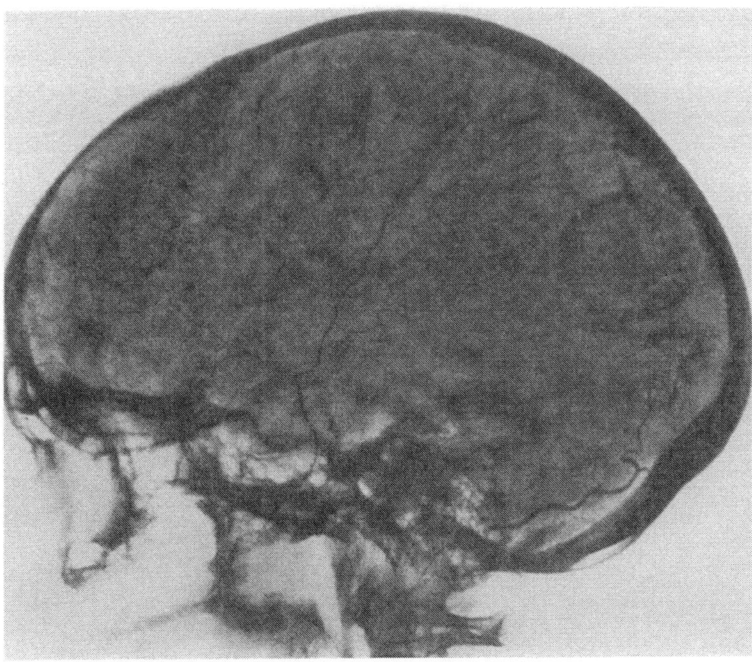

Fig. 35. Metastasis. Woman, 62 years. Mastectomy 1 year previously: carcinoma solidum. This late arterial phase shows a 4 cm large ring-shaped occipital tumor with shunts and surrounding edema. (In other pictures from the same patient two other tumors were detected.) No operation. No autopsy

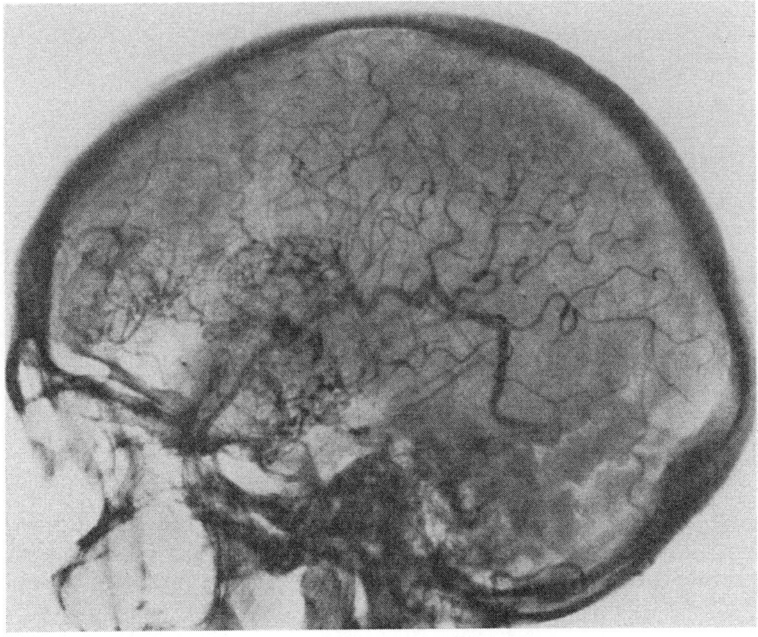

Fig. 36. Glioblastoma multiforme. Woman, 52 years. Highly vascularized glioblastoma simulating two tumors. (Note "bizzare pattern" of WICKBOM.) Multiple a–v shunts. Necropsy showed necrotic areas in tumor (between the "two tumors")

than in meningiomas, and the location of the mass may be decisive. In the highly vascularized glioblastomas the tumor vessels are usually coarser and more irregular and the arterio-venous shunts more abundant than in the metastases. To mention all the other decisive data would be a repetition.

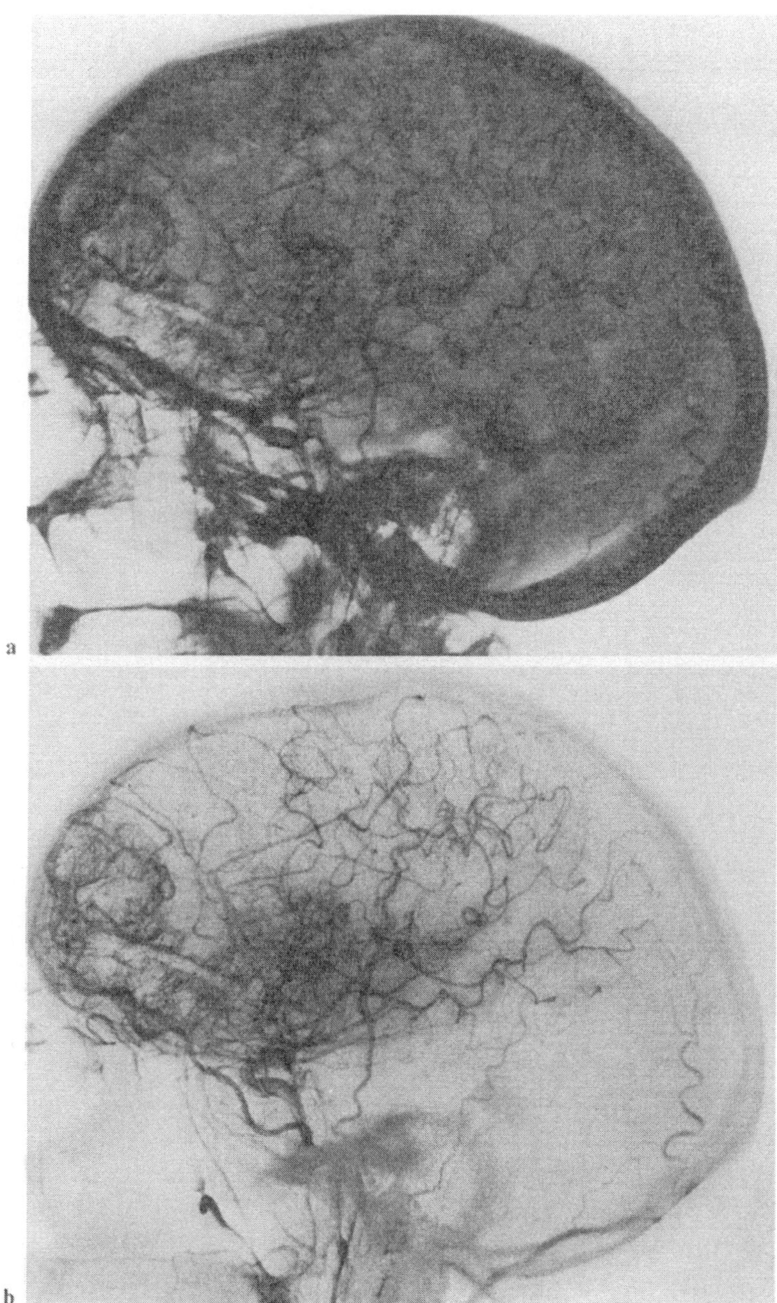

Fig. 37a and b. Glioblastoma multiforme. Man, 48 years. Technetium-scan and original films gave the impression of two separate tumors, but subtraction (**b**) disclosed the connection between them. Most irregular tumor vessels; no sharp borderline, modest dislocation. Operation: highly vascularized typical glioblastoma with bleedings and necrotic areas. Histology: glioblastoma multiforme

---

Fig. 38a–c. Glioblastoma multiforme. Two tumors. Woman, 53 years. Posterior branches of middle cerebral artery spread about a highly vascularized tumor with irregular vessels and shunts, extending wedge-shaped from the surface to midline (**c**). Besides highly malignant-looking tumor, another smaller tumor with similar vascular architecture was found in frontal lobe – in a later phase (**b**). No operation. Autopsy showed, in correspondence with angiogram, two separate tumors with same histology: glioblastoma multiforme angionecroticum. In area between tumors no pathologic changes, other than edema, were found. No tumor was found in right hemisphere ▶

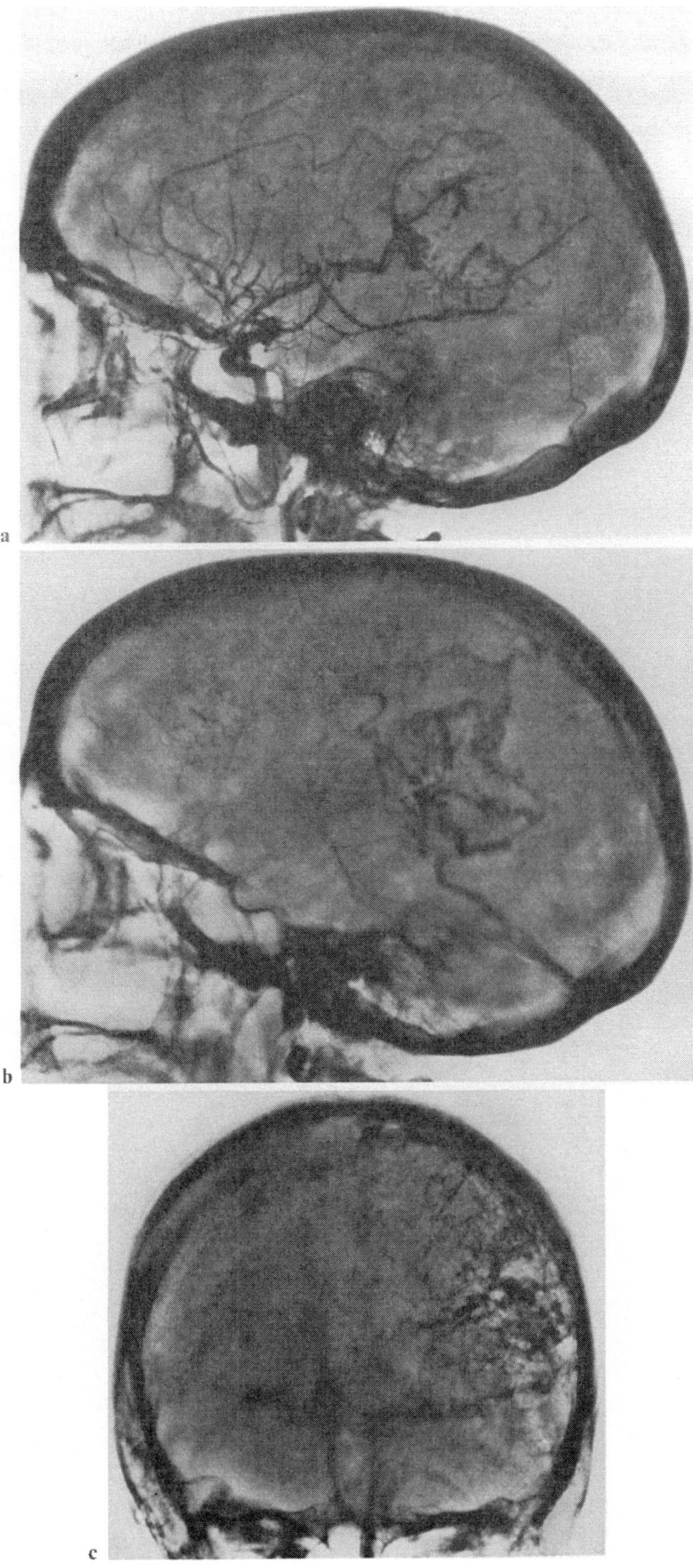
a
b
c

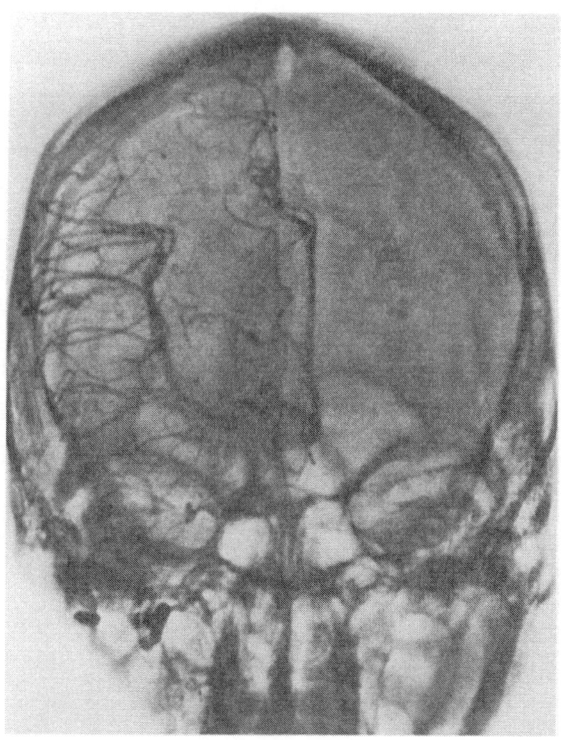

Fig. 39. Metastasis?/Glioblastoma? Man, 53 years. Operated upon for cancer coli 8 years previously; 5 years later reoperated for recurrence. 3 weeks before examination a trauma of right temple. Torpid and somnolent for 10 days without neurologic signs. Right carotid: medial dislocation of middle cerebral artery; square shift of pericallosal artery with callosomarginal sign. Stretching of lateral branches of middle cerebral artery. Operation: soft tumor, size of a hen's egg in temporal lobe. Histology: malignant, anaplastic tumor, probably glioblastoma, improbably metastasis

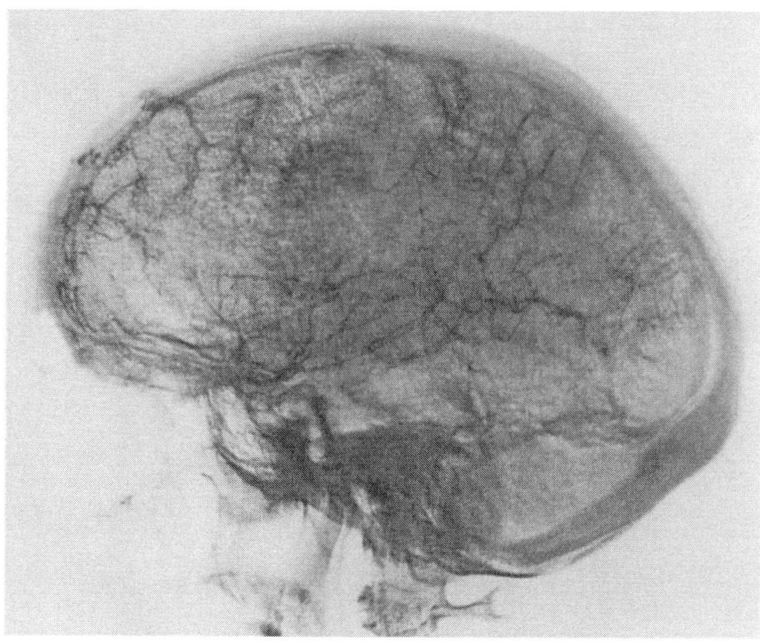

Fig. 40. Metastasis. Woman, 55 years. Cancer colli uteri stadii II 1 year previously. CAT-scanning revealed a process in middle of right hemisphere. Diffuse stain shown in the angiogram was barely visible in original film. Operation: walnut-sized tumor, infiltrating in some places. Histology: anaplastic carcinoma

About 50% of the cerebral metastases have their origin in bronchogenic carcinomas, but a multitude of primary tumors may be represented, also sarcomas. Especially in cases where no primary tumor is known, it would be most valuable if the metastatic picture could render information about the maternal tumor. Most authors agree that this is not so; only NEWTON and POOTS (1974) tell us that the metastases from hypernephromas are often highly vascularized with an abundance of wide, tortuous vessels in the arterial phase and a more or less homogeneous staining in late phases.

Having discussed the most important neoplastic supratentorial tumors, we should describe some more rarely occurring tumors in the following passage, disregarding any systematic order and omitting certain tumors which we have found less interesting from an angiographic point of view.

The *angioblastomas* (hemangioblastomas, angioreticulomas, Lindau tumors) according to ZÜLCH (1975) total 1.3% of intracranial tumors but only very few of them have been seen over the tentorium. Among the 67 Lindau tumors of KRAYENBÜHL and YAŞARGIL (1965) only five were supratentorial. ALBRECHTSEN (1971) collected 15 from the literature and added to this one patient who died without operation (Fig. 41). The carotid angiography showed a vasculated tumor in the basal ganglia; a definite angiographic diagnosis could not be made. The necropsy showed a 5×4×4 cm large, gray-red tumor situated medial to the left internal capsule, extending from hypothalamus to corpus callosum. Nothing was found in the cerebellum nor in the eyes. According to the description the tumor was not cystic. Histologic diagnosis: angioreticuloma.

WYLIE et al. (1973) presented one case in a frontal lobe; angiography showed a dense stain with arterio-venous shunt. The operation revealed a cyst of 40-ml volume with a small tumor in the wall. Histologic diagnosis: capillary hemangioblastoma, not different from the usual cerebellar hemangioblastomas. As there seems to be no difference between the supra- and infratentorial Lindau tumors, we shall leave the further discussion to part B (XIV 1/B), p. 124.

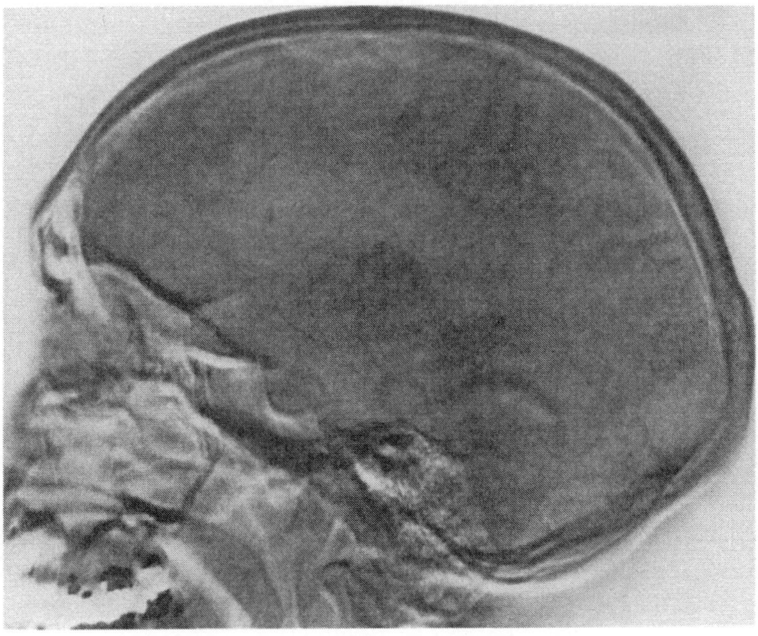

Fig. 41. Supratentorial hemangioblastoma. Man, 34 years. Increasing headache for few weeks; was unconscious at admission. Left carotid: diffuse stain and a few tortuous vessels in the region of basal ganglia. No angiographic suggestion of the nature of tumor. Patient died the day after he was admitted. Autopsy: medial to the left internal capsula a well-delineated gray-red tumor. Histology: typical angioreticuloma. Nothing was found in cerebellum

Neurinomas (neurilemmomas, Schwannomas) are smooth, encapsulated tumors of varying consistency. In Recklinghausen's neurofibromatosis they may occur on every cranial, spinal, or peripheral nerve (ZÜLCH, 1975); in the same disease they may undergo a malignant course; LIN et al. (1974) collected 120 cases of trigeminal neurinomas from the literature. It may originate from the root of the fifth nerve or from the ganglion of Gasser, and may as a dumb-bell tumor extend into the posterior and the middle fossa, thus narrowing the tentorial incisure. Destruction of the apex of the pyramid may be seen (WESTBERG, 1963). LIN et al. (1974) observed a neurinoma penetrating as an hour-glass tumor through the foramen ovale. Angiographically they are seen to be supplied from small branches of the carotid siphon as well as from branches of the middle meningeal artery; they show a regular network of delicate arteries, and they may have some resemblance to meningiomas. However, the vessels of neurinomas are more slender, the opacification less dense; veins in the capsule may be seen (NEWTON and POTTS, 1974). Extending forward they may dislocate the extradural part of the internal carotid artery – as a rule forward and medially; they may elevate the anterior choroidal artery and possibly the Sylvian group of arteries. Extending into the posterior fossa they may elevate the posterior cerebral artery and push it backward, at the same time depressing the superior cerebellar artery.

The general vascular dislocations caused by supra- and parasellar tumors of different kinds have been discussed, but here we would like to add some remarks on the vascular architecture of these different tumors.

Pituitary adenomas. The chromophobe adenomas may extend upward penetrating the sellar diaphragm (Fig. 3). The eosinophilic adenomas produce their characteristic clinical symptoms before breaking through to the optic chiasm. HATAM and GREITZ (1972) studied 13 acromegalic patients with eosinophilic or mixed adenomas; 10 of them showed suprasellar growth of the tumor. In most of the patients they were able to demonstrate a significant enlargement of the cerebral arteries; in 30 patients with chromophobe adenomas such changes were not found. The basophilic adenomas are extremely rare and rarely of any surgical significance.

The adenomas are well encapsulated; they only grow expansively without infiltration (ZÜLCH, 1975). Internal degeneration, especially in the chromophobe adenomas, may give rise to smaller or larger cysts. TAVERAS and WOOD (1964) found calcification in a few per cent of the chromophobe adenomas. In CUSHING's material (1935), of 338 pituitary adenomas 260 were chromophobe, 67 eosinophilic adenomas, and 11 carcinomas. In ZÜLCH's material (1975) of 9000 intracranial tumors the pituitary adenomas amounted to 6.6%. They are almost never seen in children; the majority of cases are between 37 and 55 years of age; this is identical for the three types. WESTBERG and ROSS (1967) in their 31 patients with chromophobe adenomas found increased vascularization in 5 cases, they found no cases with diffuse stain. POWELL et al. (1974) using magnification and subtraction were able to identify the small meningo-pituitary supplying arteries in all of their 36 cases; in all their patients they could see tumor vessels, arteries and/or veins or diffuse stain. The more or less diffuse staining indicated whether the tumor was cystic or not.

Craniopharyngiomas cause vascular dislocations which have already been described (in a rare case TAVERAS and WOOD (1964) demonstrated a 3–4-cm large craniopharyngioma only giving angiographic changes corresponding to dilatation of the lateral ventricles). In the papers of CHASE and TAVERAS (1961), KRAMER et al. (1973), HATAM and GREITZ (1972), and BACKLUND (1974) there is no reference to tumor vessels nor vascular stain. This corresponds to our own experience.

Among the supra- or parasellar tumors are mentioned the *epidermoids*. This location is second most common for this tumor. It is most frequently found in the cerebello-pontine cistern, though it may be seen in many different cisterns as well as in the ventricles. These tumors and the *dermoids* (differing from the epidermoids in that they contain hair follicles, possibly hairs, together with the glands of the skin) share in common the ability to cause dislocation of the vessels

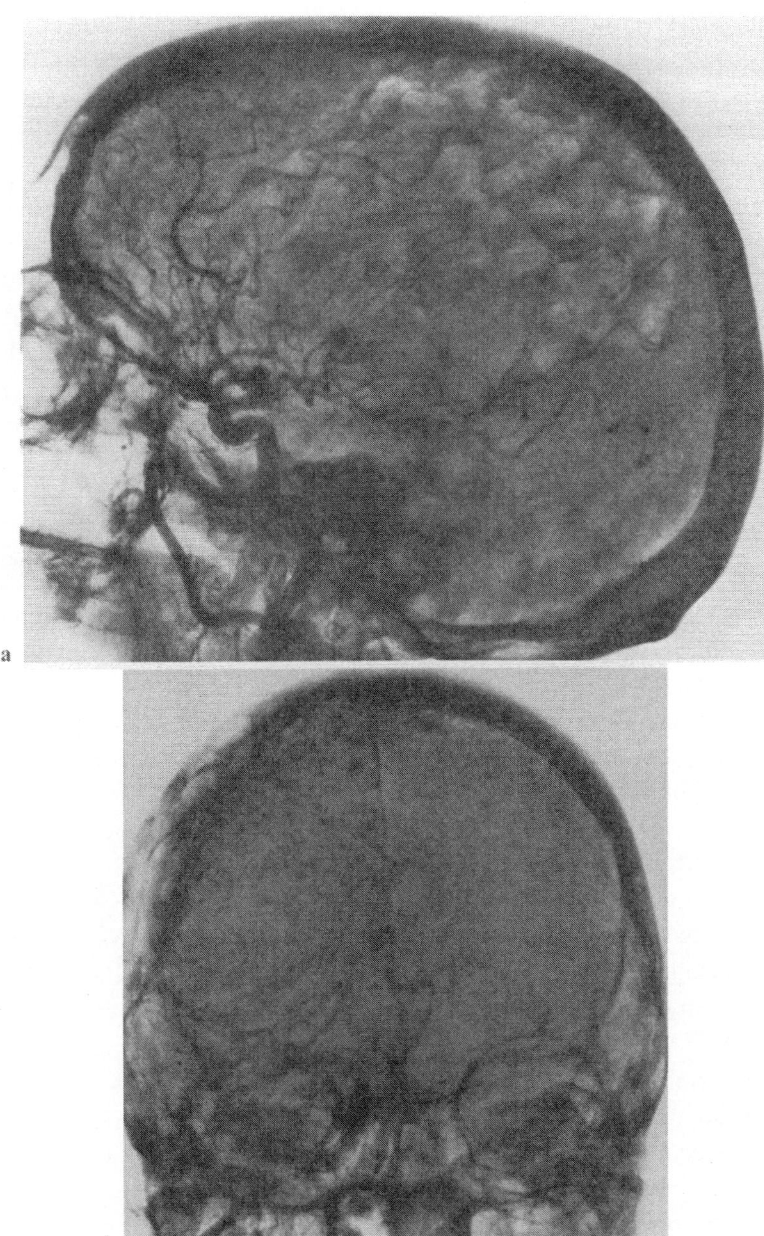

Fig. 42a and b. Cystis epidermoides regionis parietalis dx. Man, 73 years. Slight paresis of the left arm for some years. Admitted after focal seizures. Multiple internal erosions of theca several cms big. Branches of middle cerebral artery are pressed down and medially, leaving avascular zone between theca and brain. No stain or tumor vessels. Operation: large orange tumor. Histology: typical epidermoid

corresponding to their site and size; however, it must be added that the epidermoids may have a sponge-like soft structure and may find their way creeping through the cisterns without causing much vascular dislocation. They are detected easier by encephalography or – as in one of our cases – through ventriculography where the sponge-like structure was evident with the water-soluble contrast-medium (Dimer-X). The tumors show no tumor vessels or stain (Fig. 42a and b).

The *meningiomas* of the planum sphenoidale, tuberculum sellae, or the anterior clinoid processes behave like other tumors near the sella regarding dislocations and herniation. The architecture of these tumors are described on page 441.

Some rarely occurring tumors in this region are left for brief discussion. Among them the *chordoma* (ZÜLCH: 0.2%) should be mentioned. Originating from the notochord it may appear from the sacro-coccygeal region to the dorsum sellae; it is seen along the clivus, in the suboccipital region, and in the sacrococcygeal region, but in other areas of the spine we have only seen it in one patient. On the middle part of its way from Basion to dorsum sellae the notochord lies very near to the fornix pharyngis, and so the tumor may appear intracranially in the posterior fossa, extracranially in the nasopharynx, and finally again intracranially, either in the posterior fossa or near to the sella in the middle fossa. From here it may be directed backward to the tentorial notch, laterally into the temporal region, and forward to the greater wing of the sphenoid bone, which may be eroded (DECKER, 1966). In our own department we have seen a chordoma choking the middle cerebral artery. SCHECHTER et al. (1974) collected 30 intracranial chordomas, 11 of them extending into the nasopharynx, 15 showed calcification. The vascular dislocation will depend on location and size. Tumor vessels or stain are not observed; the tumor is poorly vascularized.

Among 30 extradural parasellar tumors CHASE and TAVERAS (1963) found some *carcinomas* penetrating the base of the skull from the rhinopharynx. In our own similar cases we have seen malignant-looking arteries and veins, but no diffuse stain.

Optic and chiasmatic gliomas have been described (p. 459) as polar spongioblastomas. It is difficult to decide whether the *juvenile nasal or nasopharyngeal angiofibroma* should be regarded as a tumor or as a vascular malformation, but as in certain respects it behaves like a neoplasm we feel it ought to be mentioned here together with other tumors near the sella. All the cases we know of were male patients. THIBAUT (1963) published three cases penetrating the base of the skull and extending intracranially. From our department we have published one of our cases (SIEMSSEN et al., 1967) on account of its large extension extra- and intracranially and on account of the dramatic circumstances connected to the operation. Before the operation it was shown that the right internal carotid did not take part in the supply. The tumor was fed by both external carotid arteries, the left internal, and numerous branches from the basilar artery. Tumor vessels of benign character and a certain degree of diffuse stain were noted in the extra- as well as in the intracranial portion of the tumor. No arteriovenous shunts were observed.

Lipomas are rarely occurring tumors which may be seen in different places. Most commonly it is found in connexion with total or partial agenesis of the corpus callosum as a sharply delineated mass in the midline. In cases where the pneumoencephalography or the carotid angiography show the characteristic signs of an agenesia, one will often find a thin, medially concave line of calcification symmetrically on either side of the midline. Tumor vessels are not described.

Intracranial primary sarcomas are rarely occurring tumors, some of them originating from the meninges, some in the brain cells and some in the borderlands, the periadventitial reticulo-endothelial cells in the Virchow-Robin spaces. There seems to be a great variability in the macro- and microscopic appearance, so that it has been as yet impossible to establish a constant nomenclature. Some of these extra- or intracerebral sarcomas are hard and macroscopically well-delineated tumors; others are more infiltrative than space-occupying; so some of them will show dislocations of the vessels depending on their location, others will not. In the same way the vascular architecture will differ from case to case. LEEDS et al. (1971) published two cases of what they called cerebral malignant lymphoma. Using magnification technique they demonstrated fine, wavy vessels located around bigger vessels because the tumor originates from the perivascular histiocytes. KRAYENBÜHL and YAŞARGIL (1965) have one picture which corresponds exactly to these two cases. WECHSLER and TOMIYASU (1974) had two cerebral sarcomas showing a very active uptake in gamma-scintigraphy, but negative or equivocal responses in pneumoencephalography and angiography.

With this we do not pretend to have mentioned all neoplasms occurring in the cranial cavity; some of them are beyond angiographic interest, others occur so rarely that they may be said to have been hardly classified till now.

V. Abscesses

The importance of making this diagnosis correctly was illustrated by GARFIELD (1969) who reported a mortality of 81% in patients in whom ventriculography and angiography failed to localize the abscess. The possibility of obtaining a topographic and/or histologic diagnosis varies with different materials. In a paper from our own department NIELSEN and HALABURT (1976) discussed 36 cases: one with a normal angiogram, 20 with uncharacteristic signs of a space-occupying mass, and 19 with a characteristic abscess membrane; in 5 of these 19 cases the membrane was only visualized by subtraction. In 3 cases multiple abscesses were found. (These authors, like GARFIELD, emphasized that lumbar puncture must be regarded as contraindicated, but it was still performed in 26 cases with normal fluid in 13 patients.)

The demonstration of the membrane seems to be a little more frequent in this material than in others, e.g., SEGALL et al. (1973) found capsular vasculation in 20%. Such differences may find their explanation in a fact stressed by ZÜLCH (1975): the fresh and ill-defined inflammatory phlegmon is different from the (older) well-encapsulated abscess; this is in correspondance with the findings of LECUIN et al. (1966) and JORDAN et al. (1972) who recommended that the angiography should be repeated if the first is negative. JORDAN et al. (1972) referred to four negative angiograms, two of which turned to positive findings after three weeks.

The characteristic angiographic picture is that of a space-occupying mass, often round, often the size of a walnut, dislocating the neighboring vessels. The central part is avascular; the periphery may be highly vascularized as a rule with unsharp borders to the surroundings (Fig. 43a and b – see also 44a and b). No doubt this "image en cocarde ou en anneau" (LECUIN et al., 1966) is of double origin: the abscess itself will develop its own vasculated capsule, and in the surrounding brain tissue one will meet some degree of vascular compression and some neoplastic vessels on inflammatory base. Thus it is obvious that fine arterio-venous shunts may occur (LECUIN et al., 1966; SEGALL et al., 1973; NIELSEN and HALABURT, 1976). SANCHES and CHASE (1965) reported the history of a 3-year-old girl with bad anamnestic information. Angiography showed a slight shift of the anterior cerebral artery; and many small, early occurring veins were seen in the posterior part of the frontal lobe; the diagnosis hereafter, naturally enough, was that of an infiltrating glioblastoma, but the operation disclosed an abscess containing 10 ml of pus. This abscess must have represented a transitional phase between the plegmoneous and the ripe state of development. Probably the same is the case with four abscesses showing a diffuse homogeneous blush, almost circumscribed, mentioned by LEEDS et al. (1971). In some cases abscesses are misinterpreted as metastases, this may happen particularly when more than one "tumor" is found in the same patient. JORDAN et al. (1972) performed gamma-scanning on 17 patients with brain abscesses; all the scans were positive. We are convinced we will be able to reach a similar result with CT-scanning.

VI. Edema

Little should be said about the general edematous state. It is well known that a unilateral edema, e.g., a traumatic edema, may cause a shift of the midline vessels and some spreading and stretching of the ipsilateral vessels. The edema accompanying other space-occupying processes has been discussed in the foregoing passages. What is more interesting in this connection are some reports on local, nonpurulent inflammation or local edema. MARGOLIS et al. (1972) reported on a epileptic man, 31 years of age, who after having had influenza became confused and somnolent without focal neurologic signs. Gamma-scan showed uptake in the left frontal lobe, carotid angiography gave an unsharply defined area with pathologic vessels and shunts near the frontal pole. He was operated upon; the firm, granuloma-like tissue gave the histologic diagnosis: inflam-

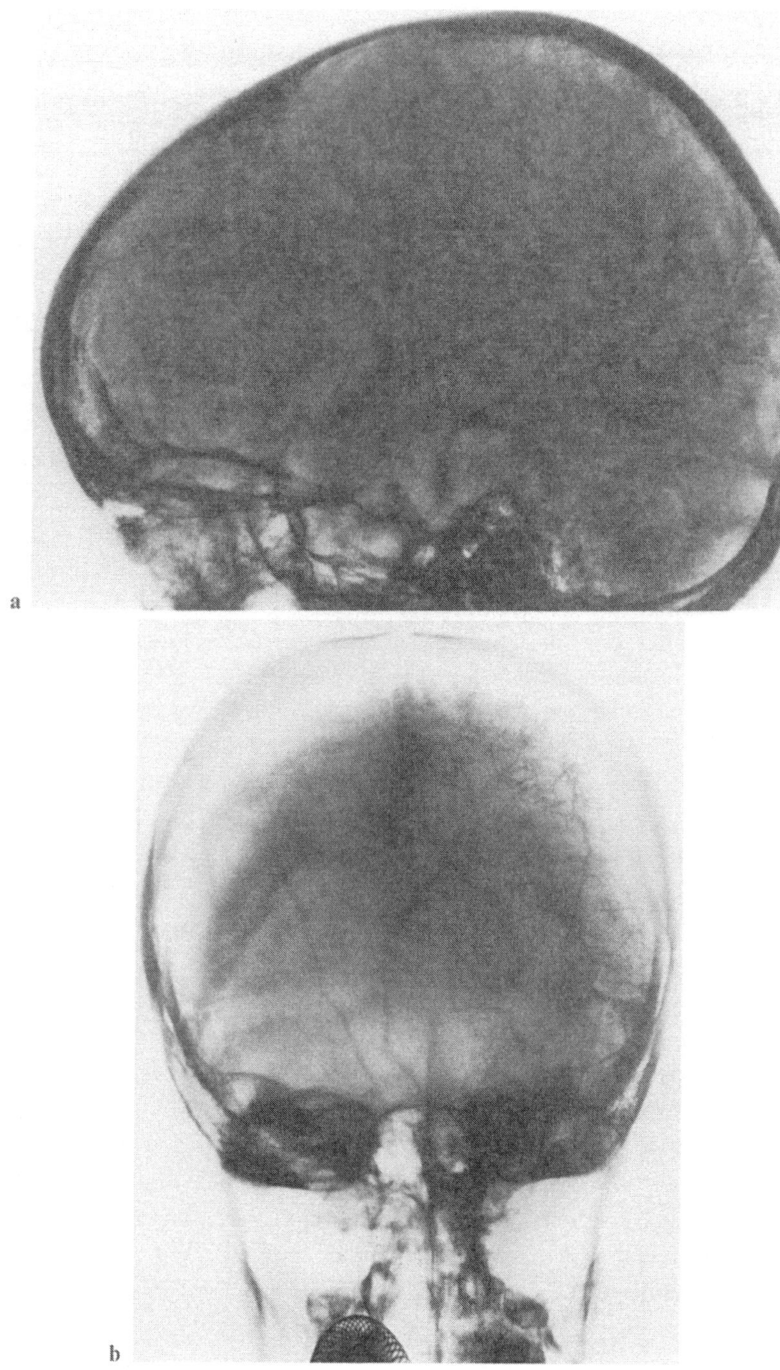

Fig. 43a and b. Cerebral abscess. Boy, $9^1/_2$ years. Treated for tonsillitis for 1 month. Increasingly torpidity, vomiting, paresis of the left oculomotor nerve. Papiledema. Admitted as urgent case. Left carotid: very large ponto-basal expanding lesion, limited by a distinct capsule. Diagnosis: abscess. 90 ml of pus was evacuated through frontal bore-hole

mation, subacute leucoencephalitis of undetermined type. Here the question concerned an inflammation, but this is not the case in the following papers: LEHRER and BHATRAHALLY VENKATESH (1973) mentioned six epileptics, examined shortly after seizures. Stretching and straightening was seen in superficial arteries in the frontal operculum; the authors interpreted the anomalies as a damage of the blood-brain barrier, followed by local edema. FARRELL and TAVERAS (1974)

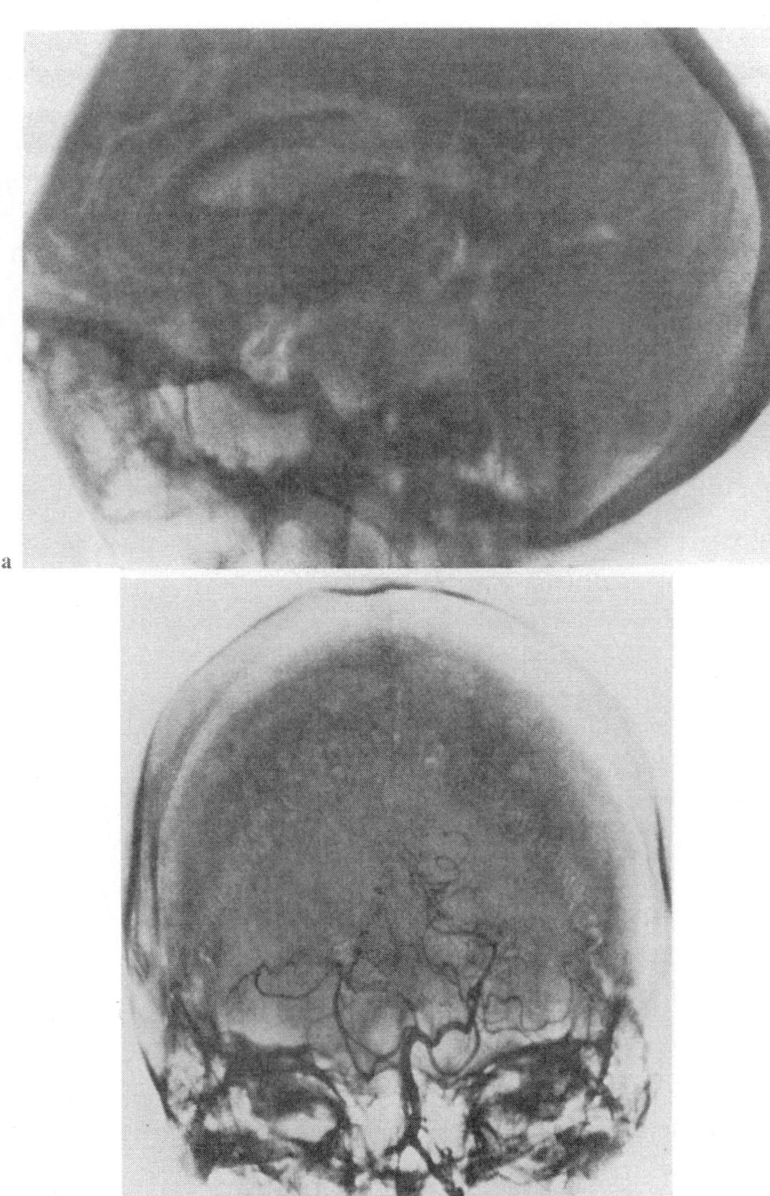

Fig. 44a and b. Abscessus extracerebralis. Man, 52 years. Paresis of right oculomotor nerve and pleocytosis of spinal fluid was found by another hospital 1 year previously. Encephalography in our department disclosed a 3 cm large round mass behind and to the right of the dorsum sellae. Carotid angiography showed nothing but an elevation of anterior choroidal artery. One tentative diagnosis was a craniopharyngioma, but considering the possibility of an aneurysm on basilar artery, a vertebral angiography was performed: a slender right posterior cerebral artery was displaced upward and medially in a bow. No aneurysm. No tumor vessels. Operation: a bull-formed mass, not adherent to any part of brain, but surrounded by leptomeningeal adhesions. Histologic diagnosis: abscess

reported the history of a woman aged 43 years. Thirteen days *post partum* she had repeated focal seizures resulting in status epilepticus. An angiography during the seizures showed an early filling of the deep veins "a pathological mixing of arterial and venous phases." Nine days later a repeated angiography was normal. The cause of the changes is supposed to have been local anoxia.

VII. Granulomas

From an angiographic point of view these lesions play a very moderate role. Tuberculomas and gummas act as space-occupying lesions, but the only statement of pathologic vessels we have seen is found in WICKBOM's dissertation (1948). In his material two gummas are included; in one of them "small irregular vessels were observed in the process." Eosinophilic granulomas from the theca may infiltrate dura and the brain; granulomas from actinomycosis and from Hodgkin's desease have been described (ZÜLCH, 1975), the same is the case with different fungi and with some parasites. Meningeal and, more rarely, intracerebral granulomas of sarcoidosis are known. They behave like other space-occupying lesions; tumor vessels or stain were not reported (SILVERSTEIN et al., 1965).

VIII. Parasites

As already mentioned, the parasites occurring in schistosomiasis, paragonomiasis, and coccidiosis may produce granulomas; the same is true for trichinosis in which the granulomas are calcified when they are discovered. Cysticercus cellulosae may be seen in the brain and in the meninges; they appear as calcifications with the form and size of a lens. *Echinococci* are solitary as a rule, but they may grow to the size of a goose egg. They are avascular, but due to their size they may cause considerable vascular dislocations. KRAYENBÜHL and YAŞARGIL (1965) presented three pictures with dislocations but no signs of pathologic vasculation; in one of the pictures the elevation of the Sylvian group of arteries is monstrous. In toxoplasmosis we have only performed very few angiographies, and apart from the hydrocephalic changes we have found nothing abnormal.

D. Auxilliary Devices

Different methods have been used to enhance the possibilities of the exact interpretation of angiograms. First among them should be mentioned the *subtraction*, which is in our opinion the most indispensable of these methods. ZIEDSES DES PLANTES invented the method in 1934 and has given an excellent account of the idea and the practical use of it in his monograph in 1961. As the correct performance depended on an efficient photographer, many departments bought the electronic television apparatuses, but the general impression was that the quality never reached that of the photographic procedure. After the appearance of simple photographic devices with special film material (COIN and MARTCHENKE, 1974) most neuroradiologic departments have returned to the photographic method – as can be seen from many of the papers quoted in this chapter, most neuroradiologists feel they cannot do without subtraction. Different methods of color subtraction have been attempted; the only reliable method seems to be that of DJINDIAN (1964) and LILIEQUIST and WELANDER (1969) which gives information of the exact time of appearance and disappearance of different groups of vessels. The same information is obtained by the sequential subtraction described by RIVOIR and HUBER (1974). The authors are very modest in saying "only in exceptional cases will this method add important facts to the diagnosis which is usually already present on the original films or the normal subtractions."

Body-section radiography (tomography) has been used by many authors. Many departments suffer from the fact that it is necessary to move the patient from one room to another during the angiographic procedure, but this is not the case in RAMELLA and ROSA (1974) who seem to have obtained excellent results with linear plesio-sectional tomography on Barazzeti's craniotome.

In some clinics body-section radiography is used in combination with the magnification technique. This for instance was the case in DECK et al. (1972) who used a 0.3 mm focus; a magnification factor of 1.5 and circular body-section radiography with multisectional cassette. Concerning the magnification per se we are not convinced that the 0.3 mm focus is small enough to give such enhanced information, that must be paid by a serious increase of the roentgen-dose. WENDE et al. (1973) worked with a 0.1 mm focus producing impressive results, partly due to the small focus, partly to the use of hypercapnia and hypertension.

Different methods of producing *stereoscopic angiograms* have been described. The most ingenious apparatus, which gives the best results is in our opinion the old apparatus found in Temple University, Philadelphia, constructed by CHAMBERLAIN in the early fifties and described by STAUFFER et al. (1955). So far as we know it has never been on the market.

The *cinematographic procedure* was made possible after the introduction of the image-amplifier. In our department we have never obtained satisfying results, but KLAUSBERGER has in his department in Vienna.

New types of films have been introduced. The *blue Medichrome film* and its use for cerebral angiographic purposes was described by BORIES (1971). We have had occasion to study the method, and corresponding to the comments made by BORIES, it is our impression that this method gives a kind of dodging and some degree of a subtraction-like effect. Recently we have started experiments with *xerography* in certain neuroradiologic examinations, but as the paper films are not available for serial angiography we have no experience in this field.

References

ALBRECHTSEN, R.: Supra-tentorial haemangioblastoma. Dan. med. Bull. **18**, 73–75 (1971)

ANDERSEN, P.E.: The lenticulostriate arteries and their diagnostic value. Acta radiol. (Stockh.) **50**, 84–91 (1958)

ANDERSEN, P.E.: Angiographic localization of small intracerebral haematomas. Acta radiol. [diagn.] (Stockh.) **1**, 173–181 (1963)

AZAMBUJA, N., LINDGREN, E., SJÖGREN, S.E.: Tentorial herniations, I Anatomy. Acta radiol. (Stockh.) **46**, 215–223 (1956a)

AZAMBUJA, N., LINDGREN, E., SJÖGREN, S.E.: Tentorial herniations, III Angiography. Acta radiol. (Stockh.) **46**, 232–241 (1956b)

AZAR-KIA, B., SARWAR, M., SCHECHTER, M., VALSAMIS, M.: Demarcated glioblastoma multiforme and prolonged angiographic tumor stain. Neuroradiol. **8**, 163–166 (1974)

BACKLUND, E.-O.: Radiographic staining of a solid craniopharyngioma in vivo. Neuroradiol. **7**, 37–39 (1974)

BANNA, M.: Angiography of malignant choroid plexus papilloma. Brit. J. Radiol. **44**, 412–415 (1971)

BATNITZKY, S., SARWAR, M., LEEDS, N., SCHECHTER, M., AZAR-KIA, B.: Colloid cysts of the third ventricle. Radiology **112**, 327–341 (1974)

BAUMGARTEN, M., KEMPERDICK, H.: Die Diagnose der Arachnoidalzysten durch die Pneumenzephalographie. Fort. Geb. Roent.-Strahlen u. Nukl. Med. **118**, 630–635 (1973)

BERNASCONI, U., CASSINARI, V.: Un segno carotidografico tipico di meningioma del tentorio. Chirurgia (Milano) **11**, 586–588 (1956)

BORIES, J.: Radiographic images on medichrome film. X-ray Bull. **18**, 14–15 (1971)

BULL, D.: Radiology of the pituitary. Proc. Aust. Ass. Neurol. **9**, 199–204 (1973)

CHASE, N., TAVERAS, J.: Cerebral angiography in the diagnosis of suprasellar tumors. Amer. J. Roentgenol. **86**, 154–165 (1961)

CHASE, N., TAVERAS, J.: Carotid angiography in the diagnosis of extradural parasellar tumors. Acta radiol. [Diagn.] (Stockh.) **1**, 214–224 (1963)

COIN, C., MARTCHENKE, E.: A technique to improve visual perception characteristics of subtracted Roentgenograms. Neuroradiol. **8**, 95–97 (1974)

CRONQVIST, S.: Radiologic changes in descending herniation over the sphenoid ridge. Acta radiol. [Diagn.] (Stockh.) **3**, 289–296 (1965)

CRONQVIST, S.: Angiography and cerebral blood flow in malignant glioma. Acta radiol. [Ther.] (Stockh.) **8**, 78–85 (1967)

CRONQVIST, S., KÖHLER, R.: Angiography in epidural haematomas. Acta radiol. [Diagn.] (Stockh.) **1**, 42–52 (1963)

CUSHING, H.: Intrakranielle Tumoren. Berlin: Springer, 1935

DECK, M., GROSSMAN, C., MOODY, D., POTTS, D.: Clinical experience with circular angiotomography. Radiology **105**, 591–595 (1972)

DECKER, K.: Clinical neuroradiology. New York: McGraw-Hill, 1966

DEE, D., WOESNER, M., SANDERS, I., BIGGERS, S.: Biloculated intracranial arachnoid cyst in a neonate. Amer. J. Dis. Child. **127**, 700–702 (1974)

DJINDIAN, R.: L'angiographie en couleurs en neuroradiologie. Atlas Radiol. clin. **72**, 1–4 (1964)

ETHELBERG, S., VAERNET, K.: The angiographic configuration of intracerebral metastatic tumors. Radiology **61**, 39–48 (1953)

FALK, B.: Radiologic diagnosis of intraventricular meningiomas. Acta radiol. (Stockh.) **46**, 171–177 (1955)

FARRELL, F., TAVERAS, J.: Angiographic stain produced by seizures. Neuroradiol. **8**, 49–53 (1974)

FERRIS, E., CIEMBRONICWICZ, J.: Subdural empyema. Report of a case demonstrating the unusual angiographic triad. Amer. J. Roentgenol. **92**, 838–843 (1964)

FITZ, C., HARWOOD-NASH, D., THOMPSON, J.: Neuroradiology of tuberous sclerosis in children. Radiology **110**, 635–642 (1974)

GALLOWAY, J., GREITZ, T.: The medial and lateral choroid arteries. An anatomic and radiographic study. Acta radiol. (Stockh.) **53**, 353–366 (1960)

GARFIELD, J.: Management of supratentorial intracranial abscess: a review of 200 cases. Brit. med. J. **2**, 7–11 (1969)

GLICKMAN, M., MCNAMAR, T., MARGOLIS, M.: Arteriographic diagnosis of subtemporal subdural hematoma. Radiology **109**, 607–615 (1973)

GREGORIUS, F., BENTSON, J.: Comparison of radiological tests in the detection of pressellar meningiomas. Neuroradiol. **8**, 267–274 (1975)

GREITZ, T.: Angiography in tuberculous meningitis. Acta radiol. [Diagn.] (Stockh.) **2**, 369–378 (1964)

GVOZDANOVIĆ, V.: Changes in the superficial veins in cases of intracranial expanding processes. Acta radiol. (Stockh.) **46**, 195–202 (1955)

HANDEL, S., KLEIN, W., YONG, WOO KIM: Intracranial epidural abscess. Radiology **111**, 117–120 (1974)

HARA, K., FUJINO, Y.: The thalamoperforate artery. Acta radiol. [Diagn.] (Stockh.) **5**, 192–200 (1966)

HATAM, A., GREITZ, T.: Ectasia of cerebral arteries in acromegaly. Acta radiol. [Diagn.] (Stockh.) **12**, 410–418 (1972)

HEISKANEN, O.: Cerebral circulatory arrest caused by acute increase of intracranial pressure: a clinical and roentgenological study of 25 cases. Acta neurol. scand. Suppl. **7**, 1–57 (1964)

HILAL, S., SOLOMON, G., GOLD, A., CARTER, S.: Primary cerebral arterial occlusive disease in children. Radiology **99**, 87–93 (1971)

HOOSHMAND, I., ROSENBAUN, A., STEIN, R.: Radiographic anatomy of normal cerebral deep medullary veins, criteria for distinguishing them from their abnormal counterparts. Neuroradiol. **7**, 75–84 (1974)

HOYT, W.: Vascular lesions of the visual cortex with brain herniation through the tentorial incisura: neuroophtalmologic considerations. Arch. Ophtal. (Chicago) **64**, 44–57 (1960)

HUANG, Y., WOLF, B.: Veins of the white matter of the cerebral hemispheres (the medullary veins), diagnostic importance in carotid angiography. Amer. J. Roentgenol. **92**, 739–755 (1964)

HUANG, Y., WOLF, B.: Precentral cerebellar vein in angiography. Acta radiol. [Diagn.] (Stockh.) **5**, 250–262 (1966)

JACOBSEN, H.H.: An interhemispherically situated haematoma. Acta radiol. (Stockh.) **43**, 235–236 (1955)

JACOBSEN, H.H., OLIVARIUS, B.: Neuroradiologically latent intracranial tumours, (Danish with English summary). Nord. Med. **76**, 940–946 (1966)

JACOBSEN, H.H., VRAA-JENSEN, G.: Fibrous dysplasia of bone. Acta radiol. (Stockh.) **31**, 1–16 (1949)

JOHNSON, R., YATES, P.: Clinico-pathological aspects of pressure changes af the tentorium. Acta radiol. (Stockh.) **46**, 242–249 (1956a)

JOHNSON, R., YATES, P.: Brain stem haemorrhages in expanding supratentorial conditions. Acta radiol. (Stockh.) **46**, 250–256 (1956b)

JORDAN, C., JAMES, E., HODGES, F.: Comparison of the cerebral angiogram and the brain radionucleide image in brain abscess. Radiology **104**, 327–331 (1972)

KALAN, C., BURROWS, E.: Calcification in intracranial gliomata. Brit. J. Radiol. **35**, 589–602 (1962)

KATZ, M., KIER, E., SCHECHTER, M.: The radiology of gangliogliomas and ganglioneuromas of the central nervous system. Neuroradiol. **4**, 69–73 (1972)

KENDALL, B.: Invasion of the facial bones by basal meningiomas. Brit. J. Radiol. **46**, 237–244 (1973)

KIEFFER, S., LARSON, D., GOLD, L., PRENTICE, W., STADLAN, E., SEYFERT, S.: Rapid circulation in intracranial meningiomas. Radiology **106**, 575–580 (1973)

KLAUSBERGER, E.: Angiographic recognition of cerebral metastases via the external carotid artery in the presence of occlusion of the internal carotid artery. Neuroradiol. **4**, 60–62 (1972)

KRAMER, R., POOLE, G., MOODY, D., NEWTON, T.: Angiography in craniopharyngiomas. Radiology **109**, 99–103 (1973)

KRAYENBÜHL, H., YASARGIL, M.: Die zerebrale Angiographie, 2nd ed. Stuttgart: Thieme, 1965

LECUIN, J., BUFFARD, P., GOUTELLE, A., THIERRY, A., DECHAUME, J., KOFMAN, J.: Considérations sur les aspects angiographiques des abscès du cerveau. Acta radiol. [Diagn.] (Stockh.) **5**, 315–319 (1966)

LEEDS, N., GOLDBERG, H.: Angiographic manifestations in cerebral inflammatory disease. Radiology **98**, 595–604 (1971)

Leeds, N., Rosenblatt, R., Zimmermann, H.: Focal angiographic changes of cerebral lymphoma with pathologic correlation; a report of two cases. Radiology **99**, 595–599 (1971)

Lehrer, H., Bhatrahally Venkatesh: Angiographic evidence for cerebral (opercular) swelling in patients with seizures. Amer. J. Roentgenol. **118**, 586–593 (1973)

Liliequist, B., Welander, U.: Colour in subtraction angiography. Preliminary report. Acta radiol. [Diagn.] (Stockh.) **8**, 1–4 (1969)

Liliequist, B., Welander, U.: Colour combination images in cerebral angiography. Neuroradiol. **1**, 39–41 (1970)

Lin, J., Siew, F.: Glioblastoma multiforme presenting angiographically as intracranial atherosclerotic vascular disease. Radiology **101**, 353–354 (1971)

Lin, S.R., Lin, Z.S., Tatoian, I.A.: Trigenimal neurinoma with extracranial extension. Neuroradiol. **8**, 183–185 (1974)

Lindblom, K.: A roentgenographic study of the vascular channels of the skull. Acta radiol. (Stockh.) Suppl. **30**, Stockholm 1936

Löfgren, F.: Vertebral angiography in the diagnosis of tumours in the pineal region. Acta radiol. (Stockh.) **50**, 108–124 (1958)

Margolis, M., Glickman, M., Hoff, J.: Focal encephalitis simulating neoplasm. Neuroradiol. **4**, 3–5 (1972)

McGrath, T., Sonderheimer, F.: How reliable is the middle meningeal artery in the diagnosis of small epidural haematomas? Brit. J. Radiol. **46**, 131–138 (1973)

Merten, D., Gooding, C., Newton, T.: The radiographic features of meningiomas in childhood and adolescense. Pediatr. Radiol. **2**, 89–96 (1974)

Meyer, A.: Herniation of the brain. Arch. Neurol. Psychiat. (Chicago) **4**, 387–400 (1920)

Newton, T., Potts, D.: Radiology of the skull and brain. Saint Louis: C.V. Mosby, 1974

Nielsen, H., Halaburt, H.: Central abscess with special reference to the angiographic changes. Neuroradiol. **12**, 73–78 (1976)

Osborn, A., Poole, G.: Angiographic signs of corpus callosum tumours: a reappraisal. Radiology **115**, 97–105 (1975)

Patriquin, H.: The bobble-head doll syndrome. A curable entity. Radiology **107**, 171–172 (1973)

Plaut, H.: Size of tentorial incisure related to cerebral herniation. Acta radiol. [Diagn.] (Stockh.) **1**, 916–928 (1963)

Potts, D., Taveras, J.: Differential diagnosis of space-occupying lesions in the region of the thalamus by cerebral angiography. Acta radiol. [Diagn.] (Stockh.) **1**, 373–384 (1963)

Powell, D., Baker, H., Laws, E.: The primary angiographic findings in pituitary adenomas. Radiology **110**, 589–595 (1974)

Ramella, G., Rosa, M.: Angiotomographic study of the normal cerebral circulation. Neuroradiol. **8**, 15–23 (1974)

Rivoir, R., Huber, P.: Sequential subtraction. Neuroradiol. **7**, 85–89 (1974)

Robinson, G.: The temporal lobe agenesis syndrome. Brain. **87**, 87–106 (1964)

Rosencrantz, M., Stattin, S.: Extradural meningiomas. Report of two cases. Acta radiol. [Diagn.] (Stockh.) **12**, 419–427 (1972)

Sackett, J., Stenswig, J., Songsirikul, P.: Meningeal and glial tumours in combination. Neuroradiol. **7**, 153–160 (1974)

Sanches, G., Chase, N.: Early venous filling in a case of well encapsulated intracerebral abscess. Acta radiol. [Diagn.] (Stockh.) **3**, 61–64 (1965)

Schechter, M., Liebeskind, A., Azar-Kia, B.: Intracranial chordomas. Neuroradiol. **8**, 67–82 (1974)

Segall, H., Rumbaugh, C., Bergeron, R., Teal, J., Gwinn, J.: Brain and meningeal infections in children. Radiologic considerations. Neuroradiol. **6**, 8–16 (1973)

Siemssen, S., Münster, E., Lester, J., Thorshauge, C., Arnfred, J., Rygg, I., Borgeskov, S., Riishede, J., Amris, J., Engel, K., Laursen, T., Andersen, M., Neukirch, F.: Langvarig dyb hypotermi med induceret kredsløbsstandsning ved eksstirpation af angiofibrom i rhinopharynx (Danish with English summary). Ugeskr. Læg. **129**, 586–600 (1967)

Silverstein, A., Feuer, M., Siltzbach, L.: Neurologic sarcoidosis, Arch. Neurol. (Paris) **12**, 1–11 (1965)

Starkman, S., Brown, P., Linell, E.: Cerebral arachnoid cysts. J. Neuropath. exp. Neurol. **17**, 484–500 (1958)

Stattin, S.: Significance of some angiographic signs of intracranial meningiomas. Acta radiol. [Diagn.] (Stockh.) **5**, 530–535 (1966)

Stauffer, H., Murtagh, F., Mokrohisky, J., Paul, R., jr.: Biplane stereoscopic cerebral angiography. Acta radiol. (Stockh.) **46**, 262–272 (1955)

Stövring, J.: Kinking of the supraclinoid segment of the internal carotia artery over neighbouring, anatomic structures in acute and subacute intracranial mass lesions. Amer. J. Roentgenol. **104**, 75–82 (1968)

Taveras, J., Wood, E.: Diagnostic neuroradiology. Baltimore, Md.: Williams and Wilkins, 1964

Telenius, R.: Angiographic appearance of angioblastic meningiomas. Acta radiol. [Diagn.] (Stockh.) **5**, 554–569 (1966)

Thibaut, A.: Angiographie carotidienne élective dans le diagnostic et le traitement des angiofibromes nasopharyngiens. Acta radiol. [Diagn.] (Stockh.) **1**, 468–480 (1963)

Tod, P., Porter, A., Jamieson, K.: Pineal tumors. Amer. J. Roentgenol. **120**, 19–26 (1974)

Traub, S.: Roentgenology of intracranial meningiomas. Springfield, Ill.: Charles C Thomas, 1961

TREVISAN, C., DETTORI, P.: Diagnostic problems of cerebral metastases. Neuroradiol. **3**, 216–223 (1972)

VESIN, S., BOHUTORA, J.: Angiographische Befunde bei entzündlichen intrakraniellen Prozessen. Fort. Geb. Roent.-Strahlen u. Nukl. Med. **117**, 250–261 (1972)

WECHSLER, A., TOMIYASU, U.: An unusual radiographical brain scan dissociation pattern with reticulum cell sarcoma (microglioma) of the brain. Bull. Los Angeles neurol. Soc. **39**, 1–8 (1974)

WELCH, K., CRAIGMILE, T.: Kinking of the internal carotid artery over the optic nerve and chiasm in acute intra-cranial mass lesions. Acta radiol. [Diagn.] (Stockh.) **1**, 509–512 (1963)

WENDE, S., NAKAYAMA, N., PALVOLGYI, R., SCHINDLER, K.: Comparison of cerebral scintigraphy with magnification angiography under hyperventilation in cerebral tumors. Neuroradiol. **6**, 78–82 (1973)

WESTBERG, G.: Angiographic changes in neurinoma of the trigeminal nerve. Acta radiol. [Diagn.] (Stockh.) **1**, 513–520 (1963)

WESTBERG, G., ROSS, R.: The vascular supply of chromophobe adenomas. Acta radiol. [Diagn.] (Stockh.) **6**, 475–480 (1967)

WICKBOM, I.: Angiography of the carotid artery. Acta radiol. (Stockh.) Suppl. **72**. Stockholm, 1948

WICKBOM, I.: Angiographic determination of tumour pathology. Acta radiol. (Stockh.) **40**, 529–546 (1953)

WOLF, B., HUANG, Y.: Diagnostic value of cerebral veins on mass lesions of the brain. Radiol. Clin. N. Amer. **4**, 117–130 (1966)

WYLIE, I., JEFFREYS, R., MAC LAINE, G.: Cerebral haemangioblastoma. Brit. J. Radiol. **46**, 472–476 (1973)

ZACHRISSON, L.: Angiography of cerebral metastases. Acta radiol. [Diagn.] (Stockh.) **1**, 521–527 (1963)

ZIEDSES DES PLANTES, B.: Subtraktion. Stuttgart: Thieme, 1961

ZIEDSES DES PLANTES, B.: Application of the roentgenographic subtraction method in neuroradiology. Acta radiol. [Diagn.] (Stockh.) **1**, 961–966 (1963)

ZÜLCH, K.: Atlas of Gross Neurosurgical Pathology. Berlin-Heidelberg-New York: Springer 1975

Zerebrale Aneurysmen und Angiome

Von

PETER HUBER

Mit 47 Abbildungen

A. Die sackförmigen Aneurysmen der Hirnarterien

I. Überblick

Die ersten klinischen Symptome eines arteriellen Aneurysmas sind gewöhnlich durch seine Ruptur und eine Subarachnoidalblutung verursacht (sog. apoplektischer Typus). Nach der großen Zusammenstellung von LOCKSLEY (1966), die auf 6368 Fällen basiert, sind sackförmige Aneurysmen mit 51% die bei weitem häufigste Ursache von Subarachnoidalblutungen. In 15% ist eine Subarachnoidalblutung durch eine hypertonische arteriosklerotische Gefäßerkrankung und in 6% durch eine arteriovenöse Mißbildung bedingt. In 6% wurden verschiedene weitere Ursachen angeschuldigt, und in 22% konnte weder klinisch noch angiographisch oder autoptisch eine Ursache für die Blutung gefunden werden.

Nach der gleichen Untersuchung ereignet sich die erste Subarachnoidalblutung in 62% aller Fälle im Alter zwischen 40 und 64 Jahren, wobei der Häufigkeitsgipfel der Aneurysmaruptur zwischen dem 50. und 54. Lebensjahr liegt. Demgegenüber erfolgt die erste Blutung aus einer arteriovenösen Mißbildung in 63% der Fälle im Alter von 20 und 49 Jahren, also bei etwas jüngeren Patienten, wobei aber kein eindeutiger Altersgipfel festzustellen ist. Die Subarachnoidalblutungen anderer Genese treffen vorwiegend etwas ältere Menschen.

1. Manifestierung der Aneurysmen. (Nach LOCKSLEY, 1966)

bis zum 20. Lebensjahr	1,6%	
zwischen 20. und 40. Lebensjahr	16,2%	
zwischen 40. und 50. Lebensjahr	24,6%	55,2%
zwischen 50. und 60. Lebensjahr	30,6%	
jenseits des 60. Lebensjahres	27,0%	

Bis zum 39. Lebensjahr überwiegen die Männer leicht, vom 40. Lebensjahr an tritt die Aneurysmaruptur etwas häufiger bei Frauen auf. Werden alle Altersgruppen zusammengefaßt, so sind 41% der Patienten Männer und 59% Frauen.

Die Mehrzahl der Abbildungen stammt aus dem Buch „Zerebrale Angiographie für Klinik und Praxis" von KRAYENBÜHL/YASARGIL/HUBER, erschienen bei Thieme, Stuttgart, 1979. (Siehe S. 562).

Die Aneurysmaruptur ist nicht selten tödlich. LOCKSLEY (1966) errechnete eine Mortalität der ersten Blutung von 10 bis 15%. Die Mortalität der ersten Rezidivblutung aus einem Aneurysma ist mit 42% ganz wesentlich höher als diejenige der Erstblutung. Das Risiko einer Rezidivblutung ist am größten zwischen dem 5. und 11. Tag nach der ersten Ruptur. Innerhalb dieser Zeitperiode kommt es bei Aneurysmen der A. carotis interna in 18,5% zu einer Rezidivblutung, bei Aneurysmen der A. communicans anterior in 26,4% und bei Aneurysmen der A. cerebri media in 13,3%.

Weniger häufig ist der sogenannte paralytische Manifestationstypus des Aneurysmas, bei welchem Hirnnerven oder Hirnstrukturen durch Druck des als raumfordernder Prozeß wirkenden Aneurysmas in Mitleidenschaft gezogen werden. Nicht selten sind diese Aneurysmen sehr groß (HEISKANEN u. NIKKI, 1962; SADIK et al., 1965; MORLEY u. BARR, 1968; BULL, 1969; PRIBRAM et al., 1969; SARWAR et al., 1976; SONNTAG et al., 1977) (siehe Abb. 12, 13, 15, 29). Nach LOCKSLEY (1966) machen nur ca. 7% der nicht rupturierten Aneurysmen Symptome, die zu einer eingehenderen Abklärung führen. Nach SARWAR et al. (1976), die über 48 sehr große Aneurysmen referieren, sind in 66% der Fälle Hirnnervenschädigungen zu beobachten, wobei der N. opticus mit 46% am häufigsten betroffen ist. Eine kombinierte Läsion der Hirnnerven II, III, IV, V und VI beobachteten diese Autoren in 12% ihrer Fälle. Große intrakavernöse Aneurysmen, die als raumfordernder Prozeß wirken, sind bei Frauen sehr viel häufiger als bei Männern. Deshalb ist bei einer Frau im mittleren Alter mit plötzlicher auftretender Diplopie und retroorbitalen Schmerzen differentialdiagnostisch immer das infraklinoidale Aneurysma in Erwägung zu ziehen. Keineswegs selten können derartige große Aneurysmen an der Schädelbasis einen Hypophysentumor mit Chiasmakompression vortäuschen (JEFFERSON, 1937; WHITE u. BALLANTINE, 1961; WHITE, 1962; GERSTENBRAND u. WEINGARTEN, 1963).

Lokalisation der Aneurysmen von apoplektischen und paralytischen Typus:

apoplektischer Typus		paralytischer Typus
31%	A. carotis interna	72%
36,1%	A. cerebri anterior	10%
20%	A. cerebri media	13%
0,9%	A. cerebri posterior	
2,8%	A. basilaris	5,7%
0,9%	A. vertebralis	
0,8%	zerebelläre Arterien	

II. Pathologie

Als Aneurysma bezeichnet man ganz allgemein eine Ausweitung des Gefäßlumens. Diese kann sich über eine mehr oder weniger lange Strecke eines Gefäßsegmentes ausdehnen (sogenanntes fusiformes Aneurysma), während das sogenannte sackförmige Aneurysma eine streng lokalisierte Ausstülpung der Gefäßwand darstellt. Die fusiformen Aneurysmen entstehen in der Regel auf der Basis von arteriosklerotischen Gefäßwandveränderungen und finden sich vorzugsweise an der A. basilaris und am intrakavernösen Abschnitt der Karotiden (Abb. 1). Sie kommen aber auch bei Jugendlichen vor und sind auch im extrakraniellen Karotisabschnitt, gelegentlich sogar bilateral, beobachtet worden (TODOROW u. NIESSEN, 1974). Sie rupturieren viel seltener als die eigentlichen sackförmigen Aneurysmen, über deren Genese zum Teil noch divergierende Ansichten vertreten werden. Nach einer häufigen Auffassung handelt es sich bei den meist an Bifurkationsstellen einer Arterie sitzenden sackförmigen Aneurysmen um kongenitale Anomalien, die sich auf

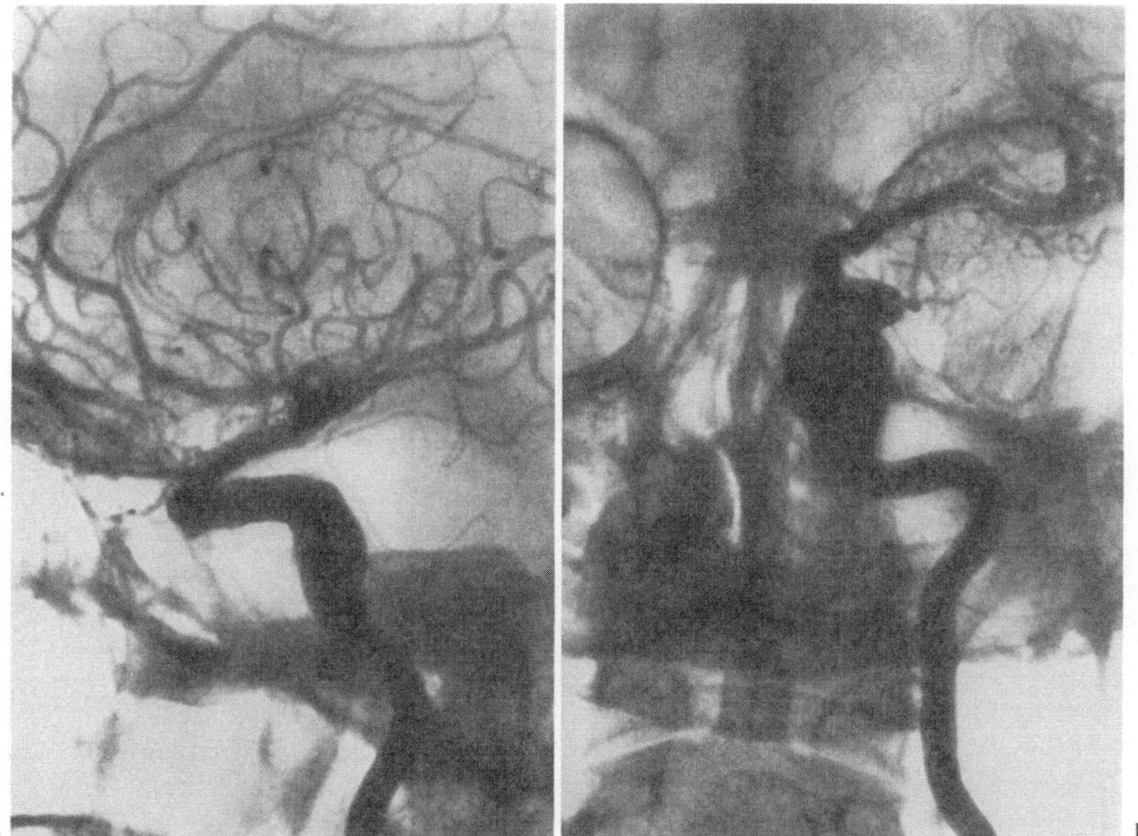

Abb. 1a u. b. Intrakavernöses fusiformes (arteriosklerotisches) Aneurysma der A. carotis interna. **a** Profilaufnahme; **b** a-p Aufnahme

dem Boden einer anlagemäßigen Schwäche der Elastica interna und der Media entwickeln. Zu einer Wandschwäche kommt es nach BREMER (1943) und BASSETT (1949) auch an Stellen, an denen sich primitive Arterien während des Embryonalstadiums zurückgebildet haben. An den Stellen dieser Wandschwäche soll es unter der Einwirkung des Blutdruckes zu einer allmählichen Dehnung der Gefäßwand kommen. Als Argument für die kongenitale Natur der Aneurysmen wird häufig die Tatsache angeführt, daß nicht selten noch andere Anomalien wie Hypoplasien und Aplasien von Teilen des Circulus Willisi, arteriovenöse Gefäßmißbildungen, Zystennieren und Koarktation der Aorta anzutreffen sind. Nach SHENKIN et al. (1964) weisen 6% der Patienten mit Zystenniere ein intrakranielles Aneurysma auf. SCHWARTZ und BARONOFSKY (1960) fanden autoptisch bei 304 Aortenkoarktationen 10mal ein Aneurysma. STEHBENS (1962a u. b) glaubt jedoch, daß bei der Koarktation und der Zystenniere das Aneurysma mit der Hypertonie und Arteriosklerose in Zusammenhang stehe.

Auf das gleichzeitige Vorkommen der fibromuskulären Dysplasie mit sackförmigen Aneurysmen der Hirngefäße oder mit arteriovenösen Mißbildungen ist mehrfach hingewiesen worden (PALUBINSKAS et al., 1966; KRAMER, 1969; ANDERSEN, 1970; HANDA et al., 1970; HARRINGTON et al., 1970; KAUFMANN, 1970; HOUSER et al., 1971; MANELFE et al., 1974). Es besteht indessen kein Zweifel darüber, daß die meisten sackförmigen Aneurysmen an Orten anzutreffen sind, wo die Muskelschicht der Media Defekte aufweist (FORBUS, 1930; GLYNN 1940; STEHBENS, 1959; DU BOULAY, 1965).

In der Diskussion um die Faktoren, die bei der Entstehung eines Aneurysmas von Bedeutung sind, spielt die Arteriosklerose eine wichtige Rolle, da die Prädilektionsstellen für arteriosklerotische Wandveränderungen mit denjenigen der sackförmigen Aneurysmen eine gewisse Übereinstimmung zeigen. In nicht wenigen sackförmigen Aneurysmen scheinen arteriosklerotische Veränderungen vorzukommen und Crawford (1959) nimmt für jeden Fall in wechselndem Ausmaß eine Kombination von kongenitalen und postnatalen arteriosklerotischen Faktoren an. Eine ähnliche Auffassung wird auch von Stehbens (1975) vertreten. Häufig ist histologisch kein eindeutiger Unterschied in der Wandbeschaffenheit von sackförmigen Aneurysmen und offensichtlich arteriosklerotischen fusiformen Dilatationen zu sehen. Die Rolle, die die Intimapolster (Hassler, 1961) bei der Entstehung der Aneurysmen spielen, ist noch nicht geklärt. Wichtig ist die von Crompton (1966b) hervorgehobene Beobachtung, daß am Gefäßsystem bei Aneurysmapatienten häufiger große Mediadefekte, Intimahyperplasien und Elastikadegenerationen gefunden werden als bei Normalen. Diese größeren Mediadefekte finden sich auch bei Hypertonie, Zystenniere und schließlich bei arteriovenösen Mißbildungen und zwar speziell an den größeren, die Mißbildung versorgenden Arterien. An der Bifurkation der A. cerebri media sind die Aneurysmen häufiger als an der Bifurkation der A. carotis interna oder der A. basilaris. An der A. cerebri media sind die Mediadefekte aber auch größer als an den beiden anderen Stellen und weniger durch Intimapolster überdeckt, die möglicherweise eine gewisse Schutzwirkung haben. Sackförmige Aneurysmen an Stellen mit ausgeprägten atheromatösen Plaques sind relativ selten. Yasargil (1977) fand bei über 600 unter dem Mikroskop operierten Aneurysmen in 80% keine Zeichen einer Arteriosklerose im Sinn einer Plaque an den entsprechenden Arterien. Es kann aber sein, daß eine beginnende arteriosklerotische Veränderung einen entscheidenden Anteil an der Schwächung der Wand im Bereiche der präexistenten Mediadefekte hat.

Mykotische Aneurysmen sind ausgesprochen selten. Sie sitzen meistens nicht am Circulus Willisi, sondern weiter in der Peripherie, besonders im Stromgebiet der A. cerebri media (Abb. 28), analog der Prädilektion für zerebrale Embolien. Infolge einer lokalen Schädigung der Gefäßwand (Angiitis) können sich auch ohne Abszeßbildung Aneurysmen entwickeln, die nicht selten fusiform sind (Ferris et al., 1968; Bell u. Butler, 1968; Leeds u. Goldberg; 1971; Wise u. Farmer, 1971; Molinari et al., 1973; Ishikawa et al., 1974; Horten et al., 1976). Mykotische Aneurysmen finden sich in 3–4% der Patienten mit subakuter bakterieller Endokarditis (McNeel et al., 1969), seltener bei Septikämien anderer Genese (Davidson u. Robertson, 1971; Sypert u. Young, 1972). Mykotische Aneurysmen machen angeblich 2,5–4% der intrakraniellen Aneurysmen aus (Cantu et al., 1966; Moskowitz u. Rosenbaum, 1974). Diese Aneurysmen wechseln unter Umständen rasch ihre Form und können thrombosieren. Mykotische Aneurysmen können sich aber auch infolge extravasaler entzündlicher Prozesse bilden, so am intrakavernösen Karotisabschnitt bei Thromophlebitis des Sinus cavernosus oder in Verbindung mit einer Mittelohrentzündung oder Meningitis (Heidelberger et al., 1968; Suwanwela et al., 1972). Nach Gefäßverletzungen können sich sowohl an der A. carotis interna und ihren Ästen (Krauland, 1955; Isfort, 1961; Brenner, 1962; Hirsch et al., 1962; Araki et al., 1965; Handa et al., 1967; 1970; Handa u. Handa, 1976; Petty, 1969; Go et al., 1971; Acosta et al., 1972; Rumbaugh et al., 1972; Burton, 1973; Bergström u. Hemmingsson, 1973; Lukin u. Chambers, 1974; Menezes u. Graf, 1974; Fleischer et al., 1975; Ludwiczak u. Fogel, 1975) als auch im Stromgebiet der A. carotis externa, speziell der A. meningea media, traumatische Aneurysmen entwickeln (Pouyanne et al., 1959; Markwalder u. Huber, 1961; Dilenge u. Wüthrich, 1962; Kuhn u. Kugler, 1964; Paillas et al., 1964; Zingesser et al., 1965; Higazi et al., 1969).

Während die einen Autoren die Auffassung vertreten, daß sich das sackförmige Aneurysma unter der Einwirkung des Blutdruckes langsam im Verlaufe der Jahre entwickle, plädieren andere für eine kurze, Tage bis Wochen dauernde, eventuell noch raschere und dramatischere Entstehung. Auffallend ist in diesem Zusammenhang, wie selten die Zufallsbefunde eines Aneurysma bei angiographischen Untersuchungen mit anderer Indikation als Subarachnoidalblutung und Lähmung von Hirnnerven sind (83 Zufallsbefunde in der über 6000 Fälle von Subarachnoidalblutungen umfaßenden Studie von Locksley, 1966). Du Boulay (1965) fand in einer Serie von 2500 Fällen mit normalen Angiogrammen oder Hirntumoren nur 5 symptomlose Aneurysmen, deren Träger alle über 30 Jahre alt waren. Auch in Autopsieserien sind die mikroskopischen Aneurysmen am Circulus Willisi eine ausgesprochene Seltenheit (Riggs u. Rupp, 1943), während sie an den feinen intrazerebralen Arterien, speziell im Bereiche des Striatum, mit zunehmendem Alter und namentlich bei Hypertonie häufig sind (Russel, 1963). Wahrscheinlich entstehen die meisten Aneurysmen als gleichmäßig rundliche Ausstülpungen. Nach Ferguson (1970, 1972) spielt die Turbulenz der Strömung beim Aneurysmawachstum eine nicht unerhebliche Rolle, da sie zu einer Vibration der Gefäßwand führt und degenerative Wandveränderungen, wie z.B. den Untergang der Elastica interna, beschleunigt.

Es ist ungewiß, warum eine Aneurysma in einem bestimmten Zeitpunkt rupturiert. Prodromalsymptome sind nicht sehr spezifisch, werden jedoch anamnestisch als Kopfschmerzen, diskretes Hemisyndrom u.a.m., nicht selten angegeben (Waga et al., 1975). Es ist in Einzelfällen durchaus möglich, daß der Anstieg des mittleren arteriellen Blutdruckes und namentlich der Pulsamplitude während einer körperlichen oder emotionellen Belastung der ausschlaggebende Faktor ist. Die Mehrzahl der Aneurysmablutungen – nahezu 70% – tritt aber in Momenten ohne besondere Belastung oder gar während des Schlafes auf.

Auftreten der Subarachnoidalblutung. (Nach Locksley, 1966)

Während des Schlafs	35,8%	Husten	2,1%
ohne besondere Umstände	32,1%	Trauma	2,8%
Heben oder Bücken	11,9%	Urinieren	2,0%
emotionelle Belastung	4,4%	chirurgische Eingriffe	0,4%
Defäkation	4,3%	Gebären	0,4%
Koitus	3,8%		

Analog sind die Prozentzahlen für das Auftreten einer Subarachnoidalblutung bei arteriovenösen Mißbildungen oder unbekannten Ursachen. Es ist nicht ausgeschlossen, daß die Ruptur nach einer bestimmten Tätigkeit oftmals mehr zufällig als kausal ist. Das seltene Zusammentreffen von Geburt und Aneurysmaruptur beruht wahrscheinlich darauf, daß die Mehrzahl der Frauen ihre Schwangerschaften und Geburten in jugendlichem Alter mit ohnehin geringer Aneurysmafrequenz haben. Subarachnoidalblutungen infolge Aneurysmaruptur treten meistens zwischen der 30. und 40. Schwangerschaftswoche oder aber kurz nach der Geburt auf und scheinen in keinem Zusammenhang mit einer besonderen kardiovaskulären Leistung zu stehen. Demgegenüber bluten arteriovenöse Mißbildungen vorwiegend zu Beginn der Schwangerschaft oder aber während der Wehentätigkeit, also in den Perioden mit der größten Veränderung des Herzminutenvolumens (Robinson et al., 1974).

Das Rupturrisiko ist offenbar besonders groß, wenn die Aneurysmen einen Durchmesser zwischen 6–15 mm erreicht haben (Crawford, 1959). Auch nach der Untersuchung von Stehbens (1963a) messen Aneurysmen, die zu einer tödlichen Blutung führten, im Durchschnitt mindestens 5 mm. Crompton (1966b) fand bei rupturierten Aneurysmen eine Durchschnittsgröße von ca. 5 mm, bei nicht rupturierten, zufällig entdeckten Aneurysmen eine solche von 2 mm.

Die Ruptur erfolgt in der Mehrzahl der Fälle am Aneurysmafundus und nur ganz selten am Aneurysmahals. Crompton (1966) fand bei 271 Aneurysmen die Rupturstelle in 83,7% an der Kuppe, in 14% am Fundus und in 2,2% im Halsabschnitt.

Die sackförmigen Aneurysmen besitzen häufig nicht eine gleichmäßig rundliche, blasenförmige Gestalt, sondern unregelmäßige Konturen mit einer oder mehreren lokalisierten Ausbuchtungen (Tochteraneurysma, Lobulus) (Hinshaw et al., 1974) (Abb. 2). Nach Crompton (1966b) kommen derartige Lobuli bei 57% der rupturierten Aneurysmen vor, während sie nur in 16% der nicht

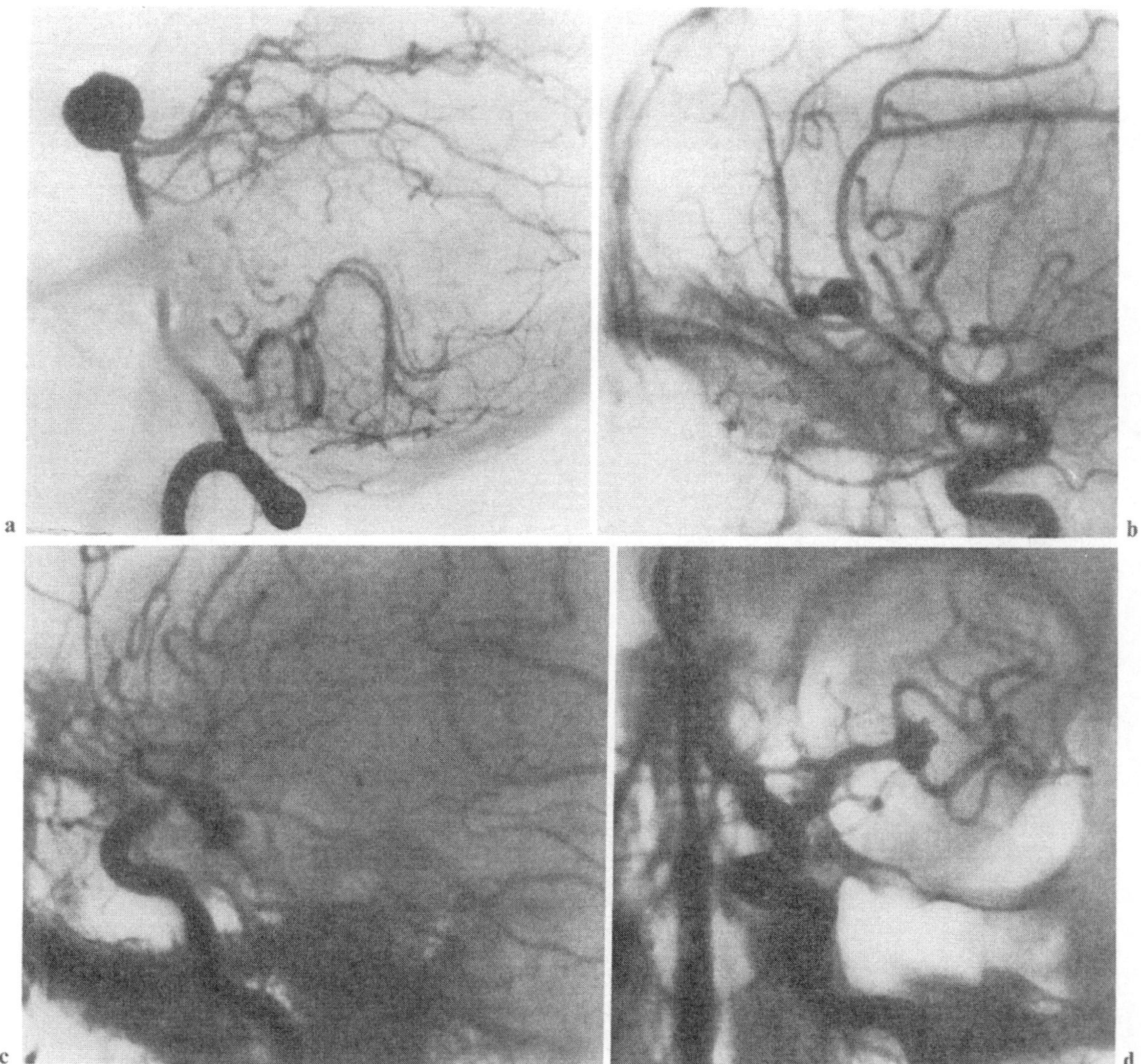

Abb. 2a–d. Verschiedene Formen der Aneurysmen. **a** Rundliches Aneurysma an der kranialen Teilungsstelle der A. basilaris. **b** Aneurysma der A. pericallosa mit deutlich abgesetztem rundlichem Lobulus. **c** Aneurysma der A. communicans posterior mit großem Lobulus. **d** Aneurysma an der Teilungsstelle der A. cerebri media mit zwei kleinen zipfelförmigen Lobuli. (Abb. 2a aus "Zerebr. Angiographic", 3. Auflage 1979, Thieme Stuttgart)

rupturierten Aneurysmen anzutreffen sind. Sowohl bei rupturierten als auch bei nicht rupturierten Aneurysmen nimmt die Häufigkeit der Lobuli mit der Aneurysmagröße zu. Besonders häufig sind sie an den Aneurysmen an der Abgangsstelle der A. communicans posterior aus der A. carotis interna zu finden. Sie sitzen meist am Aneurysmafundus, und oftmals besteht ein Zusammenhang zwischen Blutung und Lobulus, sei es, daß eine Blutung stattgefunden hat, sei es, daß eine Blutung aus dieser Ausstülpung bevorsteht. In der Regel sagen diese Lobuli aber mehr über die Vergangenheit als über die Zukunft des Aneurysmas aus (CROMPTON, 1966). Wie angiographische Kontrolluntersuchungen bei nicht operierten Aneurysmen zeigen (BJÖRKESTEN u. TROUPP, 1962; DU BOULAY, 1965; HUBER u. ROBERT, 1969), können Aneurysmen im Verlauf der Zeit ihre Form und Größe ändern (Abb. 3). Mit oder ohne klinische Symptome können Lobuli auftreten oder wieder verschwinden (thrombosieren). Die Thrombosierung eines Lobulus kann später der Aneurysmawand einen atheromatösen Aspekt verleihen, zudem sind Verkalkungen möglich.

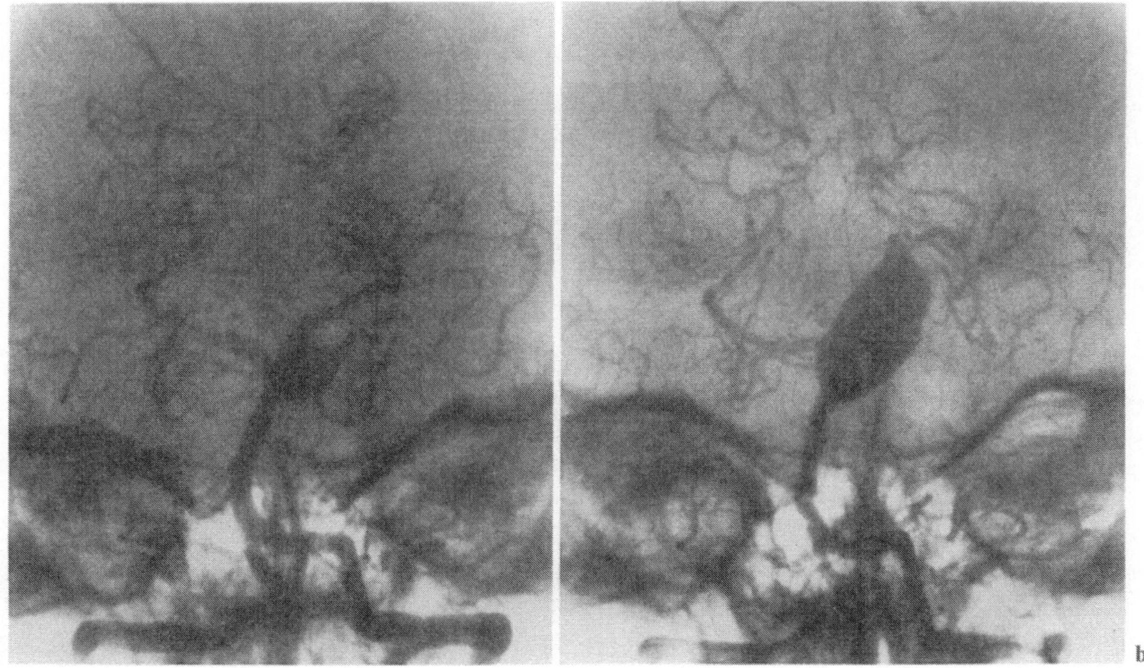

Abb. 3a u. b. Größenzunahme eines sackförmigen Aneurysmas der A. basilaris. **a** erste Untersuchung; **b** Kontrolluntersuchung 1 Jahr später

Flächenhafte Wandverkalkungen kommen aber auch ohne jegliche Lobulusbildung vor und können bei der Operation direkt gesehen werden.

Bei einer Ruptur kann die Wand des Aneurysmas im eigentlichen Sinn des Wortes platzen, wobei sich ein Loch bildet, das den freien Blutaustritt in den Liquorraum oder die Hirnsubstanz ermöglicht, oder es kann nur zu einer Dissektion mit Sickerblutung in die Wand, gegebenenfalls in die Umgebung, kommen. Letzteres dürfte eher bei größeren Aneurysmen der Fall sein, deren Wand bereits eine gewisse Dicke erreicht hat. Sofern der Patient die Blutung überlebt, kommt es zur Organisation der Blutung mit Vergrößerung des Aneurysmas und Verdickung der Adventitia. Eine murale Thrombose führt zu einer Intimaverdickung mit atheromähnlichen Veränderungen. STEHBENS (1963a) fand in den meisten Aneurysmen, die größer als 8–10 mm waren, Thrombosen, die indessen das Lumen nicht vollständig verschlossen. Durch diese Art des Aneurysmawachstums mit Blutung, Organisation und Verdickung der Adventitia kann es zu Verklebungen von Arterien im Bifurkationsbereich mit der Aneurysmaaußenwand kommen, die zum Teil so intensiv sind, daß die Arterie direkt in die Aneurysmawand einbezogen erscheint, wie z.B. bei Aneurysmen an der Teilungsstelle der A. cerebri media. Gelegentlich kann angiographisch wie bei der direkten makroskopischen Inspektion der Eindruck entstehen, daß eine Arterie aus dem Fundus des Aneurysmas hervorgehe.

Sowohl bei den sogenannten Lobuli als auch bei den sehr großen, in die Hirnsubstanz eingebetteten Aneurysmen ist es gelegentlich schwierig zu entscheiden, ob es sich um echte oder um sog. „falsche" Aneurysmen handelt, deren Wand lediglich durch Organisation eines Hämotoms entstanden ist (RAIMONDI et al., 1968). Aneurysmen der A. cerebri media führen relativ häufig zu intrazerebralen Hämatomen, und es ist durchaus wahrscheinlich, daß die von mehreren Autoren beschriebenen riesigen Aneurysmen mit unregelmäßigem kanalartigem Lumen zwischen ausgedehnten Thromben derartigen organisierten Hämatomen nach Ruptur eines kleineren Aneurysmas entsprechen (SADIK et al., 1965; TERAO u. MURAOKA, 1972; LUKIN et al., 1975). Bei 23,5% der Fälle führt die Aneurysmaruptur, neben einer Subarachnoidalblutung, zu einer Blutung in die Hirnsubstanz selbst, besonders bei den Aneurysmen der A. cerebri media (CROMPTON, 1962), und bei 37,2% kommt es zu einer intrazerebralen und intraventrikulären Blutung, besonders bei Aneurysmen der A. communicans anterior. Bei Rezidivblutung ist wegen der Verklebung des Subarachnoidalraums das Risiko einer intrazerebralen Blutung stark erhöht. Blutungen in den Subduralraum sind dagegen relativ selten (3%) (FEIN u. ROVIT, 1970) (Abb. 26).

Der bei weitem größte Anteil der eine Subarachnoidalblutung verursachenden Aneurysmen entfällt auf das Stromgebiet der A. carotis interna (ca. 95%). Unter Einschluß der multiplen Aneurysmen, der nicht rupturierten Aneurysmen, die neurologische Symptome verursachen, sowie der Zufallsbefund dürfte der wirkliche Anteil der Aneurysmen im Karotisstromgebiet um 85–90%, derjenige der vertebrobasilären Aneurysmen um 10–15% liegen. STEHBENS (1963b) gibt für die Aneurysmen im Karotisstromgebiet einen Anteil von 88,7% an und 11,3% für die Aneurysmen im vertebrobasilären Stromgebiet. Die Zahlenangaben der verschiedenen Autoren über die Lokalisation der Aneurysmen in einem größeren Krankengut schwanken etwas, was zum Teil mit der angiographischen Abklärung zusammenhängt. Nach den Berechnungen von DU BOULAY (1965) würden gut 40% der symptomatischen Aneurysmen übersehen, wenn wahlweise nur eine links- oder rechtsseitige Karotisangiographie durchgeführt würde. Die meisten Autoren sind sich jedoch einig, daß für sackförmige Aneurysmen die A. carotis interna, die A. communicans anterior und die Bifurkation der A. cerebri media die Prädilektionsstellen sind, hinter welchen die übrigen Lokalisationen eindeutig zurückstehen (KRAYENBÜHL u. YASARGIL, 1958; STEHBENS, 1963). Aufgrund der in der „cooperative study" zusammengetragenen großen Zahl von mehreren Tausend Aneurysmen gibt LOCKSLEY (1966) folgende Verteilung an:

		Einzelnes Aneurysma mit Subarachnoidalblutung
A. carotis interna	38,1%	
proximal von A. communicans posterior		4,3%
Abgang der A. communicans posterior		25,0%
distal von A. communicans posterior		4,3%
Karotisbifurkation		4,5%
A. cerebri anterior	36,1%	
präkommunikaler Abschnitt		1,5%
A. communicans anterior		30,3%
postkommunikaler Abschnitt (A. pericallosa)		2,8%
nicht spezifiziert		1,5%
A. cerebri media	20,9%	
proximaler Abschnitt		3,9%
Teilungsstelle des Hauptstammes		13,1%
distaler Abschnitt		1,4%
nicht spezifiziert		2,5%
A. cerebri posterior	0,9%	
A. basilaris	2,8%	
Bifurkation		2,0%
Stamm		0,8%
A. vertebralis	0,9%	
zerebelläre Arterien	0,8%	

Nicht selten ist ein und derselbe Patient Träger von multiplen makroskopisch sichtbaren Aneurysmen (HAMBY, 1959). Die mikroskopischen Aneurysmen dagegen sind sehr of multipel: COLE u. YATES (1967) fanden multiple Mikroaneurysmen, durchschnittlich 15–25, in 46% der Hypertoniker, dagegen nur in 7% der Normotoniker. In beiden Gruppen nehmen sie mit dem Alter

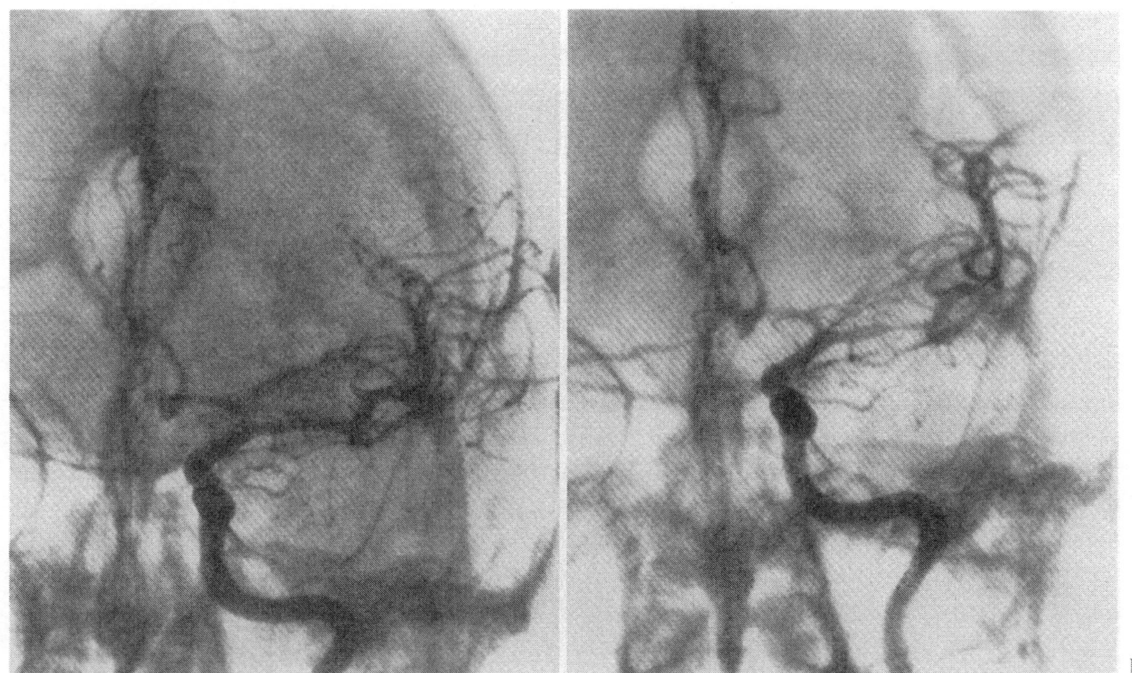

Abb. 4a u. b. Entwicklung eines Gefäßspasmus nach Aneurysmaruptur. **a** Angiographie nach der ersten Subarachnoidalblutung bei Aneurysma der linken A. communicans anterior. Kein Spasmus faßbar. **b** Angiographie nach Rezidivblutung mit Spasmen, besonders ausgeprägt an der A. cerebri media

zu (RUSSEL, 1963). Nach MCKISSOCK et al. (1964) sind 14,9% der Aneurysmen multipel, nach der Zusammenstellung von LOCKSLEY (1966) sind im klinischen Krankengut 19% der Aneurysmapatienten Träger von multiplen Aneurysmen. Im Sektionsgut erhöht sich diese Zahl auf 22%. POUYANNE et al. (1973) nehmen an, daß ungefähr 10% aller Aneurysmapatienten multiple Aneurysmen aufweisen, wobei über 90% dieser Aneurysmen im Karotisstromgebiet liegen. 39–45% der multiplen Aneurysmen sind unilateral (Abb. 16 und 20), 23–36% sitzen distal an symmetrischer Stelle, z.B. an der Teilungsstelle der A. cerebri media (Abb. 8 und 27) und 6–7% sind zwar bilateral, jedoch ganz asymmetrisch verteilt.

Von größter Bedeutung ist die Identifikation des rupturierten Aneurysmas beim Vorliegen multipler Aneurysmen. Aufgrund der klinischen Symptome ist bei multiplen Aneurysmen das rupturierte in ca. der Hälfte aller Fälle eruierbar (MCKISSOCK et al., 1964; HEISKANEN, 1965; KRAYENBÜHL, 1973). Sicherster angiographischer Hinweis auf das rupturierte Aneurysma ist das Hämatom in seiner Umgebung, welches mit Hilfe der computerisierten axialen Tomographie leicht zu erfassen ist. Spasmen und Zirkulationsstörungen sind dagegen nur von geringem lokalisatorischem Wert, da sie entfernt vom rupturierten Aneurysma, eventuell sogar auf der Gegenseite, auftreten können (WOOD, 1964) (Abb. 4). Nicht immer ist aber ein Hämatom mit entsprechenden Gefäßverlagerungen oder Spasmen vorhanden. In dieser Situation ist es in 87% (WOOD, 1964; CROMPTON, 1966) das größere, resp. größte Aneurysma, das geblutet hat. In 75% der Fälle ist es das proximalste Aneurysma, das rupturiert (BIGELOW, 1955; CROMPTON, 1966b). Nach der Erfahrung von POUYANNE et al. (1973) ist es jedoch nicht unbedingt das proximalste von multiplen Aneurysmen, das rupturiert: Sitzt eines der multiplen Aneurysmen an der A. communicans anterior, dann ist es häufig dieses, welches geblutet hat. Sind die verschiedenen Aneurysmen von gleicher Größe, so ist es das am unregelmäßigsten geformte, lobulierte Aneurysma, welches geplatzt ist (WOOD, 1964; DU BOULAY, 1965). Nach erfolgreicher Ligatur des rupturierten Aneurysmas kann jedoch später das zweite, nicht operativ versorgte Aneurysma zu einer Subarachnoidalblutung Anlaß geben (HEISKANEN u. MARTTILA, 1970).

III. Die Röntgenuntersuchungen der zerebralen Aneurysmen

Die Untersuchung von Patienten mit Subarachnoidalblutung hat nach einem genauen Plan zu erfolgen, da sonst wegen inadäquater Technik Aneurysmen übersehen werden können (KRICHEFF et al., 1964; LIN u. KRICHEFF, 1972). Wenn möglich wird die Untersuchung in Intubationsnarkose durchgeführt, namentlich bei ängstlichen oder unter heftigen Schmerzen leidenden oder nicht kooperativen Patienten. Nicht selektive Untersuchungsmethoden, wie z.B. die Arkographie und die rechtsseitige retrograde Brachialisangiographie, sind wegen zahlreicher Überlagerungen und zum Teil ungenügender Kontrastmitteldichte völlig ungeeignet. In jedem Fall ist die selektive Darstellung der Karotiden und Vertebralarterien anzustreben, sei es mit direkter Punktion des Gefäßes oder besser noch mit selektiver Katheterisierung. Falls neurologische Herdsymptome vorliegen, ist das entsprechende Gefäß zuerst darzustellen, andernfalls beginnt man die Untersuchung vorzugsweise mit der A. carotis interna der nicht dominanten, d.h. in der Regel der rechten Hemisphäre, worauf die Untersuchung der übrigen Gefäße angeschlossen wird. Der Gefäßverlauf ist auch im Hinblick auf das Vorliegen eines allfälligen Hydrocephalus internus, der nach einer Subarachnoidalblutung keineswegs selten ist, zu beurteilen (RAIMONDI u. TORRES, 1973). Zeigen die seitlichen und anteroposterioren Röntgenserien der zuerst untersuchten Seite keinen pathologischen Befund, so ist die anteroposteriore Serie unter digitaler Kompression der gegenseitigen A. carotis zu wiederholen, wobei die exakte Karotiskompression gut 2 Sekunden vor der Kontrastmittelinjektion beginnt und erst ca. eine Sekunde nach deren Beendigung aufhört. Die komprimierende Hand ist dabei selbstverständlich durch einen Bleihandschuh vor der Bestrahlung zu schützen.

Vielerorts wird für die Beurteilung der Operationsmöglichkeiten und die Wahl der Operationsmethode das Ergebnis des sogenannten gekreuzten Zirkulationstestes (SEDZIMIR, 1959) verlangt. Es wird damit die Durchgängigkeit des Circulus Willisi als potentieller Kollateralkanal beurteilt. Der Kollateralkreislauf zwischen beiden Karotiden einerseits und zwischen Karotis- und Basilarisstromgebiet andererseits muß im Hinblick auf seine Funktionstüchtigkeit abgeklärt werden, bevor ein Aneurysma oder eine zuführende Arterie verschlossen werden. Der Circulus Willisi kann infolge Fehlens oder Hypoplasie gewisser Arterien unvollständig sein. In einem Sektionsgut von 350 Normalgehirnen haben ALPERS et al. (1959) in 52,3% einen normal ausgebildeten Circulus Willisi nachgewiesen. Die häufigste Anomalie bestand in einer fadendünnen Einengung einzelner Segmente und fand sich vor allem an der A. communicans posterior (22%), wesentlich weniger häufig an der A. communicans anterior (3%) und der A. cerebri anterior (2%). Verdoppelungen der Gefäße wurden in 18,9% beobachtet und kamen hauptsächlich an der A. communicans anterior vor. Es darf jedoch nicht übersehen werden, daß Gefäßvariationen bei den Aneurysmen doch wesentlich häufiger sein dürften als in einem durchschnittlichen anatomischen Sektionsgut.

Die Wertigkeit des Kompressionstestes wurde von BEATTY und RICHARDSON (1968) an 110 Patienten eingehend überprüft. In 47 Fällen war ein Aneurysma der A. communicans anterior und in 63 Fällen ein Aneurysma der A. communicans posterior mit einer Karotisligatur behandelt worden. In 22% der Fälle traten nach der Karotisligatur ischämische Symptome auf. In der Gruppe der Aneurysmen der A. communicans anterior kam es in 28% zu einer Intoleranz, bei den Aneurysmen der A. communicans posterior in 17%. Nach Auffassung dieser Autoren ist keine besondere Konfiguration des Circulus Willisi mit einer Intoleranz verbunden. Wohl findet sich eine solche etwas häufiger bei einem asymmetrischen vorderen Circulus Willisi, doch hat diese Konfiguration keinen sicheren Voraussagewert für die Ligaturtoleranz. Einziger Befund mit konstanter Ligaturintoleranz war die doppelseitig weite (fetale) A. communicans posterior: Von 11 Patienten mit dieser Gefäßanordnung ertrugen 7 die Ligatur nicht, unabhängig von der Ausbildung des vorderen Abschnitts des Circulus Willisi. 8 von 56 Patienten mit angiographisch gutem Kollateralkreislauf zeigten nach der Karotisligatur ischämisch bedingte neurologische Ausfallserscheinungen. Umgekehrt traten bei 8 von 11 Patienten ohne Doppelfüllung beim Kompressionstest nach der Ligatur keine neurologischen Symptome auf. Offenbar ist der angiographische Kompressionstest allein somit ohne wesentlichen Wert für die Voraussage der Ligaturtoleranz (JAWAD et al., 1977).

Stellt sich auch beim Kompressionstest kein pathologischer Befund dar, so kann man in analoger Weise zur Angiographie der Gegenseite fortschreiten. Kommt aber bei der zuerst gewählten Seite ein Aneurysma oder ein aneurysmaverdächtiger Befund zum Vorschein, so sind unter Umständen Zusatzaufnahmen erforderlich, z.B. um orthograd getroffene Gefäßschlingen, die als Aneurysmen imponieren, auszuschließen oder aber die anatomischen Verhältnisse im Bereiche des Aneurysmahalses genauer darzustellen.

Ist die A. communicans anterior näher zu untersuchen, so sind Schrägaufnahmen (BOYD-WILSON, 1959b) nötig mit einer Kopfdrehung von 25–30 Grad von der injizierten Seite weg zur Gegenseite (KAMISASA, 1977). Der Zentralstrahl soll um 7 Grad von der Orbitomeatuslinie weg nach kaudal gerichtet sein, damit allfällig überdeckende Knochenstrukturen wegprojiziert werden. Zum Nachweis der frontobasalen Hämatome bei Aneurysmen der A. communicans anterior hat sich außerdem die submentovertikale Aufnahme sehr gut bewährt, da in dieser Aufsicht der Anfangsabschnitt der A. pericallosa sich über eine längere Strecke darstellt als in der anteroposterioren Aufnahme. Hinter einer relativ geringen, recht- oder spitzwinkligen Verlagerung der A. pericallosa zur Gegenseite kann sich nicht selten ein größeres frontobasales Hämatom verbergen, dessen Ausmaß aufgrund alleiniger anteroposteriorer Aufnahmen falsch eingeschätzt würde (Abb. 5). Beim Verdacht auf ein Aneurysma im Bereiche der Bifurkation der A. cerebri media wird eine transorbitale Aufnahme gemacht. Der Zentralstrahl wird parallel zur Orbitomeatuslinie durch die Orbitamitte zentriert, wobei der Kopf des Patienten, je nach Lage der Mediateilungsstelle, entweder genau gerade oder leicht zur injizierten Seite gedreht wird.

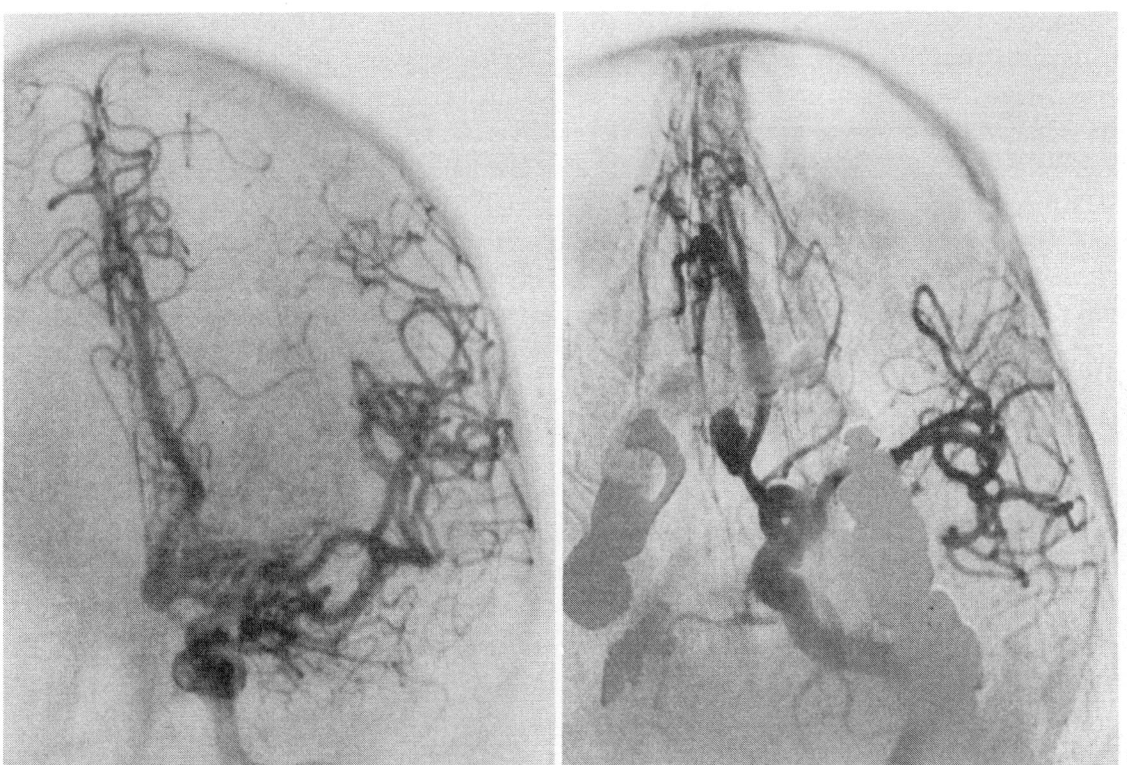

Abb. 5a u. b. Hämatom bei Aneurysma der A. communicans anterior. **a** Aufnahme nach Towne mit scheinbar winkeliger Verlagerung der A. pericallosa im infrakallösen Abschnitt. **b** Submento-vertikale Aufnahme mit bogenförmiger Ausspannung der A. pericallosa durch das Hämatom. Das Aneurysma ist besser überblickbar. (Aus „Zerebrale Angiographie", 3. Aufl. 1979, Thieme Stuttgart)

Die Abklärung der Halsverhältnisse der Aneurysmen, die von der A. carotis interna auf Höhe der Abgangsstelle der A. communicans posterior ausgehen, kann durch paraorbitale Schrägaufnahmen (AGEE, 1968) verbessert werden. Der Kopf des Patienten wird ca. 55 Grad von der injizierten Seite weg zur Gegenseite gedreht und die Röhre um 12 Grad von der Orbitomeatuslinie weg kranialwärts gerichtet. Der Zentralstrahl zielt auf einen Punkt, ca. 1 cm hinter dem lateralen unteren Orbitarand. Aneurysmen an der Karotisbifurkation und am Abgang der A. ophthalmica werden durch zusätzliche Schrägaufnahmen in gleicher Weise wie die Aneurysmen der A. communicans anterior untersucht.

Für alle Zusatzaufnahmen genügen Bilder der arteriellen Phase. Je nach Bedarf können bei verschiedenen Kopfhaltungen noch zusätzliche Aufnahmen mit horizontalem Strahlengang angefertigt werden. Wegen der eventuell notwendigen Kopfdrehungen ist die Katheteruntersuchung der direkten Gefäßpunktion vorzuziehen. In jedem Fall wird im Anschluß an die zuerst untersuchte Seite die Karotisangiographie der Gegenseite durchgeführt, sei es, um das Aneurysma überhaupt zu finden, sei es, um die keineswegs seltenen multiplen Aneurysmen nicht zu übersehen.

Keinesfalls sollten zu viele Spezialaufnahmen gemacht werden, um auf perfektionistische Weise einen Aneurysmahals darzustellen, da die benötigte Kontrastmittelmenge sonst zu groß wird. Der Untersucher muß sich darüber im klaren sein, daß er die Gefäßverhältnisse, trotz aller Bemühungen, nicht in anatomisch perfekter Weise erfassen kann, da er ja nur die freien Lumina sieht, nicht aber die Verhältnisse an der Gefäß- und Aneurysmaaußenwand. Nicht selten präsentiert sich unter dem Operationsmikroskop der Status ganz anders, als aufgrund der Angiogramme zu erwarten gewesen wäre.

Zeigen die Karotisangiogramme kein Aneurysma, so erfolgt als letzter Schritt im gleichen Untersuchungsgang die Vertebralisangiographie.

Sofern die technischen Möglichkeiten vorhanden sind, können Angiotomogramme bei der Abklärung von Aneurysmen von großem Nutzen sein (ROCCA u. ROSADINI, 1963; DU BOULAY u. JACKSON, 1965; RAMELLA et al., 1969; PIEPGRAS et al., 1968; ROSA, 1971; NADJMI et al., 1977). Um unnötige Injektionen zu vermeiden, sollen die Tomogramme jedoch nur in denjenigen Richtungen aufgenommen werden, in welchen das Aneurysma nicht auf normalem Wege von überlagernden Gefäßen frei projiziert werden kann. Bei der Abklärung der Beziehungen des Aneurysma zu umgebenden Gefäßen können stereoskopische Aufnahmen sehr hilfreich sein.

Da bei einer derartigen angiographischen Abklärung einer Subarachnoidalblutung zahlreiche Kontrastmittelinjektionen notwendig sind, ist die injizierte Menge pro Serie möglichst klein zu halten. 5–6 ml pro Injektion genügen bei richtiger Injektionstechnik und selektiver Gefäßdarstellung. Die einzelnen Injektionen sollten nicht zu rasch aufeinanderfolgen, sondern in Intervallen von 5–10 Minuten. In diesen Zeitintervallen können die Bilder der vorhergehenden Serie studiert und der weitere Schritt geplant werden.

Findet man bereits auf der zuerst untersuchten Seite ein großes intra- oder extrazerebrales Hämatom, so sollte die Untersuchung abgebrochen werden. Die Hämatomentleerung kann von wesentlich größerer Bedeutung sein als die Suche nach eventuell vorhandenen weiteren Aneurysmen. Jedenfalls ist der Neurochirurg sofort über diesen Befund zu orientieren.

Die Häufigkeit eines Aneurysmanachweises geben PERRET und NISHIOKA (1966) aufgrund ihrer Studie folgendermaßen an:

Nur einseitige Karotisangiographie	(341 Fälle)	45% pos.
Doppelseitige Karotisangiographie	(2060 Fälle)	67% pos.
3- bis 4-Gefäßangiographie	(536 Fälle)	42% pos.
total		57% pos.

Für arteriovenöse Mißbildungen ergeben sich folgende Zahlen:

Nur einseitige Karotisangiographie	(297 Fälle)	39% pos.
Doppelseitige Karotisangiographie	(819 Fälle)	27% pos.
3- bis 4-Gefäßangiographie	(632 Fälle)	49% pos.
total		34% pos.

Sie vermuten, daß die geringere Nachweisquote für Aneurysmen bei der 3- bis 4-Gefäßuntersuchung gegenüber der bilateralen Karotisangiographie dadurch bedingt ist, daß die Vertebralisangiographie nur dann durchgeführt wurde, wenn die bilaterale Karotisangiographie negativ ausgefallen war. Nach der Lokalisationsstatistik sind aber Aneurysmen im Basilarisstromgebiet relativ selten. Anders sind die Verhältnisse beim Nachweis von arteriovenösen Mißbildungen, wo die positiven Befunde bei der Totalangiographie deutlich höher sind als bei der uni- oder bilateralen Karotisangiographie.

Die Genauigkeit der Diagnose wurde von Perret und Bull (1959) anhand von 210 Fällen, die angiographisch und autoptisch untersucht worden waren, kontrolliert. Die korrekte angiographische Diagnose war in 90% gestellt worden. In 3% lag ein Irrtum des ersten Untersuchers vor, in 2,5% war das Aneurysma infolge eines ausgeprägten Spasmus nicht zur Darstellung gekommen. In 2% wurden nicht alle Aneurysmen gesehen und in weiteren 2% waren die durchgeführten Untersuchungen nicht adäquat.

Aus der Studie von Perret und Nishioka (1966) geht hervor, daß von total 2961 initial, zu verschiedenen Zeitpunkten nach der Subarachnoidalblutung, bilateral durchgeführten erstmaligen Karotisangiographien 1586 (54%) ein Aneurysma aufdeckten. In 124 Fällen kam eine arteriovenöse Mißbildung zur Darstellung. Die Blutungsquelle blieb somit in 1251 Fällen ungeklärt. Bei 207 dieser 1251 Fälle wurde zu einem späteren Zeitpunkt eine weitere Karotisangiographie durchgeführt, wobei nun in 23% (47 Fälle) ein Aneurysma gefunden wurde. Daraus ergibt sich ein Minimum von 3,8% (47/1251) initial falsch negativer Resultate. Von den restlichen Patienten mit negativem Befund verstarben später 115. Die Autopsie erbrachte 12 Aneurysmen (10,4%) im Stromgebiet der A. carotis interna und 7 Aneurysmen (6,6%) im vertebro-basilären System.

1. Spasmen

Häufig sind angiographisch in den ersten Tagen nach einer Subarachnoidalblutung Gefäßeinengungen sichtbar, die auf Spasmen zurückgeführt werden, wie schon Ecker (1945) sowie Ecker und Riemenschneider (1951) festgestellt haben. Gefäßeinengungen, die mehr als 3–4 Wochen andauern, beruhen wahrscheinlich auf organischen Veränderungen der Gefäßwand, wobei ein Ödem eine wesentliche Rolle spielen dürfte. Derartige organische Gefäßwandveränderungen nach Subarachnoidalblutungen sind von Conway und McDonald (1972) und Fein et al. (1974) histologisch verifiziert worden. Mizukami et al. (1976) haben den Ablauf der Gefäßwandveränderungen in nachfolgendem Schema dargestellt.

Röntgenologisch stellt sich der spastische Gefäßabschnitt als gleichmäßig eingeengtes Lumen mit glatter Wand dar, was die Unterscheidung gegenüber den unregelmäßig geformten, scharf begrenzten Lumeneinengungen auf atherosklerotischer Basis erlaubt (Abb. 6 und 7). Die Angaben über die Häufigkeit dieser Spasmen schwanken bei den verschiedenen Autoren, was zum Teil durch den Zeitpunkt der Angiographie bedingt ist. Die Spasmen sind in den ersten Tagen nach der Subarachnoidalblutung häufiger zu beobachten als in einem späteren Zeitpunkt. Sie dauern Tage bis wenige Wochen an. Allcock und Drake (1965) fanden keine wesentlichen

Histologische Veränderungen der Arterienwand bei Gefäßspasmen. (Nach MIZUKAMI et al., 1976)

akutes Stadium (weniger als 1 Tag)	subakutes Stadium (weniger als 2 Wochen)	chronisches Stadium (mehr als 2 Wochen)
Kontraktion der glatten Muskelzellen der Media	Kontraktion der glatten Muskelzellen der Media	Nekrose der glatten Muskelzellen der Media (Lumenerweiterung)
	↓	↓
	Verdickung der Media Fältelung der Lamina elastica interna	
	↓	
	Endothelschädigung Permeabilitätserhöhung	
	↓	
	Intimaödem Wandthrombose Organisation	Intimafibrose Verdickung (Lumeneinengung)

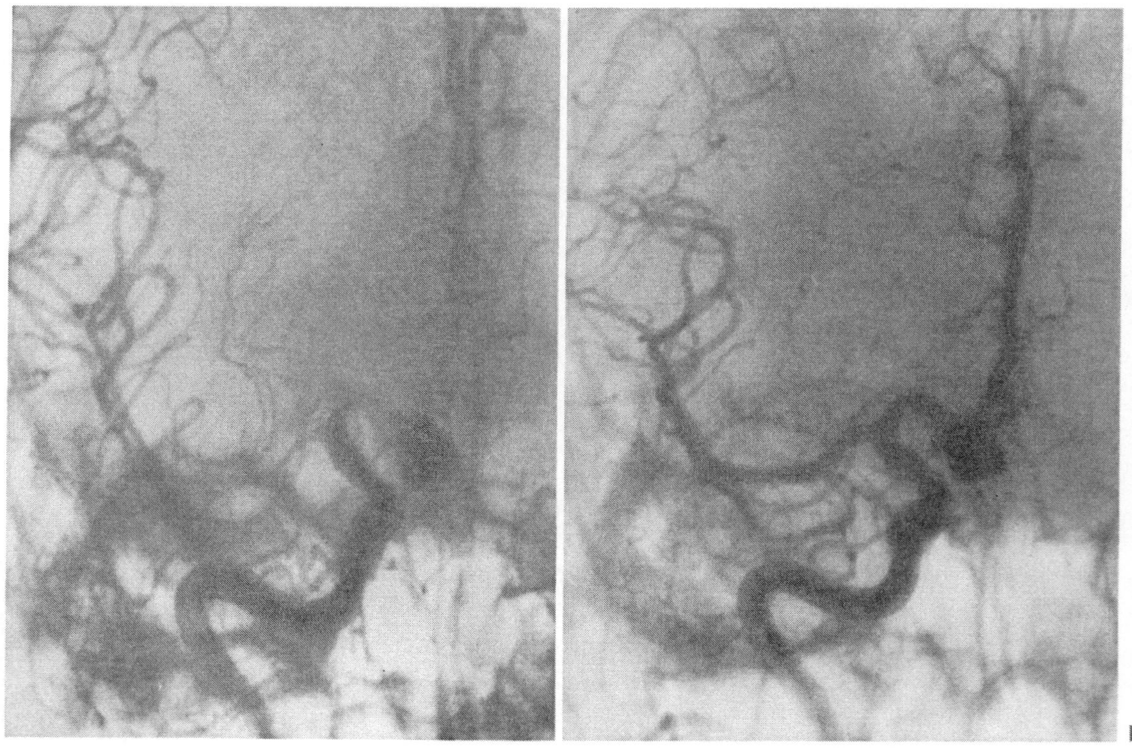

Abb. 6a u. b. Spasmus nach Subarachnoidalblutung. **a** Ausgedehnte Spasmen der A. cerebri anterior, der A. pericallosa und der A. cerebri media nach Ruptur eines Aneurysma der A. communicans anterior. **b** Kontrollaufnahme 1 Monat später, das Gefäßkaliber hat sich normalisiert. (Aus „Zerebrale Angiographie", 3. Aufl. 1979, Thieme Stuttgart)

Altersunterschiede in den Patientengruppen mit und ohne Spasmen. Die durchschnittliche Anzahl der Blutungsepisoden betrug 2,4 bei Patienten mit Spasmen und 1,8 bei Patienten ohne Spasmen. Spasmen fanden sich bei 50% der hypertonischen und bei 36% der normotonen Patienten. FLETCHER et al. (1959) geben eine Häufigkeit von 39% an, wovon 70% innerhalb der ersten drei

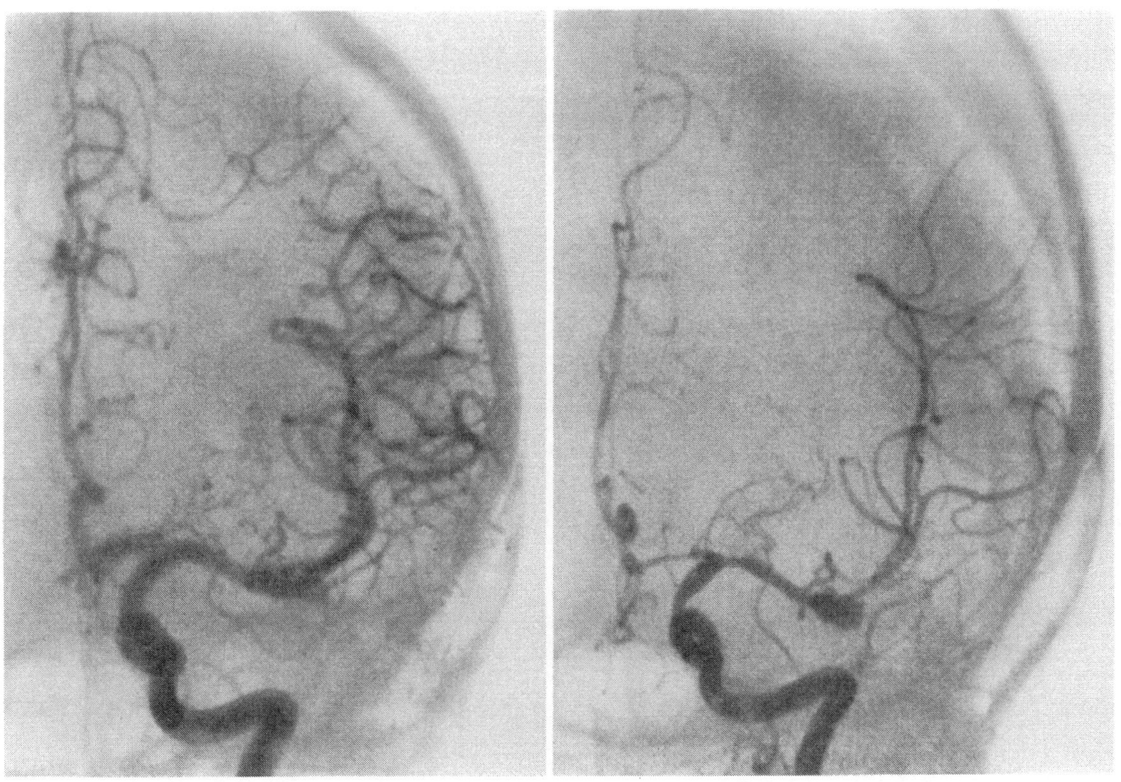

Abb. 7a u. b. Spasmus nach Subarachnoidalblutung. **a** Angiographie 1 Tag nach Subarachnoidalblutung bei 28jähriger Frau. Keine Spasmen faßbar, Aneurysma nicht deutlich dargestellt. **b** Kontrollangiographie 15 Tage später. Ausgedehnte Spasmen, das nicht mehr durch weite Gefäße verdeckte Aneurysma der A. cerebri media stellt sich gut dar. Kein raumforderndes Hämatom faßbar (mit Latenz Auftreten einer progredienten Aphasie ohne klinische Zeichen einer neuen Subarachnoidalblutung). (Aus „Zerebrale Angiographie", 3. Aufl. 1979, Thieme Stuttgart)

Wochen nach der Subarachnoidalblutung festgestellt wurden, im Durchschnitt 13 Tage nach der Blutung. Walter und Schütte (1964) fanden Spasmen in 37 von 155 Aneurysmapatienten, was 24% entspricht. Nach ihrer Beobachtung sind diese ebenfalls am häufigsten innerhalb der ersten drei Wochen nach der Blutung. Die gleiche Feststellung machten Bergvall und Galera (1969), wobei sie aber darauf hinweisen, daß beim Vorliegen eines intrazerebralen Hämatoms die Spasmen etwas früher auftreten. Wilkins et al. (1968) stellten bei 47% der Patienten mit Subarachnoidalblutung nach Aneurysmaruptur Spasmen fest, bei traumatischen Blutungen in den Subarachnoidalraum dagegen nur in 6,4%, was auch unseren Erfahrungen entspricht. Die Spasmen stehen zwar oft, jedoch keineswegs immer, in örtlichem Zusammenhang mit dem rupturierten Aneurysma. Sie können entfernt von ihm auftreten, gelegentlich sogar auf der Gegenseite, weshalb sie kein zuverlässiger Indikator zur Bestimmung des rupturierten Aneurysmas sind (Du Boulay, 1963). Spasmen finden sich besonders häufig bei Aneurysmen an der A. communicans anterior, der A. cerebri media und der Karotisbifurkation, während sie bei Aneurysmen der A. communicans posterior und im Basilarisstromgebiet weniger häufig vorkommen. Nicht mit Spasmen zu verwechseln sind hypoplastische Gefäßabschnitte im Circulus Willisi, speziell der A. cerebri anterior und der A. communicans posterior, sowie geringere Engstellungen der Karotisendstrecke, deren Lumen schon physiologischerweise distal vom Abgang der A. ophthalmica etwas abnimmt. Da die Gefäßmuskulatur zirkulär angeordnet ist, führt ein Spasmus immer nur zu einer Lumeneinengung, nie aber zu einer Verkürzung eines Gefäßabschnittes.

Die Ursache der Spasmen ist noch nicht völlig geklärt, und es werden verschiedene Faktoren diskutiert (Odom, 1975). Während einige Autoren eine neurogene Reaktion der glatten Gefäßmus-

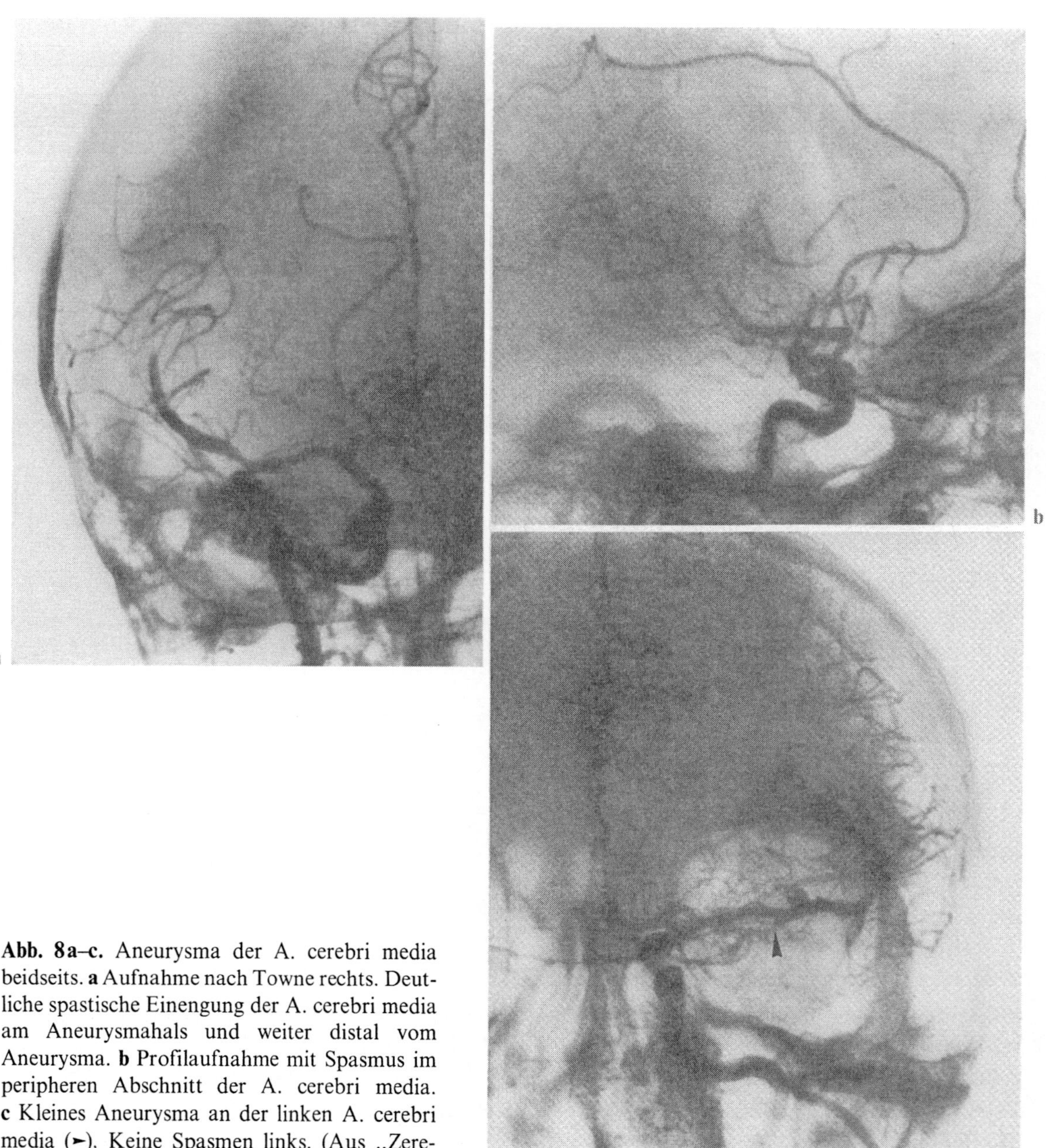

Abb. 8a–c. Aneurysma der A. cerebri media beidseits. **a** Aufnahme nach Towne rechts. Deutliche spastische Einengung der A. cerebri media am Aneurysmahals und weiter distal vom Aneurysma. **b** Profilaufnahme mit Spasmus im peripheren Abschnitt der A. cerebri media. **c** Kleines Aneurysma an der linken A. cerebri media (➤). Keine Spasmen links. (Aus „Zerebrale Angiographie“, 3. Aufl. 1979, Thieme Stuttgart)

kulatur vermuten (GURDJIAN et al., 1965), nehmen andere hormonelle und metabolische Einflüsse an. ECHLIN (1965), SIMEONE et al. (1968), KAPP et al. (1968) und ALLEN (1976) stellen sowohl die Rolle von humoralen Faktoren, die aus den Blutplättchen freigesetzt werden und sich von Serotonin und Angiotensin unterscheiden, zur Diskussion als auch rein mechanische Faktoren, wie z.B. Zerrungen oder Zerreißungen der Arachnoidea, wobei allerdings die letzteren mechanischen Faktoren nur zu kurzdauernden Vasokonstriktionen Anlaß geben.

Die Hirnarterien passieren in ihrem Verlauf durch die verschiedenen basalen Zisternen mehr oder weniger straffe Arachnoidalsepten, die u.U. durch Blutungen ausgespannt werden (YASARGIL et al., 1975, 1976), was sehr wohl zu einer mechanischen Irritation führen könnte. Von größtem Interesse sind in diesem Zusammenhang fibröse Strukturen, die sog. Chordae, welche im Subarachnoidalraum ausgespannt sind und die Arterien bis zu einem gewissen Grad in ihrer Position festhalten. Eine mechanische Irritation der Chordae, z.B. durch Zug (Anprall des in den Subarachnoidalraum einschießenden Bluts bei Aneurysmaruptur, Dehnung der Arachnoidalsepten in den basalen Zisternen), führt zu einer Gefäßwandkontraktur, wobei die nervösen Elemente in den Chordae und der Gefäßwand eine erhebliche Rolle spielen sollen (ARUTIUNOV et al., 1974).

Die Beobachtungen von BRAWLEY et al. (1968) sprechen für ein biphasisches Geschehen, wobei die erste Phase eines Spasmus durch mechanische Irritation und Serotonin verursacht werden könnte, nicht jedoch die länger dauernde zweite Phase. Ein biphasischer Verlauf ist auch von SYMON et al. (1972) und MARSHALL (1973) beschrieben worden.

Da Spasmen in relativ kurzer Zeit auftreten und wieder verschwinden können, ist es keineswegs selten, daß bei der Operation Gefäßeinengungen gefunden werden, die sich bei der Angiographie wenige Tage vorher nicht darstellten. Umgekehrt können angiographisch sichtbare Lumeneinengungen bei der Operation nicht mehr vorhanden sein.

Bei Lumeneinengungen und anterograden Zirkulationsverzögerungen distal eines Aneurysmas ist immer an die Möglichkeit zu denken, daß diese embolisch bedingt sein können, wobei das Aneurysma die Quelle für klinisch eventuell sogar symptomlos verlaufende Mikroembolien darstellt (ANTUNES u. CORELL, 1976) (Abb. 8).

Die angiographisch bestimmte zerebrale Zirkulationszeit ist nach einer Aneurysmaruptur oft etwas verlängert (OKAWARA et al., 1975). Eine Zirkulationsverzögerung findet sich namentlich dann, wenn Spasmen, ein Hydrocephalus internus oder eine Hämatom einzeln oder in Kombination vorliegen (ZINGESSER et al., 1968). Sehr hochgradige und langdauernde Spasmen können zu Infazierierung mit schweren neurologischen Störungen führen (POOL et al., 1958; CROMPTON, 1964; SCHNECK, 1964; SCHNECK und KRICHEFF, 1964; SUNDT et al., 1977). SCHNECK und KRICHEFF (1964) weisen allerdings darauf hin, daß Spasmen bei 62% der Patienten mit Infarkten vorkommen, jedoch auch bei 57% der Patienten ohne Infarkt. Von Bedeutung scheinen speziell das Ausmaß und die Dauer der Spasmen zu sein, im besonderen ihre Kombination mit einem Hämatom.

2. Der Zeitpunkt der Angiographie

Der Zeitpunkt der Angiographie ist abhängig von der Wahl des Operationstermins, falls ein operativ angehbares Aneurysma zur Darstellung kommt (HUDSON u. RAAF, 1968). Nach YASARGIL et al. (1975) ist das wesentliche Kriterium für die Wahl des Operationstermins nach einer Subarachnoidalblutung der Bewußtseinszustand des Patienten. Auf die Einhaltung einer bestimmten, willkürlich gewählten Frist zwischen Blutung und Operation wird verzichtet. Sofern es Allgemeinzustand (Alter des Patienten, Zustand des Kreislauf- und Atmungssystems, Blutdruck u.a.m.) und neurologischer Zustand (von größter Bedeutung ist die Bewußtseinslage) erlauben, wird die Angiographie sobald als möglich, eventuell schon am Tag nach der Subarachnoidalblutung, durchgeführt, damit die Operation vor der Periode mit dem größten Rezidivrisiko vorgenommen werden kann. Kommt eine allfällige Frühoperation wegen des Allgemeinzustands des Patienten nicht in Frage, so darf mit der Angiographie etwas zugewartet werden.

Eine Bewußtseinstrübung bei rupturiertem Aneurysma kann allerdings auch durch ein begleitendes raumforderndes Hämatom bedingt sein. Derartige Hämatome sind mit der computerisierten axialen Tomographie ohne jegliches Untersuchungsrisiko für den Patienten gut zu erfassen (Abb. 9). Besteht diese diagnostische Möglichkeit nicht, so kann ein Hämatom ohne Angiographie nicht sicher ausgeschlossen werden, weshalb bei bewußtlosen Patienten mit Herdsymptomen nicht allzu lange mit der Angiographie zugewartet werden sollte. Jedenfalls scheint die Angiographie in den ersten Tagen nach einer Blutung nicht gefährlicher zu sein als in einem späteren Termin, weshalb sie bei wachen oder somnolenten Patienten so rasch als möglich vorgenommen werden sollte. Es sei aber ausdrücklich davor gewarnt, daß in kleineren Spitälern mit ungenügender technischer Einrichtung und ohne notwendige neuroradiologische Erfahrung die Angiographie

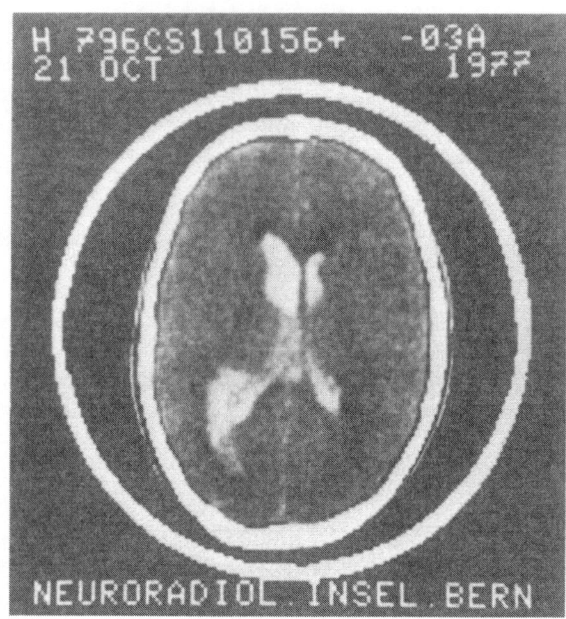

Abb. 9. Computertomogramm. Hämatocephalus internus nach Blutung aus arteriovenöser Mißbildung im linken Putamen

bei Subarachnoidalblutung überstürzt durchgeführt wird mit der Begründung, ein raumforderndes Hämatom ausschließen zu müssen. Die unter ungünstigen Verhältnissen angefertigten Angiogramme sind leider technisch oft ungenügend und geben dem Neurochirurgen nicht die erforderlichen Auskünfte, so daß sich eine Wiederholung der Angiographie aufdrängt. Besteht bei einem Patienten in schlechtem Allgemeinzustand und mit schwerer Bewußtseinstrübung der Verdacht, daß ein komplizierendes, raumforderndes Hämatom vorliegt, so sollte – wenn immer möglich – vor der Angiographie die den Patienten nicht belastende computerisierte axiale Tomographie durchgeführt werden.

3. Komplikationen der Angiographie bei Subarachnoidalblutungen

PERRET und NISHIOKA (1966) errechneten in ihrer Studie über 7165 Angiographien bei Subarachnoidalblutungen eine Komplikationsrate von 7,6%. In dieser Zahl sind selbstverständlich die Komplikationen der Angiographie allgemeiner Art eingeschlossen, und die Komplikationen, die spezifisch im Zusammenhang mit der Subarachnoidalblutung stehen, sind aus dieser Zahl schwierig herauszulösen. Von diesen Komplikationen traten 72% sofort und 28% nach einem gewissen Zeitintervall auf. In 67 Fällen kam es während oder nach der Angiographie zu einer Rezidivblutung. Es kann aber häufig nicht entschieden werden, ob eine derartige Blutung beim anerkannt hohen Risiko der Rezidivblutung nicht auch spontan, d.h. ohne Angiographie, aufgetreten wäre. SCHIEFER (1972) berichtet von einer tödlichen Rezidivblutung noch vor der Punktion bei der Lagerung des Patienten auf dem Röntgentisch.

In der Literatur finden sich Berichte über Kontrastmittelextravasate aus einem Aneurysma in den Subarachnoidalraum oder das Ventrikelsystem während der Angiographie (JAMIESON, 1954; JENKINSON et al., 1954; JACKSON et al., 1960; TRISKA, 1962; PIRKER, 1964; GOLDSTEIN, 1967; MURPHY u. GOLDBERG, 1967; BEAMER et al., 1969; FERRARI u. VIO, 1969; HOFF u. POTTS, 1969; VINES u. DAVIS, 1971; HENRY et al., 1971; LEHRER et al., 1972; TEAL et al., 1973; WAGA et al, 1973; OSGOOD u. MARTIN, 1974; GERLOCK, 1975; SOMEDA et al., 1975; LILIEQUIST et al., 1976).

Als Ursache für die Ruptur kann eine Erhöhung des intravasalen Druckes während der Kontrastmittelinjektion bei proximaler Stenose und engem Katheter oder bei peripheren Spasmen in Frage kommen (TEAL et al., 1973; LILIEQUIST et al., 1976). Leider endet die Aneurysmaruptur während einer Angiographie oft letal.

Ein Vergleich zwischen Komplikationen bei Patienten mit vorausgegangener Subarachnoidalblutung und Patienten ohne bekannte Blutung zeigt, daß bei ersteren die Häufigkeit mit 7,6% etwas höher liegt als bei letzteren mit 5,9%. Die Komplikationshäufigkeit bei Subarachnoidalblutungen ist bei Patienten mit Aneurysmen etwas höher (8,3%) als bei Patienten mit Blutung aus einer arteriovenösen Mißbildung (3,3%).

Die Komplikationsrate differiert nicht wesentlich, wenn die Gruppeneinteilung in wache, somnolente und komatöse Patienten erfolgt. Die Komplikationsrate bei der Vertebralisangiographie ist mit 4,1% geringer als diejenige bei der Karotisangiographie. Die Mortalitätsrate betrug 1,17%. Werden die Fälle mit Rezidivblutung nach der Angiographie ausgeschlossen, so verbleibt eine Mortalitätsrate von 0,82%.

IV. Das Aneurysma im angiographischen Bild

Im allgemeinen ist die angiographische Diagnose eines Aneurysmas einfach (Abb. 2). In der Mehrzahl der Fälle sind die Aneurysmen kleiner als 1 cm, besonders im Bereiche der A. communicans anterior und der A. cerebri media. Das freie Lumen dieser Aneurysmen füllt sich in der Regel während der Angiographie rasch und vollständig mit Kontrastmittel, das vom nachströmenden, kontrastmittelfreien Blut ebenso rasch wieder ausgeschwemmt wird. Gelegentlich bleibt aber etwas Kontrastmittel im Fundus liegen, was als Schichtungsphänomen bezeichnet wird (RAUSCH u. SCHIEFER, 1956; MARGUTH u. SCHIEFER, 1957; HUBER, 1961, 1966; SCHECHTER u. ELKIN, 1963; GEYER, 1965). In großen, 2 und mehr cm messenden Aneurysmen sind derartige Schichtungsphänomene relativ häufig, da das Kontrastmittel lange in den großen Aneurysmasäcken liegen bleibt (Abb. 10). Die Bestimmung der Halsweite bei sehr großen Aneurysmen, die meistens an der A. carotis interna oder an der A. basilaris sitzen, ist angiographisch häufig nicht möglich,

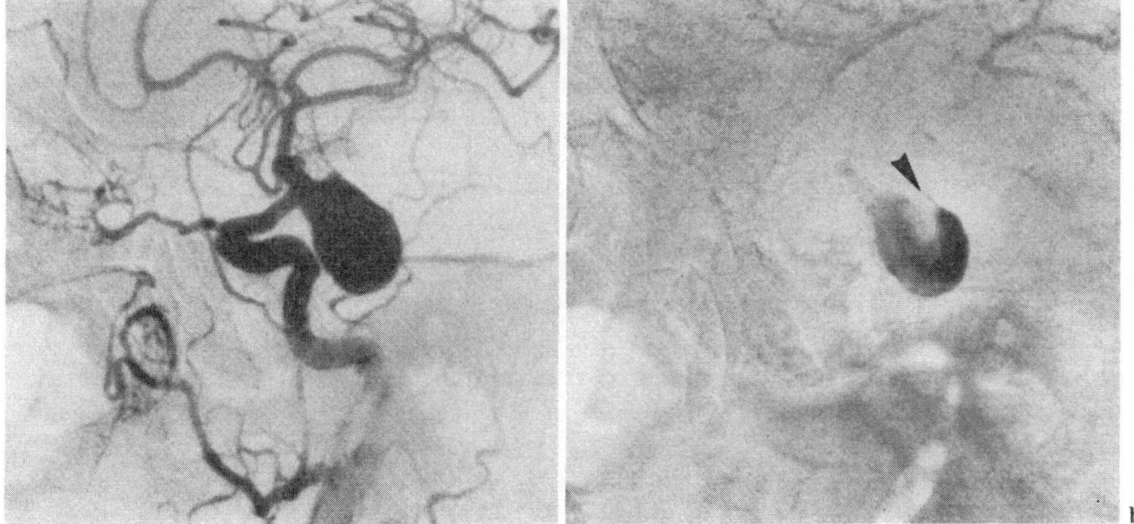

Abb. 10a u. b. Schichtungseffekt in großem Aneurysma der A. communicans posterior. **a** Arterielle Phase. **b** venöse Phase mit Schichtungseffekt. Einstrom von kontrastmittellosem Blut in das Aneurysma (►)

da die kontrastmittelgefüllten Aneurysmapartien den Hals, trotz Anwendung verschiedener Projektionsrichtungen, überdecken. Auf Serien mit einer Frequenz von 3 Aufnahmen/Sekunde kann nicht selten beobachtet werden, wie das Kontrastmittel düsenartig in das Aneurysma einschießt und der Aneurysmawand entlang fließt (Abb. 12b). Der Durchmesser des einschießenden Kontrastmittelstroms muß jedoch nicht dem Durchmesser des Aneurysmahalses entsprechen, da durch diesen gleichzeitig kontrastmittelloses Blut aus dem Aneurysma verdrängt wird. Für die unidirektionale Strömung steht wahrscheinlich nur ca. ein Drittel des Halsquerschnittes zur Verfügung (GERMAN u. BLACK, 1955).

Die Kontrastmittelmenge, die während der kurzen Passagezeit des Kontrastmittelbolus vor der Öffnung aus der Arterie in das Aneurysma übertritt, ist häufig nicht groß genug, um das kontrastmittellose Blut vollständig aus dem Aneurysma zu verdrängen. Das eingetretene Kontrastmittel wird vielmehr während einiger Zeit im Aneurysmasack herumgewirbelt, bevor es sich mit kontrastmittellosem Blut so vermischt, daß das Aneurysma sich einigermaßen homogen darstellt (PIRKER u. DIEMATH, 1969; HUBER u. RIVOIR, 1971; SATO u. KAMITANI, 1975). Zonen geringerer Kontrastmitteldichte, die Lage und Form während des Füllungs- und Entleerungsvorgangs ändern, sind nicht mit Thromben im Aneurysma zu verwechseln. Thromben in Aneurysmen mit einem Innendurchmesser von 1 cm und mehr sind allerdings häufig, doch handelt es sich meistens um murale Thromben (CROMPTON, 1966b).

Bei sehr großen Aneurysmen kommen im wesentlichen folgende Typen des Füllungs- und Entleerungsvorganges vor:

- Das Aneurysma füllt sich relativ langsam, ohne sichtbaren, düsenartig einschießenden Kontrastmittelstrahl und entleert sich wieder langsam. Die Durchmischung des kontrastmittelhaltigen mit kontrastmittellosem Blut ist relativ homogen. Es ist durchaus denkbar, daß die Pulsationen in diesen großen Aneurysmen mit starren und dicken Wänden vermindert sind, womit auch die Turbulenz im Aneurysma abnimmt und die Geschwindigkeit der Blutumsetzung verzögert wird (Abb. 11).
- Der Kontrastmittelstrom wird zur Hauptsache in das Aneurysma abgelenkt, das sich relativ rasch füllt. Das Kontrastmittel gelangt erst nach der Auswaschung aus dem Aneurysma in die Arterienabschnitte distal vom Aneurysma, was zur Folge hat, daß sich diese peripheren Gefäßabschnitte mit einer gewissen Verzögerung gegenüber den übrigen Strecken des Arteriensystems darstellen (Abb. 12). Die Strömungsgeschwindigkeit ist aber in den einzelnen Arterien nicht vermindert. Die Füllungsverzögerung ist allein durch den Umweg des kontrastmittelhaltigen Blutes durch das Aneurysma bedingt. Die vollständige Auswaschung des Kontrastmittels aus größeren Aneurysmen beansprucht u.U. mehrere Sekunden, weshalb Arterien distal vom Aneurysma noch in der venösen Phase Kontrastmittel führen können. Dieses Phänomen ist um so deutlicher, je mehr Kontrastmittel pro Serie injiziert und je vollständiger demzufolge die Füllung des Aneurysmasackes ist. Bei Verwendung kleiner Kontrastmittelmengen stellen sich die großen Aneurysmen nur unvollständig dar.

Die Analyse des Schichtungsphänomens sowohl im Modellversuch als auch in vivo zeigt indessen, daß zumindest in großen Aneurysmen keine gleichmäßig horizontale und gradlinige Begrenzung zwischen spezifisch schwerem kontrastmittelreichem und leichterem kontrastmittelarmen Blut zustande kommt, wie sie bei Spiegelbildung und Sedimentation unter statischen Verhältnissen zu beobachten ist. Die Grenzschicht ist im Gegenteil unter turbulenten Strömungsverhältnissen unregelmäßig, wobei sie meist eine mehr oder weniger deutliche Wellenlinie aufweist. Aufnahmen mit rascher Bildfolge zeigen, daß eine einigermaßen regelmäßige Grenzlinie nur kurze Zeit andauert und bereits auf der nächstfolgenden Aufnahme durch eine Wirbelbildung aufgerissen wird. Die Konfiguration des Aneurysmahalses und die Ablenkung des Blutstromes durch Intimapolster sind entscheidend für den Anteil des Blutstromes, der in das Aneurysma abgelenkt wird, und für die Lokalisation des Turbulenzmaximums.

Unter dem Einfluß des lange auf die Aneurysmawand einwirkenden hypertonischen Kontrastmittels kann es zur vollständigen Thrombosierung großer Aneurysmen innerhalb der auf die Angiographie folgenden Tage kommen (LODIN, 1966; DEVADIGA et al., 1969; SCOTT u. BALLANTINE, 1972; CARLSON u. THOMSON, 1976).

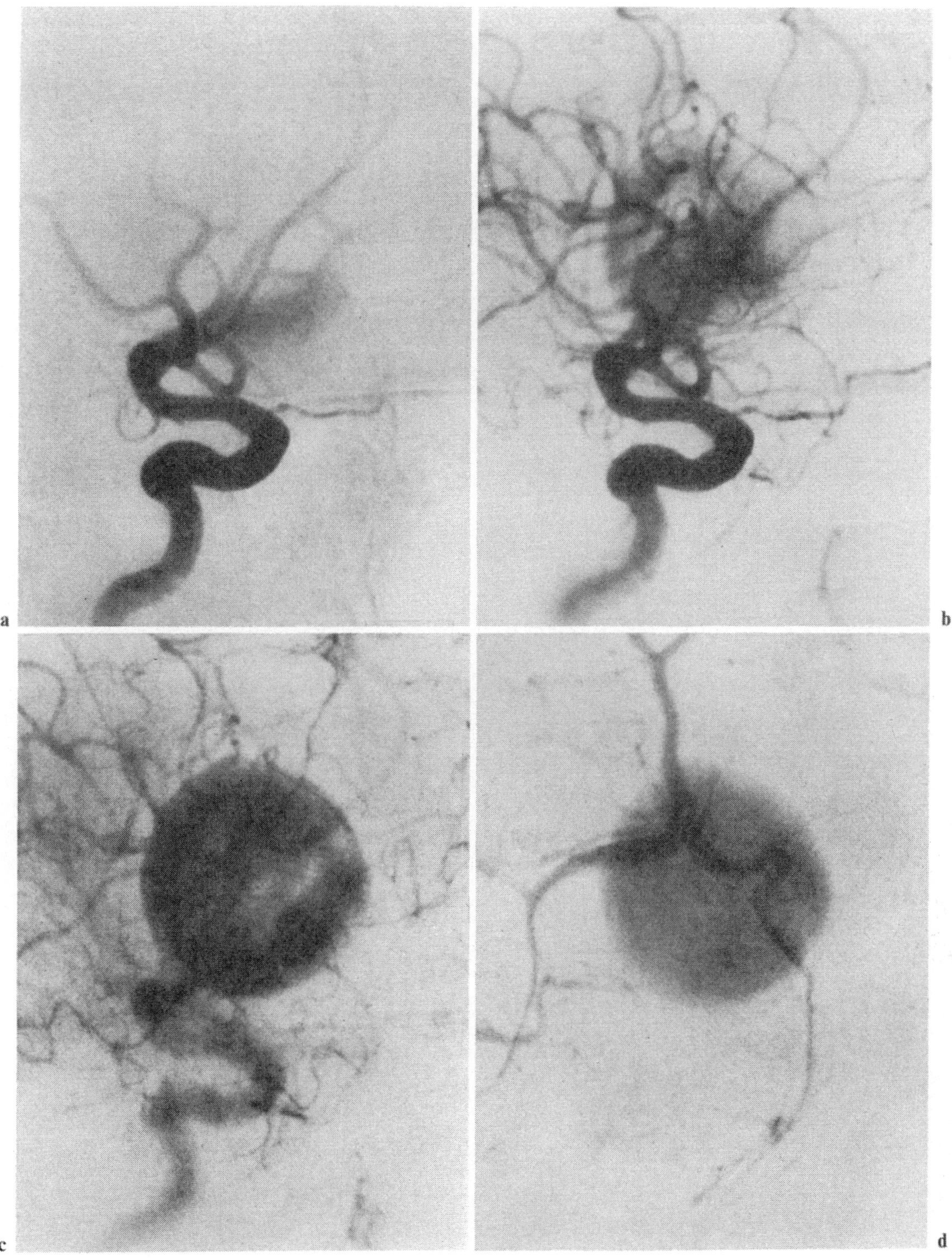

Abb. 11a–d. Füllungsablauf in großem Aneurysma an der Teilungsstelle der A. carotis interna. **a** Früharterielle Phase mit beginnendem Kontrastmitteleinstrom in das Aneurysma; **b** arterielle Phase. Das Aneurysma ist noch nicht homogen mit Kontrastmittel gefüllt; **c** spätarterielle Phase; **d** venöse Phase: Das Aneurysma ist immer noch homogen mit Kontrastmittel gefüllt. Kein Schichtungseffekt. (Aus „Zerebrale Angiographie, 3. Aufl. 1979, Thieme Stuttgart)

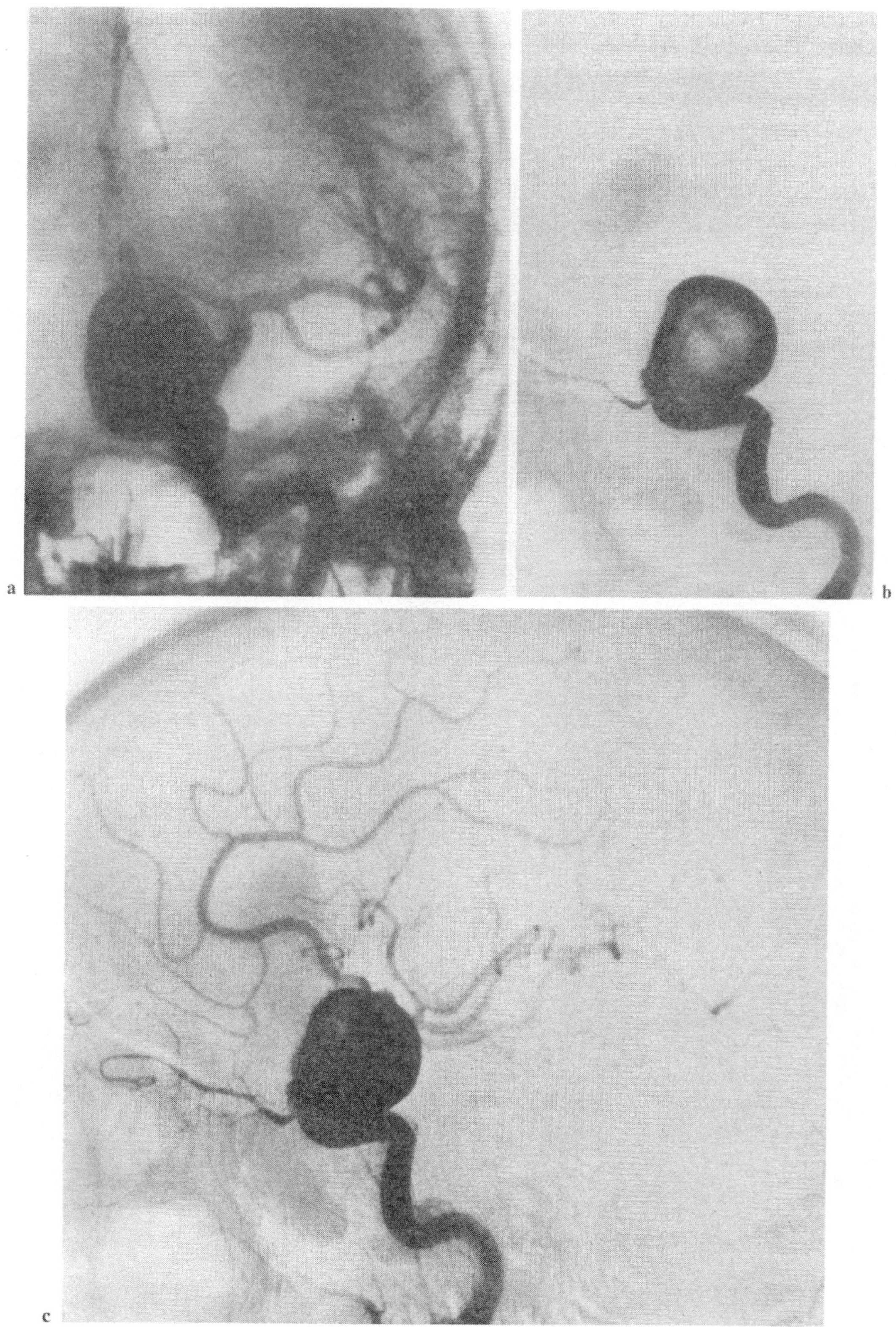

Abb. 12a–g. Füllungsablauf in großem Aneurysma der A. carotis interna. **a** a-p Aufnahme: Das Aneurysma ist nach medial gerichtet. **b–g** Profilserie: Das Kontrastmittel strömt zunächst aus der A. carotis interna der Wand entlang in das Aneurysma (**b**). In den späteren Phasen Schichtungseffekt, Kontrastmittel bleibt im Aneurysma bis in die venöse Phase (**g**) liegen. Das aus dem Aneurysma ausgeschwemmte Kontrastmittel bringt die A. pericallosa (►) auch noch in der venösen Phase zur Darstellung (**g**)

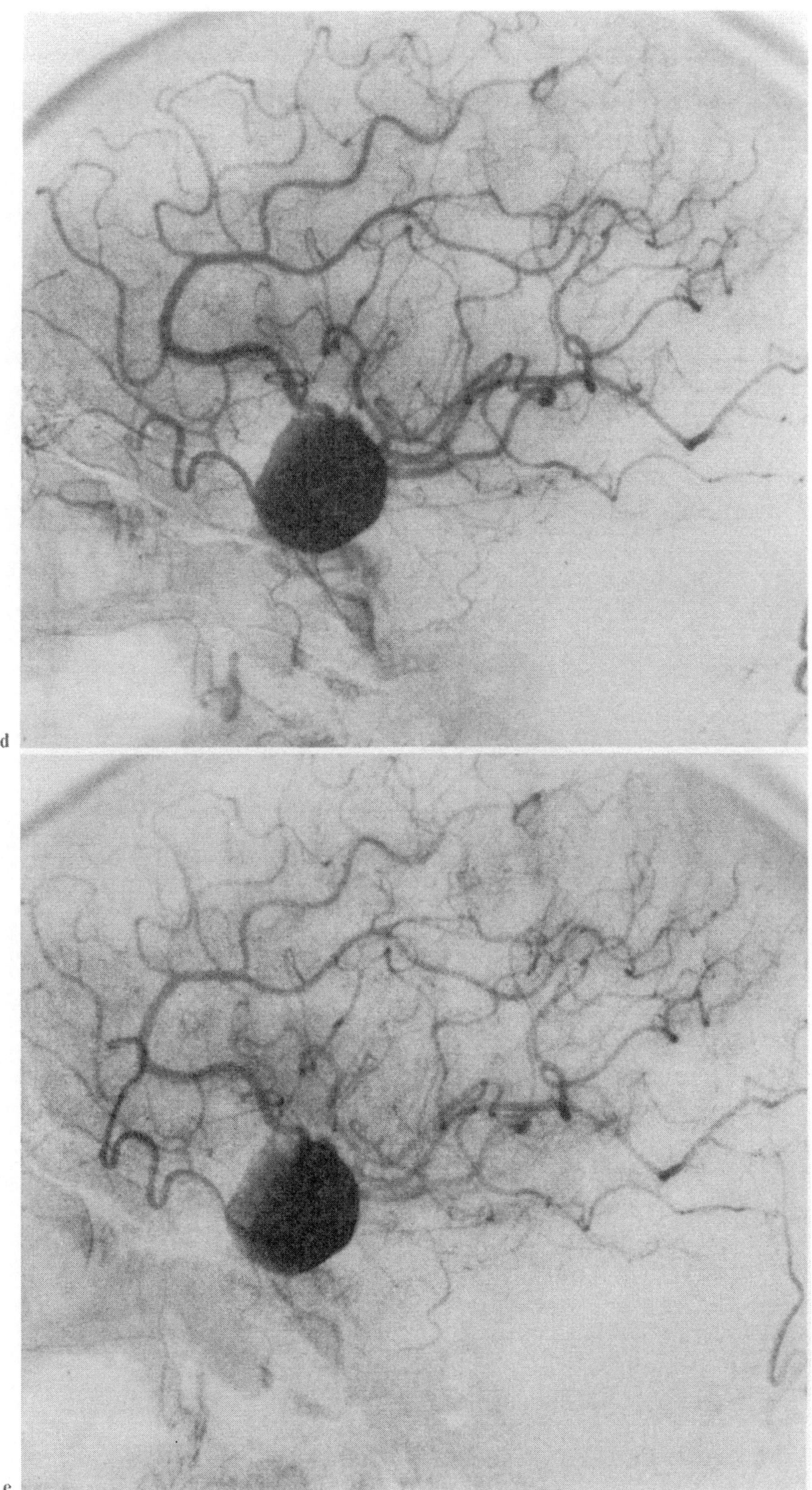

Abb. 12d u. e

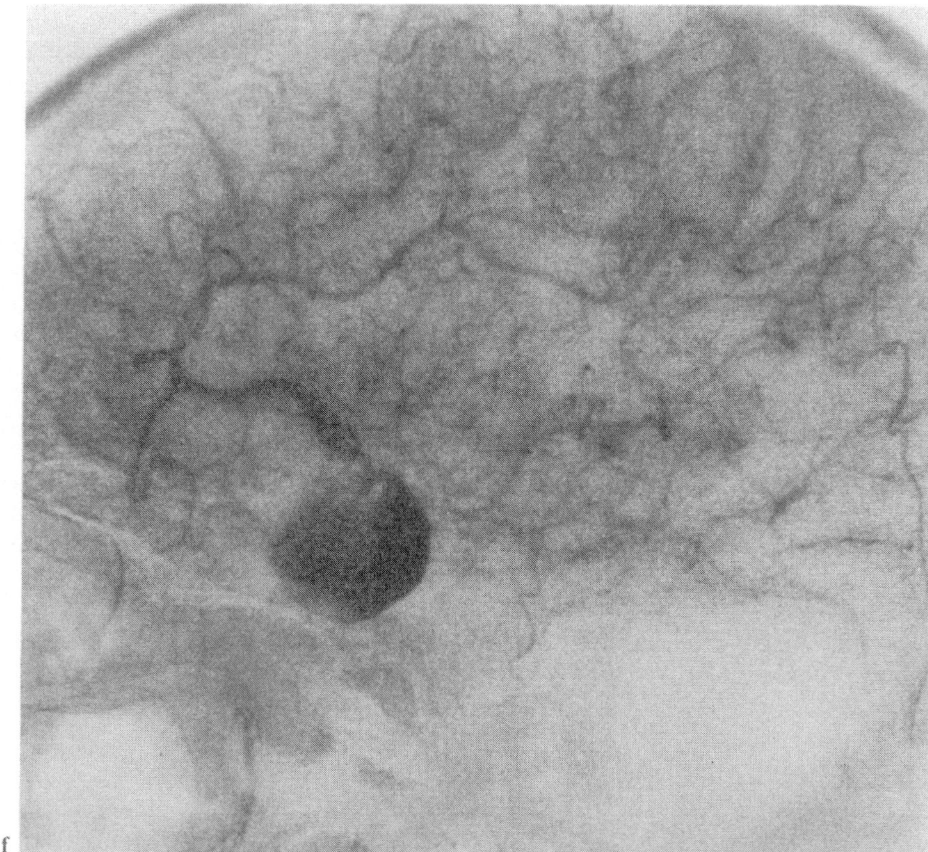
f

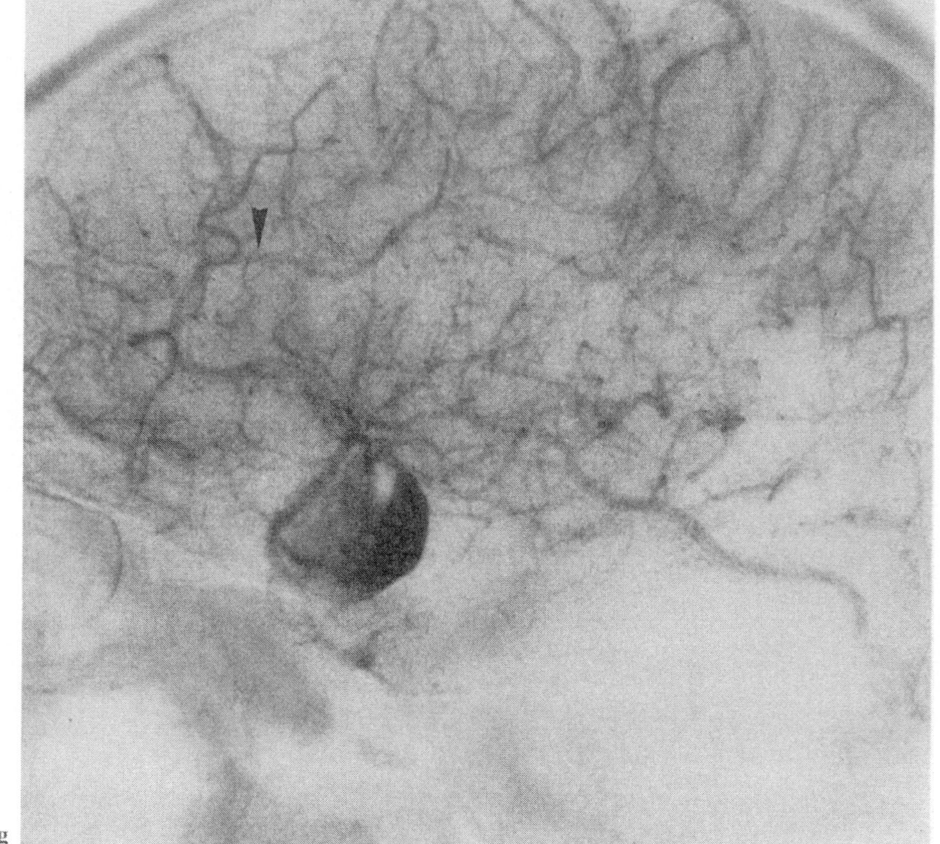
g

Abb. 12f u. g

V. Die angiographische Lokalisation der Aneurysmen

1. Extrakranielle Aneurysmen

Extrakraniell gelegene Aneurysmen der A. carotis interna sind relativ selten (MARGOLIS et al., 1972). Die Erstsymptome dieser Aneurysmen sind häufig diejenigen eines zerebrovaskulären Insults, bedingt durch die Behinderung der Strömung in der A. carotis interna oder durch Embolien aus dem Aneurysma. Von 9 extrakraniellen Aneurysmen, die GROS et al. (1970) mit diesen Initialsymptomen beobachteten, waren zwei vom fusiformen Typus, drei sackförmig und vier gehörten zur Gruppe der dissezierenden Aneurysmen. Die meisten der im extrakraniellen Karotisabschnitt gelegenen Aneurysmen entstehen auf arteriosklerotischer Basis, namentlich bei älteren Menschen, und sitzen dementsprechend häufig an der Bifurkation oder unmittelbar distal davon. 5 von 12 der von MARGOLIS et al. beschriebenen Aneurysmen waren fusiform. Ein weiterer Prädilektionsort der extrakraniellen Aneurysmen befindet sich auf Höhe der beiden obersten Halswirbel (Abb. 13). Je nach Größe und Lage kann das Aneurysma als pulsierende Schwellung im Pharynxbereich (CAMPICHE u. ZANDER, 1962) oder in der seitlichen Zervikalregion palpiert werden (ca. $^{1}/_{3}$ der Fälle). Seltener ist ein Strömungsgeräusch hörbar. Außer durch zerebrovaskuläre Symptome können sich die Aneurysmen durch Druck auf die kaudalen Hirnnerven IX–XII manifestieren.

Extrakranielle Aneurysmen können auch Folge eines perforierenden oder stumpfen Traumas sein, das zu einer Karotisruptur mit Hämatom und Bildung eines „falschen" Aneurysmas (Aneurysma spurium) geführt hat.

Die Aneurysmen auf infektiöser Grundlage stellt die kleinste Gruppe der extrakraniellen Aneurysmen dar (TOMONO et al., 1975). Sie entstehen nicht selten durch Übergreifen einer entzündlichen

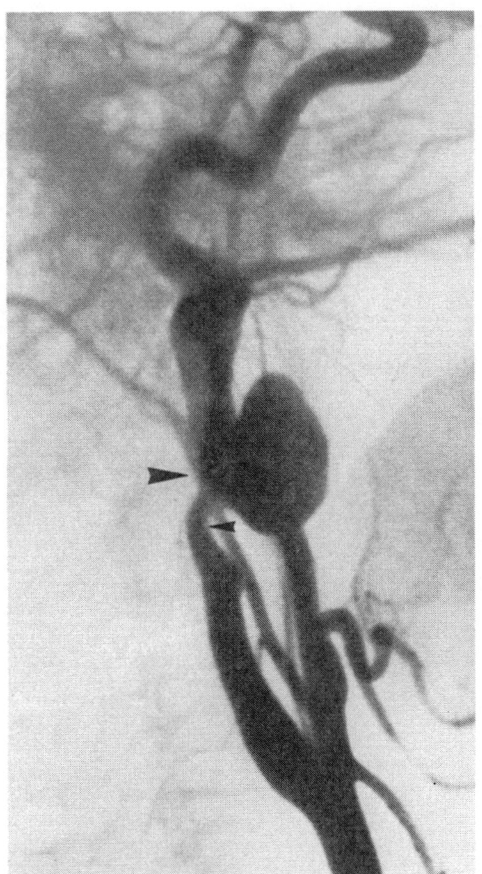

Abb. 13. Großes extrakranielles Aneurysma der A. carotis interna. Lumeneinengung der A. carotis interna unmittelbar proximal vom Aneurysma (►). Auf Höhe des Aneurysmahalses konstanter kleiner Füllungsdefekt (▶), möglicherweise durch Intimabrücke bedingt. (Aus „Zerebrale Angiographie", 3. Aufl. 1979, Thieme Stuttgart)

Pharyngealerkrankung oder einer Otitis media beim Kind auf die Karotiswand. Wichtig ist in diesen Fällen die Differentialdiagnose gegenüber Pharyngeal- oder Tonsillarabszessen.

2. Aneurysmen am intrakavernösen Abschnitt der A. carotis interna

Im Canalis caroticus und am Übergang vom intrapetrösen zum intrakavernösen Abschnitt sind Aneurysmen ausgesprochen selten (HARRISON et al., 1963; ANDERSON et al., 1972; RAVON et al., 1976).

Eine wichtigere Prädilektionsstelle bildet der intrakavernöse Abschnitt der A. carotis interna (Abb. 14): Die hier gelegenen infraklinoidalen Aneurysmen verursachen das Sinus-cavernosus-Syndrom mit Okulomotorius- und Abduzensparese sowie Schmerzen im Trigeminusgebiet (JEFFERSON, 1937, 1955; BARR et al., 1971). Bei Ruptur dieser Aneurysmen bleibt der Liquor klar. Sie können aber zu spontanen arteriovenösen Fisteln im Sinus cavernosus führen (FROMM u. HABEL, 1965; OBRADOR et al., 1974). In seltenen Fällen, wenn sie sich gegen den Sinus sphenoidalis zu ausdehnen, geben sie Anlaß zu massivem Nasenbluten (TROUPP, 1962). Häufiger allerdings ist dieses bei traumatischen Karotisaneurysmen (ARAKI et al., 1965; HANDA et al., 1967; HANDA u. HANDA, 1976). Infraklinoidale Aneurysmen können u.U. sehr groß werden (Abb. 15) und häufig schon auf Schädelröntgenbildern anhand von Knochenarrosionen, die etwa in 80% der Fälle, und Wandverkalkungen, die etwa in einem Drittel der Fälle zu sehen sind, diagnostiziert werden (RISCHBIETH u. BULL, 1958; LOMBARDI et al., 1963; JEANMART et al., 1973). Sie stellen etwa 5–6% der intrakraniellen Aneurysmen dar. Lediglich LOMBARDI et al. (1963) geben mit

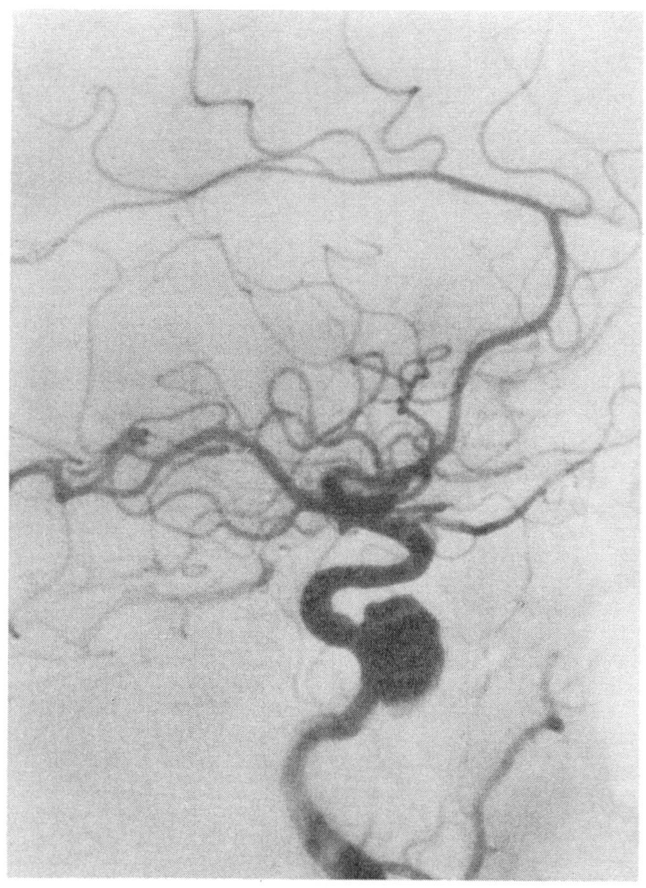

Abb. 14. Infraklinoidales Aneurysma. (Aus „Zerebrale Angiographie“, 3. Aufl. 1979, Thieme Stuttgart)

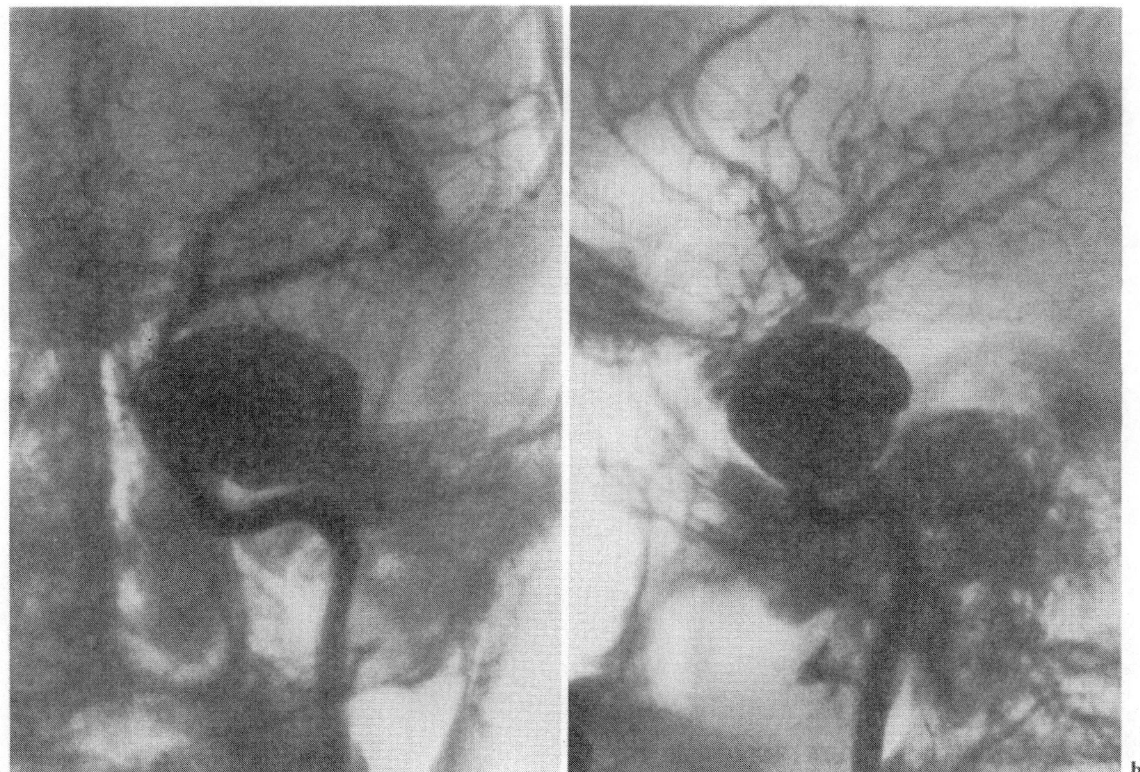

Abb. 15a u. b. Sehr großes, nach lateral gerichtetes intrakavernöses Aneurysma. **a** a-p Aufnahme; **b** Profilaufnahme

11% eine größere Häufigkeit an. Diese Aneurysmen thrombosieren wegen ihrer Größe nicht selten und sind dann angiographisch nicht mehr direkt erfaßbar.

Die intraselläre Ausdehnung eines Aneurysmas ist selten und kommt nach JEFFERSON (1937, 1955) sowie WHITE und BALLANTINE (1961) in 1,9% und nach RHONHEIMER (1959) in 2,9% der Fälle vor (GALLAGHER et al., 1956; WHITE, 1962).

Das sackförmige Aneurysma der A. ophthalmica entspringt aus der Vorderwand oder der anteromedialen Seite der A. carotis interna, unmittelbar distal, seltener proximal vom Abgang der A. ophthalmica (Abb. 16). An dieser Stelle zweigen feine, angiographisch nicht sichtbare Gefäße aus der medialen Karotiswand zum N. opticus und Chiasma ab (DAWSON, 1958; WOLLSCHLAEGER et al., 1970). LOCKSLEY (1966) gibt für diese Aneurysmalokalisation eine Häufigkeit von 5,4% an. DRAKE et al. (1968a), KOTHANDARAM et al. (1971) und THUREL et al. (1974) weisen darauf hin, daß diese Aneurysmen bei Frauen viel häufiger sind als bei Männern. Nicht selten kommen sie bilateral oder in Kombination mit Aneurysmen an anderer Stelle vor, z.B. an der A. communicans posterior. Je nach ihrer Lage oder Richtung können die Aneurysmen der A. ophthalmica in folgende Gruppen unterteilt werden:

- suboptochiasmatische Gruppe mit Aneurysmarichtung nach horizontal und medial,
- laterooptochiasmatische Gruppe mit Aneurysmarichtung nach vorne oben (seltener),
- suprachiasmatische Gruppe mit Aneurysmarichtung nach oben und
- globaler Typus

(THUREL et al., 1974; GARCIA-BENGOCHEA u. DELAND, 1975; GUIDETTI u. LA TORRE, 1975; ALMEIDA et al., 1976; YASARGIL et al., 1977). Chirurgisch am besten anzugehen sind die nach vorne oben gerichteten laterochiasmatischen Aneurysmen. Sie können zu Subarachnoidalblutungen ohne Lokalsymptome führen, während die suboptischen und subchiasmatischen Aneurysmen nicht

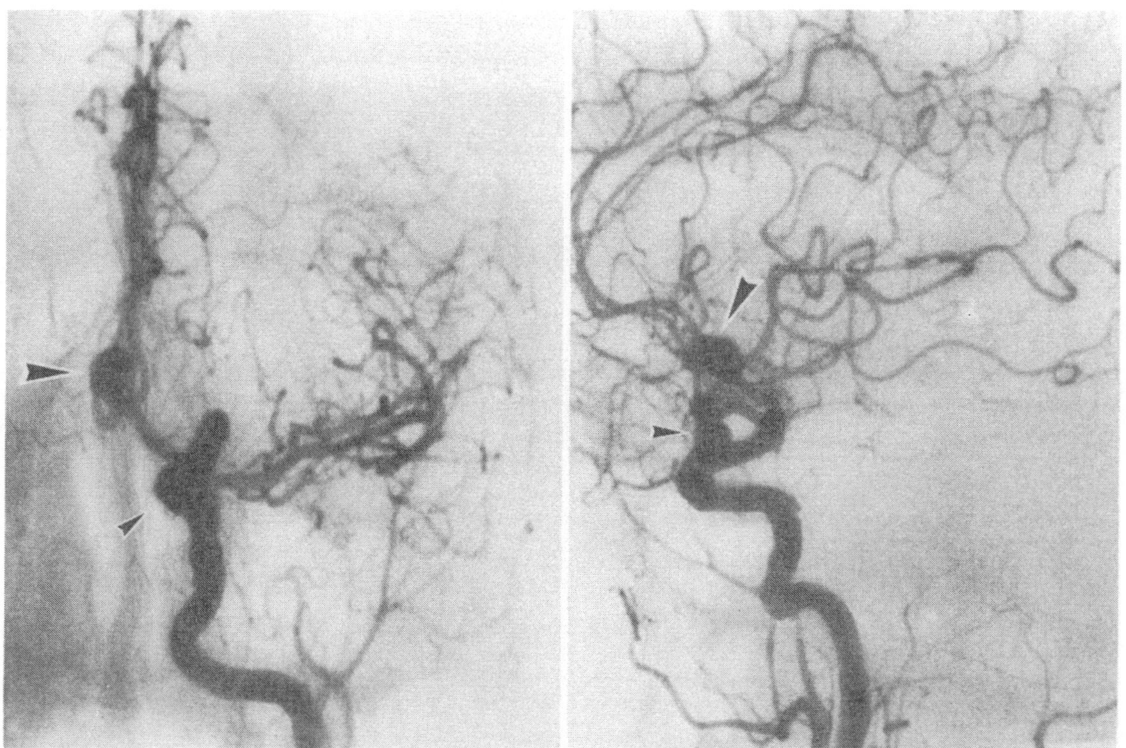

Abb. 16a u. b. Laterochiasmatisches Aneurysma der A. ophthalmica (➤) und Aneurysma der A. communicans anterior (▶), letzteres ist rupturiert (mit CT und durch Operation verifiziert). Das Aneurysma der A. communicans anterior sitzt breitbasig auf der Teilungsstelle der linken A. cerebri anterior in beide Aa. pericallosae. Eine eigentliche A. communicans anterior ist nicht vorhanden. Hypoplasie der rechten A. cerebri anterior. **a** Profilaufnahme; **b** a-p Aufnahme

selten Sehstörungen verursachen. Unter den 14 Fällen von DRAKE et al. (1968a) wies allerdings nur einer Zeichen einer Optikuskompression auf.

3. Aneurysmen der A. communicans posterior

Die A. communicans posterior weist an ihrer Abgangsstelle aus der A. carotis interna nicht selten eine infundibuläre Erweiterung auf. Derartige Erweiterungen finden sich auch am Abgang der A. choroidea anterior und der A. ophthalmica und können ein echtes sackförmiges Aneurysma vortäuschen. HASSLER und SALTZMAN (1959, 1963) haben sie am Abgang der A. communicans posterior in 6,5% bei 1020 sonst normalen Karotisanigogrammen gefunden und in 21 Fällen diese Erweiterung histologisch untersucht. In allen Fällen fanden sich Mediadefekte, die in 14 Fällen sogar sehr groß (Durchmesser über 1 mm) waren. In 6 Fällen fehlte außerdem die Elastica interna, und die Wand setzte sich wie bei einem echten sackförmigen Aneurysma nur aus Bindegewebe zusammen. Demgegenüber stellten EPSTEIN et al. (1970) bei 7 histologisch untersuchten ampullenförmigen Ausweitungen eine vollkommen normale Wandbeschaffenheit fest, weshalb sie die infundibulären Erweiterungen scharf von Präaneurysmen oder echten Aneurysmen abgrenzen. Es besteht aber kein Zweifel, daß sich am Ort infundibulärer Erweiterungen ein Aneurysma entwickeln kann (STUNTZ et al., 1970; YOUNG et al., 1971) (Abb. 17).

Die häufig recht unregelmäßig geformten und nicht selten länglichen Aneurysmen der A. communicans posterior sind nach hinten, nach hinten lateral oder lateral gerichtet, nicht aber nach medial oder vorne. Sie weisen häufig Verklebungen mit der A. communicans posterior, der A. cho-

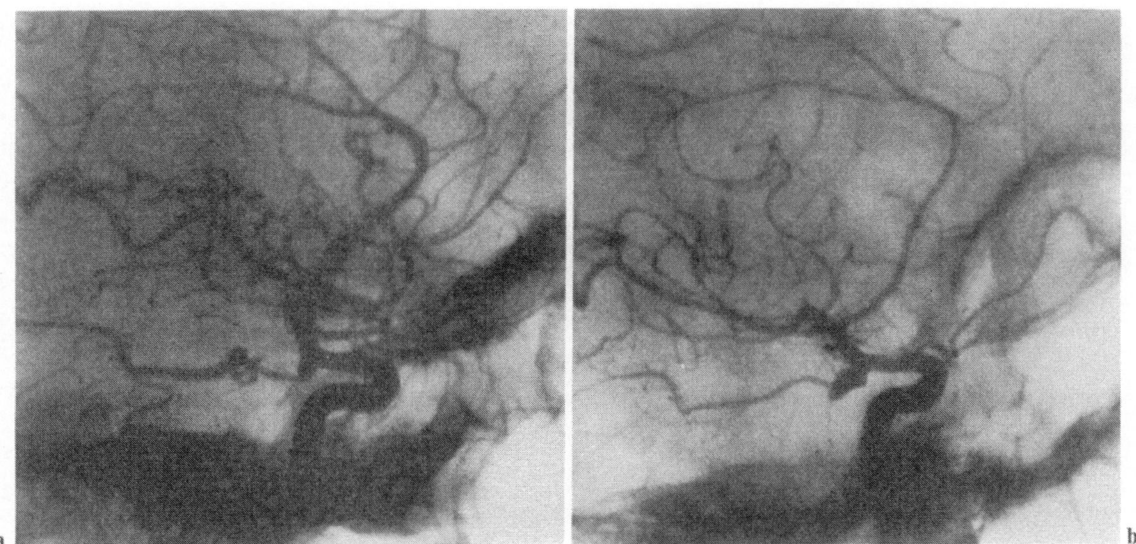

Abb. 17a u. b. Entwicklung eines sackförmigen Aneurysmas der A. communicans posterior. **a** Angiographie nach erster Subarachnoidalblutung. Ampullenförmige Ausweitung am Abgang der A. communicans posterior aus der A. carotis interna. **b** Angiographie 2 Jahre später nach zweiter Subarachnoidalblutung. Aneurysma der A. communicans posterior. (Aus „Zerebrale Angiographie", 3. Aufl. 1979, Thieme Stuttgart)

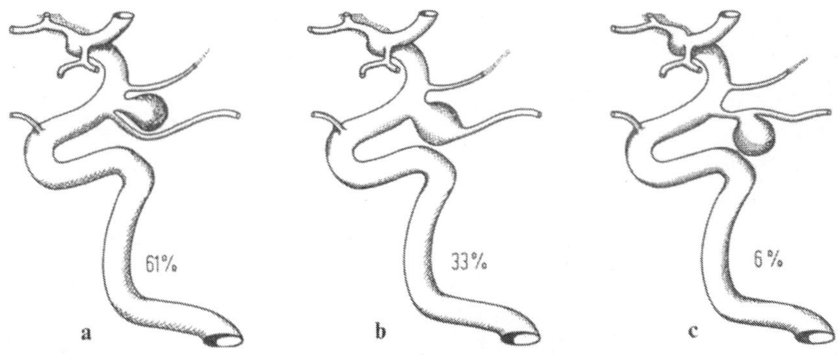

Abb. 18. Aneurysmen der A. communicans posterior. (Schematische Darstellung nach KRAYENBÜHL et al., 1972)

roidea anterior oder beiden auf, speziell auch, wenn sie nicht direkt an der Abgangsstelle der A. communicans posterior sitzen, sondern zwischen dieser und der A. choroidea anterior. Unter dem Operationsmikroskop stellen sich die Aneurysmen der A. communicans topographisch folgendermaßen dar (KRAYENBÜHL et al., 1972) (Abb. 18):

a) Am häufigsten sind die Aneurysmen zwischen der A. communicans posterior und der A. choroidea anterior gelegen (43/64, 67%) (Abb. 19 und 20).
b) In 22% (14/64) stellt das Aneurysma eine ausgeprägtere infundibuläre Erweiterung dar, aus deren Kuppe lumenmäßig deutlich abgesetzt die A. communicans posterior hervorgeht.
c) In 6% schließlich sitzt das sackförmige Aneurysma an der A. communicans posterior, kurz nach ihrem Abgang aus der A. carotis interna (Abb. 21).

Nach SACHS et al. (1968) verteilen sich die Aneurysmen der A. carotis interna folgendermaßen: Von 42 der an der A. carotis interna gefundenen Aneurysmen saßen je 4 im infraklinoidalen

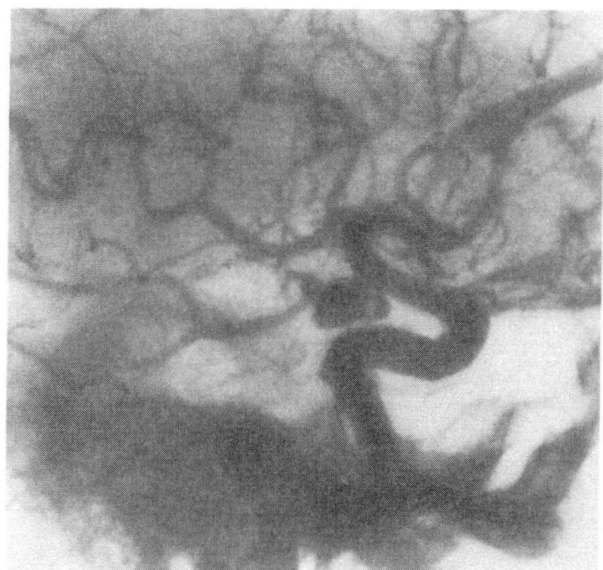

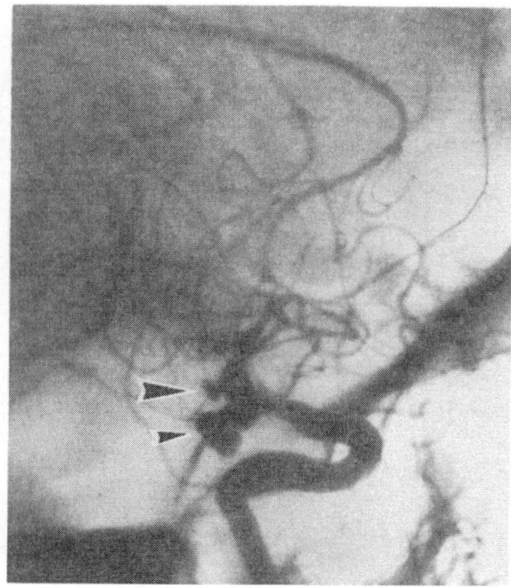

Abb. 19 **Abb. 20**

Abb. 19. Aneurysma der A. carotis interna, unmittelbar distal vom Abgang der A. communicans posterior

Abb. 20. Aneurysma am Abgang der A. communicans posterior (➤) und der A. choroidea anterior (▶). (Aus „Zerebrale Angiographie", 3. Aufl. 1979, Thieme Stuttgart)

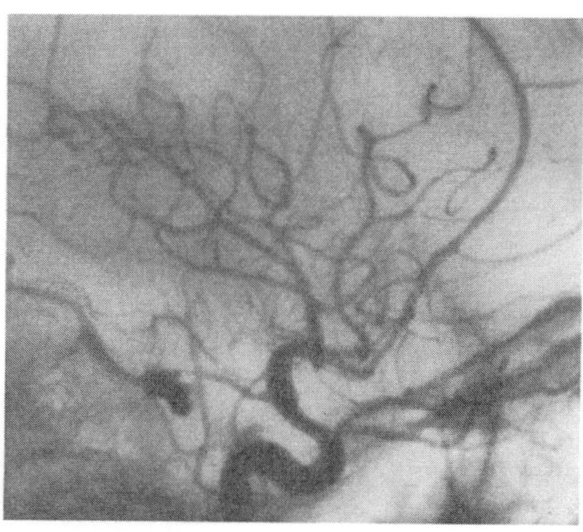

Abb. 21. Lobuliertes Aneurysma an der Einmündung der A. communicans posterior in die A. cerebri posterior. (Aus „Zerebrale Angiographie", 3. Aufl. 1979, Thieme Stuttgart)

Abschnitt und an der Teilungsstelle der A. carotis interna am Circulus Willisi. 9 Aneurysmen gingen von der Abgangsstelle der A. choroidea anterior aus. 5 Aneurysmen waren zwischen A. choroidea anterior und A. communicans posterior ausgestülpt und 20 gehörten zu den Aneurysmen der A. communicans posterior im engeren Sinn. Von diesen 20 Aneurysmen zeigten 10 keine Verwachsungen mit den benachbarten Gefäßen. 4 wiesen Verklebungen zwischen ihrer Kuppe und A. choroidea anterior auf, 3 mit der A. communicans posterior und 3 zeigten ausgedehnte Verwachsungen sowohl mit der A. choroidea anterior wie mit der A. communicans posterior.

Das Aneurysma im proximalen Abschnitt der A. communicans posterior kann aber auch mit der Vertebralisangiographie nachgewiesen werden, wenn gleichzeitig die ipsilaterale A. carotis interna komprimiert wird.

Die Chance der Nachblutung eines Aneurysmas der A. communicans posterior nach dem 40. Tag wird auf 25% geschätzt, gegenüber 10% bei Aneurysmen der A. communicans anterior (RICHARDSON et al., 1966).

4. Aneurysmen der A. choroidea anterior

Die Aneurysmen am Abgang der A. choroidea anterior sind relativ selten. Sie liegen im oberen Winkel zwischen A. choroidea anterior und A. carotis interna, sind aber angiographisch nicht immer eindeutig von den Aneurysmen der A. communicans posterior abzugrenzen. Die klinischen Symptome entsprechen weitgehend denjenigen, die durch Aneurysmen der A. communicans posterior verursacht werden (DRAKE et al., 1968b; PERRIA et al., 1969). Auch traumatische Aneurysmen sind an dieser Stelle beschrieben worden (CRESSMAN u. HAYES, 1966). Sehr selten sind Aneurysmen am intraventrikulären Abschnitt der A. choroidea anterior (STRULLY, 1955; PAPO et al., 1973).

5. Aneurysmen an der Karotisbifurkation

Die Aneurysmen an der Bifurkation der A. carotis interna am Circulus Willisi können u.U. sehr groß werden. Diese Lokalisation ist bei Kindern und Jugendlichen nicht selten. PATEL und RICHARDSON (1971) fanden bei 58 Patienten mit Aneurysmarupturen in den beiden ersten Dekaden in 35% ein Aneurysma an der Karotisbifurkation. THOMSON et al. (1973) zählten unter 15 kongenitalen Aneurysmen bei Kindern 6 an der Karotisbifurkation, die somit offenbar der Hauptsitz für Aneurysmen im Kindesalter ist (Abb. 22). Der Aneurysmahals kann gut abgegrenzt und relativ eng sein, kann aber auch breitbasig auf den Anfangsabschnitt der A. carotis anterior oder media, resp. auf beide zusammen übergreifen. Diese anatomischen Verhältnisse sind bei den meist nach oben gerichteten Aneurysmen angiographisch kaum von Verklebungen des Aneurysmasackes mit der Gefäßwand abzugrenzen. Ihre genaue Beachtung ist für den Operateur von ausschlaggebender Bedeutung beim Verschluß des Aneurysmas (DAVID u. SACHS, 1967).

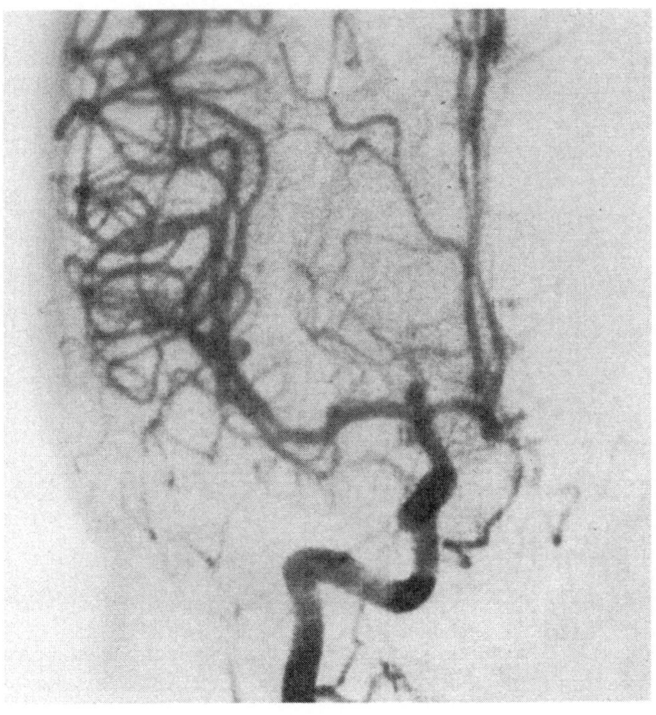

Abb. 22. Aneurysma an der Teilungsstelle der A. carotis interna bei 21j. Patienten

6. Aneurysmen der A. cerebri anterior

Die Aneurysmen der A. cerebri anterior im präkommunikalen Abschnitt sind selten und sitzen meist am Abgang der A. recurrens HEUBNER oder einer der perforierenden Arterien.

7. Aneurysmen der A. communicans anterior

Wesentlich häufiger, nach einigen Statistiken sogar am häufigsten, sind die Aneurysmen, die an der A. communicans anterior oder an der Teilungsstelle der A. cerebri anterior in A. communicans anterior und A. pericallosa sitzen (KRAYENBÜHL et al., 1959). Bei einer Asymmetrie der Aa. cerebri anteriores sitzen die Aneurysmen gewöhnlich mehr oder weniger breitbasig am Oberrand der Teilungsstelle der weiteren A. cerebri anterior in A. communicans anterior und A. pericallosa (Abb. 16 und 23). Bei symmetrisch entwickelten Aa. cerebri anteriores entspringt das Aneurysma gewöhnlich aus der A. communicans anterior. Die A. recurrens HEUBNER steht in verschiedensten Beziehungen zur A. cerebri anterior und kann, wenn letztere hypoplastisch ist, u.U. sogar mit dieser verwechselt werden (DUNKER u. HARRIS, 1976; PERLMUTTER u. RHOTON, 1976). Angiographisch muß daher dieses Gefäß, wenn irgend möglich, als solches identifiziert werden, besonders wenn es aus dem postkommunikalen Abschnitt der A. pericallosa hervorgeht, damit es nicht irrtümlicherweise mit dem Aneurysma verschlossen wird.

SACHS et al. (1968) fanden bei autoptischen Untersuchungen von 104 Patienten mit 126 operierten oder nicht operierten Aneurysmen folgende Verteilungen: 46 Aneurysmen (36,8%) waren im vorderen Abschnitt des Circulus Willisi gelegen, wovon 31 an der A. communicans anterior.

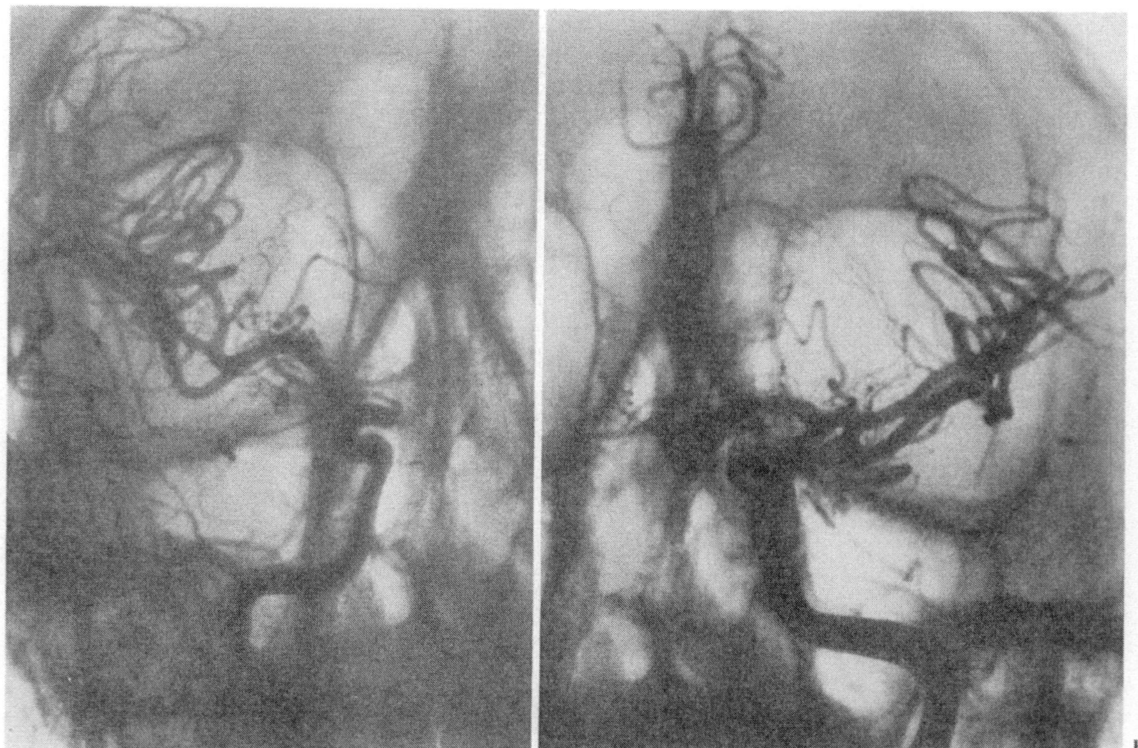

Abb. 23a u. b. Aneurysma der A. communicans anterior bei asymmetrisch angelegtem vorderen Abschnitt des Circulus Willisi. **a** Karotisangiogramm rechts mit hypoplastischer A. cerebri anterior. **b** Karotisangiogramm links. Das Aneurysma sitzt an der Teilungsstelle der weiteren linken A. cerebri anterior, die beide Aa. pericallosae versorgt

Von diesen erstreckte sich in 16 Fällen der Hals über die ganze Länge der A. communicans anterior (breitbasiges Aneurysma). In 15 Fällen zeigten die Aneurysmen einen dünneren Hals, der nur von einem kurzen Segment der A. communicans anterior ausging. 15 Aneurysmen ritten auf der Teilungsstelle der A. cerebri anterior in A. communicans anterior und A. pericallosa, wobei 14 nach oben und ein einziges nach unten gerichtet waren. Demgegenüber halten VANDERARK und KEMPE (1970) fest, daß bei den von ihnen beobachteten 100 Aneurysmen der A. communicans anterior 70 nach unten gerichtet waren. In 12 Fällen bestanden ausgedehnte Adhäsionen zwischen Aneurysma und A. pericallosa, in 16 Fällen waren keinerlei Adhäsionen nachweisbar. In 20 Fällen waren sie leicht und in 17 Fällen stark asymmetrisch. In 3 Fällen fehlte eine A. cerebri anterior vollständig. Bei stark ausgeprägter Asymmetrie stellt die A. communicans anterior oft nur eine Fortsetzung der weiteren A. cerebri anterior dar. Bei asymmetrischen Aa. cerebri anteriores saß das Aneurysma eindeutig auf der Seite der weiteren A. cerebri anterior.

YASARGIL et al. (1975) unterscheiden, aufgrund ihrer Operationsbefunde mit mikrochirurgischer Technik bei ihren 203 Fällen, folgende 3 Hauptgruppen (Abb. 24):

a) Aneurysma an der Teilungsstelle der rechten, weiteren A. cerebri anterior in A. communicans anterior und A. pericallosa bei hypoplastischer linker A. cerebri anterior: 51 Fälle (2 weitere Aneurysmen am Teilungswinkel der hypoplastischen linken A. cerebri anterior). In 5 Fällen lag eine Aplasie der A. cerebri anterior links vor.
b) Aneurysma an der Teilungsstelle der weiteren linken A. cerebri anterior bei hypoplastischer rechter A. cerebri anterior: 90 Fälle (2 weitere Aneurysmen am Teilungswinkel der hypoplastischen rechten A. cerebri anterior). Aplasie der rechten A. cerebri anterior in 4 Fällen.
   Somit waren 145 (71%) der 203 Aneurysmen im vorderen Abschnitt des Circulus Willisi mit Asymmetrien der Aa. cerebri anteriores verbunden. Von diesen 145 Aneurysmen saßen 141 (97,2%) an der Teilungsstelle der weiteren A. cerebri anterior und nur 4 an der Teilungsstelle der hypoplastischen A. cerebri anterior.
c) 58 Aneurysmen (29%) fanden sich bei symmetrisch entwickelten Aa. cerebri anteriores. Von diesen Aneurysmen saßen 54 (93%) an der A. communicans anterior und nur 4 (7%) in einem Teilungswinkel.

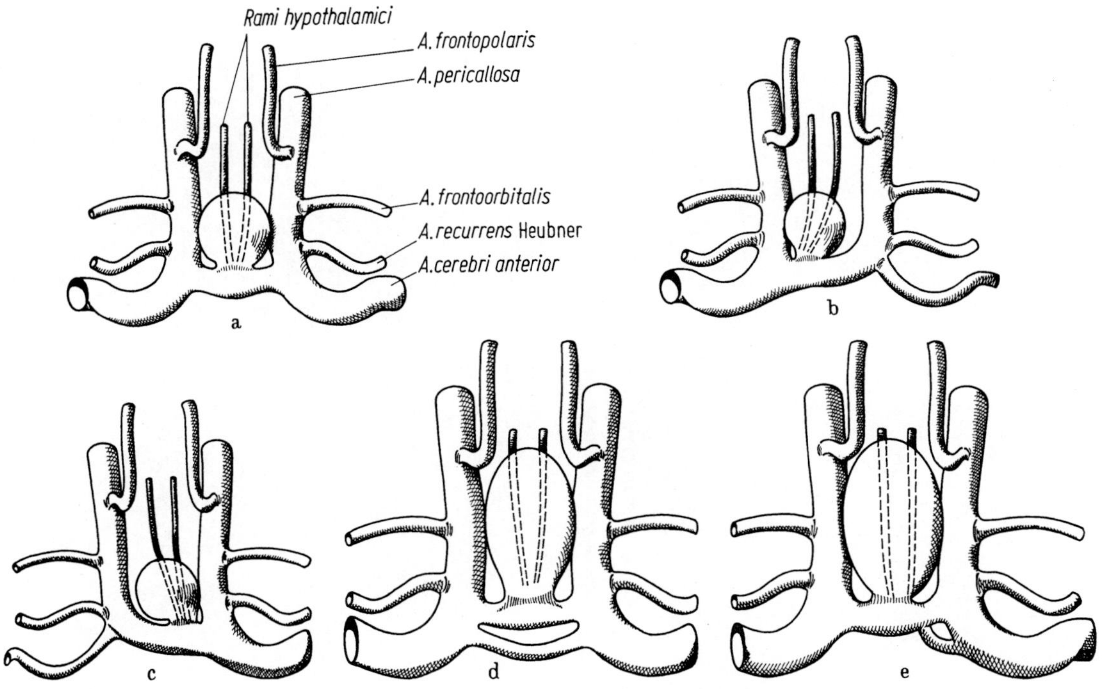

Abb. 24. Sitz der Aneurysmen an der A. communicans anterior. (Aus „Zerebrale Angiographie", 3. Aufl. 1979, Thieme Stuttgart)

Eine Duplikation der A. communicans anterior wurde in 21 Fällen (10%) gesehen, eine partielle in 15 Fällen und ein ganzes Geflecht von Gefäßen in 6 Fällen. Varianten im Bereich der A. communicans anterior lagen somit bei ca. 20% der 203 Aneurysmen vor.

KIRGIS et al. (1966) fanden unter den Varianten im vorderen Abschnitt des Circulus Willisi eine Persistenz der Mittellinienarterie über dem Corpus callosum, Verdoppelungen der A. communicans anterior und eine sehr weite A. cerebri anterior bei vorderer Trifurkation. Mit der Dominanz einer A. cerebri anterior erweitert sich auch die A. communicans anterior, was mit einer auffälligen Häufung von Aneurysmen verbunden ist. An 1000 untersuchten basalen Gefäßkränzen fanden sie 67 Aneurysmen, wovon 26 an der A. communicans anterior. Von diesen 26 waren 15 mit einer vorderen Trifurkation verbunden, also mit einem Typus des Circulus Willisi, der in ihrem Material in 10,7% der Fälle vorkam. Die 15 Aneurysmen entsprechen 22,5% der gefundenen Aneurysmen. Nach STEHBENS (1963b) ist die Hypoplasie einer A. cerebri anterior die einzige Variante in der Anlage des Circulus Willisi, die mit der Lokalisation eines Aneurysmas korreliert werden kann.

8. Aneurysmen der A. pericallosa

Aneurysmen mit dieser Lokalisation sind relativ selten, kommen aber immer noch häufiger vor als diejenigen im distalen Stromgebiet der A. cerebri media. Die meisten dieser Aneurysmen sitzen am Abgang der A. calloso-marginalis aus der A. pericallosa. An zweiter Stelle stehen die Aneurysmen an der Abgangsstelle der A. frontopolaris (LAITINEN u. SNELLMAN, 1960; DECHAUME et al., 1973; SNYCKERS u. DRAKE, 1973) (Abb. 2b). Eine bevorzugte Lokalisation ist ferner die Teilungsstelle eines unpaaren Pericallosastammes (HUBER, 1960; LAITINEN u. SNELLMAN, 1960; POOL u. POTTS, 1965) (Abb. 25). YASARGIL und CARTER (1974) betonen aufgrund ihrer Erfahrungen bei 13 Fällen, daß diese Aneurysmen wegen ihres breiten Halses und des engen Subarachnoidalraumes schwierig zu operieren sind.

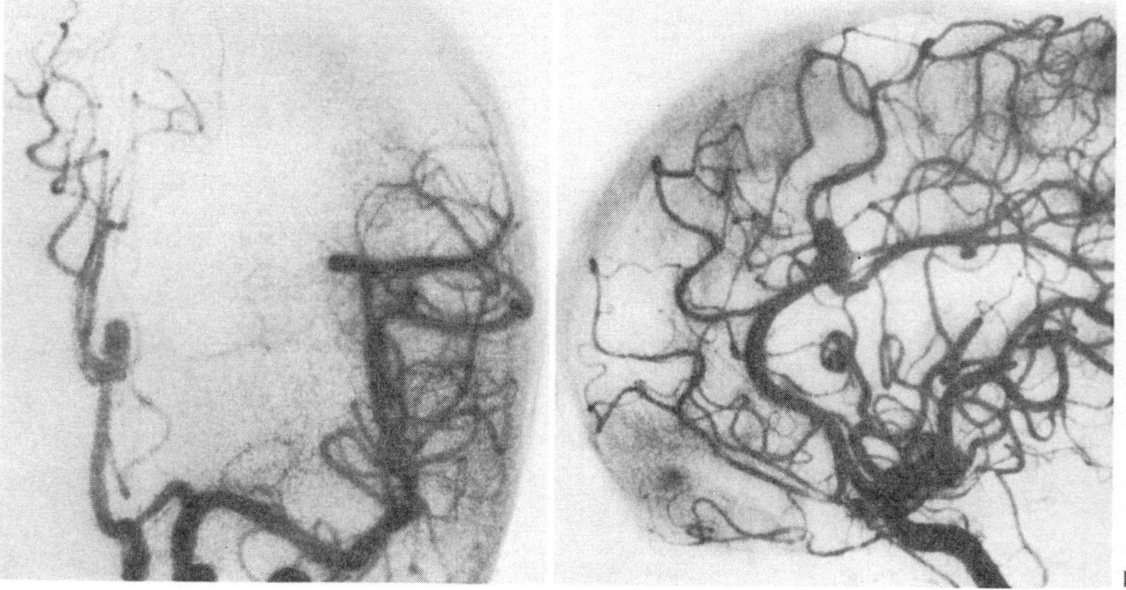

Abb. 25a u. b. Aneurysma an der Teilungsstelle eines weiten, unpaarig angelegten Pericallosa-Hauptstammes (A. pericallosa bihemisphaerica). **a** Aufnahme nach Towne. **b** Profilaufnahme

9. Aneurysmen der A. cerebri media

Die Aneurysmen der A. cerebri media sitzen wesentlich häufiger an der Teilungsstelle des Hauptstammes als am Abgang der perforierenden Arterien aus dem sphenoidalen Abschnitt oder im peripheren Stromgebiet (CROMPTON, 1962; SACHS et al., 1968) (Abb. 2d und 26). Nach LIPOVSEK (1973) gingen nur 14% von 547 Mediaaneurysmen aus dem proximalen sphenoidalen Abschnitt der A. cerebri media hervor. SACHS et al. (1968) haben 30 Aneurysmen der A. cerebri media hinsichtlich ihrer Lokalisation genauer untersucht und folgende Verhältnisse gefunden: 5 Aneurysmen saßen breit auf Gefäßteilungen, und ihre Öffnung griff zum Teil auf die Äste der Gabelungsstelle über. Der Hals von 17 Aneurysmen war auf die Teilungsstelle selbst lokalisiert. 8 Aneurysmen waren zwar auch auf die Teilungsstelle lokalisiert, doch zeigte die Außenwand der Aneurysmen ausgedehnte Verklebungen mit Ästen der Gabelungsstelle. Teilweise können diese Äste sogar in die Aneurysmawand eingemauert sein, speziell bei großen Aneurysmen, deren Wand sich aus einem organisierten Hämatom gebildet hat. In keinem Fall ging eine Arterie aus dem Aneurysma selbst hervor, was sich mit den Untersuchungen von STEHBENS (1963b) und CROMPTON (1966) deckt. Die Aneurysmen an der Teilungsstelle der A. cerebri media sind, entsprechend der Stromrichtung, häufig nach lateral gerichtet, während die Aneurysmen am Abgang der lentikulostriären Arterien nach oben, diejenigen am Abgang der A. temporo-polaris nach unten gerichtet sind (LAINE et al., 1970).

Im Gegensatz zu den Aneurysmen des A. cerebri anterior/A. communicans anterior-Komplexes besteht bei den Aneurysmen der A. cerebri media keine faßbare Beziehung zu der Weite der A. cerebri media und ihrer Äste. Dagegen scheint die von MCKISSOCK et al. (1960, 1962) festgestellte schlechtere Prognose bei Frauen auf der unterschiedlichen anatomischen Konfiguration

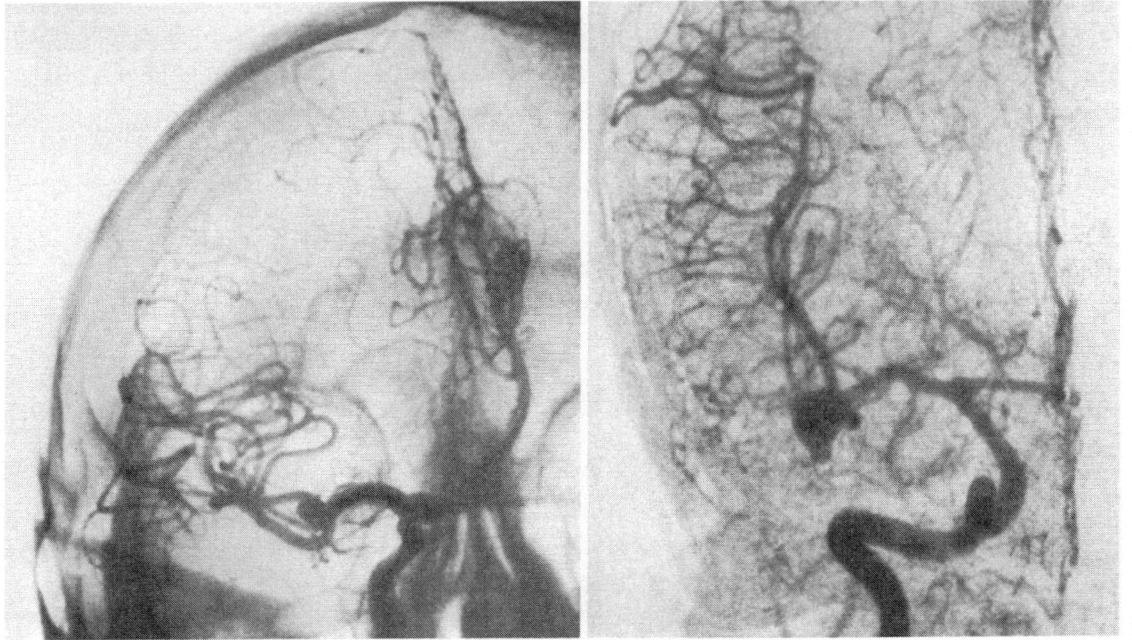

Abb. 26a. Subdurales Hämatom bei Aneurysma an der Teilungsstelle (Pseudotrifurkation) der A. cerebri media; **b** Intrazerebrales temporales Hämatom bei Aneurysma der A. cerebri media. Anhebung der Opercularschleifen. (Abb. 26a aus „Zerebrale Angiographie", 3. Aufl. 1979, Thieme Stuttgart)

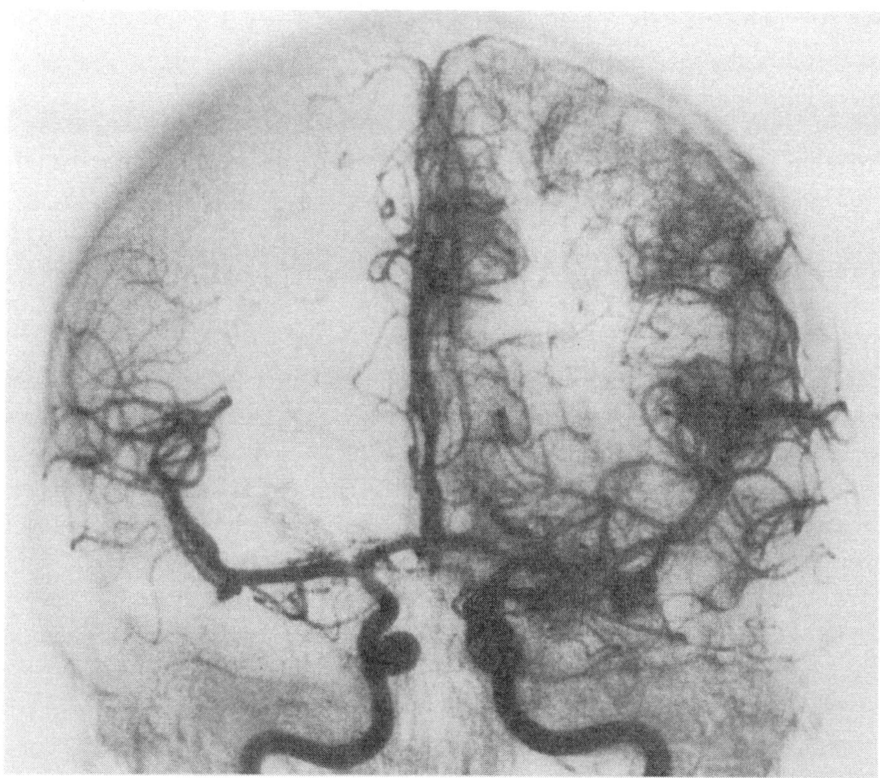

Abb. 27. Bilaterales, symmetrisch gelegenes Aneurysma an der Teilungsstelle der A. cerebri media am Mediaknie. Das größere Aneurysma links ist rupturiert (computertomographisch und operativ nachgewiesen)

dieser Aneurysmen bei beiden Geschlechtern zu beruhen (CROMPTON, 1962). Ganz allgemein scheint der Aneurysmasack bei Männern größer und der Aneurysmahals ausgeprägter zu sein als bei Frauen, weshalb die Aneurysmen bei Männern eher birnenförmig sind. Die länglichen Aneurysmen ragen deshalb mit der Kuppe stärker in die Hirnsubstanz hinein als die rundlichen, breitbasig der Teilungsstelle aufsitzenden Aneurysmen beim weiblichen Geschlecht. Das hat zur Folge, daß bei Männern intrazerebrale Hämatome, bei Frauen Hämatome in der Fossa Sylvii häufiger sind (Abb. 7 und 27). Mit den Hämatomen in der Fossa Sylvii wird die häufigere Infarzierung im Anschluß an die Aneurysmaruptur bei Frauen in Zusammenhang gebracht.

In der Peripherie des Mediastromgebietes sitzen nur selten Aneurysmen. Ein peripherer Aneurysmasitz erweckt den Verdacht auf ein mykotisches Aneurysma (Abb. 28).

10. Aneurysmen im Vertebralis- und Basilarisstromgebiet

Die Aneurysmen der A. basilaris sitzen meist an der kranialen Teilungsstelle (DRAKE 1968; YASARGIL et al., 1976b) und können u.U. sehr groß werden (Abb. 2a und 3). Sie sind nach vorne, oben oder hinten gerichtet. Weniger häufig kommen sie am Stamm der A. basilaris an den Abzweigungsstellen der Aa. cerebelli superiores oder Aa. cerebelli inferiores anteriores vor und können dann gegen den Clivus gerichtet sein (SMALTINO et al., 1972). Gelegentlich finden sie sich an der Einmündungsstelle persistierender karotido-basilärer Anastomosen, wie der A. trigemina primitiva und der A. hypoglossica primitiva (UDVARHELYI u. LAI, 1963; HUBER u. RIVOIR, 1974; SPRINGER et al., 1974). Selten sitzen die Aneurysmen an der Vereinigung der beiden Vertebralarterien zur A. basilaris und sind dann nach hinten oben und lateral gerichtet.

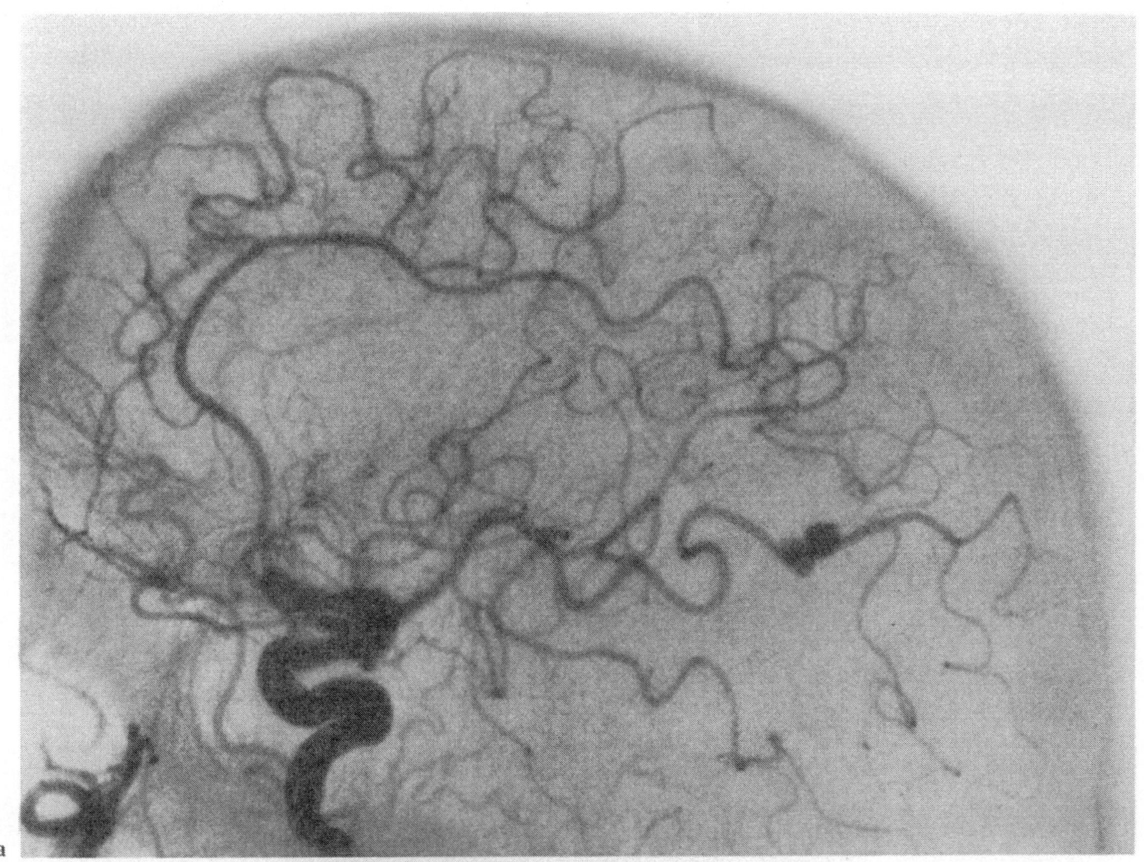
a

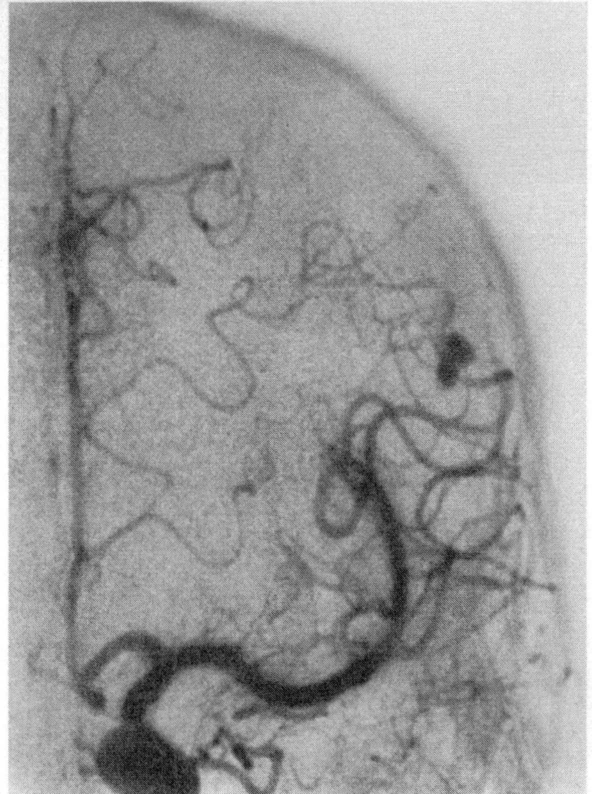
b

Abb. 28a u. b. Lobuliertes (wahrscheinlich mykotisches) Aneurysma im peripheren Stromgebiet der A. cerebri media (bekannter Infekt mit Fieberschüben und hoher Senkung, jedoch keine Operation). **a** Profilaufnahme; **b** Aufnahme nach Towne

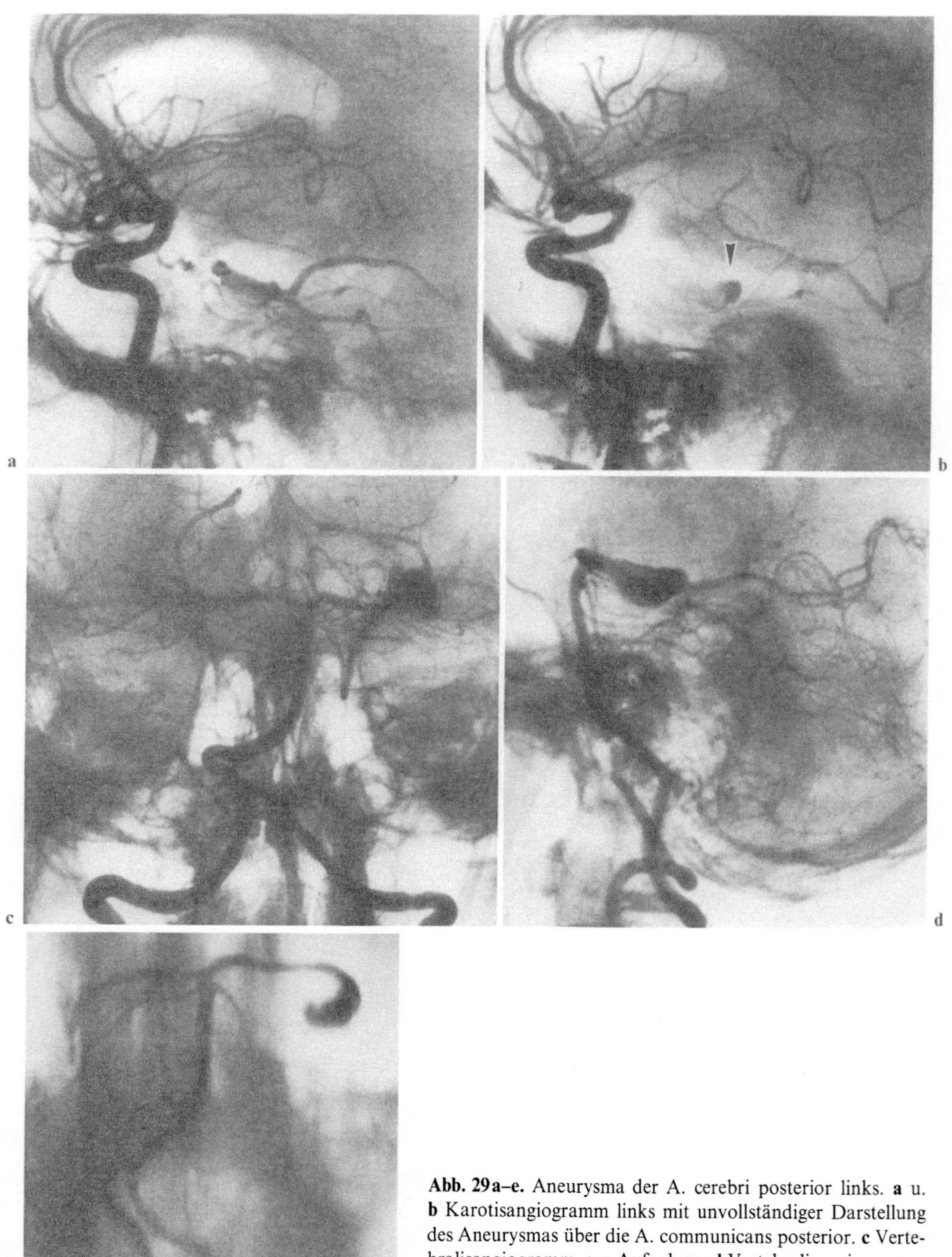

Abb. 29a–e. Aneurysma der A. cerebri posterior links. **a** u. **b** Karotisangiogramm links mit unvollständiger Darstellung des Aneurysmas über die A. communicans posterior. **c** Vertebralisangiogramm, a-p Aufnahme. **d** Vertebralisangiogramm, Profilaufnahme. **e** Angiotomogramm (Patient wegen Tumorverdacht zur Angiographie zugewiesen. Aneurysma partiell thrombosiert)

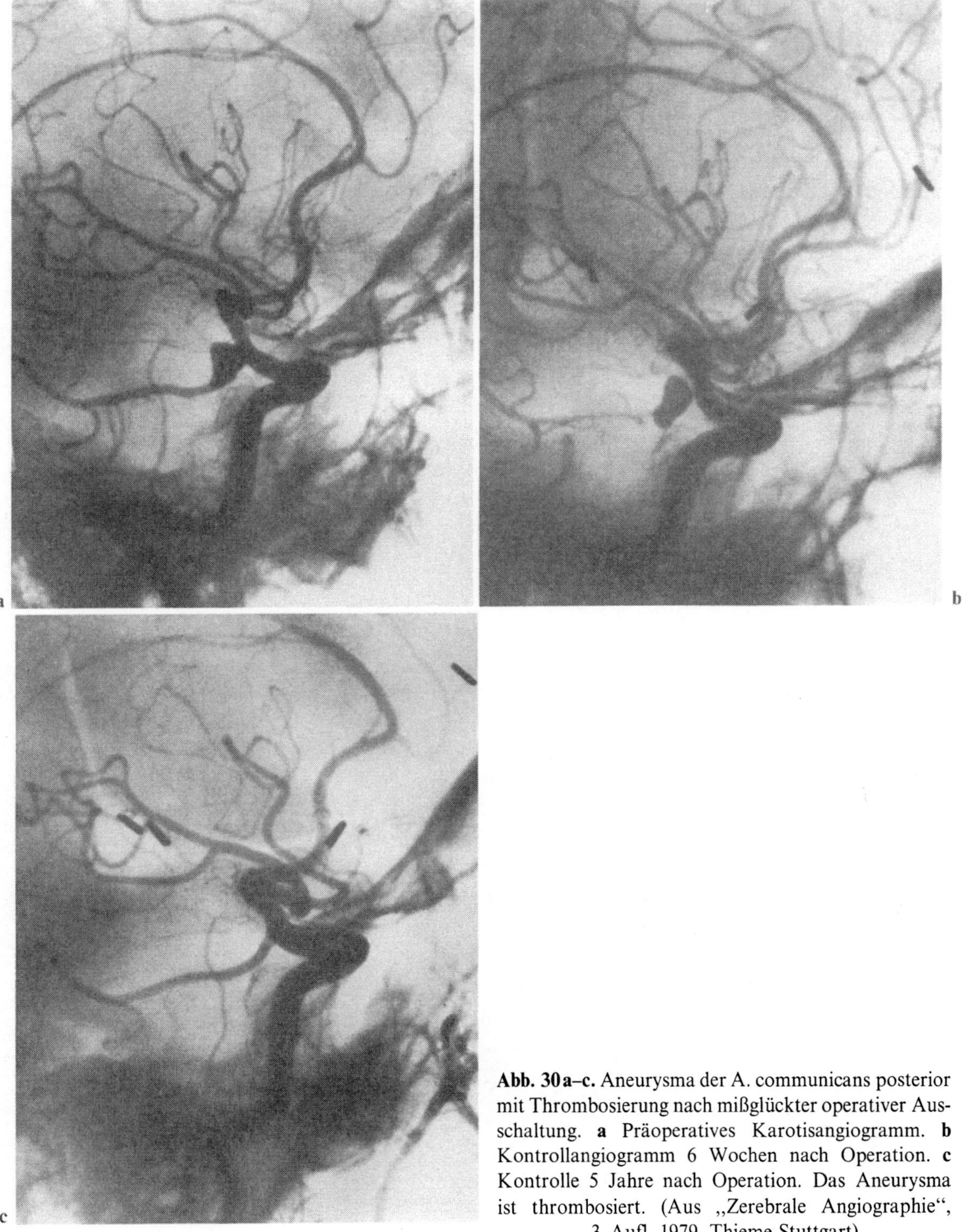

Abb. 30a–c. Aneurysma der A. communicans posterior mit Thrombosierung nach mißglückter operativer Ausschaltung. **a** Präoperatives Karotisangiogramm. **b** Kontrollangiogramm 6 Wochen nach Operation. **c** Kontrolle 5 Jahre nach Operation. Das Aneurysma ist thrombosiert. (Aus „Zerebrale Angiographie“, 3. Aufl. 1979, Thieme Stuttgart)

Aneurysmen der A. cerebri posterior sind ebenfalls selten (PIA u. FONTANA, 1977). Meistens sitzen sie an der Verbindung zwischen der A. communicans posterior und der A. cerebri posterior und sind nach lateral gerichtet. Am proximalen pedunkulären Segment der A. cerebri posterior kommen Aneurysmen nur selten vor und zeigen, entsprechend der Strömungsrichtung vorwiegend nach lateral (DRAKE u. AMACHER, 1969) (Abb. 29).

Sehr selten sind Aneurysmen an der A. cerebelli inferior anterior anzutreffen. Jedoch sind Aneurysmen im Kleinhirnbrückenwinkel und selbst im Meatus acusticus internus beschrieben worden (THIERRY et al., 1971; PORTER u. EYSTER, 1973).

VI. Per- und postoperative Angiographie

Die per- und postoperative angiographische Kontrolle wird von vielen Autoren empfohlen (ALLCOCK u. DRAKE, 1963; LOOP u. FOLTZ, 1966; CUMMINS et al., 1974; BERGER u. KYRIAZIDOU, 1975). DRAKE und ALLCOCK (1973) fanden bei angiographischen Nachkontrollen, daß bei 43 (13%) von 329 Patienten das Aneurysma nicht oder nur partiell verschlossen war. STEVEN (1966) stellte bei der angiographischen Nachkontrolle von 280 Patienten in 17,6% einen unvollständigen Aneurysmaverschluß fest. In den nur partiell verschlossenen Aneurysmen kann es zwar zu einer Thrombenbildung kommen, doch ist eine vollständige Thrombosierung relativ selten (DRAKE u. VANDERLINDEN, 1967; BONNAL u. STEVENAERT, 1969) (Abb. 30). Die partielle Thrombosierung verhütet eine Nachblutung nicht, besonders wenn sich das Restaneurysma im Verlauf der Zeit vergrößert. Bei Anwendung der mikrochirurgischen Technik können die Verhältnisse allerdings so gut überblickt werden, daß HOLLIN und DECKER (1973) sowie YASARGIL et al. (1975) eine routinemäßige postoperative Kontrollangiographie nicht mehr für nötig halten.

B. Arteriovenöse Gefäßmißbildungen

I. Überblick

Dank der Angiographie konnten Anatomie und Physiologie der Gefäßmißbildungen eingehend studiert und damit der Ausgangspunkt für die Entwicklung einer sinnvollen Operationstechnik geschaffen werden (OLIVECRONA u. LADENHEIM, 1957; POOL u. POTTS, 1965). Die superselektive angiographische Technik hat es zudem möglich gemacht, viele der Gefäßmißbildungen im Stromgebiet der A. carotis externa und z.T. sogar im Internastromgebiet im Anschluß an den diagnostischen Eingriff durch Embolisation auszuschalten (DJINDJIAN et al., 1973; DJINDJIAN, 1975; PICARD et al., 1975; MERLAND u. DJINDJIAN, 1975).

Die vaskulären Gefäßmißbildungen werden in der Literatur nach verschiedenen Gesichtspunkten klassifiziert. Am wichtigsten ist die Abgrenzung der kongenitalen, nicht neoplastischen Gefäßmißbildungen von den eigentlichen neoplastischen Gefäßgeschwülsten. Die heute am meisten verwendete Einteilung basiert auf den Arbeiten von CUSHING und BAILEY (1928) und RUSSELL und RUBINSTEIN (1959):

1. Mißbildungen
   A. Angioma cavernosum (vaskuläres Hamartom)
   B. Angioma racemosum
      a) Teleangiektasie (Angioma capillare ectaticum)
      b) Angioma capillare et venosum calcificans (Sturge-Weber)
      c) arteriovenöse Gefäßmißbildung (arteriovenöses Angiom)
2. Gefäßtumoren
   Hämangioblastom (Angioretikulom).

Die Mißbildungen bestehen aus knäuelartig angeordneten Gefäßen, die durch mehr oder weniger stark verändertes Hirngewebe, in dem die nervösen Elemente fehlen können, von einander getrennt sind. Die Hämangioblastome dagegen sind Tumoren mit embryonalem Gefäßsystem und aktiv proliferierenden Zellen, ohne zwischengeschaltetes Hirngewebe. Die arteriovenösen Gefäßmißbildungen (Angiome) stehen hinsichtlich Häufigkeit und klinischer Bedeutung an erster Stelle. Es sind Gefäßkonvolute, welche in der Regel weite, geschlängelte zu- und abführende Gefäße und dazwischen einen Gefäßknäuel von wechselnder Größe aufweisen und mit dem normalen zerebralen Gefäßsystem in Verbindung stehen. Der arterielle und venöse Anteil wechselt von Fall zu Fall. Die Mißbildungen sind meistens pial gelegen. Subkortikale und intraventrikulär gelegene arteriovenöse Mißbildungen sind selten (OJEMANN u. NEW, 1963). Die serienangiographischen Befunde zeigen, daß die Blutzirkulation durch die Mißbildung wesentlich rascher erfolgt als durch die normale Hirnsubstanz. Die großen abführenden Venen gelangen meistens schon auf den ersten Filmen der Serie zur Darstellung (Abb. 35). Deshalb ist eine sehr rasche Kontrastmittelinjektion erforderlich, und die Aufnahmen müssen in kurzen Intervallen geschossen werden. Wegen ihres geringen Strömungswiderstandes ist die Gefäßmißbildung ein Schmarotzer, der sehr viel Blut an sich zieht und das Hirngewebe einer normalen Durchblutung beraubt. Infolge dieser Zirkulationsbeeinträchtigung entwickeln sich eptileptische Störungen, Halbseitenlähmungen sowie subarachnoidale und intrazerebrale Blutungen. Die übrigen vaskulären Mißbildungen resp. Hamartome, z.B. das Angioma cavernosum, sind viel seltener. Die meistens in der Ponsregion vorkommenden Teleangiektasien entziehen sich in der Regel einem angiographischen Nachweis.

II. Entwicklung der arteriovenösen Mißbildungen

STREETER (1918) hat die Entwicklung der Hirngefäße in 5 Stadien eingeteilt:

I Aus Strängen von Angioblasten bildet sich ein primitiver Gefäßplexus.

II Diese Gefäße differenzieren sich in primitive Arterien, Kapillaren und Venen, wobei die Arterien und Venen durch Fusion einzelner Gefäßstränge entstehen.

III Das Gefäßsystem wird in ein äußeres, ein durales und ein leptomeningeales, später zerebrales System geschichtet.

IV Die einzelnen Systeme adaptieren sich an die entsprechenden, ebenfalls sich entwickelnden zerebralen und extrazerebralen Strukturen.

V Histologische Ausdifferenzierung in die definitiven Arterien, Kapillaren und Venen.

Der arteriovenösen Mißbildung liegt eine fehlende Ausdifferenzierung des primitiven Gefäßplexus in Kapillaren an einer Stelle zugrunde, weshalb die Arterien ohne dazwischen geschaltetes Kapillarnetz in die Venen übergehen, d.h. das primitive Gefäßgeflecht bleibt zwischen den sich ausdifferenzierenden Arterien und Venen bestehen. Die zur Gefäßmißbildung führenden Arterien entsprechen somit den normalerweise diese Region versorgenden Arterien, wie auch die Venen die diese Region normalerweise drainierenden Venen darstellen. Die Mißbildung wird also nicht durch neu gebildete Gefäße versorgt oder drainiert. Infolge der veränderten hämodynamischen Verhältnisse zeigen die Arterien und Venen eine starke Erweiterung und vermehrte Schlängelung, da sie ein erheblich größeres Blutvolumen zu transportieren haben. Gelegentlich finden sich an den unter erhöhtem Druck stehenden Venen zusätzliche aneurysmatische Ausweitungen (Abb. 31). Im STREETERschen Stadium III entscheidet es sich, ob die Mißbildung in der Kopfhaut, in der Dura oder pialzerebral liegt, und im Stadium IV werden die zur Mißbildung führenden Arterien determiniert. Je nach Ausdehnung führen mehrere Arterien, die eventuell sogar aus verschiedenen Irrigationsgebieten stammen, der Mißbildung Blut zu, und die venöse Drainage erfolgt – je nach Lage der Mißbildung – vorwiegend über das zentrifugale (meningeale) oder das zentripetale (innere) System. An der Blutzuleitung zu den arteriovenösen Mißbildungen sind speziell diejenigen Arterien mitbeteiligt, die sich auch bei Gefäßverschlüssen vikariierend über leptomeningeale Anastomosen ergänzen können. Bei suprasylvisch gelegenen arteriovenösen Mißbildungen sind oft,

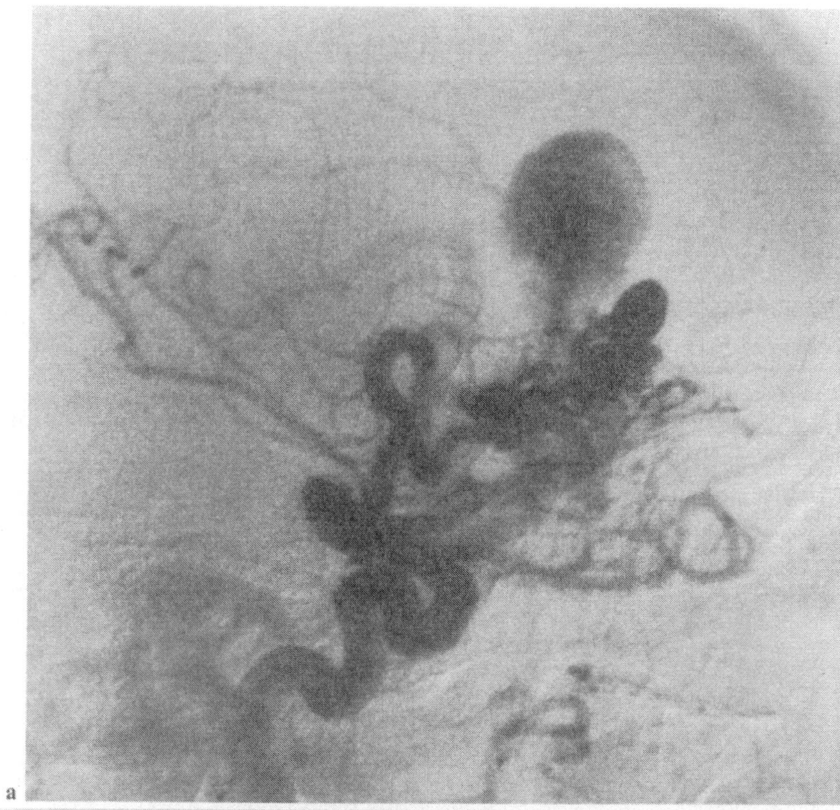

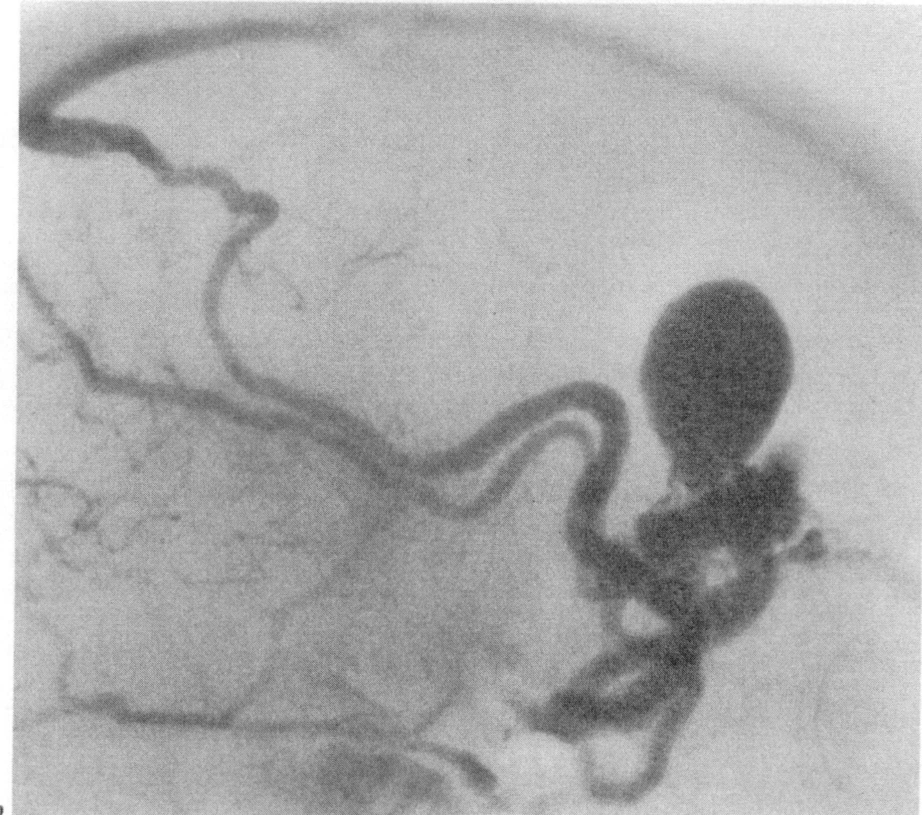

Abb. 31a u. b. Aneurysmatische Erweiterung einer Vene bei arteriovenöser Mißbildung. **a** Früharterielle Phase. Das Kontrastmittel schießt im Strahl in das venöse Aneurysma ein. **b** Venöse Phase mit homogenen gefülltem venösem Aneurysma

neben der A. cerebri media, Äste aus dem Pericallosastromgebiet mitbeteiligt, den infrasylvisch gelegenen leiten, neben der Mediagruppe, Äste der A. cerebri posterior Blut zu (KAPLAN et al., 1961).

Im Aufbau der Mißbildung wechselt der arterielle und venöse Anteil von Fall zu Fall. Häufig ist es jedoch das Konvolut der stark erweiterten drainierenden Venen, das im Gesamtbild am meisten imponiert. Die an der Hirnoberfläche gelegenen Mißbildungen weisen dementsprechend bei ausgeprägter zentripetaler Drainage durch die erweiterten Markvenen häufig Pyramiden- oder Keilform auf, wobei die breite Basis der Hirnoberfläche anliegt, die Spitze dagegen zum tiefen Venensystem gerichtet ist, was durch die Konvergenz der normalen Markvenen zu den subependymalen Venen im oberen lateralen Ventrikelwinkel bedingt ist (WICKBOM, 1950; HAMBY, 1958) (Abb. 35d).

In den Gefäßen kommen sekundäre, z.T. atheromatöse Veränderungen mit Thrombosen und Kalkeinlagerungen vor, die u.U. schon auf Schädelröntgenbildern zu erkennen sind (Abb. 36a). SUTTON (1958) sowie HOUDART und LE BESNERAIS (1963) fanden in ca. 15% der Fälle röntgenologisch Verkalkungen, PATERSON und MCKISSOCK (1956) in 24% und RUMBAUGH und POTTS (1966) sogar in 29,5%.

III. Formen und Lokalisationen der arteriovenösen Mißbildungen

Die arteriovenösen Mißbildungen präsentieren sich klinisch in einer Vielfalt von Formen, die unter teilweise verschiedenen Namen ihren Eingang in die Literatur gefunden haben. Es sei besonders auf das Syndrom verwiesen, das sich aus einer Kombination von Gefäßmißbildungen der Retina, des Gesichtes, der Dura und des Gehirns zusammensetzt (Syndrom von WYBURN-MASON der angelsächsischen, BONNET-DECHAUME-BLANC der französischen Literatur). Aus der Entwicklungsgeschichte der arteriovenösen Mißbildungen ist es durchaus verständlich, daß Kombinationen von arteriovenösen Mißbildungen in verschiedenen Schichten und an verschiedenen Orten vorkommen. Je nach der hervorstechenden Symptomatologie steht das eine oder andere pathologische Gefäßkonvolut im Vordergrund, und die übrigen werden unter Umständen als Begleiterscheinungen klassifiziert (THÉRON et al., 1974). Aus didaktischen Gründen ist allerdings eine gewisse Gruppierung erforderlich, doch muß man sich dabei immer bewußt bleiben, daß es sich im Prinzip um ein multifokales, hinsichtlich Art und Entstehung aber einheitliches Leiden handelt, mit durch lokale Gefäßanordnungen bedingten hämodynamischen Besonderheiten, die es im einzelnen angiographisch abzuklären gilt. Welche der Läsionen für die Klassifikation bestimmend ist, bleibt oft Ermessensfrage (HOYT u. CAMERON, 1968; TAMAKI et al., 1971; BROWN et al., 1973).

1. Extrakranielle arteriovenöse Mißbildungen

Am häufigsten finden sie sich in der Galea und können, sofern sie eine gewisse Größe erreichen, als pulsierende Schwellung direkt sichtbar werden (Aneurysma circoides, DANDY, 1946; ELKIN, 1946). Sie werden meist von Ästen der A. carotis externa, wie der A. temporalis superficialis, der A. occipitalis und bei der nicht so seltenen retroaurikulären Lokalisation durch die A. retroauricularis versorgt (Abb. 32), doch können auch Arterien der Dura mit Ästen, die die Kalotte durchdringen, an der Vaskularisation mitbeteiligt sein. Die venöse Drainage erfolgt entweder ausschließlich über Galeavenen oder durch die Kalotte in die duralen Sinus (VOGELSANG, 1962; OLDFIELD u. ADDISON, 1962; MALAN u. AZZOLINI, 1968; VERBIEST, 1968, 1972; THOMAS u. ANDRESS, 1971; FERNANDEZ URDANIBIA et al., 1974; WAGA et al., 1974). Sehr ausgedehnte arteriovenöse Mißbildungen können selbst über die Mittellinie von Externaästen der Gegenseite Blut beziehen.

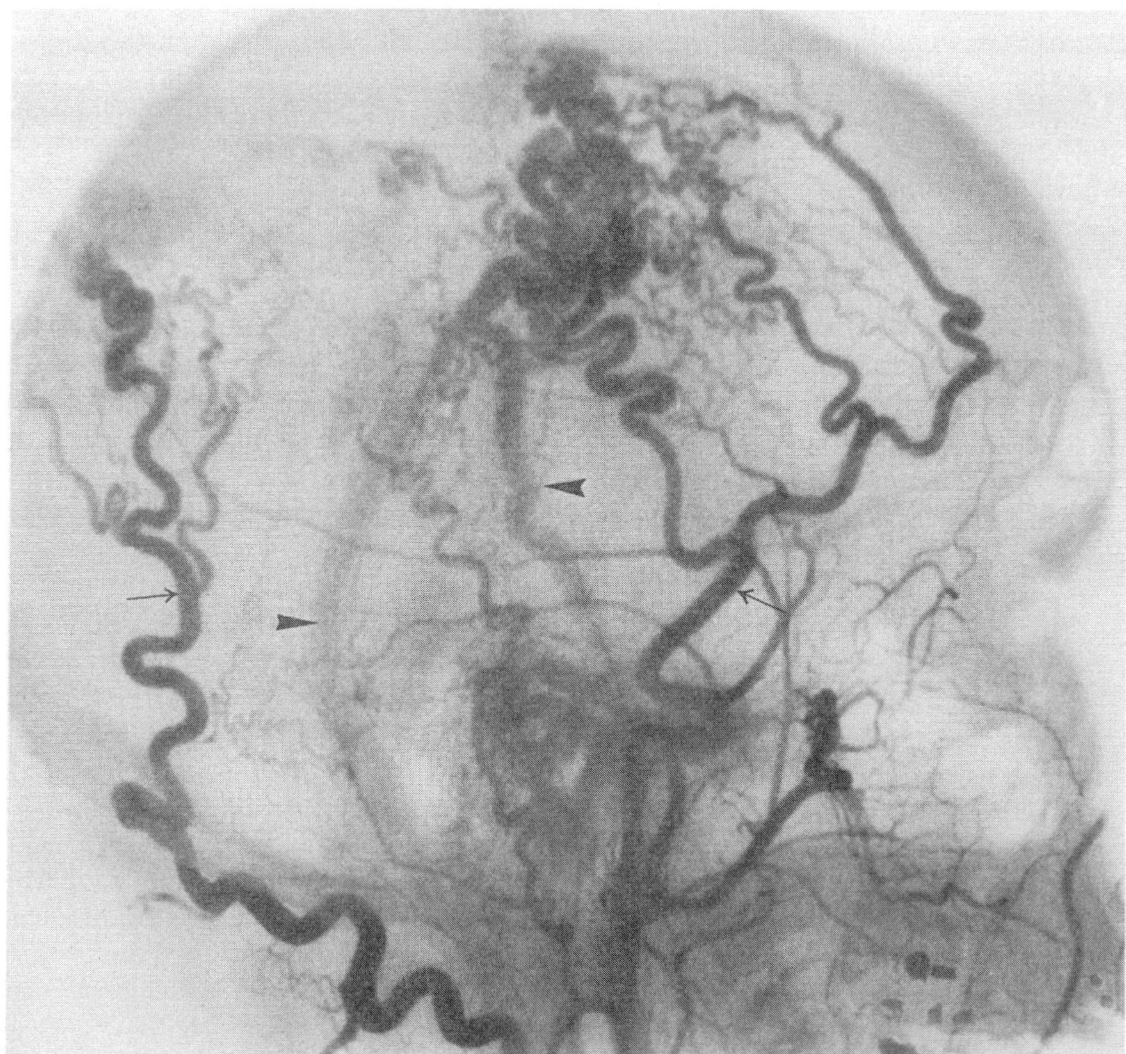

Abb. 32. Ausgedehnte arteriovenöse Mißbildung der Galea (selektive Darstellung der A. carotis externa). Die zur Mißbildung führenden Äste der A. temporalis superficialis (→) und A. occipitalis (→) sind stark erweitert. Drainierende Galeavenen (►). (Aus „Zerebrale Angiographie", 3. Aufl. 1979, Thieme Stuttgart)

Meistens ist bei diesen extrakraniellen Gefäßmißbildungen ein deutliches Geräusch zu hören. Nicht mit arteriovenösen Mißbildungen sind die ebenfalls als subkutane Schwellung imponierenden venösen Mißbildungen (Sinus pericranii) zu verwechseln.

Wegen der großen Blutungsgefahr bei Zahnextraktionen sind die arteriovenösen Mißbildungen des Ober- und Unterkiefers klinisch von Bedeutung. In Unkenntnis der Diagnose sind nach Zahnextraktion sogar tödliche Blutungen vorgekommen (PALLADINO u. DANZIGER, 1965; HOEY et al., 1970; SAILER, 1973). Die Mißbildung kann auf die Mandibula beschränkt sein (sog. zentrales Hämangiom) oder auf die umgebenden Weichteile übergreifen (WATSON u. MCCARTY, 1940; BAUM et al., 1972; POCHACZEVSKY et al., 1972; MARTIS u. KARAKASIS, 1973). Nach Mitteilung von LUND und DAHLIN (1964) ist das weibliche Geschlecht doppelt so häufig befallen wie das männliche. Eine spontane Hämorrhagie ist selten das erste Symptom. Die Röntgenaufnahmen zeigen wohl mehr oder weniger scharf begrenzte osteolytische Veränderungen, die bei ausgedehnten Prozessen die ganze Kieferregion befallen können. Aufgrund dieser Knochenveränderungen ist aber keineswegs immer eine korrekte Artdiagnose möglich, und die selektive oder superselektive Angiographie der Exteraäste ist deshalb unerläßlich (MEDELLIN u. WALLACE, 1970; MAW, 1972;

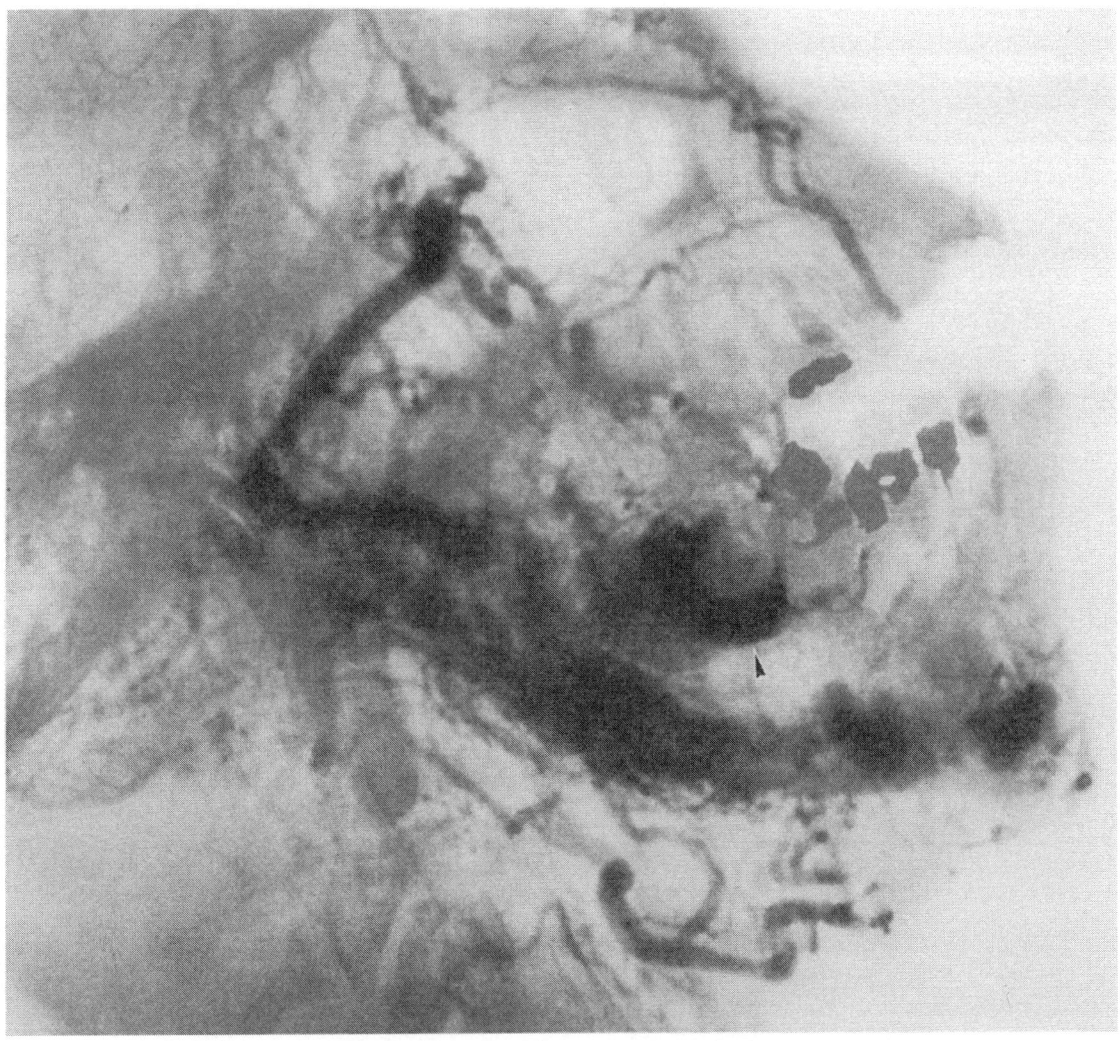

Abb. 33. Arteriovenöse Mißbildung des Unterkiefers. Retinierter Backenzahn in großer venöser Lakune (►). (Aus „Zerebrale Angiographie", 3. Aufl. 1979, Thieme Stuttgart)

DJINDJIAN et al., 1973). Dabei zeigt sich, daß einzelne Zähne in weite venöse Lakunen eingebettet sind (FODERA et al., 1976) (Abb. 33).

Gefäßmißbildungen in der Orbita sind relativ selten. Am häufigsten finden sich Hämangiome resp. Kavernome, die – entsprechend einem intraorbitalen Tumor – zu einem Exopthalmus führen. In einer eingehenden Besprechung weisen THÉRON et al. (1974) auf die Komplexität dieser Läsion hin, die in den unterschiedlichen Bezeichnungen der verschiedenen Autoren ihren Niederschlag findet. Eine Gruppe für sich bilden innerhalb der vaskulären Mißbildungen der Orbita die retrobulbären Varixknoten (WALSH u. DANDY, 1944; BRAUSTON u. NORTON, 1963).

Arteriovenöse Fisteln ohne größeres zwischengeschaltetes Gefäßkonvolut kommen in der Nakkenregion zwischen der A. vertebralis und ihren Begleitvenen vor (SVOLOS et al., 1965; EHRLICH et al., 1968; ZILKHA u. SCHECHTER, 1969; GERAUD et al., 1973). Diese Fisteln können kongenital sein oder als Folge eines Traumas auftreten (CHOU u. FRENCH, 1965; CHOU et al., 1967; WEINBERG u. FLOM, 1973), wobei das verursachende Trauma u.a. eine direkte Vertebralispunktion sein kann (ARONSON, 1961; OLSON et al., 1963; BERGSTRÖM u. LODIN, 1966; LESTER, 1966; NEWTON u. DARROCH, 1966; BERGQUIST et al., 1971) (Abb. 34).

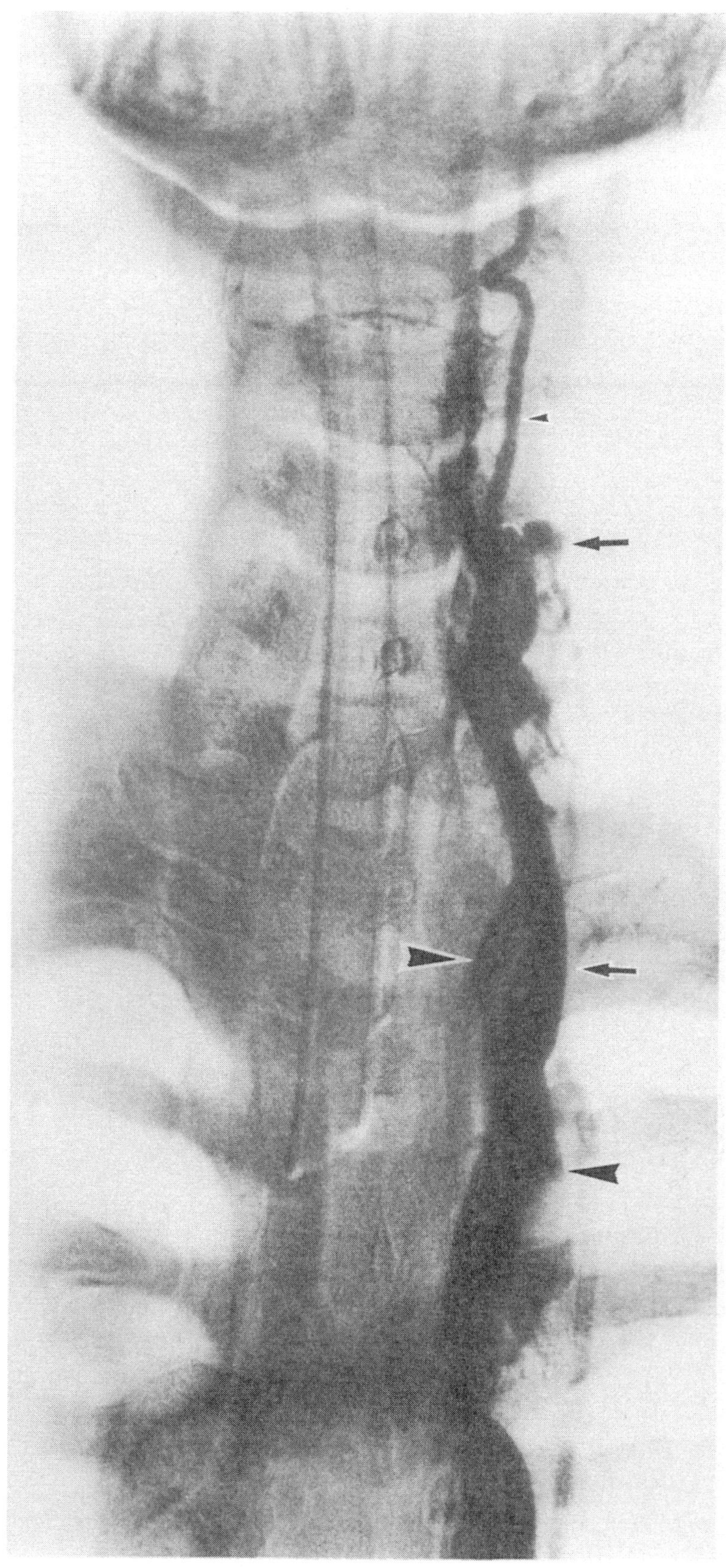

Abb. 34. Arteriovenöse Fistel zwischen A. vertebralis und Begleitvenen nach direkter Punktion der A. vertebralis. A. vertebralis, proximal von der Fistel (►) weiter als distal. (➤) Begleitvene (←)

2. Intrakranielle arteriovenöse Mißbildungen

Sie lassen sich in die auch entwicklungsgeschichtlich begründeten drei Gruppen unterteilen:

I rein pial-zerebrale Formen, die nur durch Hirnarterien versorgt werden;

II gemischt piale-durale Formen. Die Blutzufuhr erfolgt sowohl über Hirnarterien als auch über Arterien der Dura;

III rein durale Formen, die nur durch Arterien der Dura versorgt werden.

Die gemischten Formen sind früher selten beschrieben worden. Mit der Einführung der selektiven Katheterisierung der einzelnen Gefäße hat sich aber gezeigt, daß die Mitbeteiligung der Duragefäße an der Versorgung zerebraler arteriovenöser Mißbildungen keineswegs selten ist (Abb. 39 und 43). NEWTON und CRONQVIST (1969) stellten folgende Verhältnisse fest:

	supratentoriell	infratentoriell
pial	81 (79%)	13 (50%)
pial-dural	16 (15%)	4 (15%)
dural	6 (6%)	9 (35%)
	103 (80%)	26 (20%)

Wie die sackförmigen Aneurysmen, so sind auch die arteriovenösen Mißbildungen supratentoriell viel häufiger als infratentoriell. KRAYENBÜHL und YASARGIL (1958) haben aufgrund von 800 aus der Literatur und dem eigenen Krankengut zusammengestellten Fällen folgende Verteilung gefunden:

extrakraniell	8,1%	supratentoriell	85,7%
intrakraniell	91,9%	infratentoriell	6,2%

Analoge Zahlen geben PERRET und NISHIOKA (1966) an: 421 der 453 Fälle, also 93%, lagen supratentoriell, 32 (=7%) infratentoriell. Gleiche Zahlen liegen von MOODY und POPPEN (1970) vor. Das Verhältnis der supra- zu den infratentoriellen arteriovenösen Mißbildungen entspricht etwa dem Verhältnis der supratentoriellen zur infratentoriellen Hirnmasse. In ausgedehnten Gefäßgebieten ist eben auch die Wahrscheinlichkeit für das Auftreten von Mißbildungen größer.

Nach PERRET und NISHIOKA (1966) verteilen sich die arteriovenösen Mißbildungen folgendermaßen auf die einzelnen Hirnregionen:

frontal	64	14%
frontoparietal	28	6%
frontotemporal	10	2%
temporal	51	11%
temperoparietal	26	6%
tempero-okzopital	5	1%
parietal	104	23%
parieto-okzipital	18	4%
okzipital	23	5%
intraventrikulär oder paraventrikulär	81	18%
Hirnstamm	11	2%
Zerebellum	21	5%
ganze Hemisphäre	3	1%
multiple Mißbildungen	3	1%
keine Information	5	1%
	453	100%

Etwa 8% der Mißbildungen liegen in der Mittellinie.

Nach dieser Studie kommen sackförmige Aneurysmen etwa 6,5mal häufiger vor als arteriovenöse Mißbildungen. In 45 Fällen lagen arteriovenöse Mißbildungen und sackförmige Aneurysmen zusammen vor; dabei handelte es sich aber bei den Mißbildungen in 8 Fällen um arteriovenöse Fisteln im Sinus cavernosus. Bei den restlichen 37 Mißbildungen saßen in 37% der Fälle die sackförmigen Aneurysmen an der wichtigsten zur Mißbildung führenden Arterie, während in 43% die Aneurysmen an Gefäßen saßen, die keine Beziehung zur arteriovenösen Mißbildung hatten. In den restlichen Fällen gingen die Aneurysmen von einer der beiden Karotiden ab.

In 68% der arteriovenösen Mißbildungen kommen anamnestisch Subarachnoidalblutungen vor, in 32% tritt keine Blutung auf. Demgegenüber verursachen nur 9,7% der sackförmigen Aneurysmen keine Blutung. 54% der Blutungen aus arteriovenösen Mißbildungen treten bereits vor dem 30. Lebensjahr auf mit einem Gipfel zwischen dem 15. und 20. Jahr. Bis zum 40. Lebensjahr haben 42% aller blutenden arteriovenösen Mißbildungen oder 40% aller arteriovenösen Mißbildungen (blutende und nicht blutende) geblutet.

Epileptische Anfälle sind nach der Studie von Perret und Nishioka (1966) in 28% der Fälle das Leitsymptom der supratentoriellen Läsionen. 70% der Patienten mit epileptischen Anfällen erlitten nie eine Blutung. In den von Moody und Poppen (1970) zusammengestellten 105 Fällen ist die Epilepsie dagegen mit 54% deutlich häufiger.

Ein pulssynchrones Geräusch ist nach der "cooperative study" in 25%, nach Moody und Poppen in 21% auskultierbar. Geräusche bestehen – subjektiv und objektiv – namentlich bei denjenigen arteriovenösen Kurzschlüssen, die in den Sinus transversus drainieren (Kühner et al., 1976).

Die arteriovenösen Mißbildungen der Dura führen oft weniger über einen Blutentzug zu klinischen Symptomen als vielmehr über gestörte Druckverhältnisse in den Sinus, was Anlaß zur Entwicklung eines Hydrocephalus internus geben kann (Kunc u. Brat, 1969; Zingesser et al., 1969; Kosnik et al., 1974; Lamas et al., 1977). Die duralen Mißbildungen äußern sich, besonders wenn sie groß sind, schon im Säuglings- und Kindesalter nicht selten durch die Trias: vergrößerter Kopf, Strömungsgeräusche und Herzinsuffizienz oder vergrößertes Herz (Long et al., 1974), wobei sich die sekundären Veränderungen nach erfolgreicher Exstirpation der arteriovenösen Mißbildung zurückbilden können (Cronqvist et al., 1972).

IV. Angiographie der arteriovenösen Mißbildungen

1. Allgemeines

Infolge des verminderten peripheren Widerstandes ist die Zirkulation in der arteriovenösen Mißbildung, im Vergleich zur übrigen Hirnzirkulation, erheblich beschleunigt. Bildserien mit schneller Frequenz sind erforderlich, um die anatomischen und hämodynamischen Verhältnisse abzuklären. Die wesentlichen zuführenden Arterien, die meist stark erweitert und elongiert sind, lassen sich in der Regel leicht identifizieren. Trotzdem stellen sich bei der Angiographie gelegentlich nicht alle zuführenden Arterien dar. Es muß immer daran gedacht werden, daß in Grenzgebieten Zuflüsse aus nicht injizierten Gefäßen möglich sind. Zur genauen Abklärung ist deshalb die selektive Darstellung beider Karotiden und der Vertebralarterien erforderlich. Die selektive Darstellung der A. carotis externa deckt zudem nicht selten Zuflüsse aus diesem Stromgebiet auf, die bei Kontrastmittelinjektion in die A. carotis communis und natürlich auch bei selektiver Internadarstellung verborgen bleiben (Dilenge et al., 1963). Speziell bei Mißbildungen im Bereich der Hirnbasis, die bei der Darstellung der A. carotis interna einen Zufluß aus einem erweiterten

Truncus meningo-hypophyseos erkennen lassen, ist eine selektive Externadarstellung unerläßlich (PEETERS u. VROOMEN, 1970).

Die Zirkulation des Blutes durch die Mißbildungen ist so rasch, daß nahezu immer die drainierenden und in der Regel stark erweiterten Venen bereits während der arteriellen Phase auftreten (Abb. 35). Im Konvolut der dicht gelagerten Mißbildungsgefäße nehmen die arteriellen Elemente gewöhnlich einen kleineren Raum ein als die dilatierten Venen, und eine genaue Abgrenzung des arteriellen vom venösen Schenkel ist kaum oder höchstens auf sehr raschen Serien möglich. Auf Bildern der frühen arteriellen Phase ist gelegentlich innerhalb des Gefäßkonvoluts ein rundlicher oder unregelmäßig begrenzter Füllungsdefekt zu beobachten, der sich auf den nächsten Aufnahmen als weite Vene innerhalb des arteriellen Gefäßknäuels identifizieren läßt (Abb. 36).

Bei arteriovenösen Mißbildungen, die von mehreren Gefäßgebieten versorgt werden, können die Anteile, die von den einzelnen zuführenden Arterien ihr Blut beziehen, von verschiedener Größe sein. Das kann dazu führen, daß bei der Darstellung des kleineren Angiomanteils über die A. carotis interna, externa oder die A. vertebralis die drainierenden Venen nur spärlich oder überhaupt nicht sichtbar werden, da das Kontrastmittel in den Venen von kontrastmittellosem Blut aus dem größeren Angiomanteil so stark verdünnt wird, daß er röntgenologisch nicht mehr zur Darstellung kommt (KOO et al., 1970).

Erweiterte zuführende Arterien, Konvolute pathologischer Gefäße und vorzeitiges Auftreten drainierender Venen finden sich nicht nur bei arteriovenösen Mißbildungen sondern auch bei malignen Gliomen und einzelnen Metastasetypen (z.B. Metastasen des Hypernephroms). Für die keineswegs immer einfache Unterscheidung zwischen arteriovenösen Mißbildungen und malignen Gliomen haben WICKBOM (1950) sowie GOREE und DUKES (1963) folgende Kriterien aufgestellt:

	Arteriovenöse Mißbildung	*Malignes Gliom*
zuführende Gefäße:	können normal groß sein, sind aber meistens deutlich bis massiv erweitert	können normal weit bis leicht erweitert sein, zeigen aber kaum je massive Dilatationen
zuführende Gefäße in unmittelbarem Bereich der Läsion:	können auf sehr frühen arteriellen Phasen bis in die Läsion verfolgt werden, wobei sie meist eine gewisse Schlängelung beibehalten	die Gefäße können nur selten bis in die Läsion hinein verfolgt werden. Häufiger verlaufen sie in der Peripherie des Tumors und sind wegen der raumfordernden Wirkung ausgespannt und gestreckt
Gefäße in der Läsion:	nur wenig gefäßlose Zonen innerhalb des dichten Gefäßkonvolutes, Gefäße meist von regelmäßigem Kaliber	größere gefäßlose Bezirke zwischen den pathologischen, häufig unregelmäßig kalibrierten Gefäßen. Vaskularisation im Tumorzentrum häufig geringer als in den Randbezirken
wegführende Gefäße:	können normal weit sein, sind jedoch meist deutlich erweitert	meist normal weit, kaum je massive Erweiterung
Raumforderung:	meist keine wesentliche Raumforderung, es sei denn, es liege ein großes Hämatom vor, wobei dann aber die Raumforderung avaskulär ist	deutliche Raumforderung mit Gefäßverlagerungen

Raumfordernde Hämatome bei arteriovenösen Mißbildungen können zu massiven Verlagerungen führen und u.U. die Gefäße des Angioms auseinander drängen. Bei stark erhöhtem intrakraniellem Druck füllen sich die drainierenden Venen weniger rasch.

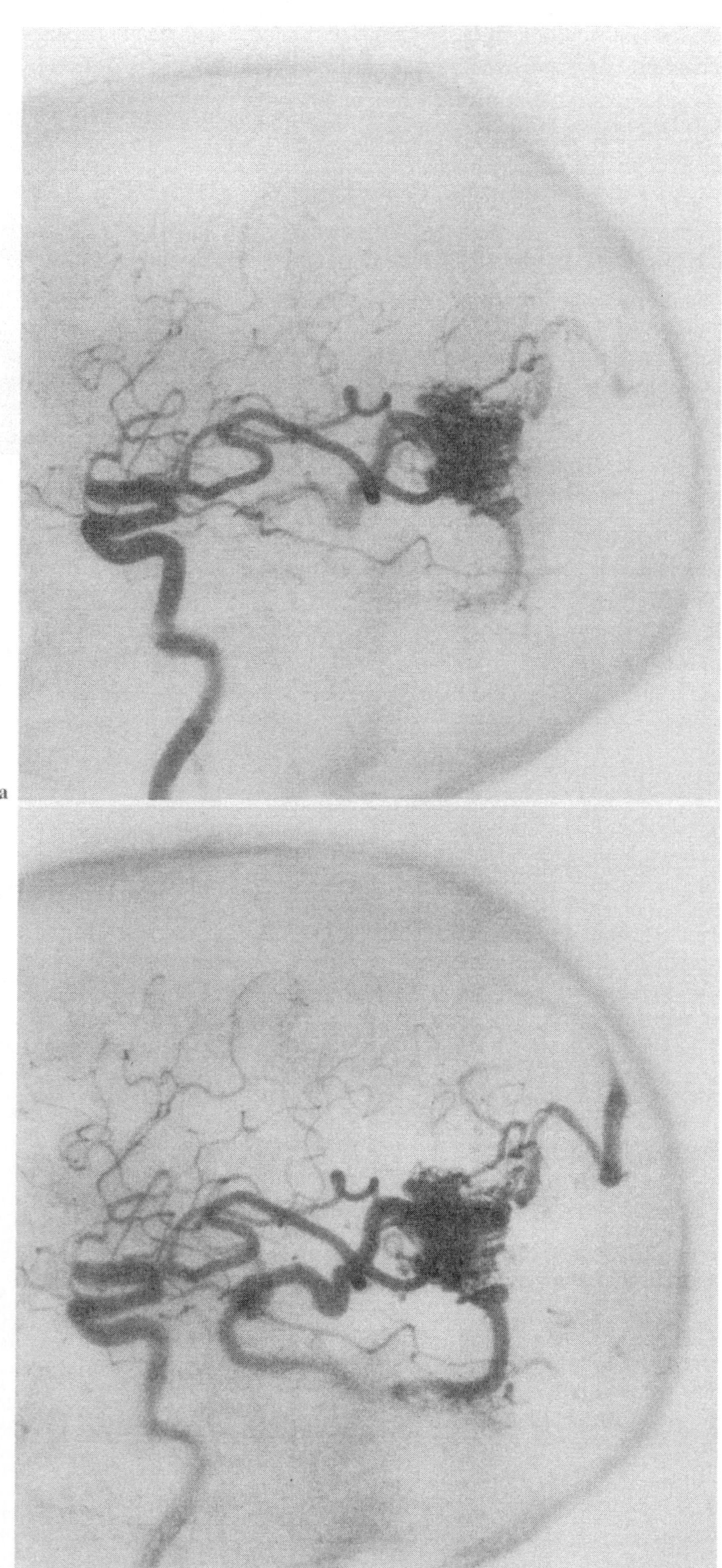

a

b

Abb. 35a u. b

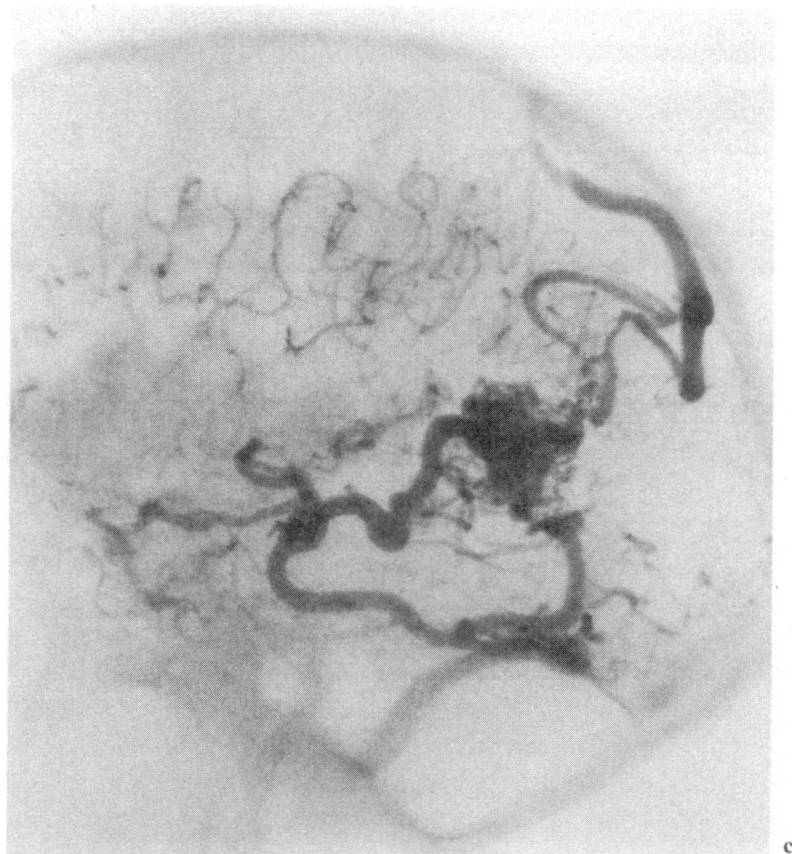
c

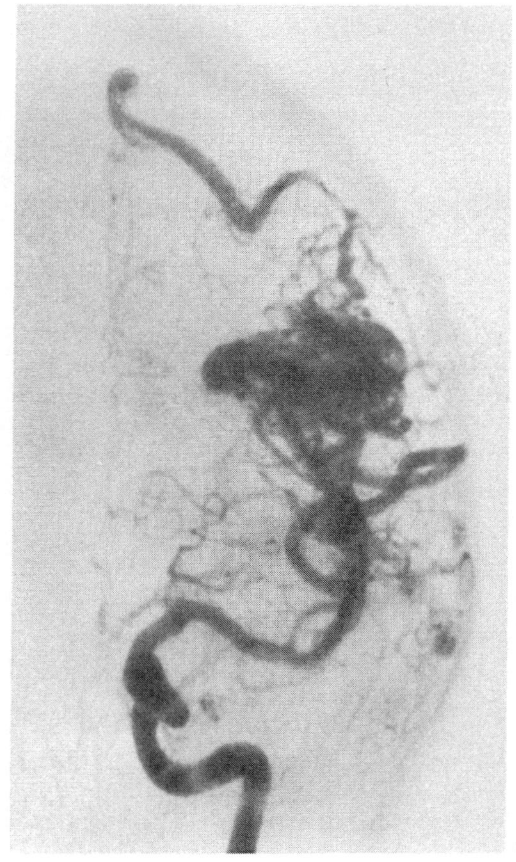
d

Abb. 35a–d. Arteriovenöse Mißbildung. **a** Profilaufnahme der früharteriellen Phase. Die zur Mißbildung führenden temporalen Mediaäste sind stark erweitert. Beginnende Darstellung der drainierenden kortikalen Venen; **b** und **c** spätere arterielle Phasen; **d** a-p Aufnahme der arteriellen Phase. Keilform der arteriovenösen Mißbildung, breite Basis dem Kortex zugewandt

Infolge der Shuntwirkung sind die Gefäße der übrigen Hemisphäre oft nur zum Teil oder überhaupt nicht sichtbar (Abb. 43 und 47), stellen sich aber nach der Angiomentfernung in normaler Weise dar. Nach operativer Ausschaltung des Angioms kehren die vorher erweiterten Gefäßabschnitte rasch zum normalen Kaliber zurück (NORLÉN, 1949; WICKBOM, 1950; AMACHER et al., 1972) (Abb. 37).

2. Untergruppen

Einzelne der arteriovenösen Mißbildungen bedürfen infolge ihrer Lage oder Form einer besonderen Besprechung:

a) Arteriovenöse Mißbildungen des Corpus callosum

Bei den arteriovenösen Mißbildungen des Corpus callosum werden nach MONTANT et al. (1971) drei Formen unterschieden

a) Mißbildungen mit Sitz im Bereich des Balkenknies werden durch die Seitenäste der A. pericallosa versorgt. Die venöse Drainage erfolgt entweder in den Sinus sagittalis inferior oder durch Septumvenen in die V. cerebri interna (Abb. 38).

b) Mißbildungen im mittleren Balkenabschnitt werden direkt oder über Seitenäste der A. pericallosa versorgt und drainieren entweder über kortikale Venen in den Sinus sagittalis superior oder durch den Balken in die V. magna Galeni.

c) Mißbildungen im Splenium werden zur Hauptsache von Ästen der A. cerebri posterior gespiesen, doch ist häufig auch der distalste Abschnitt der A. pericallosa in die Versorgung mit einbezogen. Die venöse Drainage erfolgt zur V. magna Galeni (Abb. 39).

Die Mißbildungen vom Typus a) und b) liegen oft am Balken selbst, während diejenigen vom Typus c) außerhalb des Balkens liegen und operativ dementsprechend besser anzugehen sind (YASARGIL et al., 1976).

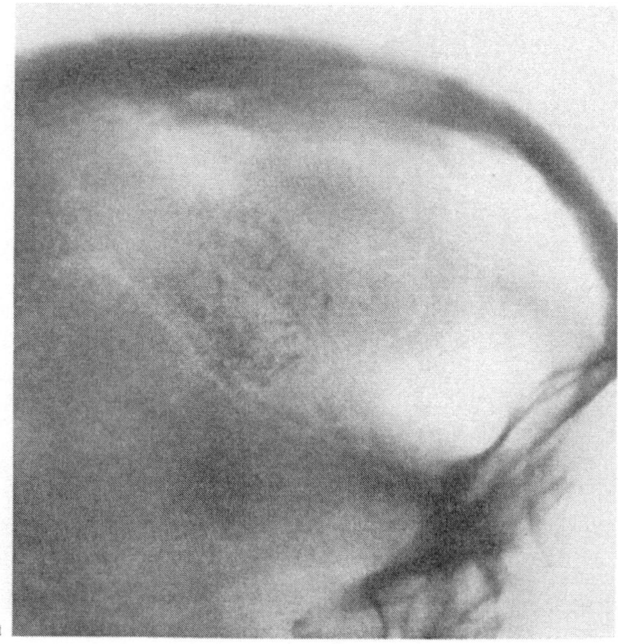

Abb. 36a–e. Frontolaterale arteriovenöse Mißbildung. **a** Verkalkungen in der arteriovenösen Mißbildung. **b–e** ► Profilserie des Karotisangiogrammes. **c** Aussparung im Gefäßkonvolut der Mißbildung, bedingt durch ausgeweitete drainierende Vene. **d** Beginnende und **e** deutliche Füllung dieser erweiterten Vene in der Mißbildung. (Aus „Zerebrale Angiographie", 3. Aufl. 1979, Thieme Stuttgart)

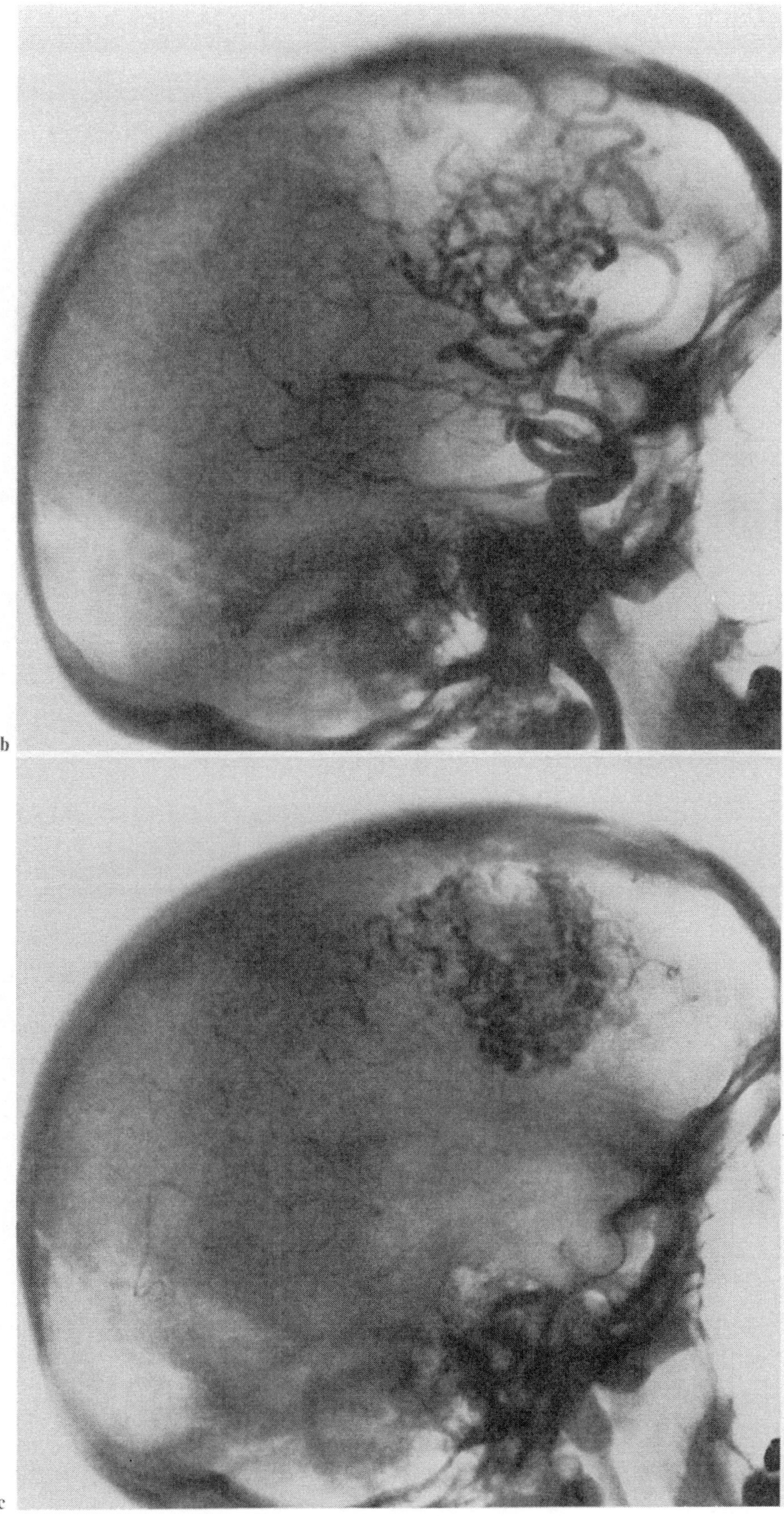

Abb. 36b u. c

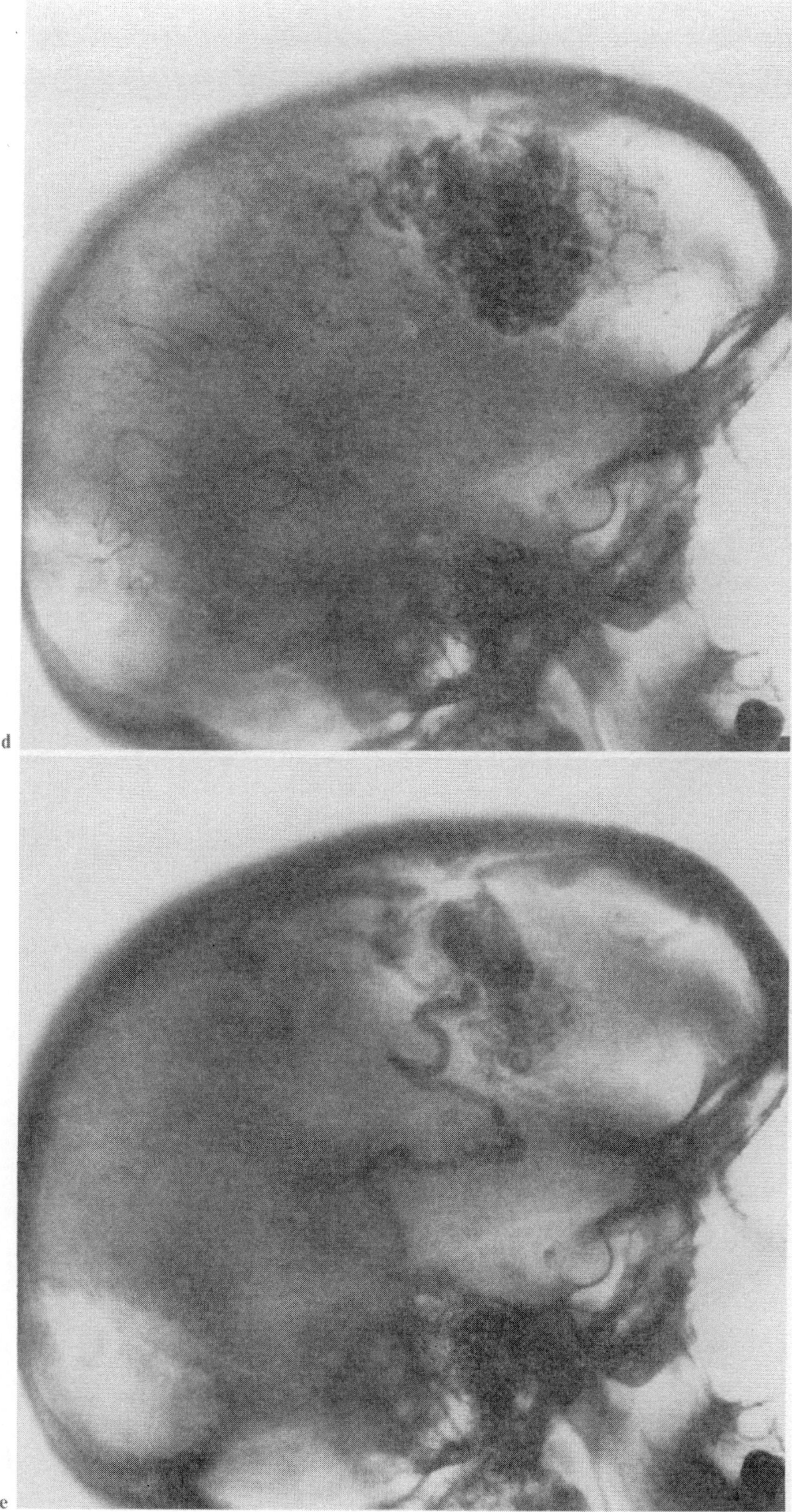

Abb. 36d u. e

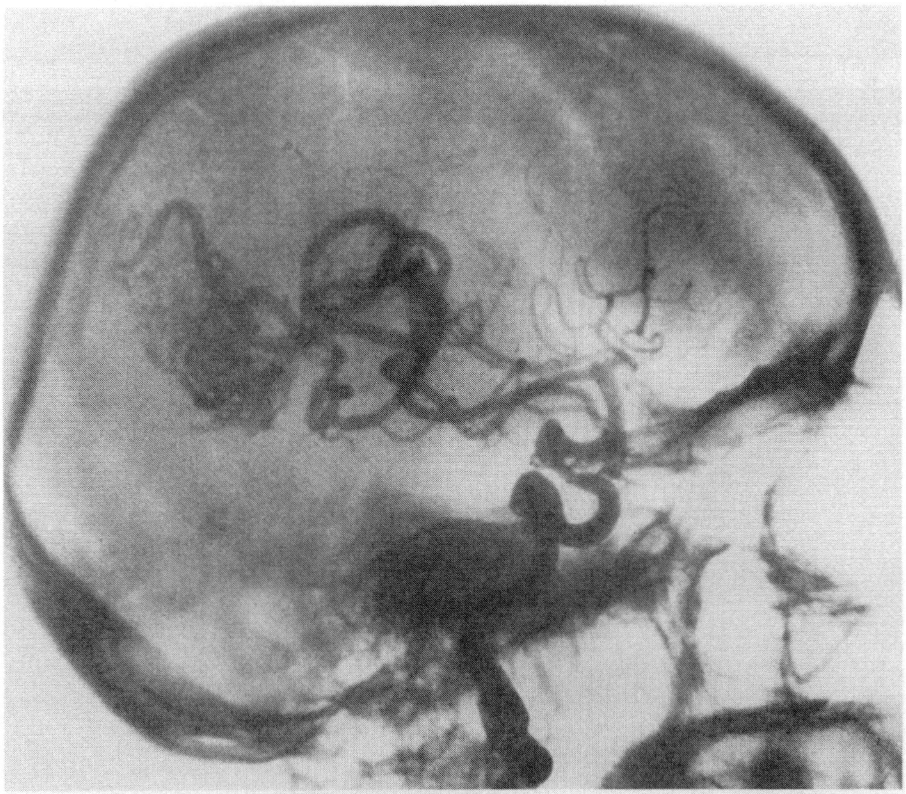

a

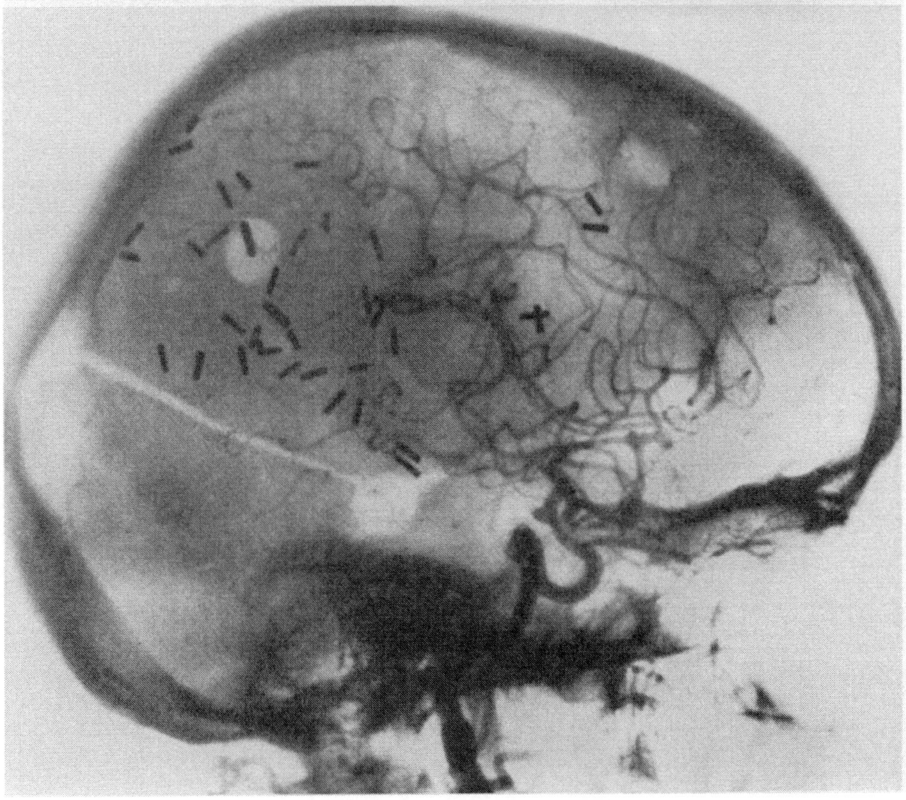

b

Abb. 37a u. b. Arteriovenöse Mißbildung. **a** Präoperative Aufnahme mit stark erweiterten, zur Mißbildung führenden Arterien. Die A. pericallosa und ihre Äste stellen sich nicht dar. **b** Kontrollangiographie 14 Tage nach Operation. Die Arterien weisen bereits wieder ein normales Kaliber auf. Die A. pericallosa und ihre Äste stellen sich gut dar. (Aus „Zerebrale Angiographie", 3. Aufl. 1979, Thieme Stuttgart)

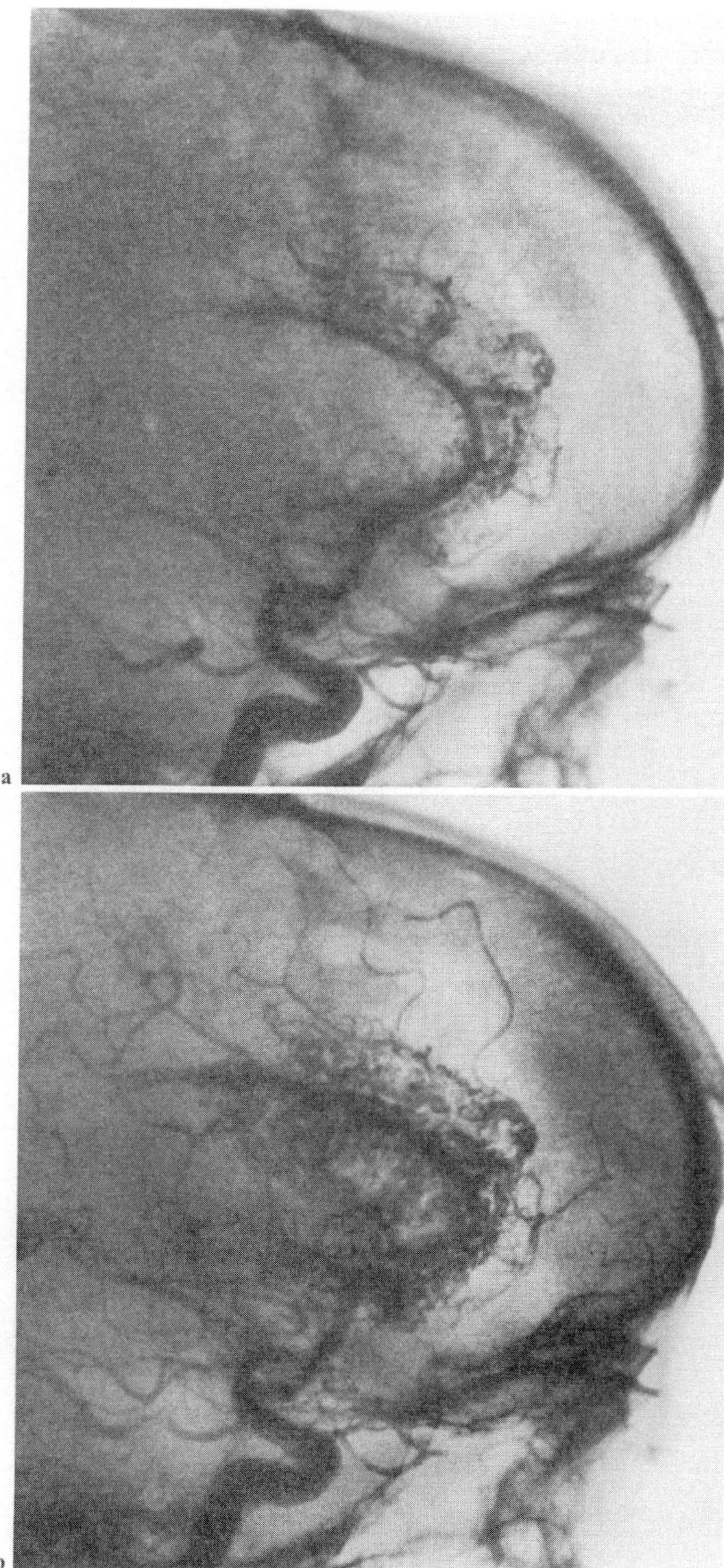

Abb. 38a–c. Arteriovenöse Mißbildungen in und um den vorderen Balkenabschnitt mit massiver Erweiterung des tiefen (zentralen) Venensystems. (Aus „Zerebrale Angiographie", 3. Aufl. 1979, Thieme Stuttgart)

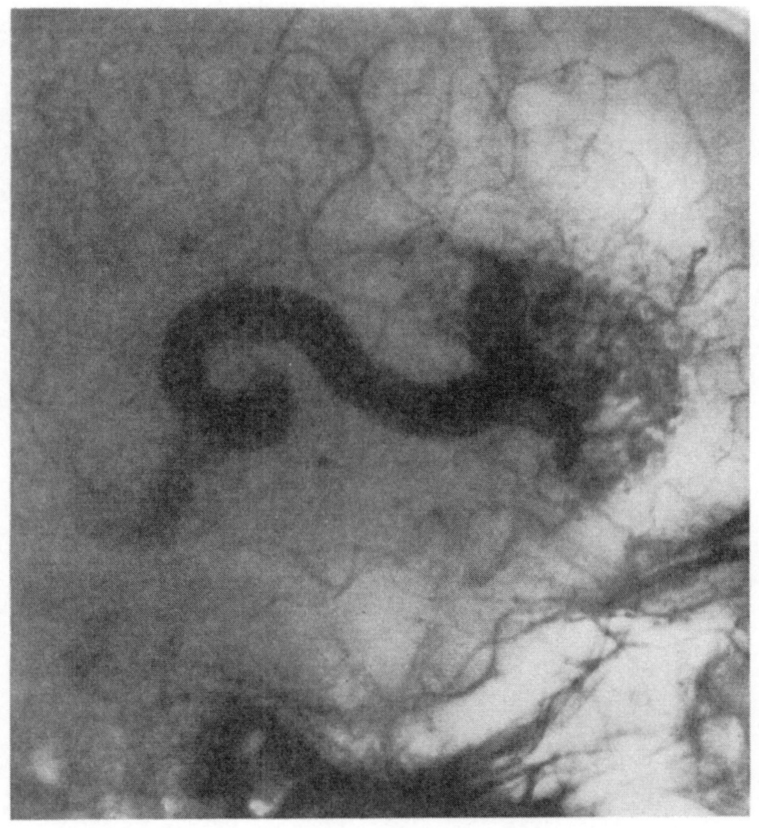

Abb. 38c

b) Arteriovenöse Mißbildungen der A. choroidea anterior und der lentikulostriären Arterien

Für die Therapie von besonderer Bedeutung ist die Unterscheidung der arteriovenösen Mißbildungen im Bereiche der A. choroidea anterior und der Arterien des Striatum (LAINE et al., 1970): Die von der A. choroidea anterior gespiesenen Mißbildungen projizieren sich auf den Aufnahmen nach TOWNE um die Karotisgabel, auf den Profilaufnahmen liegen sie basal von der Mediagruppe und folgen der Achse der A. choroidea anterior. Die venöse Drainage erfolgt über die hinteren Plexusvenen, resp. die V. basilaris (Abb. 40).

Die striären arteriovenösen Mißbildungen liegen außer- und oberhalb der Karotisteilungsstelle und reiten auf der sylvischen Achse. Operativ etwas günstiger als die übrigen arteriovenösen Mißbildungen des zentralen Graus sind diejenigen im Caput nuclei caudati, da sie vor dem Thalamus und der Capsula interna liegen (LAPRAS et al., 1972). Ihre hauptsächlichen Zuflüsse sind die A. recurrens HEUBNER und die lentikulostriären Arterien; die venöse Drainage erfolgt über die V. thalamostriata und die Vv. nuclei caudati.

c) Arteriovenöse Mißbildungen im Bereiche der V. magna Galeni

Da die V. magna Galeni den unpaaren Abschnitt des zentripetalen venösen Drainagesystems bildet, führen arteriovenöse Mißbildungen in ihrem Einzugsgebiet zu einer starken Erweiterung ihres Lumens, was als ganz besonders hervorstechendes Merkmal der Mißbildung imponiert und zur unklaren Bezeichnung eines Aneurysmas der V. magna Galeni Anlaß gegeben hat. Es handelt sich aber bei diesem Aneurysma der V. magna Galeni um einen arteriovenösen Kurzschluß, wobei der Zufluß mehr oder weniger direkt aus Ästen der A. carotis interna und/oder der A. basila-

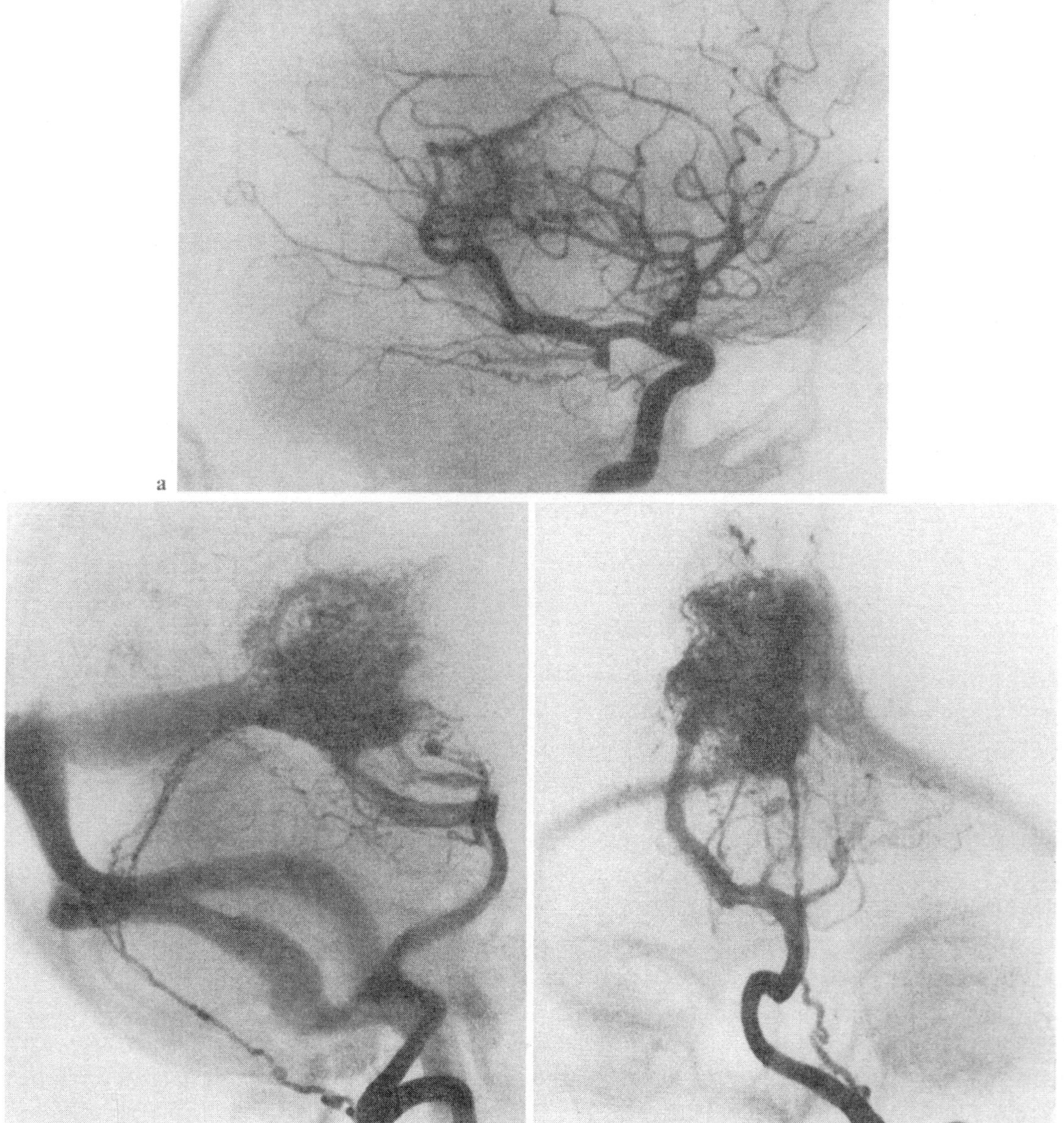

Abb. 39 a–c. Arteriovenöse Mißbildung im Spleniumbereich. **a** Karotisangiogramm rechts. Die Mißbildung wird zur Hauptsache durch die rechte A. cerebri posterior und die A. pericallosa versorgt, erhält aber auch einen geringeren Zufluß über die erweiterte A. tentorii. **b u. c** Vertebralisangiogramm: Neben der stark erweiterten A. cerebri posterior führt die erweiterte A. meningea posterior der Mißbildung Blut zu. (Aus „Zerebrale Angiographie", 3. Aufl. 1979, Thieme Stuttgart)

ris erfolgt (Abb. 41). Die direkte Fistelbildung zwischen Choroidalarterien und Ästen der A. pericallosa einerseits und der V. magna Galeni andererseits kann damit erklärt werden, daß die primitiven Gefäßplexus an der Oberfläche des Neuraltubus sehr nahe beieinander liegen und sich rechtwinklig kreuzen. Es ist deshalb möglich, daß an den Kreuzungsstellen der primitiven Gefäße, die nur durch zwei Endothelschichten getrennt sind, Fisteln auftreten (PADGET, 1956,

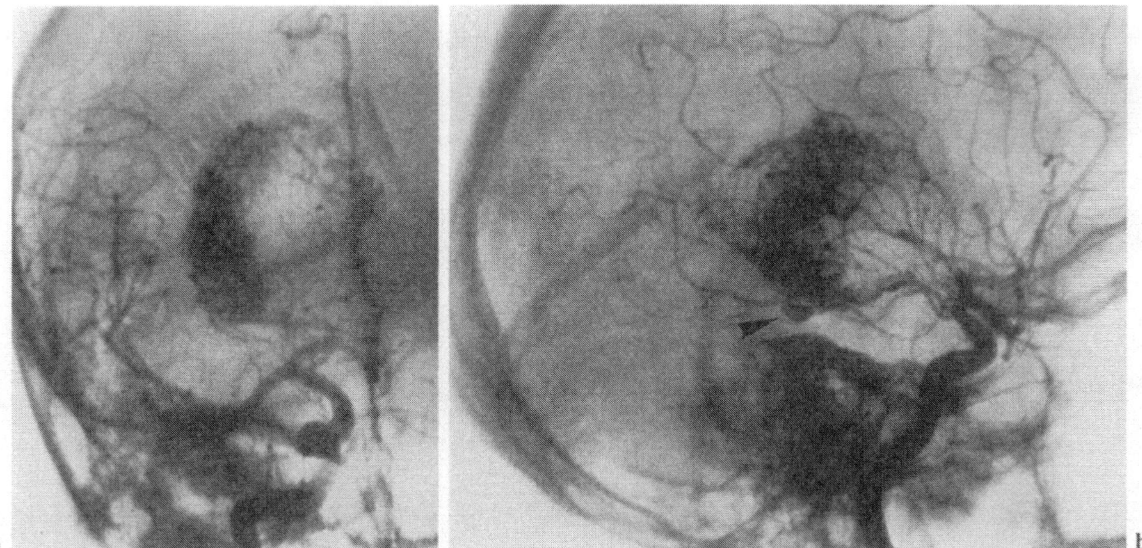

Abb. 40a u. b. Arteriovenöse Mißbildung im Stromgebiet der A. choroidea anterior (Pulvinar rechts). Die Mißbildung ist mit einem sackförmigen Aneurysma (►) kombiniert. (Aus „Zerebrale Angiographie", 3. Aufl. 1979, Thieme Stuttgart)

1957). Unter Umständen kann ein razemöses Konglomerat mit wesentlichem Abfluß in die V. magna Galeni dazwischen geschaltet sein, z.B. bei arteriovenösen Mißbildungen des Corpus callosum, die oft nur aus kleinen Ästen der A. pericallosa versorgt werden, sich aber in eine ampullenförmig erweiterte V. magna Galeni ergießen (LITVAK et al., 1960; GOLD et al., 1964; AGEE u. GREER, 1967; AGEE et al., 1969; O'BRIEN u. SCHECHTER, 1970; MONTANT et al., 1971). Diese Mißbildung verursacht häufig einen Verschluß des Aquäduktes mit Hydrocephalus internus (RUSSELL u. NEVIN, 1940; ALPERS u. FORSTER, 1945; FRENCH u. PEYTON, 1954; PAMPUS et al., 1960; POPPEN u. AVMAN, 1960; COURVILLE, 1961; AMACHER und SHILLITO, 1973; DE FEO et al., 1976) und nicht selten führt sie schon beim Neugeborenen zu Herzinsuffizienz (GLATT u. ROWE, 1960; GOMEZ et al., 1963).

d) Mikroangiome des Gehirns

Diese angiographisch oft kaum erfaßbaren Gefäßmißbildungen sind keineswegs selten Ursache von spontanen intrazerebralen Hämatomen (GERLACH u. JENSEN, 1960, 1961; MARGOLIS et al., 1951; JENSEN et al., 1963; KRAYENBÜHL u. SIEBENMANN, 1965; MCCORMICK u. NOFZINGER, 1966) (Abb. 42). MCCORMICK und NOFZINGER (1966) stellten 260 Fälle der Literatur und 48 aus dem eigenen Krankengut zusammen. 161 dieser Mißbildungen waren supratentoriell und 147 infratentoriell gelegen:

frontal	45	Basalanglien und Inselregion	25
temporal	43	Mesenzephalon, Pons, Medulla	85
parietal	23	Zerebellum	44
okzipital	9	Rückenmark	18

3. Versorgung der arteriovenösen Mißbildungen durch durale Arterien

Die Beteiligung der Duraäste an pialen arteriovenösen Mißbildungen ist im supra- und infratentoriellen Raum mit je 15% gleich häufig (Abb. 43). Dagegen sind die rein duralen Formen der arteriovenösen Mißbildungen in der hinteren Schädelgrube eindeutig häufiger als supratento-

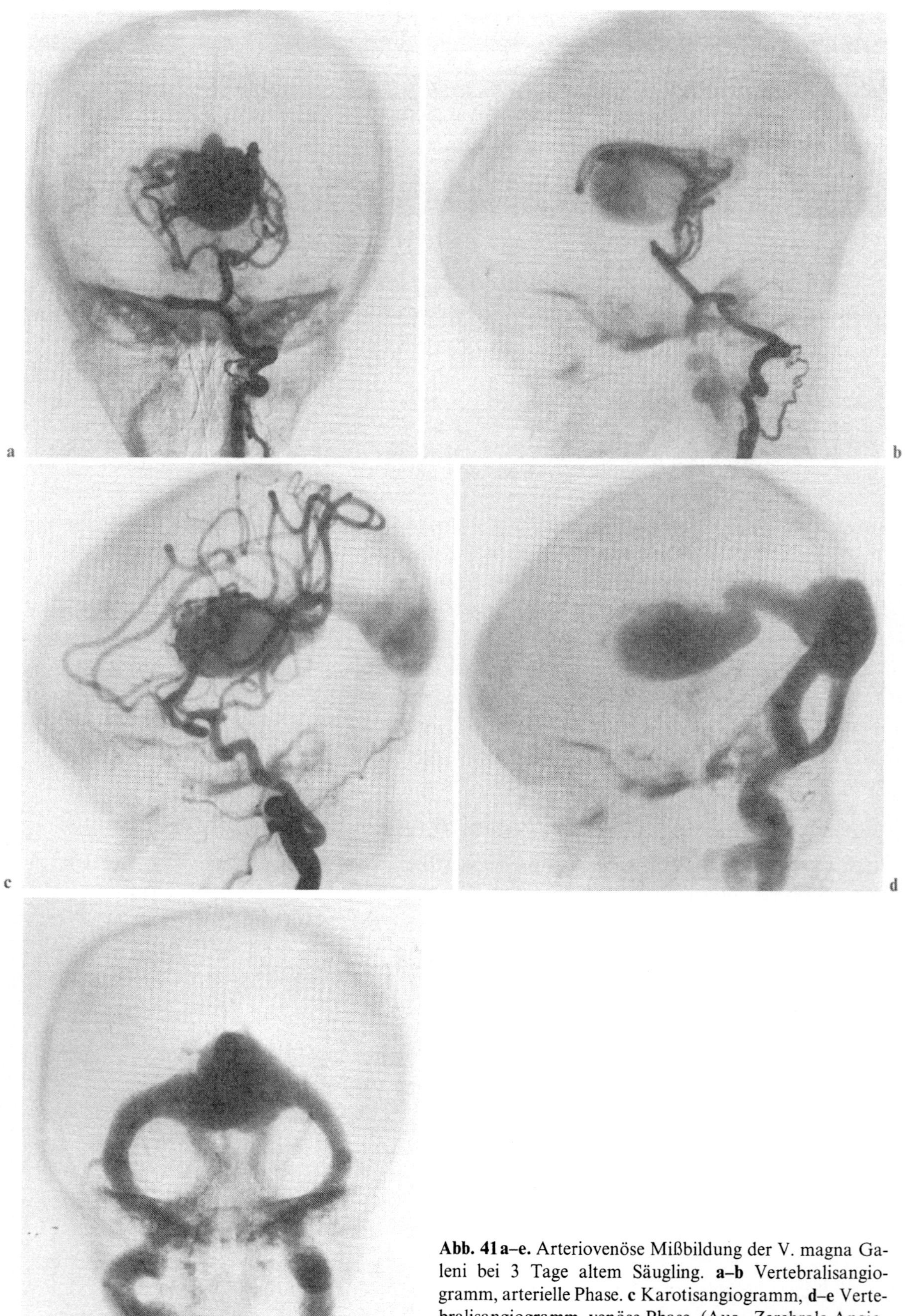

Abb. 41 a–e. Arteriovenöse Mißbildung der V. magna Galeni bei 3 Tage altem Säugling. **a–b** Vertebralisangiogramm, arterielle Phase. **c** Karotisangiogramm, **d–e** Vertebralisangiogramm, venöse Phase. (Aus „Zerebrale Angiographie", 3. Aufl. 1979, Thieme Stuttgart)

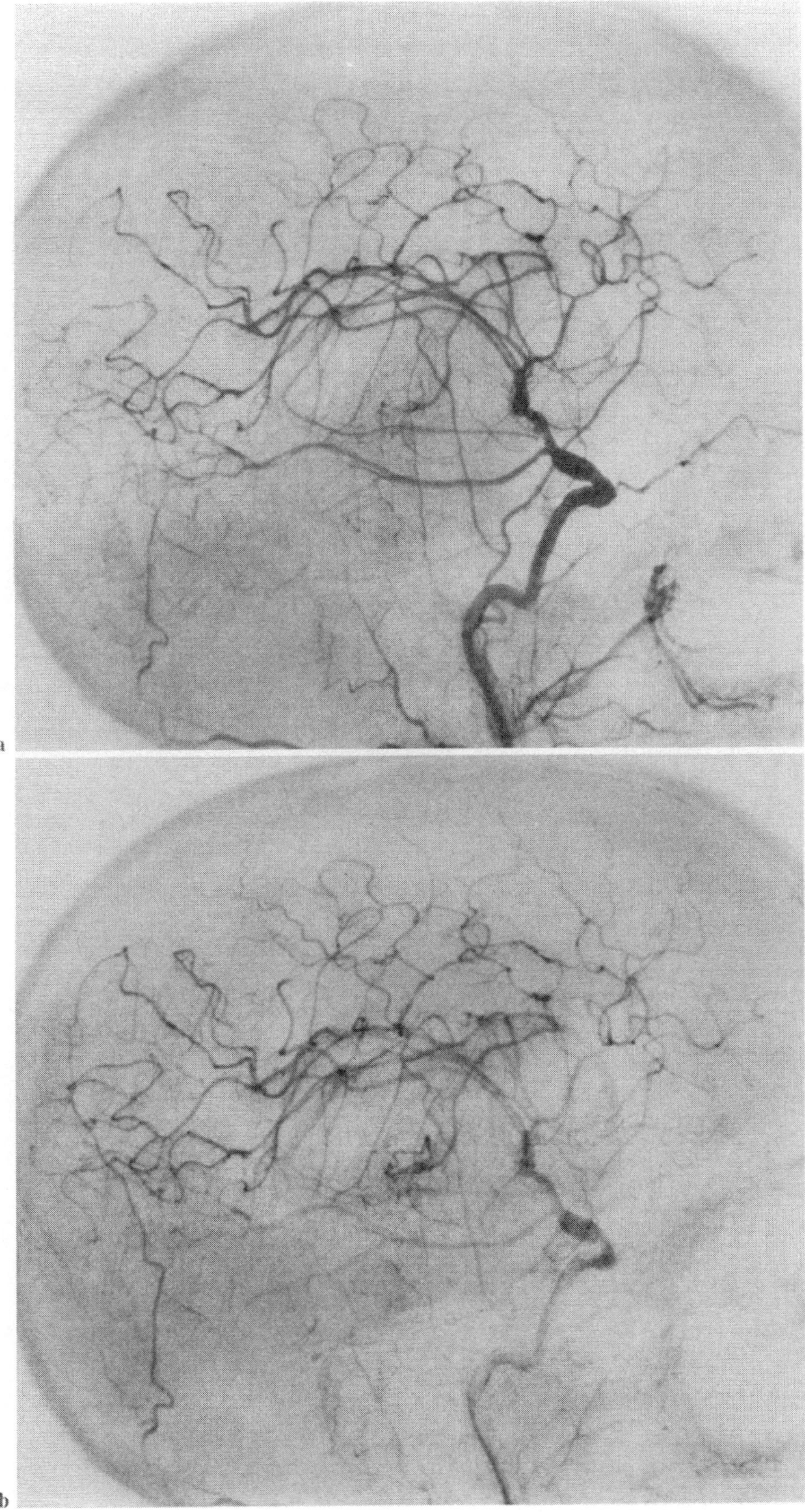

Abb. 42a–d. Mikroangiom mit intrazerebraler Blutung. **a–d** Karotisangiogramm rechts mit Anhebung des Sylvischen Dreiecks durch die Blutung aus dem Mikroangiom. **c** Beginnende Darstellung der das Mikroangiom drainierenden Vene (→)

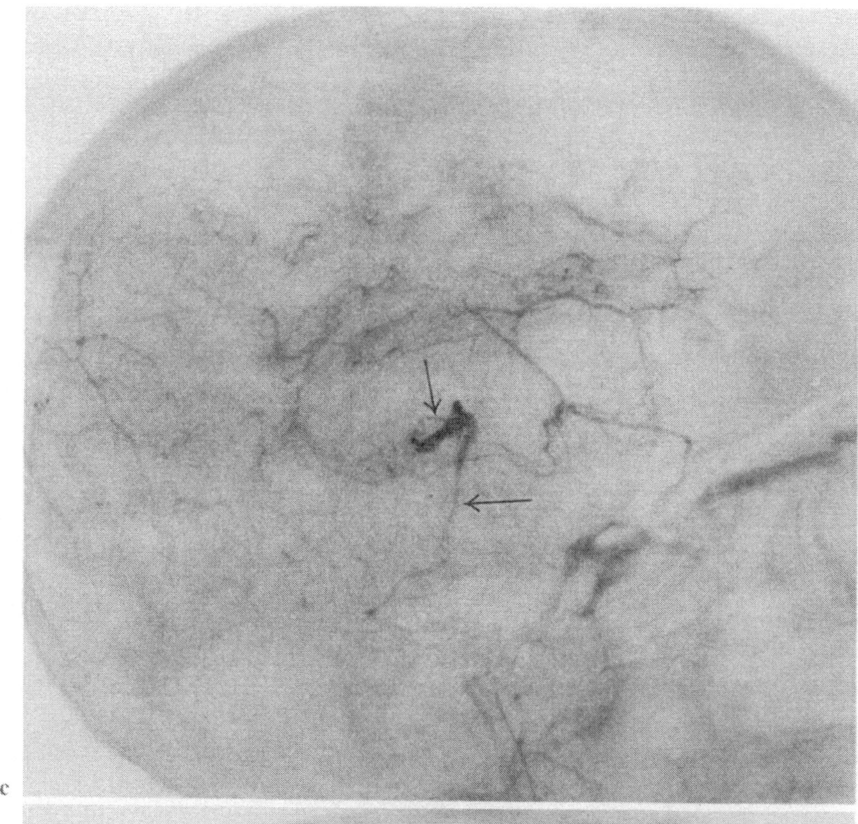
c

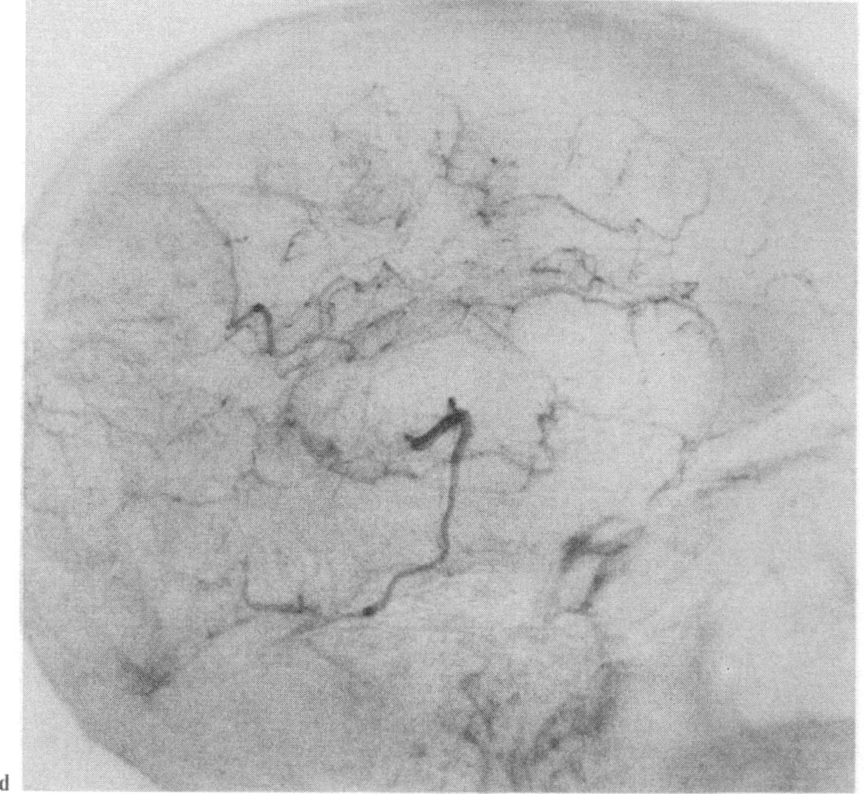
d

Abb. 42c u. d.

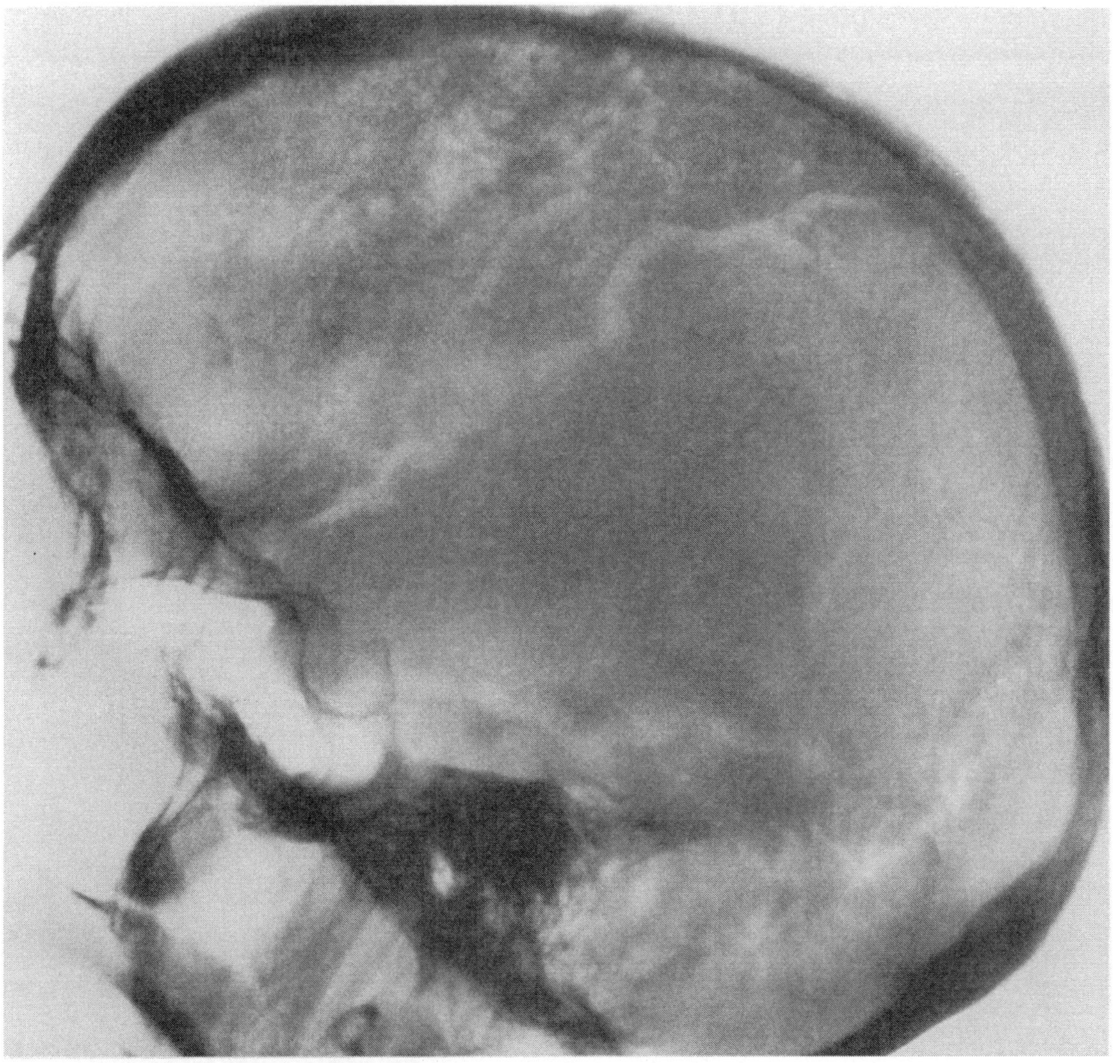

a

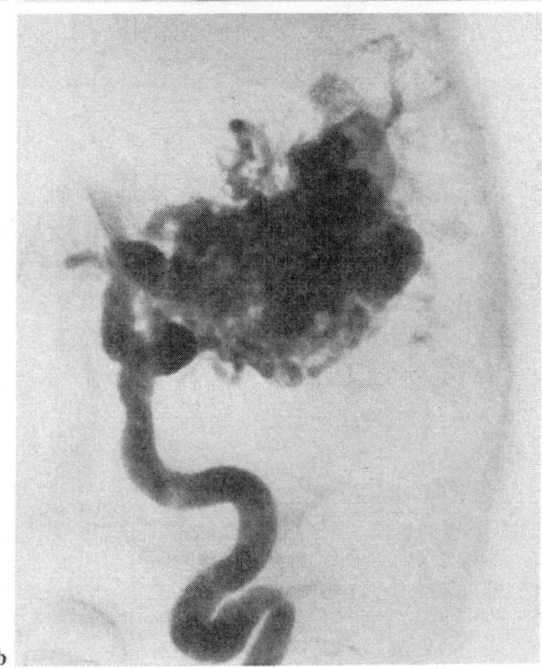

b

Abb. 43a–f. Große arteriovenöse Mißbildung temporal links mit gemischt pial-duralen arteriellen Zuflüssen. **a** Schädelröntgenbild mit erweiterter Gefäßfurche (A. meningea media, vgl. f). **b** Karotisangiogramm links, a-p Aufnahme. Sämtliches Blut aus der A. carotis interna strömt zur Mißbildung. Die A. pericallosa stellt sich nicht dar. **c–d** Karotisangiogramm rechts. Über den vorderen Abschnitt des Circulus Willisi strömt Blut zur arteriovenösen Mißbildung temporal links. Die Aa. pericallosae werden von der rechten A. carotis interna aus versorgt. Von der linken A. pericallosa ziehen ebenfalls Äste zur Mißbildung (vgl. Kollateralkreislauf bei Verschluß der A. cerebri media!). **e** Selektive Darstellung der linken A. carotis externa. Blutzustrom zur Mißbildung über die erweiterten Äste der A. meningea media. **f** Selektive Darstellung der rechten A. carotis externa, a-p Aufnahme. Die erweiterte rechte A. occipitalis greift über die Mittellinie nach links und führt der Mißbildung ebenfalls Blut zu. (Aus „Zerebrale Angiographie“, 3. Aufl. 1979, Thieme Stuttgart)

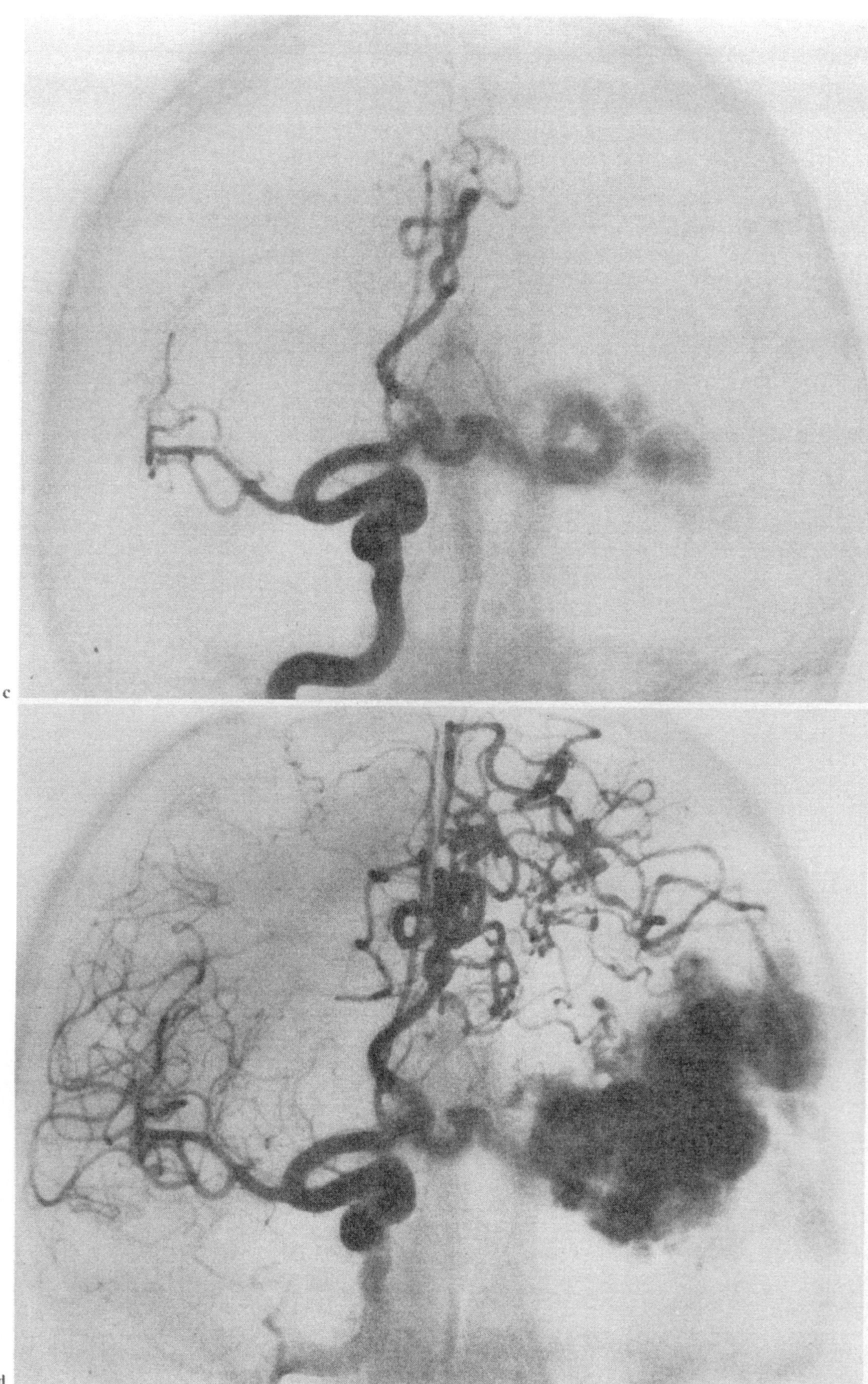

Abb. 43c u. d

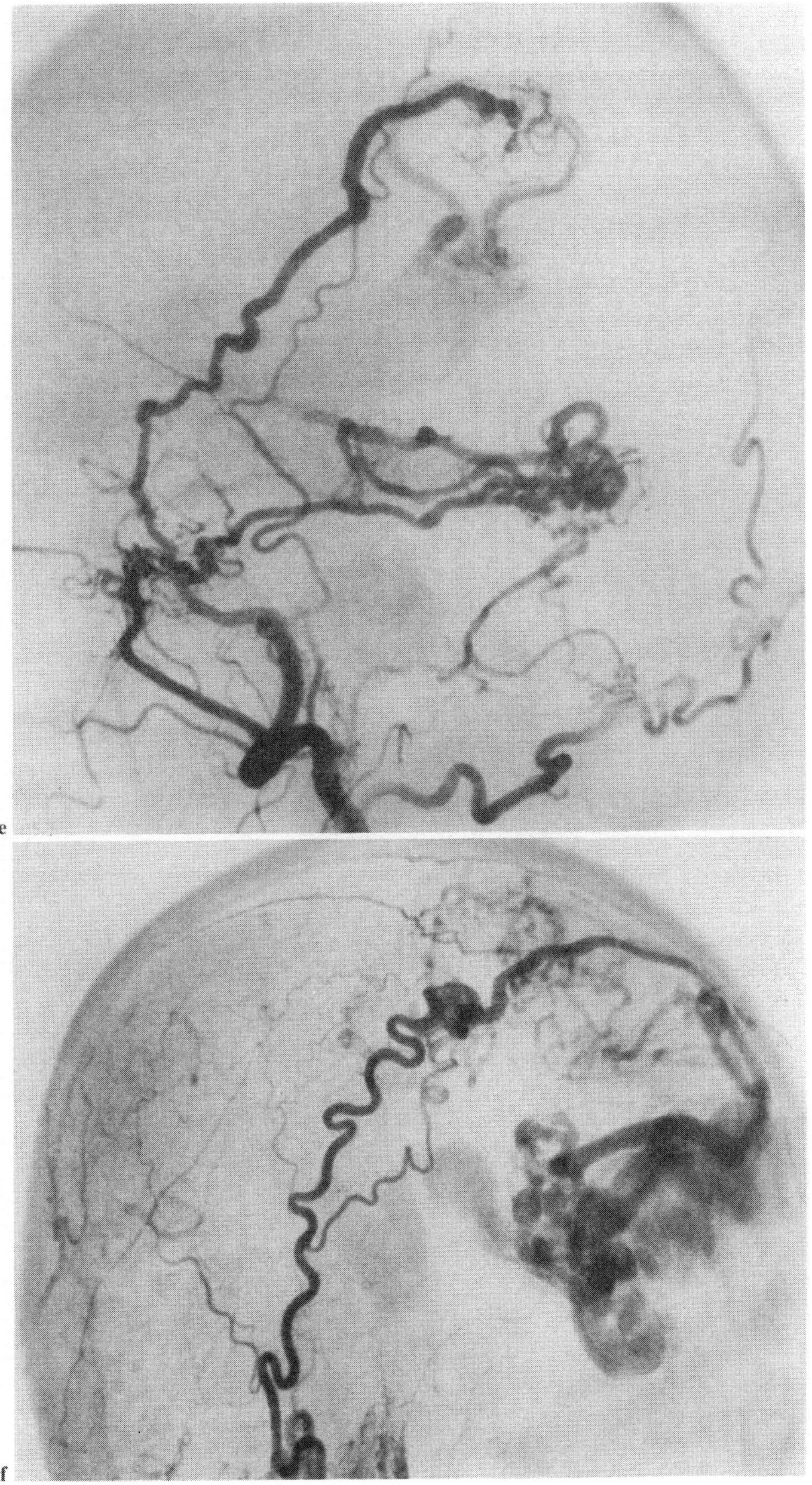

Abb. 43e u. f

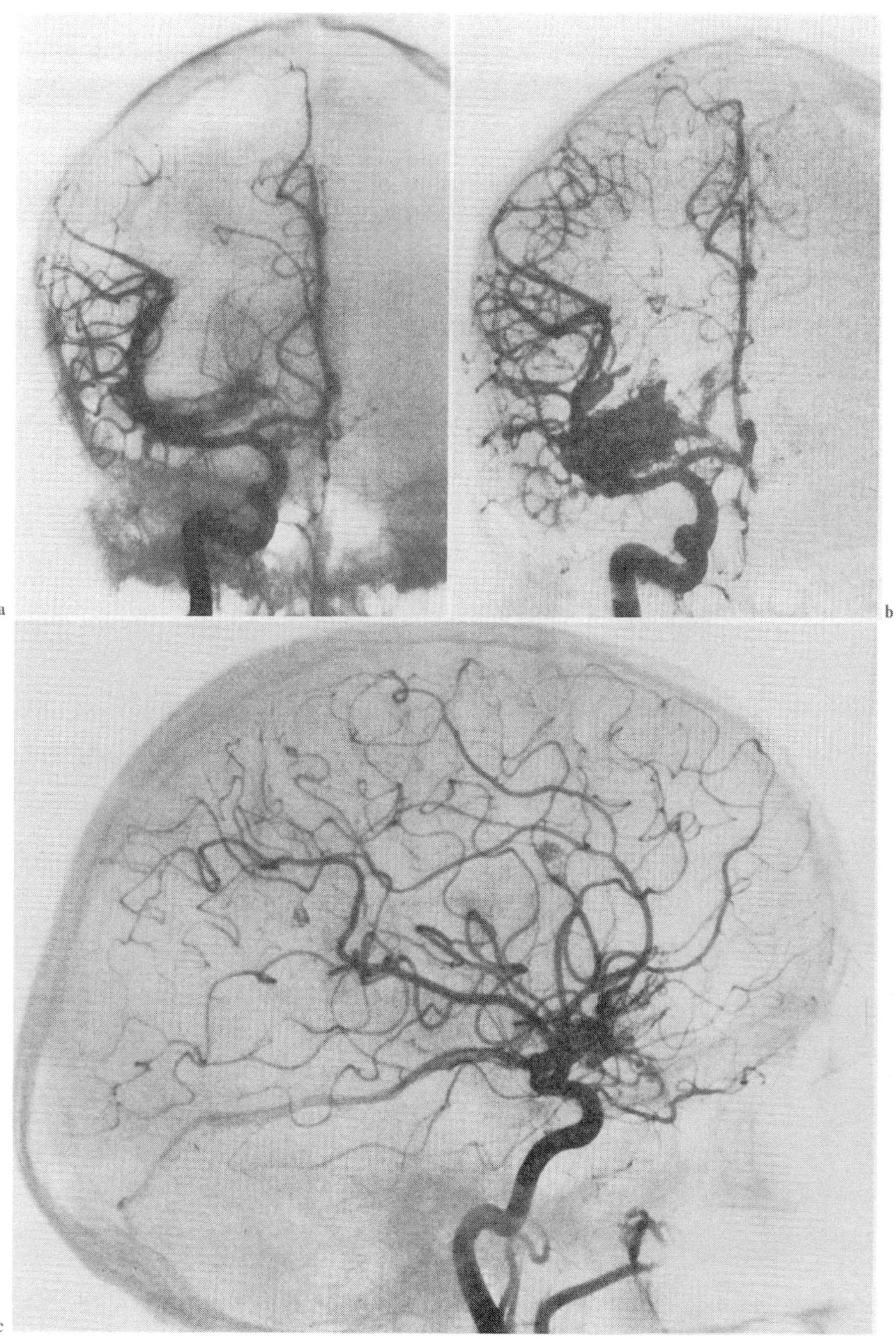

Abb. 44a–c

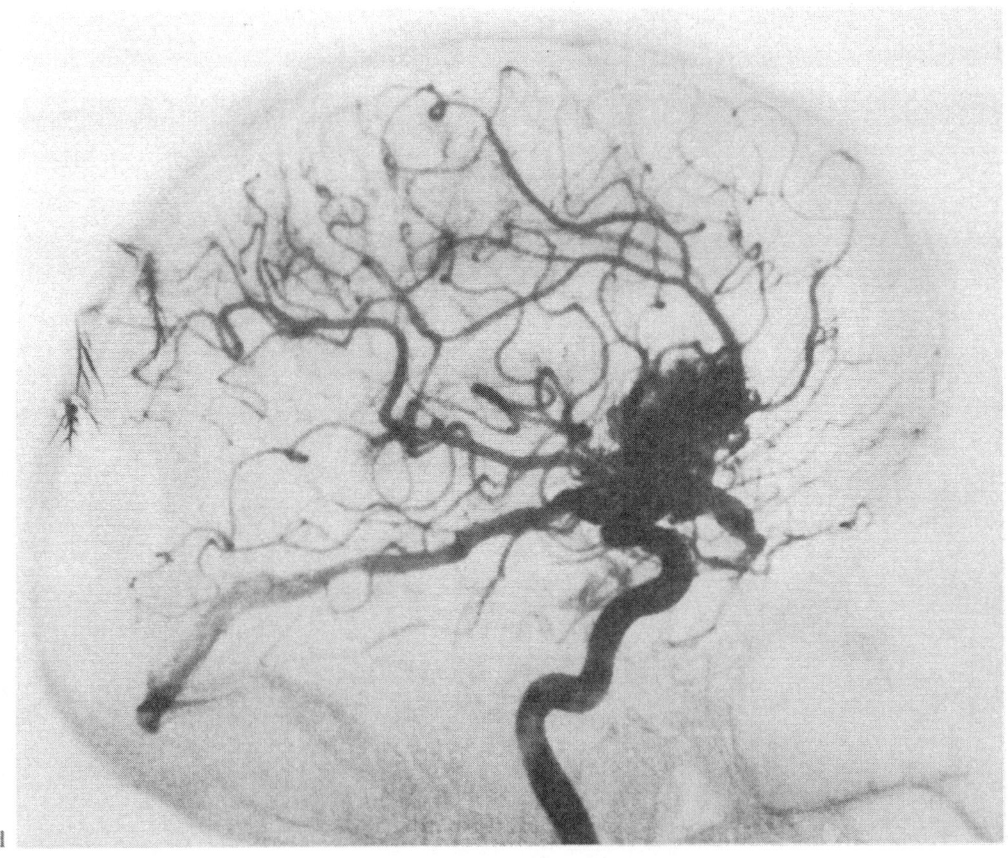

◀ **Abb. 44a–d.** Entwicklung einer arteriovenösen Mißbildung im Verlaufe von 4 Jahren. **a–b**: Carotisangiogramm rechts beim 18jährigen Patienten. **c–d**: Kontrollangiogramm 4 Jahre später: deutliche Größenzunahme der arteriovenösen Mißbildung im Striatum

riell (Newton et al., 1968; Nicola u. Nizzoli, 1968; Newton u. Cronqvist, 1969; Aminoff, 1973) (Abb. 45b und c). Für die klinische Symptomatologie scheinen weniger die zur Mißbildung führenden Arterien der Dura von Bedeutung zu sein als vielmehr die venösen Drainagewege (Houser et al., 1972; Castaigne et al., 1976). Überladungen des Sinus cavernosus durch unter erhöhtem Druck zuströmendes Blut kommen speziell bei Fisteln in der mittleren Schädelgrube vor. Doch können in größerer Entfernung gelegene arteriovenöse Fisteln – sofern sie groß genug sind – eine Rückwirkung auf den Sinus cavernosus haben.

Die zu den duralen arteriovenösen Mißbildungen oder Fisteln führenden Arterien entsprechen den Arterien, die die Dura an der betreffenden Stelle normalerweise versorgen. Die venöse Drainage kann dagegen sowohl über durale als auch über piale Venen erfolgen. Unter Umständen werden beide Abflußwege benutzt, doch scheint in der Mehrzahl der Fälle die Drainage nur über das durale System zu erfolgen, wobei die großen Sammelkanäle, wie Sinus cavernosus, Sinus transversus und Sinus petrosus superior das Blut abführen. Meistens ist die Verbindung von duralen Arteriel zu duralen Venen ziemlich direkt, analog den Fisteln, ohne Zwischenschaltung eines größeren Gefäßkonvolutes, und in diesen Fällen sind Blutungen relativ selten. Bei vorwiegend pialer venöser Drainage finden sich die charakteristischen arteriovenösen Konvolute häufiger, und diese Mißbildungen neigen eher zu Blutungen.

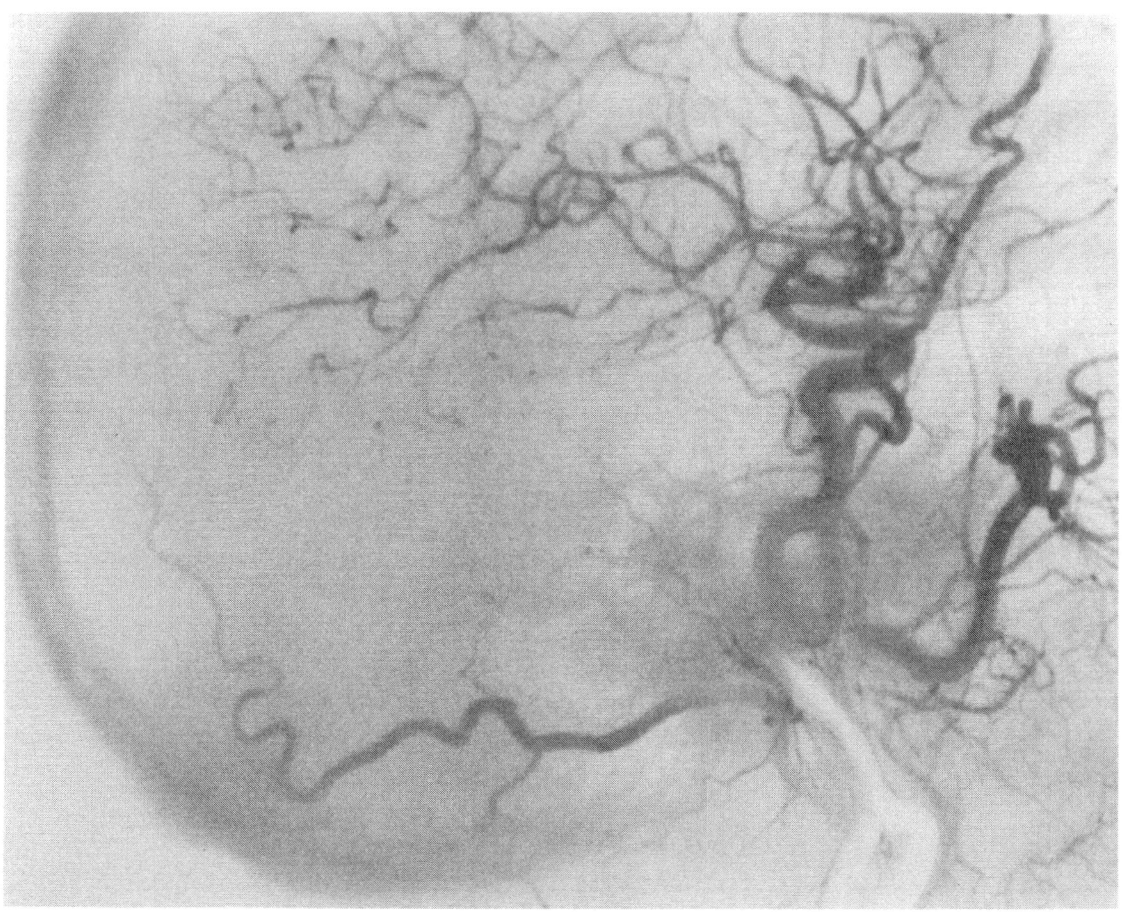

Abb. 45a–c. Entwicklung einer arteriovenösen Mißbildung der Dura der hinteren Schädelgrube. **a** Karotisangiogramm nach Subarachnoidalblutung. Kein Aneurysma und keine arteriovenöse Mißbildung sichtbar. Gegenseitige Karotisangiographie und Vertebralisangiographie normal. A. occipitalis rechts und ihre Äste gut dargestellt. **b u. c** Kontrollangiographie 6 Monate später wegen neu aufgetretenem pulssynchronem Geräusch retroaurikulär rechts. Superselektive Darstellung der A. occipitalis rechts, die sich gegenüber (**a**) deutlich erweitert hat. Arteriovenöse Mißbildung in der Dura mit Drainage in den Sinus transversus. (Aus „Zerebrale Angiographie", 3. Aufl. 1979, Thieme Stuttgart)

4. Wachstum der arteriovenösen Mißbildungen

Die arteriovenösen Mißbildungen können im Verlauf der Jahre an Größe zunehmen. Es handelt sich nicht um ein eigentliches Wachstum im Sinn der Neubildung von Gefäßen, sondern lediglich um eine Erweiterung der bereits in die Mißbildung einbezogenen Arterien und Venen (OLIVECRONA u. REEVES, 1948; SHENKIN et al., 1948; TÖNNIS u. SCHIEFER, 1955; DECKER u. FREISLEDERER, 1957; ANDERSON u. KORBIN 1958; HÖÖK u. JOHANSON, 1958; HUBER, 1959; PORTER u. BULL, 1969; ISFORT, 1972; WALTIMO, 1973; SPETZLER u. WILSON, 1975) (Abb. 44 und 45).

Spontane Verkleinerungen von arteriovenösen Mißbildungen infolge Thrombose sind von HÖÖK und JOHANSON (1958), SVIEN und PESERICO (1960), FISCHER et al. (1969), KELLY et al. (1969), KUSHNER und ALEXANDER (1970) LAKKE (1970), CONFORTI (1971), EISENMANN et al. (1972), LEVINE et al. (1973), HANSEN und SØGAARD (1976), MAGIDSON und WEINBERG (1976) mitgeteilt worden (Abb. 46).

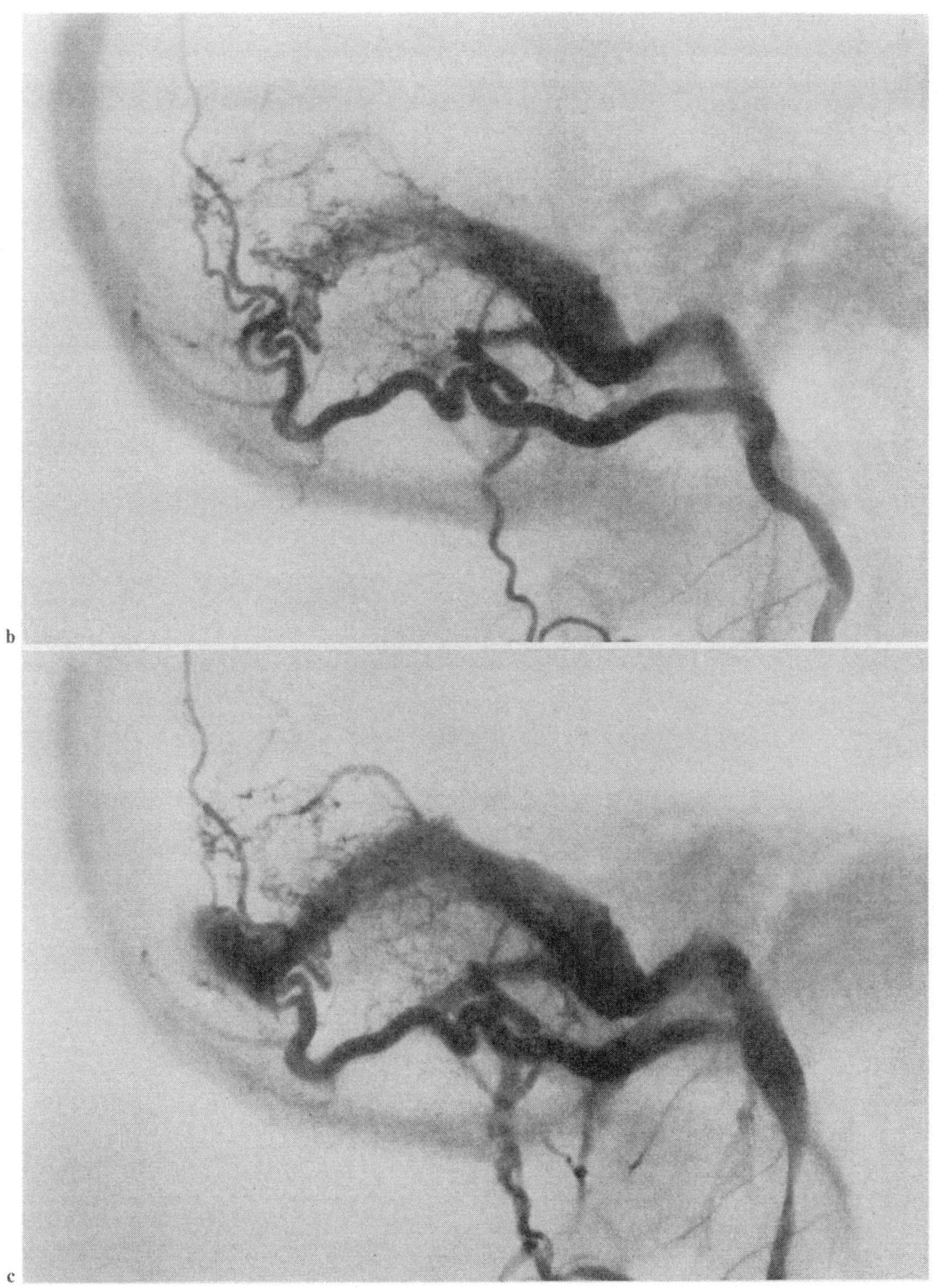

Abb. 45b u. c

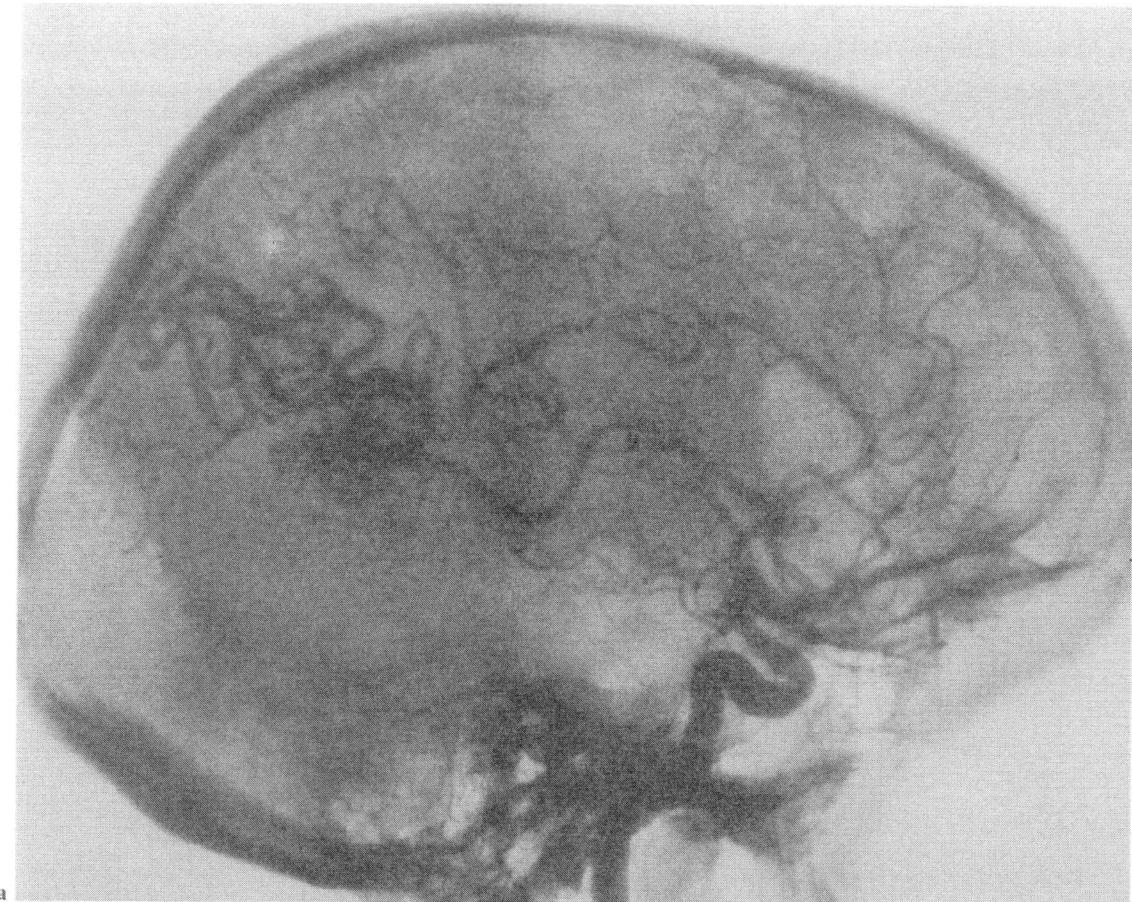

a

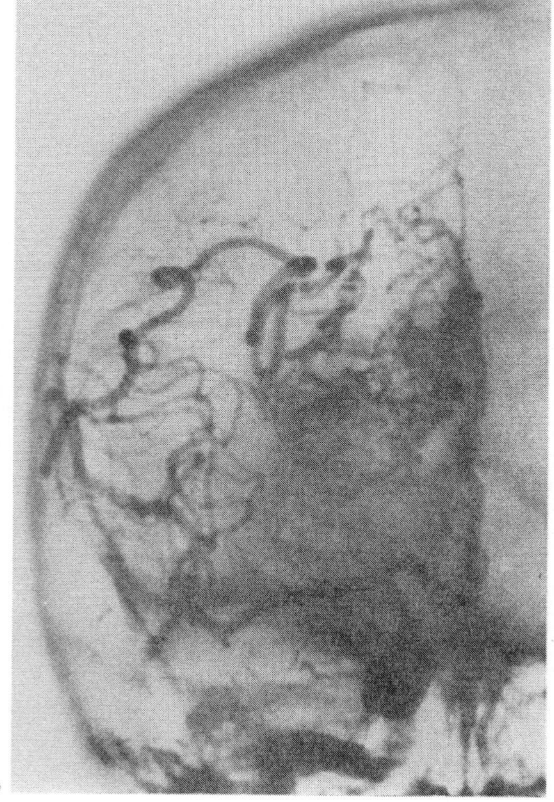

b

Abb. 46a–f. Evolution einer arteriovenösen Mißbildung im Verlauf von 20 Jahren. **a u. b** Karotisangiographie rechts nach Subarachnoidalblutung. Große arteriovenöse Mißbildung im Parietalhirn. A. pericallosa und A. gyri angularis erweitert. Keine Operation. **c u. d** Karotisangiographie rechts, 20 Jahre später, nach erneuter Blutung. Keine arteriovenöse Mißbildung mehr sichtbar **e** Vertebralisangiogramm nach 2. Blutung. Rechte A. cerebri posterior stark erweitert. Während der ganzen Serie wird jedoch weder eine arteriovenöse Mißbildung noch eine vorzeitig gefüllte Vene sichtbar. **f** Computerisierte axiale Tomographie. Parie-

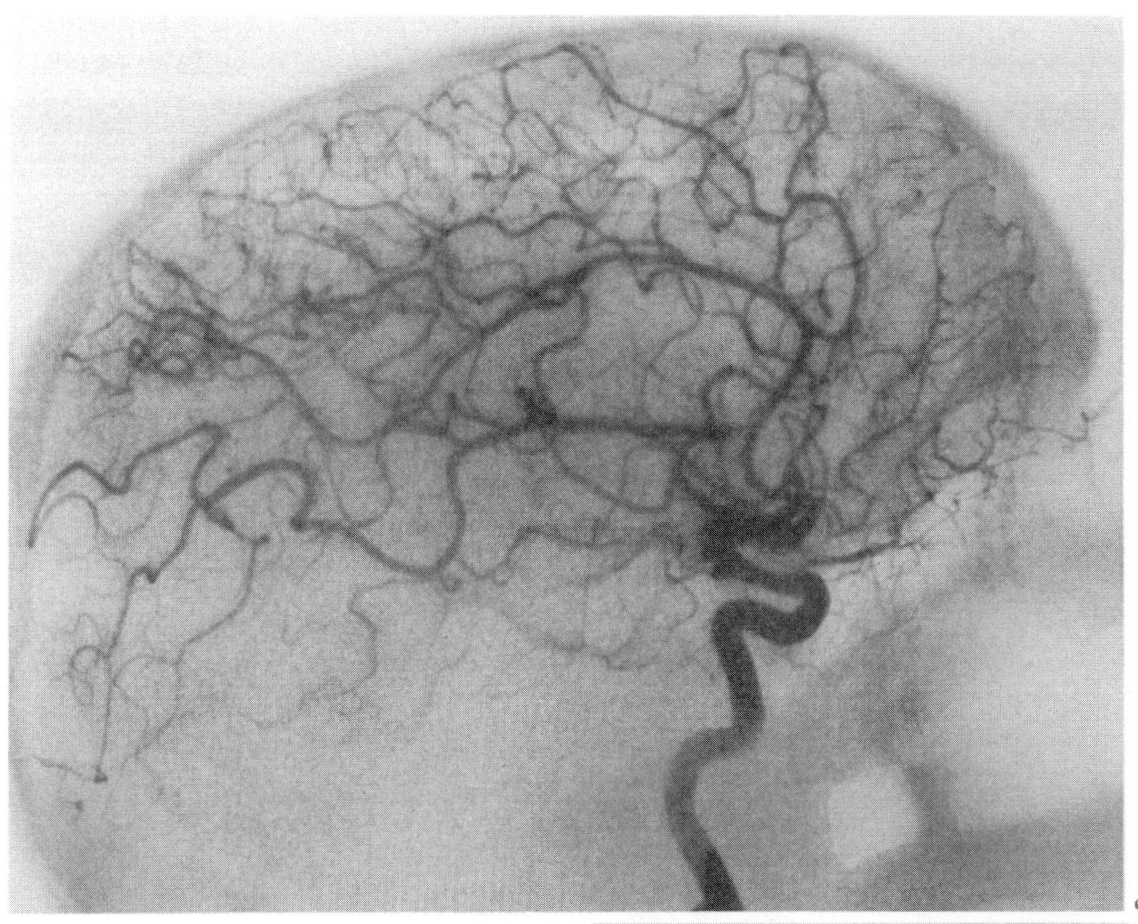

c

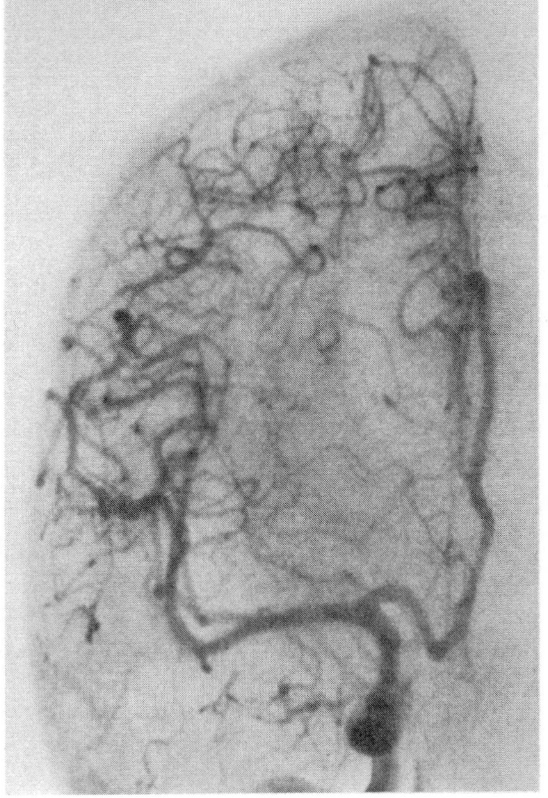

d

tales intrazerebrales Hämatom rechts mit Ventrikeleinbruch. Im Bereich des intrazerebralen Hämatoms zwei große Kalkherde, thrombosierten und verkalkten Angiomanteilen entsprechend. Bei der Operation wurde im Hämatom eine partiell thrombosierte arteriovenöse Mißbildung mit ausgedehnt verkalkten Arterien gefunden. Histologisch partiell thrombosierte und z.T. rekanalisierte arteriovenöse Mißbildung mit herdförmiger Hämosiderose und Verkalkung. Die durchgängigen Anteile der Mißbildung sind offenbar durch die Blutung zerstört worden. (Aus „Zerebrale Angiographie", 3. Aufl. 1979, Thieme Stuttgart)

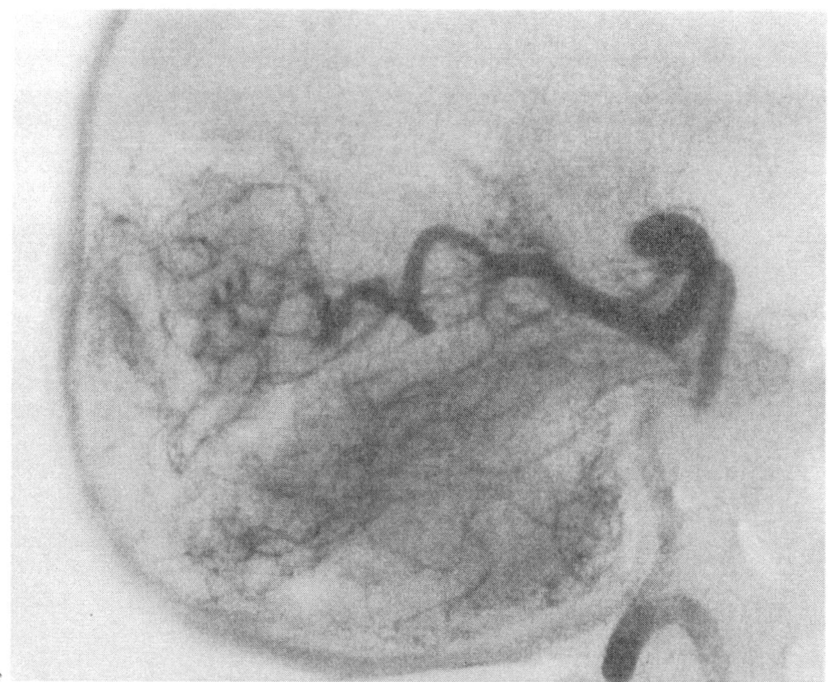

e

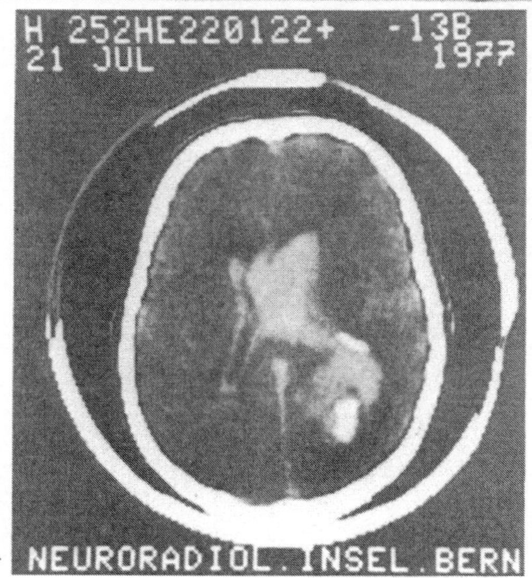

f

Abb. 46e u. f

Auf das gleichzeitige Vorkommen von arteriovenösen Mißbildungen und sackförmigen Aneurysmen ist bereits hingewiesen worden (PATERSON u. MCKISSOCK, 1956; KRAYENBÜHL u. YASARGIL, 1958; BOYD-WILSON, 1959; CRONQVIST u. TROUPP, 1966; PERRET u. NISHIOKA, 1966; WALTIMO, 1973). Die sackförmigen Aneurysmen sitzen dabei nicht selten an Arterien, die zu arteriovenösen Mißbildungen führen, im übrigen aber an klassischer Stelle (Abb. 47). Die vermehrte Strömung in den zur Mißbildung führenden Arterien mag bei der Entstehung eines sackförmigen Aneurysmas eine Rolle spielen. SHENKIN et al. (1971) haben einen Fall mitgeteilt, bei dem das sackförmige Aneurysma nach operativer Entfernung der arteriovenösen Mißbildung spontan kleiner wurde.

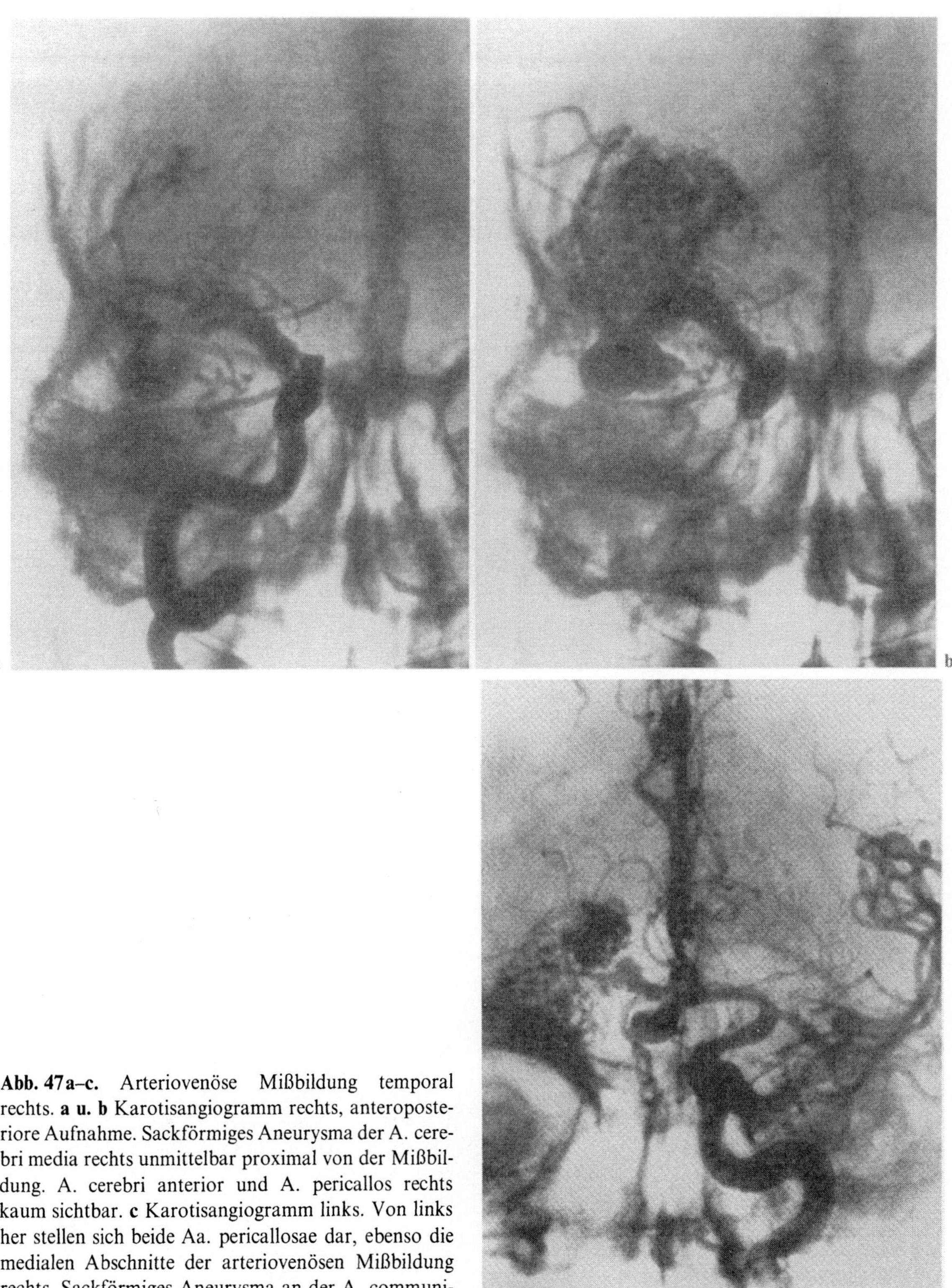

Abb. 47a–c. Arteriovenöse Mißbildung temporal rechts. **a u. b** Karotisangiogramm rechts, anteroposteriore Aufnahme. Sackförmiges Aneurysma der A. cerebri media rechts unmittelbar proximal von der Mißbildung. A. cerebri anterior und A. pericallos rechts kaum sichtbar. **c** Karotisangiogramm links. Von links her stellen sich beide Aa. pericallosae dar, ebenso die medialen Abschnitte der arteriovenösen Mißbildung rechts. Sackförmiges Aneurysma an der A. communicans anterior. (Aus „Zerebrale Angiographie", 3. Aufl. 1979, Thieme Stuttgart)

Literatur

A. Sackförmige Aneurysmen

ACOSTA, C., WILLIAMS, P.E., CLARK, K.: Traumatic aneurysma of the cerebral vessels. J. Neurosurg. **36**, 531–536 (1972)

AGEE, O.F.: The paraorbital oblique projection for the demonstration of posterior communicating area aneurysms. Radiology **90**, 797–799 (1968)

ALLCOCK, J.M.: Arterial spasm in subarachnoid haemorrhage. Acta radiol. (Diagn.) **5**, 73–83 (1966)

ALLCOCK, J.M., DRAKE, C.G.: Postoperative angiography in case of ruptured intracranial aneurysm. J. Neurosurg. **20**, 752–759 (1963)

ALLCOCK, J.M., DRAKE, C.G.: Ruptured intracranial aneurysms – the role of arterial spasm. J. Neurosurg. **22**, 21–29 (1965)

ALLEN, G.S.: Cerebral arterial spasm – part 7. Surg. Neurol. **6**, 63–70 (1976)

ALLEN, G.S.: Cerebral arterial spasm – part 8. Surg. Neurol. **6**, 71–80 (1976)

ALMEIDA, G.M., SHIBATA, M.K., BIANCO, E.: Carotid-ophthalmic aneurysms. Surg. Neurol. **5**, 41–45 (1976)

ALPERS, B.J., BERRY, R.G.: Circle of Willis in cerebral vascular disorders. The anatomical structure. Arch. Neurol. (Chic.) **8**, 398–402 (1963)

ALPERS, B.J., BERRY, R.G., PADDISON, R.M.: Anatomical studies of the circle of Willis in normal brain. Arch. Neurol. Psychiat. **81**, 409–418 (1959)

ANDERSEN, P.E.: Fibromuscular hyperplasia of the carotid arteries. Acta radiol. (Diagn.) **10**, 90–96 (1970)

ANDERSEN, P.E.: Fibromuscular hyperplasia in children. Acta radiol. (Diagn.) **10**, 203–208 (1970)

ANDERSON, R.D., LIEBESKIND, A., SCHECHTER, M.M., ZINGESSER, LH.: Aneurysms of the internal carotid artery in the carotid canal of the petrous temporal bone. Radiology **102**, 639–642 (1972)

ANDERSON, R.D., LIEBESKIND, A., ZINGESSER, L.H., SCHECHTER, M.M.: Aneurysms of the cervical internal carotid artery. Amer. J. Roentgenol. **116**, 31–36 (1972)

ANTUNES, J.L., CORRELL, J.W.: Cerebral emboli from intracranial aneurysms. Surg. Neurol. **6**, 7–10 (1976)

ARAKI, C., HANDA, H., HANDA, J., YOSHIDA, K.: Traumatic aneurysm of the intracranial extradural portion of the internal carotid artery. J. Neurosurg. **23**, 64–67 (1965)

ARUTIUNOV, A.I., BARON, M.A., MAJOROVA, N.A.: The role of mechanical factors in the pathogenesis of short-term and prolonged spasm of the cerebral arteries. J. Neurosurg. **40**, 459–472 (1974)

BARR, H.W.K., BLACKWOOD, W., MEADOWS, S.P.: Intracavernous carotid aneurysms, a clinical pathological report. Brain **94**, 607–622 (1971)

BASSETT, R.C.: Intracranial aneurysms. I. Some clinical observations concerning their development. J. Neurosurg. **6**, 216–221 (1949)

BEAMER, Y.B., CORSINO, J.F., LYNDE, R.G.: Rupture of an aneurysm of the internal carotid artery during arteriography with filling of the subarachnoid space and demonstration of a temporal lobe mass. J. Neurosurg. **31**, 224–226 (1969)

BEATTY, R.A., RICHARDSON, A.E.: Predicting intolerance to common carotid artery ligation by carotid angiography. J. Neurosurg. **28**, 9–13 (1968)

BELL, W.E., BUTLER, C.: Cerebral mycotic aneurysms in children. Two case reports. Neurology **18**, 81–86 (1968)

BERGER, E., KYRIAZIDOU, M.: Per-operative angiography in cerebral aneurysms and angiom surgery. In: Recent advance in diagnostic neuroradiology (K. Kitamura, T.H. Newton, eds). Tokyo: Igaku Shoin Ltd. 1975, pp. 124–136

BERGSTRÖM, K., HEMMINGSSON, A.: False cortical aneurysm in subdural haematoma following head injury without fracture. Acta radiol. (Diagn.) **14**, 657–661 (1973)

BERGVALL, U., GALERA, R.: Time relationship between subarachnoid hemorrhage, arterial spasm, changes in cerebral circulation and posthaemorrhagic hydrocephalus. Acta radiol. (Diagn.) **9**, 229–237 (1969)

BIGELOW, N.H.: Multiple intracranial arterial aneurysms. An analysis of their significance. Arch. Neurol. Psychiat. **79**, 76–99 (1955)

BJÖRKESTEN, G., TROUPP, H.: Changes in the size of intracranial arterial aneurysms. J. Neurosurg. **19**, 583–588 (1962)

BONNAL, J., STEVENAERT, A.: Thrombosis of intracranial aneurysms of the circle of Willis after incomplete obliteration by clip or ligature across the neck. J. Neurosurg. **30**, 158–164 (1969)

BOYD-WILSON, J.S.: The association of cerebral angiomas with intracranial aneurysms. J. Neurol. Neurosurg. Psychiat. **22**, 218–223 (1959a)

BOYD-WILSON, J.S.: Oblique views: their place in the arteriographic diagnosis of intracranial aneurysms. J. Neurosurg. **16**, 297–310 (1959b)

BRAWLEY, B.W., STRANDNESS, D.E., JR., KELLY, W.A.: The biophysic response of cerebral vasospasm in experimental subarachnoid hemorrhage. J. Neurosurg. **28**, 1–8 (1968)

BREMER, J.L.: Congenital aneurysms of cerebral arteries: embryologic study. Arch. Path. **35**, 819–831 (1943)

BRENNER, H.: Frontale Schädelspaltung mit traumatischem Aneurysma der Arteria pericallosa. Acta Neurochir. **10**, 146–152 (1962)

BULL, J.W.D.: Contribution of radiology to the study

of intracranial aneurysms. Brit. med. J. **2**, 1701–1708 (1962)

BULL, J.W.D.: Massive aneurysms at the base of the brain. Brain **92**, 535–570 (1969)

BURTON, CH., VELASCO, F., DORMAN, J.: Traumatic aneurysms of a peripheral cerebral artery. Review and case report. J. Neurosurg. **28**, 468–474 (1968)

BURTON, R.: Massive epistaxis from a ruptured traumatic internal carotid artery aneurysm. Med. J. Aust. **1**, 692–694 (1973)

CAMPICHE, R., ZANDER, E.: Anévrysme de la carotide interne dans son trajet extracranien formant une tumeur pharyngienne. Neuro-chirurgie **8**, 79–83 (1962)

CANTU, R.C., LE MAY, M., WILKINSON, H.A.: The importance of repeated angiography in the treatment of mycotic-embolic intracranial aneurysms. J. Neurosurg. **25**, 189–193 (1966)

CARLSON, D.H., THOMSON, D.: Spontaneous thrombosis of a giant cerebral aneurysm in five days. Report of a case. Neurology **26**, 334–336 (1976)

COLE, F.M., YATES, P.O.: Intracerebral microaneurysms and small cerebrovascular lesions. Brain **90**, 758–768 (1967)

CONWAY, L.W., MCDONALD, L.W.: Structural changes of the intradural arteries following subarachnoid hemorrhage. J. Neurosurg. **37**, 715–723 (1972)

CRAWFORD, T: Some observations on the pathogenesis and natural history of intracranial aneurysms. J. Neurol. Neurosurg. Psychiat. **22**, 259–266 (1959)

CRESSMAN, M.R., HAYES, G.J.: Traumatic aneurysm of the anterior choroidal artery. Case report. J. Neurosurg. **24**, 102–104 (1966)

CROMPTON, M.R.: The pathology of ruptured middle cerebral aneurysms with special reference to the differences between sexes. Lancet **II/1962**, 421–425

CROMPTON, M.R.: Hypothalamic lesions following rupture of cerebral berry aneurysms. Brain **86**, 301–314 (1963)

CROMPTON, M.R.: The pathogenesis of cerebral infarction following the rupture of cerebral berry aneurysms. Brain **87**, 491–510 (1964)

CROMPTON, M.R.: The comparative pathology of cerebral aneurysms. Brain **89**, 789–796 (1966a)

CROMPTON, M.R.: Mechanism of growth and rupture in cerebral berry aneurysms. Brit. med. J. **1**, 1138–1142 (1966b)

CUMMINS, B.H., GRIFFITH, H.B., THOMSON, J.L.G.: Per-operative cerebral angiography. Brit. J. Radiol. **47**, 257–260 (1974)

DAVID, M., SACHS, M.: Les anévrysmes de la bifurcation cartidienne. Neurochirurgia **10**, 96–105 (1967)

DAVIDSON, P., ROBERTSON, D.M.: A true mycotic (Aspergillus) aneurysm leading to fatal subarachnoid hemorrhage in a patient with hereditary hemorrhagic teleangiectasia. J. Neurosurg. **35**, 71–76 (1971)

DAWSON, B.H.: The blood vessels of the human optic chiasma and their relation to those of the hypophysis and hypothalamus. Brain **81**, 207–217 (1958)

DECHAUME, J.P., AIMARD, G., MICHEL, D., BRET, P., DESE ROGES, M., LAPRAS, C., LECUIRE, J.: Les anévrysmes de l'artère péri-calleuse. Neuro-chir. (Paris) **19**, 135–150 (1973)

DEVADIGA, K.V., MATHLA, K.V., CHARDY, J.: Spontaneous cure of intracavervous aneurysm of internal carotid artery in a 14-month old child. J. Neurosurg. **30**, 165–168 (1969)

DILENGE, D., WÜTHRICH, R.: Traumatic aneurysm of the middle meningeal artery. Neurochirurgia **4**, 202–206 (1962)

DRAKE, C.G.: Further experience with surgical treatment of aneurysms of the basilar artery. J. Neurosurg. **29**, 372–392 (1968)

DRAKE, C.G., ALLCOCK, J.M.: Postoperative angiography and the "slipped" clip. J. Neurosurg. **39**, 683–689 (1973)

DRAKE, C.G., AMACHER, A.L.: Aneurysms of the posterior cerebral artery. J. Neurosurg. **30**, 468–474 (1969)

DRAKE, C.G., VANDERLINDEN, R.G.: The late consequences of incomplete surgical treatment of cerebral aneurysms. J. Neurosurg. **27**, 226–238 (1967)

DRAKE, C.G., VANDERLINDEN, R.G., AMACHER, A.L.: Carotid ophthalmic aneurysms. J. Neurosurg. **29**, 24–31 (1968) a)

DRAKE, C.G., VANDERLINDEN, R.G., AMACHER, A.L.: Carotid. choroidal aneurysms. J. Neurosurg. **29**, 32–36 (1968b)

DU BOULAY, G.: Distribution of spasm in the intracranial arteries after subarachnoid haemorrhage. Acta radiol. (Diagn.) **1**, 257–266 (1963)

DU BOULAY, G.H.: Some observations on the natural history of intracranial aneurysms. Brit. J. Radiol. **38**, 721–757 (1965)

DU BOULAY, G.H., JACKSON, D.C.: Cranial angiotomography. Clin. Radiol. **16**, 148–153 (1965)

DUNKER, R.O., HARRIS, A.B.: Surgical anatomy of the proximal anterior cerebral artery. J. Neurosurg. **44**, 359–367 (1976)

ECHLIN, F.A.: Spasm of basilar and vertebral arteries caused by experimental subarachnoid hemorrhage. J. Neurosurg. **23**, 1–11 (1965)

ECKER, A.: Spasm of internal carotid artery. J. Neurosurg. **2**, 479–484 (1945)

ECKER, A., RIEMENSCHNEIDER, P.A.: Arteriographic demonstration of spasm of intracranial arteries: with special reference to saccular arterial aneurysms. J. Neurosurg. **8**, 660–667 (1951)

EPSTEIN, F., RANSOHOFF, J., BUDZILOVICH, G.N.: The clinical significance of junctional dilatation of the posterior communicating artery. J. Neurosurg. **33**, 529–531 (1970)

FEIN, J.M., FIOR, W.J., COHAN, S.L., PARKHURST, J.: Sequential changes of vascular ultrastructure in experimental cerebral vasospasm. Myonecrosis J. Neurosurg. **41**, 49–58 (1974)

FEIN, J.M., ROVIT, R.L.: Interhemispheric subdural hematoma secondary to hemorrhage from a calloso-marginal artery aneurysm. Neuroradiology **1**, 183–186 (1970)

FERGUSON, G.G.: Turbulence in human intracranial saccular aneurysms. J. Neurosurg. **33**, 485–497 (1970)

FERGUSON, G.G.: Direct measurement of mean and pulsatile blood pressure at operation in human intracranial saccular aneurysms. J. Neurosurg. **36**, 560–563 (1972)

FERRARI, G., VIO, M.: Radiological demonstration of rupture of a carotid aneurysm during cerebral angiography. Case report. J. Neurosurg. **31**, 462–464 (1969)

FERRIS, E.J., RUDIKOFF, J.C., SHAPIRO, J.H.: Cerebral angiography of bacterial infection. Radiology **90**, 727–734 (168)

FLEISCHER, A.S., PATTON, J.M., TINDALL, G.T.: Cerebral aneurysms of traumatic origin. Surg. Neurol. **4**, 233–239 (1975)

FLETCHER, T.M., TAVERAS, J.M., POOL, J.C.: Cerebral vasospasm in angiography for intracranial aneurysms: incidence and significance in one hundred consecutive angiograms. Amer. med. Ass. Arch. Neurol. **1**, 38–47 (1959)

FORBUS, W.D.: On the origin of miliary aneurysms of the superficial cerebral arteries. Bull. Johns. Hopk. Hosp. **47**, 239–284 (1930)

FROMM, J., HABEL, J.: Angiographischer Nachweis eines sackförmigen Aneurysmas als Ursache einer spontanen carotidocavernösen Fistel und Spontanheilung dieser Fistel nach Angiographie. Nervenarzt **36**, 170–172 (1965)

GALLAGHER, P.Q., DORSEY, J.F., STEFANINI, M.: Large intracranial aneurysms producing panhypopituitarism and frontal lobe syndrome. Neurology **6**, 829–837 (1956)

GARCIA-BENGOCHEA, F., DELAND, F.H.: Bilateral giant carotid-ophthalmic aneurysms. Case report. J. Neurosurg. **42**, 589–595 (1975)

GERLOCK, A.J., Rupture of posterior inferior cerebellar artery aneurysms into the subarachnoid space during angiography. Case report. J. Neurosurg. **42**, 469–472 (1975)

GERMAN, W.J., BLACK, S.P.W.: Intra-aneurysmal hemodynamics – jet action. Circulat. Res. **3**, 463–468 (1955)

GERSTENBRAND, F., WEINGARTEN, K.: Aneurysmen und hypophysäres Syndrom. Wien. Z. Nervenheilk. **20**, 300–310 (1963)

GEYER, K.H.: Strömungsverhältnisse im großen Karotisaneurysma. Fortschr. Röntgenstr. **103**, 440–443 (1965)

GLYNN, L.F.: Medial defects in the circle of Willis and their relation to aneurysm formation. J. Path. Bact. **51**, 213–222 (1940)

GO, K.G., PENNING, L., OEN, T.S.: Acute subdural haematoma in connection with angiographically demonstrated traumatic rupture of a cortical cerebral artery (presenting as false aneurysm). A report of 2 cases. Neuroradiology **2**, 107–110 (1971)

GOLDSTEIN, S.L.: Ventricular opacification secondary to rupture of intracranial aneurysm during angiography. J. Neurosurg. **27**, 265–267 (1967)

GROS, C., VLAHOVICH, B., LABAUGE, R., THEVENET, A., KUHNER, A., FRÈREBEAU, PH.: Les anévrysmes extra-craniens de la carotide interne. Neuro-chirurgie **16**, 367–382 (1970)

GUIDETTI, B., LA TORRE, E.: Carotid ophthalmic aneurysms. Acta Neurochir. **22**, 289–304 (1970)

GUIDETTI, B., LA TORRE, E.: Management of carotid-ophthalmic aneurysms. J. Neurosurg. **42**, 438–442 (1975)

GURDJIAN, E.S., LINDNER, D.W., THOMAS, L.M.: Experiences with ligation of the common carotid artery for treatment of aneurysms of the internal carotid artery. With particular reference to complications. J. Neurosurg. **23**, 311–318 (1965)

GURDJIAN, E.S., THOMAS, L.M., SCARTCH, G.P., DARMODY, W.R.: Cerebral vasospasm. In: Intracranial aneurysms and subarachnoid hemorrhage (Fields, W.S., Sahs, A.L., eds). Springfield III: Charles C. Thomas 1965

HAMBY, W.B.: Multiple intracranial aneurysms. J. Neurosurg. **16**, 558–563 (1959)

HANDA, J., HANDA, H.: Severe epistaxis caused by traumatic aneurysm of cavernous carotid artery. Surg. Neurol. **5**, 241–243 (1976)

HANDA, J., KAMIJYO, Y., HANDA, H.: Intracranial aneurysm associated with fibromuscular hyperplasia of renal and internal carotid arteries. Brit. J. Radiol. **43**, 483–485 (1970)

HANDA, J., KIKUCHI, H., IWAYAMA, K., TERAURA, T., HANDA, H.: Traumatic aneurysms of the internal carotid artery. Acta Neurochir. **17**, 161–177 (1967)

HARRINGTON, O.B., CROSBY, V.G., NICHOLAS, L.: Fibromuscular hyperplasia of the internal carotid artery. Ann. thorac. Surg. **9**, 516–524 (1970)

HARRISON, TH.H., ODOM, G.L., KUNKLE, E.CH.: Internal carotid aneurysm arising in carotid canal. Arch. Neurol. Psychiat. **8**, 328–331 (1963)

HASSLER, O.: Morphologic studies on the large cerebral arteries. Acta psychiat. neurol. scand. (Suppl. 154) **36**, 83–86 (1961)

HASSLER, O.: Medial defects in the menigeal arteries. J. Neurosurg. **19**, 337–340 (1962)

HASSLER, O.: On the etiology of intracranial aneurysms. In: Intracranial aneurysms and subarachnoid hemorrhage (Fields, W.S., Sahs, A.L., eds). Springfield III: Charles Thomas, Publisher 1965

HASSLER, O., SALTZMAN, G.F.: Histologic changes in infundibular widening of the posterior cummunicating artery. Acta path. microbiol. scand. **46**, 305–312 (1959)

HASSLER, O., SALTZMAN, G.F.: Angiographic and histologic changes in infundibular widening of the posterior communicating artery. Acta radiol. (Diagn.) **1**, 321–327 (1963)

HEIDELBERGER, K.P., LAYTION, W.M., FISHER, R.G.:

Multiple cerebral mycotic aneurysms complicating posttraumatic pseudomonas meningitis. J. Neurosurg. **29**, 631–635 (1968)

Heiskanen, O.: The identification of ruptured aneurysm in patient with multiple intra-cranial aneurysms. Neurochirurgia **8**, 102–107 (1965)

Heiskanen, O., Marttila, I.: Risk of rupture of a second aneurysm in patients with multiple aneurysms. J. Neurosurg. **32**, 295–299 (1970)

Heiskanen, O., Nikki, P.: Large intracranial aneurysms. Acta neurol. scand. **38**, 195–208 (1962)

Henry, P., Guerin, J., Vallat, J.M.: Extravasation per-angiographique du produit de contraste au cours de ruptures d'anévrysmes (à propos de 2 cas). Neurochirurgia **44**, 121–126 (1971)

Higazi, I., El-Banhawy, A., El-Nady, F.: Importance of angiography in identifying false aneurysm of the middle meningeal artery as a cause of extradural hematoma. J. Neurosurg. **30**, 172–169 (1969)

Hinshaw, D.B., Simmons, Ch.R., Leech, W., Minkler, J., Austin, G.: Angiography and possible etiology. Radiology **113**, 101–106 (1974)

Hirsch, J.F., David, M., Sachs, M.: Les anévrysmes artériels traumatiques intracraniens. Neurochirurgie **8**, 189–201 (1962)

Hoff, J.T., Potts, D.G.: Angiographic demonstration of hemorrhage into the fourth ventricle. Case report. J. Neurosurg. **30**, 732–735 (1969)

Hollin, S.A., Decker, R.E.: Effentiveness of microsurgery for intracranial aneurysms. Postoperative angiographic study of 50 cases. J. Neurosurg. **39**, 690–693 (1973)

Horten, B.C., Abbott, G.F., Porro, R.S.: Fungal aneurysms of intracranial vessels. Arch. Neurol. **33**, 577–579 (1976)

Houser, O.W., Baker, H.L., Sandok, B.A., Holley, K.E.: Cephalic arterial fibromuscular dysplasia. Radiology **101**, 605–611 (1971)

Huber, P.: Kombinationen von sackförmigen Aneurysmen der A. pericallosa mit Anomalien des Circulus Willisi im Carotisangiogramm. Fortschr. Röntgenstr. **93**, 178–184 (1960)

Huber, P.: Angiographische Schichtungseffekte in den sackförmigen Aneurysmen der Hirngefäße. Fortschr. Röntgenstr. **94**, 355–362 (1961)

Huber, P.: Angiographische Darstellung der Zirkulationsverhältnisse in großen sackförmigen Aneurysmen. Fortschr. Röntgenstr. **105**, 773–776 (1966)

Huber, P., Rivoir, R.: Die Zirkulation in und distal von sehr großen Aneurysmen des Circulus Willisi. Fortschr. Röntgenstr. **114**, 457–463 (1971)

Huber, P., Rivoir, R.: Aneurysms on a peristent left hypoglossal artery. Neuroradiology **6**, 277–278 (1974)

Huber, P., Robert, F.: Veränderungen von sackförmigen Aneurysmen zerebraler Arterien. Angiographische Kontrolluntersuchung bei konservativ behandelten sackförmigen Aneurysmen. Fortschr. Röntgenstr. **111**, 184–195 (1969)

Hudson, C.H., Raaf, J.: Timing of aniography and operation in patients with ruptured intracranial aneurysms. J. Neurosurg. **29**, 37–41 (1968)

Isfort, A.: Zerebrale Arterienverschlüsse durch Gefäßkompression. Fortschr. Röntgenstr. **95**, 128–135 (1961)

Ishikawa, M., Waga, S., Moritake, K., Handa, H.: Cerebral bacterial aneurysms: report of three cases. Surg. Neurol. **2**, 257–261 (1974)

Jackson, J.R., Tindall, G.T., Nashold, B.S., jr.: Rupture of an intracranial aneurysm during carotid arteriography, a case report. J. Neurosurg. **17**, 333–336 (1960)

Jamieson, K.G.: Rupture of an intracranial aneurysm during cerebral angiography. J. Neurosurg. **11**, 624–628 (1954)

Jawad, K., Miller, J.D., Wyper, D.J., Rowan, J.O.: Measurement of CBF and carotid artery pressure compared with cerebral angiography in assessing collateral blood flow supply after carotid ligation. J. Neurosurg. **46**, 185–196 (1977)

Jeanmart, L., Noterman, J., Brihaye, J., Balériaux, D.: Les anévrismes de la carotide intra-caverneuse. Neuro-chirurgie **19**, 61–73 (1973)

Jefferson, G.: Compression of the chiasma, optic nerve an optic tract by intracranial aneurysms. Brain **60**, 444–497 (1937)

Jefferson, G.: Further concerning compression of the optic pathways by intracranial aneurysms. Clin. Neurosurg. **1**, 55–103 (1955)

Jenkinson, E.L., Sugar, O., Love, H.: Rupture of an aneurysm of the internal carotid artery during cerebral angiography. Case report. Amer. J. Roentgenol. **71**, 958–960 (1954)

Kamisasa, A.: Arteriography of the anterior communicating aneurysm. Neuroradiology **12**, 227–232 (1977)

Kapp, J., Mahaley, M.S., jr., Odom, G.L.: Cerebral arterial spasm. Part 3: Purification and characterization of a spasmogenic substance in feline platelets. J. Neurosurg. **29**, 350–356 (1968)

Kaufmann, H.H.: Fibromuscular hyperplasia of the carotid artery in a case associated with an arteriovenous malformation. Arch. Neurol. **22**, 299–304 (1970)

Kirgis, H.D., Fisher, W.L., Llewellyn, R.C., Peebles, E.McC.: Aneurysms of the anterior communicating artery and gross anomalies of the circle of Willis. J. Neurosurg. **25**, 73–78 (1966)

Kothandaram, P., Dawson, B.H., Kruyt, R.C.: Carotid ophthalmic aneurysms. J. Neurosurg. **34**, 544–549 (1971)

Kramer, E.: Hyperplasie fibromusculaire et anévrysme extracranien de la carotide interne avec syndrome parapharyngien typique. Rev. Neurol. **120**, 239–244 (1969)

Krayenbühl, H.: Klassifikation und klinische Symptomatologie der zerebralen Aneurysmen. Ophthalmologica **167**, 122–164 (1973)

Krayenbühl, H., Hanhart, B., Laine, E., Lazorthes, G., Logue, V., Uehlinger, E., Weber, R.,

Yasargil, M.G.: L'anévrysme de l'artère comunicante antérieure. Paris: Masson & Cie. 1959

Krayenbühl, H., Yasargil, M.G.: Das Hirnaneurysma. Series chirurg. Geigy, Basel (1958)

Krayenbühl, H., Yasargil, M.G., Flamm, E.S., Tew, J.M.: Microsurgical treatment of intracranial saccular aneurysms. J. Neurosurg. **37**, 678–686 (1972)

Krauland, W.: Verletzungen der A. carotis interna im Sinus cavernosus und Verletzungen der großen Hirnschlagader mit Berücksichtigung der Aneurysmabildung. In: Hdb. d. spez. pathol. Anat. und Histol (Lubarsch-Henke-Roessle, Hrsg), Bd. XIII/3. Berlin: Springer 1955

Kricheff, I.I., Chase, N.E., Ransohoff, J.R.: The angiographic investigation of ruptured intracranial aneurysms. Radiology **83**, 1016–1025 (1964)

Kuhn, R.A., Kugler, H.: False aneurysms of the middle meningeal artery. J. Neurosurg. **21**, 92–96 (1964)

Laine, E., Andreussi, L., Delandsherr, J.M., Galibert, P., Christiaens, J.L., Jomin, M., Clarisse, J., Declour, J.: Anévrymes de l'artère cérébrale moyenne. Étude anatomique, clinique et thérapeutique. À propos d'une série de 116 cas dont 100 ont été opérés. Neuro-chirurgie **16**, 181–201 (1970)

Laitinen, L., Snellman, A.: Aneurysms of pericallosal artery: study of 14 cases verfied angiographically and treated mainly by direct surgial attack. J. Neurosurg. **17**, 447–458 (1960)

Leeds, N.E., Goldberg, H.I.: Angiographic manifestations in cerebral inflammatory disease. Radiology **98**, 595–604 (1971)

Lehrer, H.Z., Gross, L.A., Poon, T.P.: Ruptured intracranial aneursym. Contrast agent extravasation during brachial arteriography. Arch. Neurol. **27**, 351–354 (1972)

Liliequist, B., Lindqvist, M., Probst, T.: Rupture of intracranial aneurysm during carotid angiography. Neuroradiology **11**, 185–190 (1976)

Lin, J.P., Kricheff, I.I.: Angiographic investigation of cerebral aneurysms. Technical aspects. Radiology **1**/5, 69–76 (1972)

Lipovsek, M.: Ruptured aneurysms of the proximal middle cerebral artery. J. Neurosurg. **39**, 498–502 (1973)

Locksley, H.B.: Report on the cooperative study of intracranial aneurysms and subarachnoid hemorrhage. Natural history of subarachnoid hemorrhage, intracranial aneurysms and arteriovenous malformations based on 6368 cases in the cooperative study. J. Neurosurg. **25**, 219–239, Section V, Part I (1966)

Locksley, H.B.: Report on the cooperative study of intracranial aneurysms and subarachnoid hemorrhage. Section V, Part II. Natural history of subarachnoid hemorrhage, intracranial aneurysms and arteriovenous malformation. J. Neurosurg. **25**, 321–369 (1966)

Locksley, H.B., Sahs, A.L., Knowler, L.: Report on the cooperative study of intracranial aneurysms and subarachnoid hemorrhage. Section 2. General survey of cases in the central registry and characteristics of the sample population. J. Neurosurg. **24**, 922–932 (1966)

Locksley, H.B., Sahs, A.L., Sandler, R.: Report on the cooperative study of intracranial aneurysms and arteriovenous malformations. Section III. Subarachnoid hemorrhage unrelated to intracranial aneurysms and A-V malformation. J. Neurosurg. **24**, 1034–1056 (1966)

Lodin, H.: Spontaneous thrombosis of cerebral aneurysms. Brit. J. Radiol. **39**, 701–703 (1966)

Lombardi, G., Passerini, A., Migliavacca, F.: Intracavernous aneurysms of the internal carotid artery. Amer. J. Roentgenol. **89**, 361–371 (1963)

Loop, J.W., Foltz, E.L.: Applications of angiography during intracranial operation. Acta radiol. (Diagn.) **5**, 363–367 (1966)

Ludwiczak, R.W., Fogel, L.M.: Posttraumatic aneurysm of the cervical segment of the internal carotid artery. Neuroradiology **10**, 179 (1975)

Lukin, R., Chambers, A.: Traumatic aneurysm of peripheral cerebral artery. Neuroradiology **8**, 1–3 (1974)

Lukin, R.R., Chambers, A.A., McLaurin, R., Tew, J., jr.: Thrombosed giant middle cerebral aneurysms. Neuroradiology **10**, 125–129 (1975)

Manelfe, C., Clarisse, J., Fredy, D., Andre, J.M., Crouzet, G.: Dysplasie fibromusculaire des artères cervicocéphaliques; a propos de 70 cas. J. Neuroradiologie **1**, 149–321 (1974)

Margolis, M.T., Stein, R.L., Newton, T.H.: Extracranial aneurysms of the internal carotid artery. Neuroradiology **4**, 78–89 (1972)

Marguth, F., Schiefer, W.: Spontanheilung eines intrakraniellen Aneurysmas. Acta neurochir. **5**, 38–45 (1957)

Markwalder, H., Huber, P.: Aneurysmen der Meningealarterien. Schweiz. med. Wschr. **91**, 1344–1347 (1961)

Marshall, W.H.: Delayed arterial spasm following subarachnoid hemorrhage. Radiology **106**, 325–327 (1973)

McKissock, W., Paine, K.W., Walsh, L.S.: An analysis of the results of treatment of ruptured intracranial aneurysms. Report of 772 consecutive cases. J. Neurosurg. **17**, 762–776 (1960)

McKissock, W., Richardson, A., Walsh, L.: Middle-cerebral aneurysms. Further results in the controlled trial of conservative and surgical treatment of ruptured intracranial aneurysms. Lancet **II/1962**, 417–421

McKissock, W., Richardson, A., Walsh, L., Owen, E.: Multiple intracranial aneurysms. Lancet **I/1964**, 623–626

McNeel, D., Evans, R.A., Ory, E.M.: Angiography of cerebral mycotic aneurysms. Acta radiol. **9**, 407–412 (1969)

MENEZES, A.H., GRAF, C.J.: True traumatic aneurysm of anterior cerebral artery. Case report. J. Neurosurg. **40**, 544–548 (1974)

MIZUKAMI, M., KIN, H., ARAKI, G., MIHARA, H., YOSHIDA, Y.: Is angiographic spasm real spasm? Acta Neurochirg. **34**, 247–259 (1976)

MOLINARI, G.F., SMITH, L., GOLDSTEIN, M.N., SATRAN, R.: Pathogenesis of cerebral mycotic aneurysms. Neurology **23**, 325–332 (1973)

MORLEY, T.P., BARR, H.W.K.: Giant intracranial aneurysms: diagnosis, course and management. Clin. Neurosurg. **16**, 73–94 (1968)

MOSKOWITZ, M.A., ROSENBAUM, A.E.: Angiographically monitored resolution of cerebral mycotic aneurysms. Neurology **24**, 1103–1108 (1974)

MURPHY, D.J., GOLDBERG, R.J.: Extravasation from an intracranial aneurysm during carotid angiography. Case report. J. Neurosurg. **27**, 459–461 (1967)

NADJMI, M., MOISSL, G., RATZKA, M., PÖSCHMANN, A.: Zerebrale Gefäße im Angiotomogramm. Technik-Anatomie-Pathologie. Stuttgart: Georg Thieme 1977

NISHIOKA, H.N.: Report on the cooperative study of intracranial aneurysms and subarachnoid hemorrhage. Section VIII, Part 1. Results of the treatment of intracranial aneurysms by occlusion of the carotid artery in the neck. J. Neurosurg. **25**, 660–682 (1966)

OBRADOR, S., GOMEZ-BUENO, J., SILVELA, J.: Spontaneous carotid-cavernous fistula produced by ruptured aneurysm of the meningophypophyseal branch of the internal carotid artery. Case report. J. Neurosurg. **40**, 539–543 (1974)

ODOM, G.L.: Cerebral vasospasm. Clinical Neurosurgery, Vol. 22, 29–58 Baltimore: Williams & Wilkins Comp. 1975

OKAWARA, S., HAHN, J., KIMURA, J.: Cerebral circulation time and ruptured intracranial aneurysms. In: Recent advances in diagnostic neuroradiology (K. Kitamura, T.H. Newton eds). Tokyo: Igaku Shoin Ltd. 1975, pp. 137–141

OSGOOD, C., MARTIN, L.G.: Intraventricular constrast extravasation during carotid angiography. Surg. Neurol. **2**, 49–50 (1974)

PAILLAS, J.E., BONNAL, J., LAVIEILLE, J.: Angiographic images of false aneurysmal sac caused by rupture of middle meningeal artery in the course of traumatic extradural hematomata. Report of three cases. J. Neurosurg. **21**, 667–671 (1964)

PALUBINSKAS, A.J., PERLOFF, D., NEWTON, T.H.: Fibromuscular hyperplasia: an arterial dysplasia of increasing clinical importance. Amer. J. Roentgenol. **98**, 907–913 (1966)

PAPO, I., SALVOLINI, U., CARUSELLI, G.: Aneurysms of the anterior choroidal artery with intraventricular hematoma and hydrocephalus, case report. J. Neurosurg. **39**, 225–260 (1973)

PATEL, A.M., RICHARDSON, A.E.: Ruptured intracranial aneurysms in first two decades of life; study of 58 patients. J. Neurosurg. **35**, 571–576 (1971)

PERLMUTTER, D., RHOTON, A.L.: Microsurgical anatomy of the anterior cerebral-anterior communicating – recurrent artery complex. J. Neurosurg. **25**, 259–272 (1976)

PERRET, G., NISHIOKA, H.: Report on the cooperative study of intracranial aneurysms and subarachnoid hemorrhage. Section IV, Cerebral angiography, an analysis of the diagnostic value and complications of carotid and vertebral angiography in 5′484 patients. J. Neurosurg. **25**, 98–114 (1966)

PERRET, L.V., BULL, J.W.D.: The accuracy of radiology in demonstrating ruptured intracranial aneurysms. Brit. J. Radiol. **32**, 85–92 (1959)

PERRIA, L., VIALE, G.L., RIVANO, C.: Anévrysmes de la jonction carotide interne – choroidienne antérieure. Acta Neurochir. **21**, 153–166 (1969)

PETTY, J.M.: Epistaxis from aneurysm of the internal carotid artery due to a gunshot wound. Case report. J. Neurosurg. **30**, 741–743 (1969)

PIA, H.W., FONTANA, H.: Aneurysms of the posterior cerebral artery. Acta Neurochir. **38**, 13–35 (1977)

PIEPGRAS, U., PAMPUS, F., HANCK, F.: Der Wert der simultanen Angio-Tomographie für die Diagnostik von Hirngefäßaneurysmen. Fortschr. Röntgenstr. **108**, 170–176 (1968)

PIRKER, E.: Aneurysmaruptur während einer Karotisangiographie. Fortschr. Röntgenstr. **100**, 415–416 (1964)

PIRKER, E., DIEMATH, H.E.: Hämodynamik der sackförmigen arteriellen Aneurysmen. Acta radiol. **9**, 425–429 (1969)

POOL, J.L.: Cerebral Vasospasm. New Engl. J. Med. **259**, 1259–1264 (1958)

POOL, J.L., JACOBSON, S., FLETCHER, T.A.: Cerebral vasospasm–clinical and experimental evidence. J. Amer. med. Ass. **167**, 1599–1601 (1958)

POOL, J.L., POTTS, D.G.: Aneurysms and arteriovenous anomalies of the brain: Diagnosis and treatment. New York: Harper & Row Publishers 1965, p. 463

PORTER, R.J., EYSTER, E.F.: Aneurysm in the anterior inferior cerebellar artery at the internal acustic meatus: report of a case. Surg. Neurol. **1**, 27–28 (1973)

POUYANNE, H., BANAYAN, A., GUERIN, J., RIEMENS, V.: Les anévrysmes sacculaires multiples du système carotidien supra clinoïdien. Étude anatomoclinique et thérapeutique. Neuro-chir. (Paris) **19**, suppl. 1 (1973)

POUYANNE, H., LEMAN, P., GOT, M., GOUAZE, A.: Traumatic arterial aneurysm of the left middle meningeal artery. Rupture one month after the accident. Tempral intracerebral hematoma. Intervention/Neurochirurgie **5**, 311–315 (1959)

PRIBRAM, H.F.W., HUDSON, J.D., JOYNT, R.J.: Posterior fossa aneurysms presenting as mass lesions. Amer. J. Roentgenol. **105**, 334–340 (1969)

RAIMONDI, A.J., TORRES, H.: Acute hydrocephalus as a complication of subarachnoid hemorrhage. Surg. Neurol. **1**, 23–26 (1973)

RAIMONDI, A.J., YASHON, D., REYES, C., YARZAGARAY, L.: Intracranial false aneurysms. Neurochirurgia **11**, 219–233 (1968)

RAMELLA, G., ROSA, M., ROSSI, G.F.: Angio-tomography for the study of endocranial aneurysms. Acta Neurochir. **21**, 185–193 (1969)

RAUSCH, F., SCHIEFER, W.: Indirekte Röntgen-Kinematographie der Hirngefäße. Fortschr. Röntgenstr. **84**, 88–99 (1956)

RAVON, R., BOUQUIER, J.J., DUPUY, J.P., BOKOR, J., FEISS, P., VIDAL, J., DANY, A.: Un case d'anévrysme géant intra-pétreux et intracaverneux de la carotide interne chez l'enfant. Neuro-chirurgie **22**, 621–226 (1976)

RHONHEIMER, CH.: Zur Symptomatologie der sellären Aneurysmen. Klin. Mbl. Augenheilk. **134**, 1–34 (1959)

RICHARDSON, A.E., JANE, J.A., PAYNE, P.M.: The prediction of morbidity and mortality in anterior communicating aneurysms treated by proximal anterior cerebral ligation. J. Neurosurg. **25**, 280–283 (1966)

RIGGS, H.E., RUPP, C.: Miliary aneurysms: relation of anomalies of the circle of Willis to formation of aneurysms. Arch. Neurol. Psychiat. **49**, 615 (1943)

RISCHBIETH, R.H.C., BULL, J.W.D.: The significance of enlargement of the superior orbital (sphenoidal) fissure. Brit. J. Radiol. **31**, 125–135 (1958)

ROBINSON, J.L., HALL, CH.S., SEDZIMIR, C.B.: Arteriovenous malformations, aneurysms and pregnancy. J. Neurosurg. **41**, 63–69 (1974)

ROCCA, P., ROSADINI, G.: Cerebral angiostratigraphy, first practical results. Radiology **77**, 223–227 (1963)

ROCCA, P., ROSADINI, G.: Simultane mehrschichtige Tomographie und ihre Anwendung in der Gehirnangiographie. Acta radiol. **1**, 385–388 (1963)

ROSA, M.: Value of angio-tomography in planning operative treatment of internal carotid artery aneurysms. Neuroradiology **3**, 82–91 (1971)

RUMBAUGH, C.L., BERGERON, R.T., KURZE, T.: Intracranial vascular damage associated with skull fractures. Radiology **104**, 81–87 (1972)

RUSSEL, R.W.R.: Oberservations on intracerebral aneurysms. Brain **86**, 425–442 (1963)

SACHS, M., CABEZAS, C., POSADA, T., DAVID, M.: Recherches anatomiques sur les anévrysmes artériels intracraniens. J. neurol. Sci. **6**, 83–103 (1968)

SADIK, A.R., BUDZILOVICH, G.N., SHULMAN, K.: Giant aneurysm of middle cerebral artery. A case report. J. Neurosurg. **22**, 177–181 (1965)

SARWAR, M., BATHNITZKY, S., SCHECHTER, M.M.: Tumorous aneurysms. Neuroradiology **12**, 79–97 (1976)

SATO, O., KAMITANI, H.: Giant aneurysms of the middle cerebral artery: Surg. Neurol **4**, 27–31 (1975)

SCHECHTER, M.M., ELKIN, M.: Layering effect in cerebral angiography. Acta radiol. (Diagn.) **1**, 427–435 (1963)

SCHIEFER, W.: Zwischenfälle bei der Hirngefäßdarstellung. In: Der Hirnkreislauf (H. Gänshirt, Hrsg.), S. 781–796. Stuttgart: Georg Thieme 1972

SCHNECK, ST.A.: On the relationship between ruptured intracranial aneurysm and cerebral infarction. Neurology (Minneap) **14**, 691–702 (1964)

SCHNECK, ST.A., KRICHEFF, I.I.: Intracranial aneurysm rupture, vasospasm, and infarction. Arch. Neurol. **11**, 668–680 (1964)

SCHWARTZ, M.J., BARONOFSKY, I.D.: Ruptured intracranial aneurysm associated with coarctation of the aorta: a report of a patient treated by hypothermia and surgical repair of the coarctation. Amer. J. Cardiol. **6**, 982–988 (1960)

SCOTT, R.M., BALLANTINE, H.TH.: Spontaneous thrombosis in a giant middle cerebral artery aneurysm. J. Neurosurg. **37**, 361–363 (1972)

SEDZIMIR, C.B.: An angiographic test of collateral circulation through the anterior segment of the circle of Willis. J. Neurol. Neurosurg. Psychiat. **22**, 64–88 (1959)

SHENKIN, H.A., POLLACK, H., SOMACH, F., BIJAISORADATA, S.: Value of routine urography during cerebral angiography. J. Amer. med. Ass. **187**, 207–211 (1964)

SHIBUYA, S., IGARASHI, S., AMO, T., SATO, H., FUKUMITSU, T.: Mycotic aneurysms of the internal carotid artery. J. Neurosurg. **44**, 105–108 (1976)

SIMEONE, F.A., RYAN, K.G., COTTER, J.R.: Prolonged experimental cerebral vasospasm. J. Neurosurg. **29**, 357–366 (1968)

SMALTINO, F., BERNINI, F.P., ELEFANTE, R., FUCCI, G.: Les anévrysmes du systems vertebro-basilaire. Ann. Radiol. **15**, 725–731 (1972)

SNYCKERS, F.D., DRAKE, C.G.: Aneurysms of the distal anterior cerebral artery. A report of 24 verified cases. S. Afr. med. J. **47**, 1787–1791 (1973)

SOMEDA, K., YASUI, N., MORIWAKI, Y., KAWAMURA, Y., MATSUMURA, H.: Extravasation of contrast material into subdural space from internal carotid aneurysm during angiography. J. Neurosurg. **42**, 473–477 (1975)

SONNTAG, V.K.H., YUAN, R.H., STEIN, B.M.: Giant intracranial aneurysms. A review of 13 cases. Surg. Neurol. **8**, 81–84 (1977)

SPRINGER, TH., FISHBONE, G., SHAPIRO, R.: Persistent hypoglossal artery associated with superior cerebellar artery aneurysm. Case report. J. Neurosurg. **40**, 397–399 (1974)

STEHBENS, W.E.: Medial defects of the cerebral arteries of man. J. Path. Bact. **78**, 179–185 (1959)

STEHBENS, W.E.: Hypertension and cerebral aneurysm. Med. J. Aust. **49**, 8–10 (1962a)

STEHBENS, W.E.: Cerebral aneurysms and congenital abnormalities. Aust. Ann. Med. **11**, 102–112 (1962a)

STEHBENS, W.E.: Histopathology of cerebral aneurysms. Arch. Neurol. (Chic.) **8**, 272–285 (1963a)

STEHBENS, W.E.: Aneurysm and anatomical variation of the cerebral arteries. Arch. Path. **75**, 45–64 (1963b)

STEHBENS, W.E.: Ultrastructure of aneurysms. Arch. Neurol. **32**, 798–807 (1975)

STEVEN, J.L.: Postoperative angiography in treatment of intracranial aneurysms. Acta radiol. (Diagn.) **5**, 536–548 (1966)

STRULLY, K.J.: Successful removal of intraventricular aneurysm of the choridal artery. J. Neurosurg. **12**, 317–321 (1955)

STUNTZ, J.T., OJEMANN, G.A., ALVORD, E.C.: Radiographic and histologic demonstration of an aneurysm developing on the infundibulum of the posterior communicating artery. J. Neurosurg. **33**, 591–595 (1970)

SUNDT, T.M., SZURSZEWSKI, J., SHARBROUGH, F.W.: Physiological considerations important for the management of vasospasm. Surg. Neurol. **7**, 259–268 (1977)

SUWANWELA, C., SUWANWELA, N., CHRUCHINDA, S., HONGSAPRABHAS, C.: Intracranial mycotic aneurysms of extravascular origin. J. Neurosurg. **36**, 552–559 (1972)

SYMON, L., DU BOULAY, G.H., ACKERMAN, R.H., DORSCH, N.W.C., SHAH, S.H.: The time-course of blood induced spasm of cerebral arteries in baboons. Neuroradiology **5**, 40–42 (1972)

SYMON, L., DU BOULAY, G., ACKERMAN, R.H., DORSCH, N.W.C., SHAH, S.H.: The reactivity of spastic arteries. Neuroradiology **5**, 37–39 (1973)

SYPERT, G.W., YOUNG, H.F.: Ruptured mycotic pericallosal aneurysm with meningitis due to neisseria meningitidis infection. J. Neurosurg. **37**, 467–469 (1972)

TEAL, J.S., RUMBAUGH, C.L., SEGALL, H.D., BERGERON, R.T.: Anomalous branches of the internal carotid artery. Radiology **106**, 567–573 (1973)

TEAL, J.S., WADE, P.J., BERGERON, TH.R., RUMBAUGH, C.L., SEGALL, H.D.: Ventricular opacification during carotid angiography secondary to rupture of intracranial aneurysm. Case report. Radiology **106**, 581–583 (1973)

TERAO, H., MURAOKA, I.: Giant aneurysm of the middle cerebral artery contanining blood channel. Case report. J. Neurosurg. **37**, 352–356 (1972)

THIERRY, A., BALLIVET, J., BINNERT, D., MABILLE, J.P., HUOT, E., FOISSAC, J.C.: Les anévrysmes sacciformes de l'artére cérébelleuse moyenne (Artère cérébelleuse antérieure et inférieure) Présentation d'un cas opéré avec succès et revue de la litérature. Neuro-chirurgie **17**, 137–142 (1971)

THOMSON, J.R., HARWOOD-NASH, D.C., FITZ, C.R.: Cerebral aneurysms in children. Amer. J. Roentgenol. **118**, 163–175 (1973)

THUREL, C., REY, A., THIÉBAUT, J.B., CHAI, N., HOUDART, R.: Anévrysmes carotido-ophthalmiques. Neuro-chirurgie **20**, 25–39 (1974)

TODOROW, S., NIESSEN, K.H.: Bilaterales cervikales Aneurysma der A. carotis interna mit einseitiger intrakranieller Ausdehnung. Neurochirurgie **17**, 58–62 (1974)

TOMONO, Y., SHIRAI, S., MAKI, Y.: Aneurysm of the upper cervical portion of the internal carotid artery due to exogeneous focal arteritis. Neuroradiology **10**, 55–58 (1975)

TRISKA, H.: Ein Fall von Kontrastmittelextravasat bei einem rupturierten Aneurysma der A. cerebri media. Zbl. Neurochir. **22**, 291–295 (1962)

TROUPP, H.: Infraclinoid aneurysm of the internal carotid artery as a cause of nosebleed. Acta otolaryng. **55**, 326–330 (1962)

UDVARHELYI, G.B., LAI, M.: Subarachnoid haemorrhage due to rupture of an aneurysm on a persistent left hypoglossal artery. Brit. J. Radiol. **36**, 843–847 (1963)

VANDERARK, G.D., KEMPE, L.C.: Classification of anterior communicating aneurysms as a basis for surgical approach. J. Neurosurg. **32**, 300–303 (1970)

VINES, F.S., DAVIS, D.O.: Rupture of intracranial aneurysm at angiography. Case report and comment on causative factors. Radiology **99**, 353–354 (1971)

WAGA, S., KONDO, A., MORITAKE, K., HANDA, H.: Rupture of intracranial aneurysm during angiography. Neuroradiology **5**, 169–173 (1973)

WAGA, S., OHTSUBO, K., HANDA, H.: Warning signs in intracranial aneurysms. Surg. Neurol. **3**, 15–20 (1975)

WALTER, W., SCHÜTTE, W.: Über die Gefäßspasmen bei frisch rupturierten sackförmigen Aneurysmen der Hirnarterien. Acta Neurochir. **11**, 631–652 (1964)

WHITE, J.C.: Aneurysms mistaken for hypophyseal tumors. Clin. Neurosurg. **10**, 224–250 (1962)

WHITE, J.C., BALLANTINE, H.T.: Intrasellar aneurysms simulating hypophyseal tumors. J. Neurosurg. **18**, 34–49 (1961)

WILKINS, R.H., ALEXANDER, J.A., ODOM, G.L.: Intracranial arterial spasm: a clinical analysis. J. Neurosurg. **29**, 121–134 (1968)

WILSON, G., RIGGS, H.E., RUPP, C.: The pathologic anatomy of ruptured cerebral aneurysms. J. Neurosurg. **11**, 128–134 (1954)

WISE, G.R., FARMER, T.W.: Bacterial cerebral vasculitis. Neurology **21**, 195–200 (1971)

WOLLSCHLAEGER, P.B., WOLLSCHLAEGER, G., HART, W.M., IDE, C.H.: Eigene Beobachtungen zur Blutversorgung des Fasciculus opticus, Chiasma fasciculorum opticorum, Tractus opticus, Tuber cinereum und Infundibulum. Radiologe **10**, 433–437 (1970)

WOOD, E.H.: Angiographic identification of the ruptured lesion in patients with multiple cerebral aneurysms. J. Neurosurg. **182**–198 (1964)

YASARGIL, G.M. 1977: persönl. Mitteilung.

YASARGIL, M.G., ANTIC, J., LACIGA, R., JAIN, K.K., HODOSH, R.M., SMITH, R.D.: Microsurgical pterional approach to aneurysms of the basilar bifurcation. Surg. Neurol. **6**, 83–91 (1975b)

YASARGIL, M.G., CARTER, L.PH.: Saccular aneurysms of the distal anterior cerebral artery. J. Neurosurg. **39**, 218–223 (1974)

YASARGIL, M.G., FOX, J.L., RAY, M.W.: The operative approach to aneurysms of the anterior communicating artery. In: Advance and technical standards in Neurosurgery (Krayenbühl, H., ed), Vol. 2. Wien – New York: Springer 1975, pp. 114–170

YASARGIL, M.G., GASSER, J.C., HODOSH, R.M., RANKIN, T.V.: Carotidophthalmic aneurysms: direct microsurgial approach. Surg. Neurol. **8**, 155–165 (1977)

YASARGIL, M.G., KASDAGLIS, K., JAIN, K.K., WEBER, H.P.: Anatomical observations of the subarachnoid cisterns of the brain during surgery. J. Neursurg. **44**, 298–302 (1976a)

YASARGIL, M.G., SMITH, R.D.: Association of middle cerebral artery anomalis with saccular aneurysms and Moyamoya disease. Surg. Neurol. **5**, 39–43 (1976)

YOUNG, R., MEACHAM, W.F., ALLEN, J.H.: Documented enlargement and rupture of a small arterial sacculation. Case report. J. Neurosurg. **34**, 814–817 (1971)

ZINGESSER, L.H., SCHECHTER, M.M., DEXTER, J., KATZMAN, R., SCHEINBERG, L.C.: On the significanse of spasm associated with rupture of a cerebral aneurysm. Arch. Neurol. **18**, 520–528 (1968)

ZINGESSER, L.H., SCHECHTER, M.M., RAYPORT, M.: Truths and untruths concerning the angiographic findings in extracerebral haematomas. Brit. J. Radiol. **38**, 835–847 (1965)

B. Arteriovenöse Mißbildungen

AGEE, O.F., GREER, M.: Anomalous cephalic venous drainage in association with aneurysm of the great vein of Galen. Radiology **88**, 725–729 (1967)

AGEE, O.F., MUSELLA, R., TWEED, C.G.: Aneurysm of great vein of Galen. J. Neurosurg. **31**, 346–351 (1969)

ALPERS, B.J., FORSTER, F.M.: Arteriovenous aneurysm of great cerebral vein and arteries of circle of Willis. Arch. Neurol. Psychiat. **54**, 181–185 (1945)

AMACHER, A., SHILLITO, J.: The syndrome and surgical treatment of aneurysms of the great vein of Galen. J. Neurosurg. **39**, 89–97 (1973)

AMACHER, A.L., ALLCOCK, J.M., DRAKE, C.G.: Cerebral angiomas: the sequelae of surgical treatment. J. Neurosurg. **37**, 571–575 (1972)

AMINOFF, M.J.: Vascular anomalies in the intracranial dura mater. Brain **96**, 601–612 (1973)

ANDERSON, F.M., KORBIN, M.A.: Arteriovenous anomalies of the brain. A review and presentation of 37 cases. Neurology **8**, 89–101 (1958)

ARONSON, N.I.: Traumatic arteriovenous fistula of the vertebral vessels, angiographic demonstrations and a rationale for treatment. Neurology **11**, 817–823 (1961)

BAUM, S.M., POCHACZEVSKY, R., SUSSMAN, R.: Central hemangioma of the maxilla. J. oral. Surg. **30**, 885–892 (1972)

BERGQUIST, E., BERGSTRÖM, K., HUGOSSON, R., JORULF, H.: Complicated arteriovenous fistula after vertebral angiography. Neuroradiology **2**, 170–175 (1971)

BERGSTRÖM, K., LODIN, H.: Arteriovenous fistula as a complication of cerebral angiography. Report of three cases. Brit. J. Radiol. **39**, 263–266 (1966)

BONNET, P., DECHAUME, J., BLANC, E.: L'anévrysme cirsoide de la rétine (anévrysme racemeux), ses relations avec l'anévrysme cirsoide du cerveau. J. Méd. Lyon **18**, 165–178 (1937)

BOYD-WILSON, J.S.: The association of cerebral angiomas with intracranial aneurysms. J. Neurol. Neurosurg. Psychiat. **22**, 218–223 (1959)

BRAUSTON, B.B., NORTON, E.W.D.: Intermittent exophthalmos. Amer. J. Ophthalmol. **55**, 701–708 (1963)

BROWN, D.G., HILAL, S.K., TENNER, M.S.: Wyburn-Mason-syndrome – report of two cases Arch. Neurol. **28**, 67–68 (1973)

CASTAIGNE, P., BORIES, J., BRUNET, P., MERLAND, J.J., MEINIGER, V.: Les fistules artério-veineuses méningées pures à drainage veineux cortical. Rev. Neurol. **132**, 169–181 (1976)

CHOU, S.N., FRENCH, L.A.: Arteriovenous fistula of vertebral vessels in the neck. J. Neurosurg. **22**, 77–80 (1965)

CHOU, S.N., STROY, J.L., SELJESKOG, E., FRENCH, L.A.: Further experience with arteriovenous fistulas of the vertebral artery in the neck. Surgery **62**, 779–788 (1967)

CONFORTI, P.: Spontaneous disappearance of cerebral arteriovenous angioma. J. Neurosurg. **34**, 432–434 (1971)

COURVILLE, C.B.: Obstructive internal hydrocephalus incident to a small vascular anomaly of the midbrain. Bull. Los Angeles neurol. Soc. **26**, 41–45 (1961)

CRONQVIST, S., GRANHOLM, L., LUNDSTRÖM, N.R.: Hydrocephalus and congestive heart failure caused by intracranial arteriovenous malformations in infants. J. Neurosurg. **36**, 249–254 (1972)

CRONQVIST, S., TROUPP, H.: Intracranial arteriovenous malformation and arterial aneurysm in the same patient. Acta neurol. scand. **42**, 307–316 (1966)

CUSHING, H., BAILEY, P.: Tumors arising from the blood vessels of the brain: angiomatous malformations and hemangioblastoma. Springfield, Ill.: Charles C. Thomas 1928

DANDY, W.E.: Arteriovenous aneurysms of the scalp and face. Arch. Surg. **52**, 1–32 (1946)

DE FEO, D.R., KUSSKE, J.A., RUSH, J.L., PRIBRAM, H.: Aqueductal occlusion by midline arteriovenous malformation. Surg. Neurol. **5**, 59–62 (1976)

DECKER, K., FREISLEDERER, W.: Arteriovenöse Angiome des Gehirns im Kindesalter. Arch. Kinderheilk. **155**, 34–43 (1957)

DILENGE, D., DAVID, M., ROESER, J., ABOULKER, J.:

Anévrysmes artério-veineux cérébraux opacifiés par l'angiographie de l'artère carotide externe. Neurochirurgie **9**, 365–370 (1963)

Djindjian, R.: Supercelective internal carotid arteriography and embolization. Neuroradiology **9**, 145–156 (1975)

Djindjian, R.: Indications, contre-indications, accidents, incidents dans l'embolisation de la carotide externe. J. Neuroradiol. **2**, 173–200 (1975)

Djindjian, R., Cophignon, J., Rey, A., Theron, J., Merland, J.J., Houdart, R.: Superselective embolisation by the femoral route in Neuroradiology. Neuroradiology Part I **6**, 20–26 (1973, Part II **6**, 132–142 (1973), Part III **6**, 143–152 (1973)

Djindjian, R., Merland, J.J., Rey, A., Thurel, J., Houdart, R.: Arteriographie supersélective de la carotide externe. Interêt de cette nouvelle téchnique dans la diagnostic neurologique et dans les embolisations en neurochirurgie. Neurochirurgie **19**, 165–171 (1973)

Ehrlich, F.E., Carey, L., Kitrinos, N.P.: Congenital arteriovenous fistula between the vertebral artery and vertebral vein; case report. J. Neurochirurg. **29**, 929–930 (1968)

Eisenmann, J.I., Alekoumbides, A., Pribram, H.: Spontaneous thrombosis of vascular malformations of the brain. Acta radiol. **13**, 77–85 (1972)

Elkin, D.C.: Cirsoid aneurysm of the scalp. Report of four cases. Ann. Surg. **123**, 591–600 (1946)

Fernandez Urdanibia, J., Silvela, J., Soto, M.: Occipital dural arteriovenous malformations. Neuroradiology **7**, 57–64 (1974)

Fischer, G., Brunon, J., Thierry, A., Aimard, G., Rochet, M., Mansuy, L.: Thrombose au cours de l'évolution des anévrysmes artério-veinneux cérébreaux (à propos de 2 observations). J. méd. Lyon **3**, 613–625 (1969)

Fodera, L., Rivoir, R., Huber, P.: Die angiographische Darstellung einer arteriovenösen Mißbildung der Mandibula. Fortschr. Röntgenstr. **124**, 86–88 (1976)

French, L.A., Peyton, W.T.: Vascular malformations in the region of the great vein of Galen. J. Neurosurg. **11**, 448–498 (1954)

Geraud, J., Manelfe, G., Caussanel, J.P., Stallenave, J.: Fistule artério-veineuse spontanée de l'artère vertébrale. Rôle éventuel de la dysplasie fibromusculaire dans sa pathogénie. Rev. Neurol. **128**, 206–213 (1973)

Gerlach, J., Jensen, H.P.: Mikroangiome des Gehirns. Langenbecks Arch. klin. Chir. **293**, 481–493 (1960)

Gerlach, J., Jensen, H.P.: Die intrazerebralen Hämatome bei Mikroangiomen. Acta neurochir. Suppl. VII, 367–373 (1961)

Glatt, B.S., Rowe, R.D.: Cerebral arteriovenous fistula associated with congestive heart failure in the newborn; report of two cases. Pediatrics **26**, 596–603 (1960)

Gold, A.P., Ransohoff, J., Carter, S.: Vein of Galen malformation. Acta neurol. scand. **40**, 1–31 (Suppl. 11) (1964)

Gomez, M.R., Whitten, C.F., Nolke, A., Bernstein, J., Meyer, J.S.: Aneurysmal malformation of the great vein of Galen causing heart failure in early infancy; report of live cases. Pediatrics **31**, 400–411 (1963)

Goree, J.A., Dukes, H.T.: The angiographic differential diagnosis between the vascularized malignant glioma and the intracranial arteriovenous malformation. Amer. J. Roentgenol. **90**, 512–521 (1963)

Hamby, W.B.: The pathology of the supratentorial angioma. J. Neurosurg. **15**, 65–75 (1958)

Hansen, J.H., Søgaard, I.: Spontaneous regression of an extra-and intracranial arteriovenous malformation. J. Neurosurg. **45**, 338–341 (1976)

Hoey, M.F., Courage, G.R., Newton, T.H., Hoyt, W.F.: Management of vascular malformations of the mandible and maxilla: review and report of two cases treated by embolization and surgical obliteration. J. oral Surg. **28**, 696–706 (1970)

Höök, O., Johanson, C.: Intracranial arteriovenous aneurysms; a follow-up study with particular attention to their growth. Arch. Neurol. Psychiat. **80**, 39–54 (1958)

Houdart, R., Le Besnerais, Y.: Les anévrysmes artérioveineux des hémishères cérébraux. Paris: Masson & Cie. 1963

Houser, O.W., Baker, H.L., Rhoton, A.L., Jr., Okazaki, H.: Intercranial dural arteriovenous malformations. Radiology **105**, 55–64 (1972)

Hoyt, W.F., Cameron, R.B.: Racemose angioma of the mandible, face, retina and brain, Report of a case. J. oral. Surg. **26**, 296–301 (1968)

Huber, P.: Ein Beitrag zur Problematik des zerebralen arteriovenösen Aneurysmas beim Kind. Dtsch. Z. Nervenheilk. **179**, 510–522 (1959)

Isfort, A.: Zum Wachstum der arteriovenösen Angiome der Hirngefäße. Arch. Röntgenstr. **116**, 772–775 (1972)

Jensen, H.P., Brumlik, J., Boshes, B.: The application of serial angiography to diagnosis of the smallest cerebral angiomatous malformations. J. nerv. ment. Dis. **136**, 1–4 (1963)

Kaplan, H.A., Aronson, S.M., Browder, E.J.: Vascular malformations of the brain; an anatomical study. J. Neurosurg. **18**, 630–635 (1961)

Kelly, D.L., Alexander, E., Davis, C.H., Maynard, D.C.: Intracranial arteriovenous malformations; clinical review and evaluation of brain scans. J. Neurosurg. **31**, 422–428 (1969)

Koo, A.H., Ferris, E.J., Shapiro, J.H.: Cerebral straight sinus "jet phenomenon" in arteriovenous malformations. Radiology **95**, 577–579 (1970)

Kosnik, E.J., Hunt, W.E., Miller, C.A.: Dural arteriovenous malformations. J. Neurosurg. **40**, 322–329 (1974)

Krayenbühl, H.A.: Angiographic contribution to the problem of enlargement of cerebral arteriovenous malformations. Acta Neurochir. **36**, 215–242 (1977)

KRAYENBÜHL, H., SIEBENMANN, R.: Small vascular malformations as a cause of primary intracerebral hemorrhage. J. Neurosurg. **22**, 7–20 (1965)

KRAYENBÜHL, H., SIEGFRIED, J.: Der neurochirurgische Beitrag zur Behandlung der intrazerebralen Blutung. Wien. klin. Wschr. **23**, 401–404 (1964)

KRAYENBÜHL, H., YASARGIL, M.G.: Das Kleinhirnangiom. Schweiz. med. Wschr. **88**, 99–104 (1958)

KÜHNER, A., KRASTEL, A., STOLL, W.: Arteriovenous malformations of the transversal dural sinus. J. Neurosurg. **45**, 12–19 (1976)

KUNC, Z., BRAT, J.: Congenital arterio-sinusal fistulae. Acta Neurochir. **20**, 85–103 (1969)

KUSHNER, J., ALEXANDER, E.: Partial spontaneous regressive arteriovenous malformation. Case report with angiographic evidence. J. Neurosurg. **32**, 360–366 (1970)

LAINE, E., DELANDTSHEER, J.M., PRUVOT, P., JOMIN, M., CHRISTIAENS, J.L., ANDREUSSI, L., CLARISSE, J., DELCOUR, J.: Les anévrysmes circoides choroidiens antérieurs et les anévrysmes circoides striés. Étude anatomo-clinique et thérapeutique. Neurochirurgie **16**, 383–396 (1970)

LAKKE, J.P.W.F.: Regression of an arteriovenous malformations of the brain. J. Neurol. Sci. **11**, 489–496 (1970)

LAMAS, E., LOBATO, R.D., ESPARZA, J., ESCUDERO, L.: Dural posterior fossa AVM producing raised sagittal sinus pressure. Case report. J. Neurosurg. **46**, 804–810 (1977)

LAPRAS, C., BOCHU, M., RUSSEL, F., SINDOU, M.: Les angiomes de la tête du noyau caudé. (A propos de 8 cas opérés). Neurochirurgie **18**, 471–483 (1972)

LESTER, J.: Arteriovenous fistula after percutaneous vertebral angiography. Acta radiol. **5**, 337–340 (1966)

LEVINE, J., MISKO, J.C., SERES, J.L., SNODGRASS, R.G.: Spontaneous angiographic disappearance of a cerebral arteriovenous malformation. Third reported case. Arch. Neurol. **28**, 195–196 (1973)

LITVAK, J., YAHR, M.D., RANSOHOFF, J.: Aneurysms of the great vein of Galen and midline cerebral arteriovenous anomalies. J. Neurosurg. **17**, 945–954 (1960)

LONG, D.M., SELJESKOG, PH.D., CHOU, S.N., FRENCH, L.A.: Giant arteriovenous malformations of infancy and childhood. J. Neurosurg. **40**, 305–312 (1974)

LUND, B.A., DAHLIN, D.C.: Hemangiomas of the mandible and maxilla. J. oral. Surg. **22**, 234–242 (1964)

MAGIDSON, M.A., WEINBERG, P.E.: Spontaneous closure of a dural arteriovenous malformation Surg. Neurol. **6**, 107–110 (1976)

MALAN, E., AZZOLINI, A.: Congenital arteriovenous malformations of the face and scalp. J. cardiovasc. Surg. **9**, 109–140 (1968)

MARGOLIS, G., ODOM, G.L., WOODHALL, B., BLOOR, B.M.: The role of small angiomatous malformations in the production of intracerebral hematomes. J. Neurosurg. **8**, 564–575 (1951)

MARTIS, C., KARAKASIS, D.: Central hemangioma of the mandible; report of case. J. oral. Surg. **31**, 613–616 (1973)

MAW, R.A.: Some features of arteriovenous malformations in the head and neck. Laryngoscope **82**, 5, 785–795 (1972)

MCCORMICK, W.F., NOFZINGER, J.D.: "Cryptic" vascular malformation of the central neorvous system. J. Neurosurg. **24**, 865–875 (1966)

MEDELLIN, H., WALLACE, S.: Angiography in neoplasms of the head and neck. Radiol. clin. N. Amer. **8**, 307–321 (1970)

MERLAND, J.J., DJINDJIAN, R.: Technique et résultats de l'embolisation des angiomes du territoire carotidien externe. J. Neuroradiol. **2**, 201–232 (1975)

MONTANT, J., VITTINI, F., HEPNER, H., PICARD, L., LEPOIRE, J.: Les anévrysmes artério-veineux du corps calleux. A propos de 4 observations d'A.A.V. de la péricalleuse. Neurochirurgie **17**, 379–394 (1971)

MOODY, R.A., POPPEN. J.L.: Arteriovenous malformations. J. Neurosurg. **32**, 503–511 (1970)

NEWTON, T., DARROCH, J.: Vertebral arteriovenous fistula complication vertebral angiography. Acta radiol. (Diagn.) **5**, 428–440 (1966)

NEWTON, T.H., CRONQVIST, S.: Involvement of dural arteries in intracranial arteriovenous malformations. Radiology **93**, 1071–1078 (1969)

NEWTON, T.H., HOYT, W.F.: Dural arteriovenous shunts in the region of the cavernous sinus. Neuroradiology **1**, 71–81 (1970)

NEWTON, T.H., WEIDNER, W., GREITZ, T.: Dural anteriovenous malformation in the posterior fossa. Radiology **90**, 27–35 (1968)

NICOLA, G.C., NIZZOLI, V.: Dural arteriovenous malformations of the posterior fossa. J. Neurol. Neurosurg. Psychiat. **31**, 514–519 (1968)

NORLÉN, G.: Arteriovenous aneurysms of the brain. Report of lo cases of total removal of the lesion. J. Neurosurg. **6**, 475–495 (1949)

O'BRIEN, M.S., SCHECHTER, M.M.: Arteriovenous malformations involving the galenic system. Amer. J. Roentgenol. **110**, 50–55 (1970)

OJEMANN, R.G., NEW, P.F.J.: Spontanous resolution of an intraventricular hematoma. J. Neurosurg. **20**, 899–902 (1963)

OLDFIELD, M.C., ADDISON, N.V.: Cirsoid aneurysms of the scalp. Brit. med. J. **2**, 23–24 (1962)

OLIVECRONA, H., LADENHEIM, G.: Congenital arteriovenous aneurysms of the carotid and vertebral arterial system. Berlin: Springer Verlag 1957

OLIVECRONA, H., REEVES, J.: Arteriovenous aneurysms of the brain. Their diagnosis and treatment. Arch. Neurol. Psychiat. **59**, 567–602 (1948)

OLSON, R.W., BAKER, H.L., SVIEN, H.J.: Arteriovenous fistula. A complication of vertebral angiography. J. Neurosurg. **20**, 73–75 (1963)

PADGET, D.H.: Cranial venous system in man in reference to development. adult configuration and relation to arteries. Amer. J. Anat. **98**, 307–355 (1956)

PADGET, D.H.: Development of cranial venous system in man from viewpoint of comparative anatomy. Contr. Embryol. **36**, 81–140 (1957)

PALLADINO, V.S., DANZIGER, A.E.: Hemangioma of the maxilla. J. Amer. derm. Ass. **70**, 636–641 (1965)

PAMPUS, F., GÖTT, H., KERSTING, G.: Das Aneurysma der Vena Galeni als Ursache des Hydrocephalus occlusivus internus and apoplektischer Blutungen im Säuglings-, Kindes- und Jugendalter. Neurochirurgia **3**, 203–222 (1960)

PATERSON, J.H., MCKISSOCK, W.: A clinical survey of intracranial angiomas with special reference to their mode of progression and surgical treatment: a report of 110 cases. Brain **79**, 233–266 (1956)

PEETERS, F.L.M., VROOMEN, J.G.H.: Die meningeale Versorgung intrakranieller arteriovenöser Mißbildungen. Fortschr. Röntgenstr. **113**, 303–311 (1970)

PERRET, G., NISHIOKA, H.: Report on the cooperative study of intracranial aneurysms and subarachnoid hemorrhage. Section IV. Cerebral angiography, an analysis of the diagnostic value and complications of carotid and vertebral angiography in 5'484 patients. J. Neurosurg. **25**, 98–114 (1966)

PERRET, G., NISHIOKA, H.: Report on the cooperative study of intracranial aneurysms and subarachnoid hemorrhage. Section VI. Arteriovenous malformations. An analysis of 545 cases of cranio-cerebral arteriovenous malformations and fistulae reported to the cooperative study. J. Neurosurg. **25**, 467–490 (1966)

PICARD, L., ANDRÉ, J.M., ROLAND, J., SIGIEL, M., MONTAUT, J., LEPOIRE, J.: L'embolisation dans les malformations vasculaires méningo-cranio-cutanées complexes. J. Neuroradiol. **2**, 233–256 (1975)

POCHACZEVSKY, R., SUSSMAN, R., STOOPACK, J.: Arteriovenous fistulas of the maxillofacial region. J. canad. Ass. Radiol. **23**, 201–206 (1972)

POOL, J.L., POTTS, D.G.: Aneurysms and arteriovenous anomalies of the brain. Diagnosis and treatment. Hoeber medical Division. New York: Harper & Row Publ. 1965

POPPEN, J.L., AVMAN, N.: Aneurysms of the great vain of Galen. J. Neurosurg. **17**, 238–244 (1960)

PORTER, A.J., BULL, J.: Some aspects of the natural history of cerebral arteriovenous malformation. Brit. J. Radiol. **42**, 667–675 (1969)

RUMBAUGH, C.L., POTTS, D.G.: Skull changes associated with intracranial arteriovenous malformations. Amer. J. Roentgenol. **98**, 525–534 (1966)

RUSSEL, D.S., NEVIN, S.: Aneurysm of the great vein of Galen causing internal hydrocephalus. J. Path. Bact. **51**, 375–385 (1940)

RUSSELL, D.S., RUBINSTEIN, L.J.: Pathology of tumours of the nervous system. London: Edward Arnold 1959, pp. 72–92

SAILER, H.F.: Perimandibuläre kavernöse Hämagiome. Schweiz. Mschr. Zahnheilk. **83**, 1267–1273 (1973)

SHENKIN, H.A., JENKINS, F., KIM, K.: Arteriovenous anomaly of the brain associated with cerebral aneurysm. Case report. J. Neurosurg. **34**, 225–228 (1971)

SHENKIN, H.A., SPITZ, E.B., GRANT, F.C., KETY, S.S.: Physiologic studies of arteriovenous anomalies of the brain. J. Neurosurg. **5**, 165–172 (1948)

SPETZLER, R.F., WILSON, CH.B.: Enlargement of an arteriovenous malformation documented by angiography. J. Neurosurg. **43**, 767–769 (1975)

STREETER, G.L.: The development alterations in the vascular system of the brain of the human anbryo. Contr. Embryol. **8**, 5–38 (1918)

SUTTON, D.: Radiology of cerebral angiomas with special reference to neuro-ophthalmology. J. Fac. Radiol. (Lond.) **9**, 90–96 (1958)

SVIEN, H.J., PESERICO, L.: Regression in size of arteriovenous anomaly. J. Neurosurg. **17**, 493–496 (1960)

SVOLOS, D., NOMIKOS, N., TZOULIADIS, V.: Congenital arteriovenous aneurysm in the neck; a case report. J. Neurosurg. **23**, 68–71 (1965)

TAMAKI, N., FUMITA, K., YAMASHITA, H.: Multiple arteriovenous malformation involving the scalp, dura, retina, cerebrum and posterior fossa. J. Neurosurg. **34**, 95–98 (1971)

THÉRON, J., NEWTON, T.H., HOYT, W.F.: Unilateral retinocephalic vascular malformations. Neuroradiology **7**, 185–196 (1974)

THOMAS, M.L., ANDRESS, M.R.: Angiography in angiomas of the face. Amer. J. Roentgenol. **112**, 332–338 (1971)

TÖNNIS, W., SCHIEFER, K.: Zur Frage des Wachstums arteriovenöser Aneurysmen. Zbl. Neurochir. **15**, 145–150 (1955)

VERBIEST, H.: Arteriovenous aneurysms of the posterior fossa. Prof. Brain. Res. **30**, 383–396 (1968)

VERBIEST, H.: Results of artifical slow angiography with arteriovenous aneurysms in the supply area of the external or internal carotid arteries. Amer. J. Roentgenol. **116**, 1–15 (1972)

VOGELSANG, H.: Die arteriovenösen Angiome im extrakraniellen Karotis- und Vertebralisbereich. Dtsch. Z. Nervenheilk. **184**, 83–97 (1962)

VOGELSANG, H.: Angioma racemosum arteriale demonstated by serial angiography. Acta radiol. **57**, 232–236 (1962)

WAGA, S., OHTSUBO, K., HANDA, J., HANDA, H.: Extracranial congenital arterio-venous malformations. Surg. Neurol. **2**, 241–245 (1974)

WALSH, F.B., DANDY, W.E.: Pathogensis of intermittent exophthalmos. Arch. Ophthalmol. **32**, 1–10 (1944)

WALTIMO, O.: The relationship of size, density and localization of intracranial arteriovenous malformations to the type of initial symptom J. neurol. Sci. **19**, 13–19 (1973)

Waltimo, O.: The change in size of intracranial arteriovenous malformations. J. neurol. Sci. **19**, b) 21–27 (1973)

Watson, W.L., McCarty, W.D.: Blood and lymph vessel tumours, a report of 1056 cases. Surg. Gynee. Obstet. **71**, 569 (1940)

Weinberg, P.E., Flom, R.A.: Traumatic vertebral arteriovenous fistula. Surg. Neurol. **1**, 162–167 (1973)

Wickbom, I.: Angiographic examination of intracranial arteriovenous aneurysms. Acta radiol. **34**, 384–398 (1950)

Wyburn-Mason, R.: Arteriovenous aneurysm of mid-brain and retina, facial naevi and mental changes. Brain **66**, 163–203 (1943)

Yasargil, M.G., Jain, K.K., Antic, J., Laciga, R.: Arteriovenous malformations of the splenium of the corpus callosum: microsurgical treatment. Surg. Neurol. **5**, 5–14 (1976)

Zilkha, A., Schechter, M.: Arteriovenous fistulas of the major vessels of the neck. Acta radiol. (Diagn.) **9**, 560–572 (1969)

Zingesser, L.H., Schechter, M.M., Kier, E.L., O'Brien, M.S.: Vascular malformations of the posterior fossa including the tentorial hiatus. Amer. J. Roentgenol. **105**, 341–347 (1969)

Die relativ große Anzahl der Abbildungen, die aus der *„Zerebralen Angiographie für Klinik und Praxis"*, Krayenbühl/Yasargil, 3. vollständig neubearbeitete Auflage von P. Huber, Georg Thieme Verlag, Stuttgart 1979 (ISBN 3-13-366003-9) übernommen wurde, erklärt sich durch den Umstand, daß in einer einzigen Neuroradiologischen Abteilung innerhalb weniger Jahre nur wenige Fälle von gewissen selteneren Befunden anzutreffen sind, von welchen zudem nicht alle typisch und für eine Abbildung geeignet sind. Wir sind deshalb dem Verlag Georg Thieme für die großzügige Erlaubnis zur Übernahme der Abbildungen, die aber alle aus der Neuroradiologischen Abteilung (Chefarzt Prof. Dr. P. Huber) des Institutes für diagnostische Radiologie der Universität Bern stammen, zu größtem Dank verpflichtet.

P. Huber

Stenosierende und obliterierende zerebrale Gefäßprozesse

Von

Peter Huber

Mit 63 Abbildungen und 2 Tabellen

A. Allgemeiner Überblick über das angiographische Bild der Gefäßkrankheiten

I. Die klinischen Formen der zerebralen Ischämie und ihre Ursachen

Der Schlaganfall ist wegen seiner Häufigkeit die wichtigste zerebrovaskuläre Erkrankung. Er kann sowohl durch eine Behinderung des Blutzustromes zum Hirngewebe als auch durch eine Blutung verschiedenster Genese ausgelöst werden. Im Folgenden werden nur die angiographischen Befunde bei denjenigen zerebralen Insulten besprochen, die durch stenosierende oder obstruierende Prozesse der extra- und intrakraniellen Arterien verursacht werden.

Unter diesen lumeneinengenden Gefäßprozessen kommt der Atherosklerose und ihren embolischen Komplikationen die größte Bedeutung zu.

Der durch eine zerebrale Ischämie ausgelöste Schlaganfall kann sich klinisch in verschiedener Weise manifestieren:

- Die ischämische Attacke oder der transitorische ischämische Insult (transient ischemic attack, TIA der angelsächsischen Literatur) äußert sich in akuten kurzdauernden, meist brachiofazial betonten Lähmungen mit oder ohne Sensibilitätsstörungen, die sich vollständig zurückbilden, in flüchtigen Sprachstörungen oder selten einmal in fokalen Anfällen. In die gleiche Kategorie gehört die Amaurosis fugax, die für sich allein oder kontralateral zu den Lähmungserscheinungen auftreten kann. Diese ischämischen Attacken können sich mehrmals wiederholen und sind oft die Vorboten einer schweren Zirkulationsstörung, die zu bleibenden Lähmungen führt (Baker et al., 1968).
- Bilden sich die Lähmungen nicht oder nur unvollständig zurück, so weist dies darauf hin, daß als Folge der Zirkulationsstörung ein Erweichungsherd (Hirninfarkt) eingetreten ist. Die Symptome des Hirninfarktes können sich innerhalb Sekunden bis Minuten einstellen oder aber sich schubweise oder kontinuierlich über Stunden oder Tage entwickeln.
  Die protrahiert entstehenden Hirninfarkte (progressive stroke, stroke in evolution) sind weniger häufig als die akut auftretenden Infarkte.
- Ein mit bleibender Lähmung abgeschlossener Gewebsuntergang wird als kompletter Hirninfarkt (completed stroke) bezeichnet, wobei es keine Rolle spielt, ob die Lähmung akut oder protrahiert aufgetreten ist.

Ein Teil der Abbildungen stammt aus dem Buch „Zerebralen Angiographie für Klinik und Praxis“ Von Krayenbühl/Yasargil/Huber, erschienen bei Thieme Stuttgart, 1979. (S. Seite 661.)

Verschlußstelle im Gefäßsystem und Lokalisation des Infarktes im Gehirn müssen keineswegs enge topographische Beziehungen aufweisen, ebensowenig ist die Art und der Ort der Gefäßerkrankung allein entscheidend für den zeitlichen Ablauf und das Ausmaß der Hirnparenchymschädigung, sondern es spielen noch eine ganze Reihe hämodynamischer und metabolischer Faktoren eine Rolle, unter welchen dem Kollateralkreislauf und seiner augenblicklichen Suffizienz nach der Gefäßblockierung die hervorragendste Bedeutung zukommt (MEYER u. DENNY-BROWN, 1957; MEYER, 1961; MEYER u. GOTOH, 1961; ZÜLCH, 1961; DICKINSON, 1961; MEYER et al., 1962; MÜLLER et al., 1964; ZÜLCH et al., 1964; CRONQVIST, 1966; INGVAR, 1967; PAULSON, 1971). Arterienverschlüsse ohne nachweisbaren Infarkt einerseits und Infarkte ohne faßbare Arterienverschlüsse andererseits sind keine Seltenheit.

80% der Hirninfarkte werden durch Arterienverschlüsse verursacht, wobei 90% dieser Arterienverschlüsse durch Atherosklerose und ihre embolischen Komplikationen hervorgerufen werden (WYLIE u. EHRENFELD, 1970). Die von verschiedenen Autoren behaupteten Rassenunterschiede in der Krankheitsanfälligkeit für Atherosklerose (KIEFER et al., 1967) scheinen nach KURTZKE (1969) einer näheren Prüfung nicht standzuhalten. Wie das Beispiel der Neger in Amerika zu zeigen scheint, spielen Umwelteinflüsse und Lebensgewohnheiten wahrscheinlich eine größere Rolle als die Rasse (WILLIAMS et al., 1969, 1970, 1975). Die Atherosklerose allein führt allerdings relativ selten zum vollständigen Gefäßverschluß, sondern dieser ist meist die Folge eines zusätzlich auf die atheromatöse Läsion aufgepfropften Abscheidungsthrombus. Neben der Atherosklerose spielen andere Schädigungen oder Erkrankungen der Gefäßwand wie Entzündungen der verschiedensten Ätiologie, Gefäßkompressionen durch raumfordernde Prozesse, Traumafolgen, Dysplasien und Mißbildungen eine untergeordnete Rolle.

Beim Kind sind Gefäßverschlüsse nicht selten. BANKER (1961) fand in 8% der Autopsien einer großen Kinderklinik Gefäßverschlüsse, wobei die Atherosklerose naturgemäß nur eine kleine Rolle spielt. Beim Kind ist die klinische Symptomatologie oft nicht so eindeutig bei beim Erwachsenen, da wegen wirksamer Kollateralkreisläufe ein Gefäßverschluß besser ertragen wird. Nicht selten sind uncharakteristische psychische Veränderungen das einzige Symptom eines Gefäßverschlusses.

Auf die pathologische Anatomie der Atherosklerose und der übrigen Gefäßwanderkrankungen wird hier nicht eingetreten, eine ausführliche Darstellung haben ULE und KOLKMANN (1972) gegeben.

Unabhängig von lokalen Gefäßwanderkrankungen können Verschlüsse oder Stenosen durch Embolien verursacht werden, die zumeist aus dem Herzen stammen (KANE u. ARONSON, 1970). Keineswegs selten ist aber auch ein extrakardialer Ursprung des Embolus. Man unterscheidet zwischen Thromboembolien, d.h. Verschleppung von thrombotischem Material aus Abscheidungsthromben an atheromatösen Plaques des Arcus aortae, des Truncus brachiocephalicus (A. anonyma) und der Karotiden, thrombotischen (und evtl. septischen) Embolien aus Lungenvenen einerseits und anderen Formen von Embolien wie atheromatösen Embolien (z.B. nach Aufbruch einer atheromatösen Plaque in die Blutbahn), Fett- und Gasembolien und Geschwulstembolien (z.B. beim seltenen Myxom des Herzens; STOANE et al., 1966).

Schließlich können Gefäßverschlüsse durch Veränderungen der Blutzusammensetzung (Polyzythämie, Sichelzellanämie, thrombotische Thrombozytopenie) und Störungen im Gerinnungssystem wie während der Schwangerschaft und der Einnahme von Ovulationshemmern (JENNETT u. CROSS, 1967; ALTSCHULER et al., 1968; BERGERON u. WOOD, 1969; MUMENTHALER et al., 1970) verursacht werden.

Zerebrale Ischämien, die auf einem vorübergehend ungenügenden Blutangebot an das Hirn beruhen, z.B. bei Herzrhythmusstörungen (MCHENRY et al., 1961), werden hier nicht näher besprochen, da sie keiner neuroradiologischen Abklärung zugeführt werden müssen.

II. Die röntgenologischen Befunde

1. Verkalkungen der Gefäßwand

Bereits auf den Übersichtsaufnahmen nachweisbare Wandverkalkungen der größeren Gefäße sind praktisch immer auf eine Atherosklerose zurückzuführen, beweisen aber noch nicht das Vorliegen einer Stenose (TAVERAS u. WOOD, 1964). Häufigster Sitz dieser Gefäßwandverkalkungen sind der Karotisabschnitt im Sinus cavernosus (DI CHIRO u. LIBOW, 1971), der Arcus aortae und der Karotissinus (HAYLER u. FISCHER, 1963), ferner die Abgangsstelle der Vertebralarterien aus der A. subclavia und ihre Durchtrittsstelle durch die Dura. Bei Verkalkungen im intrakavernösen Karotisabschnitt und an den Durchtrittsstellen der Vertebralarterien durch die Dura finden sich oft keine wesentlichen Lumeneinengungen, an den übrigen Stellen dagegen kommen die Verkalkungen nur in Verbindung mit atheromatösen Plaques vor (BOSTRÖM u. HASSLER, 1965).

2. Die Veränderungen des Gefäßlumens im Angiogramm

Die angiographische Untersuchung des Patienten ist z.Zt. diejenige Methode, welche die genaueste Information über Lokalisation und Ausdehnung eines Strömungshindernisses erlaubt. Die Erkrankungen der Hals- und Hirnarterien lassen sich dabei auf verschiedene Weise erfassen (TÖNNIS u. SCHIEFER, 1959; TAVERAS u. WOOD, 1964; KRAYENBÜHL u. YASARGIL, 1965; LEE u. HODES, 1967; NEWTON u. POTTS, 1974):

- In anatomischen Kriterien wie in Verschmälerungen, Abbrüchen oder Verbreiterungen des dem freien Gefäßlumen entsprechenden Kontrastmittelbandes, wobei aber auf Grund des röntgenologischen Befundes allein eine artdiagnostische Charakterisierung des die Lumenveränderung verursachenden pathologischen Gefäßprozesses oft nicht möglich ist.
- In hämodynamischen Kriterien wie Strömungsumleitungen durch Kollateralsysteme und Abweichungen von der normalen Passagezeit des Kontrastmittels durch die einzelnen Gefäßterritorien, d.h. in lokalen oder allgemeinen Strömungsverzögerungen, in gewissen Fällen aber auch in lokalen Beschleunigungen.
- In Veränderungen der kapillären Anfärbungen (avaskuläre Zonen oder verstärkte kapilläre Anfärbung, sog. capillary blush).

Daneben gibt es aber auch zerebrovaskuläre Erkrankungen, die angiographisch nicht faßbar sind. Sie spielen sich entweder in Abschnitten der Strombahn ab, die durch die makroskopische Röntgenmethode nicht mehr dargestellt werden können wie z.B. im Bereich der sehr feinen perforierenden Arterien im Hirnstammgebiet (GILLILAN 1964) oder aber die Strömungsbeeinträchtigung im darstellbaren Abschnitt des Gefäßsystems ist nur kurzdauernd gewesen und im Augenblick der Angiographie bereits wieder behoben (z.B. Lyse eines frischen Thromboembolus).

a) Die Stenose

Die Form der Gefäßstenose, wie sie sich im Angiogramm präsentiert, kann bis zu einem gewissen Grad Aufschluß über die Art des stenosierenden Prozesses geben. Ein scharf und unregelmäßig begrenzter und zudem exzentrisch gelegener Füllungsdefekt weist auf eine atheromatöse Plaque hin. Konzentrische Stenosen ohne scharf abgrenzbare Ausdehnung in der Längsrichtung und mit glatter Kontur bieten differentialdiagnostisch größere Schwierigkeiten. Sie können auf Spasmen der Gefäßwand beruhen, die im extrakraniellen Abschnitt die Folge der direkten Gefäßpunktion (DECKER, 1956; RAYNOR u. ROSS, 1960) oder eines anderen, auch indirekten Traumas sein können (ECKER, 1945). Aber auch bei der Katheteruntersuchung können im extrakraniellen Karotisabschnitt Spasmen auftreten (SCHECHTER, 1963). Traumatische oder spontane Dissektionen der Gefäßwand sowie partielle Thrombosen sind aufgrund eines etwas unregelmäßigeren Gefäßlumens auf Höhe der Stenose in der Regel von funktionellen Engerstellungen unterscheidbar.

An den intrakraniellen Gefäßabschnitten ist meist eine Subarachnoidalblutung der auslösende Faktor für Spasmen (Ecker u. Riemenschneider, 1951; Pool, 1958; Pool et al., 1958; Fletcher et al., 1959; Maspes u. Marini, 1962; Walter u. Schütte, 1964; Wood, 1964; Taveras u. Wood, 1964; Krayenbühl u. Yasargil, 1965). Konzentrische Gefäßeinengungen der basalen und leptomeningealen Arterien können aber auch die Folge von Arteritiden verschiedenster Genese sein (s.u.) und selten einmal durch ein Trauma ausgelöst werden (Freidenfeld u. Sundström, 1963; Huber, 1964). Infolge eines Spasmus kommt es kaum je zu einem vollständigen Abbruch der Kontrastmittelfüllung.

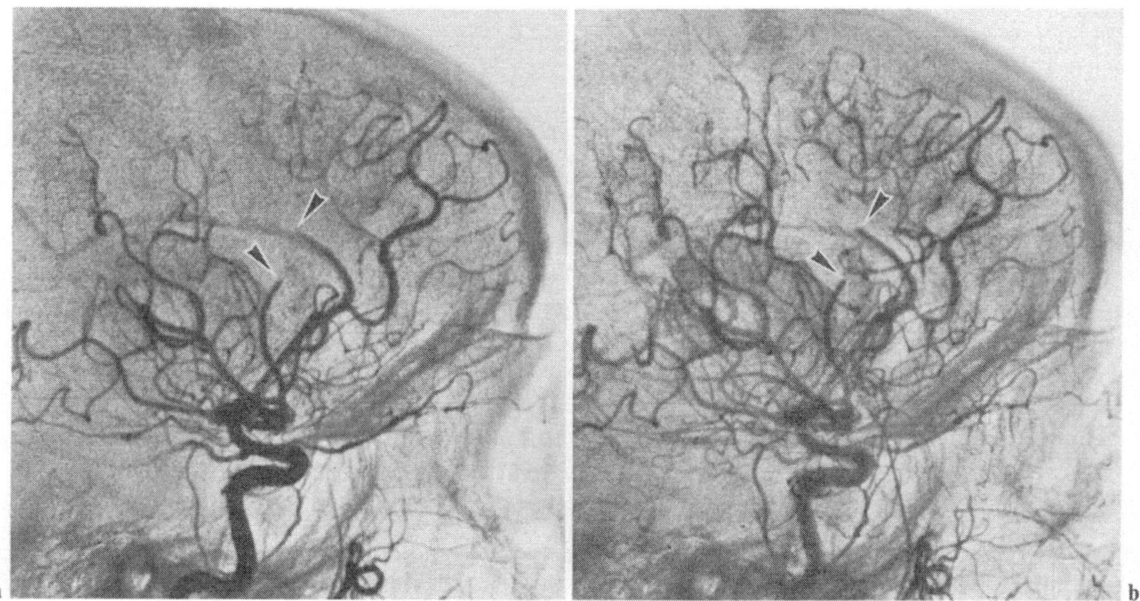

Abb. 1 a u. b. Multiple Gefäßverschlüsse. In der früheren arteriellen Phase fadenförmiges Auslaufen der Kontrastmittelsäule vor dem Verschluß **a**, später Auffüllung des Gefäßlumens proximal vom Verschluß mit querem Abbruch der Kontrastmittelsäule **b**. (Aus „Zerebrale Angiographie", Thieme Stuttgart, 1979)

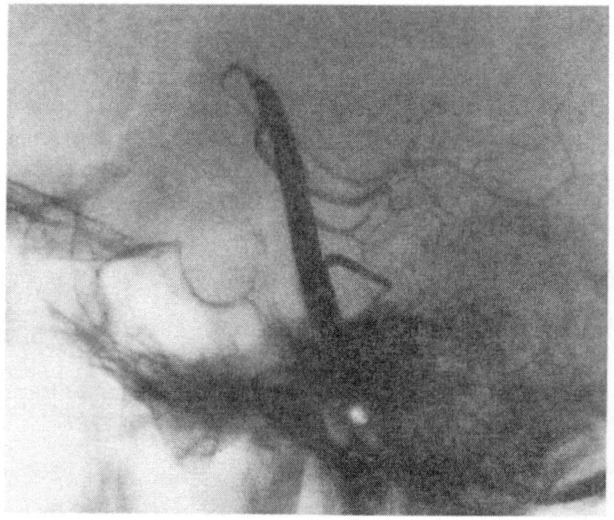

Abb. 2. Elongation der A. basilaris. (Aufnahme von Prof. K.J. Zülch, Köln)

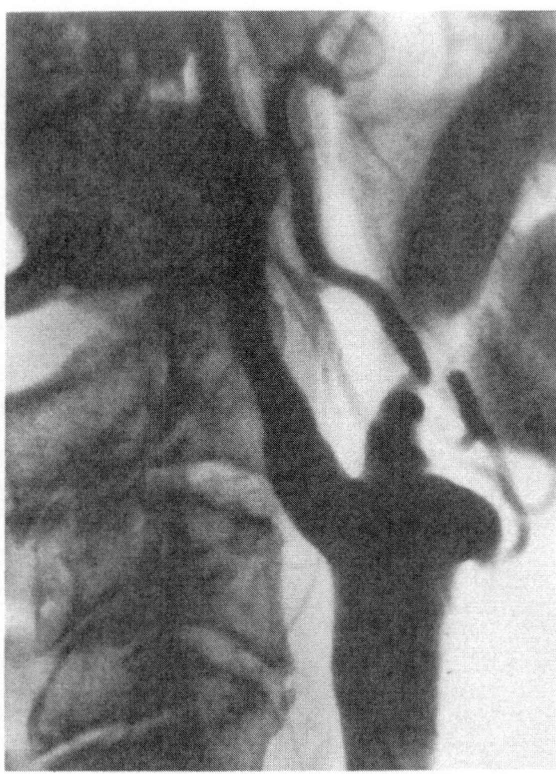

Abb. 3. Dilatation des distalen Abschnittes und der Teilungsstelle der A. carotis communis; Profilansicht

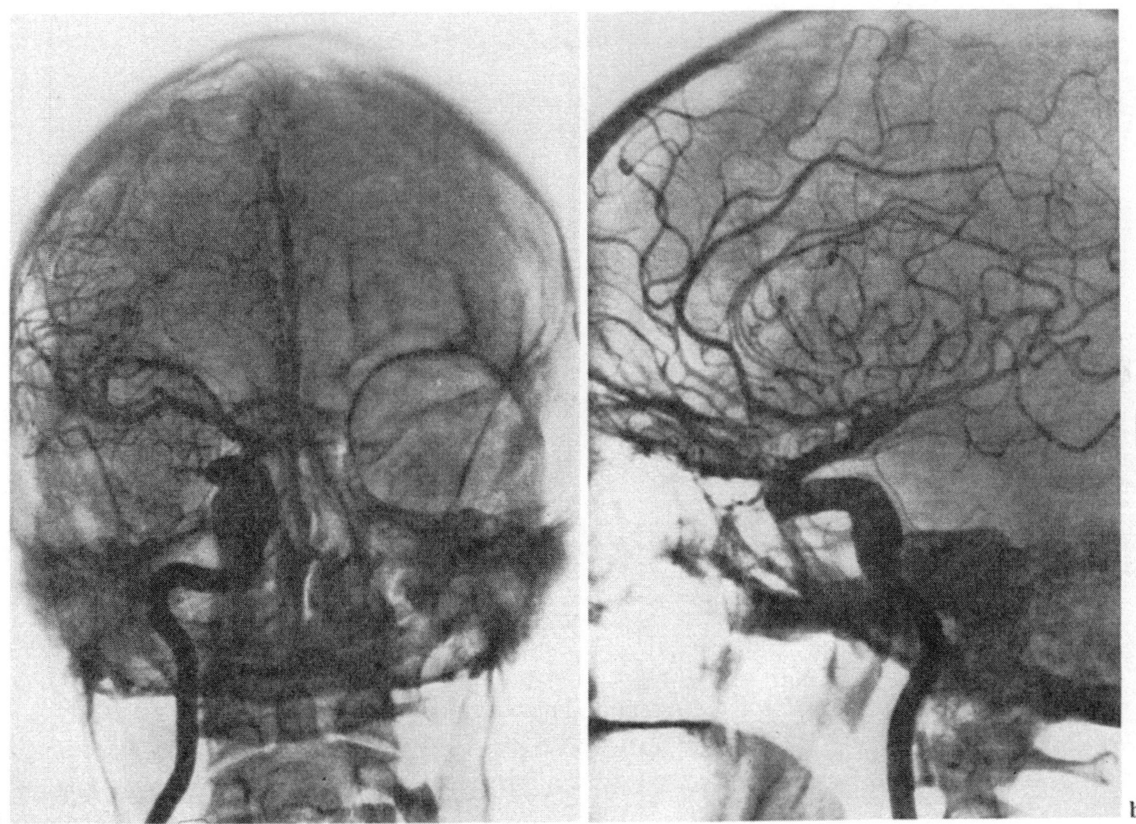

Abb. 4a u. b. Fusiforme Erweiterung der A. carotis interna bei Arteriosklerose; a-p Aufnahme **a** und Profilansicht **b**

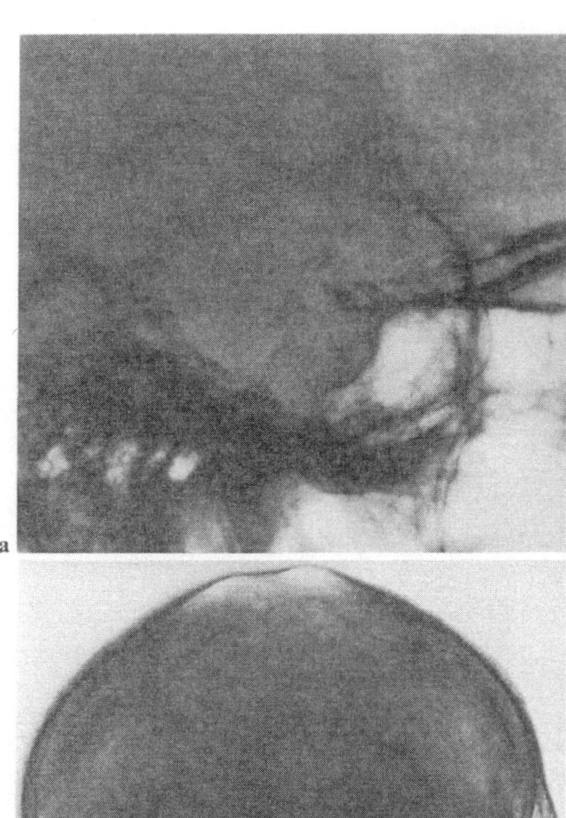

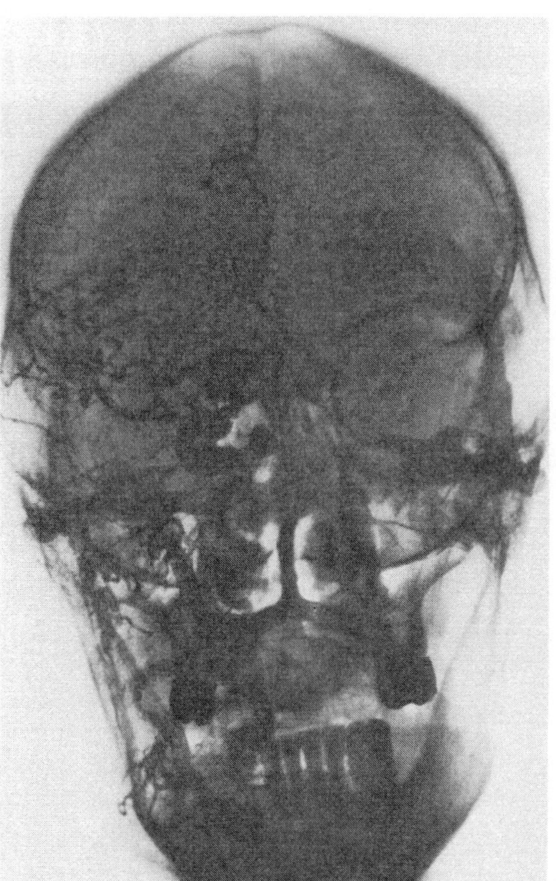

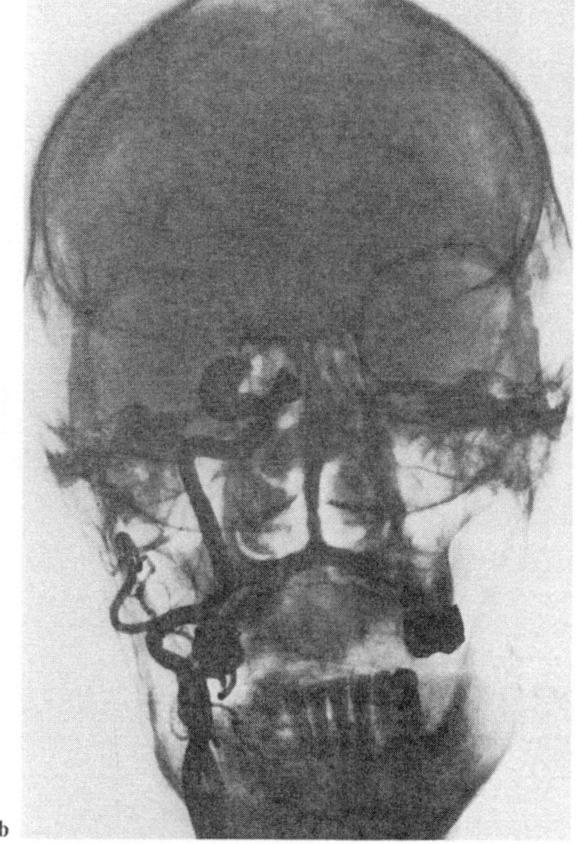

Abb. 5a–d. Wandverkalkungen **a** bei arteriosklerotischem Aneurysma im Bereiche des Karotissiphons; **d** Arteriosklerose der Hirnarterien mit multiplen Stenosen (Pfeile). (Aus „Zerebrale Angiographie", Thieme Stuttgart, 1979)

b) Der Verschluß

Der Gefäßverschluß ist am vollständigen Abbruch des Kontrastmittelfadens gut erkennbar, doch kann die Form der Kontrastmittelsäule unmittelbar proximal vom Verschluß verschiedene Formen aufweisen (IVAN u. MARIAN, 1969), weshalb Rückschlüsse auf die Ursache des Verschlusses nur ganz bedingt abgeleitet werden können. Die Höhe des Kontrastmittelabbruches muß mit dem primären Verschluß topographisch nicht übereinstimmen, da sich auf den obstruierenden Prozeß Stagnations- oder Propagationsthromben bis in die Nähe der nächsten Gefäßteilungsstelle

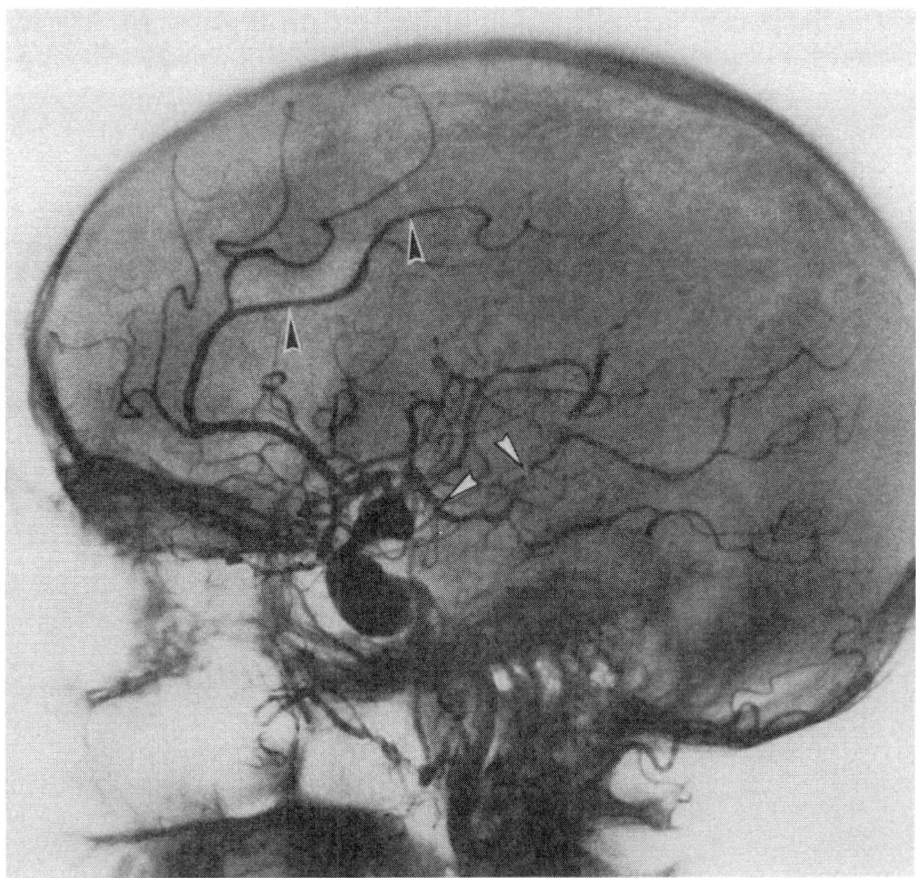

Abb. 5d

aufpflanzen können. Wegen der verminderten Strömung im restlichen Blindsack und der dadurch bedingten verminderten Kontrastfüllung imponiert gelegentlich ein noch offenes Gefäßlumen als verschlossen (CLARK et al., 1971).

Eine partielle Thrombosierung des Gefäßlumens proximal von einem Verschluß kann durch das fadenförmige Auslaufen des Kontrastmittelbandes vorgetäuscht werden, da sich das kontrastmittelhaltige Blut nur noch langsam in das noch offene Gefäßlumen proximal vom Verschluß vorschiebt. Spätere Aufnahmen der angiographischen Serien zeigen in diesen Fällen nicht selten eine vollständige Ausfüllung eines an sich normal weiten Gefäßlumens proximal vom Stop mit scharfem, quer zum Gefäß verlaufenden Kontrastmittelabbruch (Abb. 1). Das Phänomen des sich langsam vorschiebenden Kontrastmittelbolus während der Dauer der Angiographie mit der erst spät erfolgenden Auffüllung des Gefäßlumens etwa auf Höhe des Abganges der A. ophthalmica aus der A. carotis interna ist charakteristisch für den Zirkulationsstillstand infolge enorm erhöhtem intrakraniellem Druck und Behinderung des venösen Abflusses in die Sinus (PRIBRAM, 1961; MITCHELL et al., 1962; TROUPP u. HEISKANEN, 1963; HUBER, 1964; LANGFITT u. KASSEL, 1966).

c) Ektasien und Elongationen

Die durch Alterunsprozesse, eventuell in Kombination mit Arteriosklerose verursachten Strukturveränderungen der Gefäßwand und der damit verbundene Elastizitätsverlust können auch zu Gefäßerweiterungen (Ektasien) und Elongationen führen, hauptsächlich im Bereiche des Karotissiphons, der basalen Hirnarterien und namentlich der A. basilaris (Megalodolichobasilaris; Abb. 2), die bei gleichzeitigem Vorliegen einer Hypertonie besonders ausgeprägt sind (GREITZ u. LÖFSTEDT,

1954; BOERI u. PASSERINI, 1964; KRAYENBÜHL u. YASARGIL, 1965). Derartige Ektasien (Abb. 3) sind jedoch wahrscheinlich ohne wesentlichen Einfluß auf die Strömungsgröße im betroffenen Gefäß (RYTTMAN, 1972). Die nicht seltenen Abweichungen der A. basilaris von der Mittellinie sind aber häufig keineswegs der Ausdruck eines altersbedingten Elastizitätsverlustes und einer damit verbundenen Elongation, sondern können bereits bei gefäßgesunden Jugendlichen beobachtet werden. Sie beruhen auf einer ungleich großen Strömung in asymmetrisch angelegten Vertebralarterien, wobei der größere Strom in der weiteren A. vertebralis die Abweichung der A. basilaris nach der Gegenseite zu bewirkt. Dabei spielt aber auch noch der Einmündungswinkel der beiden Ae. vertebrales eine Rolle (HAVERLING, 1974).

Gelegentlich kann die Ektasie auf einen kürzeren Gefäßabschnitt lokalisiert sein und zu einer eigentlichen, meist fusiformen aneurysmatischen Ausweitung führen, wie denn überhaupt die Arteriosklerose bei der Entstehung der zerebralen Aneurysmen eine Rolle zu spielen scheint. (DU BOULAY 1965; Abb. 4 u. 5).

Kaliberunregelmäßigkeiten mit eng aufeinander folgendem Wechsel von Erweiterungen und Verengerungen über ein längeres Gefäßsegment, meist im oberen Zervikalabschnitt der A. carotis interna, gelegentlich aber auch an den Vertebralarterien, sind charakteristisch für die fibromuskuläre Dysplasie (s. daselbst).

III. Das Angiogramm bei normalen und gestörten zerebralen Zirkulationsverhältnissen

Neben der rein morphologischen Betrachtung des Kontrastmittelbandes in den Gefäßen spielt seit der Einführung der Serienangiographie auch die Beachtung der Durchgangsgeschwindigkeit des Kontrastmittelbolus durch das zerebrale Gefäßsystem eine wichtige Rolle in der Diagnostik der zerebralen Gefäßerkrankungen.

1. Die normale Strömungsgeschwindigkeit

Korrekterweise spricht man von arteriellen und venösen Füllungs- und Entleerungsphasen, die GREITZ (1956) folgendermaßen definiert hat:

arterielle Füllungsphase = Zeitintervall zwischen Eintritt des Kontrastmittels in den Karotissiphon und Erreichen der periphersten, angiographisch noch sichtbaren Arterien.

arterielle Entleerungsphase = Zeitintervall zwischen beginnender Entleerung des Karotissyphons und Entleerung der peripheren Arterien.

venöse Füllungsphase = Zeitintervall zwischen beginnender Venenfüllung und maximaler Kontrastmittelkonzentration in den Venen.

venöse Entleerungsphase = Zeitintervall zwischen maximaler Kontrastmittelkonzentration in den Venen und Verschwinden des Kontrastmittels aus dem Venensystem.

Aus diesen Definitionen geht hervor, daß sich Füllungs- und Entleerungsphase überschneiden können. Abgesehen von vorwiegend technisch bedingten Artefakten an der Punktionsstelle (partiell intramurale oder perivasale Injektion und punktionsbedingte Spasmen) werden durch zu große Kontrastmittelmengen oder inadäquaten Injektionsdruck, resp. inadäquate Injektionsgeschwindigkeit, Verlängerungen speziell der arteriellen Zirkulationszeit vorgetäuscht, da die arterielle Füllungszeit nie kürzer sein kann als die Injektionszeit. Bei normalem arteriellem Kohlensäurepartialdruck (p art. CO_2 von ca. 40 mm Hg) und Injektion von nicht mehr als 6.0 ml Kontrastmittel ist eine Dauer der arteriellen Phase über 2,5 s als pathologisch zu bezeichnen.

Füllungs- und Entleerungsphasen der einzelnen Gefäßterritorien lassen sich mit Hilfe der fraktionierten Subtraktion (sequential subtraction) nach RIVOIR und HUBER (1974) eindeutig abgrenzen:

Das Prinzip der Methode beruht darauf, daß für die Subtraktion eines Filmes das unmittelbar vorhergehende Bild der angiographischen Serie zur Herstellung der Maske verwendet wird. Demzufolge stellen sich Gefäße, deren Kontrastgehalt sich im Vergleich zur vorhergehenden Aufnahme erhöht hat, schwarz dar. Gefäße mit unverändertem Kontrastmittelgehalt werden subtrahiert und sind deshalb nicht sichtbar, Gefäße mit abnehmendem Kontrastmittelgehalt stellen sich in weißer Tönung dar.

Die kapilläre Phase ist auf Serienangiogrammen mit langsamer Bildfolge und Verwendung von mehr als 6,0 ml Kontrastmittel wegen der Überschneidung von arterieller Entleerungs- und venöser Füllungsphase schlecht sichtbar und deshalb nicht näher zu definieren. Auf Serien mit schneller Bildfolge und geringen Kontrastmittelmengen (ca. 3,0 ml) kommt die kapilläre Phase, also die Phase ohne sichtbare Arterien und Venen, meist gut zur Darstellung und dauert normalerweise 0,5 bis höchstens 1 s.

Die frontalen und temporalen Venen stellen sich in der Regel zuerst dar, gefolgt von den parietalen und zentralen Venen, während die okzipitalen Venen und die drainierenden Sinus zuletzt sichtbar werden (GREITZ, 1956). Diese Sequenz ist weitgehend durch die Wegstrecke bedingt, die das Blut vom Karotissiphon zum Parenchym zurückzulegen hat. Für die zentralen, speziell die subependymalen Venen spielt es aber auch eine Rolle, ob die Venen vorwiegend graue oder weiße Substanz drainieren, indem die Zirkulation durch die graue Substanz rascher ist als durch die weiße (WHITE u. GREITZ, 1972). Aus diesen Gründen ist bei der Beurteilung der venösen Füllungs- und Entleerungsphase auch das drainierte Territorium zu berücksichtigen. Unter Normalbedingungen erreicht das Kontrastmittel die parietalen Venen nicht vor den frontalen und die okzipitalen nicht vor den parietalen. Eine Füllung parietaler oder okzipitaler Venen vor den frontalen ist pathologisch. Am längsten bleibt das Kontrastmittel in den zentralen Venen sichtbar, auch in Normalfällen nicht selten bis 10 s nach Beginn der Kontrastmittelinjektion.

Die arteriovenöse zerebrale Zirkulationszeit, definiert als Zeitintervall zwischen maximaler Füllung des Karotissyphons und der parietalen Venen (GREITZ, 1956), beträgt ca. 4 s (Tabellen 1 und 2). Im Vertebralisstromgebiet beträgt die arteriovenöse Zirkulationszeit durchschnittlich 3,6 s

Tabelle 1. Arteriovenöse Zirkulationszeit im Karotisstromgebiet beim gesunden Erwachsenen

Autoren	Mittelwert (s)	Minimum (s)	Maximum (s)
GREITZ (1956)	4,13	2,7	5,5
GILROY et al., (1963)	3,5 s		4,2
FERREL, DAVIS, CARTER (1972)	3,5–5,5		
HUBER (1972)	4,4		

Tabelle 2. Dauer der arteriellen, kapillären und venösen Phase im normalen Karotisangiogramm des Erwachsenen

Autoren	arterielle Phase (s)	kapilläre Phase (s)	venöse Phase (s)	total (s)
FROWEIN (1956)	3,0	0,5	4,5–5,0	7–8
TAVERAS und WOOD (1964)	1,5	0,5–1,0	4–5	
TÖNNIS und SCHIEFER (1959)	2,3	0,5	3,5	6,3
WORINGER et al., (1956)	2–3	1–2	3–6	7–10
HUBER (1972)	2,0	1 max	1,0–6 [a]	7–9

[a] venöse Füllungsphase in Parietalregion 1,0–1,5 s, venöse Entleerungsphase in Parietalregion 4–6 s

(GREITZ, 1969). Diese im Vergleich zum Karotisangiogramm etwas kürzere arteriovenöse Zirkulationszeit dürfte in erster Linie durch die kürzeren Wegstrecken bedingt sein.

Bei Kindern mit der normalerweise höheren Hirndurchblutung (ca. 100 ml/100 g/min) sind die arteriovenösen Zirkulationszeiten etwas kürzer: TAVERAS und POSER (1959) fanden einen Wert von 3,3 s, in unserem eigenen Krankengut bei Personen unter 15 Jahren liegt er mit 3,0 s ($\pm$1,10 s) in der gleichen Größenordnung.

Zum Studium der Physiologie der Hirndurchblutung sei der Leser auf die Arbeiten von BATSON (1944), LASSEN (1959) und LÜBBERS (1972) verwiesen. An dieser Stelle kann nur erwähnt werden, daß die Größe der Hirndurchblutung sehr stark vom Kohlensäurepartialdruck im arteriellen Blut abhängig ist (MEYER u. GOTOH, 1961; MEYER et al., 1962; WYKE, 1963): Bereits eine Zunahme des arteriellen Kohlensäurepartialdruckes von 5 mm Hg führt zu einer Vermehrung der Hirndurchblutung und umgekehrt reduziert eine Senkung des arteriellen Kohlensäurepartialdruckes um 10 mm durch Hyperventilation die Hirndurchblutung auf ca. $^2/_3$ des Ausgangswertes (PATTERSON, 1960). Dementsprechend findet man angiographisch bei Hyperkapnie Verkürzungen, bei Hypokapnie dagegen Verlängerungen der arteriovenösen Zirkulationszeit (HUBER u. HANDA, 1967; FERREL et al., 1972).

Erfahrungsgemäß sind die meisten Patienten, die in Intubationsnarkose angiographiert werden, mehr oder weniger stark hyperventiliert, ein Umstand, dem bei der Beurteilung der Zirkulationsgeschwindigkeit Rechnung zu tragen ist.

Zu einer ganz erheblichen Zirkulationsverzögerung kommt es während des VALSALVA-Versuches (HAWKINS u. POWELL, 1972; HUBER, 1972), was u.U. bei Untersuchungen in Lokalanästhesie berücksichtigt werden muß.

Bei erhaltener Autoregulation beeinflussen Änderungen des Blutdruckes die Strömung (MEYER et al., 1965) und die Zirkulationszeit (HUBER et al., 1971) im Stromgebiet der A. carotis interna nicht.

Nach CRONQVIST und GREITZ (1969) besteht innerhalb gewisser Grenzen eine recht gute Korrelation zwischen globaler Hirndurchblutung und arteriovenöser Zirkulationszeit, die sich in der Formel

$$\text{Hirndurchblutung (in ml/100 g/min)} = 110 - (8 \times \text{Zirkulationszeit})$$

ausdrücken läßt. Eine exakte quantitative Erfassung der regionalen Hirndurchblutung ist dagegen angiographisch nicht möglich.

2. Laminäre Strömung

Unter Normalbedingungen ist die Strömung in den Gefäßen laminär. Dieses Phänomen spielt namentlich dort eine Rolle, wo Gefäße aus verschiedenen Systemen mit gleicher Strömungsrichtung in ein einziges Gefäß einmünden, wie z.B. die beiden A. vertebrales, die sich zur A. basilaris vereinigen oder die A. communicans posterior, die die Verbindung zwischen A. carotis interna und der aus der A. basilaris hervorgehenden A. cerebri posterior herstellt. Die gleiche Anordnung findet sich auch an den karotidobasilären Anastomosen wie der A. trigemina primitiva und der A. hypoglossica primitiva. An der Vereinigungsstelle dieser Kollateralwege unterbleibt nicht selten die vollständige Durchmischung der beiden Blutströme, weshalb bei der Angiographie das Gefäßlumen distal von der Vereinigungsstelle nicht vollständig mit kontrastmittelhaltigem Blut ausgefüllt wird und deshalb enger erscheint, als es in Wirklichkeit ist. Bei der A. basilaris ist deshalb nur dann mit einer vollständigen Füllung zu rechnen und das Gefäßlumen sicher zu beurteilen, wenn ein Kontrastmittelreflux in die kontralaterale Vertebralarterie erfolgt, der dann ebenfalls in die A. basilaris eingeschwemmt wird.

3. Zirkulationsverhältnisse bei allgemeinen Hirngefäßerkrankungen und beim Hirninfarkt

a) Zirkulationsverzögerungen bei der Arteriosklerose

Allgemeine Zirkulationsverzögerungen findet man sehr oft bei der Arteriosklerose der Hirnarterien und zwar sowohl beim normotonen als auch beim hypertonen Arteriosklerotiker, ohne daß sich morphologisch an den größeren Gefäßen lokalisierte Stenosen nachweisen lassen. In Einzelfällen haben wir bei hypertonischen Arteriosklerotikern eine Dauer der arteriellen Phase bis zu 7 s gefunden und ähnlich lange Zeiten sind von DECKER (1960) mitgeteilt worden. Bei Patienten mit einem Durchschnittsalter von 60 Jahren und zerebrovaskulären Erkrankungen ohne angiographisch faßbare Gefäßverschlüsse oder Stenosen ist der Durchgang eines Kontrastmittelbolus von 3,0 ml durch den Karotissiphon von einem Normalwert von 1,82 s (SD$\pm$0,11″) auf 2,25″ (SD$\pm$0,3″) verlängert (HUBER, 1967b). Bei diesen Zirkulationsverzögerungen können in der A. carotis interna gelegentlich sogar Schichtungseffekte auftreten (DEBAENE, 1973). Die Verlängerung der arteriellen Phase bei normalem oder sogar erhöhtem arteriellem Kohlensäurepartialdruck ohne Karotisstenose oder raumfordernden intrakraniellem Prozeß ist beim morphologisch wenig auffälligen Gefäßbild oft der einzige, allerdings unzuverlässige Hinweis auf eine zerebrale Arteriosklerose. Die Zirkulationsverzögerung ist weniger durch einen Druckabfall in den größeren Arterien oder ein vermehrtes Volumen des arteriellen Schenkels der Strombahn zu erklären als vielmehr durch eine Erhöhung des peripheren Widerstandes, der schon normalerweise zum größten Teil in den leptomeningealen und perforierenden Arterien lokalisiert ist (KANZOW u. DIECKHOFF, 1969). Das gesamte zerebrale Blutvolumen beträgt ca. 132 ml (NYLIN et al., 1961; FAZIO et al., 1963), das Volumen der A. carotis interna und der leptomeningealen Arterien einer Hemisphäre beträgt an der Leiche ca. 4,0 ml (GREITZ, 1956). Eine engere Korrelation zwischen Strömung einerseits und Hypertonie und Alter andererseits, wie sie von GOTOH (1959) und AIZAWA et al. (1961) aufgrund von Strömungsmessungen festgestellt wurde, läßt sich bei der an sich möglichen angiographischen Strömungsmessung (HILAL, 1966, 1974; HUBER, 1967a; RUTISHAUSER et al., 1967) nicht mit Sicherheit feststellen. Bei Subarachnoidalblutungen mit oder ohne Spasmen ist nach ZINGESSER et al. (1968) die Korrelation zwischen angiographisch geschätzter Strömung und regionaler Strömungsmessung mit Isotopen sogar schlecht.

Die Bestrebung, angiographisch quantitative Hirndurchblutungsmessungen durchzuführen, sind zwar wissenschaftlich interessant, praktisch aber für die Diagnostik und Therapieplanung von beschränktem Nutzen, da sich die Durchblutung im zeitlichen Ablauf eines Infarktgeschehens ändert und von zahlreichen Faktoren wie Autoregulation (JOHANNSON, 1964; HÄGGENDAL, 1965; HÄGGENDAL u. JOHANNSON, 1965; HARPER, 1965, 1966), Hirnstoffwechsel (MEYER u. GOTOH, 1961) Schwankungen des Blutdruckes und des Herzminutenvolumens, Fortschreiten der Thrombosen, Rekanalisierungen und dementsprechende Beeinflussungen des Kollateralkreislaufs abhängig ist.

Nicht unbedingt als Verzögerung im Sinn einer Verlängerung der Zirkulationszeit, sondern eher als Phasenverschiebung ist die Beobachtung von BOCZKO und CAPLAN (1967) zu werten, wonach bei 75% der Patienten mit einer einseitigen extrakraniellen Karotisstenose von mehr als 50% der Kontrastmitteleinstrom in die Hemisphärengefäße auf der Seite der Stenose während der Arkographie ca. 0,5 s später erfolgt als auf der gesunden Seite. Bei Gefäßgesunden oder geringerer Karotisstenose ist dieses Phänomen nicht zu beobachten.

Nach einem Gefäßverschluß, der die Strömung im distalen Stromgebiet um mindestens ein Drittel reduziert und zu einem Infarkt geführt hat (FIESCHI, 1970), laufen die hämodynamischen Veränderungen im wesentlichen in 3 Stufen ab:

- Hyperämische Phase im Sinn der „luxury perfusion“ (LASSEN, 1966). Diese Phase dauert nur einige Tage.
- Auf diese erste Phase folgt ein Stadium der fokalen Ischämie mit verzögerter Zirkulation und verminderter kapillärer Anfärbung (CRONQVIST et al., 1965; CRONQVIST, 1968).

– Das letzte Stadium äußert sich in einer verzögerten und verminderten Zirkulation im Bereich der ganzen erkrankten Hämisphäre (BETETA et al., 1965; TAVERAS et al., 1969).

b) Die lokale Hyperämie mit Zirkulationsbeschleunigung

Bei Patienten mit zerebralen Insulten zeigen die Serienangiogramme und die Messungen der regionalen Hirndurchblutung mit radioaktiven Isotopen, daß im Infarktbezirk nicht dauernd eine Zirkulationsverzögerung und Mangeldurchblutung bestehen muß, sondern vorübergehend eine Mehrdurchblutung, sog. luxury perfusion (LASSEN, 1966) mit Zirkulationsbeschleunigung, zumindest in den Randbezirken, bestehen kann. Die Zirkulationsbeschleunigung und Mehrdurchblutung äußern sich weniger in einer raschen Füllung und Entleerung der Arterien, als vielmehr in einer verstärkten lokalen kapillären Anfärbung (capillary blush) und dem vorzeitigen Auftreten einer oder mehrerer diesen Bezirk drainierenden Venen (Abb. 6); WORINGER et al., 1958; LANNER u. ROSENGREN, 1964; TAVERAS u. WOOD, 1964; FERRIS et al., 1966; HØEDT-RASMUSSEN et al.,

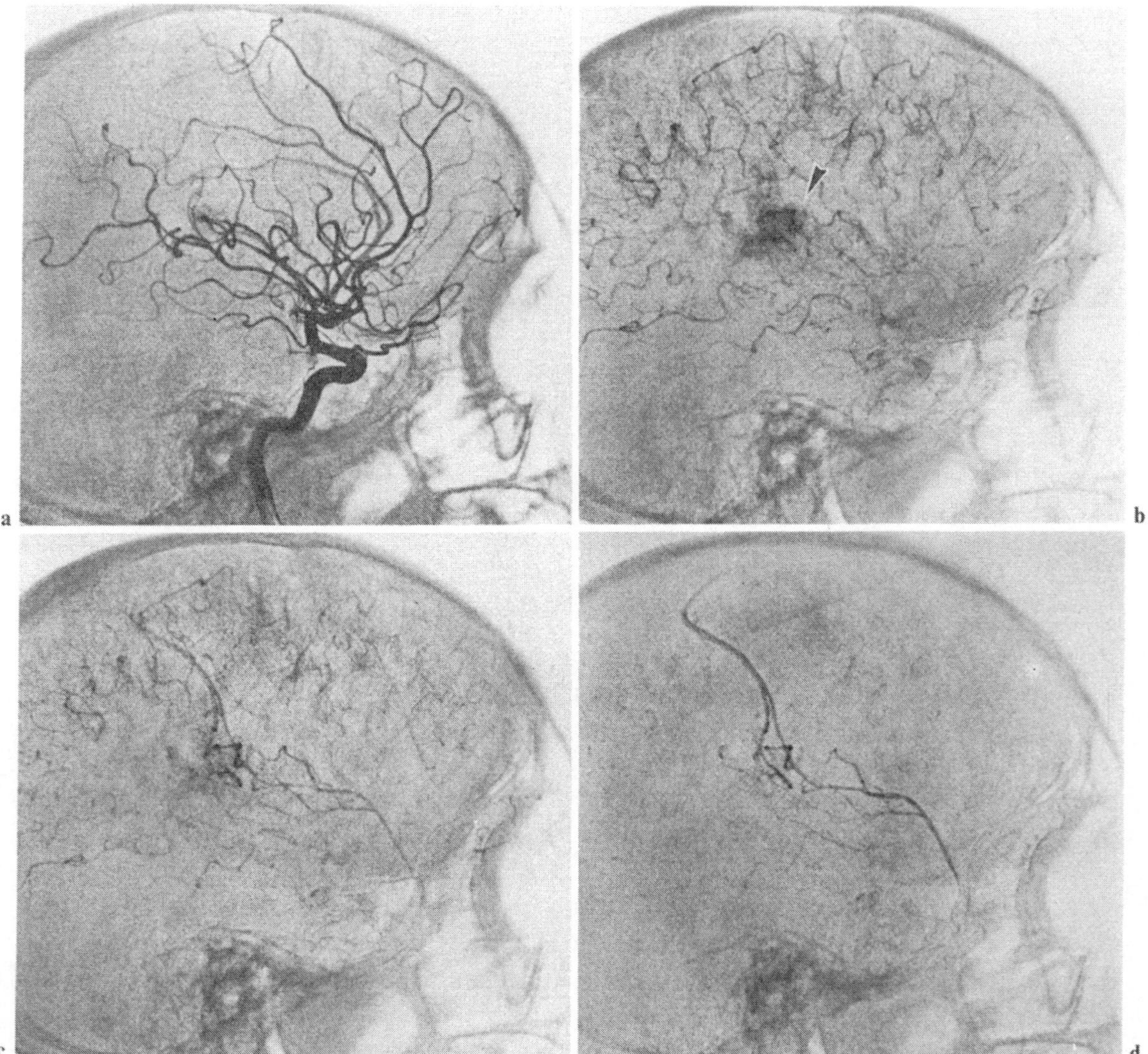

Abb. 6a–d. Vorzeitige Venenfüllung im frischen Stadium eines Infarktes. Deutlicher kapillärer blush **b**, der mit dem Auftreten der drainierenden Venen abklingt **c**

1967; CRONQVIST u. LAROCHE, 1967; FERRIS et al., 1968a; HUBER, 1968). Unter einer vorzeitigen Venenfüllung verstehen wir eine isolierte Venendarstellung in einem Zeitpunkt, da allgemein noch die arterielle Phase andauert und/oder eine Venenfüllung, die nicht phasengerecht auftritt, wie z.B. die Füllung der okzipitalen vor den frontalen Venen. Die fraktionierte Subtraktion zeigt, daß die Venenfüllung mit dem Ablassen der kapillären Anfärbung auftritt. Verstärkte kapilläre Anfärbung und vorzeitige Venenfüllung beruhen auf einer azidotischen Gefäßerweiterung und Vasoparalyse, derzufolge der periphere Widerstand vermindert ist. Sie stellt somit eine funktionelle Störung der Zirkulation dar und ist nicht mit der vorzeitigen Venenfüllung bei arteriovenösen Kurzschlüssen in Gefäßmißbildungen oder Tumoren gleichzusetzen, die eine anatomische Grundlage haben. Infolge der funktionellen Genese ist die vorzeitige Venenfüllung nur während einer kürzeren Phase im Infarktablauf zu beobachten und verschwindet bei Normalisierung der Stoffwechsellage, d.h. beim Abklingen der Azidose, wieder. Meist tritt sie in der Frühphase, unter Umständen schon wenige Minuten nach dem Gefäßverschluß, auf und dauert Stunden bis Tage. Bei Astverschlüssen sind es in der Regel die regionalen kortikalen Venen, die sich vorzeitig darstellen, bei Verschlüssen des Mediahauptstammes dagegen die zentralen Venen.

Die Angaben über die Häufigkeit der vorzeitigen Venenfüllung nach Infarkten schwanken bei den einzelnen Autoren zwischen 14 und 33%, was z.T. mit dem zeitlichen Intervall zwischen Insult und Angiographie zusammenhängt, da mit zunehmendem zeitlichen Abstand der Angiographie vom Infarkt die vorzeitige Venenfüllung seltener zu beobachten ist.

Bei der Beurteilung von Venen, die bereits in der spätarteriellen Phase auftreten, ist immer zu bedenken, daß die Arterien zumindest solange sichtbar sind, als Kontrastmittel injiziert wird. Bei der Injektion von 8–10 ml Kontrastmittel ist die Injektionsdauer mindestens 1–2 s länger, als wenn nur 4–5 ml injiziert werden. (Bei höherem Injektionsdruck kommt es zu einer stärkeren retrograden Füllung der A. carotis interna oder communis und beim Aufhören des Injektionsdrukkes wird das nach proximal gepresste Kontrastmittel mit dem Blutstrom wieder in die Peripherie transportiert.) Da das Kontrastmittel den arteriellen Schenkel der Strombahn in ca. 1,5–2,0 s passiert, ist es bei verlängerter Injektionsdauer ohne weiteres möglich, daß die Spitze des Kontrastmittelbolus den venösen Schenkel bereits erreicht hat, während die Injektion in die A. carotis noch andauert oder erst abgeschlossen worden ist. Die relativ großen V. Trolard und Rolandi mit der entsprechend dickeren Säule kontrastmittelführenden Blutes stellen sich besser dar als die dünneren frontalen Venen, während die initiale Füllung durch die kapilläre Anfärbung überdeckt werden kann. Demzufolge kann bei Verwendung größerer Kontrastmittelmengen der Eindruck entstehen, daß die parietalen Venen nicht nur in der spätarteriellen Phase, sondern auch vor den frontalen Venen auftreten, womit an sich die Kriterien der vorzeitigen Venenfüllung erfüllt wären.

Mit Hilfe der fraktinierten Subtraktion kann diese pseudovorzeitige Venenfüllung von der echten vorzeitigen Venenfüllung unterschieden werden: Da bei Verwendung größerer Kontrastmittelmengen der Kontrastmittelgehalt in den Arterien während der artifiziell verlängerten arteriellen Phase nicht mehr zunimmt, sondern gleichbleibt oder sogar abnimmt, kommt es zu einer weitgehenden Subtraktion der Arterien. In schwarzer Tönung stechen aber bereits gefüllte kortikale Venen hervor, die in der Frontal- und Präzentralregion ein geringeres Kaliber besitzen und deshalb auf Originalfilmen oder Subtraktionen zwischen den kleinen peripheren Arterien schwer identifizierbar sein können (Abb. 7).

Wegen der aufgehobenen Autoregulation im frischen Infarktstadium kann unter pharmakologischer Blutdrucksteigerung während der Angiographie eine derartige vorzeitige Venenfüllung noch stärker in Erscheinung treten (Abb. 8). In Einzelfällen verschwindet jedoch die vorzeitige Venenfüllung unter Blutdrucksteigerung (HUBER, 1970). Auch durch Hyperventilation kann eine vorzeitige Venenfüllung zum Verschwinden gebracht werden, möglicherweise infolge einer Wiederherstellung der chemischen Regulationsvorgänge und Verminderung der lokalen Azidose (PAULSON et al., 1972).

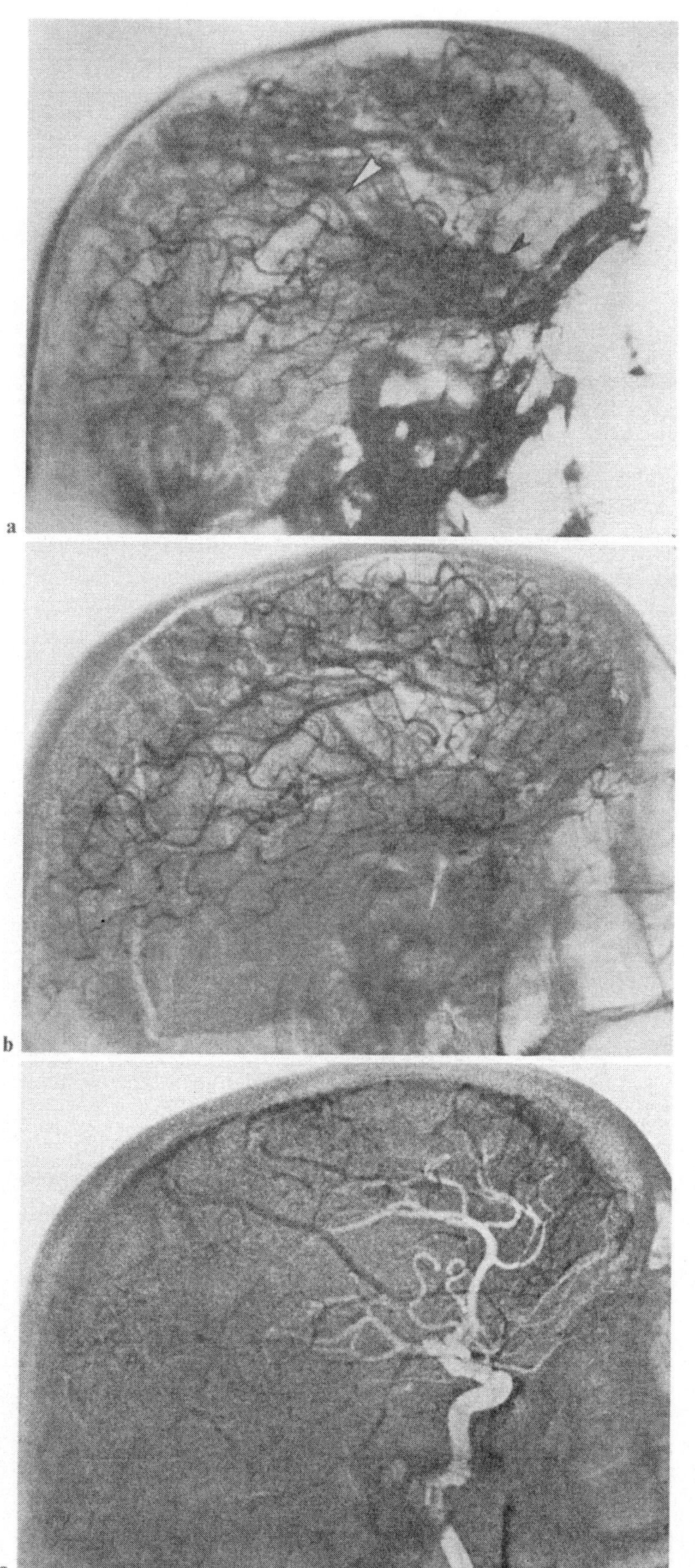

Abb. 7. a Kortikale aszendierende Vene (V. Trolard, großer Pfeil) und Vene der Fossa Sylvii (kleiner Pfeil) während der arteriellen Phase sichtbar. **b** Subtraktionsaufnahme derselben Phase. Die beiden Venen sind deutlich erkennbar, weitere Venen sind jedoch nicht sicher identifizierbar. **c** Fraktionierte Subtraktion derselben Phase. A. pericallosa und proximaler Abschnitt der Mediagruppe in Entleerungsphase (weiß). Die peripheren Arterienabschnitte sind nicht sichtbar: sie sind subtrahiert, da sich ihr Kontrastmittelgehalt gegenüber der Voraufnahme nicht verändert hat. Die sich füllenden (schwarzen) übrigen kortikalen Venen kommen jetzt gut zur Darstellung. (Aus HUBER et al.: Neuroradiology **10**, 35–41 (1975))

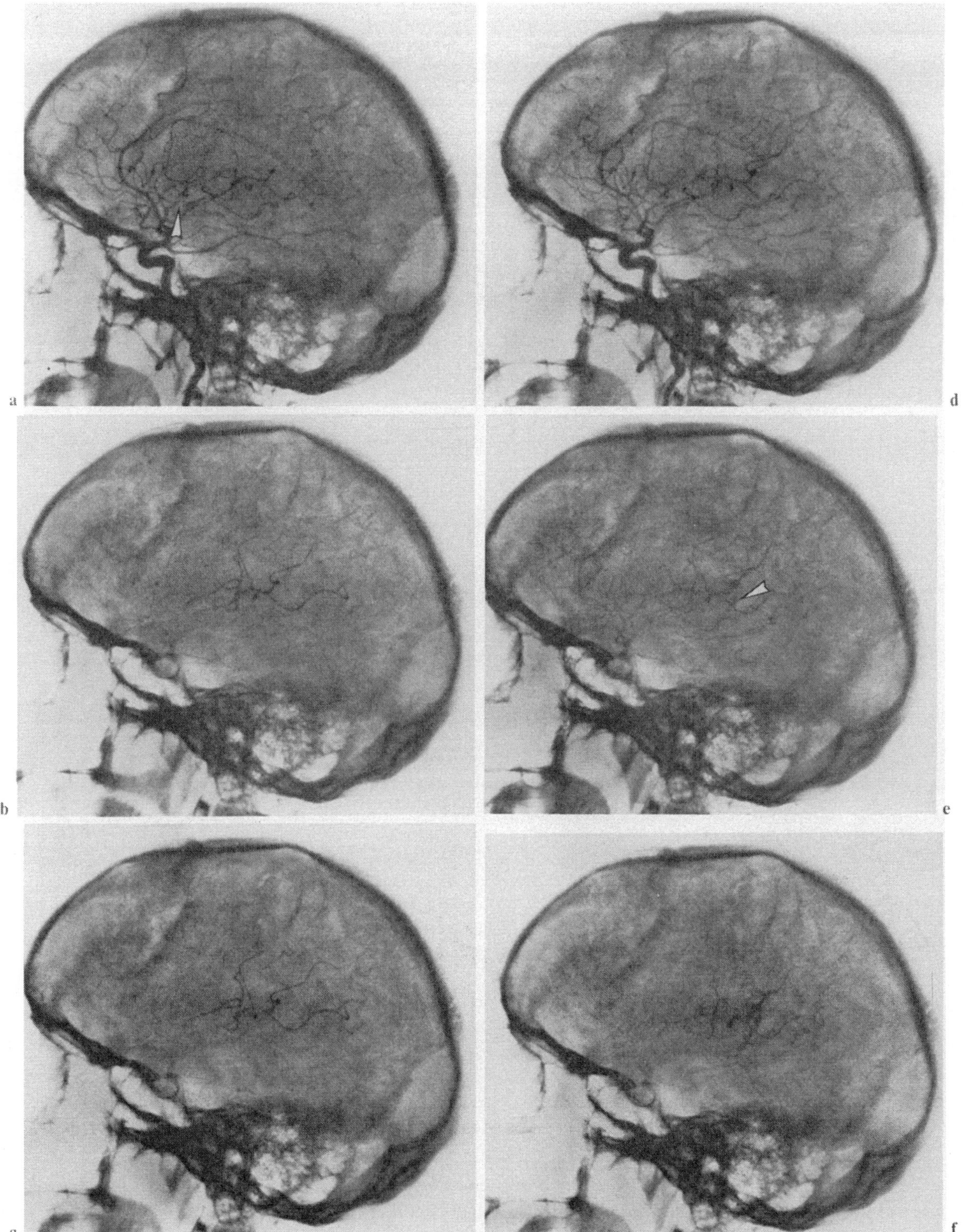

Abb. 8a–f. Verzögerte anterograde Füllung von Mediaseitenästen bei proximaler Stenosierung durch Embolus an Gefäßteilungsstelle (**a**, Pfeil). Blutdruck 155/90 mm Hg, **a**–**c**. Beschleunigung der Zirkulation distal von der Stenose durch Steigerung des Blutdruckes auf 200/105 mm Hg, **d**–**f**. Auftreten einer vorzeitigen Venenfüllung (**e**, Pfeil)

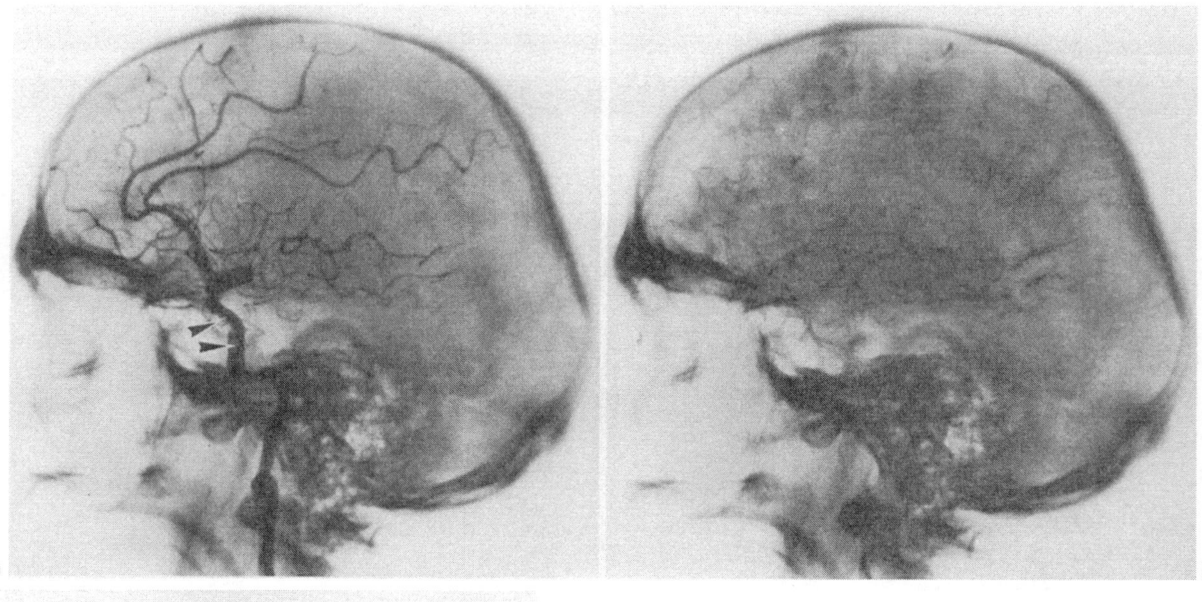

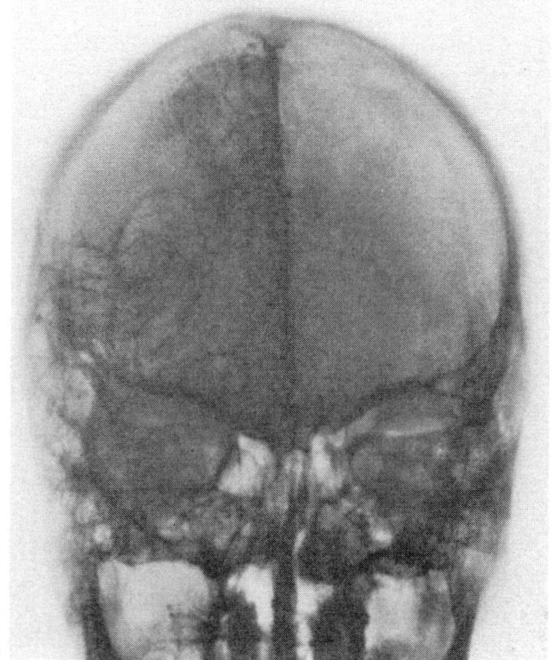

Abb. 9a–c. Karotisstenose im proximalen Siphonschenkel durch atheromatöse Plaque mit Appositionsthrombus (Pfeil) und Verschluß der parietalen Mediaseitenäste. Kein nennenswerter Kollateralkreislauf sichbar **a** u. **b**. In der venösen Phase (**c**, Towne-Projektion) dreieckförmige Zone in der Parietalregion mit vollständig fehlender Gefäßzeichnung. (Aus „Zerebrale Angiographie", Thieme Stuttgart, 1979)

c) Die lokale Zirkulationsverzögerung

Bei den lokalisierten Zirkulationsverzögerungen muß zwischen verzögerter Füllung einerseits und verzögerter Entleerung resp. Stase in den verzögert gefüllten Gefäßen unterschieden werden. Die verzögerte lokale Füllung und die Stase können im wesentlichen durch zwei Faktoren verursacht werden, die einzeln oder in Kombination wirksam sind:

– Die verzögerte Füllung beruht entweder auf einer Stenose, die mindestens 70–80% des Gefäßquerschnittes ausmacht (BRICE et al., 1964), oder aber auf einer Verlängerung der Wegstrecke bei retrogradem Kontrastmitteleinstrom über Anastomosen in Gefäßabschnitte distal von einem Verschluß: Einflußverzögerung. An kleinen Gefäßen kann sich die Stenose einer direkten Beobachtung entziehen, gelegentlich aber mit Hilfe der Vergrößerungstechnik erfaßt werden (WENDE u. SCHINDLER, 1970).

– Abflußbehinderung oder Stase durch Blockierung der kleinen, angiographisch meist nicht mehr sichtbaren intraparenchymatösen (penetrierenden oder perforierenden) Arterien oder der drainierenden Venen (Sinus- und kortikale Venenthrombose). Eine Behinderung des Abflusses distal von einer Stenose mit erheblichem Druckgradienten kann aber auch durch eine Verminderung der vis a tergo verursacht werden.

Eine Blockierung der Parenchymzirkulation kann mit einiger Wahrscheinlichkeit nur bei gleichzeitigem Fehlen eines retrograden Kontrastmitteleinstromes über Anastomosen distal vom Verschluß und einer Verminderung der kapillären Anfärbung angenommen werden. Zum Nachweis der verminderten kapillären Anfärbung ist die Subtraktionstechnik oft unerläßlich (Abb. 9).

d) Die allgemeine Strömungsverminderung und Zirkulationsverzögerung im Spätstadium nach einem Infarkt

Der angiographische Befund und die Zirkulationsverzögerung unterscheiden sich nicht wesentlich vom Befund bei der allgemeinen Arteriosklerose. Ob es sich im Einzelfall um eine Zirkulationsverzögerung bei einer Arteriosklerose oder um eine solche im Spätstadium nach einem Infarkt handelt, kann – falls größere Gefäßverschlüsse fehlen – nur aufgrund der Anamnese entschieden werden.

4. Der Kollateralkreislauf

Zwischen den verschiedenen Gefäßterritorien des Gehirns bestehen anlagemäßig Verbindungen, die als arterio-arterielle Anastomosen an der Hirnbasis (Circulus Willisi) relativ weit, als arteriolo-arterioläre oder kapilläre Anastomosen dagegen eng sind. Anastomosen zwischen leptomeningealen Gefäßen mit einem Durchmesser von 0,2–0,6 mm kommen mit Ausnahme der Medulla überall an der Oberfläche des Zentralnervensystems vor (VAN DEN BERGH u. VANDER EECKEN, 1968). Da unter normalen Umständen in den einzelnen, unter sich in Verbindung stehenden Gefäßabschnitten weitgehend gleiche Druckverhältnisse herrschen, erfolgt durch diese Anastomosen kein konstanter unidirektionaler Blutdurchfluß, sondern die Strömung pendelt von einer Richtung zur anderen, je nachdem, in welcher Richtung ein kurzdauerndes Druckgefälle besteht. Derartige kurze Druckunterschiede sind unter physiologischen Bedingungen innerhalb der größeren basalen Anastomosen (Circulus Willisi und Vertebralis- Basilarissystem) ziemlich häufig, so z.B. bei Kopfdrehungen, Inklinationen und Reklinationen. Bei der angiographischen Untersuchung sind unidirektionale Strömungen, die die Anastomosen überhaupt erst zur Darstellung bringen, nicht selten zu beobachten. Während Sekundenbruchteilen erfolgt während der frühen arteriellen Phase ein Durchfluß kontrastmittelhaltigen Blutes durch die A. communicans anterior zu der kontralateralen Hemisphäre oder durch die A. communicans posterior zur A. cerebri posterior, evtl. sogar zu den obersten Abschnitten der A. basilaris (WOLLSCHLAEGER et al., 1971). In analoger Weise kann es bei der Vertebralisangiographie zu einem kurzdauernden Reflux in die kontralaterale A. vertebralis kommen oder über die A. communicans posterior in die Karotisendstrecke. Die unmittelbar nachfolgenden Aufnahmen der Serie zeigt diese Kommunikation nicht mehr, obgleich das injizierte Gefäß noch kontrastmittelhaltiges Blut führt. Diese kurzdauernden unidirektionalen Flußrichtungen sind dagegen unter normalen Verhältnissen fast nie an den leptomeningealen Anastomosen über den Groß- oder Kleinhirnhemisphären nachweisbar. Es ist deshalb sehr wahrscheinlich, daß es bei selektiver Darstellung der A. carotis interna oder der A. vertebralis unter dem Injektionsdruck zu einer kurzdauernden Störung des Druckgleichgewichtes auf Höhe der Verbindungsstelle am basalen Gefäßkranz kommt, wobei möglicherweise auch die Herzzyklusphase eine Rolle spielt. Eine kurzdauernde Injektion unter hohem Druck am Ende der Systole oder zu Beginn der Diastole könnte dazu führen, daß der diastolische Druckabfall in der injizierten Arterie etwas verzögert eintritt, wodurch es während eines kurzen Momentes zu einem hämodynamischen

Ungleichgewicht auf Höhe der Anastomosenstelle kommt, das aber bereits bei der nächsten Systole nicht mehr besteht. Deshalb vermag die selektive Angiographie wenig über die tatsächlichen hämodynamischen Verhältnisse auszusagen obgleich sie – wie auch die postmortale Angiographie (WOLLSCHLAEGER u. WOLLSCHLAEGER, 1966) – die Existenz dieser Anastomosen besser zeigt.

Die Füllung der kontralateralen A. pericallosa über die A. communicans anterior stellt den häufigsten Typus einer derartigen Anastomosendarstellung zu Beginn der Kontrastmittelinjektion dar und findet sich nahezu in einem Drittel aller Fälle (SALTZMAN, 1959; KRAYENBÜHL u. YASARGIL, 1965). In ungefähr einem Viertel aller Karotisangiographien fließt durch die A. communicans posterior kontrastmittelhaltiges Blut in die ipsilaterale A. cerebri posterior (SALTZMAN, 1963), die kontralaterale A. cerebri posterior wird dagegen nur in ca. 3% sichtbar. In ungefähr gleicher Seltenheit (1–2%) stellen sich die kontralaterale A. cerebri media und die A. basilaris dar. Im Krankengut von KRAYENBÜHL und YASARGIL (1965) ist eine komplette Doppelfüllung in weniger als 1% sichtbar. Zu einer etwas längeren Darstellung der Gefäße der kontralateralen Hemisphäre kommt es auch ohne Gefäßverschlüsse, wenn die Untersuchung in Intubationsnarkose mit Hyperventilation durchgeführt wird (AMUNDSEN et al., 1966) oder wenn ein mehr oder weniger kräftiger Valsalva-Versuch durchgeführt wird (HUBER, 1970).

Eine über die ganze Dauer der Serie sich erstreckende Doppelfüllung weist auf ein organisch bedingtes Druckgefälle an der Anastomosenstelle hin und erweckt Verdacht auf hochgradige Stenose oder Verschluß der kontralateralen A. carotis interna oder eine arteriovenöse Fistel im kontralateralen Sinus cavernosus, resp. auf eine Erhöhung des peripheren Widerstand im ipsilateralen Karotissystem (z.B. ipsilateraler Mediaverschluß, schwere Arteriosklerose, Hirnödem).

Bei einem organischen Gefäßverschluß oder einer sehr hochgradigen Stenose mit erheblichen Druckgradienten kommt es augenblicklich zu einem hämodynamischen Ungleichgewicht an den Anastomosenstellen des verschlossenen Gefäßterritoriums zu den Nachbargebieten (SYMON et al., 1963; ISHIKAWA et al., 1965). Das augenblickliche Einspringen der Zirkulation über die Anastomosen des basalen Gefäßkranzes kann angiographisch auch bei digitaler Kompression der nicht injizierten Gefäßen während der Kontrastmittelinjektion belegt werden (GRYSPEERDT, 1963). Diese arterio-arteriellen Anastomosen des basalen Gefäßkranzes und die leptomeningealen Anastomosen erweitern sich in der Regel im Verlauf der Zeit kaum mehr wesentlich, wie u.a. Experimente an Affen gezeigt haben (HANDA et al., 1965b). Demgegenüber sind die transkraniellen und transduralen sowie die feinen intraparenchymatösen Anastomosen zu einer langsamen Weiterentwicklung fähig.

Bei selektiver Injektion der A. carotis externa und Kompression der ipsilateralen A. carotis interna gelingt es, den Anastomosenweg über die A. ophthalmica, welche in der Regel einen Innendurchmesser von wenig mehr als 1 mm aufweist, darzustellen. Bei akuten Karotisverschlüssen mit Halbseitenlähmung ist die A. ophthalmica meist dünn, kann sich aber bei insuffizientem Einspringen des basalen Gefäßkranzes infolge Hypoplasien im Verlauf der Zeit deutlich erweitern. Ein Umgehungsweg über eine weite A. ophthalmica spricht somit für ein ungenügendes Einspringen des Circulus Willisi (PITTS, 1962).

Das Anastomosensystem zwischen A. carotis externa und A. carotis interna ist praktisch immer angelegt, wird aber bei einem Karotisverschluß proximal vom Abgang der A. ophthalmica keineswegs immer benützt. Dies ist dann der Fall, wenn der Bluteinstrom in die A. carotis interna distal vom Verschluß über den Circulus Willisi so kräftig ist, daß es zu keinem Druckabfall an der Abgangsstelle der A. ophthalmica kommt und somit an den Anastomosen zwischen den Ästen der A. ophthalmica einerseits und der A. basalis, A. lacrimalis und A. infraorbitalis ein Druckgleichgewicht bestehen bleibt. Es sind dies in der Regel die Fälle mit fehlender oder sehr geringer ophthalmo-dynamometrischer Seitendifferenz (PACH et al., 1971).

Im gewöhnlichen Sprachgebrauch bezeichnet man den Blutstrom über Anastomosen in das Gefäßterritorium distal von einem Verschluß als Kollateralkreislauf. ZÜLCH (1969) hat auf die Ungenauigkeit dieser Bezeichnung hingewiesen:

Kollateralen sind definitionsgemäß parallel verlaufende Gefäße, in welchen das Blut in gleicher Richtung zu einem Gefäß oder Organ strömt, wie z.B. in den beiden Aa. vertebrales, die in die A. basilaris einmünden. Beim Ausfall des einen Systems strömt entsprechend mehr Blut im andern System ohne Richtungsänderung. Unter Anastomosen dagegen versteht man Verbindungen von mehr netzartigem Charakter zwischen zwei oder mehr funktionell getrennten Systemen, über die beim Ausfall eines Systems Blut in das Territorium distal vom Verschluß einströmen kann. Gewisse Gefäßstrecken werden dabei in umgekehrter Richtung durchströmt. Bei vielen der in der Literatur als Kollateralkreisläufe beschriebenen Umwegskreisläufen (VANDER EECKEN u. ADAMS, 1953; MOUNT u. TAVERAS, 1957; VANDER EECKEN, 1959; ALAJOUANINE et al., 1959; GILLILAN, 1959; TATELMAN, 1960; GALATIUS-JENSEN u. RINGBERG, 1963; TAVERAS u. WOOD, 1964; FIELDS et al., 1965; KRAYENBÜHL u. YASARGIL, 1965; SCHECHTER u. ZINGESSER, 1965; WEIDNER et al., 1965a, b; HAWKINS, 1966; LOVE et al., 1966; SINDERMANN, 1967; LAZORTHES u. GOUAZE, 1968) handelt es sich, streng genommen, eigentlich um Anastomosensysteme. Da sich der Ausdruck Kollateralkreislauf als Synonym für Anastomosenkreislauf eingebürgert hat, wird er im Folgenden beibehalten, um Unklarheiten zu vermeiden.

Es sind zahlreiche Versuche unternommen worden, die sehr große Zahl von Anastomosen und die theoretisch nahezu unbegrenzte Zahl von Kombinationen beim Aufbau eines Umwegkreislaufes zu ordnen. Prinzipiell gibt es zwei verschiedene Möglichkeiten für den Blutzustrom in ein Territorium distal von einem Verschluß:

α) Systeme, bei denen der Blutstrom durch mehr oder weniger komplizierte Umleitungen schließlich wieder in das ursprüngliche Gefäß distal vom Verschluß zurückgeleitet wird, ohne daß ein Nachbarsystem angezapft werden muß (Prinzip des Kollateralkreislaufs). Zu dieser Gruppe gehören:
- Die Umwegbahn über die Äste der A. carotis externa zur A. ophthalmica bei Verschlüssen der A. carotis interna (Circulus arteriosus transcranialis und transduralis).
- Die Umwegbahn A. vertebralis – A. cerebellaris inferior posterior – A. cerebellaris superior (ipsi- oder kontralateral) – A. basilaris bei Verschlüssen der A. basilaris in ihrem mittleren Abschnitt (KRAYENBÜHL u. YASARGIL, 1957; SCHECHTER u. ZINGESSER, 1965).
- Die Umwegbahn A. vertebralis – A. spinalis anterior – A. vertebralis bei kranialen Vertebralisverschlüssen (SCHECHTER, 1964; SCHECHTER u. ZINGESSER, 1966).
- Die Umwegbahn A. pericallosa – A. callosomarginalis – A. pericallosa bei Pericallosaverschlüssen distal vom Abgang der A. callosomarginalis.
- In seltenen Fällen können sich bei einem Verschluß der A. cerebri media distal vom Abgang der lentikulostriären Arterien die zu den Basalganglien führenden Arterien erweitern, so daß sich ein Kollateralkreislauf von diesen Gefäßen zu den Inselarterien und dem distalen Mediastromgebiet entwickeln kann.

In diese Gruppe gehören auch die Anastomosen zwischen den Duragefäßen der A. carotis externa und den Duraästen, die aus dem Truncus meningohypophyseos der A. carotis interna auf Höhe des Karotissyphon entspringen (PARKINSON, 1964; WALLACE et al., 1967; MARGOLIS u. NEWTON, 1969). Bei Karotisverschlüssen können auch über andere Gefäße der Dura Kreisläufe zum Internastromgebiet hergestellt werden (HANDA et al., 1971; PITON et al., 1971), speziell auch über die A. meningea anterior und ihre Äste (POLLOCK u. NEWTON, 1968).

Diese Verbindungen zum intrakraniellen Karotisendabschnitt über Duragefäße bei extrakraniellen Gefäßverschlüssen sind von zahlreichen Autoren (MOUNT u. TAVERAS, 1957; LEEDS u. ABBOTT, 1965; HAWKINS, 1966; MINAGI u. NEWTON, 1966; HAWKINS u. SCOTT, 1967; JONES u. WETZEL, 1970; NICOLA, 1970; PRENSKY u. DAVIS, 1970) als Rete mirabile bezeichnet worden.

Ein Rete mirabile, wie es beim Schwein, Schaf und anderen Tieren von ASK-UPMARK (1935), DU BOULAY und VERITY (1973), DU BOULAY et al. (1973) beschrieben worden ist, existiert beim Menschen in dieser Form nicht, und deshalb sollte dieser Ausdruck für die Bezeichnung der transduralen Anastomosen über Meningealarterien nicht verwendet werden (DE GUTIÉRREZ-MAHONEY u. SCHECHTER, 1972).

β) Systeme, bei denen der Blutzufluß zum Gefäßterritorium distal vom Verschluß durch benachbarte Gefäßsysteme erfolgt, wobei aus dem Nachbarsystem Blut über Anastomosen abgezweigt wird. Unter Umständen kann es im angezapften System wegen des Blutabflusses zu einer Mangeldurchblutung kommen (Steal-Syndrom).

Zu dieser Gruppe gehören als wichtigste:

- Der Circulus Willisi (Circulus arteriosus cerebralis basilaris) mit seinen Verbindungen zwischen den beiden Karotissystemen über die A. communicans anterior und denjenigen zwischen Karotis- und Basilarissystem über die A. communicans posterior, resp. in ganz seltenen Fällen über den Circulus arteriosus primitivus (persistierende A. trigemina primitiva, persistierende A. hypoglossica primitiva u.a.). Im Bereich des Circulus Willisi sind Variationen mit Hypoplasien einzelner Segmente sehr häufig (ALPERS et al., 1959; ALPERS u. BERRY, 1963; WOLLSCHLAEGER u. WOLLSCHLAEGER, 1974). In ca. 50% aller Fälle fehlen einzelne kommunizierende Arterien, Hypoplasien im vorderen Abschnitt des Circulus Willisi (A. cerebri anterior, A. communicans anterior) kommen in 36% vor (RIGGS u. RUPP, 1963). Durch den Ausfall einzelner Segmente wird die Leistungsfähigkeit des Circulus Willisi unter Umständen ganz erheblich beeinträchtigt.
- Circulus arteriosus inter- und intrahemisphäricus corticalis et subcorticalis. Es handelt sich hier um feinere leptomeningeale Anastomosen zwischen den Seitenästen der A. pericallosa und Seitenästen der A. cerebri media sowie der A. cerebri posterior. In gleicher Weise bestehen Verbindungen zwischen den einzelnen Ästen der A. cerebri media untereinander. Die beiden Ae. pericallosae stehen über ein feines Gefäßnetz auf dem Balken untereinander in Verbindung.

Die Verbindungen zwischen A. chorioidea anterior und posterior, Verbindungen zwischen A. pericallosa und A. corporis callosi posterior und schließlich Verbindungen zwischen den Aa. cerebellares superiores und der A. cerebri posterior sind an anatomischen Präparaten (STEPHENS u. STILWELL, 1969) sowie im postmortalen Angiogramm (WOLLSCHLAEGER u. WOLLSCHLAEGER, 1966) sehr schön nachzuweisen. Diese auch angiographisch faßbaren Verbindungen sind aber wegen ihrer Feinheit bei akuten Verschlüssen häufig insuffizient. Bei langsam auftretenden Gefäßobliterationen sind sie aber einer Erweiterung fähig und können dann beim schließlich eingetretenen Verschluß voll wirksam sein. Die intraparenchymatösen Verbindungen auf präkapillärem und kapillärem Niveau sind angiographisch wegen ihrer Kleinheit nicht mehr darstellbar. Sie manifestieren sich höchstens als verstärkte kapilläre Anfärbung in der Umgebung von ischämischen Zonen.

Retrograd über leptomeningeale Anastomosen dargestellte Gefäßabschnitte distal von Verschlüssen sind nicht selten erweitert. Zumindest im Frühstadium nach einem akuten Gefäßverschluß ist ein Umbau der Gefäßwand mit Erweiterung des Gefäßlumens weniger wahrscheinlich als eine rein funktionelle Dilatation, die über verschiedene Mechanismen zustande kommen kann:

Wahrscheinlich genügt der Druckgradient an den Anastomosestellen für sich allein unmittelbar nach einem Gefäßverschluß nicht, um ein Kollateralkreislauf voll wirksam werden zu lassen (GREEN et al., 1943; MEYER u. BENNY-BROWN, 1957). Ob der verminderte intravasale Druck bereits zu einer angiographisch faßbaren Gefäßerweiterung führt (BAYLISS, 1902; FOG, 1939; LUNDBERG et al., 1968) kann nicht entschieden werden. Dagegen ist die lokale Azidose, wie sie in ischämischen Bezirken auftritt (MEYER u. GOTOH, 1961; MEYER et al., 1962) durchaus in der Lage, die Gefäße erheblich zu erweitern, wodurch der periphere Widerstand vermindert und der Druckgradient an den Anastomosestellen noch erhöht wird. Ausmessungen der Gefäßlumina auf Angiogrammen, die unter verschiedenem Kohlensäurepartialdruck angefertigt worden sind, haben röntgenologisch eindeutig faßbare Kaliberveränderungen gezeigt (HUBER u. HANDA, 1967). Der Verlust der Autoregulation im Bereiche eines frischen Infarktes ist ebenfalls ein Faktor, der zu einer Vasodilatation führen kann, indem die Gefäßwand wegen des verminderten Bolus dem Blutdruck etwas nachgibt (HÄGGENDAL u. JOHANSSON, 1965; HARPER, 1966; EKSTRÖM-JODAL et al., 1969; LASSEN u. PAULSON, 1969; PAULSON, 1971). Versuche mit Blutdrucksteigerung während angiographischer Serien haben eine meßbare Erweiterung der Gefäßabschnitte in frischen Infarktbezirken ergeben (HUBER et al., 1971). Bei Infarkten, die älter als ein Monat sind, läßt sich diese Gefäßerweiterung unter Blutdrucksteigerung nicht mehr nachweisen, ebensowenig in Gefäßgebieten außerhalb des Infarktbezirks, wo die Blutdrucksteigerung zu einer Vasokonstriktion führt. Bei der oft deutlich verlangsamten Strömung in den retrograd gefüllten Gefäßabschnitten führt das vasoaktive Kontrastmittel selbst infolge der längeren Kontaktzeit mit der Gefäßwand zu einer Vasodilatation (ROBERT, 1969), ein Umstand, der die Abschätzung der effektiven Gefäßerweiterung erschwert bis verhindert.

5. Das Anzapf- (Steal-) Phänomen

Die Anastomosierung verschiedener Gefäßterritorien mit der Möglichkeit des vikariierenden Blutzuflusses in das Stromgebiet distal von Arterienverschlüssen hat zur Folge, daß demjenigen Arteriensystem, das den vikariierenden Stromkreis speist, Blut entzogen wird. Unter Umständen kann es deshalb zu Ischämien in Regionen kommen, die in keiner Weise zum Versorgungsgebiet der verschlossenen Arterien gehören. Prototyp dieser Anzapfung benachbarter Gefäßgebiete ist das sogenannte Subclavia-Steal-Syndrom, das erstmals von CONTORNI (1960) beschrieben worden ist. Seither sind zahlreiche Publikationen über dieses Krankheitsbild erschienen (EDITORIAL, 1961;

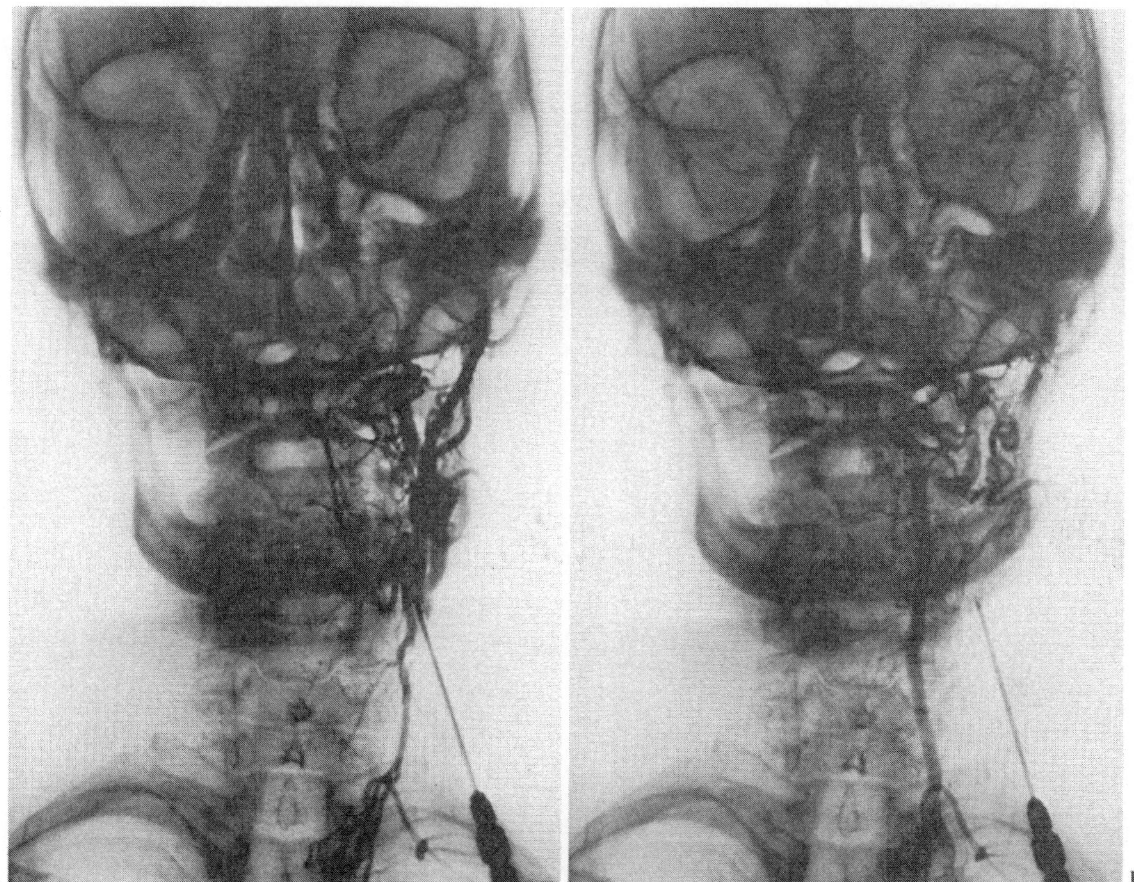

Abb. 10a u. b. Subclavia-Verschluß links und Verschluß der linken A. carotis interna. Kollateralkreislauf von der A. carotis externa aus über Muskeläste zur A. vertebralis und über die A. ophthalmica zur A. carotis interna. Stromumkehr in der linken A. vertebralis. (Aus „Zerebrale Angiographie“, Thieme Stuttgart, 1979)

NORTH et al., 1962; ASHBY et al., 1963; FISCHER u. MATTEY, 1963; STEINBERG u. HALPERN, 1963; BÜCHELER et al., 1964; VOLLMAR et al., 1965; SANTSCHI et al., 1966; WEIBEL u. FIELDS, 1969; zusammenfassende Darstellung von DÜHMKE et al., 1974). Nach SANTSCHI et al. (1966) liegt der Subclaviaverschluß in 75% der Fälle links und in 50% der Fälle sind zusätzliche Strömungsbehinderungen im Bereiche der Halsarterien vorhanden, wodurch es zur Ausbildung von recht komplizierten Umwegskreisläufen kommen kann (Abb. 10). VOLLMAR et al. (1965) unterscheiden aufgrund der Beobachtung an 40 Patienten 4 verschiedene Typen von Umgehungswegen, wovon 3 eine Stromumkehr in der Vertebralarterie aufweisen:

– vertebro-vertebraler Weg	66%
– karotido-basilärer Weg	26%
– externo-vertebraler Weg	6%
– karotido-subklavialer Weg (Innominata steal)	2%

Da es sich hierbei nicht um eine primäre Erkrankung einer zum Hirn führenden Arterie handelt, wird auf eine eingehendere Besprechung des röntgenologischen Befundes verzichtet. Es sei lediglich darauf hingewiesen, daß bei einer gezielten Angiographie, bei der auf dem Röntgenfilm die obere Thoraxapertur und der Arcus aortae ja nicht sichtbar sind, ungewöhnlich weite und stark geschlängelte Nackengefäße, die direkt an eine Mißbildung erinnern, ohne daß aber vorzeitig gefüllte Venen zu Darstellung kommen, Verdacht auf einen derartigen Kollateralkreislauf (Typus III externo-vertebraler Weg nach VOLLMAR et al., 1965) erwecken müssen und eine entsprechende Abklärung erfordern (Abb. 11).

Zahlreiche Autoren (FAZIO, 1964; LASSEN u. PALVÖLGYI, 1968; SYMON, 1968; FAZIO, 1970; VAN DER DRIFT u. KOK, 1970; ZÜLCH u. ESCHBACH, 1972) haben auf das intrazerebrale Steal-

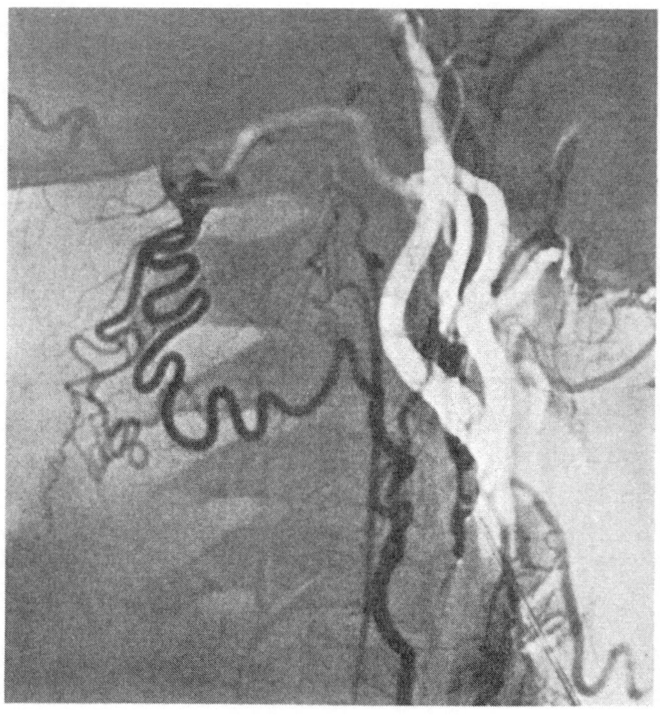

Abb. 11. Subclaviaverschluß. Kollateralkreislauf von der A. carotis externa aus über A. occipitalis und girlandenförmig erweiterte Muskeläste zur A. cervicalis ascendens und in geringerem Maße zur A. vertebralis. (Fraktionierte Subtraktion. Die Stromrichtung von der A. carotis externa (bereits in Entleerung, weiß) zur A. cervicalis ascendens (in Füllung, deshalb schwarz) und A. vertebralis kommt gut zur Darstellung

Phänomen bei zerebrovaskulären Erkrankungen aufmerksam gemacht. Der Mechanismus dieses Steal-Phänomens beruht darauf, daß im Rahmen der Umverteilung des Blutes (Hämometakinese) der Abfluß in das Stromgebiet distal von einem Verschluß umso stärker wird, je größer die Druckdifferenz an der Anastomosenstelle ist. Da die Gefäße im anzapfenden System zumindest in den frühen Stadien nach dem Gefäßverschluß ihre normale Regulationsfähigkeit verloren haben, bestimmt weitgehend der Druck im Donatorsystem die Menge des abgegebenen Blutes. Eine Erhöhung des peripheren Gefäßwiderstandes im Donatorsystem, z.B. durch Hyperventilation, wird diese Blutmenge erhöhen, eine Verminderung des peripheren Gefäßwiderstandes durch Vasodilatation dagegen verringern.

Die angiographische Sichtbarkeit eines derartigen vikariierenden Bluteinstromes über Anastomosen in ein benachbartes Territorium allein berechtigt nun keineswegs, bereits von einem Stealphänomen zu sprechen. Das Wesentliche an diesem Begriff ist die als Folge des Blutabflusses in der Peripherie des angezapften Gebietes auftretende Mangeldurchblutung, also die klinische Symptomatologie, gegebenenfalls der pathologisch-anatomische Nachweis eines Infarktes im Irrigationsgebiet des Donatorsystems oder aber die regionale Strömungsmessung mit radioaktiven Isotopen. Es ist nämlich erwiesen, daß beim Subklavia-Steal-Syndrom unter Normalbedingungen in vielen Fällen dem Hirn überhaupt kein Blut entzogen wird, sondern erst bei verstärkter Muskelarbeit mit dem Arm auf der Seite der verschlossenen A. subclavia (Erweiterung des peripheren Stromgebietes). Experimente an Affen haben gezeigt, daß die Strömung in der A. carotis interna trotz Subklaviaverschluß und Stromumkehr in der ipsilateralen A. vertebralis keineswegs vermindert sein muß, sondern erhöht sein kann und die Hemisphäre trotz dem Blutabfluß über die A. vertebralis eine normale Blutmenge erhält (Handa et al., 1965a). Nach Vollmar et al. (1965) treten beim Subklavia-Steal zerebrale Durchblutungsinsuffizienzen in der Regel erst dann auf, wenn auch in der zerebralen Strombahn hämodynamisch signifikante Strömungshindernisse vorliegen. Analoge Verhältnisse sind für die intrazerebralen Blutumleitungen sehr wahrscheinlich, meßtechnisch jedoch nicht unbedingt leicht zu erfassen. Beim etablierten Kollateralkreislauf kommt es erst zu einem Steal-Phänomen, wenn unter besonderen Bedingunggen die Kompensation in der Peripherie des angezapften Gebietes nicht gelingt, was z.B. der Fall sein kann, wenn distal von den Anastomosestellen der Widerstand infolge von Stenosen oder raumfordernden Prozessen (Tumoren, Hirnkontusionen mit Ödem, Hämatom) erhöht oder aber durch einen Blutdruckabfall das Blutangebot an das vergrößerte Versorgungsgebiet ungenügend wird. Auf das Steal-Phänomen bei arteriovenösen Gefäßmißbildungen oder Fisteln wird an dieser Stelle nicht eingetreten.

6. Die pharmakologische Beeinflussung der Hirnzirkulation speziell des Kollateralkreislaufes bei Verschlußkrankheiten

Durch vasoaktive, im speziellen gefäßerweiternde Medikamente kann eine Erweiterung der Arterien in normal perfundierten Hirnabschnitten erzielt werden, wobei sich die Kohlensäure und intraarteriell verabreichtes Papaverin als besonders wirksam erwiesen haben (Sokoloff, 1959; Gottstein, 1965; Erikson u. Lodin, 1967; Huber u. Handa, 1967; Olesen u. Paulson, 1971). Durch diese medikamentös herbeigeführte Vasodilatation wird die Kollateralzirkulation aber nicht verbessert. Im ischämischen Gebiet sind die Arterien infolge der Azidose und Vasoparalyse erweitert und eine wesentliche zusätzliche Dilatation ist mit therapeutisch möglichen Dosen kaum zu erreichen (Paulson, 1971). Da der Widerstand in den normal perfundierten Gebieten infolge der dort stattfindenden Gefäßerweiterung sinkt, wird die Druckdifferenz an den Anastomosestellen geringer, womit auch der Bluteinstrom in das Kollateralsystem geringer wird. Es ist deshalb nicht korrekt, unter diesen Bedingungen von einem umgekehrten Steal zu sprechen, da kein Blutabstrom aus dem Infarktgebiet in das normale Territorium erfolgt, sondern lediglich ein geringeres Blutangebot an den Kollateralkreislauf zur Infarktzone.

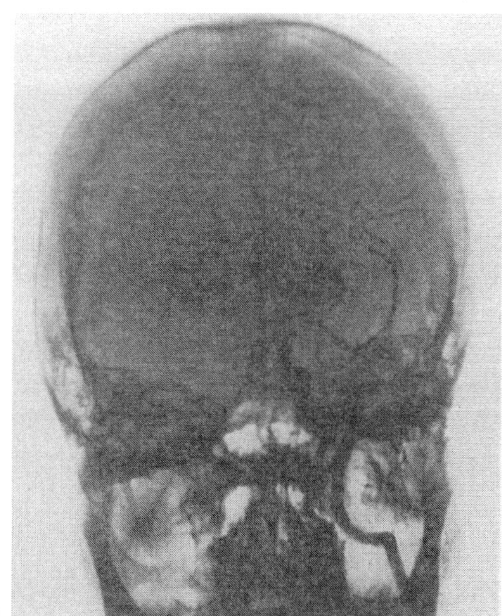

Abb. 12. a Hochgradige Stenosierung der Karotisteilungsstelle am Circulus Willisi. Frischer Infarkt. **b–e** Verzögerte und unvollständige Darstellung des Stromgebietes der A. cerebri media. Blutdruck 130/70 mm Hg (Blutdruckabfall bei vorbestehender Hypertonie). **f–i** Zirkulationsbeschleunigung in den noch offenen Mediaästen nach Anhebung des Blutdruckes auf 190/110 mm Hg. Während der akuten medikamentösen Blutdrucksteigerung sind die Externaäste enger, die Mediaäste dagegen weiter geworden. (Aus HUBER et al.: Neuroradiology **3**, 68–74 (1971))

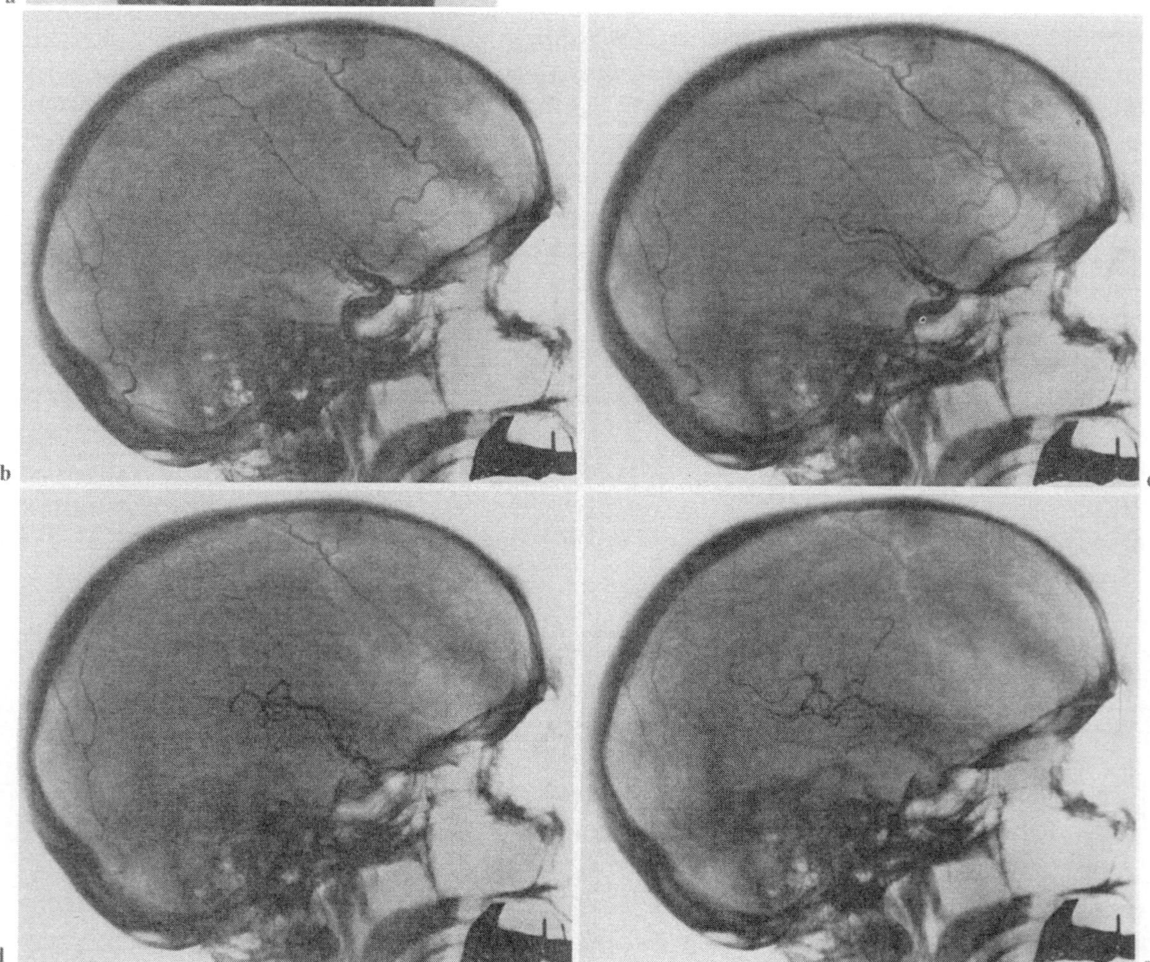

Bei einer Vasokonstriktion, z.B. infolge Hyperventilation und entsprechender Erhöhung des Widerstandes im normal reagierenden Gefäßterritorium kann es zu einer Zunahme des Blutabstromes in das Kollateralsystem kommen. (BRAWLEY et al., 1967; BATTISTINI et al., 1969). Die häufig zu beobachtende kontrastreichere Darstellung auch im Kollateralkreislauf unter Hyperventilation

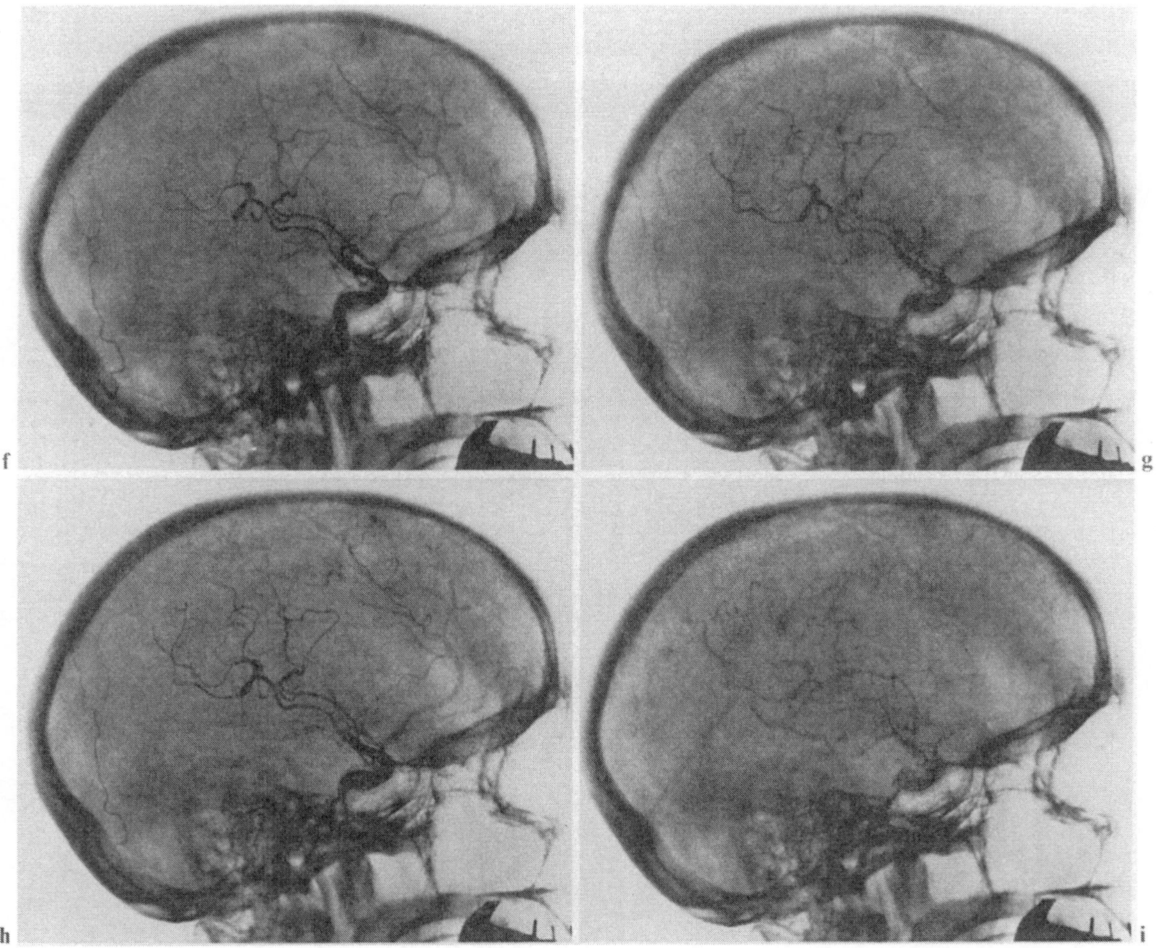

Abb. 12f–i

beweist aber keine Störmungsverbesserung, sondern ist lediglich der Ausdruck einer geringeren Verdünnung des Kontrastmittels in der A. carotis interna, da die Störung durch Hyperventilation etwas reduziert wird (KRUEGER et al., 1963; ROCKOFF et al., 1966; HUBER u. HANDA, 1967; DALLAS u. MOXOU, 1969; DU BOULAY et al., 1970; DU BOULAY u. SYMON, 1971).

Unter medikamentöser Blutdrucksteigerung verändert sich die angiographisch meßbare Zirkulationsgeschwindigkeit in normalen Hirnabschnitten nicht, die Arterien zeigen eine leichte bis mittelmässige Konstriktion (HUBER et al., 1971). In Hirnabschnitten mit Blutversorgung über Anastomosen oder bei Behinderung des anterograden Bluteinstromes durch Stenosen lassen sich bei gestörter Autoregulation unter medikamentöser Blutungssteigerung folgende Veränderung der Hämodynamik feststellen:

- Die Konstrastmittelpassage die über Anastomosen gefüllten Gefäßabschnitte erfolgt schneller, was dafür spricht, daß die Mikrozirkulation nicht blockiert ist. In diesen Fällen liegt eine effektive Strömungszunahme vor, worauf auch gelegentliche Therapieerfolge hinweisen (FARHAT u. SCHNEIDER, 1967).
- Unter Blutdrucksteigerung kann das Kontrastmittel in den retrograd gefüllten Gefäßabschnitten weiter nach der Verschlußstelle vorgetrieben werden. Diese Tatsache allein spricht aber nicht für eine Verbesserung der Zirkulation, sofern nicht auch die Kontrastmittelpassage beschleunigt wird. Eine auch unter Blutdrucksteigerung unveränderte Stase weist auf eine Blockierung der Mikrozirkulation hin, die retrograd gefüllten Abschnitte entsprechen unter diesen Bedingungen eher Sackgassen als echten Kollateralkreisläufen. Eine Blutdrucksteigerung in

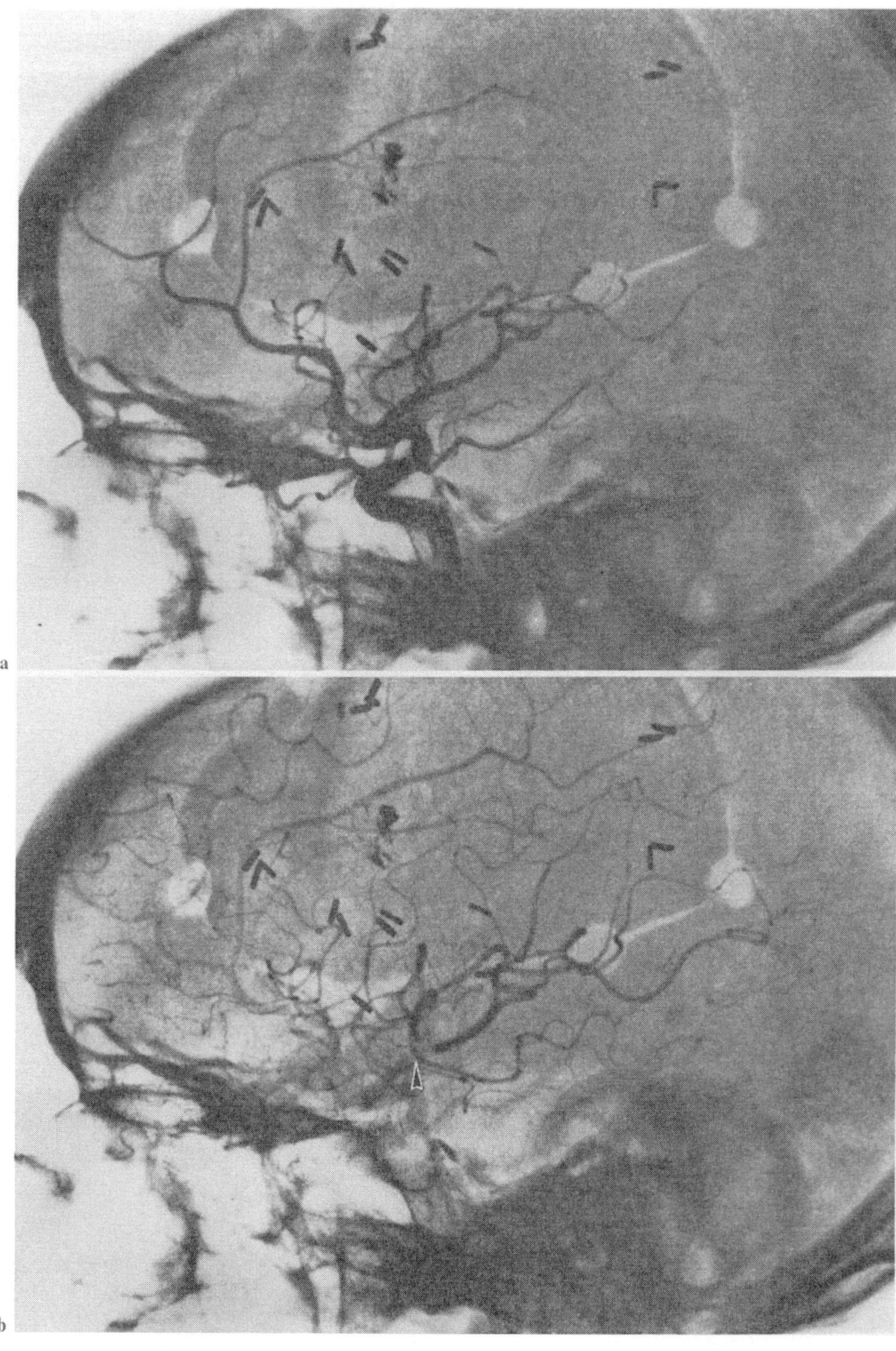

Abb. 13a–d. Iatrogener Embolus (frisches Fibringerinnsel) während der Kontrastmittelinjektion. Der Embolus sitzt an einer Gefäßteilungsstelle (**b**, Pfeil). Wegen der Gefäßblockierung wird die arterielle Entleerungsphase im Stromgebiet distal vom Embolus sehr stark verzögert **c–d**. Kontrollangiographie 90 Minuten später ohne jegliche therapeutische Maßnahme im Intervall: keine Füllungsdefekte mehr erkennbar, Zirkulationsgeschwindigkeit vollkommen normal. (Aus HUBER et al.: Z. Neurol. **200**, 248–266 (1971))

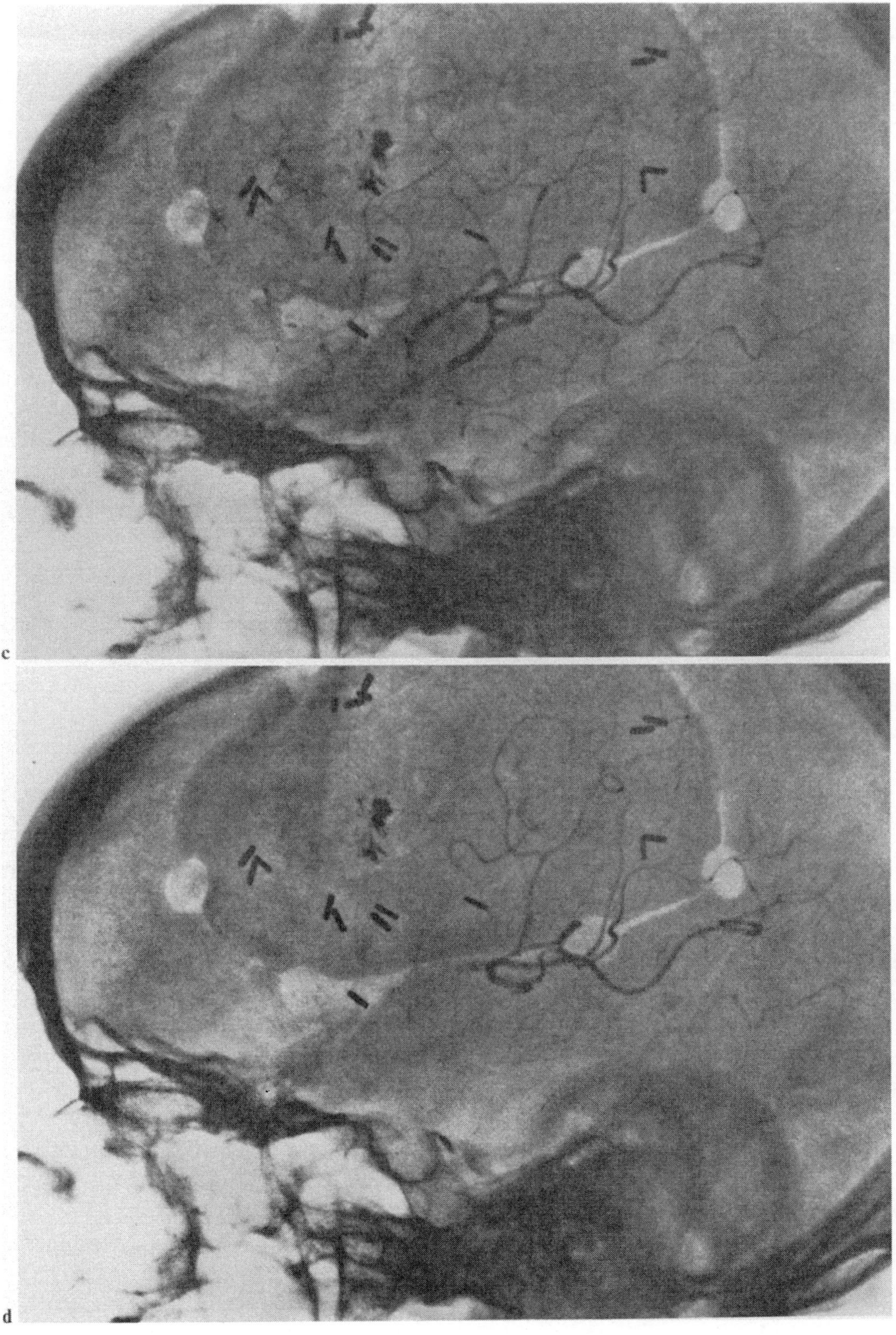

Abb. 13c u. d

dieser Situation birgt die Gefahr einer Blutung im Infarktbereich in sich (WALTZ u. SUNDT, 1967, 1969).

– Bei hämodynamisch signifikanten Stenosen kann die anterograde Zirkulation während eines Blutdruckabfalles stark behindert und verzögert werden. Unter Blutdrucksteigerung kann sich eine raschere und bessere Darstellung der peripheren Gefäßabschnitte einstellen, was auf eine echte Zirkulationsverbesserung hinweist (Abb. 12).

IV. Die Bedeutung der angiographischen Befunde. Korrelation zwischen Angiogramm und klinischer Symptomatologie

Das angiographische Bild hält die Kontrastmittelpassage in Momentaufnahmen fest und ist somit kein sehr zuverläßiger Indikator für die effektive Hirndurchblutung. Dies umso weniger, als sich die Mikrozirkulation einer angiographischen Beurteilung weitgehend entzieht. Darauf ist die nicht selten unbefriedigende Korrelation zwischen angiographischem Bild und klinischer Symptomatologie zurückzuführen. Die Messung der Passagezeit für das Kontrastmittel durch die Hirngefäße, eventuell mit Hilfe der fraktionierten Subtraktion nach RIVOIR und HUBER (1974) und die Beachtung der kapillären Anfärbung mit Hilfe des normalen Subtraktionsverfahrens erlauben indessen gewisse Rückschlüsse auf die Zirkulation im Parenchym, sofern die Injektionsdauer kurz gehalten wird. (TÖNNIS u. SCHIEFER, 1959; TAVERAS u. WOOD, 1964; FISCHGOLD et al., 1968).

Der Kontrastmittelgehalt in einem Gefäß ist jedoch ein unzuverläßiger Maßstab für die Beurteilung der Strömungsgröße, da an Anastomosestellen immer Beimischungen von kontrastmittellosem Blut aus nicht primär injizierten Gefäßabschnitten möglich sind, speziell im Bereiche des Circulus Willisi.

Die Korrelation zwischen neurologischen Störungen und Angiogramm ist relativ gut bei Verschlüssen der A. cerebri anterior und der A. pericallosa sowie der A. cerebri posterior, relativ schlecht bei Symptomen, die durch eine Schädigung von Bezirken im Mediastromgebiet liegen. BALOW et al. (1966) fanden bei Mediasymptomen einen Mediaverschluß nur in 13% der Fälle, in 37% lag ein Karotisverschluß vor und in 50% der Fälle konnte überhaupt kein Verschluß festgestellt werden. Diese schlechte Korrelation ist zum Teil dadurch zu erklären, daß ein Verschluß der lentikulostriären Arterien zwar zu Hemiparesen führt, daß diese feinen Arterien aber oft schlecht erkennbar und namentlich in ihrer Zahl variabel sind, weshalb ein Ausfall von einem oder zweien dieser Gefäße sich einem Nachweis entziehen kann. Wird die Angiographie erst einige Zeit nach dem akuten zerebralen Insult durchgeführt, so besteht die Möglichkeit, daß durch Lyse eines Embolus die Gefäße wieder rekanalisiert sind und der angiographische Befund somit trotz Halbseitenlähmung normal ist (GANNON u. CHAIT, 1962; FIESCHI u. BOZZOA, 1969). Nach SINDERMAN et al. (1969) kommt eine Rekanalisation in 24% der Fälle vor, oft schon innerhalb weniger Tage. Artifizielle Embolien während der Angiographie, namentlich bei der Verwendung von Punktionsnadeln mit offenem Hub, sind keineswegs selten (BATES u. BOOKSTEIN, 1966; ZATZ u. IANNONE, 1966; DAVIS et al., 1969; CRONQVIST et al., 1970; HUBER et al., 1971) und können vorbestehende Gefäßverschlüsse vortäuschen. Diese artifiziellen Embolien können gelegentlich nur durch Kontrollaufnahmen als solche erkannt werden, da sie sich in der Regel innerhalb weniger Minuten auflösen (HUBER et al., 1971; Abb. 13). FOIX und LEVY (1927) haben die klinischen Symptome bei Mediaverschlüssen in Beziehung zu den ischämischen Herden gesetzt und dabei eine recht gute Korrelation gefunden. Rein angiographisch läßt sich zwischen dem Verschluß der A. cerebri media oder ihren Ästen und der klinischen Symptomatologie in vielen Fällen zweifellos eine recht gute Korrelation feststellen (FROWEIN, 1956, 1961). Nicht selten ist aber die Übereinstimmung unbefriedigend. Ganz abgesehen davon, daß der Ausfall peripherer Mediaseitenäste u.U. schwierig zu erkennen ist (WADDINGTON u. RING, 1968; GERAUD et al., 1970; SALAMON et al., 1971) hängt dies auch damit zusammen, daß wir angiographisch die Infarktzone nicht abgrenzen können. Die regionale Strömungsmessung mit radioaktiven Isotopen vermag hier sehr oft bessere Auskunft zu geben (PAULSON, 1970; PAULSON et al., 1970). Die Darstellbarkeit von Kollateralkreisläufen an sich ist kein Beweis dafür, daß dieser Kollateralkreislauf auch suffizient ist. Umgekehrt ist es möglich, daß ein Kollateralkreislauf zu einem kleinen Infarktgebiet mit geringer, jedoch suffizienter Strömung nicht zur Darstellung kommt, weil das in ihm fließende Blut nicht genügend Kontrastmittelmengen mit sich führt.

Besondere Vorsicht ist bei der Interpretation diskreter angiographischer Befunde geboten, wie BULL et al. (1960) dargelegt haben. Bei Blindversuchen wurde festgestellt, daß die Beurteilung nicht nur zwischen verschiedenen erfahrenen Untersuchern erheblich schwanken kann, sondern daß auch ein und derselbe Untersucher bei wiederholten Befundungen zu unterschiedlichen Beurteilungen kommt. Dabei hat sich gezeigt, daß Gefäßschlängelungen und die Form der Aufteilung der A. carotis interna am Circulus Willisi kein Maß für den Elastizitätsverlust von Gefäßen bei Arteriosklerose sind und somit nicht als Hinweis für das Vorliegen einer zerebrovaskulären Erkrankung gelten können. Wandunregelmäßigkeiten kleinerer Gefäße sind an sich diagnostisch schon wertvoller, für sich allein jedoch häufig auch ungenügend. Ein Mikrobefund gewinnt an Zuverläßigkeit, wenn er durch andere Befunde gestützt wird, so z.B. der Füllungsabbruch in einem kleinen Gefäß, der mit einer lokalen Zirkulationsverzögerung oder einem retrograden Kontrastmitteleinstrom verbunden ist.

B. Stenosen und Verschlüsse der zum Hirn führenden Arterien proximal vom Circulus Willisi

I. Prädilektionsstellen

Aufgrund der klinischen Symptomatologie kann zwar die Stenose oder der Verschluß eines Gefäßes vermutet werden, doch kann nur die Angiographie den Beweis und Auskunft über morphologische Einzelheiten liefern. Die Gefäßpalpation am Hals ergibt unzuverläßige Resultate und auch das Strömungsgeräusch über den Halsarterien ist trügerisch (MCDOWELL et al., 1966). ZIEGLER et al. (1971) fanden bei 73% der Stenosen kein Geräusch, und umgekehrt konnte bei 10% der Fälle mit einem Geräusch keine Stenose nachgewiesen werden.

Atheromatöse Wandveränderungen, die zu Stenosen oder Verschlüssen führen, finden sich vorzugsweise an Biegungs- und Teilungsstelle der Arterien, also an Stellen mit besonders starker Wandbeanspruchung. BAKER und IANNONE (1961) bezeichnen, gestützt auf die Befunde an 1175 Autopsien, die Hypertonie als wichtigsten Faktor, wogegen die Wandbeanspruchung an Teilungsstellen nur eine kleine Rolle spiele. Die Bedeutung der Hypertonie als Risikofaktor wird auch von MCDOWELL et al. (1961) und RESCH und BAKER (1964) unterstrichen. Nach MEYER et al. (1960) und MCGEE et al. (1962) ist die Korrelation zwischen Erkrankungen des vertrebro-basilären Systems und Hypertonie besonders hoch. Die Verschlüsse im Vertebralisstromgebiet sind dabei besonders häufig, treten aber im Durchschnitt etwa eine Dekade später auf als im Karotisstromgebiet (MCDOWELL et al., 1961).

In Übereinstimmung mit Statistiken, die auf pathologisch-anatomischer Basis beruhen (BAKER u. IANNONE, 1959; BAKER et al., 1960; TORVIK u. JÖRGENSEN, 1964, 1966; JÖRGENSEN u. TORVIK, 1969) ergeben angiographische Untersuchungen eines größeren Krankengutes als am häufigsten befallene Stelle die Bifurkation der A. carotis communis, resp. die Anfangsstrecke der A. carotis interna (ELVIDGE u. WERNER, 1951; FISHER, 1951, 1954; JOHNSON u. WALKER, 1951; GURDJIAN u. WEBSTER, 1953; LIVINGSTON et al., 1955; WEBSTER et al., 1956; HUTCHINSON u. YATES, 1957; TATELMAN, 1958; GURDJIAN et al., 1959; PETERSON et al., 1960; GURDJIAN et al., 1961; MUMEN-

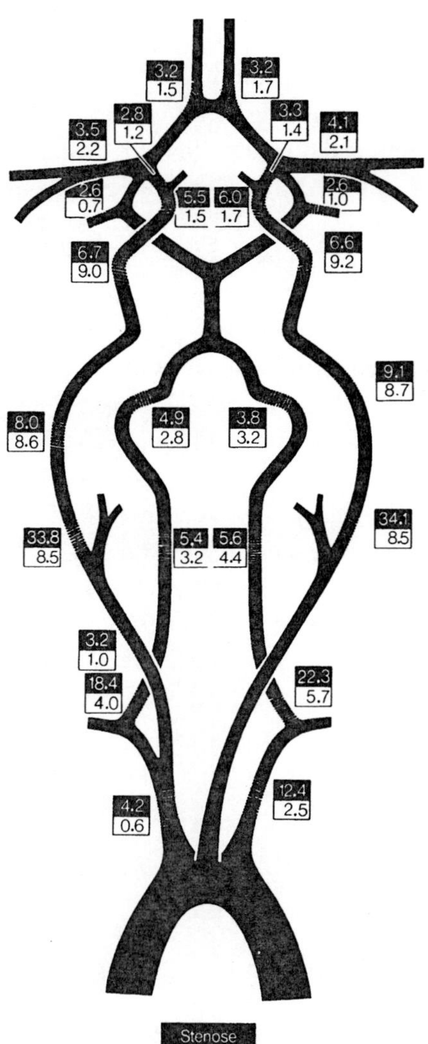

Abb. 14. Prädilektionsstellen der Stenosen und Verschlüsse. (Nach HASS et al.: Joint study of extracranial arterial occlusion. J.A.M.A. 203, 961–968 (1968))

THALER et al., 1961; YATES u. HUTCHINSON, 1961; MÜLLER et al., 1964; TAVERAS u. WOOD, 1964; KRAYENBÜHL u. YASARGIL, 1965; CHASE u. KRICHEFF, 1966; DORNDORFF u. GÄNSHIRT, 1972), gefolgt von der Abgangsstelle der A. vertebralis aus der A. subclavia. Aufgrund der American Joint Study (HASS et al., 1968), die 4748 Patienten mit zerebrovaskulären Erkrankungen erfaßt, wovon 3788 (80%) mit Vier-Gefäß-Angiographie untersucht wurden, verteilen sich die Läsionen folgendermaßen (Abb. 14):

- 41,2% der Patienten zeigen Gefäßerkrankungen (Stenosen oder Verschlüsse) nur im extrakraniellen Arteriensystem, wobei die Stenosen an allen Lokalisationen wesentlich häufiger sind als die Verschlüsse. An erster Stelle stehen dabei die Veränderungen im Bereiche der Karotisbifurkation.
- 67,3% der Patienten aus der gleichen Serie, jedoch nach einer früheren Auswertung, zeigen multiple Läsionen im chirurgisch angehbaren extrakraniellen Abschnitt (LYONS, 1965).
- 33,3% der Patienten weisen sowohl Läsionen im extra- wie im chirurgisch nicht angehbaren extra- oder intrakraniellen Abschnitt auf.
- Bei 6,1% der Patienten liegen nur chirurgisch nicht angehbare Läsionen vor und
- bei 19,4% der Patienten sind angiographisch keine Gefäßveränderungen faßbar.

In der älteren Literatur wird öfters darauf hingewiesen, daß die einem angiographisch nachgewiesenen Karotisverschluß zugrundeliegende Gefäßerkrankung häufig nicht näher bestimmt werden können (Riechert, 1938; Krayenbühl u. Weber, 1944; Decker u. Holzer, 1954). Viele dieser Autoren ziehen als Verschlußursache die Thrombangiitis obliterans in Erwägung (Krayenbühl u. Weber, 1944; Krayenbühl u. Richter, 1952; Elvidge u. Werner, 1951), wobei der Gefäßverschluß bei der Arteriosklerose für seltener gehalten wird als bei der Thrombangiitis obliterans (Decker u. Holzer, 1954; Tönnis u. Schiefer, 1959). Nach neueren Auffassungen (Blackwood, 1963) sollte diese Diagnose im Bereiche des Hirngefäßsystems nur mit größter Zurückhaltung gestellt werden, es sei denn, die folgenden drei Kriterien seien erfüllt:

1. akute entzündliche Reaktion der Hirnarterien mit Epitheloid- und Riesenzellen im Thrombus oder der Intima und Verschonung der Media (im Gegensatz zur Riesenzellarteriitis);
2. Obliteration von langen Gefäßstrecken und kortikalen Nekrosen bei nicht arteriosklerotischen oder syphilitischen Patienten;
3. gleichzeitiges Vorkommen der charakteristischen Thrombangiitis obliterans in den Gliedmaßengefäßen. Wahrscheinlich handelt es sich bei den früher zahlreich mitgeteilten Fällen von Thrombangiitis obliterans um Atherosklerosen mit Gefäßthrombosen und sekundärer entzündlicher Reaktion in der Gefäßwand.

Die Feststellung, daß Patienten mit Hirninfarkten häufig Stenosen oder Verschlüsse im extrakraniellen Gefäßabschnitt aufweisen und die Möglichkeit, durch einen chirurgischen Eingriff wiederum ein normales Gefäßlumen herzustellen (Hutchinson u. Yates, 1957; Lyons u. Galbraith, 1957; Luessenhop, 1959; Gurdjian et al., 1960), haben das Interesse vorwiegend auf diese Regionen gelenkt, wobei sich aber bald herausstellte, daß noch lange nicht jede in diesem Bereich festgestellte Stenose das klinische Bild zu erklären vermag (Fazekas et al., 1963; Millikan, 1963), da die Blutströmung offensichtlich nicht dem Gesetz von Poiseuille folgt (Barnett, 1965). Auch die postmortalen Untersuchungen vermochten nicht wesentlich weiter zu helfen, obgleich an einer Serie von 130 Autopsien Stein et al., (1963) zeigen konnten, daß alle Patienten mit klinischen Symptomen Gefäßstenosen aufgewiesen haben. 20% der Patienten aus dieser Serie waren aber trotz Stenosen symptomfrei geblieben. Faris et al. (1963) fanden sogar bei der Hälfte von angiographisch untersuchten Patienten ohne zerebrovaskuläre Symptome als Zufallsbefunde Lumeneinengungen an Karotiden und Vertebralarterien. Es zeigte sich, daß die chirurigsche Korrektur einer Stenose, die den Gefäßdurchmesser um weniger als 50% eingeengt hatte, postoperativ zu keiner wesentlichen Strömungszunahme führte (Crawford et al., 1962; Delin et al., 1968). Es sind offensichtlich embolische Komplikationen der atheromatösen Plaques, die in der Mehrzahl der Fälle – ganz unabhängig vom Ausmaß der Stenosierung – die neurologischen Ausfälle verursachen.

II. Stenosen durch atherosklerotische Wandveränderungen

Atheromatöse Wandveränderungen – die bei weitem häufigste Ursache der Stenosen – sind auf einen Sektor des Gefäßquerschnittes beschränkt, sofern sie nicht sehr ausgedehnt sind. Demzufolge können sie in einer Strahlenrichtung sichtbar werden, in einer anderen aber verborgen bleiben. Bei der angiographischen Abklärung der verschiedenen Formen des zerebralen Schlaganfalles sind die typischen Prädilektionsstellen der atheromatösen Wandveränderungen, speziell die Karotisbifurkation, in verschiedenen Strahlenrichtungen darzustellen, zumindest aber in anterioposteriorem und seitlichem Strahlengang.

1. Die atheromatösen Wandveränderungen an der A. carotis interna

Auf Höhe der Karotisbifurkation sitzen die atheromatösen Plaques häufig an der Gefäßhinterwand (Kishore 1974) und nur bei stärkerer Ausdehnung wird das Gefäßlumen allseitig eingeengt,

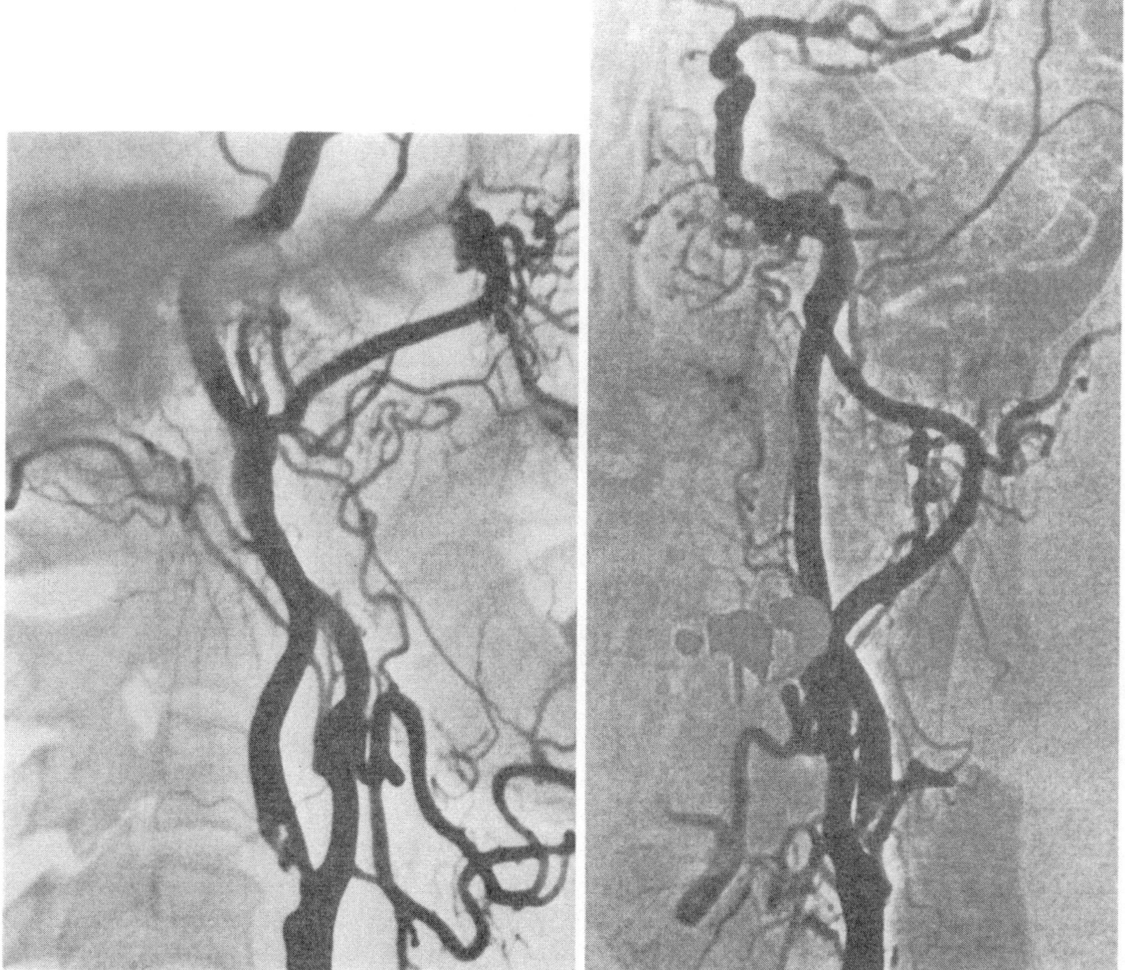

Abb. 15. Stenose der A. carotis interna im Anfangsabschnitt. Die atheromatöse Plaque sitzt an der Gefäßhinterwand und weist in der Mitte ein Ulcus auf, das auf der anteroposterioren Aufnahme nicht zur Darstellung kommt. (Aus „Zerebrale Angiographie", Thieme Stuttgart, 1979)

wobei aber trotzdem meist der exzentrische Ausgangspunkt der Stenosierung deutlich erkennbar bleibt. Der durch die Plaques verursachte Füllungsdefekt ist meist scharf begrenzt und unregelmäßig geformt (Abb. 15). Völlig konzentrische Lumeneinengungen mit glatter Gefäßwand entsprechen eher einem Prozeß, der die äußeren Wandschichten befallen hat, so z.B. entzündliche Veränderungen. Die konzentrische Gefäßeinengung schließt jedoch die Atherosklerose keineswegs aus. Von differentialdiagnostischer Bedeutung kann der Nachweis von Wandverkalkungen an dieser Stelle sein (Abb. 16).

a) Das atheromatöse Ulkus; die zerebrale Embolie

Im Zusammenhang mit den flüchtigen Insulten (transient ischemic attacks), die nach neueren Ansichten weniger auf einer Drosselung der Strömung durch die Stenose an sich als vielmehr durch Embolien, die von einer atheromatösen Plaque oder einem Appositionsthrombus abgehen (PICKERING, 1948; FISHER, 1959; JULIAN et al., 1963; BLADIN, 1964; GUNNIG et al., 1965; MILLIKAN, 1965; EHRENFELD et al., 1966; MOORE u. HALL, 1968; MADDISON u. MOORE, 1969; WOOD u. CORREL, 1969; KISHORE et al., 1971b; KISHORE, 1974) ist die sorgfältige Suche nach Ulzera,

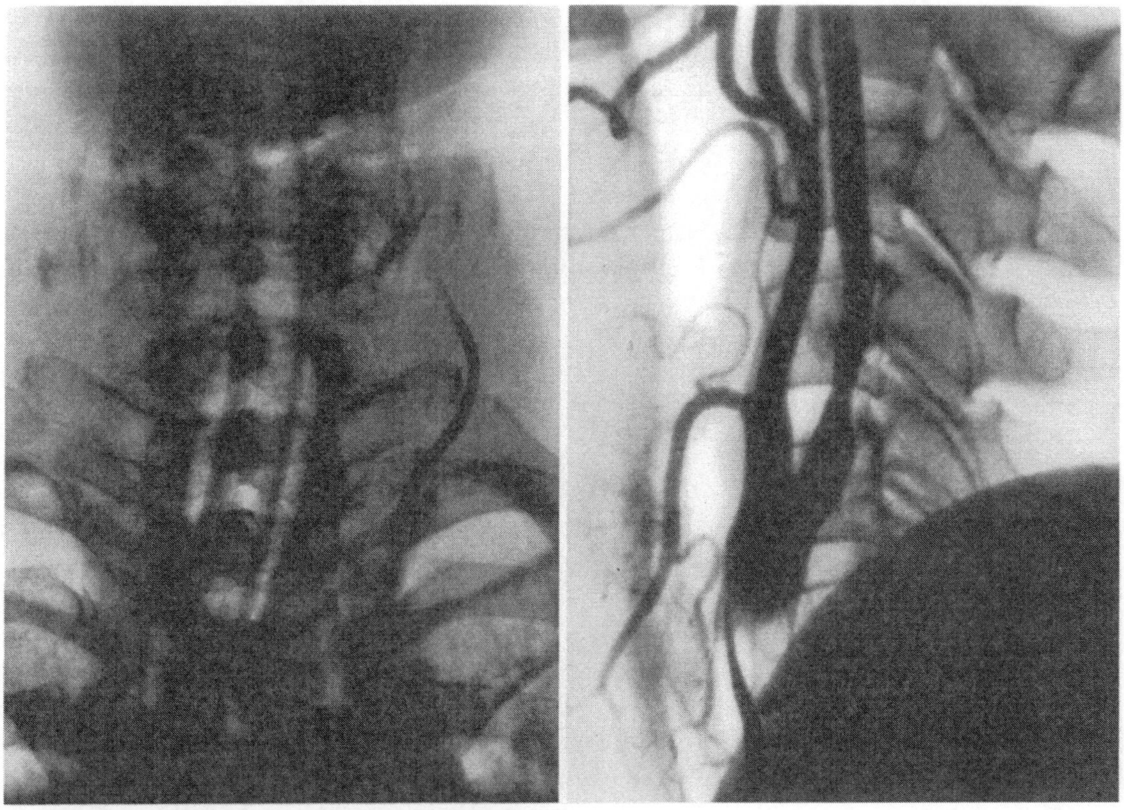

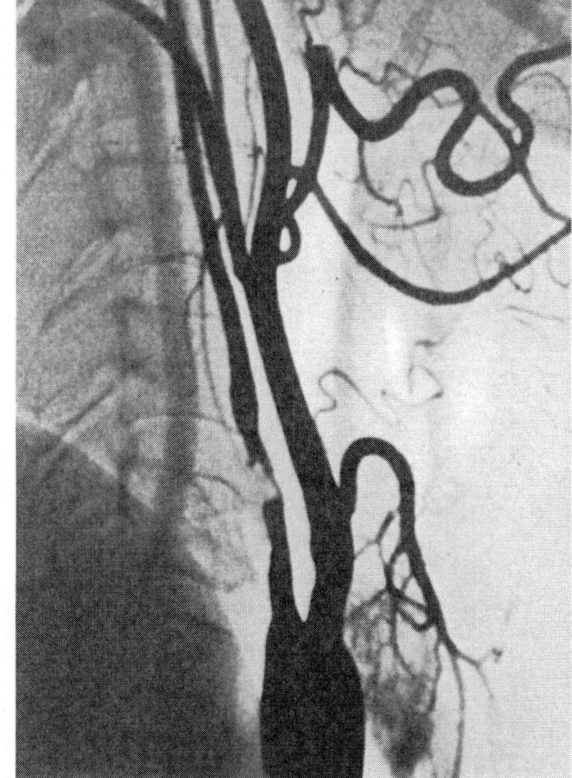

Abb. 16a. a-p-Aufnahme des Halses mit Wandverkalkungen der A. carotis interna beidseits. **b** Konzentrische und glattwandige Stenose im Anfangsabschnitt der A. carotis interna links. **c** Hochgradige Stenose der A. carotis interna rechts durch atheromatöse Plaque an der Gefäßhinterwand. Relativ dünne A. carotis interna, möglicherweise als Folge der verminderten Strömung. (Unter dem Injektionsdruck retrograder Kontrastmittelfluß in der A. carotis communis, so daß auch die A. vertebralis dargestellt wird). (Abb. 16b aus „Zerebrale Angiographie", Thieme Stuttgart, 1979)

die auch in kleinen Plaques auftreten können, von besonderer Wichtigkeit. Diese Ulzera sind die häufigste bedeutungsvolle Komplikation der Atherosklerose der großen Halsgefässe. Durch Aufbrechen der Plaques entleert sich Atherombrei in den Blutstrom (MCBRIEN et al., 1963), wodurch es zur Entstehung des Ulkus kommt. Das ausgeschwemmte Material gelangt mit dem Hauptblutstrom zum gößten Teil in das Stromgebiet der A. cerebri media. LUESSENHOP (1969) wies nach, daß von 100 Emboli, die artifiziell in die A. carotis interna eingebracht wurden, um eine arteriovenöse Mißbildung zu verschliessen, 90 in die A. cerebri media und nur 10 in die A. cerebri anterior gelangten, obgleich die Mißbildung in gleicher Weise von A. cerebri anterior und media versorgt wurde. Nach KISHORE (1974) zeigen 17% der Patienten mit zerebrovaskulärer Insuffizienz Ulzera an den Karotiden und weitere 17% weisen unregelmäßig aufgerauhte Oberflächen der Plaques auf. Nach WOOD und CORREL (1969) kommen in 54% der atheromatösen Plaques Ulzera vor, wobei aber offenbar keine Korrelation zwischen Ausmaß der Stenose und Häufigkeit der Ulzera besteht. Nicht selten sind die Stenosen bei gleichzeitigem Ulkus sogar geringer, möglicherweise infolge der Entleerung von Atherombrei aus der Plaque. Glatte Stenosen zeigen nach KISHORE et al. (1971 b) nur in 16% noch zusätzliche Mediaverschlüsse oder Stenosen, während bei unregelmäßigen Stenosen oder Ulzera in 33% der Fälle zusätzliche Mediaverschlüsse vorliegen. Im Vertebralisstromgebiet sind derartige Ulzera offenbar wesentlich seltener und transitorische Basilarisinsuffizienzen scheinen sich eher auf hämodynamischer Basis abzuspielen (RUSSEL, 1970).

Die Entwicklung einer atheromatösen Plaque ist mit einer Atrophie der darunterliegenden Muskularis und Elastika verbunden, was zu einer Wandschwächung führt. Die Ulzera können sich nach Ausschwemmung des Atherombreies deshalb fuchsbauartig bis zur Adventitia erstrecken, überragen aber die normale äußere Gefäßlinie nicht. Durch Aufrauhung der Gefäßinnenwand nach der Ulkusbildung kann es ferner zur Ablagerung von frischen, leicht ablösbaren Thromben kommen, so daß z.B. durch ein äußeres Trauma der Halsregion weitere Embolien abgesprengt werden können. Die meisten Ulzera sitzen nicht weiter als 2,5 cm von der Karotisbifurkation entfernt an der Karotishinterwand (MADDISON u. MOORE, 1969), selbst wenn diese auch noch weiter distal atheromatöse Veränderungen aufweist. Arkogramme und gewöhnliche Profilaufnahmen bringen diese Ulzera nur in etwa 30% zur Darstellung, wogegen mit einer gezielten Exploration der Karotisbifurkation in 70% der Fälle mit flüchtigen Insulten sichere ulzeröse Läsionen dargestellt werden können (WIGGLI u. OBERSON, 1973). Diese Autoren empfehlen deshalb als

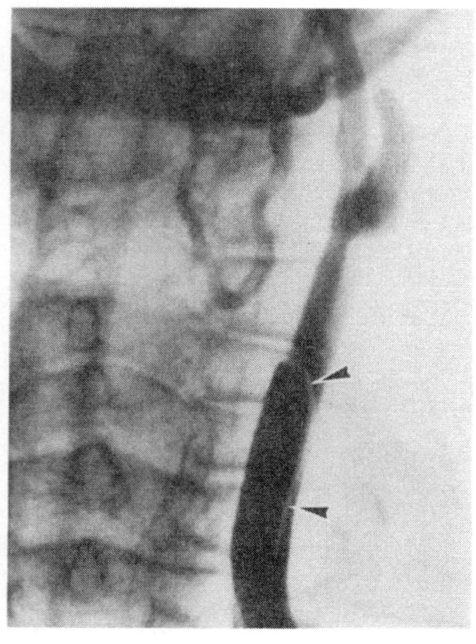

Abb. 17. Subintimale Kontrastmittelinjektion. Die abgehobene Intima ist deutlich erkennbar (Pfeile)

Untersuchungsgang bei den flüchtigen Insulten nach transfemoraler Kathetrisierung die gezielte Exploration der statistisch am häufigsten von gefäßdegenerativen Prozessen betroffenen Karotisbifurkation. Bei negativem Befund wird die Arkographie angeschlossen. Sind diese Abklärungen negativ, so steigt die Wahrscheinlichkeit einer kardiogenen oder pulmogenen Embolusquelle. Nach BARRON et al. (1960) stammen ca. 10% der zerebralen Embolien aus dem Herzen (bakterielle oder rheumatische Endokarditiden ausgeschlossen). Die am häufigsten bei dieser Endokarditisform anzutreffende weitere Krankheit ist das Karzinom.

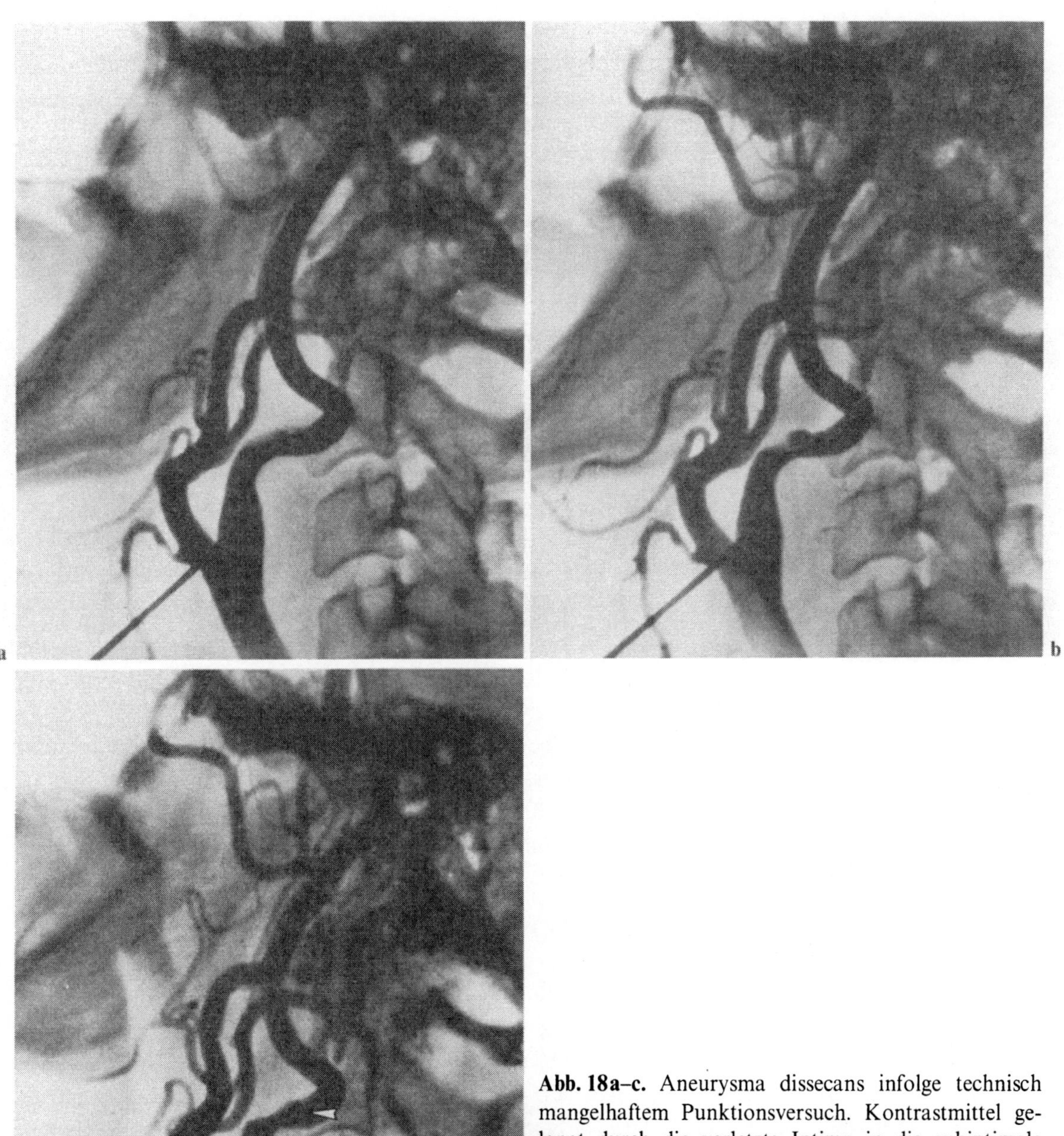

Abb. 18a–c. Aneurysma dissecans infolge technisch mangelhaftem Punktionsversuch. Kontrastmittel gelangt durch die verletzte Intima in die subintimale Tasche (**a** u. **b**). **c** Kontrollangiographie: das subintimale Hämatom wölbt sich noch gegen das Gefäßlumen vor, füllt sich aber nicht mehr mit Kontrastmittel. Faltenbildung der Intima als heller Streifen (Pfeil) immer noch erkennbar (ähnlich wie "clamp defect"). (Aus „Zerebrale Angiographie“, Thieme Stuttgart, 1979)

Das typische Bild der Ulzeration besteht in einem oft etwas langgezogenen, unregelmäßig begrenzten intramuralen Hohlraum im Bereich einer Plaque, wobei die Öffnung des Ulkus gegen das Gefäßlumen zu etwas exzentrisch in der Plaque liegt, meist in Strömungsrichtung. Mikroulzera sind trichterartige, nur wenige Millimeter tiefe, intramurale Defekte. In den größeren Ulzera, deren Grund als normale Gefäßwand zwischen zwei Stenosen imponieren kann, ist bei rascher Serienangiographie nicht selten ein Schichtungseffekt zu beobachten.

b) Differentialdiagnostik

Differentialdiagnostisch sind die Ulzera aufgrund folgender Kriterien leicht von intramuralen Kontrastmittelinjektionen zu unterscheiden.:

- im iatrogen entstandenen Aneurysma dissecans bleibt das Kontrastmittel sehr lange liegen.
- Die Kontrastmitteldichte ist bei der subintimalen und intramuralen Injektion wesentlich höher als im Gefäßlumen oder in einem Ulkus, da das Kontrastmittel ohne Verdünnung durch den Blutstrom direkt in die Gefäßwand injiziert worden und vom strömenden Blut abgeschlossen ist.
- Bei der intramuralen Injektion stellt sich die abgehobene Intima als feine, strahlendurchläßige Linie dar (Abb. 17).
- Schwierigkeiten in der Diagnose können subintimale Hämatome nach vorausgegangenen schwierigen Punktionsversuchen bedeuten, wenn sich der Hohlraum unter der abgehobenen Intima nicht mehr mit Kontrastmittel füllt (Abb. 18).

2. Die Atherosklerose der A. vertebralis

Während sich an der A. carotis interna die atheromatösen Wandveränderungen und die dadurch bedingten Stenosen zur Hauptsache auf zwei Stellen, den Anfangsabschnitt der A. carotis interna und den Karotissiphon konzentrieren, sind sie an der A. vertebralis neben der Hauptlokalisation am untersten Abschnitt (Abb. 19) über die ganze Gefäßstrecke verteilt. Die Verhältnisse werden zudem an der A. vertebralis dadurch kompliziert, daß durch Osteophyten (Unkarthrose) das Gefäß verlagert wird (Abb. 20). Eine eigentliche Gefäßkompression mit Stenosierung wird durch die Osteophyten allerdings von CHASE und KRICHEFF (1966) und LEGRÉ et al. (1967) als ungewöhnlich bezeichnet, während andere Autoren (TATLOW u. BAMMER, 1957; MEYER et al., 1960; SHEEHAN et al., 1960; BAUER et al., 1961) sie besonders bei Extrembewegungen des Kopfes für bedeutungsvoll halten, indem sie, zusammen mit arteriosklerotischen Veränderungen, im Endstromgebiet über den Mechanismus der Strömungsreduktion zu klinischen Symptomen führen. In der A. vertebralis sind Ulzera im Bereich von atheromatösen Plaques eine Seltenheit (RUSSEL, 1970).

3. Die Atherosklerose der A. basilaris

Nach der American Joint study (HASS et al., 1968) finden sich Stenosen der A. basilaris in 7.7% der wegen zerebrovaskulären Erkrankungen untersuchten Patienten. Bei 41% der Patienten mit Basilarisinsuffizienzsyndromen konnten BALOW et al. (1966) angiographisch atheromatöse Veränderungen der A. basilaris nachweisen. LEGRÉ et al. (1967) unterscheiden fünf verschiedene Typen der Atherosklerose der A. basilaris, wovon nur einer durch erhebliche filiforme Lumeneinengungen charakterisiert ist (stenosierender Typus). Die Stenosierung erstreckt sich vorwiegend über das mittlere und kraniale Drittel der A. basilaris und kann zu einer Mangeldurchblutung der Ae. cerebellares superiores und der Ae. cerebri posteriores führen. Eine zweite Form zeichnet sich durch deutliche Wandunregelmäßigkeiten aus, die durch eine oder mehrere atheromatöse Plaques bedingt sind. Derartige Plaques können außerdem auch an der A. cerebri posterior sitzen, wodurch die Strömung so stark reduziert wird, daß es zu einem thrombotischen Verschluß kommt.

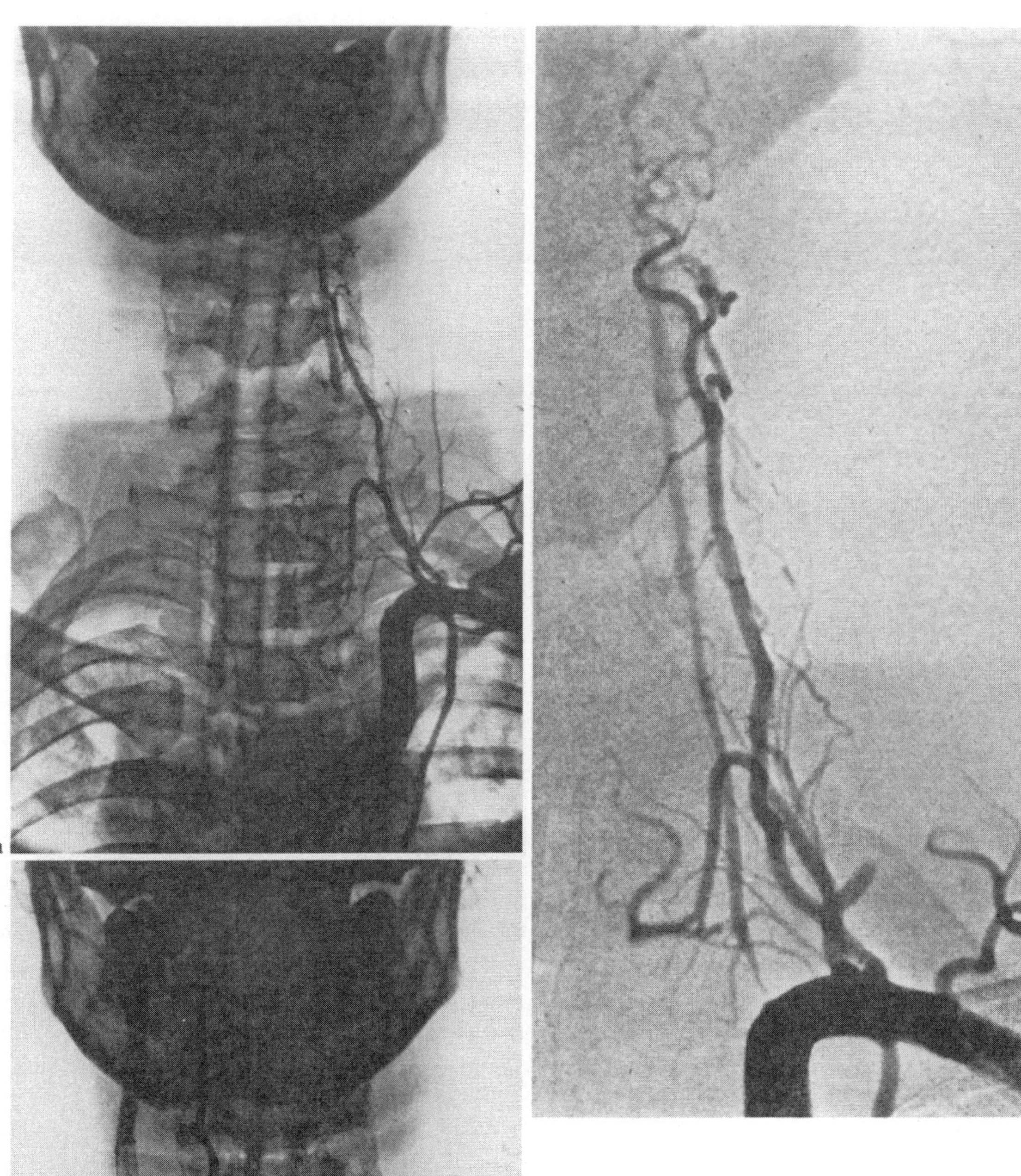

Abb. 19. a Verschluß der linken A. vertebralis an der Abgangsstelle aus der A. subclavia. Kollateralkreislauf zum distalen Vertebralisabschnitt über die A. cervicalis ascendens. **b** Kontrollaufnahme 1 Jahr später: Die A. vertebralis stellt sich bis zur A. subclavia dar, der Anfangsabschnitt ist aber sehr eng, die Verbindung zur A. subclavia kann angiographisch nicht bewiesen werden. Der Kollateralkreislauf über die A. cervicalis ascendens ist immer noch funktionstüchtig, die Arterie hat sich sogar etwas erweitert (Ausmessung auf Originalfilm). **c** Stenose an der Abgangsstelle der A. vertebralis rechts. (Abb. 19a und c aus „Zerebrale Angiographie", Thieme Stuttgart, 1979)

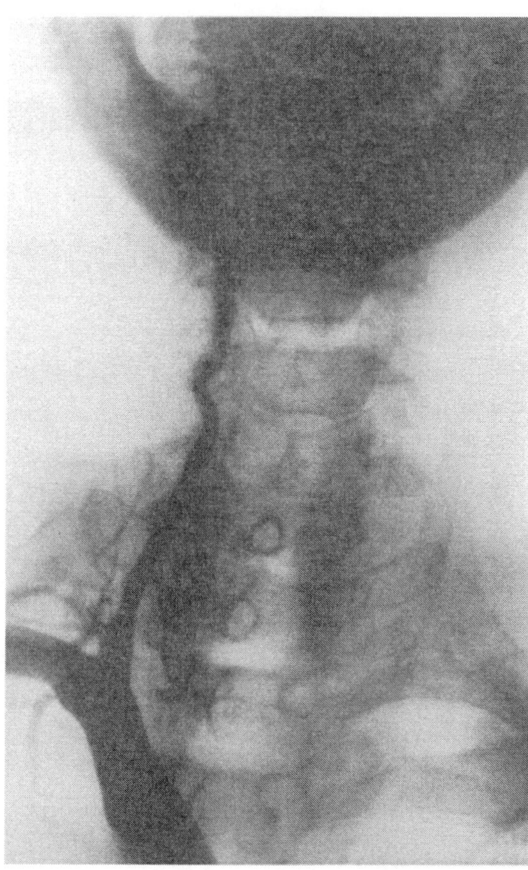

Abb. 20. Verlagerung der A. vertebralis durch Osteophyten (Uncarthrose). Das Gefäßlumen ist nicht eingeengt

Füllungsdefekte in der A. basilaris sind aber nur dann mit Sicherheit zu diagnostizieren, wenn bei der Vertebralisangiographie ein Reflux von kontrastmittelhaltigem Blut in die kontralaterale A. vertebralis erfolgt, da sonst die Beimischung von kontrastmittelfreiem Blut aus der kontralateralen A. vertebralis und fehlender Durchmischung der Blutströme (laminäre Strömung) in der A. basilaris Füllungsdefekte vorgetäuscht werden können. Dies tritt besonders dann auf, wenn zufälligerweise die engere A. vertebralis kathetrisiert und durch einen zu weiten Katheter das Lumen stark eingeengt wird, so daß der Bluteinstrom aus der kontralateralen weiteren A. vertebralis eindeutig dominiert. Das gleiche Phänomen tritt bei direkter Vertebralispunktion und nicht ganz korrekter Nadellage auf und kann sogar einen Basilarisverschluß vortäuschen (SCHECHTER u. ZINGESSER, 1965).

Daneben existieren Formen der Basilarisatherosklerose, die zu einer Gefäßlongation, vermehrten Schlängelung und allgemeinen Dilatation, der sog. Megalodolichobasilaris (BOERI u. PASSERINI, 1964) führen. Durch diese Wandveränderungen wird weniger die Strömung in der A. basilaris selbst als vielmehr diejenige in ihren Seitenästen zur Pons beeinträchtigt. Die verschiedenen Formen der Basilarissklerose können kombiniert vorkommen und finden sich besonders häufig bei der Hypertonie.

4. Die Entwicklung der Atherosklerose

Trotz der Vielzahl von Arbeiten über die angiographischen Untersuchungsbefunde bei Patienten mit atheromatösen Gefäßläsionen ist über die Entwicklung der Plaque bis zum Auftreten von zerebralen Mangeldurchblutungen und die Veränderungen der einmal festgestellten Läsionen im

Verlaufe der Zeit im Einzelfall relativ wenig bekannt. BAUER et al. (1968) haben bei 48 Patienten die Prädilektionsstellen für die Entwicklung von atherosklerotischen Gefäßwandschädigungen nach einem durchschnittlichen Intervall von 36,2 Monaten nachkontrolliert und dabei festgestellt, daß 77,8% der zur Überprüfung ausgewählten Stellen bei der Primäruntersuchung unauffällig gewesen waren. 94% dieser initial unauffälligen Stellen zeigten auch bei der späteren Kontrolle keine angiographisch faßbaren Veränderungen. Von den restlichen 22,2% der bei der Erstuntersuchung bereits einen pathologischen Befund aufweisenden Stellen waren später 77,7% unverändert und 22% zeigten eine Progression der Atherosklerose. 9,3% der untersuchten Stellen zeigten in einem durchschnittlichen Zeitintervall von 24,9 Monaten somit eine Progression von normal zu pathologisch oder von pathologisch zu stärker pathologisch, wobei allerdings die intrakraniellen Gefäße mit einem Innendurchmesser von weniger als 2 mm in dieser Studie nicht eingeschlossen sind. Ferner werden nur die Größe der Plaques, resp. das Ausmaß der Stenose berücksichtigt, nicht aber die morphologischen Veränderungen bereits bestehender Plaques, resp. das Auftreten von Ulzera und deren eventuelle Veränderungen.

III. Nicht durch Atherosklerose bedingte Stenosen

1. Spasmen und Entzündungen

Als Folge der direkten Gefäßpunktion können Spasmen auftreten, die das Gefäßlumen ganz erheblich einengen (DECKER, 1965). Ähnliche spastische Lumeneinengungen kommen aber auch nach Katheteruntersuchungen vor (SCHECHTER, 1963). Diese spastischen Lumeneinengungen dehnen sich in der Regel nicht bis in den intrakraniellen Karotisabschnitt aus. Die Stenosierung erfolgt im Unterschied zu den atheromatösen Plaques ganz allmählich ohne scharfe Abgrenzung und ist konzentrisch und glattwandig.

Ein ähnliches Bild kann nach stumpfem Trauma der A. carotis interna im extra- oder intrakraniellen Abschnitt zustande kommen, wobei in schweren Fällen eine Verletzung der Gefäßintima oder die Entwicklung eines Hämatoms in der Gefäßwand sogar den vollständigen Verschluß der A. carotis interna verursachen kann (ECKER, 1945; FRANTZEN et al., 1961; FREIDENFELT u. SUNDSTRÖM, 1963; GURDJIAN et al., 1963; HUBER, 1964; FLEMING u. PETRIC, 1968; HUGHES u. BROWNELL, 1968; JANON, 1970; GURDJIAN et al., 1971; SULLIVAN et al., 1973).

Ein im wesentlichen gleiches angiographisches Bild wird durch das seltene spontane Aneurysma dissecans der A. carotis interna verursacht, dessen Ursache eine Degeneration der Gefäßmedia (Elastika oder Muskularis) ist (ANDERSON u. SCHECHTER, 1959; ISLER, 1960; SPUDIS et al., 1962; BROWN u. ARMITAGE, 1973; Abb. 21).

Bei Kindern kommen hochgradige Stenosierungen oder Verschlüsse im Bereiche des Endabschnittes der A. carotis interna vor, die sich auf die A. cerebri media ausdehnen können. Diese Stenosen sitzen meist distal vom Abgang der A. ophthalmica und die A. chorioidea anterior ist meist noch durchgängig, was wichtig für die Entwicklung eines Kollateralkreislaufes ist. Die lentikulostriären Arterien sind von der Stenosierung häufig in Mitleidenschaft gezogen, was zu einer Ischämie im Bereiche der Basalganglien und der Capsula interna führt. Rekanalisationen der verschlossenen oder stenosierten Abschnitte kommen aber vor (HILAL et al., 1971a). Häufig bleibt die Ursache dieser Stenosierungen oder Verschlüsse ungeklärt, doch kommt aufgrund von histologischen Befunden eine Vaskulitis in Frage (BAKER, 1961; BICKERSTAFF, 1964; SHILLITO, 1964). Auch ein Aneurysma dissecans, eventuell auf der Grundlage einer Arteritis kommt als Ursache in Betracht (NORMAN u. ULRICH, 1957; WOLMAN, 1959; SCOTT et al., 1960; NEDWICH et al., 1963; DONROV et al., 1964; ROBERT et al., 1964; KUNZE u. SCHIEFER, 1971).

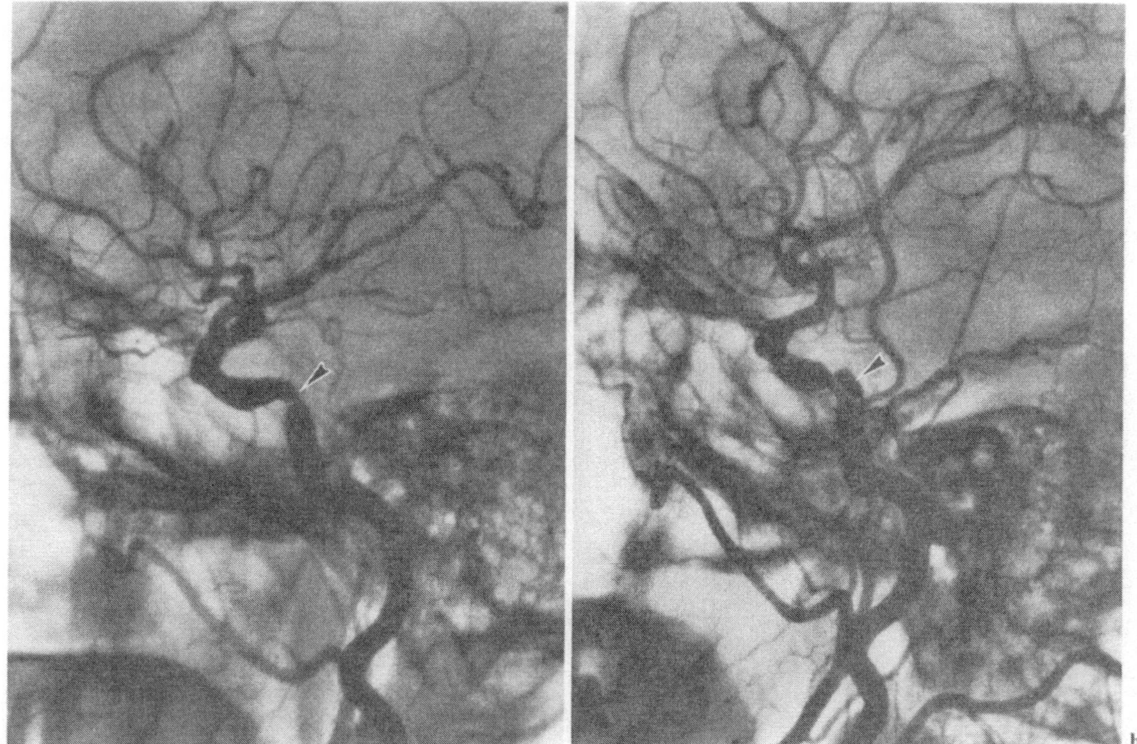

Abb. 21. a Carotisangiogramm nach Insult. Hochgradige Stenose im Anfangsabschnitt des Karotissiphons. Ursache der Stenose ungeklärt, Atherosklerose? **b** Carotisangiogramm 1 Jahr später nach erneutem Insult. Unverändert hochgradige Stenose, an deren Dorsalseite jetzt ein lokalisiertes Aneurysma dissecans sichtbar ist. (Der Patient wurde nach dem 1. Insult wegen der Stenose mit Antikoagulantien behandelt.) (Aus „Zerebrale Angiographie", Thieme Stuttgart, 1979)

MOMOSE und NEW (1973) zählten unter 7000 Angiogrammen 1440 Fälle von Stenosen oder Verschlüssen der A. carotis interna, die nicht durch eine Atherosklerose verursacht waren. Abgesehen von den am häufigsten vorkommenden fehlenden Darstellungen der intrakraniellen Gefäße infolge eines sehr stark erhöhten intrakraniellen Druckes spielen unter diesen zu Stenosen oder Verschlüssen führenden Prozessen die Tumoren der Schädelbasis eine wichtige Rolle, speziell die parasellären Meningiome (ISFORT, 1961; CONSTANS et al., 1967). Daneben kommen als Ursache auch entzündliche Affektionen primärer oder sekundärer Art in Betracht, wie Riesenzellarteritis, Meningitis purulenta, Osteomyelitis der Schädelbasis, Tuberkulose, Mukormykose beim Diabetiker und Phykomykosen (CARPENTER et al., 1968; COUREY et al., 1973).

2. Die fibromuskuläre Dysplasie

Bei der fibromuskulären Dysplasie handelt es sich um eine Angiopathie unbekannter Aetiologie, die hauptsächlich die Arterien mittlerer Größe befällt, wobei es im wesentlichen zu segmentären Stenosen kommt. Der pathologische Prozeß besteht in einer Wandfibrose und einer Destruktion der elastischen Fasern, der vorwiegend die Media betrifft, jedoch auch auf die anderen Wandschichten übergreifen kann. Er kann mit oder ohne Hyperplasie der muskulären Fasern einhergehen und da er gleichzeitig hyperplastisch und destruktiv ist, ist die Bezeichnung fibromuskuläre Dysplasie dem ursprünglichen Ausdruck fibromuskuläre Hyperplasie, der von MCCORMACK et al. (1958) bei der Beschreibung dieser Affektion an den Nierenarterien geprägt worden ist, vorzuziehen (HUNT et al., 1965; KINCAID et al., 1968). Nachdem diese Erkrankung auch an anderen extrarena-

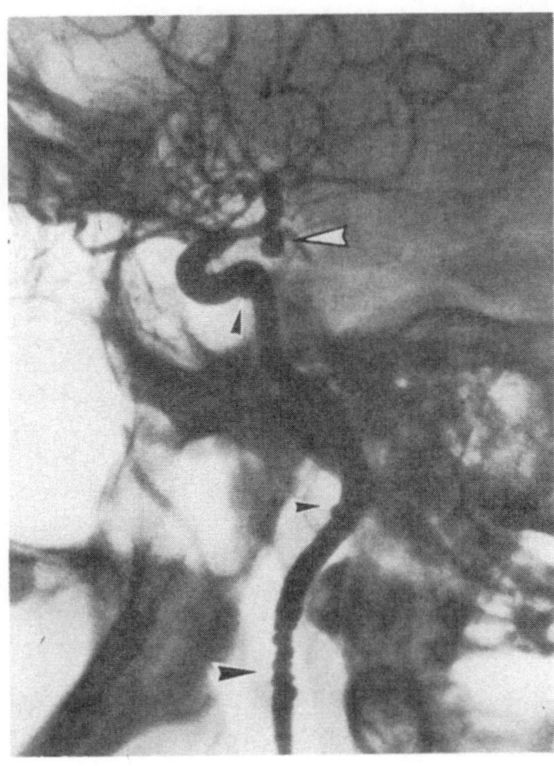

Abb. 22

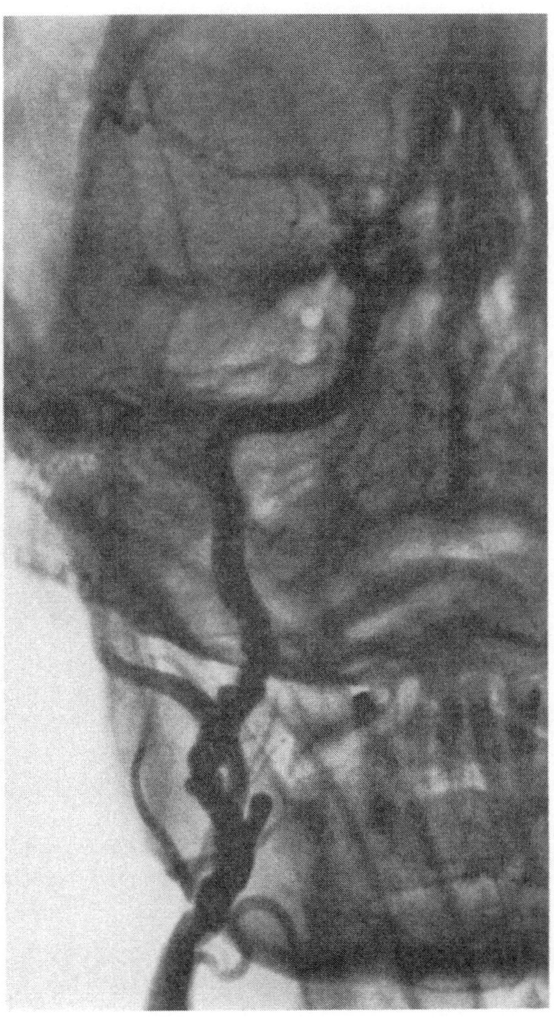

Abb. 23

Abb. 22. Gleichzeitiges Vorkommen eines sackförmigen Aneurysmas (offener Pfeil) und der fibromuskulären Dysplasie. Neben dem typischen Wechsel von Stenosen und Lumenerweiterungen im oberen Zervikalbereich (großer Pfeil) finden sich noch 2 Mikroaneurysmen an der A. carotis interna (kleine Pfeile)

Abb. 23. Fibroplasie der Media mit Wandaneurysmen auf Höhe der Halswirbel C1–C3. Der Gefäßabschnitt mit den angiographisch sichtbaren Wandveränderungen (Aspekt der "Chaussettes en accordéon") erscheint eher etwas weiter als die übrigen Gefäßstrecken

len Arterien beobachtet worden war, veröffentlichten PALUBINSKAS und RIPLEY (1964) die erste Beschreibung eines Befalles des extrakraniellen Karotisabschnittes, der in rascher Folge zahlreiche weitere Publikationen folgten (u.a. HILL u. ANTONIUS, 1965; EHRENFELD et al., 1967; HOUSER u. BAKER, 1968; ANDERSEN, 1970; HOUSER et al., 1971; KISHORE et al., 1971a; SUKOFF et al., 1971). Veränderungen an intrakraniellen Arterien, die dem angiographischen Bild der fibromuskulären Dysplasie entsprechen könnten, wurden von HUBER und FUCHS (1967) und IOSUE et al. (1972) mitgeteilt, allerdings ohne histologische Verifikation.

Auf das gleichzeitige Vorkommen der fibromuskulären Dysplasie mit sackförmigen Aneurysmen der Hirngefäße (PALUBINSKAS et al., 1966; KRAMER, 1969; ANDERSEN, 1970; HANDA et. al., 1970; HARRINGTON et al., 1970; HOUSER et al., 1971; Abb. 22) oder mit arteriovenösen Mißbildungen

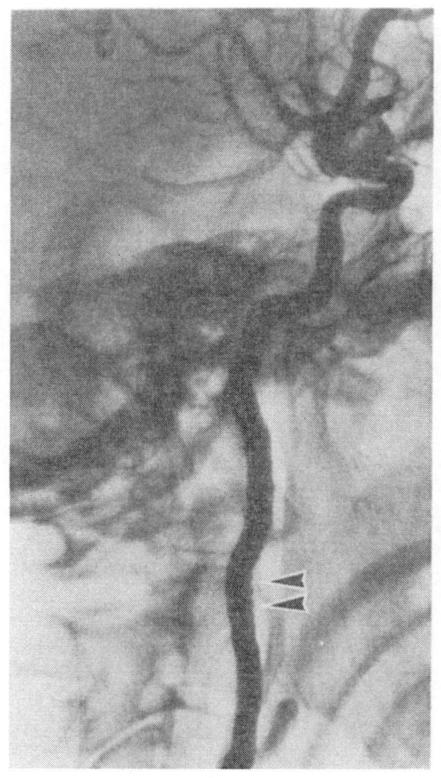

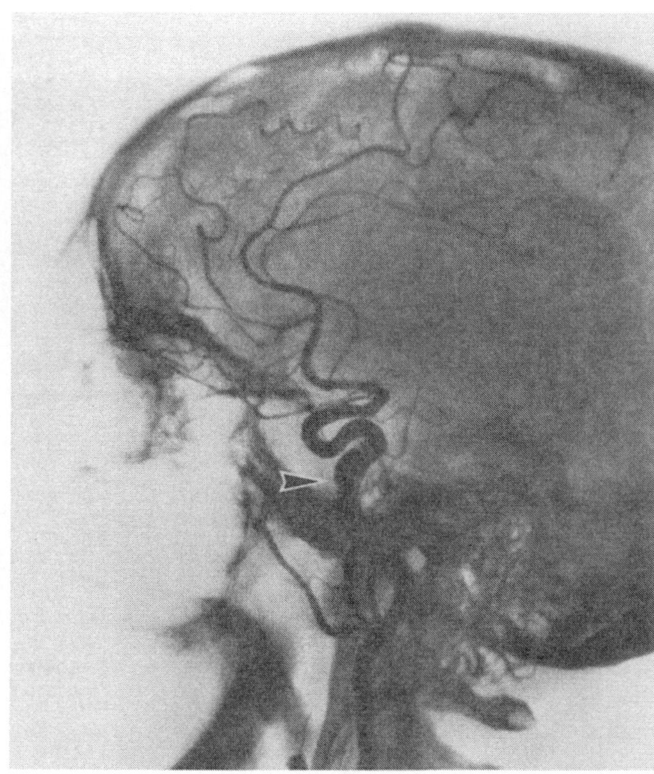

Abb. 24 **Abb. 25**

Abb. 24. Aufeinanderfolge von einigen Mikroaneurysmen an der Gefäßvorderwand auf Höhe des 2. Halswirbels (Pfeile), jedoch keine Stenosen. Die vollkommen glatte Gefäßhinterwand macht „stehende Wellen" unwahrscheinlich

Abb. 25. Infraklinoidales lokalisiertes Aneurysma dissecans an der Karotisvorderwand (Pfeil) und Verschluß der A. cerebri media. Die übrigen Abschnitte der A. carotis interna zeigen keine pathologischen Veränderungen. Ob es sich um ein Aneurysma dissecans im Rahmen der fibromuskulären Dysplasie handelt, kann aufgrund des Angiogrammes allein nicht mit Sicherheit entschieden werden. (Aus „Zerebrale Angiographie", Thieme Stuttgart, 1979)

(KAUFMANN, 1970) ist mehrfach hingewiesen worden. Bei 50 Patienten mit fibromuskulärer Dysplasie fanden HARRINGTON et al. (1970) in 15 Fällen (26%) ein Aneurysma der Hirnarterien, HOUSER et al. (1971) stellten unter 52 Fällen 10mal (19%) eine Subarachnoidalblutung mit Aneurysma fest. In der umfassenden Zusammenstellung von MANELFE et al. (1974) zeigen 27 von 70 Patienten (39%) ein Hirnaneurysma. Nach diesen Autoren kommen bei 28% der 200 aus der Literatur zusammengestellten Fällen von fibromuskulärer Dysplasie Aneurysmen vor. Die Häufigkeit der sackförmigen Aneurysmen ist bei dieser Gefäßaffektion somit ganz erheblich höher als in einer allgemeinen Population, wo sie nach STEHBENS (1972) ungefähr 0,5–1,5% beträgt.

In der pathologisch-anatomischen Klassifizierung der verschiedenen Formen der fibromuskulären Dysplasie folgen MANELFE et al. (1974) dem Vorschlag, den HARRISON und MCCORMACK (1971) an den Nierenarterien ausgearbeitet haben:

α) Fibroplasie der Intima mit segmentärer konzentrischer oder exzentrischer Stenose der Arterie. Diese Form ist mit 1–2% selten.

β) Fibromuskuläre Dysplasie der Media, mit 60–70% der häufigste Typus.
- Fibroplasie der Wand mit Wandaneurysmen. Über eine Gefäßstrecke hin folgen im Wechsel Stenosen mit Wandverdünnungen (Aneurysmen), was angiographisch dem Gefäß ein perlschnurartiges Aussehen verleiht. Die Muskularis ist mehr oder weniger vollständig durch fibroplasti-

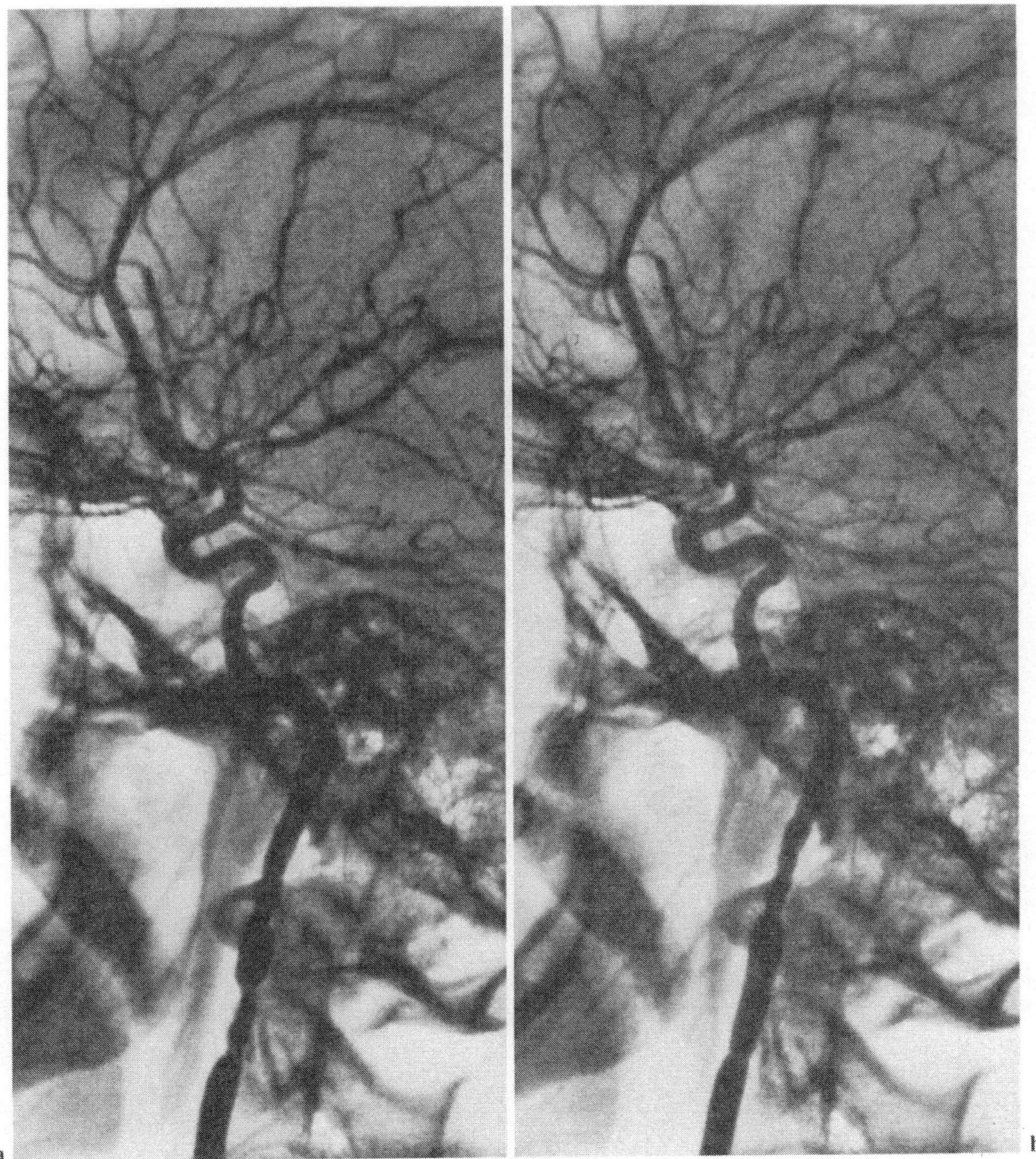

Abb. 26. a Kaliberunregelmäßigkeiten der A. carotis interna im oberen Zervikalabschnitt bei großem Balkengliom. **b** Die Kontrollaufnahme einige Minuten später zeigt ein anderes Bild der Kaliberunregelmäßigkeiten im oberen Zervikalabschnitt. Dieser Wechsel innerhalb kurzer Zeit spricht für spastische Veränderungen und gegen eine fibromuskuläre Dysplasie. (Aus „Zerebrale Angiographie", Thieme Stuttgart, 1979)

sches Gewebe ersetzt, die Lamina elastica ist immer gestört (Verdoppelungen, Fragmentationen). Die hochgradige Verdünnung oder das vollständige Schwinden der Media führt zu den Wandaneurysmen.

- Mediahyperplasie (5–15%). Infolge einer Hyperplasie der Muskularis ohne Mediaruptur und Wandaneurysmen kommt es zu einer Stenose der Arterie.
- Perimediale Fibroplasie (15–25%). Die Fibroplasie der äußeren Mediaschicht kann gelegentlich unregelmäßig sein und deshalb dem Gefäß einen perlschnurartigen Aspekt verleihen. Bei der Fibroplasie der Media mit Wandaneurysmen soll das Gefäß allerdings allgemein weiter sein als eine normale Arterie, während es bei der perimedialen Fibroplasie enger ist.
- Dissektion der Media (5–10%). In den äußeren Mediaschichten, jedoch noch innerhalb der Lamina elastica externa kommt es zur Bildung eines neuen Lumens (vergl. Abb. 25 und Abb. 28).

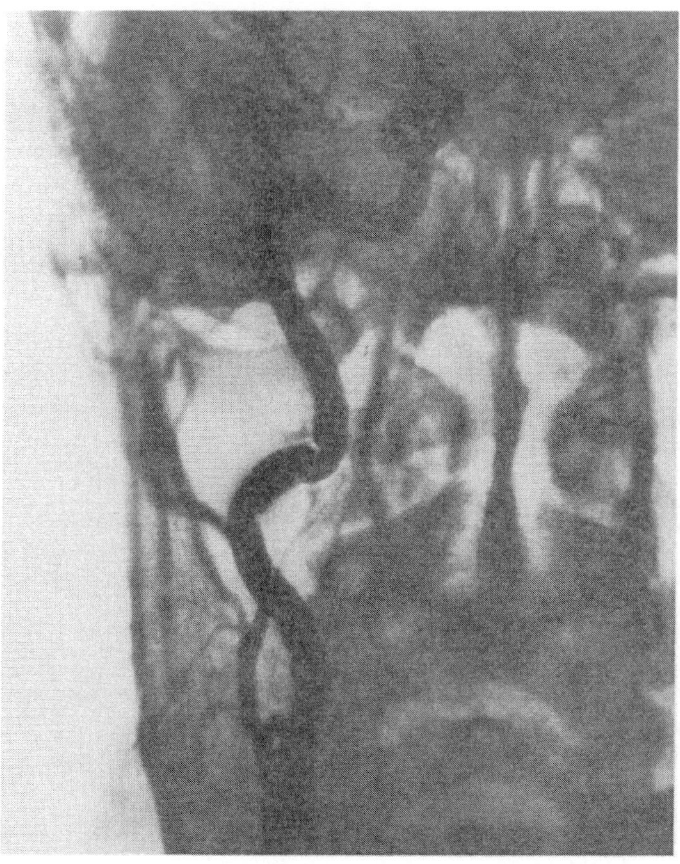

Abb. 27. Faltenartig gegen das Gefäßlumen vorspringende Füllungsdefekte auf der konkaven Seite von Gefäßbiegungsstellen im oberen Zervikalabschnitt. Ob es sich dabei um eine Faltenbildung der Intima, Spasmen oder eine Form der fibromuskulären Dysplasie handelt, kann ohne Kontrollaufnahmen und Histologie nicht entschieden werden

δ) Die Fibroplasie der Adventitia ist sehr selten (weniger als 1%) und führt zu einer Stenosierung des Gefäßlumens.

Die fibromuskuläre Dysplasie wird nach MANELFE et al. (1974) in ca. 1% der zerebralen Angiographien gefunden. Nach HOUSER et al. (1971) ist in ca. 60% der doppelseitig angiographierten Patienten ein Befall beider Karotiden anzutreffen. Die Krankheit kann in jedem Lebensalter auftreten, wird aber meist im mittleren Lebensalter diagnostiziert. Sie ist bei Frauen ungefähr 5mal häufiger als bei Männern.

Die häufigsten Symptome, die zur zerebralen Angiographie und damit zur Entdeckung der Krankheit führen, sind flüchtige oder dauernde Lähmungserscheinungen auf der Basis von Ischämien oder intrazerebralen Hämatomen, ferner Subarachnoidalblutungen bei Aneurysmarupturen, fokale oder generalisierte epileptische Anfälle, Kopfschmerzen und schließlich Strömungsgeräuschen über den Halsarterien.

Das angiographische Bild der häufigsten Form der Mediafibroplasie mit Wandaneurysmen, ist charakteristisch: meist vor den Halswirbelkörpern C2–C3 unter Aussparung des Segmentes unmittelbar distal von der Carotisbifurkation, zeigt die A. carotis interna über eine Strecke von 3–5 cm Länge in ganz enger Folge unregelmäßig begrenzte Stenosen und Erweiterungen, was ihr den Aspekt von schlaff herabhängenden Strümpfen verleiht („Chaussettes en accordéon" MANELFE et al., 1974 ; Abb. 23). Der erkrankte Abschnitt erscheint indessen allgemein weiter als die normalen proximalen und distalen Gefäßabschnitte. Die Mikroaneurysmen der Gefäßwand müssen sorgfältig gesucht werden (Abb. 24), da sie in einem Strahlengang u.U. verborgen bleiben

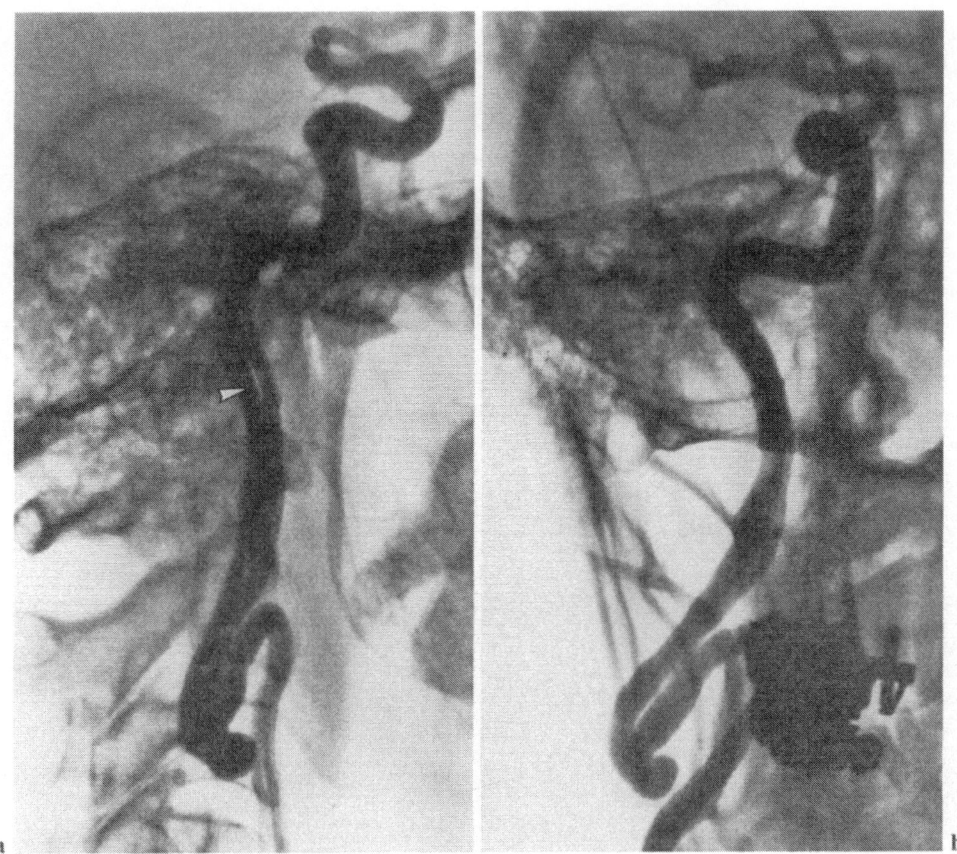

Abb. 28. a Doppeltes Lumen der A. carotis interna im oberen Zervikalabschnitt (Pfeil) und **b** sackförmiges Aneurysma auf der Höhe des 3. Halswirbels

können. Sie sind häufig von postpunktionellen Narben kaum zu unterscheiden (vergl. auch Abb. 22).

Die übrigen Formen stellen sich als mehr oder weniger eng umschriebene und mehr oder weniger glattwandige Stenosen dar, die unter Umständen sehr schwer von anderen stenosierenden Läsionen zu unterscheiden sind (Abb. 25, 27). Besonders schwierig ist die Abgrenzung gegenüber Spasmen im extrakraniellen Karotisabschnitt, wie sie gelegentlich bei intrakraniellen Tumoren zu beobachten sind. Die Differentialdiagnose ist praktisch nur durch Kontrollaufnahmen zu stellen (Abb. 26).

Die extrakraniellen Aneurysmen der A. carotis interna sitzen häufig auf der Höhe des ersten Halswirbels, somit dem typischen Sitz der fibromuskulären Dysplasie. Ob es sich in diesen Fällen, besonders wenn sie mit weiteren Anomalien wie Diastematoarterie gekoppelt sind, um die klassischen sackförmigen Aneurysmen oder um Wandaneurysmen im Rahmen der fibromuskulären Dysplasie handelt, kann ohne histologische Untersuchung nicht entschieden werden (Abb. 28).

3. Stehende Wellen (stationary arterial waves)

Die regelmäßige Aufeinanderfolge von schnürringartigen Gefäßeinengungen ist zuerst von Wickbom und Bartley (1957) und Theander (1960) an den peripheren Arterien beschrieben

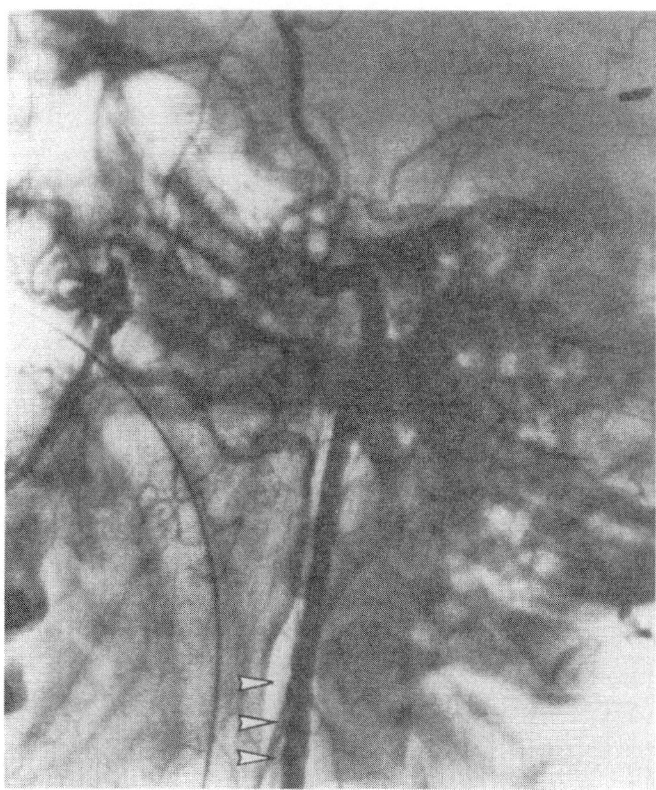

Abb. 29. Stehende Wellen (Pfeile). Status nach Operation eines traumatischen intrakraniellen Hämatoms. Die präoperative Angiographie zeigte eine völlig unauffällige A. carotis interna. Die Kontrollangiographie wegen Verdacht auf Arrêt circulatoire läßt bei fehlender Darstellung der intrakraniellen Gefäße auf Höhe des 2. Halswirbels an der A. carotis interna stehende Wellen erkennen

worden, sie kommen aber auch an den Halsarterien vor (NEW, 1966; LEHRER, 1967). Der Abstand zwischen den einzelnen Schnürringen ist gleich groß wie der Gefäßdurchmesser oder kleiner, nimmt also bei sich verjüngenden Gefäßen gegen die Peripherie zu ab. Die Veränderung erstreckt sich nur über kürzere Gefäßsegmente, selten ist ein Abschnitt von mehreren Zentimetern Länge betroffen. Nach LEHRER (1967) stehen diese stehenden Wellen mit den Pulswellen in Zusammenhang und treten dann auf, wenn die Oszillationen der Strömungsgeschwindigkeit in antero- und retrograder Richtung gleich sind. Obgleich diese Wellen unter variablen hämodynamischen Bedingungen veränderlich sind (z.B. Zurückziehen des Katheters, Veränderung des Injektionsdruckes), weisen sie nicht selten auf ein peripheres Strömungshindernis hin (Abb. 29).

4. Schlängelung, Schleifenbildung und Knickung der A. carotis interna

Abweichungen der A. carotis interna vom relativ geradlinigen Verlauf sind im extrakraniellen Abschnitt nicht selten. Es werden drei verschiedene Formen dieser Verlaufsabweichungen unterschieden, deren Häufigkeit und Abhängigkeit vom Alter von WEIBEL und FIELDS (1965) untersucht worden sind. Bei der Schlängelung (tortuosity) weist die A. carotis interna innerhalb der ersten 4 cm einen S- oder C-förmigen Verlauf auf. Diese Verlaufsform kommt bei Jugendlichen und Erwachsenen unter 50 Jahren keineswegs selten vor, ist aber nach dem 50. Lebensjahr häufiger.

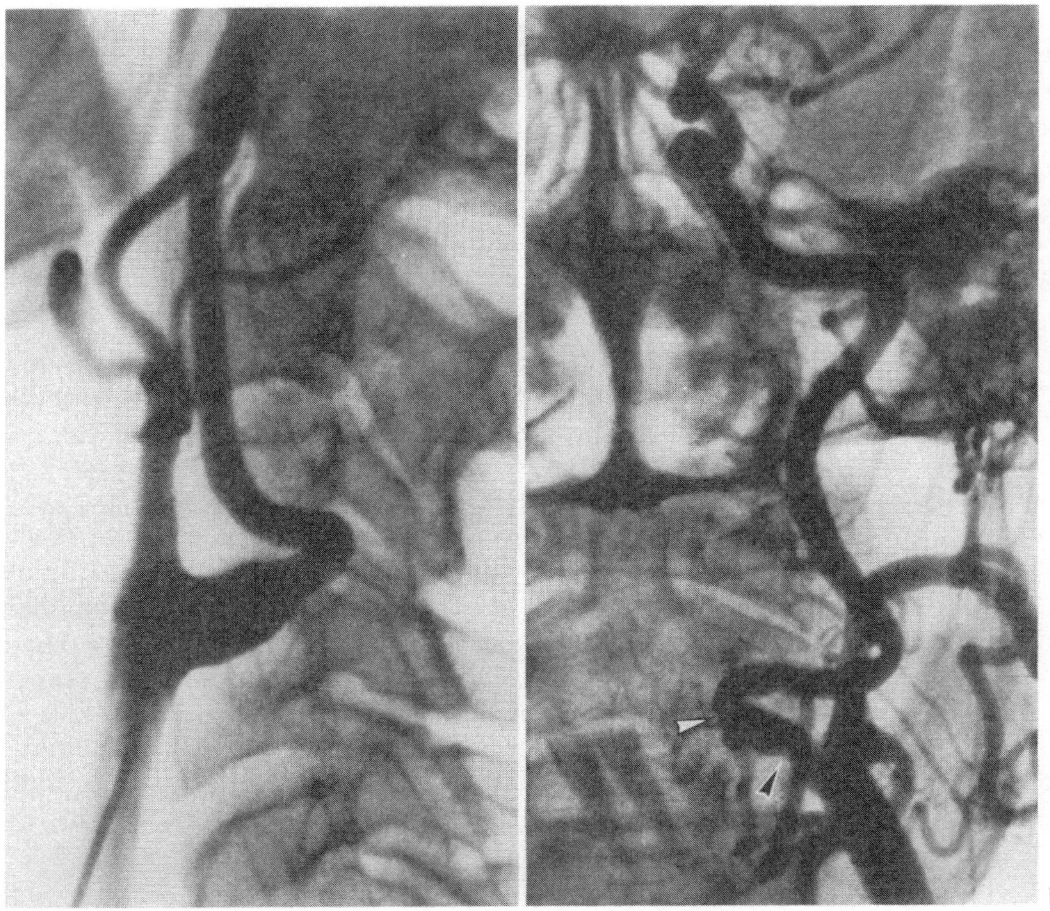

Abb. 30. a Knickbildung ("kinking") der A. carotis interna ohne Stenosierung. Dilatation des Karotisabschnittes vor der Knickbildung. **b** Knickbildung mit deutlicher Stenosierung (Pfeil) und atherosklerotischer Lumeneinengung vor der Knickbildung. (Aus „Zerebrale Angiographie", Thieme Stuttgart, 1979)

Bei beidseitig untersuchten Fällen ist sie bilateral etwa doppelt so häufig wie unilateral. Wahrscheinlich handelt es sich um eine kongenitale Anlage, die infolge Alterung und Arteriosklerose stärker zum Ausdruck kommt.

Die Schlingenbildung (coiling) ist wesentlich seltener und kommt in den beiden Altersgruppen unter und über 50 Jahren nahezu in gleicher Häufigkeit vor, was für eine kongenitale Anlage spricht. Sie bevorzugt den Abschnitt zwischen 4 und 8 cm distal von der Bifurkation, liegt also im oberen Zervikalbereich. Sie ist bilateral fast gleich häufig anzutreffen wie unilateral.

Die Knickbildung der A. carotis interna (kinking) findet sich innerhalb der ersten 2–4 cm distal von der Bifurkation. Durch die Knickbildung kommt es oft zu einer Stenosierung, die aber die Zirkulationsgeschwindigkeit, soweit sich dies angiographisch beurteilen läßt, nicht wesentlich beeinträchtigt. Die Knickbildung ist unilateral mehr als doppelt so häufig wie bilateral und findet sich bei der Altersgruppe über 50 Jahren etwas häufiger als bei jüngeren Patienten. Nicht selten ist die Knickung mit einer Dilatation des proximalen und einer Schleifenbildung des distalen Segmentes verbunden. Wahrscheinlich handelt es sich bei dieser Verlaufsform um eine durch Alter, Arteriosklerose und eventuell Hypertonie verstärkte Schleifenbildung (Abb. 30).

5. Lumeneinengungen bei Gefäßmißbildungen

Hämodynamisch sind die segmentalen Verdoppelungen (Diastematoarterie) oder Fenestrationen, die an den Vertebralarterien, speziell auf der Höhe des ersten Halswirbels öfters anzutreffen sind (MIZUKAMI et al., 1972; KOWADA et al., 1972) als an der A. basilaris (TAKAHASHI et al., 1973), an der A. carotis interna oder an den intrakraniellen Gefäßen (TEAL et al., 1973; WOLLSCHLAEGER u. WOLLSCHLAEGER, 1974) wahrscheinlich von geringer Bedeutung.

Hypoplasien der A. carotis interna sind selten (LAGARDE et al., 1957; TURNBULL, 1962; LAVAURS et al., 1963; HILLS u. SAMENT, 1968; LIE, 1968; SMITH et al., 1968; LHERMTTE et al., 1968; STEIMLE et al., 1969; AUSTIN u. STEARS, 1971; ROSEN et al., 1975). Nach einem normal weiten oder sogar erweiterten Abschnitt verjüngt sich das Gefäß mehr oder weniger abrupt, kann aber nicht selten noch bis zur Schädelbasis oder gar bis zum Circulus Willisi verfolgt werden. Dieses Bild könnte differentialdiagnostisch auch an Spasmen, an ein Aneurysma dissecans oder eine Thrombose, die sich vom Karotissiphon aus retrograd gegen die Bifurkation zu erstreckt, denken lassen, während eine Lumeneinengung infolge Atherosklerose wegen der glatten Wand weniger in Frage kommt. Angiographische und autoptische Befunde zeigen aber, daß bei Karotishypoplasien Varianten am Circulus Willisi vorliegen, die einen genügenden Blutzufluß zum Hemisphäre auf der Seite der hypoplastischen A. carotis interna gewährleisten, so z.B. eine stark erweiterte und eventuell sogar elongierte A. communicans anterior oder posterior. In einigen Fällen sitzen an diesen strömungsmäßig stark belasteten Gefäßabschnitten sackförmige Aneurysmen, wie sie auch an den zu einer arteriovenösen Gefäßmißbildung führenden Arterie bekannt sind. In analoger Weise kommen Aneurysmen im vorderen Abschnitt des Circulus Willisi auch häufig an der weiteren A. cerebri anterior vor, die wegen einer Hypoplasie der kontrolateralen A. cerebri anterior beide Ae. pericallosae zu versorgen hat. Die weite kommunizierende Gefäßstrecke kann deshalb ein wichtiges Kriterium in der Differentialdiagnose zu den oben erwähnten Affektionen sein, da sich bei diesen akuten Ereignissen die kommunizierenden Arterien am Circulus Willisi kaum erweitern. Die Aneurysmaruptur kann das Erstsymptom einer Karotishypoplasie sein, weshalb bei ungenügender Darstellung der Halsabschnitte fälschlicherweise die Hypoplasie als Spasmus nach Subarachnoidalblutung interpretiert werden könnte.

Hypoplasien der Vertebralarterien sind relativ häufig, in 4–6% der Fälle ist nach KRAYENBÜHL und YASARGIL (1957) eine Vertebralarterie sehr dünn.

Bei der Persistenz embryonaler karotido-basilärer Anastomosen sind ebenfalls Hypoplasien der großen Arterien bekannt, so z.B. der ipsilateralen A. vertebralis bei Persistenz der A. hypoglossica primitiva. Die richtige Deutung dieser Lumeneinengung bietet indessen keine besonderen Schwierigkeiten.

IV. Angiographische Kontrolluntersuchungen nach gefäßchirurgischen Eingriffen

MADDISON (1970) stellte die Resultate von 118 Patienten mit total 155 Operationen zusammen, von denen, mit Ausnahme von 11, alle nachangiographiert wurden und zwar im Durchschnitt 2 Wochen nach der Operation. Bei durchgängigem Gefäß können folgende Befunde erhoben werden:

- Am distalen Ende der Endarterektomiestelle ragt ein freies Intimaende klappenartig in das Gefäßlumen vor (Intimaflap). Dieses freie Ende kann durch den Blutstrom weiter abgehoben werden und schließlich zum Gefäßverschluß führen. Ähnliche Befunde sind beim spontanen Aneurysma dissecans bekannt.
- Bildung falscher Aneurysma bei Nahtdehiszenz,
- gestielte Thromben,
- rezidivierende Stenosen.

Ohne wesentliche Bedeutung dagegen sind die sog. „clamp defects“. Infolge der instrumentellen Gefäßabklemmung während der Endarterektomie findet man parallel verlaufende, feine Aufhellungszonen, die Intimadefekten entsprechen und in relativ kurzer Zeit abheilen. Wandunregelmäßigkeiten, die wahrscheinlich durch an der Wand haftende und eine Pseudointima bildende Thrombozyten bedingt sind, werden einen Monat nach der Operation nicht mehr angetroffen.

V. Gefäßverschlüsse

Der Verschluß der großen Gefäße durch eine atheromatöse Plaque ist an sich relativ selten, in der Regel führt erst ein Abscheidungsthrombus zum vollständigen Verschluß. Die nächsthäufige Verschlußursache ist der Embolus, während zahlenmäßig Verschlüsse infolge Trauma, Aneurysma dissecans oder entzündlichen Wandveränderungen in den Hintergrund treten.

1. Karotisverschluß

Entsprechend der Lokalisation der Stenosen ist auch der häufigste Sitz des Karotisverschlusses unmittelbar distal von der Karotisbifurkation oder dann im Karotisendabschnitt, wobei der Abgang der A. communicans posterior oder der A. cerebri posterior noch verschont bleibt. Zwischen diesen beiden Prädilektionsstellen sind atheromatöse oder embolische Gefäßverschlüsse ausgesprochen selten. Beim proximalen Verschluß kann sich ein Stagnationsthrombus nach distal ausdehnen, beim distalen Verschluß dagegen nach proximal zu. Beim nach distal wachsenden Stagnationsthrombus bleibt die Karotisendstrecke nicht selten wegen des Kollateralkreislaufs über die A. ophthalmica und die A. communicans posterior offen. Die Propagation des Stagnationsthrombus von distal nach proximal kann zu einer falschen Lokalisation des primären Verschlusses führen.

Das angiographische Bild des Internaverschlusses mit dem vollständigen Abbruch der Kontrastmittelfüllung ist seit langem bekannt (Moniz et al., 1937; Johnson u. Walker, 1951; Krayenbühl

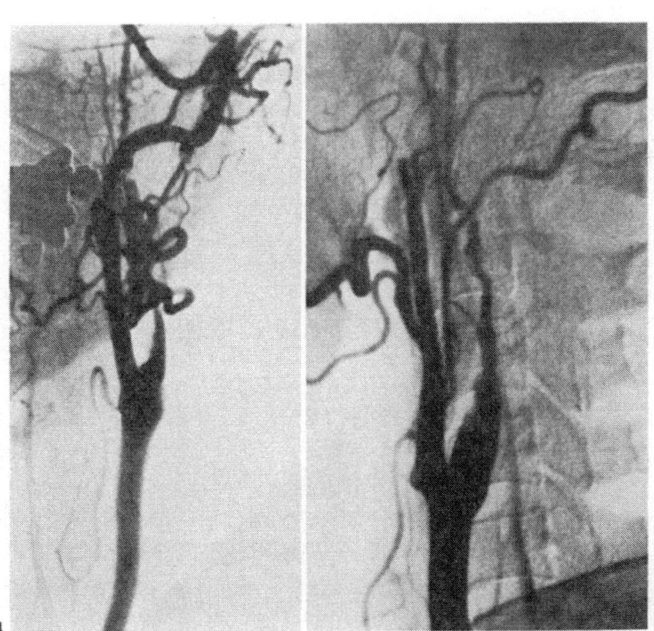

Abb. 31a u. b. Partieller Verschluß der A. carotis interna durch Stagnationsthrombus. Höhe der primären Gefäßwanderkrankung nicht mehr eindeutig bestimmbar

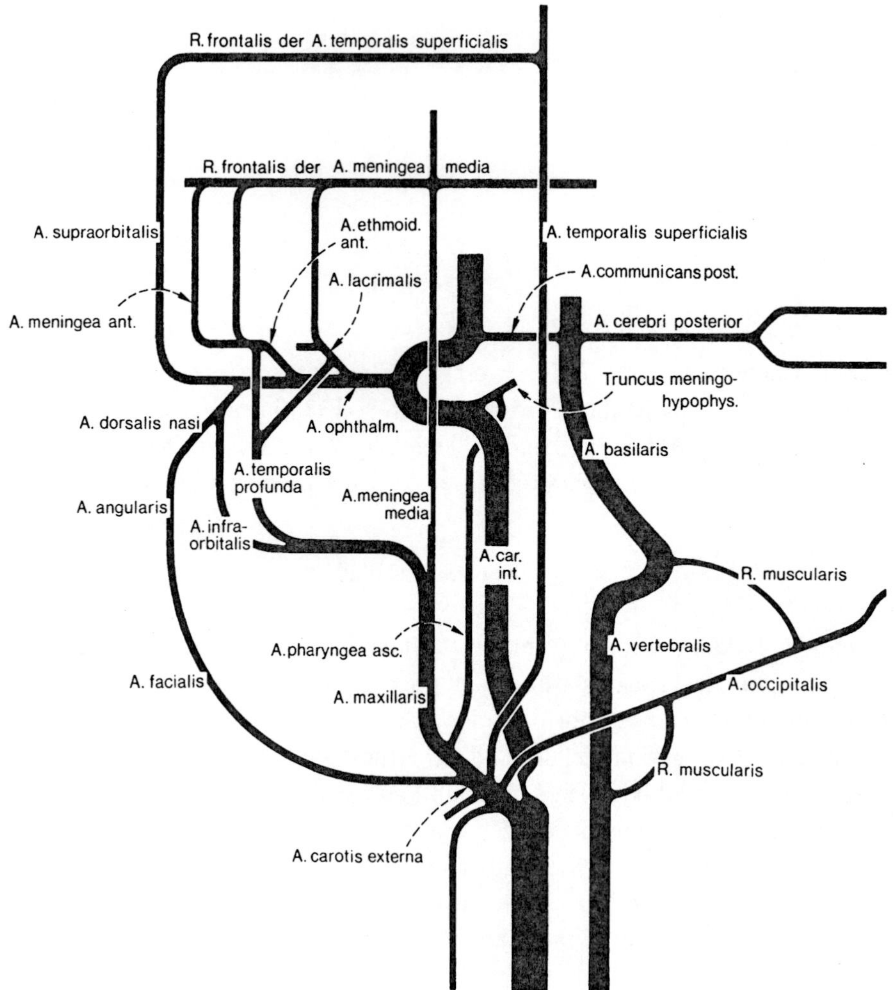

Abb. 32. Schematische Darstellung der Anastomosemöglichkeiten beim Verschluß der A. carotis interna (vorderer Abschnitt des Circulus Willisi nicht eingezeichnet)

u. RICHTER, 1952; GURDJIAN u. WEBSTER, 1953; RIISHEDE, 1957; TÖNNIS u. SCHIEFER, 1959; TAVERAS u. WOOD, 1964). Aus der Form des Kontrastmittelabbruches ist kein zuverlässiger Schluß auf die Verschlußursache (atheromatöse plaque oder Embolus) möglich (Abb. 31). Eine kegelförmig auslaufende Kontrastmittelsäule spricht indessen in der Regel für einen primären Verschluß weiter distal mit oder ohne proximalwärts wachsenden Stagnationsthrombus, wie FROWEIN (1961) auch im Modellversuch gezeigt hat. Gelegentlich setzt sich ein dünner und z.T. unreglmäßiger Kontrastmittelfaden zwischen Stagnationsthrombus und Gefäßwand nach distal zu fort.

Beim Karotisverschluß springen Kollateralkreisläufe ein, die u.U. den Ausfall vollständig kompensieren können (HARDY et al., 1962). Es sind selbst doppelseitig Karotisverschlüsse bekannt geworden, die wegen der guten Kompensation zu keinen neurologischen Ausfallserscheinungen geführt haben.

Die größte Bedeutung kommt in der Regel dem vikariierenden Blutzustrom über den Circulus Willisi zu. Genügt dieses System nicht, z.B. bei Hypoplasie einzelner Segmente des basalen Gefäßkranzes, so gewinnt der Kollateralkreislauf von der A. carotis externa her an Bedeutung, wobei zahlreiche Verbindungswege zur A. carotis interna möglich sind und z.T. auch in verschiedenen Kombinationen benutzt werden, wobei allerdings die Regel gilt, daß das Blut den kürzesten Weg wählt (Abb. 32, 33, 34). Die wichtigste Gefäßverbindung ist die A. ophthalmica, die sich im Verlaufe weniger Tage bis Wochen erheblich erweitern kann. Schließlich ist ein Bluteinstrom

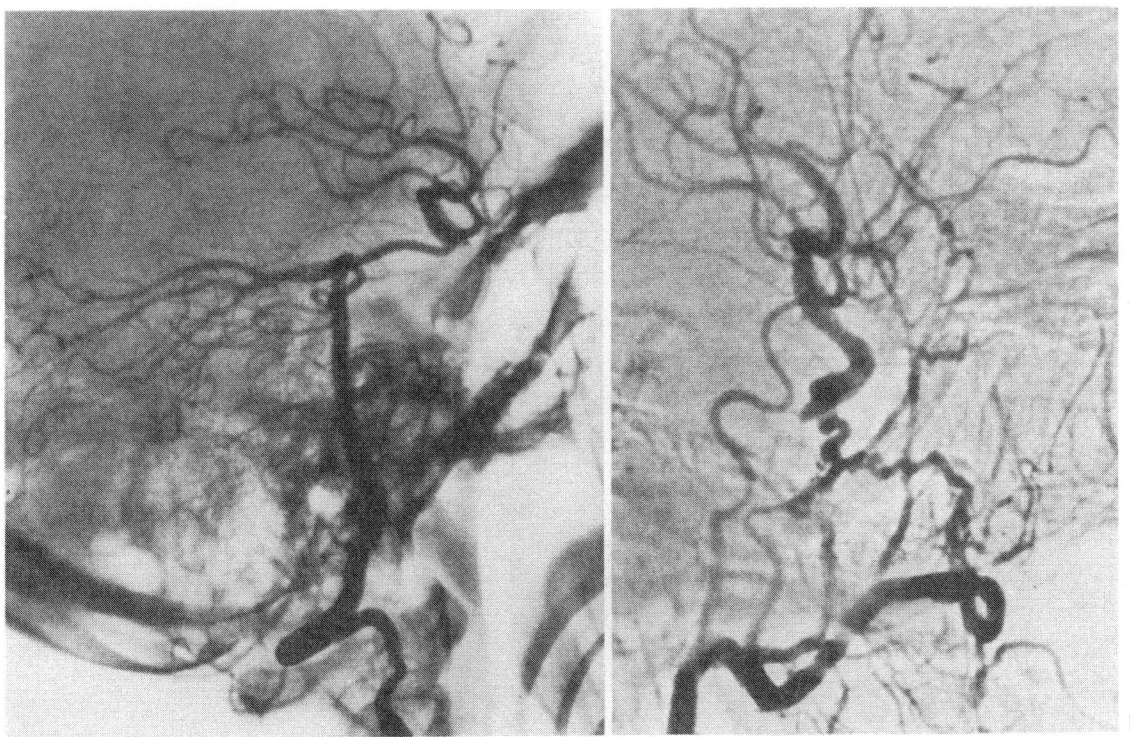

Abb. 33a u. b. Infraclinoidaler Verschluß der A. carotis interna bei Kraniopharyngeom. **a** Vertebralisangiographie. Darstellung der Karotisendstrecke und der Mediagruppe über die A. communicans posterior. **b** Injektion der A. carotis externa. Kollateralkreislauf von der A. maxillaris aus über eine erweiterte A. temporalis profunda zum Karotissiphon. (Der Karotissiphon stellt sich bei der Vertebralisangiographie nicht dar, weil er über diese Kollateralen mit kontrastmittellosem Blut durchströmt wird.) (Abb. 33a aus „Zerebrale Angiographie", Thieme Stuttgart, 1979)

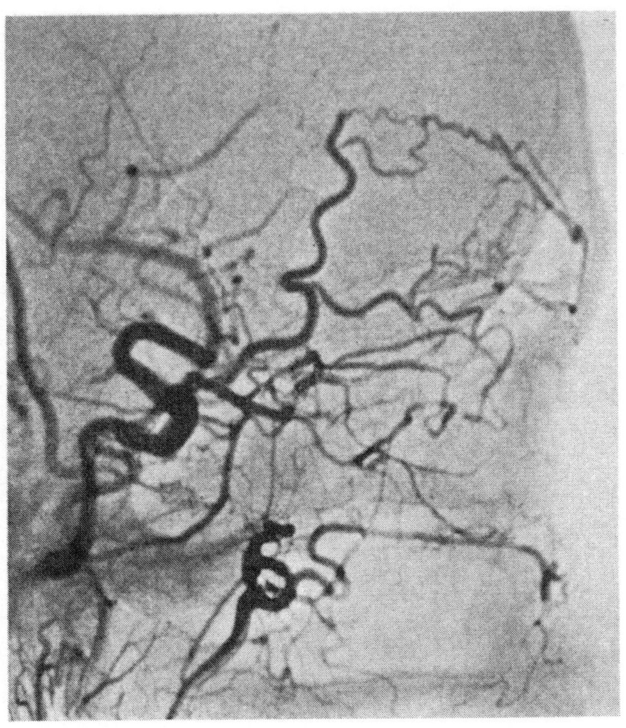

Abb. 34. Kollateralkreislauf über den R. frontalis der A. temporalis superficialis und die A. supraorbitalis zur A. ophthalmica sowie über die A. infraorbitalis bei Karotisverschluß

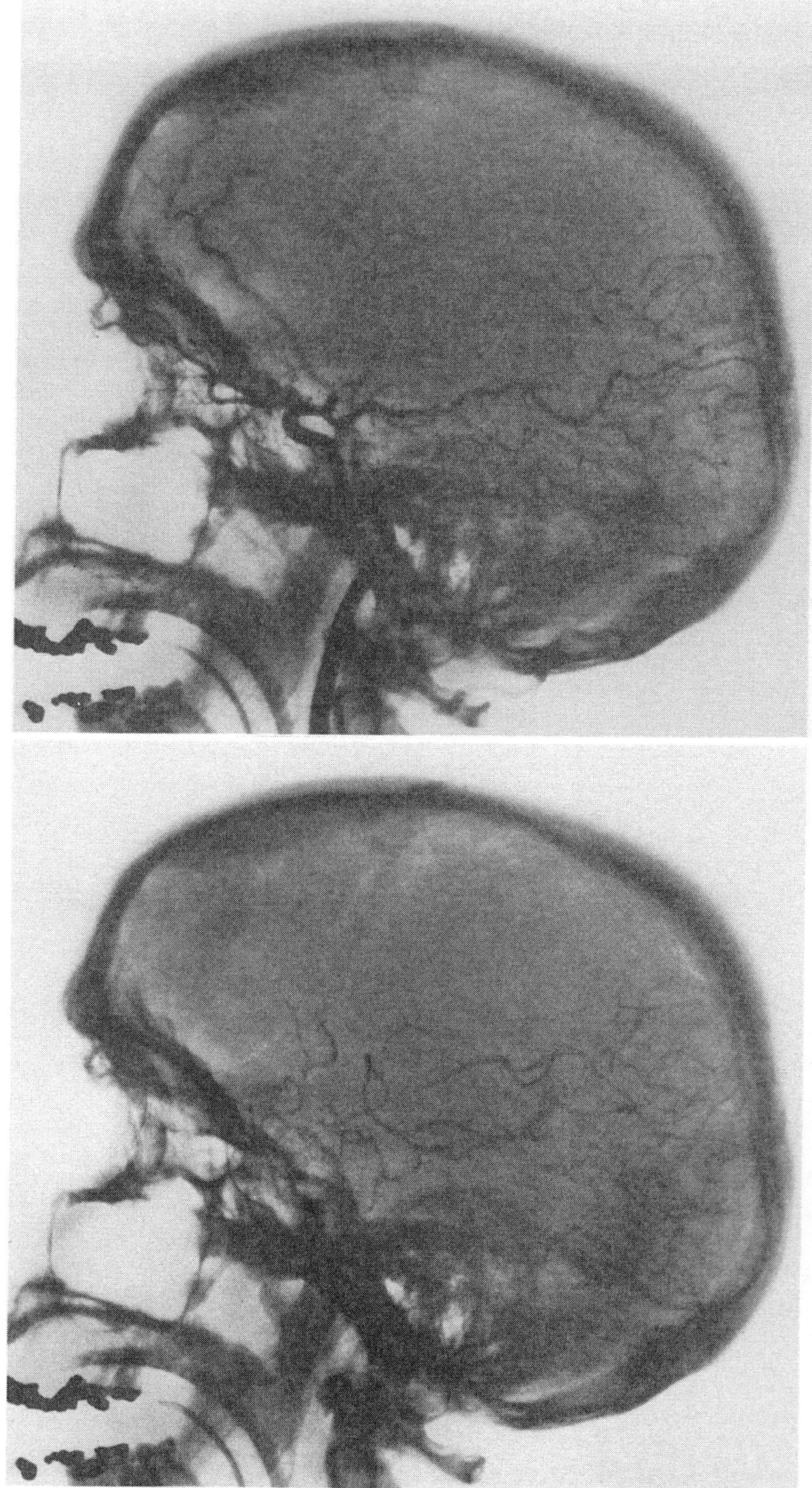

Abb. 35. Karotisverschluß distal von der A. cerebri posterior. Über leptomeningeale Anastomosen stellen sich von der A. cerebri posterior aus retrograd die A. temporalis posterior und die A. gyri angularis dar. (Aus „Zerebrale Angiographie", Thieme Stuttgart, 1979)

in das Territorium der verschlossenen A. carotis interna über leptomeningeale Anastomosen von der A. cerebri posterior zur ipsilateralen A. pericallosa und A. cerebri media möglich oder aber über die interhemisphärischen Verbindungen zwischen den beiden Ae. pericallosae über dem Balken (Abb. 35).

Die Verschlüsse der A. carotis communis sind selten, am ehesten finden sie sich am Abgang der A. carotis communis aus der Aorta resp. dem Truncus brachiocephalicus. Neben den Kollateralkreisläufen, die beim Internaverschluß wirksam werden, kann zudem Blut von der A. vertebralis her über Muskeläste vorwiegend zur A. occipitalis und von da aus über die A. carotis externa zur Karotisbifurkation fließen.

2. Vertebralisverschlüsse

Die Verschlüsse der A. vertebralis finden sich am häufigsten an der Abgangsstelle aus der A. subclavia. Kollateralkreisläufe über Muskeläste von der A. occipitalis, der A. cervicalis profunda und der A. cervicalis ascendens zu der A. vertebralis sowie über die Rami spinales der kontralateralen A. vertebralis sind gewöhnlich vorhanden, z.T. aber wegen der Überlagerung durch die Halswirbelsäule nur mit Hilfe der Subtraktionsmethode angiographisch nachweisbar (Abb. 36). Ein wesentlicher Zustrom erfolgt über den Circulus Willisi via Ae. communicantes posteriores, so daß auch bilaterale Vertebralisverschlüsse ertragen werden können (NIZZOLI et al., 1970). Eine weitere Prädilektionsstelle für Verschlüsse ist der Vertebralisabschnitt zwischen Atlas und A. basilaris (KRAYENBÜHL u. YASARGIL, 1957; RESCH u. BAKER, 1964; SCHOTT et al., 1965), wobei namentlich bei Kindern Traumen der oberen Halswirbelsäule ein wichtiger auslösender Faktor sind (GURDJIAN et al., 1963; DEVIVO u. FARRELL, 1972; MARKS u. FREED, 1973; LATCHAV et al., 1974). Die Diagnose eines derartigen Verschlusses ist allerdings mit Vorsicht zu stellen: Sowohl bei Verwendung eines zu weiten Katheters als auch bei direkter Punktion (punktionsbedingter Spasmus, perivasale Kontrastmittelinjektion) kann es zu einer Strömungsbehinderung mit

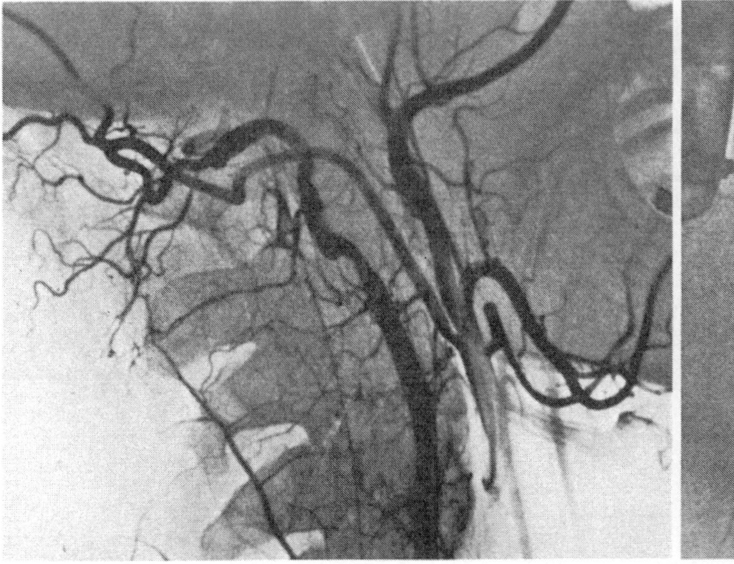

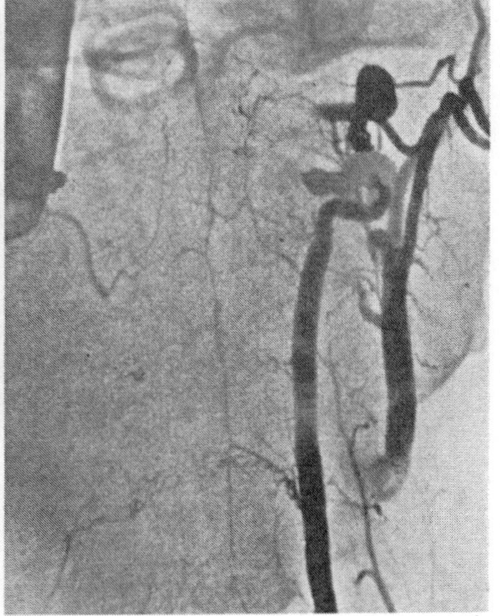

Abb. 36. Verschluß der linken A. vertebralis auf Höhe des Atlas. (Hypoplasie der rechten A. vertebralis. Versorgung des Basilarisstromgebietes über die Aa. communicantes posteriores.) Kathetrisierung der linken A. vertebralis. Unter dem Injektionsdruck stellen sich die Anastomosen zur A. occipitalis und das Externastromgebiet dar. Das kontrastmittelhaltige Blut in der A. carotis externa wird von proximal her durch kontrastmittelloses Blut ausgewaschen. A. spinalis anterior und Rami radiculares beidseits gut sichtbar. (Aus „Zerebrale Angiographie", Thieme Stuttgart, 1979)

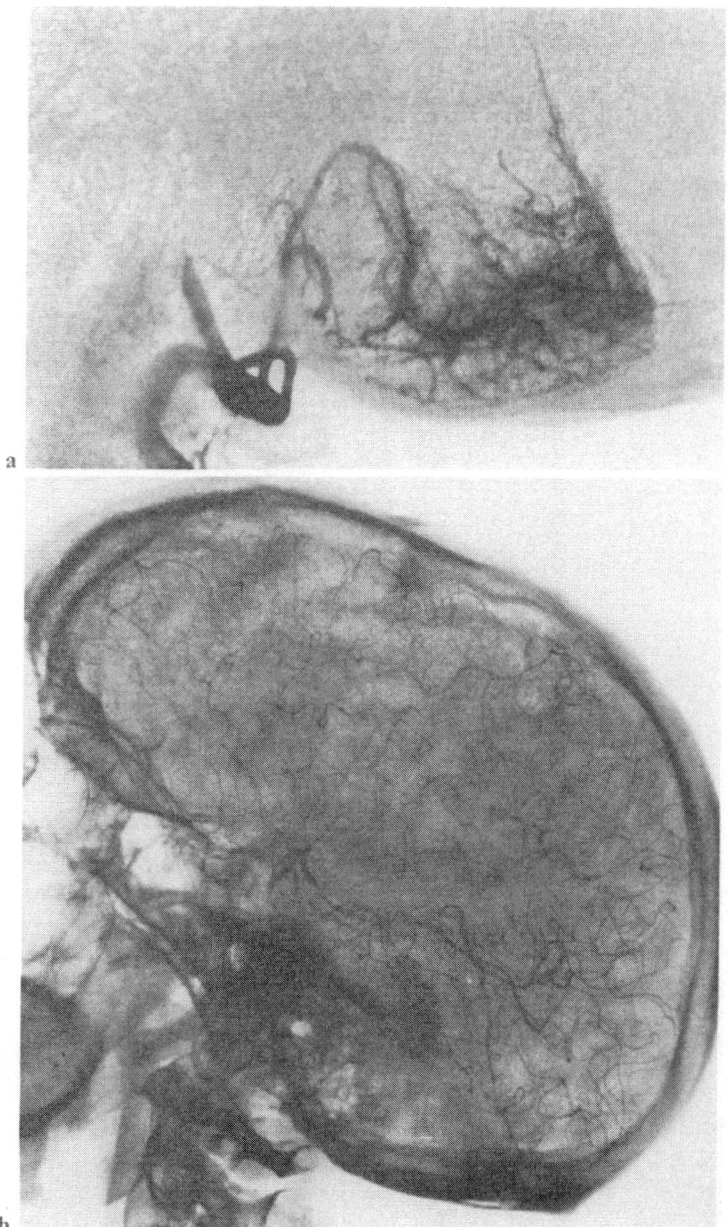

Abb. 37a u. b. Verschluß der A. basilaris. **a** Vertebralisangiogramm. Die A. cerebellaris inferior posterior ist frei durchgängig und gut gefüllt. **b** Karotisangiogramm. Über die A. communicans posterior haben sich neben der A. cerebri posterior auch der obere Abschnitt der A. basilaris und die A. cerebellaris superior dargestellt. Das kontrastmittelhaltige Blut bleibt in diesen Gefäßabschnitten liegen, da es nicht durch den normalen Blutstrom in der A. basilaris ausgeschwemmt wird

Druckabfall im distalen Vertebralissegment kommen, was den Einstrom von kontrastmittellosem Blut aus der kontralateralen A. vertebralis in das distale ipsilaterale Vertebralissegment erleichtert. Mit Sicherheit ist ein derartiger Verschluß nur zu diagnostizieren, wenn die erwähnten technischen Fehler ausgeschlossen und ein Kollateralkreislauf nachgewiesen sind.

Sowohl bei den Verschüssen der A. carotis interna als auch denjenigen der A. vertebralis ist eine Rekanalisation möglich (SINDERMAN et al., 1974).

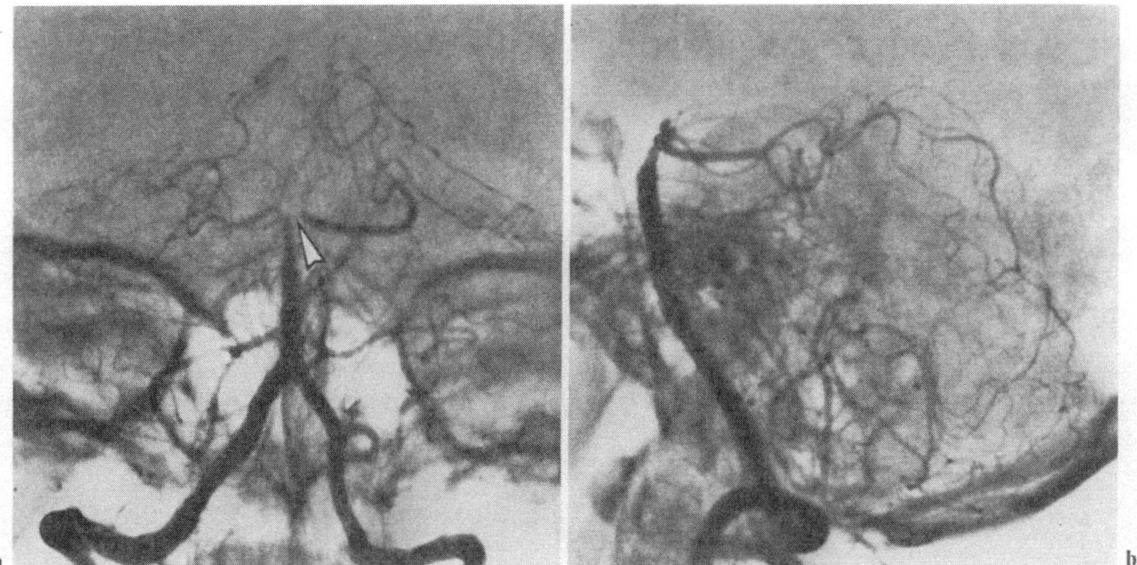

Abb. 38a u. b. Fehlende Darstellung der Basilarisendstrecke mit Aufteilung in die Aa. cerebri posteriores. **a** Der Füllungsdefekt im Anfangsabschnitt der linken A. cerebellaris superior (Pfeil), **b** spricht gegen eine Hypoplasie der Basilarisendstrecke. (Aus „Zerebrale Angiographie", Thieme Stuttgart, 1979)

3. Basilarisverschluß

Verschlüsse der A. basilaris sind keineswegs selten (KRAYENBÜHL u. YASARGIL, 1957, 1961; SCHECHTER u. ZINGESSER, 1965; SUTTON u. DAVIES, 1966; CASTAIGNE et al., 1973). MOSCOW und NEWTON (1973) stellten bei 4834 unselektionierten Autopsien einen Basilarisverschluß in 0,2% fest. Der Verschluß erfolgt meist auf der Basis einer Atherosklerose, seltener aufgrund eines Aneurysma dissecans bei Medianekrose. In der Mehrzahl der Fälle erstreckt sich der Verschluß über das Segment zwischen Abgang der Ae. cerebellares inferiores posteriores und Ae. cerebellares superiores (Abb. 37). Es handelt sich somit auch hier sehr oft um einen Stagnationsthrombus in einem Abschnitt, von dem praktisch keine Gefäße abgehen, über die ein Kollateralkreislauf etabliert werden könnte. Vom distalen Basilarisverschluß sind die Fälle einer distalen Hypoplasie der A. basilaris oder des basilären Abschnittes der A. cerebri posterior zu unterscheiden (GRÜTER u. HERRMANN, 1963; SZDZUY u. LEHMANN, 1972; Abb. 38).

Auch beim Basilarisverschluß kann sich ein Kollateralkreislauf entwickeln (KRAYENBÜHL u. YASARGIL, 1957; SCHECHTER u. ZINGESSER, 1965; WEIDNER et al., 1965a; MOSCOW u. NEWTON, 1973; Abb. 39).

Der oberste Abschnitt der A. basilaris stellt sich sehr oft über die A. communicans posterior von der A. carotis interna her dar, wobei das Kontrastmittel in diesem Abschnitt stagniert. Die Anlage dieses Kollateralkreislaufes sowie die Ausbildung der Vertebralarterien und der Aa. cerebellares inferiores posteriores sind für das Schicksal dieser Patienten von größter Bedeutung (FIELDS et al., 1966).

Ein retrograder Kontrastmitteleinstrom in den obersten Basilarisabschnitt bis zum Abgang der Aa. cerebellares superiores und eventuell noch weiter gegen die Vertebralarterien zu kann aber auch unter normalen Bedingungen vorkommen und erlaubt noch keinen Rückschluß auf eine Basilaristhrombose, besonders wenn das Kontrastmittel von der A. basilaris her rasch wieder ausgeschwemmt wird.

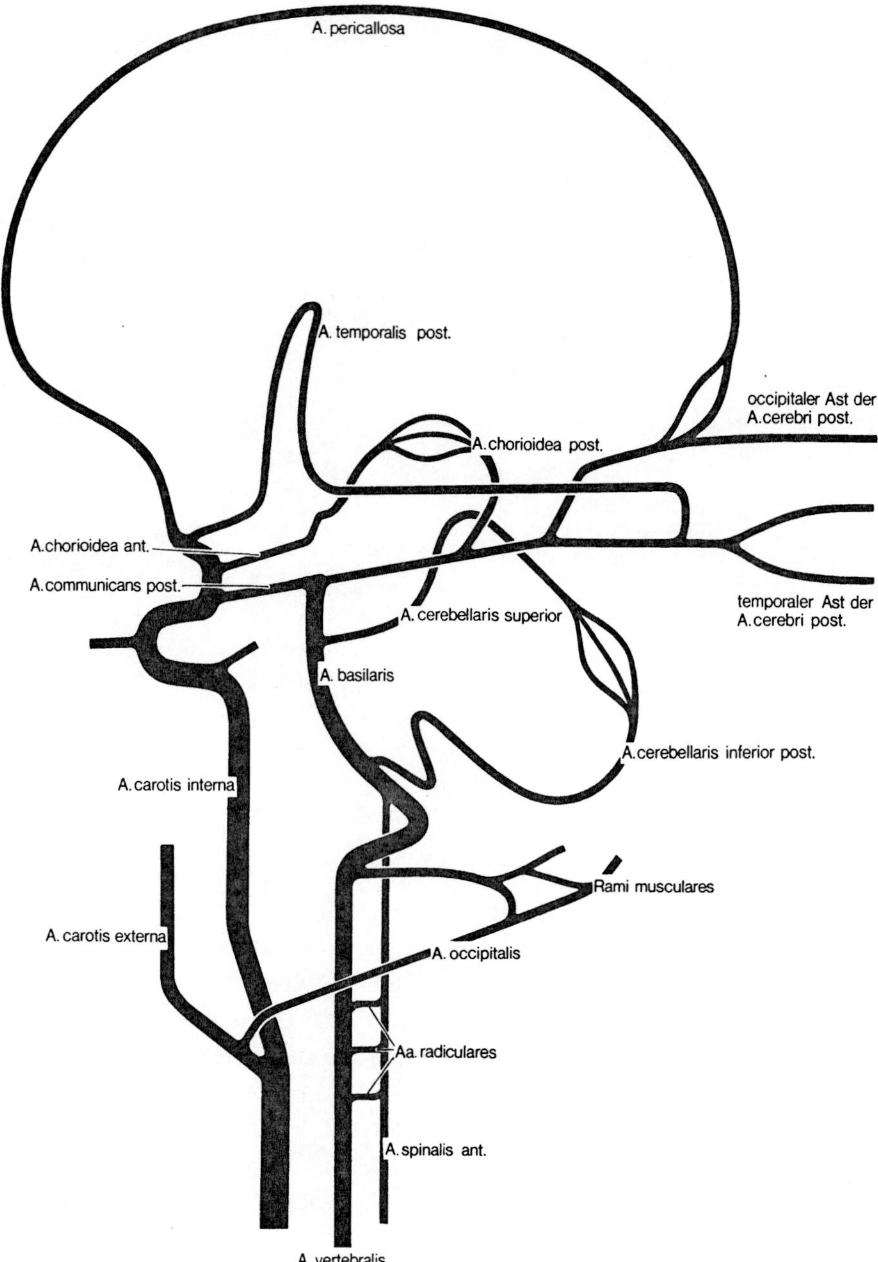

Abb. 39. Schematische Darstellung der Anastomosemöglichkeiten bei Verschlüssen der A. vertebralis und der A. basilaris

4. Nicht durch Atherosklerose oder Thromboembolien bedingte Verschlüsse

a) Artifiziell bedingte und falsche Verschlüsse

Das Bild des artifiziellen Verschlusses durch technisch fehlerhafte Kontrastmittelinjektion ist von KLINGLER (1952) und DECKER und NAGEL (1954) beschrieben worden. Durch die perivasale oder subintimale Injektion kann es zu einer Blockierung der Kontrastmittelsäule in der A. carotis interna auf Höhe des supraklinoidalen Abschnittes kommen, wobei das Kontrastmittel im Gefäß lange stehen bleibt, ohne daß sich die A. ophthalmica, die A. chorioidea anterior und die A. communicans posterior darstellen (LEE und HODES (1967)). Wegen des Druckabfalles in der A. carotis interna verschiebt sich das Druckgleichgewicht an diesen Anastomosestellen in der Richtung

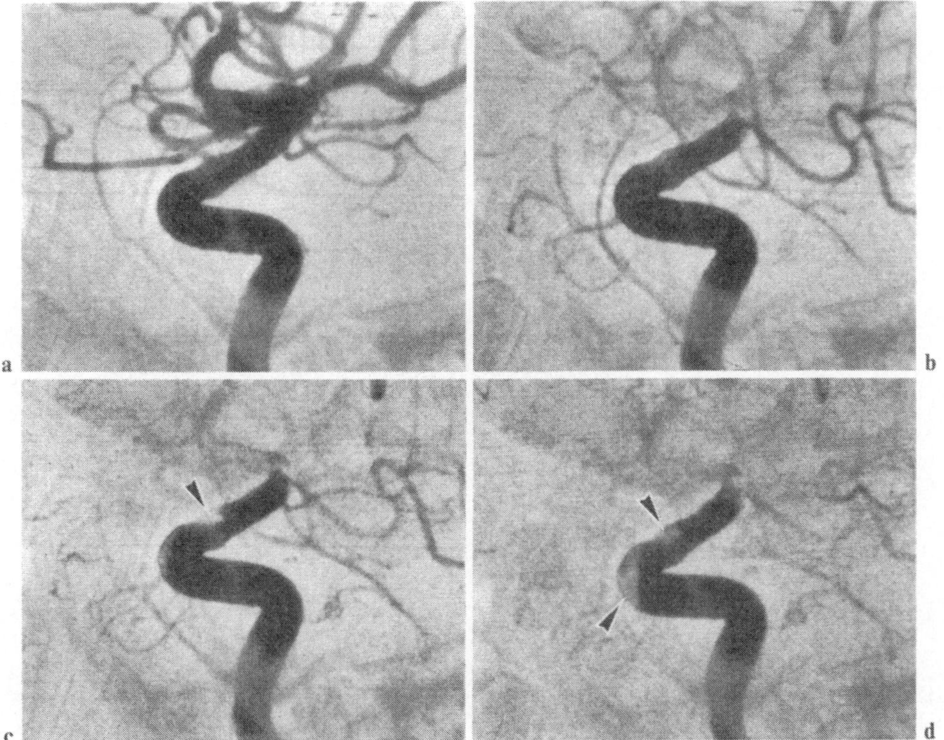

Abb. 40a–d. Strömungsbehinderung in der A. carotis interna. Durch einen zu weit vorgeschobenen Katheter ist das Gefäßlumen blockiert worden. Unter dem Injektionsdruck zunächst gut Darstellung der A. carotis interna und der Hemisphärengefäße **a**. Nach Aufhören des Injektionsdruckes bleibt die Kontrastmittelsäule in der A. carotis interna stehen, die A. ophthalmica führt kein kontrastmittelhaltiges Blut mehr. In den Arterien distal vom Circulus Willisi wird das Kontrastmittel durch kontrastmittelloses Blut von der Gegenseite her ausgeschwemmt **b**. Durch Stromumkehr in der A. ophthalmica wird durch kontrastmittelloses Blut von der A. carotis externa her das Kontrastmittel in der A. carotis interna langsam ausgeschwemmt. (**c** u. **d**, Pfeil)

A. carotis, und die genannten Gefäße werden mit kontrastmittellosem Blut durchspült (Abb. 40). Ein falscher Block der A. carotis interna ist von GANNON (1961) auch bei massivem Blutdruckabfall während der Kontrastmittelinjektion beobachtet worden. Das Phänomen, das von GANNON auf den Karotissinusreflex zurückgeführt wird, dürfte heute bei entsprechender Vorbereitung des Patienten nur noch selten zu beobachten sein.

Auch bei einer fehlenden Darstellung der A. vertebralis sind, sofern keine Hypoplasie vorliegt, Artefakte anzunehmen, wenn kein Kollateralkreislauf sichtbar wird (THOMAS et al., 1962; MOSELEY u. SONDHEIMER, 1974). Ausgedehnte Stagnationsthromben, die das Lumen der Vertebralarterien vollständig ausfüllen, sind nämlich im Zervikalbereich wegen der zahlreichen Seitenäste der A. vertebralis wesentlich seltener als in der A. carotis interna.

b) Verschiedene Verschlußursachen

Neben den bereits erwähnten Gefäßkompressionen oder Durchwachsungen durch Tumoren sind Gefäßverschlüsse auch beim Lupus erythematodes bekannt geworden, wobei der Verschluß mit den neurologischen Ausfallserscheinungen oft das erste Symptom darstellt (ADAMS u. GRAHAM, 1967).

Verschlüsse der extra- und intrakraniellen Arterien können bei Frauen durch Gerinnungsstörungen während der Schwangerschaft, des Wochenbettes und der Einnahme von Ovulationshemmern (JENNETT u. CROSS, 1967; ALTSCHULER et al., 1968; BERGERON u. WOOD, 1969; MUMENTHALER et al., 1970) verursacht werden.

VI. Der progressive zerebrale Gefäßverschluß (Moyamoya)

Bei dieser besonderen Form einer progressiven Stenosierung des Karotisendabschnittes und des Circulus Willisi, die schließlich zum Verschluß führt, handelt es sich um eine klinisch und radiologisch wohl definierte einheitliche Krankheit, deren Ursache aber noch nicht abgeklärt

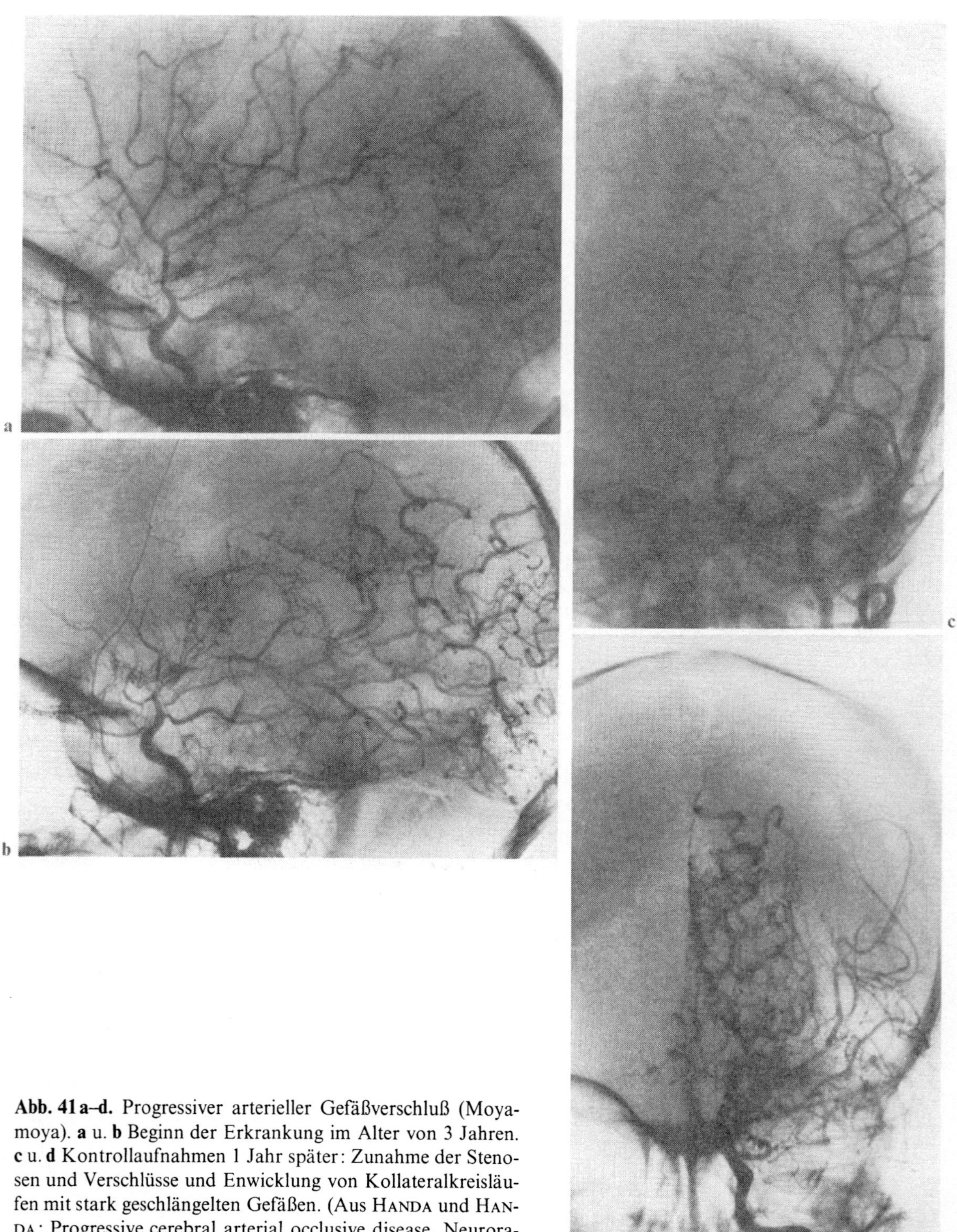

Abb. 41 a–d. Progressiver arterieller Gefäßverschluß (Moyamoya). **a** u. **b** Beginn der Erkrankung im Alter von 3 Jahren. **c** u. **d** Kontrollaufnahmen 1 Jahr später: Zunahme der Stenosen und Verschlüsse und Enwicklung von Kollateralkreisläufen mit stark geschlängelten Gefäßen. (Aus HANDA und HANDA: Progressive cerebral arterial occlusive disease. Neuroradiology 3, 119–133 (1972))

ist (ANDRÉ u. PICARD, 1974). Auch an den histologisch untersuchten Gefäßen konnten bisher keine spezifischen pathologisch-anatomischen Befunde erhoben werden (PICARD et al., 1974). Das Leiden ist in Japan offenbar besonders häufig und wurde auch von japanischen Autoren zuerst beschrieben und studiert (FUKUYAMA et al., 1965; KUDO, 1965, 1968; MORIYASU, 1965; NISHIMOTO et al., 1965; SUZUKI et al., 1965, 1966; TAKEUCHI u. KOBAYASHI, 1965; NISHIMOTO et al., 1966; YAMAMOTO et al., 1966; NISHIMOTO u. TAKEUCHI, 1968; SUZUKI u. TAKAKU, 1969; HANDA et al., 1971; HANDA u. HANDA, 1972; NISHIMOTO u. TAKEUCHI, 1972). Die Krankheit kommt aber überall und auch außerhalb der japanischen Rasse vor und scheint im außerjapanischen Gebiet keine besondere geographische Häufung aufzuweisen (LEEDS u. ABBOTT, 1965; KRAYENBÜHL u. YASARGIL, 1968; ISLER, 1969; LEPOIRE et al., 1969; TAVERAS, 1969; GALLIGIONI et al., 1971; HILAL et al., 1971a; CALLIAUW, 1972; LEVESQUE et al., 1973, 1974; PICARD et al., 1974). Die Krankheit wird bei Kindern und Jugendlichen häufiger gefunden als bei Erwachsenen, indem es sich bei 60% der beschriebenen Fälle um Jugendliche handelt. Das weibliche Geschlecht scheint bei der jüngeren Altersgruppe häufiger befallen zu sein als das männliche, während beim Erwachsenen keine eindeutige Geschlechtsbevorzugung mehr vorhanden ist. Beim Kind äußert sich die Krankheit in erster Linie in rezidivierenden Hemiparesen, die sich in der Regel wieder zurückbilden, doch können sensorische oder visuelle Störungen sowie Ausfälle der Hirnnerven oder Krampfanfälle zurückbleiben. In 30–50% der Fälle ist auch ein psychomotorisches Syndrom festzustellen (LEVESQUE et al., 1974). Ein tödlicher Ausgang ist bei Kindern relativ selten und dann meist auf eine subarachnoidale oder intrazerebrale Blutung zurückzuführen. Beim Erwachsenen manifestiert sich die Krankheit in der überwiegenden Mehrzahl der Fälle in Subarachnoidalblutungen.

Angiographisch ist das wesentliche Merkmal der Affektion eine supraklinoidale Stenosierung der A. carotis interna, wobei in den doppelseitig angiographierten Fällen die Affektion immer doppelseitig zu beobachten ist, das Ausmaß der Veränderungen aber nicht unbedingt symmetrisch sein muß. Als Folge dieser Stenosierung, die langsam bis zum Verschluß fortschreitet, kommt es zur Entwicklung eines Kollateralsystems in der Gegend der Stammganglien, des Thalamus und Hypothalamus und eventuell des Mesenzephalons über die lentikulostriären Arterien, die vorderen Chorioidalarterien, die A. recurrens Heubner, die A. communicans posterior (A. hypo-

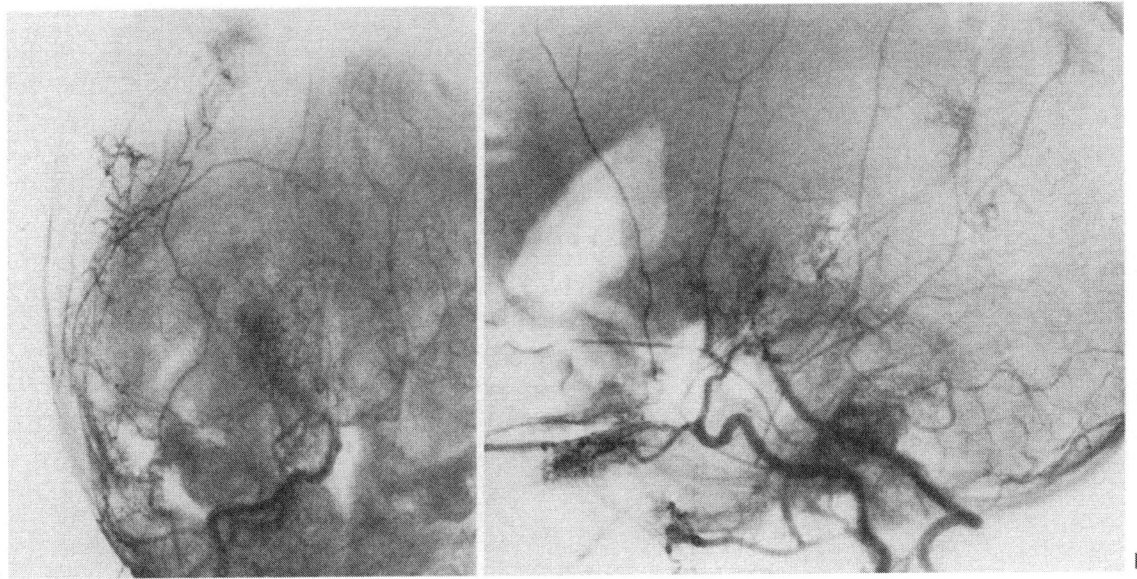

Abb. 42a u. b. Progressiver arterieller Gefäßverschluß (Moyamoya). Ausgedehnte Verschlüsse der Hirnarterien. Neben dem Kollateralennetzwerk im Bereiche der Basalganglien findet sich auch ein orbitales Moyamoya. Ausgeprägte transdurale Anastomosennetze. (Aus HANDA und HANDA: Progressive cerebral arterial occlusive disease. Neuroradiology 3, 119–133 (1972))

thalami, Ae. thalami und A. chorioidea posterior) sowie über die in Abb. 32 dargestellten Kollateralwege von der A. carotis externa her über die A. ophthalmica zum Stromgebiet der A. carotis interna distal vom Circulus Willisi (Ethmoidalarterien, Meningealarterien; HANDA u. HANDA, 1972; CROUZET et al., 1974). Diese Kollateralen erweitern sich im Verlaufe der Zeit und bilden ein dichtes Netzwerk, das sogenannte Moyamoya, das der Krankheit den Namen gegeben hat (Abb. 41 u. 42).

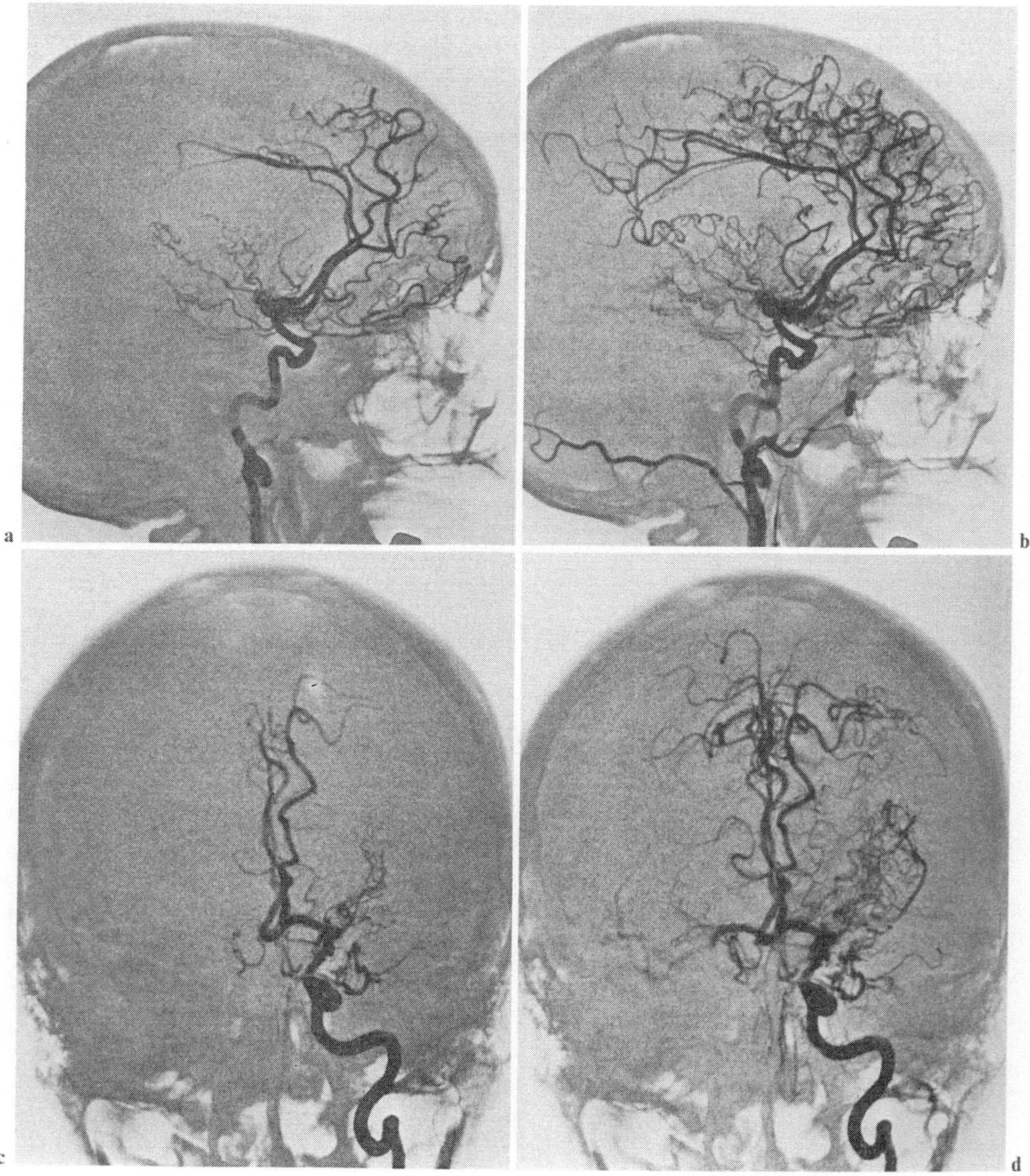

Abb. 43a–d. Kontrollangiogramm bei Verschluß der A. cerebri media links vor mehreren Jahren. Die lentikulostriären Arterien sind z.T. erweitert und stark geschlängelt. Von diesen Gefäßen aus hat sich ein Kollateralkreislauf zu den Arterien der Inselregion und zu den Mediaseitenästen im hinteren Abschnitt des Sylvischen Dreieckes entwickelt. (Verzögerte anterograde Darstellung der Kandelaberarterie). (Aus „Zerebrale Angiographie", Thieme Stuttgart, 1979)

Mit dem Fortschreiten der Krankheit greift die Stenosierung und Obliteration auf den Circulus Willisi und dessen Äste über, wodurch es zum Ausfall von Kollateralnetzen kommt und sich weiter in der Peripherie neue Kollateralgeflechte, z.B. meningo-kortikale oder transdurale Anastomosen entwickeln.

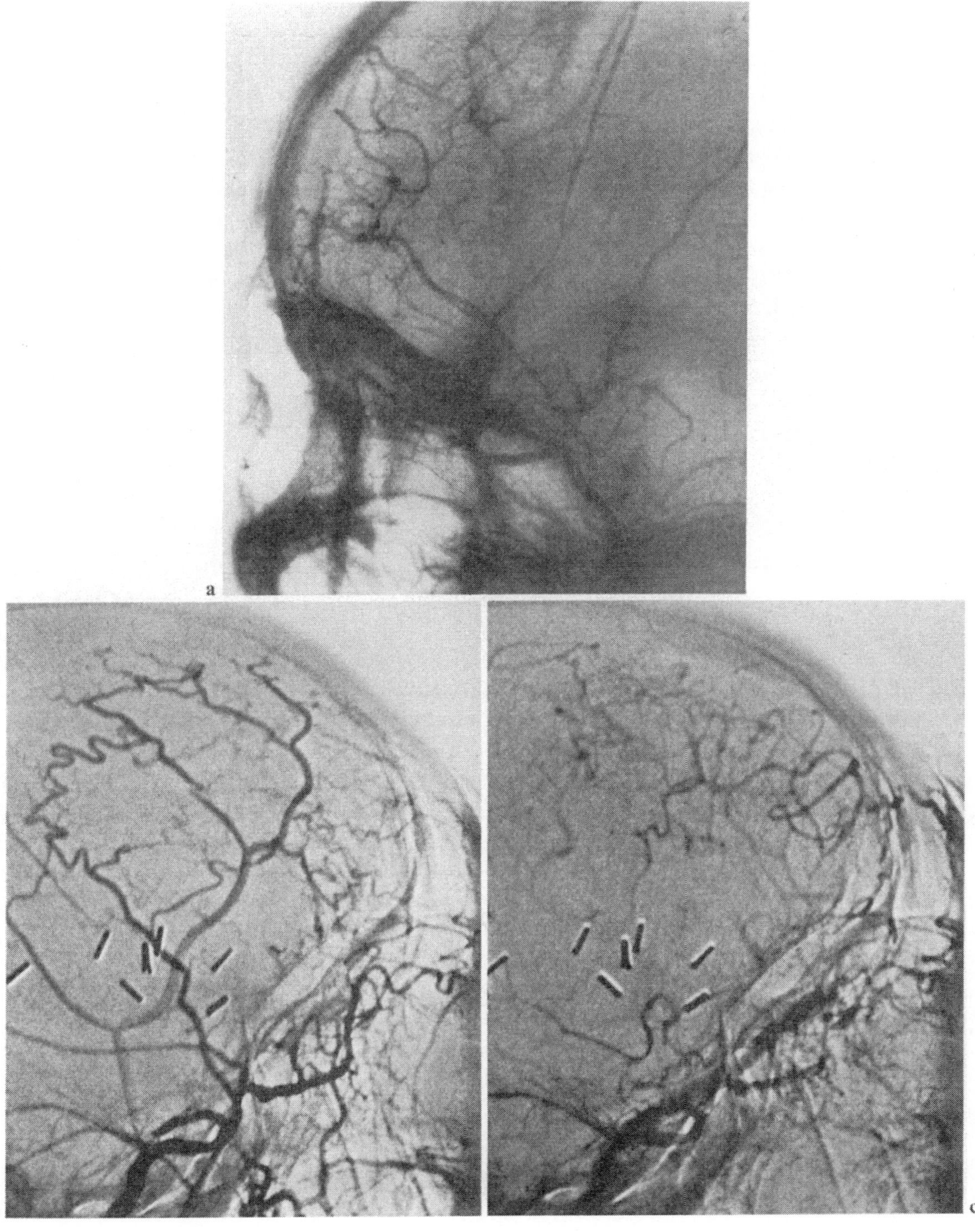

Abb. 44. a Progressiver arterieller Gefäßverschluß (Moyamoya). Darstellung der Pericallosaäste über die A. meningea anterior (aus HANDA und HANDA: Neuroradiology 3, 119–133 (1972)). **b** u. **c** Postoperativer Verschluß der A. carotis interna und beider Aa. pericallosae bei sehr großem Hypophysentumor. Darstellung der frontalen Pericallosaseitenäste über transdurale frontale Anastomosen

Nach dem Vorschlag von SUZUKI und TAKAKU (1969) wird die Krankheit in 6 Stadien unterteilt:
I. Stadium: isolierte Stenose der Karotisendstrecke.
II. Stadium: Auftreten eines feinen Kollateralgeflechtes und Erweiterung der distalen Hirnarterien.
III. Stadium: volle Entwicklung des Kollateralgeflechtes (Moyamoya) mit verminderter Darstellung der A. cerebri anterior und media.
IV. Stadium: Das basale Gefäßgeflecht verschwindet allmählich und wird durch ein gröberes Geflecht ersetzt. Die Stenosen der Karotisendstrecke dehnen sich aus und greifen auf die Hirnarterien über. Es stellt sich jetzt ein transduraler Kollateralkreislauf ein, u.a. kommt es zur Entwicklung eines orbitalen und ethmoidalen Moyamoya. Die A. cerebri anterior und die A. pericallosa sowie die A. media sind nur noch dünn und stellen sich schlecht dar.
V. Stadium: Das basale Moyamoya ist nur noch spärlich entwickelt, die A. cerebri anterior und media sind kaum mehr erkennbar. Die intrazerebralen Anastomosen von der A. cerebri posterior und die transduralen Kollateralwege verstärken sich. Die Obliteration der A. carotis interna dehnt sich proximalwärts aus.
VI. Stadium: Die Vaskularisation des Anterior-/Pericallosa- und Mediastromgebietes findet praktisch nur noch über Externaäste (transdurale Anastomosen) und vom Vertebralis/Basilarisstromgebiet her statt. Dieses Stadium wird bei Kindern kaum je beobachtet.

Es ist wiederholt bezweifelt worden, daß es sich beim Moyamoya um ein Krankheitsbild sui generis handle, da bei isolierten Gefäßverschlüssen in der Nähe des Circulus Willisi oder weiter in der Peripherie im Verlauf der Zeit sich ebenfalls ein dichtes, moyamoyaähnliches Anastomosennetz entwickeln kann (PECKER et al., 1973; PICARD et al., 1974; ZÜLCH et al., 1974; DEBRUN et al., 1975; Abb. 43 u. 44).

Ausgeprägte basale Anastomosengeflechte sind z.B. auch nach Bestrahlung von Gliomen des Chiasmas und des Hypothalamus beschrieben worden, wobei es durch die Tumorkompression und/oder Bestrahlung zum Karotisverschluß gekommen ist (LEE u. HODES, 1967; DEBRUN et al., 1975). Derartige Beobachtungen sind aber lediglich ein Beleg dafür, daß beim Jugendlichen nach Gefäßverschlüssen embolischer, entzündlicher oder kompressiver Genese infolge der noch bestehenden Adaptionsfähigkeit des Gefäßsystems eine besonders ausgiebige Entwicklung von Kollateralkreisläufen möglich ist. Diese Entwicklung eines kräftigen Kollateralkreislaufes ist zweifellos auch beim Moyamoya der wesentliche Faktor. Im Gegensatz zu diesen aufgeführten moyamoyaähnlichen Bildern beinhaltet das eigentliche Moyamoya-Syndrom aber die doppelseitige Karotisstenose und namentlich die Progression der Verschlüsse im Bereiche des Circulus Willisi mit rezidivierenden, eventuell alternierenden Hemiparesen und Subarachnoidalblutungen.

Differentialdiagnostische Schwierigkeiten zu diesem Moyamoya-Syndrom können allenfalls bilaterale Karotishypoplasien (LANCIEN, 1971), arteriovenöse Mißbildungen der zentralen Kerne und Glioblastome mit starker pathologischer Vasularisation dieser Region bilden (SIMON et al., 1974).

C. Stenosen und Verschlüsse der Gefäße distal vom Circulus Willisi

I. Diffuse Arteriosklerose der Hirngefäße

Die Angiographie ist zum Nachweis einer allgemeinen Arteriosklerose der Hirngefäße nicht indiziert. Sie kommt nur dann in Frage, wenn aufgrund der klinischen Befunde und der Ergebnisse der übrigen Hilfsuntersuchungen differentialdiagnostische Probleme bestehen (in ungefähr 5–10% der Fälle mit klinischem Verdacht auf eine Arteriosklerose der Hirngefäße liegen den neurologischen Störungen raumfordernde Prozesse zugrunde, nicht selten das chronische Subduralhämatom). Die Diagnose einer allgemeinen Arteriosklerose der Hirngefäße stellt bei strenger Indikationsstellung gewissermaßen nur ein Beiprodukt der angiographischen Abklärung dar.

In der älteren Literatur werden verschiedene Kriterien als pathognomonisch für die Arteriosklerose aufgeführt:

- z.T. gradlinig verlaufende Arterien mit Kaliberunregelmäßigkeiten
- fehlende Verzweigungen der starren eckigen Gefäße, häufig verbunden mit arteriosklerotischen Mikroaneurysmen (LÖHR, 1936).
- Darstellung der A. carotis externa vor dem Gefäßbaum der A. carotis interna.
- ANDERSEN (1955) unterscheidet aufgrund einer Studie über die Korrelation zwischen pathologischer Anatomie und Angiographie zwischen der Arteriosklerose der größeren Gefäße (Mediasklerose), die an steifen eckigen Gefäßen mit Ektasien erkennbar ist und einer diffusen hyperplastischen Sklerose (Arteriosklerose) mit Lumeneinengungen und nackten Hauptästen.

Später hat man vor der Überbewertung einzelner Befunde als Kriterien für die Arteriosklerose wie z.B. vermehrte Gefäßschlängelung, Form der Teilungsstelle der A. carotis interna am Circulus Willisi, steifer und eckiger Verlauf der Gefäße gewarnt (BULL et al., 1960).

Die Einführung der raschen Serienangiographie hat gezeigt, daß die oft als Füllungsdefekt interpretierten Befunde auf späteren Aufnahmen der Serie nicht mehr zu erheben waren und somit lediglich aussagten, daß im Moment der inkrimierten Aufnahme die Füllung noch nicht bis in die Peripherie vorgedrungen war.

Dagegen haben ihre Bedeutung für die Diagnose der Arteriosklerose nicht eingebüßt:

- Kaliberunregelmäßigkeiten der Gefäße, die sich z.T. mit der Vergrößerungstechnik wesentlich besser darstellen lassen (WENDE u. SCHINDLER, 1970; WENDE et al., 1974).
- Die spärlichen peripheren Gefäßverzweigungen. Der eckige Gefäßverlauf ist nicht selten dadurch verursacht, daß an Teilungsstellen der eine Seitenast verschlossen ist (Abb. 45).
- Die Zirkulationsverzögerung im arteriellen Schenkel, in welchem bereits ein erheblicher Druckabfall stattfindet.

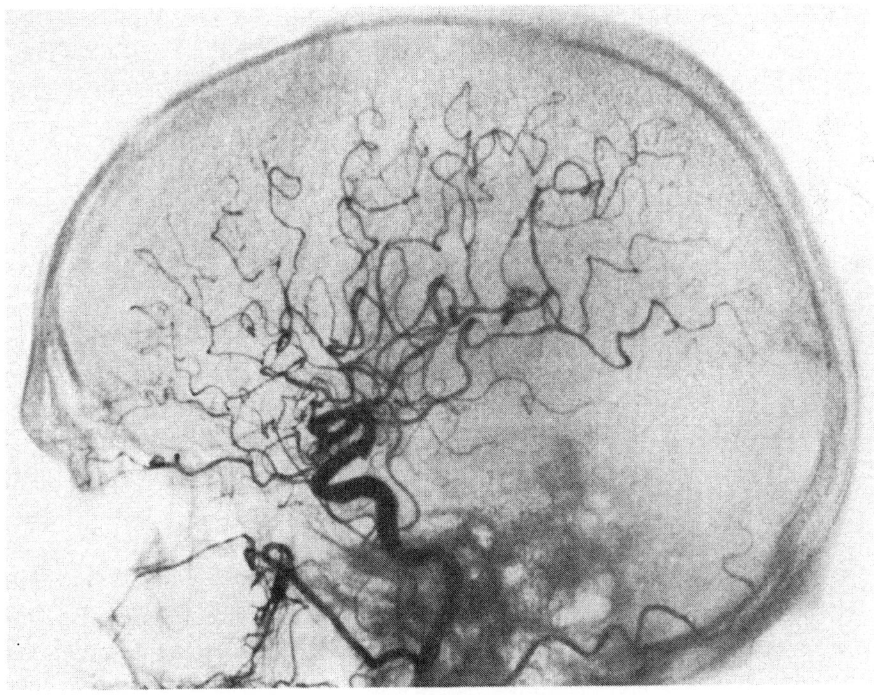

Abb. 45. Arteriosklerose der Hirngefäße

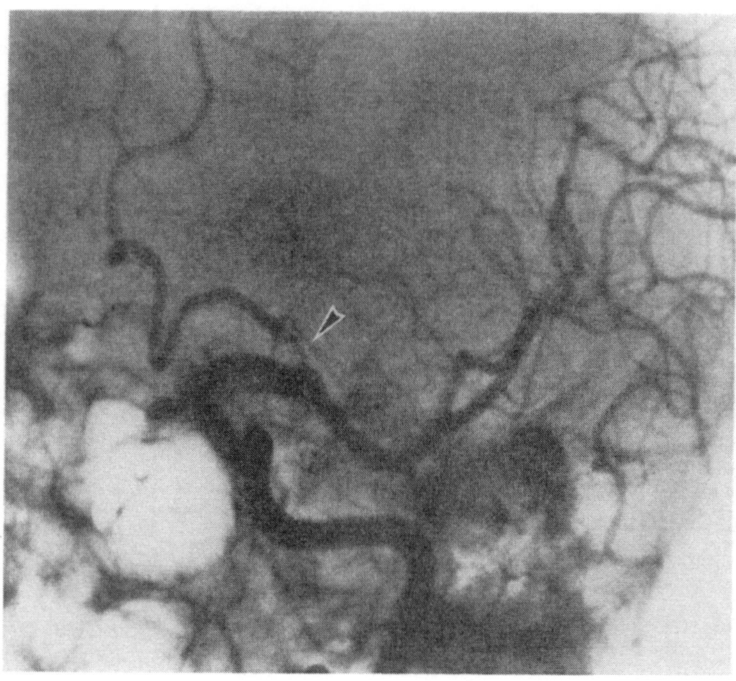

Abb. 46. Stenose am Anfangsabschnitt der A. cerebri anterior (Pfeil)

- Von geringer Bedeutung ist eine verstärkte Schlängelung, die sich unter Umständen nur schwer gegenüber den normalen Variationen abgrenzen läßt. Durch diese Schlängelungen sind die früher erwähnten Mikroaneurysmen vorgetäuscht worden.

Die Kaliberunregelmäßigkeiten der Gehirnarterien infolge Arteriosklerose können ganz verschiedene Verteilungsmuster aufweisen (ROVIRA, 1969):
- Lokalisierte Stenose an einer einzigen Hirnarterie (Abb. 46).
- Im Verlaufe einer Arterie finden sich verschiedene Lumeneinengungen, wobei gelegentlich zwischen den einzelnen Stenosen oder auch hinter der distalsten Stenose eine Dilatation zu beobachten ist.
- Ein ganzes Gefäßterritorium wie das Stromgebiet der A. cerebri media oder der A. pericallosa oder sogar Gefäße in verschiedenen Territorien weisen Stenosierungen und Verschlüsse auf (Abb. 47).

In stenosierten Arterien kommt es häufig zu einer verzögerten anterograden Füllung. Die angiographisch faßbare Entwicklung eines Kollateralkreislaufes ist in dieser Situation aber selten. In Einzelfällen sind im peripheren Stromgebiet der meist mit Kaliberunregelmäßigkeiten behafteten Arterien feine, z.T. unregelmäßig geschlängelte Arterien zu sehen, die normalerweise zumindest in dieser regellosen geflechtartigen Form nicht vorkommen. Es ist nicht ausgeschlossen, daß es sich dabei um eine Art Kollateralkreislauf als Kompensationsmechanismus bei hochgradiger Stenosierung handelt, wie er in stärker ausgeprägter Form bei Moyamoya zu sehen ist. Gleichartige feine Gefäßnetze finden sich auch distal von embolischen Gefäßverschlüssen, selbst wenn das ursprünglich verschlossene Gefäß wieder rekanalisiert ist (TAVERAS u. WOOD, 1964; RING, 1966). Auch nach Rekanalisation und klinischer Restitution bleibt die regionale Durchblutung aber vermindert (KOHLMEYER, 1971). Aufgrund des angiographischen Befundes allein und ohne die Möglichkeit des Vergleiches mit früheren Stadien der Erkrankung dürfte eine Unterscheidung zwischen arteriosklerotischer Stenose und partieller Rekanalisation nach embolischem Verschluß bei diesen kleinen Gefäßen kaum möglich sein.

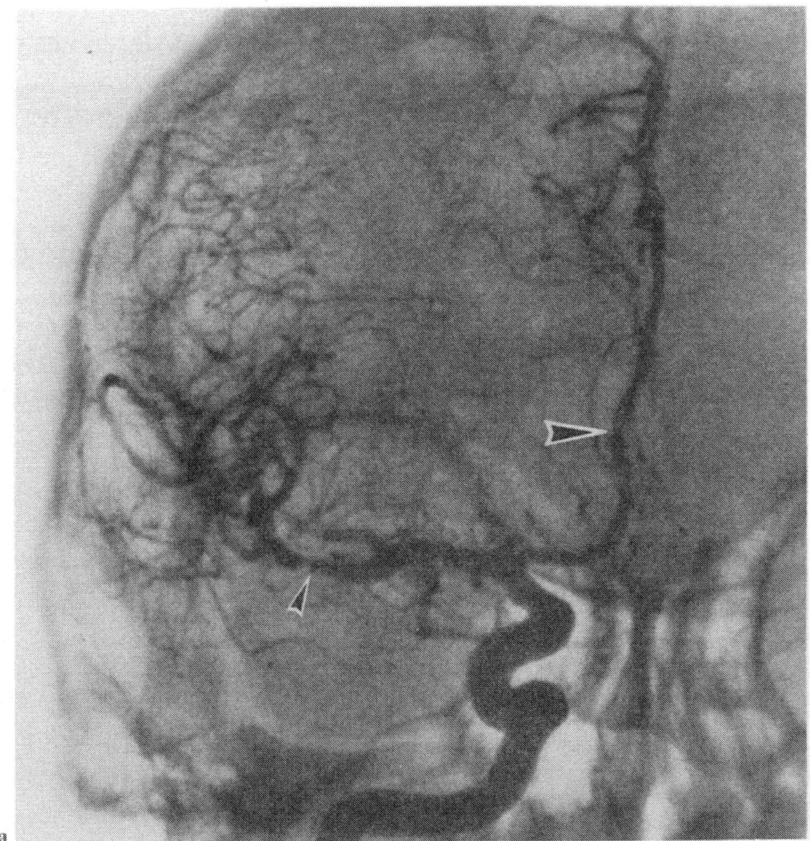

a

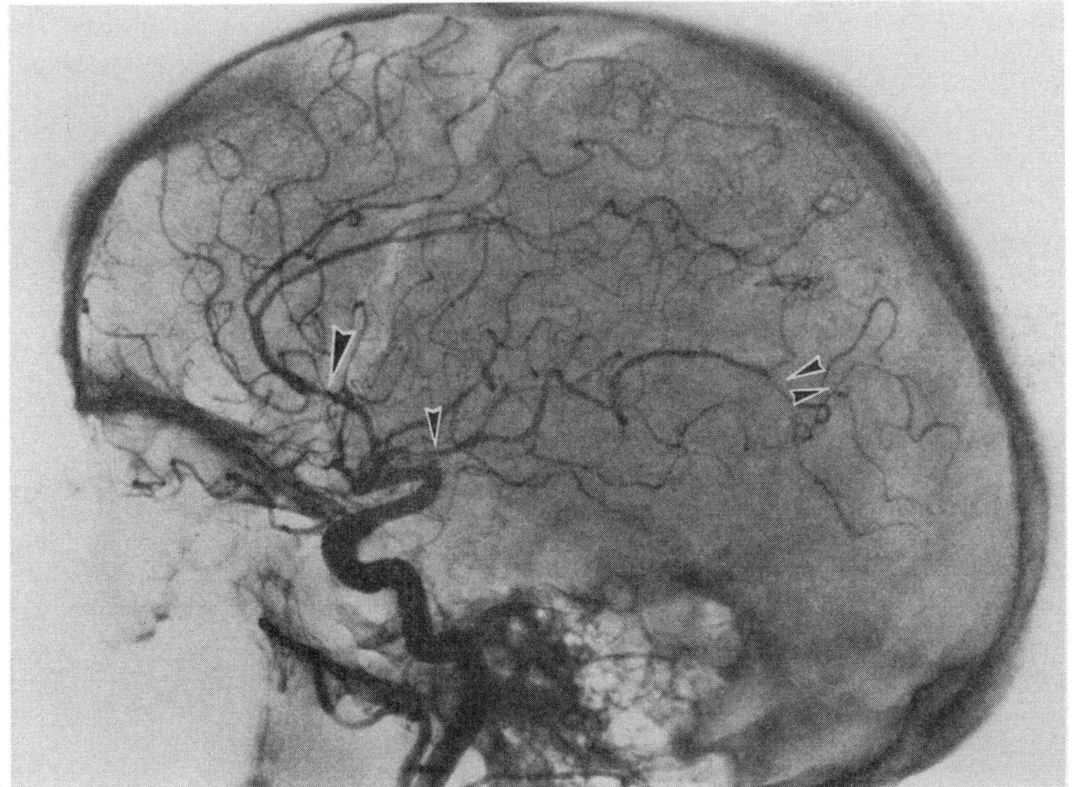

b

Abb. 47a u. b. Multiple Stenosen an der A. pericallosa (großer Pfeil), dem sphenoidalen Abschnitt der A. cerebri media und den peripheren Mediaästen (kleine Pfeile)

II. Lokalisierte Stenosen

Atheromatöse Plaques verursachen meist exzentrische und unregelmäßige Stenosen der Hirnarterien, die denjenigen an den großen Gefäßen proximal vom Circulus Willisi vollkommen entsprechen, doch sind die morphologischen Details wegen der Feinheit der Gefäße oft nicht mehr mit Sicherheit zu beurteilen. RESCH und BAKER (1964) fanden atheromatöse Gefäßwandveränderungen distal vom Circulus Willisi hauptsächlich an den Anfangsabschnitten der A. cerebri media und posterior.

Von den atherosklerotischen Stenosen sind die Stenosen anderer Genese abzugrenzen, was aufgrund des Röntgenbildes allein und ohne zusätzliche weitere Angaben aus Klinik oder Laboratorium aber häufig nicht möglich ist.

1. Stenosierung durch Gefäßkompression

Relativ einfach ist die Diagnose einer Stenosierung oder Obliteration durch einen raumfordernden Prozeß, der sich als solcher an Verlagerungen und pathologischen Gefäßen erkennen läßt. Die Einengungen erfolgen meist durch Anpressung des Gefäßes an starre Strukturen der Schädelbasis oder freie Ränder der Dura, z.B. in Fällen einer Herniation in den Tentoriumschlitz oder unter der Falx hindurch. Nicht mit atheromatösen Plaques zu verwechseln sind die bei starken Verlagerungen durch Hämatome auftretenden Eindellungen der Karotisendstrecke durch die Processus clinoidei anteriores, das Chiasma, das Ligamentum interclinoideum und das Dorsum sellae (WELCH u. CRAIGMILE, 1963). Einschnürungen der A. carotis interna kommen auch durch Zug der in den Tentoriumschlitz eingepreßten A. communicans posterior zustande (Abb. 48–50).

Bei Subarachnoidalblutungen infolge Aneurysmaruptur auftretende Spasmen sind als solche wegen der konzentrischen Gefäßeinengung mit glatter Wand meist leicht zu identifizieren, ebenso die im frischen Stadium von Hirnverletzungen gelegentlich zu beobachtenden Kaliberunregelmäßigkeiten (FREIDENFELT u. SUNDSTRÖM, 1963; HUBER, 1964).

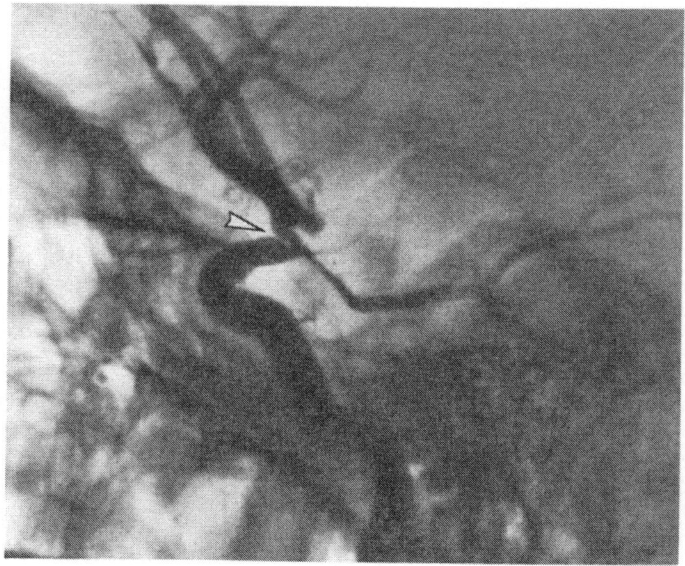

Abb. 48. Einengung der Karotisendstrecke durch Zug der in den Tentoriumschlitz eingepreßten A. communicans posterior bei temporalem Epiduralhämatom. (Aus „Zerebrale Angiographie", Thieme Stuttgart, 1979)

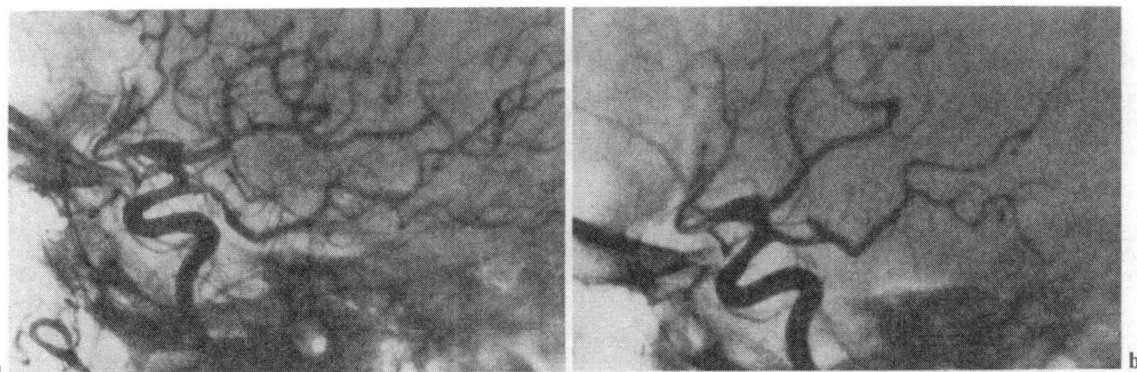

Abb. 49a u. b. Einengung der tiefgedrängten A. communicans posterior bei temporalem Hämatom **a**. Normalisierung des Verlaufes und des Kalibers der A. communicans posterior nach operativer Hämatomausräumung **b**

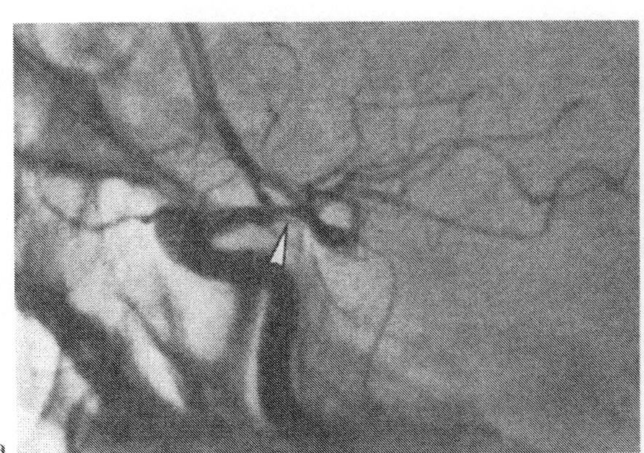

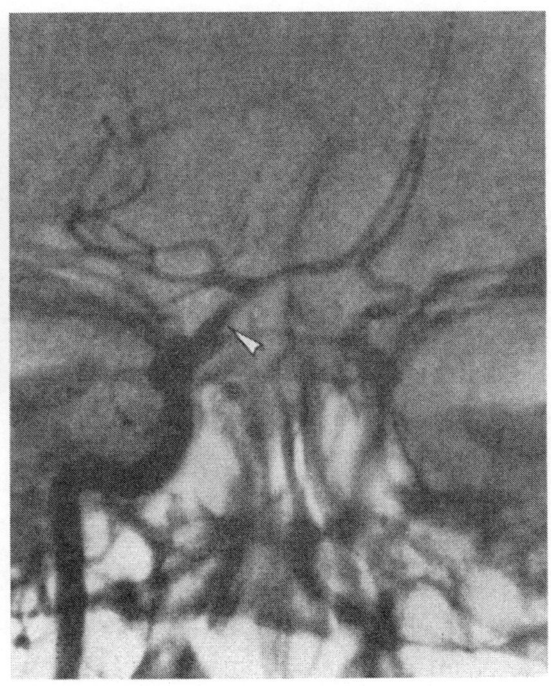

Abb. 50a u. b. Starke Verlagerung der A. carotis interna bei großem Epiduralhämatom und Eindellung der Karotisendstrecke durch Dorsum sellae (Pfeil). (Aus „Zerebrale Angiographie", Thieme Stuttgart, 1979)

2. Stenosen bei entzündlichen Gefäßerkrankungen

Entzündungen infektiöser und nicht infektiöser Art können zu Gefäßeinengungen führen und zwar über den Weg einer Arteriitis mit Wandinfiltraten, evtl. in Kombination mit Spasmen, Exsudaten oder Wandödemen (FERRIS, 1974). Auf die Einengung der basalen Gefäße bei der Meningitis tuberculosa wurde von GREITZ (1964), DAVIS und TAVERAS (1966), LEHRER (1966), WADIA und SINGKAL (1968) und LEEDS und GOLDBERG (1971) hingewiesen. Ähnliche Veränderungen kommen bei der Lues (RABINOV, 1963; SUCHENWIRTH, 1967) und der purulenten Meningitis (LYONS u. LEEDS, 1967) oder Abszessen (RAIMONDI et al., 1965) vor. Die Einengungen finden sich vorwiegend an den größeren Arterien, während die kleinkalibrigen peripheren Gefäßabschnitte verschlossen werden. Wie bei den Verschlüssen anderer Genese können sich Kollateralkreisläufe entwickeln und im Frühstadium des Verschlusses kann eine vorzeitige Venenfüllung beobachtet

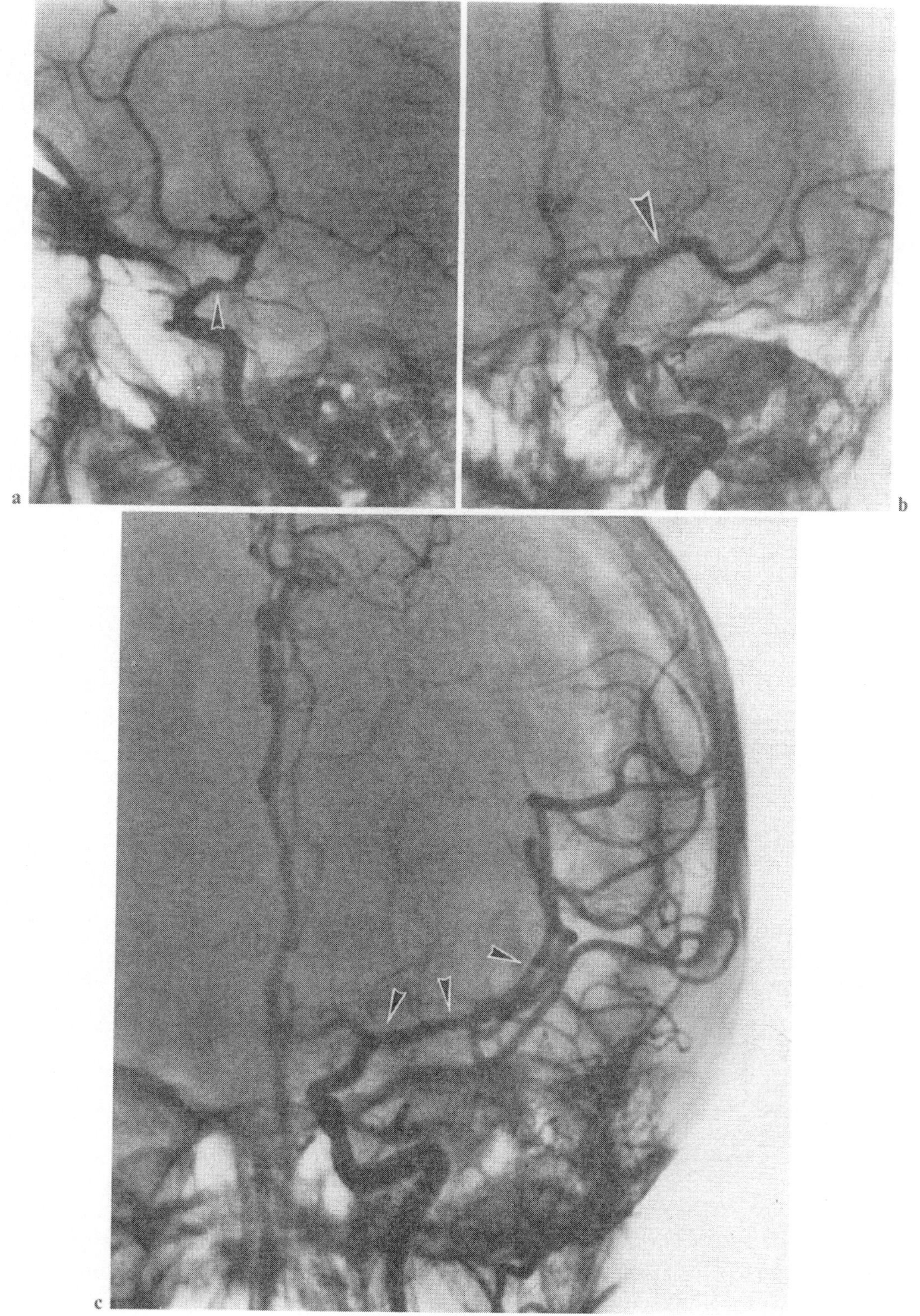

Abb. 51 a–c. Ringförmige Stenose der Karotisendstrecke (Pfeil) und gezähnelte Wandunregelmäßigkeiten an der Anfangsstrecke der A. cerebri media (großer Pfeil) bei partiellem Mediaverschluß. Ätiologie ungeklärt, keine infektiöse Erkrankung bekannt **a, b**. Perlschnurartige A. cerebri media, Ätiologie unklar. Arteriitis? Fibromuskuläre Dysplasie? **c**

werden als Zeichen einer fokalen Hyperämie. Als charakteristisch für den Gefäßverschluß bei einer Perivaskulitis wird das fadenförmige Auslaufen des Kontrastmittels bezeichnet im Gegensatz zum abrupten Verschluß beim Embolus (FERRIS et al., 1968b; vgl. Abb. 1).

Bei septischen Embolien kann es zur Bildung eines Abszesses im Infarktbereich kommen. Infolge einer lokalen Schädigung der Gefäßwand können sich auch mykotische Aneurysmen entwickeln, die nicht selten fusiform sind (FERRIS et al., 1968b; BELL u. BUTLER, 1968; WISE u. FARMER, 1971; MOLINARI et al., 1973).

Unter den zahlreichen weiteren Krankheiten, die gelegentlich auch im Bereich der Hirngefäße zu Stenosierungen oder Verschlüssen führen, sich im wesentlichen aber nicht von Verschlüssen und Stenosen auf arteriosklerotischer oder thromboembolischer Basis unterscheiden, finden sich Aktinomykose (WICKBOM u. DAVIDSON, 1967), Sichelzellanämie (STOCKMAN et al., 1972), Riesenzellsarkome (LIEBESKIND et al., 1973), Lupus erythematodes (SILVERSTEIN, 1963; TREVOR et al., 1972), Periarteriitis nodosa (FORD u. SIEKERT, 1965; ROOS, 1969), Riesenzellarteriitis (WILKINSON u. RUSSEL, 1972) sowie zahlreiche weitere Affektionen.

Der perlschnurartige Aspekt von Hirnarterien, der meist im Anfangsabschnitt der A. cerebri media beobachtet wird, ist schwierig zu deuten, da er offenbar bei den verschiedensten Gefäßleiden vorkommen kann. Ob es sich dabei um eine fibromuskuläre Dysplasie der intrakraniellen Gefäße handelt (HUBER u. FUCHS, 1967; IOSUE et al., 1972; MANELFE et al., 1974) oder um eine Arteriitis im Gefolge von nasopharyngealen Infekten (HARWOOD-NASH et al., 1971), läßt sich häufig nicht entscheiden, da die histologische Verifikation nicht erbracht werden kann. Namentlich beim Fehlen jeglicher Begleiterkrankung wird man sich deshalb mit der morphologischen Beschreibung des Bildes begnügen müssen (Abb. 51).

3. Drogenangiopathie

Nekrotisierende Angiitiden mit lokalen Lumeneinengungen und Erweiterungen, eventuell verbunden mit Mikroaneurysmen, die zu Infarkten und Blutungen führen können, sind beim Drogenmißbrauch beschrieben und auch tierexperimentell erzeugt worden (CITRON et al., 1970; GOODMAN u. BECKER, 1970; KURTZMAN, 1970; WEISS et al., 1970; MARGOLIS u. NEWTON, 1971; RUMBAUGH et al., 1971a, b; SOBEL et al., 1971; SYPERT u. YOUNG, 1972; WOODS u. STREWLER, 1972; GILROY et al., 1973). Ob dem Amphetamin dabei eine besondere Bedeutung zukommt oder ob es sich um drogenunspezifische Wirkungen, wie Sepsis, Embolien und Thrombosen, handelt, dürfte im Einzelfall jeweils schwierig zu entscheiden sein.

Stenosen und Verschlüsse sind aber auch bei medikamentöser Verwendung anderer Substanzen beobachtet worden, so z.B. beim Ergotamin (RICHTER u. BANKER, 1973) und der Epsilonaminokapronsäure (SONNTAG u. STEIN, 1974).

4. Angiodysplasien

Bei zahlreichen Phakomatosen, Bindegewebsdysplasien und angeborenen Stoffwechselstörungen sind ebenfalls Stenosen und Verschlüsse kleinerer Gefäße zu beobachten (WESENBERG et al., 1969; HILAL et al., 1971b; ANDRÉ et al., 1974). Die Bilder der Verschlüsse, eventuell verbunden mit Ektasien und vermehrten Gefäßschlängelungen, wie sie z.B. bei neurokutanen Syndromen (DI CHIRO u. LINDGREN, 1951; POSER u. TAVERAS, 1957; CHAO, 1959; HILAL et al., 1971b) und beim Kinky-hair-Syndrom (WESENBERG et al., 1969) beschrieben werden, sind für die einzelnen Syndrome nicht pathognomisch, sondern weisen lediglich auf die Angiodysplasie hin. Die Zuordnung zu einem bestimmten Syndrom ist erst aufgrund der Klinik und genetischen Untersuchungen, resp. Stoffwechseluntersuchungen (Kupferstoffwechsel beim erwähnten Kinky-hair-Syndrom), möglich.

III. Verschlüsse von Hirnarterien distal vom Circulus Willisi

Die Infarkte infolge thrombotischer Gefäßverschlüsse verteilen sich ziemlich gleichmäßig über das ganze Gehirn, während die durch einen Embolus verursachten Gefäßverschlüsse und Infarkte zur Hauptsache im Mediastromgebiet zu finden sind (JÖRGENSEN u. TORVIK, 1969).

Beim Verschluß der größeren und mittleren Hirnarterien kommt es meist in ganz unterschiedlichem Ausmaß zur Darstellung eines Kollateralkreislaufes. Dieser Kollateralkreislauf ist naturgemäß an den größeren Gefäßen leichter zu erkennen als an den feinen Seitenästen. Rein angiographisch sind deshalb zuverlässige Zahlen über die Häufigkeit der Verschlüsse der peripheren kleinen Äste nicht erhältlich. Namentlich beim proximalen Verschluß von Hirnarterien sind trotz Kollateralkreislauf weiter in der Peripherie gelegene segmentale Verschlüsse häufig entweder schwer zu erkennen oder können aber dadurch vorgetäuscht werden, daß kontrastloses Blut aus anderen Gefäßterritorien über Anastomosen in das Verschlußgebiet einströmt.

Die Korrelation zwischen neurologischen Störungen und dem angiographischen Befund ist relativ gut bei Verschlüssen der A. cerebri anterior, A. pericallosa und der A. cerebri posterior, etwas schlechter dagegen bei Infarkten, die im Stromgebiet der A. cerebri media gelegen sind (BALOW et al., 1966; WADDINGTON u. RING, 1968). Diese schlechte Korrelation ist z.T. dadurch bedingt, daß ein Verschluß der lentikulostriären Arterien zwar zu Hemiparesen führt, daß diese feinen Arterien aber oft schlecht erkennbar und namentlich in ihrer Zahl variabel sind, weshalb ein Ausfall von einem oder zweien dieser Gefäße sich dem Nachweis entziehen kann. Wird die Angiographie erst einige Zeit nach dem akuten zerebralen Insult durchgeführt, so besteht die Möglichkeit, daß sich das Gefäß rekanalisiert hat und der angiographische Befund somit trotz Halbseitenlähmung normal ist (GANNON u. CHAIT, 1962; FIESCHI u. BOZZAO, 1969; SINDERMANN et al., 1969).

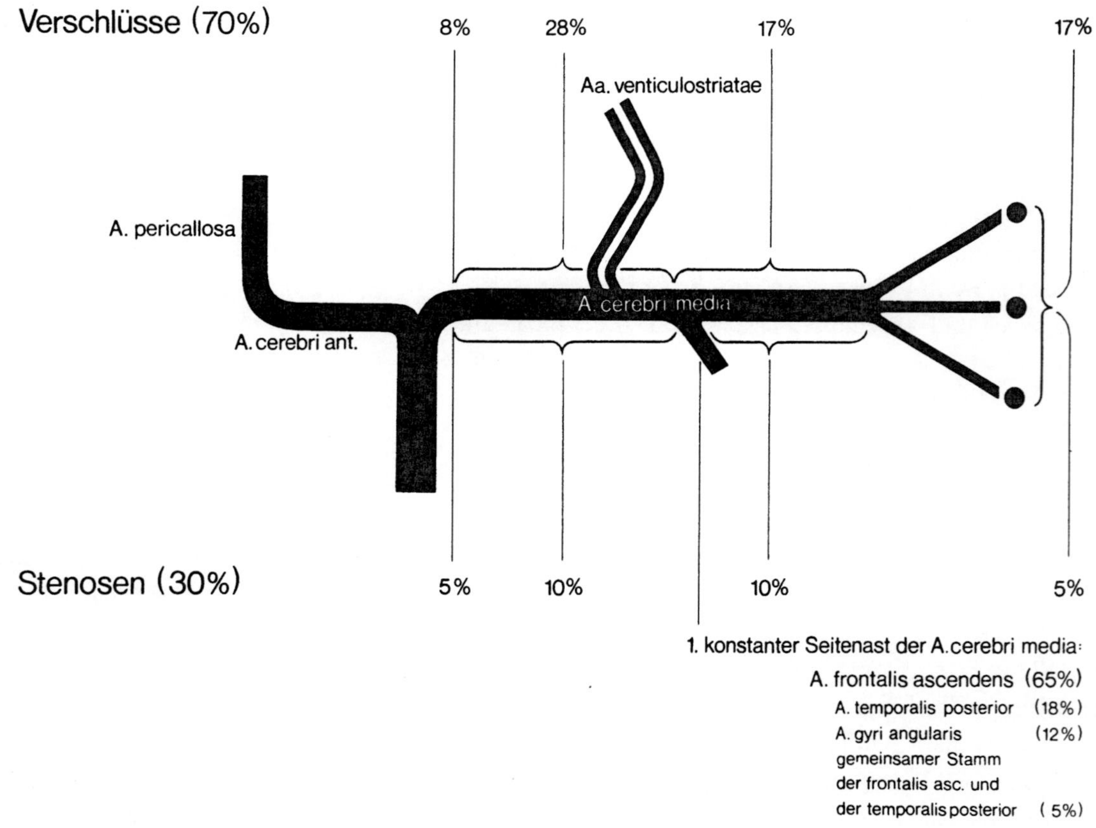

Abb. 52. Topographische Verteilung der Stenosen und Verschlüsse der A. cerebri media (nach BURROWS u. LASCELLES, 1965)

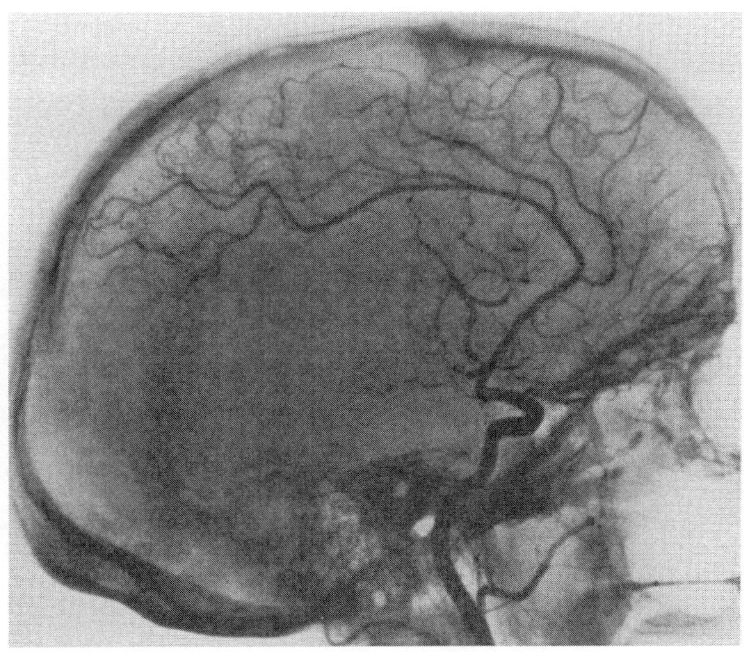

Abb. 53. Verschluß der A. cerebri media distal vom Abgang des ersten größeren Seitenastes (A. frontalis ascendens). Lentikulostriäre Arterien gut sichtbar

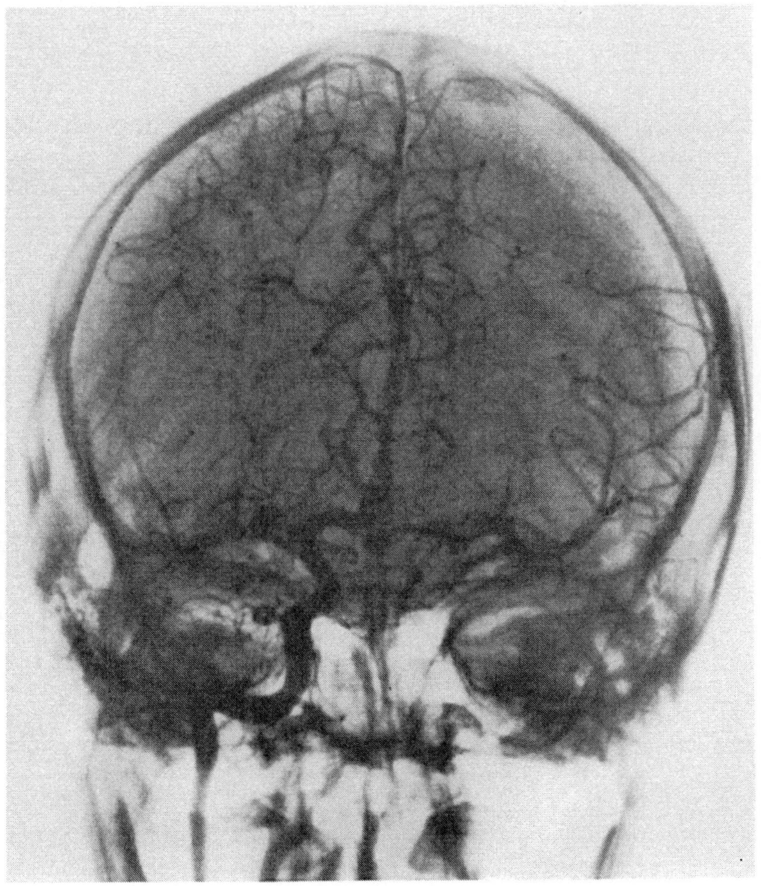

Abb. 54. Darstellung der kontralateralen Hemisphärengefäße über den vorderen Abschnitt des Circulus Willisi bei Verschluß der A. cerebri media rechts

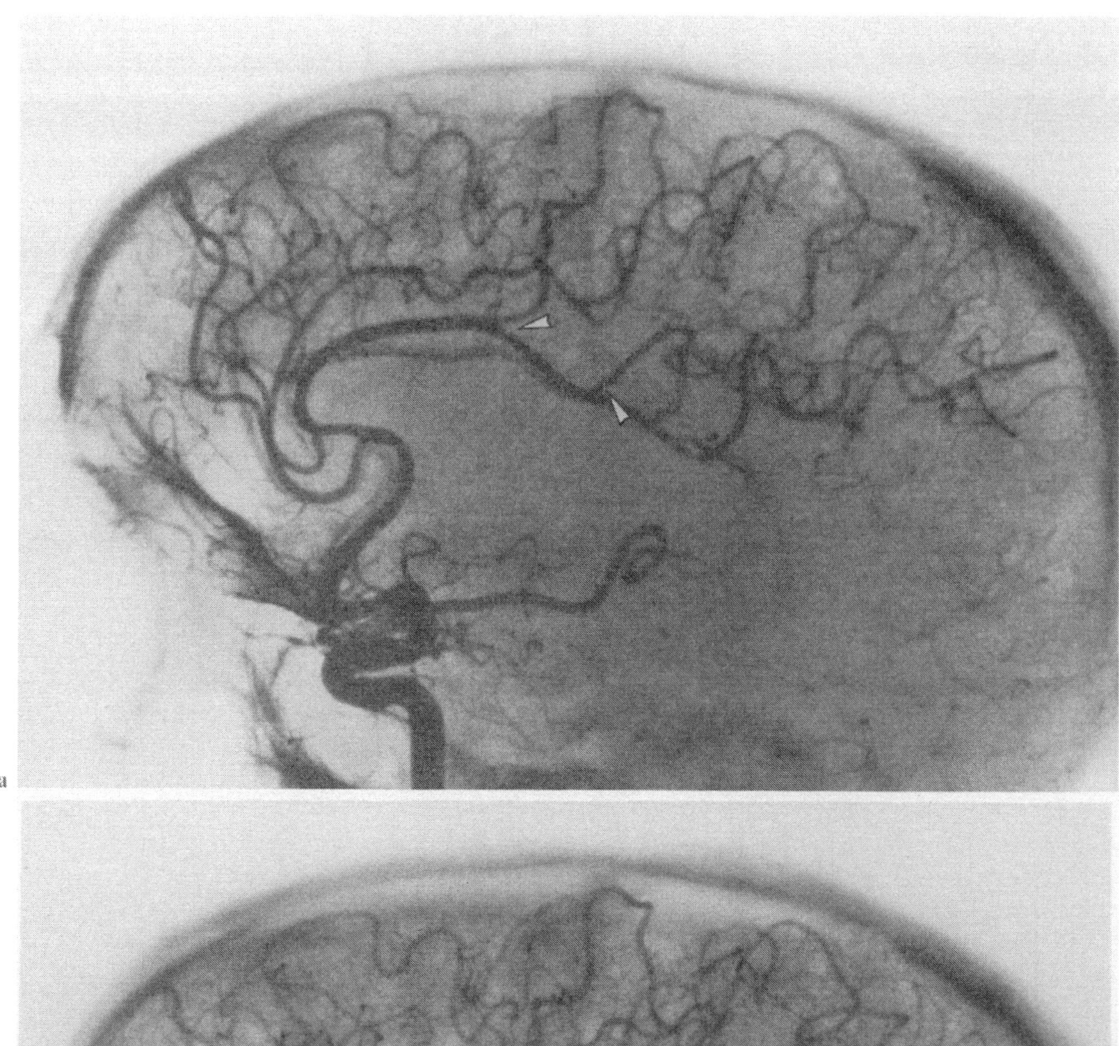

a

b

Abb. 55a–d. Verschluß der A. cerebri media mit gut entwickeltem Kollateralkreislauf über leptomeningeale Anastomosen von der A. pericallosa her. Das Mediastromgebiet stellt sich retrograd bis nahe an die Verschlußstelle dar. Kleine lokalisierte Stenosen an der A. pericallosa (**a**, Pfeile). Embolusfragmente? Kleine Plaques?

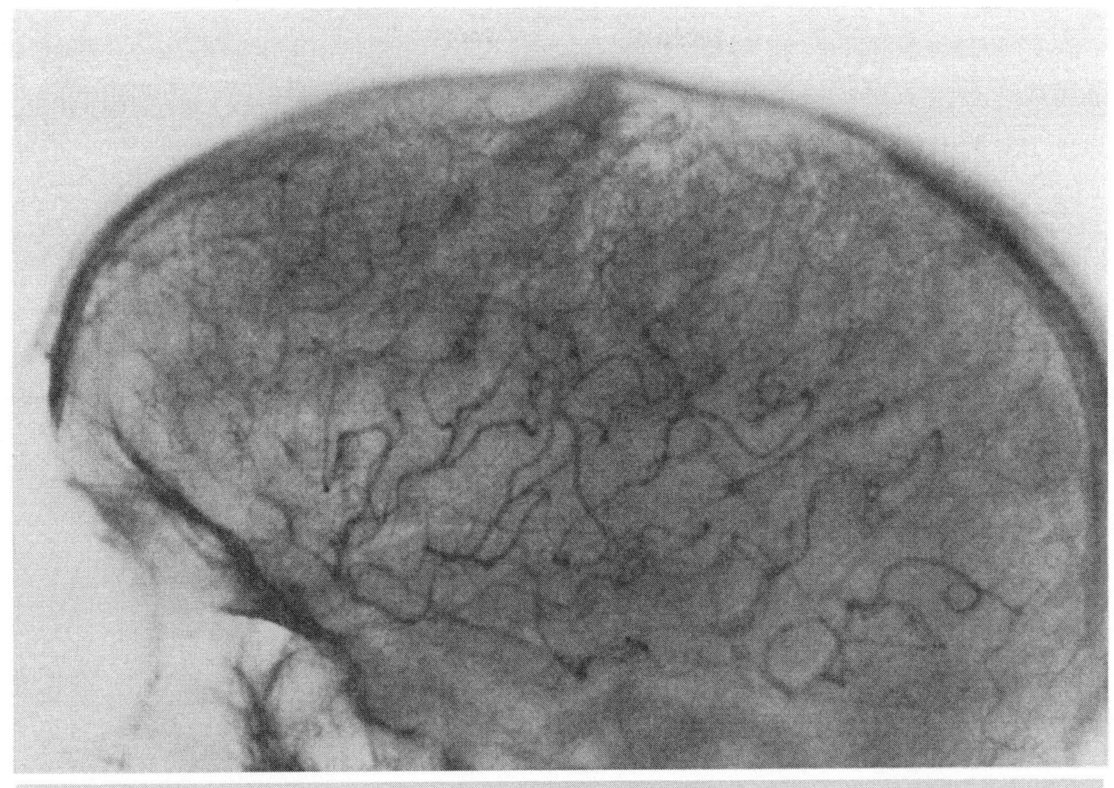

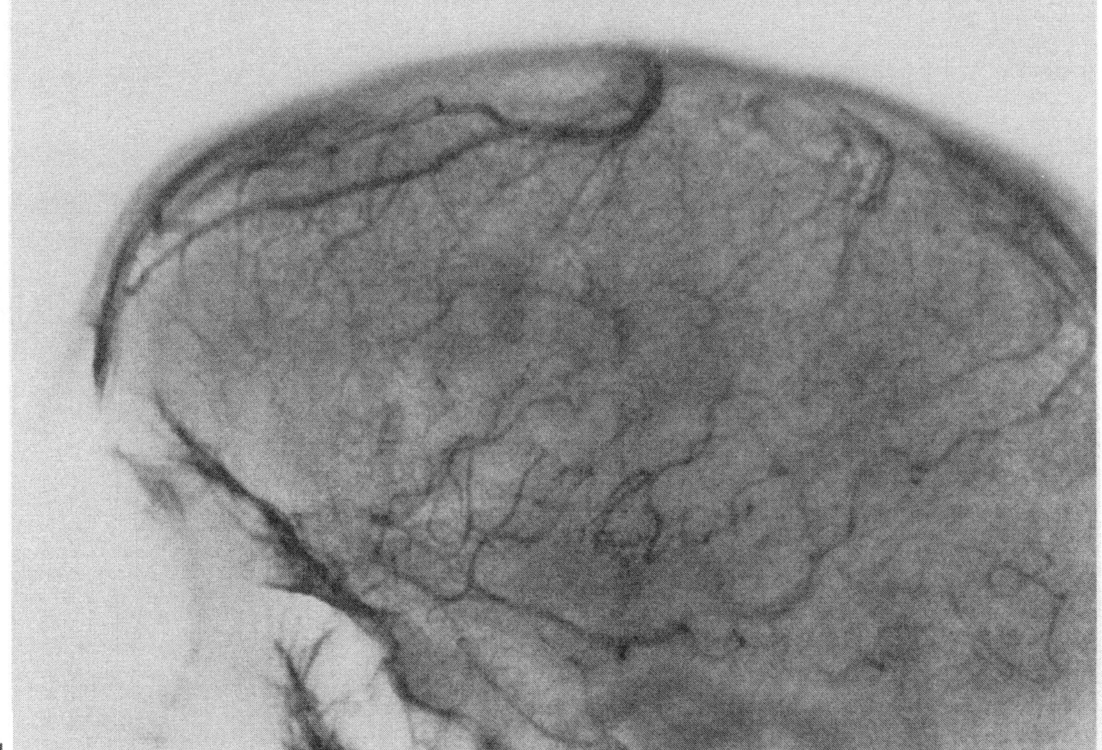

d

Abb. 55c u. d

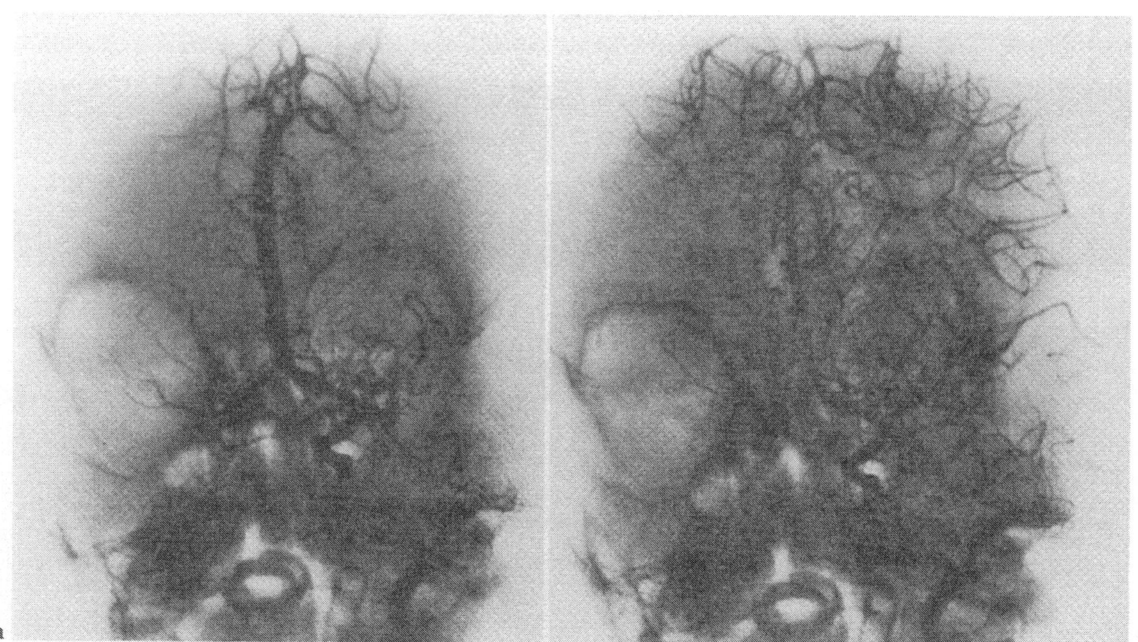

Abb. 56a u. b. Doppelseitiger Mediaverschluß. Die beiden Aa. pericallosae versorgen über leptomeningeale Anastomosen die peripheren Abschnitte des Mediastromgebietes

1. Verschlüsse der A. cerebri media und ihrer Äste

Am häufigsten finden sich Verschlüsse der A. cerebri media und ihrer Seitenäste (78% der intrakraniellen Gefäßverschlüsse nach DORNDORF u. GÄNSHIRT, 1972). Da die A. cerebri media in hämodynamischer Hinsicht die direkte Fortsetzung der A. carotis interna darstellt, ist es verständlich, daß gerade das Stromgebiet der A. cerebri media so häufig von Verschlüssen durch Embolien befallen ist (BLADIN, 1964; LUESSENHOP, 1969). Die Verschlußstelle liegt dabei sehr häufig im horizontalen Abschnitt der A. cerebri media zwischen A. carotis interna und Teilungsstelle des Mediahauptstammes am Mediaknie (BURROWS u. LASCELLES, 1965; Abb. 52). Liegt der Verschluß nicht im Anfangsabschnitt der A. cerebri media, sondern auf Höhe ihrer Teilungsstelle, so sind die orbitofrontalen Mediaäste oft noch frei durchgängig, da sie in einem relativ spitzen Winkel aus dem Mediahauptstamm abgehen können (Abb. 53). In diesen Fällen sind auch die lentikulostriären Arterien gut sichtbar. Nicht selten findet sich beim totalen Mediaverschluß angiographisch eine Darstellung der kontralateralen Hemisphärengefäße über den Circulus Willisi, da das Blut unter dem Injektionsdruck vor dem Hindernis zur Gegenseite ausweicht (Abb. 54). Der Kollateralkreislauf zum Mediastromgebiet findet meist über kortikale Anastomosen aus dem Perikallosastromgebiet zu den frontalen, präzentralen und parietalen Mediaästen, aus der A. cerebri posterior zur A. temporalis posterior und zur A. gyri angularis statt (Abb. 55–57). Bei sehr proximalen Mediahauptstammverschlüssen können sich über diese Kollateralen auch die lentikulostriären Arterien noch füllen. Bei Verschlüssen im Bereich der Ursprungsstelle der lentikulostriären Arterien sind Kollateralkreisläufe aus der A. cerebri anterior via A. recurrens Heubneri, aus der A. chorioidea anterior via deren zisternale Äste, aus der A. communicans posterior via prämammilare Arterien und aus der A. cerebri posterior via Aa. thalamoperforantes möglich, angiographisch jedoch nur selten sicher faßbar. Diese Kollateralkreisläufe können angio-

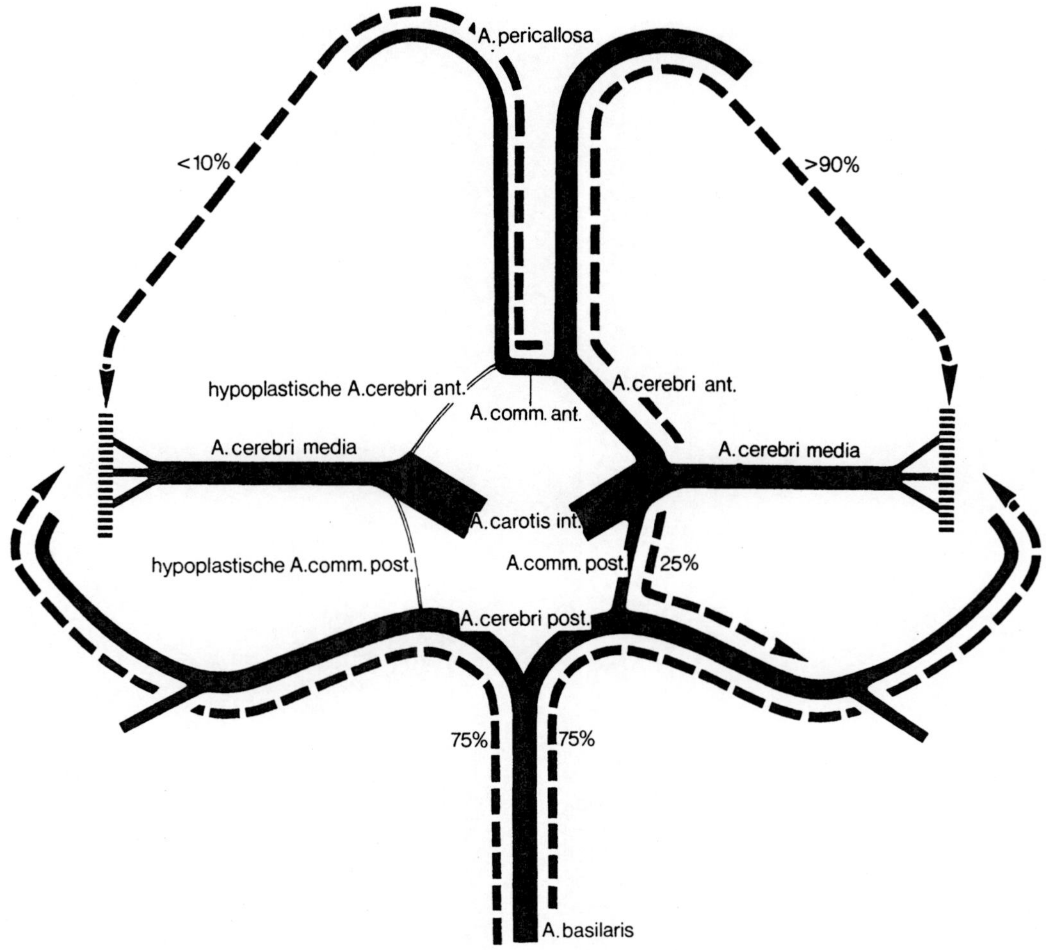

Abb. 57. Die Bedeutung der Anastomosensysteme beim Mediaverschluß

graphisch schon in kürzester Zeit nach dem Verschlußereignis sichtbar werden (Dichgans u. Voigt, 1969).

Beim Stammverschluß der A. cerebri media kommt es in ca. 25% der Fälle infolge eines Ödems zu einer Seitenverlagerung der A. pericallosa (Sindermann et al., 1969). Beim ungenügenden Kollateralkreislauf und fehlender Gefäßzeichnung kann, speziell bei offenen orbito-frontalen Ästen, auf den anteroposterioren Aufnahmen der Eindruck eines subduralen Hämatoms entstehen (Lee u. Hodes, 1967; Lehrer et al., 1967; Abb. 58, vgl. auch Abb. 9).

Die meisten Autoren sind sich einig, daß aufgrund des angiographisch sichtbaren Kollateralkreislaufes keine sichere Prognose hinsichtlich der Erholungsfähigkeit gestellt werden kann. Patienten mit gutem Kollateralkreislauf während der Ödemphase sind – statistisch gesehen – vielleicht etwas besser dran als Patienten mit fehlendem oder kaum nachweisbarem Kollateralkreis (Burrows u. Lascelles, 1965; Larson et al., 1965; Shenkin et al., 1965; Huber, 1966; Allcock, 1967).

Während der Verschluß größerer Mediaäste in der Regel keine diagnostischen Schwierigkeiten bietet, ist die Diagnose kleiner Astverschlüsse keineswegs immer augenfällig und sicher, da Anzahl und Verlauf dieser kleinen Äste variabel sind. Ring (1966, 1969) hat ein topographisches Schema ausgearbeitet, mit dessen Hilfe sich der Ausfall der kleineren Mediaseitenäste leichter erfassen läßt (Geraud et al., 1970). Für einen peripheren Astverschluß spricht das Auftreten eines retrograden Kontrastmitteleinstromes über Anastomosen, der sich mit der fraktionierten Subtraktion (Rivoir u. Huber, 1974) im dichten Netz der peripheren Gefäße leichter erfassen läßt als auf den Originalaufnahmen. Bei peripheren Gefäßverschlüssen kann jedoch auch ein verzögerter

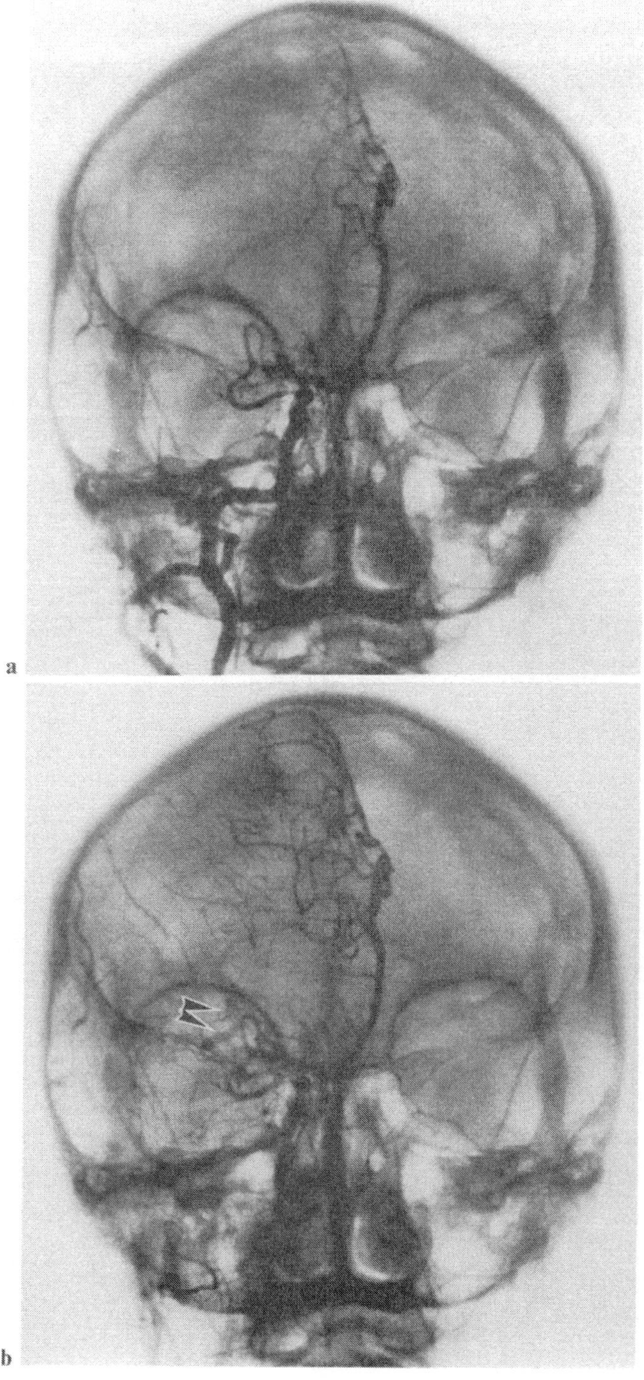

Abb. 58a u. b. Massive Verlagerung der A. pericallosa nach links bei Hirnödem rechts nach Mediaverschluß rechts. Vorzeitige Darstellung der V. ophthalmica superior (**b**, Pfeile). (Aus „Zerebrale Angiographie", Thieme Stuttgart, 1979)

anterograder Strom proximal und ein retrograder Strom distal vom Verschluß beobachtet werden (SINDERMANN et al., 1974; Abb. 59, 60).

Bei diesen kleinen Astverschlüssen, die meist embolisch bedingt sind (STURGILL u. NETSKY, 1963; SOLOWAY u. ARONSON, 1964; RING, 1966) ist immer auch in Betracht zu ziehen, daß artifizielle Embolien während der Angiographie das gleiche Bild verursachen (vgl. Abb. 13).

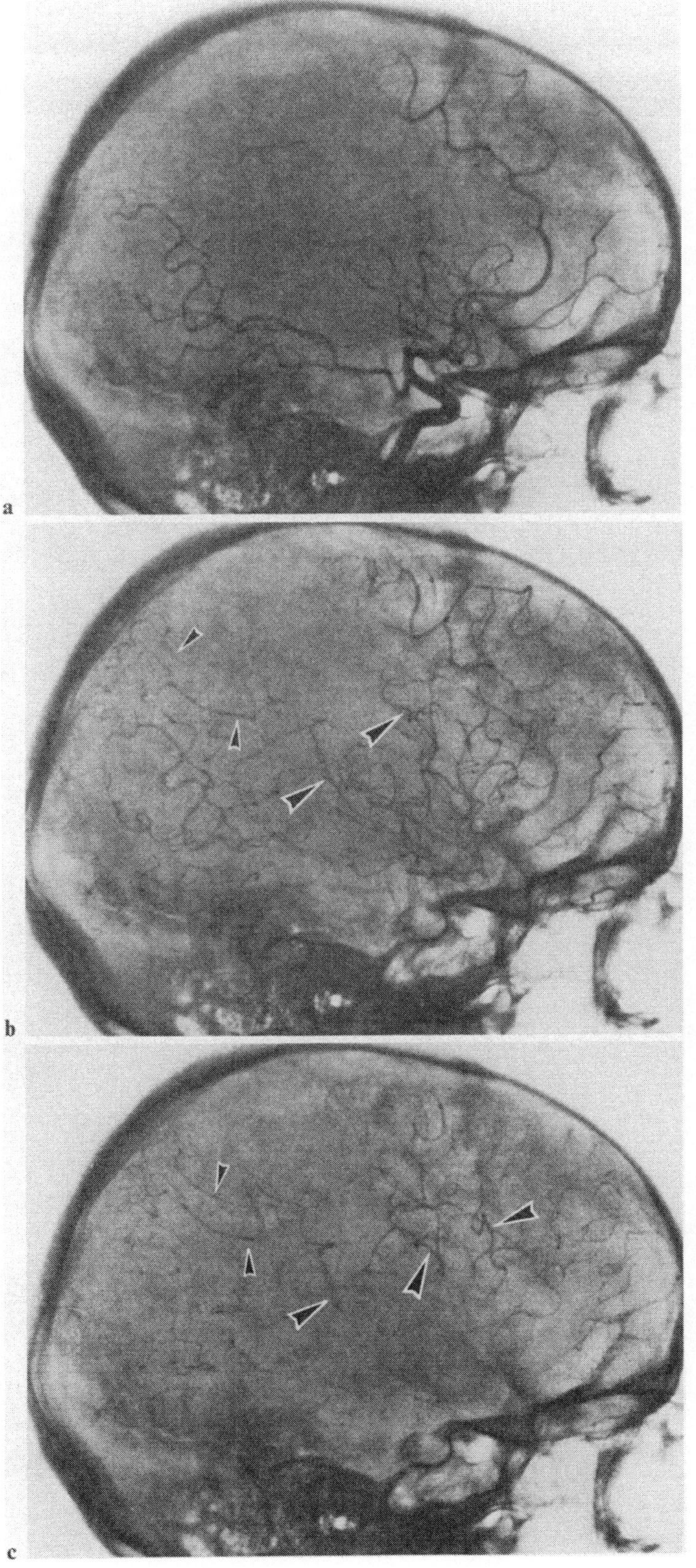

Abb. 59a–c. Verschluß eines postzentralen Mediaseitenastes. Verzögerte anterograde und retrograde Füllung. Anterograd gefüllter Abschnitt: große Pfeile. Retrograd gefüllte Abschnitte: kleine Pfeile

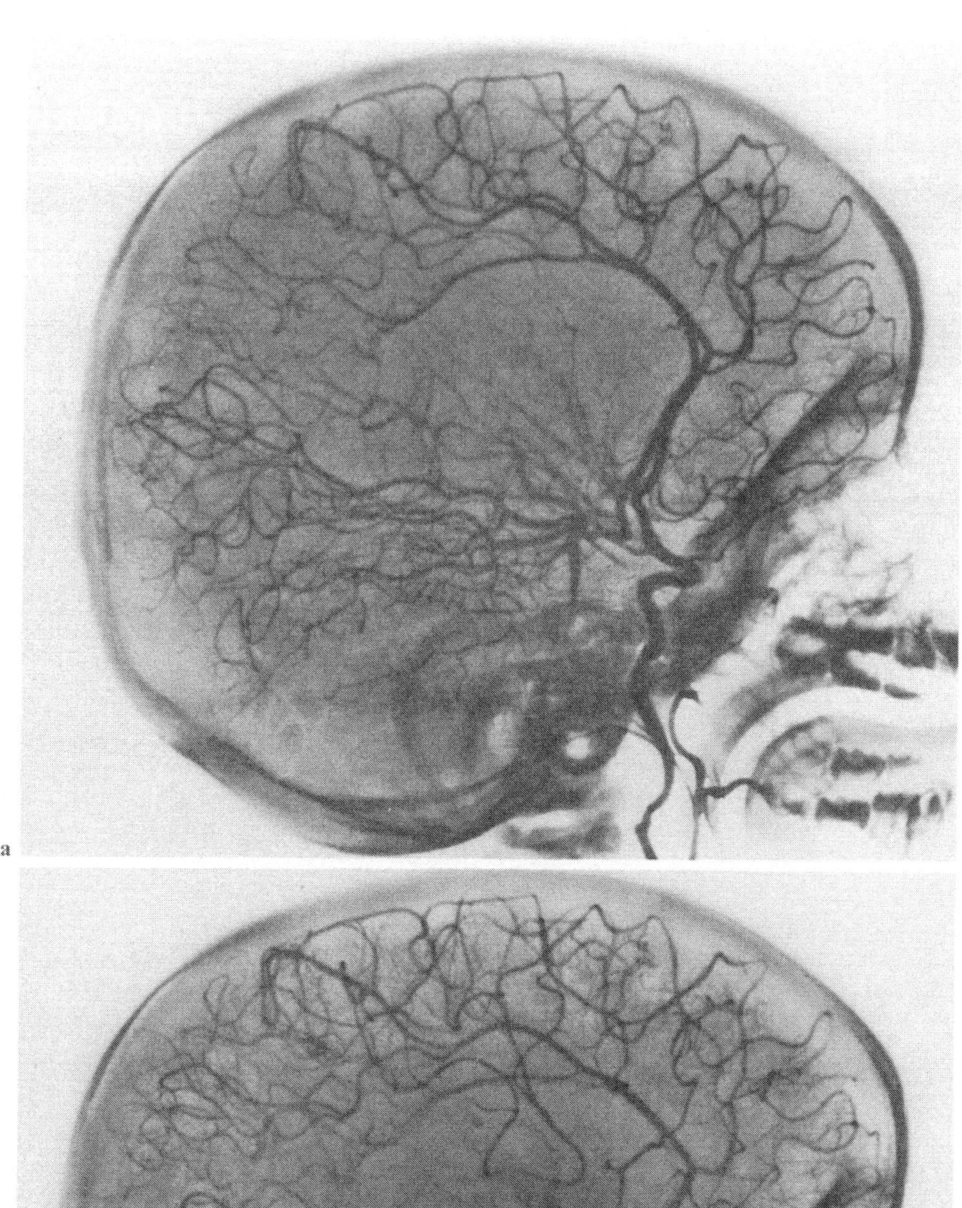

Abb. 60a–c. Embolischer Mediaverschluß (bei Herzvitium) mit massiver Doppelfüllung und Darstellung des oberen Basilarisabschnittes unter dem Injektionsdruck. Kollateralkreislauf über leptomeningeale Anastomosen in das Mediastromgebiet von der A. pericallosa und der A. cerebri posterior her. Zusätzliche weitere Verschlüsse von Mediaästen (**c**, Pfeile). Embolusfragmente oder Stagnationsthrombose? (Aus „Zerebrale Angiographie“, Thieme Stuttgart, 1979)

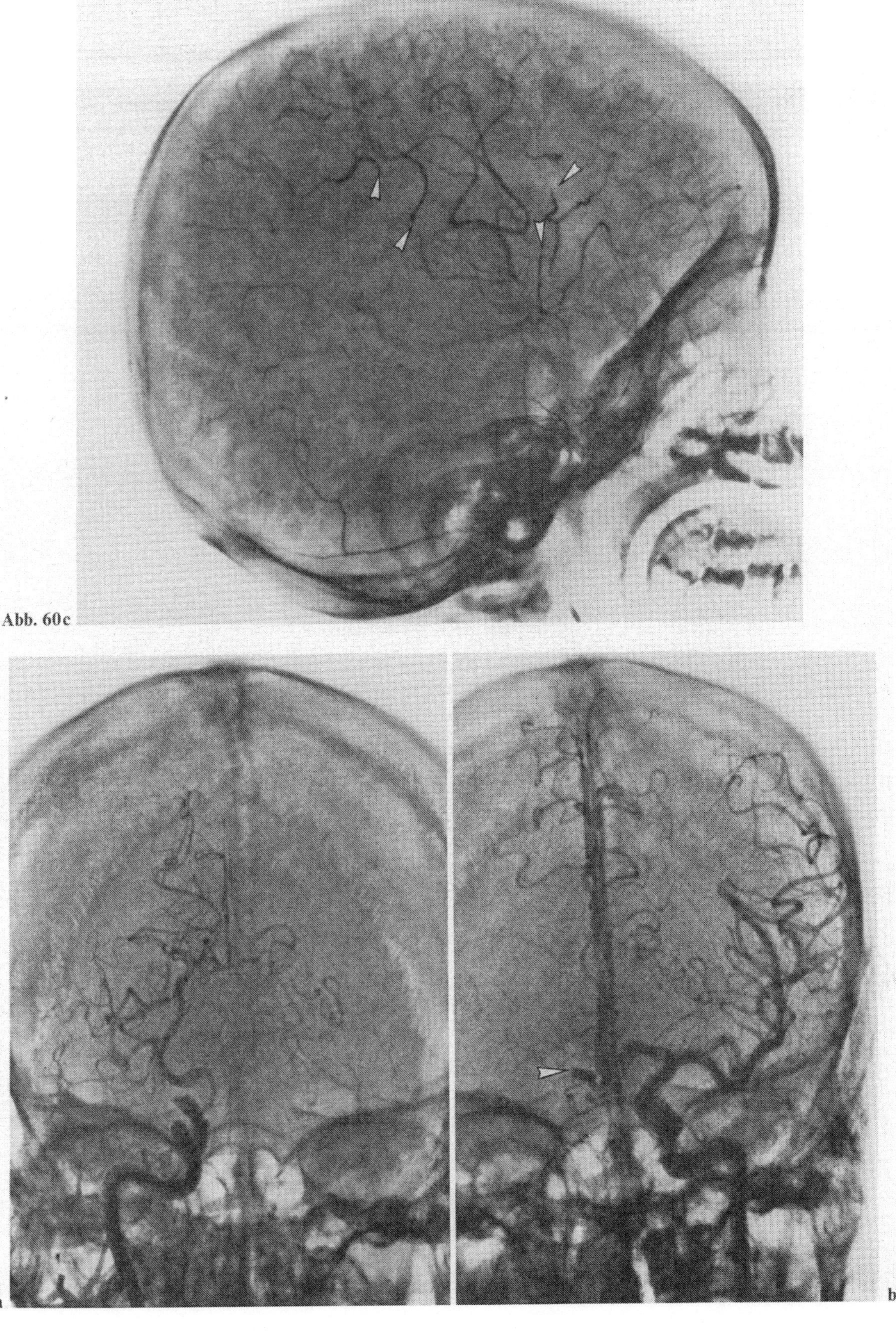

Abb. 61 a u. b. Embolischer Verschluß der A. carotis interna rechts distal vom Abgang der A. communicans posterior (**a**). Bei der Karotisangiographie links Darstellung des distalen Segmentes der A. cerebri anterior rechts über die A. communicans anterior. Verschluß des proximalen Segmentes der A. cerebri anterior (Pfeil). Keine Hypoplasie (**b**)

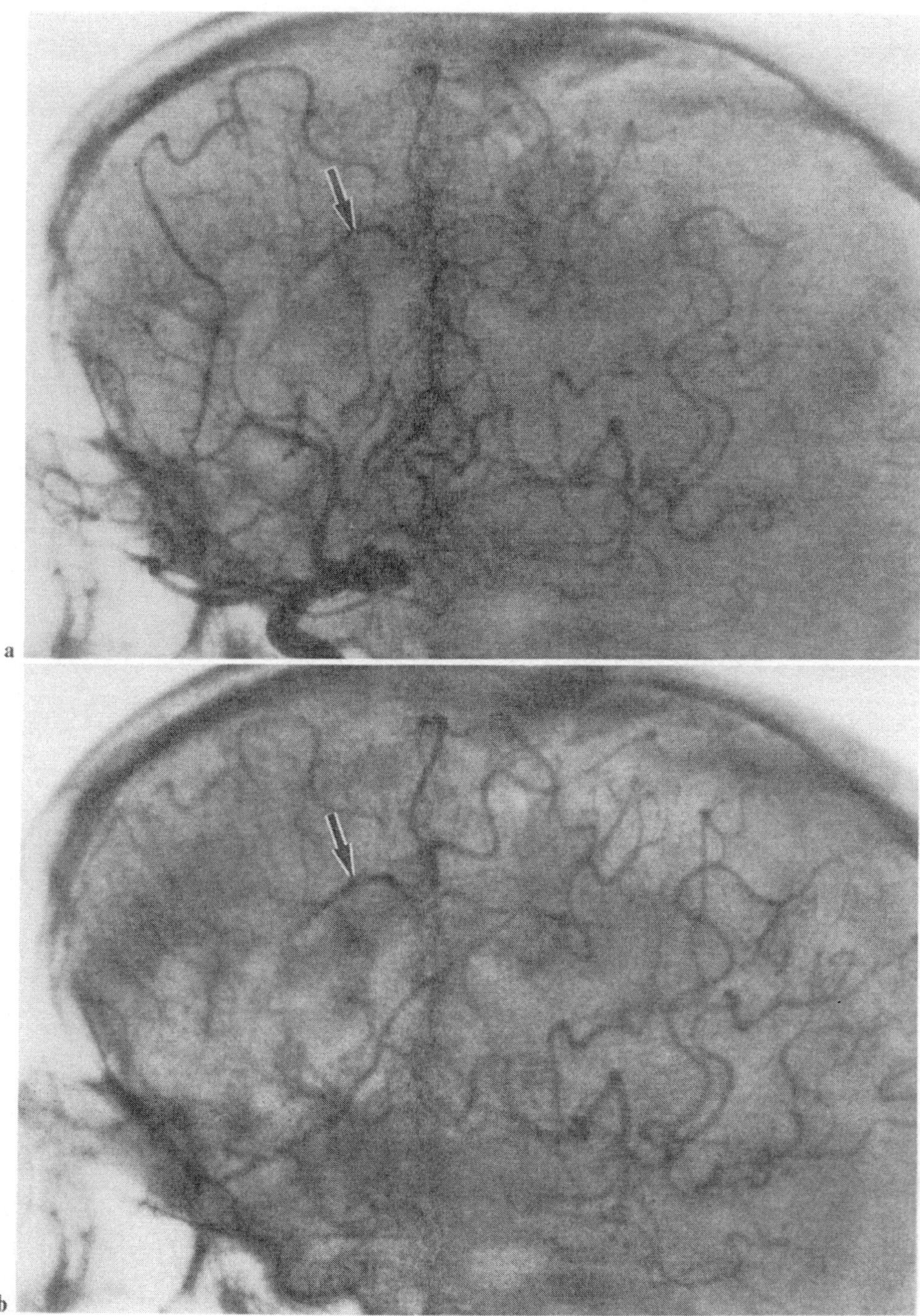

Abb. 62a–c. Verschluß der A. pericallosa mit Kollateralkreislauf von der A. cerebri media her (Pfeile). **a** und **b**: Profilaufnahmen der arteriellen Phase. **c**: a.-p. Aufnahme mit Verschluß der A. pericallosa (Pfeil)

Von einem präexistenten Verschluß sind diese artifiziellen Embolien nahezu nur durch die Kontrollangiographie zu unterscheiden, da sich diese frischen artifiziellen Fibrinembolien spontan innerhalb kurzer Zeit wieder auflösen (DALAL et al., 1965; HUBER et al., 1971), während die Embolien aus atheromatösem oder organisiertem thrombotischen Material längere Zeit unverändert bleiben.

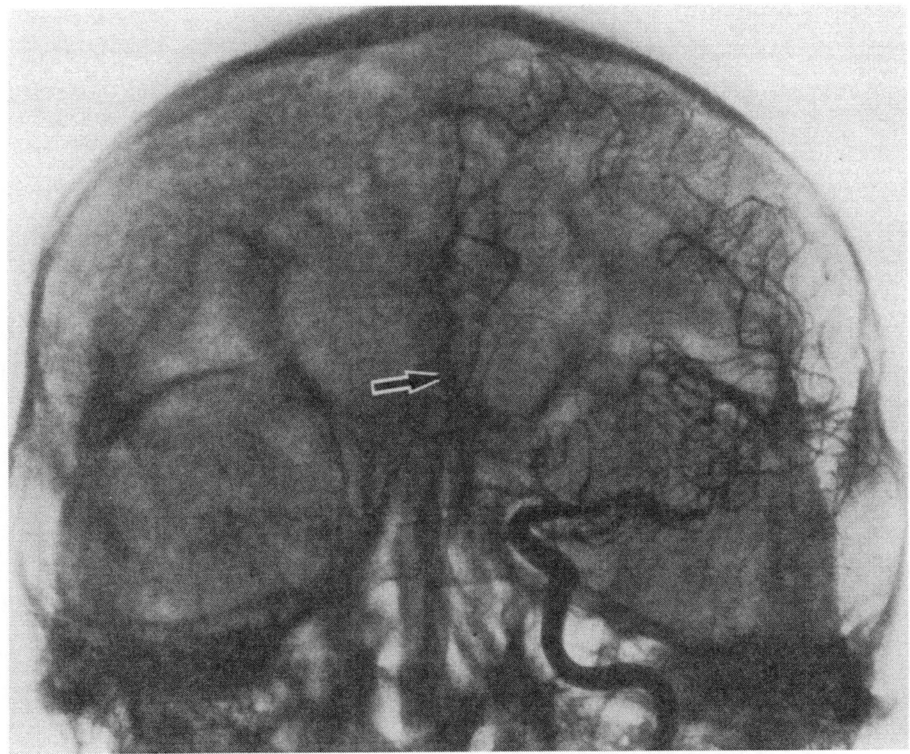

Abb. 62c

Zuverlässige Angaben über die Häufigkeit kleinerer Gefäßverschlüsse fehlen. RING (1966) fand in ca. 15% der Insultpatienten kleinere Gefäße mitverschlossen, wobei in einigen Fällen ein Thrombus in der A. carotis interna als Emboliequelle sichergestellt werden konnte. Im Krankengut von HUBER und SIEGENTHALER (1973) lagen in einem noch höheren Prozentsatz kleine Astverschlüsse in der Peripherie bei Verschlüssen oder Stenosen der größeren proximalen Gefäße vor.

2. Verschlüsse im Stromgebiet der A. cerebri anterior / A. pericallosa

Die Verschlüsse der A. cerebri anterior und der A. pericallosa sind seltener als die Mediaverschlüsse und im Unterschied zu diesen weniger embolisch als vielmehr arteriosklerotisch bedingt. WEBSTER et al. (1960) geben höhere Zahlen an als DORNDORF und GÄNSHIRT (1972), die annehmen, daß Verschlüsse in diesem Stromgebiet nur 7% aller intrakraniellen und nur 2,25% aller Hirnarterienverschlüsse ausmachen. Eine fehlende Darstellung der A. cerebri anterior darf noch nicht mit einem Verschluß gleichgesetzt werden, da Hypoplasien im vorderen Abschnitt des Circulus Willisi keineswegs selten sind (ALPERS et al., 1959; WOLLSCHLAEGER u. WOLLSCHLAEGER, 1974). Die Angiographie der Gegenseite wird in der Regel erforderlich sein, um die Verhältnisse abzuklären, wobei sich bei digitaler Kompression auf der Seite der primär nicht sichtbaren A. cerebri anterior diese doch noch als hypoplastisches Gefäß darstellen kann. Stellen sich beide Aa. pericallosae dar und ist die A. communicans anterior relativ weit, so ist ein Anteriorverschluß auf der Gegenseite weniger wahrscheinlich als eine Hypoplasie (Abb. 61).

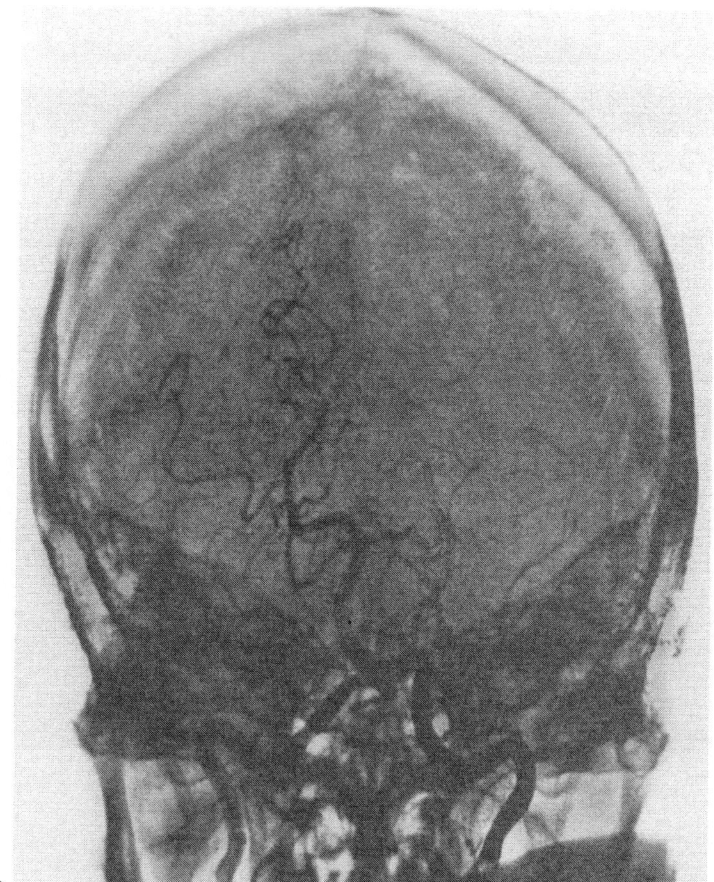

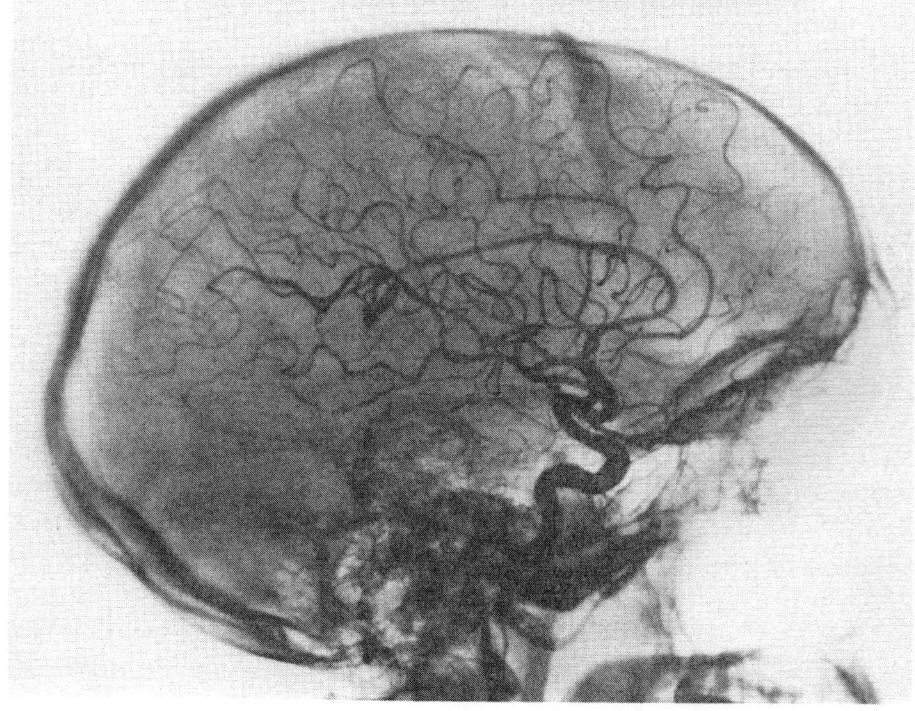

Abb. 63a–d. Verschluß der linken A. cerebri posterior. (**a**) Vertebralisangiogramm. (**b–d**) Karotisangiogramm. Retrograde Darstellung der A. cerebri posterior von der A. cerebri media aus

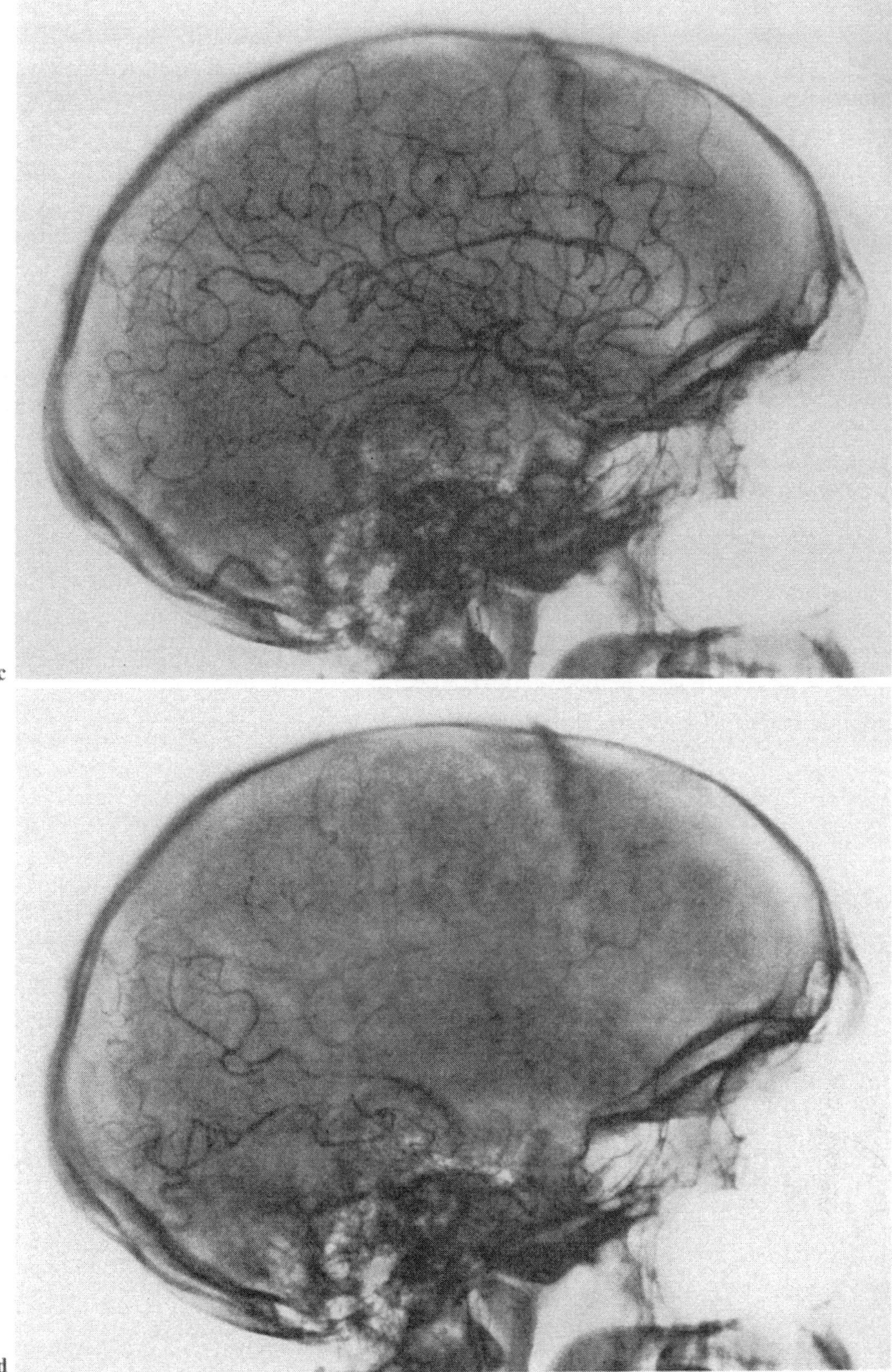

Abb. 63c u. d

Der Perikallosaverschluß sitzt meist nicht an der Abgangsstelle aus der A. cerebri anterior, sondern etwas weiter distal, etwa auf Höhe des Balkenknies oder im oberen Perikallosa-Abschnitt und ist angiographisch deshalb auch leichter zu belegen als der Anteriorverschluß. Es kann sich dabei ein Kollateralkreislauf von Ästen der A. cerebri media (Abb. 62) oder posterior einstellen sowie von der gegenseitigen A. pericallosa her über das auf dem Corpus callosum gelegene

Anastomosennetz. Ist der Verschluß der A. pericallosa distal vom Abgang der A. calloso-marginalis gelegen, so kann auch über dieses Gefäß ein Kollateralkreislauf in das periphere Perikallosastromgebiet zustande kommen. In seltenen Fällen treten transdurale Anastomosen von der A. meningea media oder anterior her auf, die sich unter Umständen kräftig erweitern.

Nicht mit einem Verschluß zu verwechseln ist die unpaare Anlage der A. pericallosa (LEMAY u. GOODING, 1966; SZDZUY et al., 1972). Diese Variante ist durch das Fehlen einer A. communicans anterior und die Aufteilung des unpaaren Pericallosahauptstammes nach kürzerem oder längerem Verlauf in zwei meist gleich stark entwickelte Äste charakterisiert.

3. Der Verschluß der A. cerebri posterior

Der Verschluß der A. cerebri posterior tritt in ungefähr gleicher Häufigkeit auf wie der Verschluß der A. cerebri anterior (KRAYENBÜHL u. YASARGIL, 1957; MONES et al., 1961; SCHOTT et al., 1965; DAVID et al., 1968; DORNDORF u. GÄNSHIRT, 1972), wurde früher aber zu Unrecht als seltenes Ereignis bezeichnet (MILLETTI, 1954; BILLEWICZ et al., 1970). Wegen der verschiedenen anatomischen Varianten im hinteren Abschnitt des Circulus Willisi ist ein Posteriorverschluß nur dann mit Sicherheit nachgewiesen, wenn sich das Gefäß weder mit der Karotis- noch mit der Vertebralisangiographie darstellen läßt und ein Kollateralkreislauf zur Darstellung kommt. Dieser erfolgt meist über die hinteren Äste der A. cerebri media, speziell die A. temporalis posterior und die A. gyri angularis (Abb. 63). Daneben sind auch Umgehungskreisläufe über die terminalen Äste der A. pericallosa, die Chorioidalarterien sowie über die A. cerebellaris superior möglich (GALATIUS-JENSEN u. RINGBERG, 1963).

IV. Das Hirnödem bei Gefäßverschlüssen

Im Infarktbereich kommt es häufig zur Entwicklung eines Ödems, dessen Höhepunkt auf den dritten bis fünften Tag nach dem Infarkt fällt und das dann im Verlauf der folgenden zwei Wochen wiederum abklingt (ADAMS u. GRAHAM, 1967; SHAW et al., 1967; SINDERMANN et al., 1969). Die ödembedingten Verlagerungen sind um so ausgeprägter, je ausgedehnter der Infarkt ist, d.h. sie finden sich vorzugsweise bei Verschlüssen des Mediahauptstammes oder der A. carotis interna und fehlendem oder ungenügendem Kollateralkreislauf. Bei einer massiven Seitenverlagerung der A. pericallosa oder der zentralen Venen um 12–15 mm und der fehlenden Darstellung der Gefäße distal vom Verschluß ist es u.U. sehr schwierig, die Verlagerung richtig zu interpretieren, wenn das Infarktgeschehen selbst durch einen Sturz mit Schädeltrauma kompliziert war. Es besteht dann, zumindest in der Frühphase, immer der Verdacht, daß die Verlagerung nicht allein durch ein Ödem, sondern durch ein zusätzliches intra- oder extrazerebrales Hämatom bedingt sein könnte.

Literatur

ADAMS, J.H., GRAHAM, D.I.: 12 cases of fatal cerebral infarction due to arterial occlusion in the absence of atheromatous stenosis or embolism. J. Neurol. Neurosurg. Psychiat. **30**, 479–488 (1967)

AIZAWA, T., TAZAKI, Y., GOTOH, F.: Cerebral circulation in cerebrovascular disease. Wld. Neurol. **2**, 635–648 (1961)

ALAJOUANINE, T., CASTAIGNE, P., LHERMITTE, F., GAUTIER, J.C.: Les anastomoses des artères. Leur rôle de suppléance. Sem. Hôp. Paris **35**, 1133–1141 (1959)

ALLCOCK, J.M.: Occlusion of the middle cerebral artery: serial angiography as a guide to conservative therapy. J. Neurosurg. **27**, 353–363 (1967)

ALPERS, B.J., BERRY, R.G.: Circle of Willis in cerebral vascular disorders. Arch. Neurol. 8, 338–402 (1963)

ALPERS, B.J., BERRY, R.G., PADDISON, R.M.: Anatomical studies of the circle of Willis in normal brain. Amer. med. Ass. Arch. Neurol. 81, 409–418 (1959)

ALTER, M., KIEFFER, S., RESCH, J., ANSARI, K.: Cerebral infarction. Clinical and angiographic correlations. Neurology 22, 590–602 (1972)

ALTSCHULER, J.H., LAUGHLIN, R.A., NEUBURGER, K.T.: Neurological catastrophe related to oral contraceptives. Arch. Neurol. 19, 264–273 (1968)

AMUNDSEN, A.K., AMUNDSEN, O., REFSUM, H.: Circulation time and pattern in cerebral angiography using different techniques for general anesthesia. Acta radiol. 5, 84–90 (1966)

ANDERSEN, P.E.: Arteriosklerose der zerebralen Arterien. Über die Korrelation zwischen den arteriographischen und postmortalen Befunden. Fortschr. Röntgenstr. 82, 491–495 (1955)

ANDERSEN, P.E.: Fibromuscular hyperplasia of the carotid arteries. Acta radiol. Diagn. 10, 90–96 (1970)

ANDERSEN, P.E.: Fibromuscular hyperplasia in children. Acta radiol. Diagn. 10, 203–208 (1970)

ANDERSON, R. MC D., SCHECHTER, M.M.: A case of spontaneous dissecting aneurysm of the internal carotid artery. J. Neurol. Neurosurg. Psychiat. 22, 195–201 (1959)

ANDRÉ, J.M., PICARD, L.: Moyamoya: syndrome ou maladie? Étude étio-pathogénique. Déductions thérapeutiques. J. Neuroradiol. 1, 133–139 (1974)

ANDRÉ, J.M., PICARD, L., KISSEL, P.: Les angiodysplasies systematisées. J. Neuroradiol. 1, 3–45 (1974)

ASHBY, R.N., KARRAS, B.G., CANNON, A.H.: Clinical and roentgenographic aspects of the subclavian steal syndrome. Amer. J. Roentgenol. 90, 535–545 (1963)

ASK-UPMARK, E.: The carotid sinus and the cerebral circulation. An anatomical, experimental and clinical investigation including some observations on the rete mirabile caroticum. Acta psychiat. scand. Suppl. VI Kopenhagen 1935

AUSTIN, J.H., STEARS, J.C.: Familial hypoplasia of both internal carotid arteries. Arch. Neurol. 24, 1–10 (1971)

BAKER, A.B., IANNONE, A.: Cerebrovascular disease. I. The large arteries of the circle of Willis. Neurology (Minneap.) 9, 321–332 (1959)

BAKER, A.B., IANNONE, A.: A study of etiologic mechanisms. Neurology 11, 23–31 (1961)

BAKER, A.B., REFSUM, S., DAHL, E.: Cerebrovascular disease. IV. A study of a Norwegian population. Neurology (Minneap.) 10, 525 (1960)

BAKER, H.L.: Angiographic investigation of cerebrovascular insufficiency. Radiology 77, 399–405 (1961)

BAKER, R.N., RAMSEYER, J.C., SCHWARTZ, W.S.: Prognosis in patients with transient cerebral ischemic attacks. Neurology 18, 1157–1165 (1968)

BALOW, J., ALTER, M., RESCH, J.A.: Cerebral thromboembolism. A clinical appraisal of 100 cases. Neurology (Minneap.) 16, 559–564 (1966)

BANKER, B.Q.: Cerebral vascular disease in infancy and childhood. I. Occlusive vascular disease. J. Neuropathol. exp. Neurol. 20, 127–140 (1961)

BARNETT, G.O.: Factors influencing pulsatile flow in individual vessels. In: Cerebral Vascular Disease. Transactions of the forth Princeton conference. (Millikan C.H., Sieckert, R.G., Whisnant J.P., eds). New York & London: Grune & Stratton, 1965, pp. 32–36

BARRON, K.D., SIQUEIRA, E., HIRANO, A.: Cerebral embolism caused by nonbacterial thrombotic endocarditis. Neurology 10, 391–397 (1960)

BATES, B.F., BOOKSTEIN, J.J.: Intercurrent embolization during cerebral arteriography. Clinical and experimental observations. Invest. Radiol. 1, 107–112 (1966)

BATSON, O.V.: Anatomical problems concerned in the study of cerebral blood flow. Fed. Proc. 3, 139–144 (1944)

BATTISTINI, N., CASACCHIA, M., BARTOLINI, A., BAVA, G., FIESCHI, C.: Effects of hyperventilation on focal brain damage following middle cerebral artery occlusion. In: Cerebral blood flow. Berlin-Heidelberg-New York: Springer Verlag 1969, pp. 249–253

BAUER, R., SHEEHAN, S., MEYER, J.S.: Arteriographic study of cerebrovascular disease. II. Cerebral symptoms due to kinking, tortuosity and compression of carotid and vertebral arteries in the neck. Arch. Neurol. 4, 119–131 (1961)

BAUER, R.B., BOULOS, R.S., MEYER, J.S.: Natural history and surgical treatment of occlusive cerebrovascular disease evaluated by serial arteriography. Amer. J. Roentgenol. 104, 1–17 (1968)

BAUER, R.B., SHEEHAN, S., WECHSLER, N., MEYER, J.S.: Arteriographic study of sites, incidence and treatment of arteriosclerotic cerebrovascular lesions. Neurology 12, 698–711 (1962)

BAYLISS, W.M.: On the local reactions of the arterial wall to changes of internal pressure. J. Physiol. (Lond.) 28, 220–231 (1902)

BELL, W.E., BUTLER, C.: Cerebral mycotic aneurysms in children. Two case reports. Neurology 18, 81–86 (1968)

BERGERON, R.TH., WOOD, E.H.: Oral contraceptives and cerebrovascular complications. Radiology 92, 231–238 (1969)

BETETA, E., SCHEINBERG, P., REINMUTH, O., SKAFEY, S., SHINYYO, S.: Simultaneous bilateral cerebral blood flow and metabolism with arteriographic correlation in unilateral brain infarction or hemorrhage. J. Neurol. Neurosurg. Psychiat. 28, 335–343 (1965)

BICKERSTAFF, E.R.: Aetiology of acute hemiplegia in childhood. Brit. med. J. 2, 82–87 (1964)

BILLEWICZ, O., BABIN, E., MASSOT, R., BEN AMOR, M., SCHMELTZER, A.: Thrombosis of the posterior cerebral artery. Neuroradiology 1, 99–100 (1970)

BLACKWOOD, W.: Thrombo-angiitis obliterans (Winiwarter-Buerger's disease). In: Greenfield's Neuropathology. Baltimore: Williams and Wilkins Comp. 1963, pp. 112–114

BLADIN, P.F.: A radiologic and pathologic study of embolism of the internal carotid middle cerebral arterial axis. Radiology **82**, 615–625 (1964)

BOCZKO, M.L., CAPLAN, L.H.: Alteration of flow dynamics in the carotid artery system of "stroke" patients. Clinical and arteriographic study. Invest. Radiol. **2**, 33–40 (1967)

BOERI, R., PASSERINI, A.: The megadolichobasilar anomaly. J. neurol. Sci. **1**, 475–484 (1964)

BOSTRÖM, K., HASSLER, O.: Radiological study of arterial calcification. 1. Aortic arch and large cervical vessels. Neurology **15**, 941–950 (1965)

BRAWLEY, B.W., STRANDNESS, D.E., KELLY, W.A.: The physiologic response to therapy in experimental cerebral ischemia. Arch. Neurol. **17**, 180–187 (1967)

BRICE, J.G., DOWSETT, D.J., LOVE, R.D.: Haemodynamic effects of carotid artery stenosis. Brit. med. J. **2**, 1363–1366 (1964)

BROWN, O.L., ARMITAGE, J.L.: Spontaneous dissecting aneurysms of the cervical internal carotid artery. Two case reports and a survey of the literature. Amer. J. Roentgenol. **118**, 648–653 (1973)

BÜCHELER, E., DUEX, A., THURN, P.: Die retrograde Durchströmung der Arteria vertebralis (Subclavian Steal-Syndrom). Fortschr. Röntgenstr. **101**, 607–618 (1964)

BULL, J.W.D., COUCH, R.S.C., JOYCE, D., MARSHALL, J., ROTTS, D.G., SHAER, D.A.: Observer variation in cerebral angiography: An assessment of the value of minor angiographic change in the radiological diagnosis of cerebrovascular disease. Brit. J. Radiol. **33**, 165–170 (1960)

BURROWS, E.H., LASCELLES, R.G.: The contribution of radiology to the diagnosis and prognosis of occlusions of the middle cerebral artery and its branches. Brit. J. Radiol. **38**, 481–493 (1965)

CALLIAUW, L.: Moyamoya. Neurochirurgie **18**, 383–390 (1972)

CARPENTER, D.F., BURBAKER, L.H., POWELL, R.D., VALSAMIS, M.P.: Phycomycotic thrombosis of the basilar artery. Neurology **18**, 807–812 (1968)

CASTAIGNE, P., LHERMITTE, F., GAUTIER, J.C., ESCOUROLLE, R., DEROUESNE, C., DER AGOPIAN, P., POPA, C.: Arterial occlusions in the vertebrobasilar system. A study of forty-four patients with post-mortem data. Brain **96**, 133–154 (1973)

CHAO, D.H.: Congenital neurocutaneous syndromes in childhood. I. Neurofibromatosis. J. Pediat. **55**, 189–199 (1959). II. Tuberous sclerosis, J. Pediat. **55**, 447–459 (1959). III. Sturge-Weber disease, J. Pediat. **55**, 635–649 (1959)

CHASE, N.E., KRICHEFF, I.I.: Cerebral angiography in the evaluation of patients with cerebrovascular disease. Radiol. Clin. N. Amer. **6**, 131–144 (1966)

CITRON, B.P., HALPERN, M., MCCARRON, M., LUNDBERG, G.P., MCCORMICK, R., PINCUS, I.J., TATTER, D., HAVERBACH, B.J.: Necrotizing angiitis associated with drug abuse. New Engl. J. Med. **283**, 1003–1011 (1970)

CLARK, O.H., MOORE, W.S., HALL, A.D.: Radiographically occluded, anatomically patent carotid arteries. Arch. Surg. **102**, 604–606 (1971)

CONSTANS, J.P., DILENGE, D., POUYANNE, H.: Occlusions artérielles par compression tumorale intracrânienne. Neurochirurgie **13**, 701–710 (1967)

CONTORNI, L.: Il circolo collaterale vertebro-vertebrale nella obliterazione dell'arteria succlavia alla sua origine. Minerva chirg. **15**, 268–271 (1960)

COUREY, W.R., NEW, P.F.J., PRICE, D.L.: Angiographic manifestations of craniofacial Phycomycosis. Radiology **103**, 329–334 (1973)

CRAWFORD, E.S., WUKASCH, D.W., DEBAKEY, M.E.: Hemodynamic changes associated with carotid artery occlusion: an experimental and clinical study. Cardiovasc. Res. **1**, 3–10 (1962)

CRONQVIST, S.: Total angiography in evaluation of cerebro-vascular disease: a correlative study of aorto-cervical and selective cerebral angiography. Brit. J. Radiol. **39**, 805–810 (1966)

CRONQVIST, S.: Regional cerebral blood flow and angiography in apoplexy. Acta radiol. **7**, 521–534 (1968)

CRONQVIST, S., EFSING, H.O., PALACIOS, E.: Embolic complications in cerebral angiography with the catheter technique. Acta radiol. Diagn. **10**, 97–107 (1970)

CRONQVIST, S., EKBERG, R., INGVAR, D.: Regional cerebral blood flow related to neuroradiological findings. Acta neurol. scand. Suppl. **14**, 176–178 (1965)

CRONQVIST, S., GREITZ, T.: Cerebral circulation time and cerebral blood flow. Acta radiol. Diagn. **8**, 296–304 (1969)

CRONQVIST, S., LAROCHE, F.: Transitory hyperaemia in focal cerebral vascular lesions studies by angiography and regional cerebral blood flow measurements. Brit. J. Radiol. **40**, 270–274 (1967)

CROUZET, G., AGNETTAZ, G., PELLAT, J., BARGE, M.: Les voies de suppléance au cours de Moyamoya. J. Neuroradiol. **1**, 87–101 (1974)

DALAL, P.M., SHAH, P.M., SHETH, J.C., DESHPANDE, C.K.: Cerebral embolism. Angiographic observations on spontaneous clot lysis. Lancet **I/1965**, 61–64

DALLAS, S.H., MOXOU, G.P.: Controlled ventilation for cerebral angiography. Brit. J. Anaesth. **41**, 597–602 (1969)

DAVID, M., MOSSING, R., DILENGE, D., HARSPE, L., METZGER, J.: Le problème des sténoses et thromboses vertébrobasilaires. A propos de cinquante observations. Presse méd. **72**, 147–150 (1968)

DAVIS, D.O., RUMBAUGH, C.L., GILSON, J.M.: Angiographic diagnosis of small-vessel cerebral emboli. Acta radiol. Diagn. **9**, 264–271 (1969)

DAVIS, D.O., TAVERAS, J.M.: Radiological aspects of inflammatory conditions affecting the central nervous system. Clin. Neurosurg. **14**, 192–210 (1966)

DEBAENE, A.: Layering of contrast in the internal carotid artery related to angiographic circulation time and cerebral blood flow. Neuroradiology **6**, 71–77 (1973)

Debrun, G., Sauvegrain, J., Aicardi, J., Goutieres, F.: Moyamoya, a nonspecific radiological syndrome. Neuroradiology **8**, 241–244 (1975)

Decker, K.: Der Spasmus der A. carotis interna. Acta radiol. **46**, 351–356 (1956)

Decker, K.: Klinische Neuroradiologie. Stuttgart: Thieme 1960

Decker, K., Holzer, E.: Gefäßverschlüsse im Carotis- und Vertebralisangiogramm. Fortschr. Röntgenstr. **80**, 565–575 (1954)

Decker, K., Nagel, H.: Gefäßverschlüsse im Carotis- und Vertebralisgebiet. Mschr. Psychiat. **126**, 365–377 (1954)

De Gutiérrez-Mahoney, C.G., Schechter, M.M.: The myth of the rete mirabile in man. Neuroradiology **4**, 141–158 (1972)

Delin, N.A., Ekerström, S., Telenius, R.: Relation of degree of internal carotid artery stenosis to blood flow and pressure gradient. Invest. Radiol. **3**, 337–344 (1968)

DeVivo, D.C., Farrell, F.W.: Vertebrobasilar occlusive disease in children. A recognizable clinical entity. Arch. Neurol. **26**, 278–281 (1972)

Dichgans, J., Voigt, K.: Rasches Erscheinen leptomenigealer Anastomosen nach embolischen Astverschlüssen der A. cerebri media. Fortschr. Röntgenstr. **110**, 651–655 (1969)

Di Chiro, G., Libow, L.S.: Carotid siphon calcification and cerebral blood flow in the healthy aged male. Radiology **99**, 103–107 (1971)

Di Chiro, G., Lindgren, E.: Radiographic findings in 14 cases of Sturge-Weber syndrome. Acta radiol. **35**, 387–399 (1951)

Dickinson, C.J.: Functional efficiency of the circle of Willis. Implications for reconstructive surgery of main cerebral arteries. Brit. med. J. **1**, 858–859 (1961)

Donrov, N., Locoge, M., Themelin, G., De Rede, J.: Étude anatomo-clinique et radiologique d'un cas d'hématome disséquant d'une artère cérébrale chez un sujet jeune. Rev. belge Path. **30**, 265–281 (1964)

Dorndorf, W., Gänshirt, H.: Die Klinik der arteriellen zerebralen Gefäßverschlüsse. In: Der Hirnkreislauf. Physiologie, Pathologie, Klinik (H. Gänshirt, Hrsg.), S. 512–650. Stuttgart: Thieme Verlag 1972

Du Boulay, G., Edmonds-Seal, J., Bostick, T.: Effect of intermittent positive pressure ventilation upon cerebral angiography: quality of film and diameter of vessels including those in spasm. In: Recent advances in the study of cerebral circulation (J.M. Taveras, H. Fischgold, D. Dilenge et al., eds). Springfield, Ill.: Charles C. Thomas 1970

Du Boulay, G.H.: Some observations on the natural history of intracranial aneurysms. Brit. J. Radiol. **38**, 453–455 (1965)

Du Boulay, G.H., El Gammal, T., Trickey, S.E.: True and false carotid retia. Birt. J. Radiol. **46**, 205–212 (1973)

Du Boulay, G.H., Symon, L.: The anaesthesist's effect upon cerebral arteries. Proc. roy. soc. Med. **64**, 77–80 (1971)

Du Boulay, G.H., Verity, P.M.: The cranial arteries of mammals. London: W. Heinamann 1973

Dühmke, E., Gremmel, H., Schulte-Brinkmann, W.: Erkrankung der thorakalen Aorta (ausser Fehlbildungen). In: Handbuch der med. Radiologie, Bd. X/2b, S. 389–405. Berlin-Heidelberg-New York: Springer Verlag 1974

Ecker, A., Riemenschneider, P.A.: Arteriographic demonstration of spasm of the intracranial arteries with special reference to saccular arterial aneurysms. J. Neurosurg. **8**, 660–667 (1951)

Ecker, A.D.: Spasm of the internal carotid artery. J. Neurosurg. **2**, 479–484 (1945)

Editorial: New vascular syndrom "The subclavian steal". New Engl. J. Med. **265**, 912 (1961)

Ehrenfeld, W.K., Hoyt, W.F., Wylie, E.J.: Embolization and transient blindness from carotid atheroma. Surgical considerations. Arch. Surg. **93**, 787–794 (1966)

Ehrenfeld, W.K., Stoney, R.J., Wylie, E.J.: Fibromuscular hyperplasia of the internal carotis artery. Arch. Surg. **95**, 284–287 (1967)

Ekström-Jodal, B., Häggendal, E., Nilsson, N.J., Norbäck, B.: Changes of the transmural pressure – the probable stimulus to cerebral blood flow autoregulation. In: Cerebral blood flow (M. Brock, C. Fieschi, D.H. Ingvar, N.A. Lassen, K. Schürmann, eds). Berlin-Heidelberg-New York: Springer 1969

Elvidge, A.R., Werner, A.: Hemiplegia and thrombosis of the internal carotid system. Amer. med. Ass. Arch. Neurol. Psychiat. **66**, 752–782 (1951)

Erikson, U., Lodin, H.: Bradykinin in cerebral angiography. Clin. Radiol. **18**, 454–459 (1967)

Farhat, S.M., Schneider, R.C.: Observations on the effect of systemic blood pressure on intracranial circulation in patients with cerebrovascular insufficiency. J. Neurosurg. **27**, 441–445 (1967)

Faris, A.A.,, Poser, C.M., Wilmore, D.W., Agnew, C.H.: Radiologic visualization of neck vessels in healthy men. Neurology **13**, 386–396 (1963)

Fazekas, J.F., Alman, R.W., Sullivan, J.F.: Prognostic uncertainities in cerebral vascular disease. Arch. intern. Med. **58**, 93–101 (1963)

Fazio, C.: Observations sur la Pathogénése de l'infarctus cerebral. In: Kongreßband des II. Internat. Salzburger Symposiums Ed.: Der Hirnkreislauf in Forschung und Klinik (O. Eichhorn, H. Lechner, K.-H. Auel, Hrsg.), S. 117–123. Wien: Verlag Brüder Hollinek 1964

Fazio, C.: The importance of the "intracerebral steal" in the pathogenesis of focal brain ischemia. In: IV. Internat. Salzburg Conference (J.S. Meyer, H. Lechner, M. Reivich, O. Eichhorn, eds). Springfield: Charles C. Thomas 1970, pp. 57–59

Fazio, C., Fieschi, C., Agnoli, A.: Direct common carotid injection of radioisotopes for the evaluation of cerebral circulatory disturbances. Neurology **13**, 561–574 (1963)

Ferrel, F.W., Davis, D.O., Carter, C.C.: Correlation of cerebral angiographic circulation times with arterial paCO2 levels. Acta radiol. Diagn. **13**, 86–93 (1972)

Ferris, E.J.: Arteritis. In: Radiology of the skull and brain. Angiography, Vol. 2, Book 4 Chapter 84 (Newton T.H., Potts D.G., eds). Louis: C.V. Mosby Comp. 1974, pp. 2566–2597

Ferris, E.J., Gabriele, O.F., Hipona, F.A., Shapiro, J.H.: Early venous filling in cranial angiography. Radiology **90**, 553–557 (1968a)

Ferris, E.J., Rudikoff, J.C., Shapiro, J.H.: Cerebral angiography of bacterial infection. Radiology **90**, 727–734 (1968b)

Ferris, E.J., Shapiro, J.H., Simeone, A.: Arteriovenous shunting in cerebrovascular occlusive disease. Amer. J. Roentgenol. **98**, 631–636 (1966)

Fields, W.S., Bruetman, M.E., Weibel, J.: Collateral circulation of the brain. Monogr. Surg. Sci. **2**, 183–259 (1965)

Fields, W.S., Ratinov, G., Weibel, J., Campos, R.J.: Survival following basilar artery occlusion. Arch. Neurol. **15**, 463–471 (1966)

Fields, W.S., Sharkey, P.C., Crawford, E.St., Morris, G.C.: Correlation of neurologic syndromes with lesions found angiographically. Neurology **10**, 431–438 (1960)

Fieschi, C.: Some considerations on the problem of hyperemia and loss of autoregulation in brain infarcts. In: Taveras J.M., Fischgold, H., Dilenge, D., Recent advance in the study of cerebral circulation. Springfield, Ill.: Charls C. Thomas 1970

Fieschi, C., Agnoli, A.: The "intercerebral steal": A phenomenon in the pathogenesis of focal brain ichemia. In: Cerebral Circulation and Stroke (K.J. Zülch, ed). Berlin-Heidelberg-New York: Springer 1971

Fieschi, C., Agnoli, A., Battistini, N., Bozzao, L., Prencipe, M.: Derangement of regional cerebral blood flow and its regulatory mechanisms in acute cerebrovascular lesions. Neurology **18**, 1166–1179 (1968)

Fieschi, C., Bozzao, L.: Transient embolic occlusion of the middle cerebral and internal carotid arteries in cerebral apoplexy. J. Neurol. Neurosurg. Psychiat. **32**, 236–240 (1969)

Fischer, M.J., Mattey, W.E.: The subclavian steal syndrome. Amer. J. Roentgenol. **90**, 532–534 (1963)

Fischgold, H., Dilenge, D., Metzger, J.: Quantitative and qualitative methods in the study of cerebral blood flow. In: Pregress in Brain Research, Vol. 30 Cerebral Circulation (W. Luydendijk, ed). Amsterdam-London-New York: Publishing Company 1968, pp. 171–180

Fisher, M.: Occlusion of the internal carotid artery. Amer. med. Ass. Arch. Neurol. Psychiat. **65**, 346–377 (1951)

Fisher, M.: Occlusion of the carotid arteries. Further experiences. Arch. Neurol. Psychiat. **72**, 187–204 (1954)

Fisher, M.G.: Observations of the fundus oculi in transient monocular blindness. Neurology **9**, 333–347 (1959)

Fleming, S.F., Petric, D.: Traumatic thrombosis of the internal carotid artery with delayed hemiplegia. Canad. J. Surg. **11**, 166–172 (1968)

Fletcher, T.M., Taveras, J.M., Pool, J.L.: Cerebral vasospasm in angiography for intracranial aneurysms. Incidence and significance in one hundred consecutive myograms. Amer. med. Ass. Arch. Neurol. **1**, 38–47 (1959)

Fog, M.: Cerebral Circulation. II. Reaction of pial arteries to increase in blood pressure. Arch. Neurol. Psychiat. **41**, 260–268 (1939)

Foix, C., Lévy, M.: Les ramollissements sylviens. Syndromes des lésions en foyer du territoire de l'artère sylvienne et de ses branches. Rev. neurol. **2**, 1–51 (1927)

Ford, R.G., Siekert, R.G.: Central nervous system manifestations of periarteritis nodosa. Neurology **15**, 114–122 (1965)

Frantzen, E., Jacobson, H.H., Therhelsen, J.: Cerebral artery occlusion in children due to trauma to the head and neck. Neurology **11**, 695–700 (1961)

Freidenfelt, H., Sundström, R.: Local and general spasm in the internal carotis system following trauma. Acta radiol. Diagn. **1**, 278–283 (1963)

Frowein, R.: Angiographische Befunde bei cerebralen Gefäßerkrankungen und ihre Beziehungen zu den klinischen Syndromen. Acta radiol. **46**, 381–389 (1956)

Frowein, R.: Klinische Syndrome der arteriellen Gefäßverschlüsse im Lichte funktioneller Angiographie. Acta neurochir. Suppl. **7**, 224–247 (1961)

Fukuyama, Y., Suzuki, Y., Segawa, M.: Acute recurrent transient hemiplegia in children with special reference to cases with teleangiectasis, like anomalous vascularity at the base of brain. Brain Nerve (Tokyo) **17**, 757–760 (1965)

Galatius-Jensen, F., Ringberg, V.: Anastomosis between the anterior choroidal artery and the posterior cerebral artery demonstrated by arteriography. Radiology **81**, 942–944 (1963)

Galligioni, F., Andrioli, G.C., Marin, G., Briani, S., Iraci, G.: Hypoplasia of the internal carotid artery associated with cerebral pseudoangiomatosis. Report of 4 cases. Amer. J. Roentgenol. **112**, 251–262 (1971)

Gannon, W.E.: False block of the internal carotid artery during angiography. Radiology **76**, 748–754 (1961)

Gannon, W.R., Chait, A.: Occlusion of the middle cerebral artery with recanalization. Amer. J. Roentgenol. **88**, 24–26 (1962)

GERAUD, J., RASCOL, A., BES, A., MANELFE, C., GUIRAUD, B., DAVID, J., CAUSSANEL, J.P., GERAUD, G., CROGUENNE, Y.: La méthod de Ring dans le diagnostic des occlusions des branches de l'artère cérébrale moyenne. Etude neuroradiologique. Corrélations radio-cliniques. Rev. Neurol. **123**, 387–413 (1970)

GILLILAN, L.A.: Significant superficial anastomoses in arterial blood supply to human brain. J. comp. Neurol. **112**, 55–74 (1959)

GILLILAN, L.A.: The correlation of the blood supply to the human brain stem with clinical brain stem lesions. J. Neuropath. exp. Neurol. **23**, 78–108 (1964

GILLILAN, L.A., MARKESBERY, W.R.: Arteriovenous shunts in the blood supply to the brains of some common laboratoty animals – with special attention to the rete mirabile conjugatum in the cat. J. comp. Neurology **121**, 305 (1963)

GILROY, J., ANDAYS, L., THOMAS, V.J.: Intracranial myotic aneurysms and subacute bacterial endocarditis in Heroin addiction. Neurology **23**, 1193–1198 (1973)

GILROY, J., BAUER, R.B., KRABBENHOFT, K.L., MEYER, J.S.: Cerebral circulation time in cerebral vascular disease measured by serial angiography. Amer. J. Roentgenol. **90**, 490–505 (1963)

GOODMAN, S.J., BECKER, D.P.: Intracranial hemorrhage associated with amphetamine abuse. J. Amer. med. Ass. **212**, 480 (1970)

GOTOH, F.: Effects of blood pressure in cerebral circulation. Keio J. Med. **8**, 13–29 (1959)

GOTTSTEIN, U.: Der Hirnkreislauf unter dem Einfluß vasoaktiver Substanzen. Heidelberg: Hüthig 1962

GOTTSTEIN, U.: Pharmacological studies of total cerebral blood flow in man with comments in the possibility of improving regional cerebral blood flow by drugs. Acta neurol. scand. Suppl. **14**, 74–79 (1965)

GREEN, H.D., COSBY, R.S., RADZOW, K.H.: Dynamics of collateral circulation. Amer. J. Physiol. **140**, 726–736 (1943)

GREITZ, T.: A radiologic study of the brain circulation by rapid serial angiography of the carotid artery. Acta radiol. Suppl. 140 (1956)

GREITZ, T.: Angiography in tuberculous meningitis. Acta radiol. Diagn. **2**, 369–378 (1964)

GREITZ, T.: Evaluation of circulation time in angiography of the vertebral artery. Acta radiol. Diagn. **9**, 300–309 (1969)

GREITZ, T., LÖFSTEDT, S.: The relationship between the third ventricle and the basilar artery. Acta radiol. **42**, 85–100 (1954)

GROLLMAN, J.H., HANAFEE, W.: The roentgen diagnosis of Takayasu's arteritis. Radiology **83**, 387–395 (1964)

GRÜTER, W., HERRMANN, E.: Eine Fehlbildung der A. basialis. Fortschr. Röntgenstr. **99**, 418–420 (1963)

GRYSPEERDT, G.L.: Angiographic studies of the blood flow in the circle of Willis. The value of various arteriel compression tests. Acta radiol. **1**, 298–313 (1963)

GUNNING, A.J., PICKERING, G.W., ROBB-SMITH, A.H., ROSS RUSSEL, R.: Mural thrombosis of the internal carotid artery and subsequent embolism. Quart. J. Med. **33**, 155–195 (1965)

GURDJIAN, E.S., AUDET, B., SIBAYAN, R.W., THOMAS, L.M.: Spasm of the extracranial carotid artery resulting from blunt trauma demonstrated by angiography. J. Neurosurg. **35**, 742–747 (1971)

GURDJIAN, E.S., HARDY, W.G., LINDNER, D.W., WEBSTER, J.E.: Neurosurgical diagnostic evaluation of the patient with cerebrovascular disease (stroke syndrome). J. nerv. ment. Dis. **129**, 273–290 (1959)

GURDJIAN, E.S., HARDY, W.G., LINDNER, D.W.: The surgical consideration of 258 patients with carotid artery occlusion. Surg. Gynec. Obstet. **110**, 327–338 (1960)

GURDJIAN, E.S., HARDY, W.G., LINDNER, D.W., THOMAS, L.M.: Closed cervical cranial trauma associated with involvement of carotid and vertebral arteries. J. Neurosurg. **20**, 418–427 (1963)

GURDJIAN, E.S., LINDNER, D.W., HARDY, W.G., THOMAS, L.M.: "Completed stroke" due to occlusive cerebrovascular disease. An analysis of 409 cases. Neurology **11**, 724–733 (1961)

GURDJIAN, E.S., WEBSTER, J.E.: Stroke resulting from internal carotid artery thrombosis in the neck. J. Amer. med. Ass. **151**, 541–545 (1953)

HÄGGENDAL, E.: Blood flow autoregulation of the cerebral grey matter with comments on its mechanism. Acta neurol. scand. Suppl. **14**, 104–110 (1965)

HÄGGENDAL, E., JOHANSSON, B.: Effects of arterial carbon dioxide tension and oxygen saturation on cerebral blood flow autoregulation in dogs. Acta physiol. scand. suppl. **258**, 27–53 (1965)

HÄGGENDAL, E., WINSÖ, I.: Influence of hypoxia on the response of CBF to hypnocapnia. In: Cerebral blood flow (M. Brock, C. Fieschi, D.H. Ingvar, N.A. Lassen, K. Schürmann, eds). Berlin-Heidelberg-New York: Springer 1969

HALSEY, J.H., CLARK, L.C.: Some regional circulatory abnormalities following experimental cerebral infarction. Neurology **20**, 238–246 (1970)

HANDA, J., HANDA, H.: Progressive cerebral arterial cocclusive disease: Analysis of 27 cases. Neuroradiology **3**, 119–133 (1972)

HANDA, J., ISHIKAWA, S., HUBER, P., MEYER, J.S.: Experimental production of the "subclavian steal". Electromagnetic flow measurements in the monkey. Surgery **58**, 703–712 (1965a)

HANDA, J., KAMIJYO, Y., HANDA, H.: Intracranial aneurysm associated with fibromuscular hyperplasia of renal and internal carotid arteries. Brit. J. Radiol. **43**, 483–485 (1970)

HANDA, J., MEYER, J.S., HUBER, P., YOSHIDA, K.: Time course of development of cerebral collateral circulation. Vasc. dis. **2**, 271–282 (1965b)

HANDA, J., WAGA, S., HANDA, H.: Dural cortical arterial anastomosis as a collateral channel in carotid occlusive disease. Clin. Radiol. **22**, 302–307 (1971)

HARDY, W.G., LINDNER, D.W., THOMAS, L.M., GURDJIAN, E.S.: Anticipated clinical course in carotid artery occlusion. Arch. Neurol. **6**, 138–150 (1962)

HARPER, A.M.: The inter-relationship between $apCO_2$ and blood pressure in the regulation of blood flow through the cerebral cortex. Acta neurol. scand. Suppl. **14**, 94–103 (1965)

HARPER, A.M.: Autoregulation of cerebral blood flow: Influence of the arterial blood pressure on the blood flow through the cerebral cortex. Neurosurg. Psychiat. **29**, 398–403 (1966)

HARRINGTON, O.B., CROSBY, V.G., NICHOLAS, L.: Fibromuscular hyperplasia of the internal carotid artery. Ann. Thorac. Surg. **9**, 516–524 (1970)

HARRISON, E.G., MCCORMACK, L.J.: Pathologic classification of renal arterial disease in renovascular hypertension. Mayo Clin. Proc. **46**, 161–167 (1971)

HARWOOD-NASH, D.C., MCDONALD, P., ARGENT, W.: Cerebral arterial disease in children: an angiographic study of 40 cases. Amer. J. Roentgenol. **111**, 672–686 (1971)

HASS, W.K., FIELDS, W.S., NORTH, R.R., KRICHEFF, I.I., CHASE, N.E., BAUER, R.B.: Joint study of extracranial arterial occlusion. II. Arteriography, technique, sites and complications. J. Amer. med. Ass. **203**, 961–968 (1968)

HAVERLING, M.: The tortuous basilar artery. Acta radiol. Diagn. **15**, 241–249 (1974)

HAWKINS, T.D.: The collateral anastomoses in cerebro-vascular occlusion. Clin. Radiol. **17**, 203–219 (1966)

HAWKINS, T.D., POWELL, D.: Cerebral angiography during a modified valsalva manoeuvre under general anaesthesia. Acta radiol. Diagn. **13**, 97–104 (1972)

HAWKINS, T.D., SCOTT, W.C.: Bilateral rete carotidis in man. Clin. Radiol. **18**, 163–165 (1967)

HAYLER, K., FISCHER, E.: Karotisverkalkungen im Halsgebiet. Fortschr. Röntgenstr. **99**, 765–772 (1963)

HILAL, S.K.: Human carotid artery flow determination using a radiographic technique. Invest. Radiol. **1**, 113–122 (166)

HILAL, S.K.: Cerebral hemodynamics assessed by angiography. In Radiography of the skull and brain. In: Angiography, Vol. 2, Book 1, Chapter 54 (Newton, T.H., Potts, D.G., eds). St. Louis: C.V. Mosby Comp. 1974, pp. 1049–1085

HILL, L.D., ANTONIUS, J.I.: Arterial dysplasia. An important surgical lesion. Arch. Surg. **90**, 585–595 (1965)

HILAL, S.K., SOLOMON, G.E., GOLD, A.P., CARTER, S.: Primary cerebral arterial occlusive disease in children. Part I: acute acquired syndromes. Radiology **99**, 71–86 (1971a)

HILAL, S.K., SOLOMON, G.E., GOLD, A.P., CARTER, S.: Primary cerebral arterial occlusive disease in children. Part II: Neurocutaneous syndromes. Radiology **99**, 87–93 (1971b)

HILLS, J., SAMENT, S.: Bilateral agenesis of the internal carotid artery associated with cardiac and other anomalies. Case report. Neurology **18**, 142–146 (1968)

HØEDT-RASMUSSEN, K., SKINHOJ, E., PAULSON, O., EWALD, J., BJERRUM, J.K., FAHRENKRUG, A., LASSEN, N.A.: Regional cerebral blood flow in acute apoplexy. Arch. Neurol. **17**, 271–281 (1967)

HOUSER, O.W., BAKER, H.L.: Fibromuscular dysplasia and other uncommun diseases of the cervical carotid artery: angiographic aspects. Amer. J. Roentgenol. **104**, 201–212 (1968)

HOUSER, O.W., BAKER, H.L., SANDOK, B.A., HOLLEY, K.E.: Cephalic arterial fibromuscular dysplasia. Radiology **101**, 605–611 (1971)

HUBER, P.: Zerebrale Angiographie beim frischen Schädel-Hirntrauma. Fortschr. Röntgenstr. **42**, Ergänzungsband. Stuttgart: Thieme (1964)

HUBER, P.: Die prognostische Bedeutung des angiographisch sichtbaren Kollateralkreislaufs bei Verschlüssen der A. carotis media. Fortschr. Röntgenstr. **104**, 82–89 (1966)

HUBER, P.: Die angiographische Beurteilung der Hirndurchblutung: der klinische Wert der Densitometrie. Schweiz. Arch. Neurol. Neurochir. Psychiat. **100**, 1–37 (1967a)

HUBER, P.: Angiographic evaluation of internal carotid blood flow in patients with cerebrovascular disease. Radiol. clin. biol. **36**, 82–90 (1967b)

HUBER, P.: Die hyperämische Phase bei zerebralem Infarkt. Schweiz. Rundschau Med. (Praxis) **57**, 9–19 (1968)

HUBER, P.: Functional test in angiography of cerebrovascular disease. Neuroradiology **1**, 122–131 (1970)

HUBER, P.: Angiographische Funktionsdiagnostik des Hirnkreislaufes. In: Der Hirnkreislauf (H. Gänshirt, Hrsg.), S. 270–298. Stuttgart: Verlag Thieme 1972

HUBER, P., FUCHS, W.A.: Gibt es eine fibromuskuläre Hyperplasie zerebraler Arterien? Fortschr. Röntgenstr. **107**, 119–126 (1967)

HUBER, P., HANDA, J.: Effect of contrast material, hypercapnia, hyperventilation, hypertonic glucose and papaveriine on the diameter of cerebral arteries. Invest. Radiol. **2**, 17–32 (1967)

HUBER, P., MAGUN, H., RIVOIR, R.: The effect of pharmacologically increased blood pressure on the brain circulation. Angiographic investigation of arterial diameter and blood flow in patients with normal and pathologic angiogramms. Neuroradiology **3**, 68–74 (1971)

HUBER, P., RIVOIR, R., MAGUN, M.: Embolism during cerebral angiography. Z. Neurol. **200**, 248–266 (1971)

HUBER, P., RIVOIR, R., MAGUN, H.: Investigation of early filling veins by sequential subtraction. Neuroradiology **10**, 35–41 (1975)

HUGHES, J.T., BROWNELL, B.: Traumatic thrombosis of the internal carotid artery in the neck. J. Neurol. Neurosurg. Psychiat. **31**, 307–314 (1968)

HUNT, J.C., HARRISON, E.G., SHEPS, S.G., BERNATZ, P.E., DAVIS, G.D.: Hypertension caused by fibromuscular dysplasia of renal arteries. Postgrad. Med. **38**, 53–63 (1965)

HUTCHINSON, E.C., YATES, P.O.: Caroticovertebral stenosis. Lancet **I/1957**, 2–8

INGVAR, D.H.: The pathophysiology of occlusive cerebrovascular disorders. Acta neurol. scand. **43**, 93–107 (1967)

IOSUE, A., KIER, E.L., OSTROW, D.: Fibromuscular dysplasia involving the intracranial vessels. Case report. J. Neurosurg. **37**, 749–752 (1972)

ISFORT, A.: Zerebrale Arterienverschlüsse durch Gefäßkompression. Fortschr. Röntgenstr. **95**, 128–135 (1961)

ISHIKAWA, S., HANDA, J., MEYER, J.S., HUBER, P.: Haemodynamics of the circle of Willis and the leptomeningeal anastomoses: an electromagnetic flowmeter study of intracranial arterial occlusion in the monkey. J. Neurol. Neurosurg. Psychiat. **28**, 124–136 (1965)

ISLER, W.: Aneurysma dissecans und entzündliches Aneurysma mit Angiospasmen bei Kindern. Schweiz. Arch. Neurol. Neurochir. Psychiat. **85**, 210–212 (1960)

ISLER, W.: Akute Hemiplegien und Hemisyndrome im Kindesalter. Stuttgart: Thieme 1969

IVAN, L.P., MARIAN, J.J.: Angiographic occlusive patterns of the internal carotid artery. J. Neurosurg. **30**, 233–237 (1969)

JANON, E.A.: Traumatic changes in the internal carotid artery associated with basal skull fractures. Radiology **96**, 55–59 (1970)

JENNETT, W.B., CROSS, J.N.: Influence of pregnancy and oral contraception on the incidence of strokes in women of childbearing age. Lancet **I/1967**, 1019–1023

JÖRGENSEN, L., TORVIK, A.: Ischaemic cerebrovascular diseases in an autopsy series. Part 2: Prevalence, location, pathogenesis and clinical course of cerebral infarcts. J. neurol. Sci. **9**, 285–320 (1969)

JOHANNSON, P.C.: Review of previous studies and current theories of autoregulation. Circulat. Res. **15**, 2–9 (1964)

JOHNSON, H.C., WALKER, A.E.: The angiographic diagnosis of spontaneous thrombosis of the internal and common carotid arteries. J. Neurosurg. **8**, 631–659 (1951)

JONES, R.R., WETZEL, N.: Bilateral carotid vertebrobasilar rete mirabile. Case report. J. Neurosurg. **33**, 581–586 (1970)

JULIAN, O.C., DYE, W.S., JAVID, H., HUNTER, J.A.: Ulcerative lesions of the carotid artery bifurcation. Arch. Surg. **86**, 808–809 (1963)

KANE, W.C., ARONSON, S.M.: Cardiac disorders predisposing to embolic stroke. Stroke 1, 164–172 (1970)

KANZOW, E., DIECKHOFF, D.: On the location of the vascular resistance in the cerebral circulation. In: Cerebral Blood Flow (Brock, M., Fieschi, C., Ingvar, D.H., Lassen, N.A., Schürmann, K., eds). Berlin-Heidelberg-New York: Springer 1969, pp. 96–97

KAUFMANN, H.H.: Fibromuscular hyperplasia of the carotid artery in a case associated with an arteriovenous malformation. Arch. Neurol. **22**, 299–304 (1970)

KIEFFER, ST.A., TAKEYA, Y., RESCH, J.A., AMPLATZ, K.: Racial differences in cerebrovascular disease. Angiographic evaluation of japanese and american populations. Amer. J. Roentgenol. **101**, 94–99 (1967)

KINCAID, O.W., DAVIS, G.D., HALLERMAN, F.J., HUNT, J.C.: Fibromuscular dysplasia of the renal arteries. Arteriographic features, calssification and observations in natural history of the disease. Amer. J. Roentgenol. **104**, 271–282 (1968)

KISHORE, P.R.S.: The significance of the ulcerative plaque. Radiol. Clin. N. Amer. **12**, 343–351 (1974)

KISHORE, P.R.S., CHASE, N.E., KRICHEFF, I.I.: Carotid stenosis and intracranial emboli. Radiology **100**, 351–356 (1971 b)

KISHORE, P.R.S., LIN, J.P., KRICHEFF, I.I.: Fibromuscular hyperplasia and stationary waves of the internal carotid artery. Acta radiol. Diagn. **11**, 619–625 (1971 a)

KLINGLER, M.: Zur Diagnose der Carotisthrombose; irreführende arteriographische Bilder. Acta neurochir. **2**, 197–209 (1952)

KOHLMEYER, K.: Rekanalisation intrakranieller Gefäßverschlüsse und vergleichende Messungen der regionalen Hirndurchblutung (r CBF). Radiologe **11**, 479–485 (1971)

KOWADA, M., YAMAGUCHI, K., TAKAKASHI, H.: Fenestration of the vertebral artery with a review of 23 cases in Japan. Radiology **103**, 343–346 (1972)

KRAMER, W.: Hyperplasie fibromusculaire et anévrysme extracrânien de la carotide interne et syndrome parapharyngien typique. Rev. Neurol. **120**, 239–244 (1969)

KRAYENBÜHL, H., RICHTER, H.H.: Die zerebrale Angiographie. Stuttgart: Thieme 1952

KRAYENBÜHL, H., WEBER, G.: Die Thrombose der A. carotis interna und ihre Beziehung zur Endangitis obliterans. Helv. med. Acta **11**, 289–333 (1944)

KRAYENBÜHL, H., YASARGIL, M.G.: Die vaskulären Erkrankungen im Gebiet der A. vertebralis und A. basilaris. Fortschr. Röntgenstr. Suppl. **80**, Stuttgart: Thieme 1957

KRAYENBÜHL, H., YASARGIL, M.G.: Die zerebrale Angiographie. 2. Aufl. Stuttgart: Thieme 1965

KRAYENBÜHL, H., YASARGIL, M.G.: Cerebral angiography. London: Butterworths 1968

KRAYENBÜHL, H., YASARGIL, M.G.: Die Angiographie der Thrombose der A. basilaris. Schweiz. med. Wschr. **91**, 1504–1507 (1961)

KRUEGER, T.P., ROCKOFF, D., THOMAS, L.J., OMMAYA, A.: The effect of changes of end expiratory carbon dioxide tension on the normal cerebral angiogramm. Amer. J. Roentgenol. **90**, 506–511 (1963)

KUDO, T.: Juvenile occlusion of the circle of Willis. Clin. Neurol. **5**, 607–627 (1965)

KUDO, T.: Spontaneous occlusion of the circle of Willis. Neurology **18**, 485–496 (1968)

KUNZE, ST., SCHIEFER, W.: Angiographic demonstration of a dissecting aneurysm of the middle cerebral artery. Neuroradiology **2**, 201–206 (1971)

KURTZKE, J.F.: Epidemiology of cerebrovascular disease. Berlin-Heidelberg-New York: Springer 1969

KURTZMAN, R.S.: Complication of narcotic addition. Radiology **96**, 23–30 (1970)

LAGARDE, C., VIGOUROUX, R., PERRONTY, P.: Angénésie terminale de la carotide interne et anévrisme de la communicante antérieure. Documents radiologiques. J. radiol. électr. **38**, 939–941 (1957)

LANCIEN, G.: Une anomalie vasculaire rare: l'hypoplasie bilatérale des carotide interne. A propos d'un cas. Academie thesis. Université de Rennes. 1971

LANGFITT, T.W., KASSEL, N.F.: Non-filling of cerebral vessels during angiography: correlation with intracranial pressure. Acta Neurochir. **14**, 96–104 (1966)

LANNER, L.O., ROSENGREN, H.: Angiographic diagnosis of intracerebral vascular occlusions. Acta radiol. Diagn. **2**, 129–137 (1964)

LARSON, S.J., LOVE, L., TIMMONS, C.: Segmental occlusion of the middle cerebral artery. Amer. J. Roentgenol. **94**, 223–229 (1965)

LASCELLES, R.G., BURROWS, E.H.: Occlusion of the middle cerebral artery. Brain **88**, Part I, 85–96 (1965)

LASSEN, N.A.: Cerebral blood flow and oxygen consumption in man. Physiol. Rev. **39**, 183–238 (1959)

LASSEN, N.A.: The luxury-perfusion syndrom and its possible relation to acute metabolic acidosis within the brain. Lancet **II/1966**, 1113–1115

LASSEN, N.A., PALVÖLGYI, R.: Cerebral steal during hypercapnia and the inverse reaction during hypnocapnia observed by the 133-Xenon technique in man. Scand. J. clin. Lab. Invest. Suppl. **102**, p. XIII-D (1968)

LASSEN, N.A., PAULSON, O.B.: Partial cerebral vasoparalysis in patients with apoplexy. In: Cerebral blood flow (M. Brock, C. Fieschi, D.H. Ingvar, N.A. Lassen, K. Schürmann, eds). Berlin-Heidelberg-New York: Springer 1969

LATCHAV, R.E., SEEGER, J.F., GABRIELSEN, T.O.: Vertebrobasilar arterial occlusions in children. Neuroradiology **8**, 141–147 (1974)

LEVAURS, G., BONNAL, J., HUGUET, J.F., SEDAN, R.: Les ischémies cérébrales d'origine congénital (à propos de 2 cas d'absence de carotide) Ann. Radiol. **6**, 81–85 (1963)

LAZORTHES, G., GOUAZE, A.: Les voies anastomotiques de suppléance (ou système de securité) de la vascularisation artérielle de l'axe cérébromédullaire. Nancy: Georges Thomas 1968

LEE, K.F., HODES, PH.J.: Intracranial ischemic lesions. Radiol. Clin. N. Amer. **5**, 363–393 (1967)

LEEDS, M.E., ABBOTT, K.H.: Collateral circulation in cerebro-vascular disease in childhood via rete mirabile and perforating branches of anterior choroidal and posterior cerebral arteries. Radiology **85**, 628–634 (1965)

LEEDS, N.E., GOLDBERG, H.I.: Angiographic manifestations in cerebral inflammatory disease. Radiology **98**, 595–604 (1971)

LEGRÉ, J., ATLAN, D., GIUDICELLI, G., LAVIEILLE, J., DUFOUR, M.: Aspects radiologiques de l'athérosclérose du tronc vertébro-basilaire. Ann. Radiol. **10**, 837–849 (1967)

LEHRER, H.: The angiographic triad in tuberculous meningitis. Radiology **87**, 829–835 (1966)

LEHRER, H.: The physiology of angiographic arterial waves. Radiology **89**, 11–19 (1967)

LEHRER, H., DE PALMA, N., FERRIS, E.: Cerebrovascular occlusive disease as a differential diagnosis in subdural hematomas. Radiology **88**, 85–89 (1967)

LEMAY, M., GOODING, C.A.: The clinical significance of the azygos anterior cerebral artery. Amer. J. Roentgenol. **98**, 602–610 (1966)

LEPOIRE, J., TRIDON, P., MONTANT, J., HEPNER, H., RENARD, M., PICARD, L.: Malformations angiomateuses artério-artérielles du système carotidien. Neuro-chirurgie **15**, 5–18 (1969)

LEVESQUE, M., BORIES, J., LEFEBVRE, J.: Moya-Moya. A propos de six observations. Ann. Radiol. **16**, 27–40 (1973)

LEVESQUE, M., LEFEBVRE, J., BORIES, J., LEGRE, J.: Les formes infantiles du syndrome de sténose progressive des branches du polygone de Willis. J. Neuroradiol. **1**, 55–68 (1974)

LHERMITTE, F., GUATIER, J.C., POIRIER, J., TYRER, J.: Hypoplasia of the internal carotid artery. Neurology **18**, 439–446 (1968)

LIE, T.A.: Congenital anomalies of the carotid arteries. An angiographic study and a review of the literatur. Excerpta med. Amst. (1968)

LIEBESKIND, A., COHEN, ST., ANDERSON, R., SCHECHTER, M.M., ZINGESSER, L.H.: Unusual segmental cerebrovascular changes. Radiology **106**, 119–122 (1973)

LIVINGSTON, K.E., ESCOBAR, A., NICHOLS, G.D.: Hemiplegia caused by cerebrovascular thrombosis. An arteriographic study. J. Neurosurg. **12**, 336–344 (1955)

LÖHR, W.: Erkrankungen der Hirngefäße in arteriographischer Darstellung. Arch. klin. Chir. **186**, 298–316 (1936)

LOVE, L., HILL, B.J., LARSON, S.J., RAIMONDI, A.J., LESCHER, A.J.: Cranial collateral pathways in stroke syndrome. Amer. J. Roentgenol. **98**, 637–646 (1966)

LÜBBERS, D.W.: Physiologie der Gehirndurchblutung. In: Der Hirnkreislauf (H. Gänshirt, Hrsg.), S. 214–260. Stuttgart: Thieme 1972

LUESSENHOP, A.J.: Occlusive disease of the carotid artery: observations on the prognosis and surgical treatment. J. Neurosurg. **16**, 705–730 (1959)

LUESSENHOP, A.J.: Artificial embolization for cerebral arteriovenous malformations. Progr. Neurol. Surg. **3**, 320–362 (1969)

LUNDBERG, N., CRONQVIST, S., KJÄLLQVIST, A.: Clinical investigations on interrelations between intracranial pressure and intracranial hemodynamics. In: Progress in Brain Research, Vol. 30, Cerebral Circulation (W. Luyendijk, ed). Amsterdam-London-New York: Elsevier Publishing Company 1968, pp. 69–75

LYONS, C.: Progress report of the joint study of extracranial arterial occlusion. In: Cerebral vascular diseases (C.H. Millikan, R.G. Siekert, J.P. Whisnant, eds). New York: Grune & Stratton 1965

LYONS, C., GALBRAITH, G.: Surgical treatment of atherosclerotic occlusion of the internal carotid artery. Ann. Surg. **146**, 487–498 (1957)

LYONS, E.L., LEEDS, N.E.: The angiographic demonstration of arterial vascular disease in purulent meningitis. Radiology **88**, 935–938 (1967)

MADDISON, F.E.: Arteriographic evaluation of carotid artery surgery. Amer. J. Roentgenol. **109**, 121–126 (1970)

MADDISON, F.E., MOORE, W.S.: Ulcerated atheroma of the carotid artery: arteriographic appearance. Amer. J. Roentgenol. **107**, 530–534 (1969)

MANELFE, C., CLARISSE, J., FREDY, D., ANDRE, J.M., CROUZET, G.: Dysplasie fibromusculaire des artère cervico-céphaliques. A propos de 70 cas. J. Neuroradiol. **1**, 149–321 (1974)

MARGOLIS, M.T., NEWTON, T.H.: Collateral pathways between the cavernous portion of the internal carotid and external carotid arteries. Radiology **93**, 834–836 (1969)

MARGOLIS, M.T., NEWTON, TH.H.: Methamphetamine arteritis. Neuroradiology **2**, 179–182 (1971)

MARKS, R.L., FREED, M.M.: Nonpenetrating injuries of the neck and cerebrovascular accident. Arch. Neurol. **28**, 410–414 (1973)

MASPES, P.E., MARINI, G.: Intracranial arterial spasm related to supraclinoid ruptured aneurysms. Acta neurochir. **10**, 630–638 (1962)

MCBRIEN, D.J., BRADLEY, R.D., ASHTON, N.: The nature of retinal emboli in stenosis of the internal carotid artery. Lancet **I/1963**, 697–699

MCCORMACK, L.J., HAZARD, J.B., POUTASSE, E.F.: Obstructive lesions of the renal artery associated with remediable hypertension. Amer. J. Roentgenol. **34**, 582 (1958)

MCCORMACK, L.J., NOTO, T.J., POUTASSE, E.F., DUSTAN, H.P.: A radiologic-pathologic correlation of occlusive renal arterial disease. Clin. Res. **12**, 363–369 (1964)

MCDOWELL, F., RENNIE, L., EJRUP, B.: Arterial bruit in cerebrovascular disease. In: Cerebro Vascular Disease. Transaction of the fifth Princeton conference (Millikan, C.H., Siekert, R.G., Whisnant, J.P., eds). New York: Grune & Stratton 1966, pp. 124–136

MCDOWELL, F.H., POTES, J., GROCH, S.: The natural history of internal carotid and vertebral-basilar artery occlusion. Neurology **11**, 153–157 (1961)

MCGEE, D.A., MCPHEDRAN, R.S., HOFFMANN, H.J.: Carotid and vertebral artery disease. Neurology **12**, 848–859 (1962)

MCHENRY, L.C., FAZEKAS, J.F., SULLIVAN, J.F.: Cerebral hemodynamics of Synocope. Amer. J. med. Sci. **80**, 173–178 (1961)

MEYER, J.S.: Changes in cerebral blood flow resulting from vascular occlusion. In: Pathogenesis and treatment of cerebrovascular disease (Fields, W.S., ed). Springfield, Ill.: Charles C. Thomas 1961, pp. 80–105

MEYER, J.S., GOTOH, F.: Interaction of cerebral hemodynamics and metabolism. Neurology **11**, 46–65 (1961)

MEYER, J.S., GOTOH, F., TAZAKI, Y., HAMAGUCHI, K., ISHIKAWA, S., NOUAIHAT, F., SYMON, L.: Regional cerebral blood flow and metabolism in vivo. Arch. Neurol. **7**, 560–581 (1962)

MEYER, J.S., HANDA, J., HUBER, P., YOSHIDA, K.: Effect of hypotension on internal and external carotid blood flow. J. Neurosurg. **23**, 191–198 (1965)

MEYER, J.S., SHEEHAN, S., BAUER, R.B.: An arteriographic study of cerebrovascular disease in man. I – Stenosis and occlusions of the vertebral-basilar arterial system. Arch. Neurol. **2**, 27–45 (1960)

MEYER, S.J., DENNY-BROWN, D.: The cerebral collateral circulation. Part I (Factors influencing collateral blood flow). Neurology **7**, 447–458 (1957)

MILLETTI, M.: Angiographic demonstration of an isolated thrombosis of the posterior cerebral artery. Acta Neurochir. **3**, 301 (1954)

MILLIKAN, C.H.: Editorial: Perplexities in cerebrovascular diesease. Ann. intern. Med. **58**, 191–192 (1963)

MILLIKAN, C.H.: The pathogenesis of transient focal cerebral ischemia. Circulation **32**, 438–450 (1965)

MINAGI, H., NEWTON, T.H.: Carotid rete mirabile in man. A case report. Radiology **86**, 100–102 (1966)

MITCHELL, O.CH., DE LA TORRE, E., ALEXANDER, E., DAVIS, C.H.: The nonfilling phenomenon during angiography in acute intracranial hypertension. J. Neurosurg. **19**, 766–774 (1962)

MIZUKAMI, M., TOMITA, T., MINE, T., MIHARA, H.: Bypass anomaly of the vertebral artery associated with cerebral aneurysm and arteriovenous malformation. J. Neurosurg. **37**, 204–209 (1972)

MOLINARI, G.F., SMITH, L., GOLDSTEIN, M.N., SATRAN, R.: Pathogenesis of cerebral mycotic aneurysms. Neurology **23**, 325–332 (1973)

MOMOSE, K.J., NEW, P.F.J.: Non-atheromatous stenosis and occlusion of the internal carotid artery and its main branches. Amer. J. Roentgenol. **118**, 550–566 (1973)

MONES, R.J., CHRISTOFF, N., BENDER, M.B.: Posterior cerebral artery occlusion. A clinical and angiographic study. Arch. Neurol. **5**, 68–76 (1961)

MONIZ, E., LIMA, A., DE LACERDA, R.: Hémiplégies par thrombose de la carotide interne. Presse méd. **45**, 977–980 (1937)

MOORE, W.S., HALL, A.D.: Ulcerated athreroma of the carotid artery. A cause of transient cerebral ischemia. Amer. J. Surg. **116**, 237–242 (1968)

MOOSSY, J.: Cerebral infarcts and complicated lesions of intracranial and extracranial atherosclerosis. In: Cerebral Vascular Diseases. Fourth Conference (Millikan, C.H., Siekert, R.G., Whisnant, J.P., eds). New York-London: Grune & Stratton 1965, p. 162–167

MORIYASU, N.: On five cases presenting malformation of the bilateral internal carotid arteries at the base of the brain. Brain Nerve (Tokyo) **17**, 777–778 (1965)

MOSCOW, N.P., NEWTON, T.H.: Angiographic implications in diagnosis and prognosis of basilar artery occlusion. Amer. J. Roentgenol. **119**, 597–604 (1973)

MOSELEY, I.F., SONDHEIMER, F.K.: Artefactual absence of the vertebral artery: a previously unrecorded phenomenon of axillary catheterisation. Neuroradiology **7**, 45–47 (1974)

MOUNT, L.A., TAVERAS, J.M.: Arteriographic demonstration of the collateral circulation of the cerebral hemispheres. Amer. med. Ass. Arch. Neurol. Psychiat. **78**, 235–353 (1957)

MÜLLER, R., GREITZ, T., LILIQVIST, B., HELLSTRÖM, L.: Aortocervical angiography in occlusion cerebrovascular disease. Neurology **2**, 136–146 (1964)

MUMENTHALER, M., HUBER, P., GRANDJEAN, PH.: Cerebrovasculäre Insulte bei jungen Frauen. Aetiologische Analyse. Pathogene Rolle von Ovulationshemmern? Z. Neurol. **198**, 46–64 (1970)

MUMENTHALER, M., WELLAUER, J., SCHAMAUN, M.: Apoplexie bei vollständigen Carotisverschlüssen. Klinik, Diagnostik und gefäßchirurgische Therapie. Helv. med. Acta **28**, 705–740, 808–830 (1961)

NEDWICH, A., HAFT, H., TELLEM, M., KAUFFMAN, L.: Dissecting aneurysms of cerebral arteries. Arch. Neurol. **9**, 477–484 (1963)

NEW, P.F.J.: Arterial stationary waves. Amer. J. Roentgenol. **97**, 488–499 (1966)

NEWTON, TH.H., WYLIE, E.J.: Collateral circulation associated with occlusion of the proximal subclavian and innominate arteries. Amer. J. Roentgenol. **91**, 394–405 (1964)

NEWTON, T.H., MANI, R.L.: The vertebral artery. In: Radiology of the skull and brain. Angiography Vol. 2, Book 2, Chapter 67 (Newton, T.H., Potts, D.G., eds). St. Louis: C.V. Mosby Comp. 1974, pp. 1659–1709

NEWTON, T.H., POTTS, D.G.: Radiology of the skull and brain. Angiography, Vol. 2, Book 4. St. Louis: C.V. Mosby Comp. 1974

NICOLA, G.: The rete mirabile in man. Vasc. Surg. 4, 156–160 (1970)

NISHIMOTO, A., SUGIN, R., MANNAMI, T.: Hemangiomatous malformation of bilateral internal carotid artery at the base of the brain. Brain Nerve (Tokyo) **17**, 750–756 (1965)

NISHIMOTO, A., SUGIN, R., TAKEUCHI, S.: Malformations of the circle of Willis presenting a peculiar cerebral angiographic picture. Cases encountered in Japan. Brain Nerve (Tokyo) **18**, 508–513 (1966)

NISHIMOTO, A., TAKEUCHI, S.: Abnormal cerebrovascular network related to the internal carotid arteries. J. Neurosurg. **29**, 255–260 (1968)

NISHIMOTO, A., TAKEUCHI, S.: Moyamoya disease. Abnormal cerebrovascular network in the cerebral basal region. Handbook of Clinical Neurology (Winken u. Bruyn, eds), Vol. 12. Amsterdam: North-Holland Publishing Co. 1972, pp. 352–383

NIZZOLI, V., SOLIME, F., REGGIANI, R., NICOLA, G.C.: Bilateral obstruction of the vertebral arteries. Europ. Neurol. **3**, 28–37 (1970)

NORMAN, R.M., ULRICH, H.: Dissecting aneurysm of the middle cerebral artery as a cause of acute infantile hemiplegia. J. Path. Bact. **73**, 580–583 (1957)

NORTH, R.R., FIELDS, W.S., DE BAKEY, M., CRAWFORD, E.ST.: Brachial-basilar insufficiency syndrome. Neurology **12**, 810–820 (1962)

NYLIN, G., HEDLUND, S., REGNSTRÖM, O.: Cerebral circulation studied with labelled red cells in healthy males. Acta radiol. **55**, 281–304 (1961)

OLESEN, J., PAULSON, O.B.: The effect of intra-arterial papverine on the regional cerebral blood flow in patients with stroke or intracranial tumor. Stroke **2**, 148–159 (1971)

PACH, J., DORNDORF, W., GÄNSHIRT, H.: Ophthalmodynamographie beim Carotisverschluß. Z. Neurol. **199**, 224–233 (1971)

PALUBINSKAS, A.J., NEWTON, T.H.: Fibromuscular hyperplasia of the internal carotid arteries. Radiol. clin. **34**, 365–370 (1965)

PALUBINSKAS, A.J., PERLOFF, D., NEWTON, TH.H.: Fibromuscular hyperplasia. An arterial dysplasia of increasing clinical importance. Amer. J. Roentgenol. **98**, 907–913 (1966)

PALUBINSKAS, A.J., RIPLEY, H.R.: Fibromuscular hyperplasia in extracranial arteries. Radiology **82**, 451–454 (1964)

PARKINSON, D.: Collateral circulation of cavernous carotid artery: anatomy. Canad. J. Surg. **7**, 251–268 (1964)

PATTERSON, J.L.: Circulation through the brain. In: Medical Physiology and Biophysics (T. Ruch, J.F. Fulton, eds. Philadelphia: Saunders 1960, p. 741

PAULSON, O.B.: Regional cerebral blood flow in apoplexy due to occlusion of the middle cerebral artery. Neurology (Minneap.) **20**, 63–77 (1970)

PAULSON, O.B.: Cerebral apoplexy (Stroke): Pathogenesis, pathophysiology and therapy as illustrated by regional blood flow measurements in the brain. Stroke **2**, 327–360 (1971)

PAULSON, O.B., LASSEN, N.A., SKINHOJ, E.: Regional cerebral blood flow in apoplexy without arterial occlusion. Neurology **20**, 125–138 (1970)

PAULSON, O.B., OLESEN, J., CHRISTENSEN, S.: Restoration of autoregulation of cerebral blood flow by hypocapnia. Neurology **22**, 286–293 (1972)

PECKER, J., SIMON, J., GUY, G., HERRY, J.F.: Nishimoto's disease: Significance of its angiographic appearances. Neuroradiology **5**, 223–230 (1973)

PETERSON, R.E., LIVINGSTON, K.E., ESCOBAR, A.: Development and distribution of gross atherosclerotic lesions at cervical carotid bifurcation. Neurology **10**, 955–959 (1960)

PICARD, L., ANDRÉ, J.M., ROLAND, J., ARNOULD, G., LEPOIRE, J., CROUZET, G., DJINDJIAN, R.: "Moyamoya" de l'adulte. Formes de passage. J. Neuroradiol. **1**, 69–86, (1974)

PICARD, L., ANDRÉ, J.M., TRIDON, P.: Introduction, Historique du syndrome "Moyamoya". J. Neuroradiol. **1**, 47–54 (1974)

PICARD, L., FLOQUET, J., ANDRÉ, J.M., MONTANT, J., SALAMON, G.: Syndrome Moyamoya. Étude anatomo-pathologique. J. Neuroradiol. **1**, 113–132 (1974)

PICKERING, G.W.: Transient cerebral paralysis in hypertension and in cerebral embolism. J. Amer. med. Ass. **137**, 423–430 (1948)

PITON, J., CAILLE, J.M., BROUSSIN, J.: Anastomoses carotido-carotidiennes chez l'homme. J. Radiol. Électrol. **52**, 447–450 (1971)

PITTS, F.W., Variations of collateral circulation in internal carotid occlusion. Comparison of clinical and X-ray findings Neurology **12**, 467–471 (1962)

POLLOCK, J.A., NEWTON, T.H.: The anterior falx artery; normal and pathologic anatomy Radiology **91**, 1089–1095 (1968)

POOL, J.L.: Cerebral Vasospasm. New Engl. J. Med. **259**, 1259–1264 (1958)

POOL, J.L., JACOBSON, S., FLETCHER, T.M.: Cerebral vasospasm. Clinical and experimental evidence. J. Amer. med. Ass. **167**, 1599–1601 (1958)

POSER, C.M., TAVERAS, J.M.: Cerebral angiography in encephalotrigeminal angiomatosis. Radiology **68**, 327–336 (1957)

PRENSKY, A.L., DAVIS, C.D.: Obstruction of major cerebral vessels in early childhood without neurological signs. Neurology **20**, 945–953 (1970)

PRIBRAM, H.F.W.: Angiographic appearances in acute intracranial hypertension. Neurology **11**, 10–21 (1961)

RABINOV, K.R.: Angiographic findings in a case of brain syphilis. Radiology **80**, 622–624 (1963)

RAIMONDI, A.J., MATSUMOTO, S., MILLER, R.A.: Brain abscess in children with congenital heart disease. J. Neurosurg. **23**, 588–595 (1965)

RAYNOR, R.B., ROSS, G.: Arteriography and vasospasm. J. Neurosurg. **17**, 1055–1061 (1960)

REIVICH, M., HOLLING, H.E., ROBERTS, B., TOOTE, J.F.: Reversal of blood flow through vertebral artery and its effect on cerebral circulation. New Engl. J. Med. **265**, 878–885 (1961)

RESCH, J.A., BAKER, A.B.: Etiologic mechanisms in cerebral atherosclerosis. Preliminary study of 3839 cases. Arch. Neurol. **10**, 617–628 (1964)

RICHTER, A.M., BANKER, V.P.: Carotid ergotism. A complication of migraine therapy. Radiology **106**, 339–340 (1973)

RIECHERT, T.: Die Arteriographie der Hirngefässe bei einseitigem Verschluß der Carotis interna. Nervenarzt **11**, 290–297 (1938)

RIGGS, H.E., RUPP, C.: Variation in form of circle of Willis. The relation of the variations to collateral circulation: anatomic analysis. Arch. Neurol. **8**, 8–14 (1963)

RIISHEDE, J.: Cerebral apoplexy. An arteriographical and clinical study of 100 cases. Acta psychiat. scand. **32** (Suppl.), 118 (1957)

RING, B.A.: Diagnosis of embolic occlusions of smaller branches of the intracerebral arteries. Amer. J. Roentgenol. **97**, 575–582 (1966)

RING, B.A.: The neglected cause of stroke: occlusion of the smaller intracranial arteries and their diagnosis by cerebral angiography. St. Louis: Warren H. Green, Inc. 1969

RIVOIR, R., HUBER, P.: Sequential subtraction. Neuroradiol. **8**, 85–90 (1974)

ROBERT, F.: Der Einfluß des Kontrastmittels auf den Kollateralkreislauf beim Verschluß der A. cerebri media. Radiol. clin. biol. **38**, 357–371 (1969)

ROBERT, F., MALTAIS, R., GIROUX, J.C.: Dissecting aneurysm or middle cerebral artery. J. Neurosurg. **21**, 413–415 (1964)

ROCKOFF, S.D., DOPPMAN, J., KRUEGER, D.P., THOMAS, T.J., OMMAYA, A.K.: Altered opacification of the external carotid circulation by changes of end expiratory carbon dioxide tension. Invest. Radiol. **1**, 123–128 (1966)

ROOS, W.: Die Periarteritis nodosa im Carotisangiogramm. Radiologe **9**, 3–5 (1969)

ROSEN, I.W., MILLS, D.F., NADEL, H.I., KAISERMAN, D.D.: Angiographic demonstration of congenital absence of both internal carotid arteries. Case report. J. Neurosurg. **42**, 478–482 (1975)

ROVIRA, M.: Angiographie dans les lésions athéromateuses nonobstructives des artéres cérébrales. Acta radiol. Diagn. **9**, 445–449 (1969)

RUMBAUGH, C.L., BERGERON, R.TH., FANG, H.C.H., MCCORMICK, R.: Cerebral angiographic changes in the drug abuse patient. Radiology **101**, 335–344 (1971 a)

RUMBAUGH, C.L., BERGERON, R.TH., SCANLAN, R.L., TEAL, J.S., SEGALL, H.D., FANG, H.C.H., MCCORMICK, R.: Cerebral vascular changes secondary to amphetamine abuse in the experimental animal. Radiology **101**, 345–351 (1971 b)

RUMBAUGH, C.L., DAVIS, D.O., GILSON, J.M.: Experimental cerebral emboli: angiographic evaluation of autologous emboli in the dog. Invest. Radiol. **3**, 330–336 (1968)

RUMBAUGH, C.L., DAVIS, D.O., GILSON, J.M.: Fate of experimental autologous emboli. Acta radiol. **9**, 450–454 (1969)

RUSSEL, R.W.R.: The origin and effects of cerebral emboli. In: Modern Trends in Neurology (Williams, D., ed). London: Butterworths 1970

RUTISHAUSER, W., SIMON, H., STUCKY, J.P., SCHAD, N., NOSEDA, G., WELLAUER, J.: Evaluation of roentgen cinedensitometry for flow measurement in models and in the intact circulation. Circulation **36**, 951–963 (1967)

RYTTMAN, A.: Influence of arterial ectasia and ventricular size on cerbral blood flow. Neuroradiology **4**, 185–189 (1972)

SALAMON, G., GONZALES, J., RAYBAUD, CH., GRISOLI, F., MICHOTEY, P.: Analyse angiographique des branches corticales de l'artère sylvienne. A propos d'un nouveau procédé de repérage. Neurochirurgie **17**, 177–189 (1971)

SALTZMAN, G.F.: Circulation through the anterior communicating artery studied by carotid angiography. Acta radiol. **52**, 194–208 (1959)

SALTZMAN, G.F.: Circulation through the posterior communicating artery in different tests. Acta radiol. Diagn. **1**, 298–313 (1963)

SANTSCHI, D.R., FRAHM, J.C., PASCALE, L.P.; DUMANIAN, A.V.: The subclavian steal syndrome. Clinical and angiographic considerations in 74 cases in adults. J. thorac. cardiovasc. Surg. **51**, 103–112 (1966)

SCHECHTER, M.M.: Percutaneous carotid catheterization. Acta radiol. Diagn. **1**, 417–426 (1963)

SCHECHTER, M.M.: The occipital-vertebral anastomosis. J. Neurosurg. **21**, 758–762 (1964)

SCHECHTER, M.M., ZINGESSER, L.H.: The radiology of basilar thrombosis. Radiology **85**, 23–32 (1965)

SCHECHTER, M.M., ZINGESSER, L.H.: The spinal arteries. Acta radiol. **5**, 1124–1131 (1966)

SCHOTT, B., BOURRAT, CH., TRILLET, M., GOUTELLE, A.: Pathologie artérielle du systéme vertébro-basilaire. Paris; Masson 1965

SCOTT, G.E., NEUBUERGER, K.T., DENST, J.: Dissecting aneurysms of intracranial arteries. Neurology **10**, 22–27 (1960)

SHAW, CH., ALVORD, E.C., BERRY, R.G.: Swelling of the brain following ischemic infarction with arterial occlusion. Brain **90**, 681–696 (1967)

SHEEHAN, S., BAUER, R.B., MEYER, J.S.: Vertebral artery compression in cervical spondylosis; arteriographic demonstration during life of vertebral artery insufficiency due to rotation and extension of the neck. Neurology **10**, 968–986 (1960)

SHENKIN, H.A., HAFT, H., SOMACH, F.M.: Prognostic significance of arteriography in nonhemorrhagic strokes. J. Amer. med. Ass. **194**, 612–616 (1965)

SHILLITO, J.: Carotid arteritis: a cause of hemiplegia in childhood. J. Neurosurg. **21**, 540–551 (1964)

SILVERSTEIN, A.: Cerebrovascular accidents as the initial major manifestation of lupus erythematosus. N.Y. J. Med. **63**, 2942–2948 (1963)

SIMON, J., GIUDICELLI, G., SIGNARGOUT, J.: Diagnostic différentiel du syndrome Moyamoya. J. Neuroradiol. **1**, 102–112 (1974)

SINDERMANN, F.: Krankenbild und Kollateralkreislauf bei einseitigem und doppelseitigem Carotisverschluß. J. neurol. Sci. **5**, 9–25 (1967)

SINDERMANN, F., BRUEGEL, R., GIEDKE, H.: Spontaneous recanalisation of internal carotid artery occlusions. Neuroradiology **7**, 53–56 (1974)

SINDERMANN, F., DICHGANS, J., BERGLEITER, R.: Occlusion of the middle cerebral artery and its branches: Angiographic and clinical correlates. Brain **92**, 607–620 (1969)

SINDERMANN, F., GIEDKE, H., KRIEBEL, J.: Bidirectional flow of contrast material in middle cerebral artery branches. Neuroradiology **8**, 113–117 (1974)

SMITH, K.R., NELSON, J.S., DOOLEY, J.M.: Bilateral "hypoplasia" of the internal carotid arteries. Neurology **18**, 1149–1156 (1968)

SOBEL, J., ESPINAS, O.E., FRIEDMAN, S.A.: Carotid artery obstruction following LSD capsule ingestion. Arch. intern. Med. **127**, 290–291 (1971)

SOKOLOFF, L.: Action of drugs on the cerebral circulation. Pharmacol. Rev. **11**, 1–85 (1959)

SOLOMON, G.E., HILAL, S.K., GOLD, A.P., CARTER, S.: Natural history of acute hemoplegia of childhood. Brain **93**, 107–120 (1970)

SOLOWAY, H., ARONSON, S.: Atheromatous emboli to central nervous system. Neurology **11**, 657–668 (1964)

SONNTAG, V.K.H., STEIN, B.M.: Arteriographic complications during treatment of subarachnoid hemorrhage with epsilon-amino-caproic acid. J. Neurosurg. **40**, 480–485 (1974)

SPUDIS, E.V., SCHARYJ, M., ALEXANDER, E., MARTIN, J.F.: Dissecting aneurysms in the neck and head. Neurology **12**, 867–875 (1962)

STEHBENS, W.E.: Pathology of the cerebral blood vessels. 1. Bd. St. Louis: Mosby 1972

STEIMLE, R., ROYER, S., ACHARD, M., SEINT-HILLIER, Y.: Agénésie de la carotide interne. Neuro-chirurgie **15**, 147–152 (1969)

STAIN, B.M., MCCORMICK, W.F., RODRIGUEZ, J.N., TAVERAS, J.M.: Radiography of atheromatous disease involving the extracranial arteries as seen at postmortem. Acta radiol. **1**, 455–467 (1963)

STEINBERG, I., HALPERN, M.: Roentgen manifestations of the subclavian steal syndrom. Amer. J. Roentgenol. **90**, 528–531 (1963)

STEPHENS, R.B., STILWELL, D.L.: Arteries and veins of the human brain. Charles C. Springfield, Ill.: Thomas 1969

STOANE, L., ALLEN, J.H., COLLINS, H.A.: Radiologic observations in cerebral embolization from left heart myxomas. Radiology **87**, 262–266 (1966)

STOCKMAN, J.A., NIGRO, M.A., MISHKIN, M.M., OSKI, F.A.: Occlusion of large cerebral vessels in sickle-cell anemia. New Engl. J. Med. **287**, 846–849 (1972)

STURGILL, B.C., NETSKY, M.G.: Cerebral infarction by atheromatous emboli. Amer. med. Ass. Arch. Path. **76**, 189–196 (1963)

SUCHENWIRTH, R.: Hirntumorsyndrom bei luischer Arterititis. Dtsch. Z. Nervenheilk. **190**, 338–348 (1967)

SUKOFF, M.H., DORSEY, T.J., JOHNSON, D.A., HEPPS, S.A., BERGGREN, R.L.: Intimal fibroplasia of the internal carotid arteries. Stroke **2**, 483–486 (1971)

SULLIVAN, H.G., VINES, F.S., BECKER, D.P.: Sequelae of indirect internal carotid injury. Radiology **109**, 91–98 (1973)

SUTTON, D., DAVIES, E.R.: Arch aortography and cerebrovascular insufficiency. Clin. Radiol. **17**, 330–345 (1966)

SUZUKI, J., TAKAKU, A., ASAHI, M.: Study of disease presenting fibrille – like vessels at the base of brain. (frequently found in the Japanese). Brain Nerve (Tokyo) **17**, 767–776 (1965)

SUZUKI, J., TAKAKU, A., ASAHI, M.: The disease showing the abnormal vascular network at the base of brain, particularly found in Japan. A following-up study. Brain Nerve (Tokyo) **18**, 897–908 (1966)

SUZUKI, J., TAKAKU, A.: Cerebrovascular "Moyamoya" disease. Disease showing abnormal net-like vessels in base of brain. Arch. Neurol. **20**, 288–299 (1969)

SYMON, L.: Experimental evidence for "intracerebral steal". Following CO_2 – inhalation. Scand. J. clin. Lab. Invest. **22** (Suppl. 102), XIII-A (1968)

SYMON, L., ISHIKAWA, S., MEYER, J.S.: Cerebral arterial pressure changes and development of leptomeningeal collateral circulation. Neurology (Minneap.) **13**, 237–250 (1963)

SYPERT, G.W., YOUNG, H.F.: Ruptured mycotic pericallosal aneurysm with meningitis due to Neisseria meningitidis infection. J. Neurosurg. **37**, 467–469 (1972)

SZDZUY, D., LEHMANN, R.: Hypoplastic distal part of the basilar artery. Neuroradiology **4**, 118–120 (1972)

SZDZUY, D., LEHMANN, R., NICKEL, B.: Common trunk of the anterior cerebral arteries. Neuroradiology **4**, 51–56 (1972)

TAKAHASHI, M., TAMAKAWA, Y., KISHIKAWA, T., KOWADA, M.: Fenestration of the basilar artery. Radiology **109**, 79–82 (1973)

TAKEUCHI, K., KOBAYASHI, S.: Arterial occlusion at the base of brain in children. Brain Nerve (Tokyo) **17**, 779–780 (1965)

TATELMAN, M.: The angiographic evaluation of cerebral atherosclerosis. Radiology **70**, 801–810 (1958)

TATELMAN, M.: Pathways of cerebral collateral circulation. Radiology **75**, 349–362 (1960)

TATLOW, W.F.T., BAMMER, H.G.: Syndrome of vertebral artery compression. Neurology **7**, 331–340 (1957)

TAVERAS, J.M.: Multiple progressive intracranial arterial occlusion: a syndrom of children and young adults (Caldwell lecture 1968). Amer. J. Roentgenol. **106**, 235–268 (1969)

TAVERAS, J.M., GILSON, J.M., DAVIS, D.O., KILGORE, B., RUMBAUGH, C.L.: Angiography in cerebral infarction. Radiology **93**, 549–558 (1969)

TAVERAS, J.M., POSER, C.M.: Roentgenologic aspects of cerebral angiography in children. Amer. J. Roentgenol. **82**, 371–391 (1959)

TAVERAS, J.M., WOOD, E.H.: Diagnostic neuroradiology. Baltimore: Williams & Wilkins Company 1964

TEAL, J.S., RUMBAUGH, C.L., BERGERON, R.TH., SEGALL, H.D.: Angiographic demonstration of fenestrations of the intradural intracranial arteries. Radiology **106**, 123–126 (1973)

THEANDER, G.: Arteriographic demonstration of stationary arterial waves. Acta radiol. Diagn. **53**, 417–425 (1960)

THOMAS, L.M., HARDY, W.A., LINDNER, D.W., GURDJIAN, E.S.: Retrograde brachial angiography in cerebro-vascular disease. Arch. Neurol. **7**, 339–346 (1962)

TÖNNIS, W., SCHIEFER, W.: Zirkulationsstörungen des Gehirns im Serienangiogramm. Berlin-Göttingen-Heidelberg: Springer 1959

TORVIK, A., JÖRGENSEN, L.: Thrombotic and embolic occlusions of the carotid arteries in an autopsy series. Part 2: cerebral lesions and clinical course. J. neurol. Sci. **3**, 410–432 (1966)

TORVIK, A., JÖRGENSEN, L.: Thrombotic and embolic occlusions of the carotid arteries in an autopsy material. Part I. Prevalence, location and associated diseases. J. neurol. Sci. **I**, 24–39 (1964)

TREVOR, R.P., SONDHEIMER, F.K., FESSEL, W.J., WOLPERT, S.M.: Angiographic demonstration of major cerebral vessel occlusion in systemic lupus erythematosus. Neuroradiology **4**, 202–207 (1972)

TROUPP, H., HEISKANEN, O.: Cerebral angiography in cases of extremely high intracranial pressure. Acta neurol. scand. **30**, 213–223 (1963)

TURNBULL, I.: Agenesis of the internal carotid artery. Neurology **12**, 588–590 (1962)

ULE, G., KOLKMANN, F.W.: Pathologische Anatomie. S. 47–160 In: Der Hirnkreislauf. Physiologie, Pathologie, Klinik. (H. Gänshirt, Hrsg.). Stuttgart: Thieme 1972

VAN DEN BERGH, R., VANDER EECKEN, H.: Anatomy and embryology of cerebral circulation. Progr. Brain Res. **30**, 1–25 (1968)

VAN DER DRIFT, J.H.A., KOK, N.K.D.: "Intracerebral Steal" in cerebrovascular occlusion, vascular malformation, and brain tumor: clinical EEG, angiographic, and circulatory findings. In: IV. International Salzburg Conference (J.S. Meyer, H. Lechner, M. Reivich, O. Eichhorn, eds). Springfield, see.: Charles C. Thomas 1970

VANDER EECKEN, H., ADAMS, R.D.: The anatomy and funcional significance of the meningeal arterial anastomoses of the human brain. J. Neuropath. exp. Neurol. **12**, 132–157 (1953)

VANDER EECKEN, H.H.: The anastomoses between the leptomeningeal arteries of the brain. Springfield, Ill.: Charles C. Thomas 1959

VOLLMAR, J., EL BAYAR, M., KOLMAR, D., PFLEIDERER, TH., DIETZEL, P.B.: Zerebrale Durchblutungsinsuffizienz bei Verschlußprozessen der A. Subclavia. (Subclavian steal effect) Dtsch. med. Wschr. **90**, 8–14 (1965)

WADDINGTON, M.M., RING, B.A.: Syndromes of occlusions of middle cerebral artery branches. Angiographic and clinical correlation. Brain, **91**, 685–696 (1968)

WADIA, N.H., SINGKAL, B.S.: Vascular changes in tuberculous meningitis. An arteriographic study in 33 patients. Proc. Aust. Ass. Neurol. **5**, 623–629 (1968)

WALLACE, S., GOLDBERG, H., LEEDS, N.E., NISHKIN, M.M.: The cavernous branches of the internal carotid artery. Amer. J. Roentgenol. **101**, 34–46 (1967)

WALTER, W. SCHÜTTE, W.: Über die Gefäßspasmen bei frisch rupturierten sackförmigen Aneurysmen der Hirnarterien. Acta Neurochirg. **11**, 631–652 (1964)

WALTZ, A.G., SUNDT, TH.M.: The microvascular and microcirculation of the cerebral cortex after arterial occlusion. Brain **90**, 681–696 (1967)

WALTZ, A.G., SUNDT, TH.M.: Influence of systemic blood pressure on blood flow and microcirculation of ischemic cerebral cortex: a failure of autoregulation. In: "Cerebral Circulation", Progress in Brain Research, Vol. 30 (W. Luyendijk, ed). Amsterdam-London-New York: Elsevier 1969, pp. 107–112

WEBSTER, J.E., GURDJIAN, E.S., LINDNER, D.W., HARDY, W.G.: Proximal occlusion of the anterior cerebral artery. Amer. med. Ass. Arch. Neurol. **2**, 19–26 (1960)

WEBSTER, J.E., GURDJIAN, E.S., MARTIN, F.A.: Carotid artery occlusion. Neurology **6**, 491–502 (1956)

WEIBEL, J., FIELDS, W.S.: Tortuosity, coiling, and kinking of the internal carotid artery. I. Etiology and radiographic anatomy. Neurology (Minneap.) **15**, 7–18 (1965)

WEIBEL, J., FIELDS, W.S.: Atlas of arteriography in occlusive cerebrovascular disease. Stuttgart: Thieme 1969

WEIDNER, W., CRANDALL, P., HANAFEE, W., TOMIYASU, U.: Collateral circulation in the posterior fossa via leptomeningeal anastomoses. Amer. J. Roentgenol. **95**, 831–836 (1965a)

WEIDNER, W., HANAFEE, W., MARKHAM, CH.H.: Intracranial collateral circulation via leptomeningeal and rete mirabile anastomoses. Neurology (Minneap.) **15**, 39–48 (1965b)

WEISS, S.R., RASKIND, R., MORGENSTERN, N.L., PYTLYK, P.J., BAIZ, T.C.: Intracerebral and subarachnoid hemorrhage following use of methamphetamine ("speed"). Int. Surg. **53**, 123–127 (1970)

WELCH, K., CRAIGMILE, T.K.: Kinking of the internal carotid artery over the optic nerve and chiasm in acute intracranial mass lesions. Acta radiol. Diagn. **1**, 509–512 (1963)

WENDE, S., SCHINDLER, K.: Technique and use of X-ray magnification in cerebral arteriography. Neuroradiology **1**, 117–120 (1970)

WENDE, S., ZIELER, E., NAKAYAMA, N.: Cerebral magnification angiography. Berlin-Heidelberg-New York: Springer 1974

WESENBERG, R.L., GWINN, J.L., BARNES, G.R.: Radiological findings in the kinky-hair syndrome. Radiology **92**, 500–506 (1969)

WESTBERG, G.: Arteries of the basal ganglia Acta radiol. **5**, 581–596 (1966)

WHITE, E., GREITZ, T.: Subependymal venous filling sequence at cerebral angiography. Influence of grey and whit matter distribution. Acta radiol. Diagn. **13**, 272–285 (1972)

WICKBOM, I., BARTLEY, O.: Arterial "spasm" in peripheral angiography using the catheter method. Acta radiol. **47**, 433–448 (1957)

WICKBOM, G.I., DAVIDSON, A.J.: Angiographic findings in intracranial actinomycosis. Radiology **88**, 536–537 (1967)

WIGGLI, U., OBERSON, R.: Wert und Resultate von Zielaufnahmen der Karotisbifurkation bei Patienten mit transitorischen ischämischen Attacken. Schweiz. med. Wschr. **103**, 1282–1288 (1973)

WILKINSON, I.M.S., RUSSEL, R.W.R.: Arteries of the head and neck in giant cell arteritis. Arch. Neurol. **27**, 378–391 (1972)

WILLIAMS, A.O.: Atherosclerosis of cerebral arteries in African and American negroes and American caucasians. 5. Salzburg conference on cerebral blood flow. Salzburg 1970

WILLIAMS, A.O., LOEWENSON, R., LIPPERT, D.M., RESCH, J.A.: Cerebral atherosclerosis and its relationship to selected diseases in Nigerians: a pathological study. Stroke **6**, 395–401 (1975)

WILLIAMS, A.O., RESCH, J.A., LOEWENSON, R.B.: Cerebral atherosclerosis – a comparative autopsy study between Nigerian negroes and American negroes and Caucasians. Neurology **19**, 205–210 (1969)

WILLIAMS, A.O., RESCH, J.A., LOEWENSON, R.B.: Atherosclerosis of cerebral arteries in African and American negroes and Caucasians. In: Research on the cerebral Circulation. Fifth international Salzburg conference (Meyer, J.S., Reivich, M., Lechner, H., eds). Springfield, Ill.: Charles C. Thomas 1972, pp. 61–70

WISE, G.R., FARMER, T.W.: Bacterial cerebral vasculitis. Neurology **21**, 195–200 (1971)

WISOFF, H.S., ROTHBALLER, A.B.: Cerebral arteriel thrombosis in children. Arch. Neurol. **4**, 258–267 (1961)

WOLLSCHLAEGER, G., WOLLSCHLAEGER, P.B.: Arterial anastomoses of the human brain. Acta radiol. **5**, 604–614 (1966)

WOLLSCHLAEGER, G., WOLLSCHLAEGER, P.B.: The Circle of Willis. In Radiology of the skull and brain. Angiography Vol. 2, Book 2, Chapter 58 (Newton, T.H., Potts, D.G., eds). St. Louis: C.V. MOSBY Comp. 1974, pp. 1171–1201

WOLLSCHLAEGER, P.B., WOLLSCHLAEGER, G., LOPEZ, V.F., METHEWS, C.L., HOLLY, J.J., BLACK, S.P.W.: The reflux from internal carotid artery to posterior circulation: Variation of anatomy versus pathology. Neuroradiology **2**, 65–75 (1971)

WOLMAN, L.: Cerebral dissecting aneurysms. Brain **82**, 276–291 (1959)

WOOD, E.H.: Angiographic identification of the ruptured lesion in patients with multiple cerebral aneurysms. J. Neurosurg. **21**, 182–198 (1964)

WOOD, E.H., CORREL, J.W.: Atheromatosous ulceration in major neck vessels as a cause of cerebral embolism. Acta radiol. **9**, 520–536 (1969)

WOODS, B.T., STREWLER, G.J.: Hemiparesis occuring six hours after intravenous heroin injection. Neurology **22**, 863–870 (1972)

WORINGER, E., BAUMGARTNER, J., BRAUN, J.P.: Le signe de l'opacification veineuse loco-régionale précoce au cours de la sério-angiographie rapide carotidienne. Acta radiol. **50**, 125–131 (1958)

WORINGER, E., LANGS, A., BRAUN, J.B., BAUMGARTNER, J.: Étude sérioangiographique de la dynamique circulatoire du cerveau. Acta radiol. **46**, 357–363 (1956)

WYKE, B.: Brain function and metabolic disorders. London: Butterworhs 1963

WYLIE, E.J., EHRENFELD, W.K.: Extracranial occlusive cerebrovascular disease: diagnosis and management. Philadelphia: W.B. Saunders & Co., 1970

YAMAMOTO, T., KAGAMI, T., TAMEGIWA, A., KAWANDA, Y.: Physiologic aspects of vascular network at brain base of newborn and its correlation with cerebral juxta-basal teleangiectasia. Nippon Acta Neuroradiol. **7**, 12–15 (1966)

YATES, P.O., HUTCHINSON, E.C.: Cerebral infarction: The role of stenosis of the extracranial cerebral arteries. Medical Research Report Nr. 300, Her majesty's stationary office, London 1961

ZATZ, L.M., IANNONE, A.M.: Cerebral emboli complicating cerebral angiography. Acta radiol. Diagn. **5**, 621–630 (1966)

ZIEGLER, D.K., ZILELI, T., DICK, A., SEBAUGH, J.L.: Correlation of bruits over the carotid artery with angiographically demonstrates lesions. Neurology **21**, 860–865 (1971)

ZINGESSER, L.H., SCHECHTER, M.M., DEXTER, J., KATZMAN, R., SCHEINBERG, L.C.: Relationship between cerebral angiographic circulation time and regional cerebral blood flow. Invest. Radiol. **3**, 86–91 (1968)

ZÜLCH, K.J.: Die Pathogenese von Massenblutungen und Erweichungen unter besonderer Berücksichtigung klinischer Gesichtspunkte. Acta neurochir. Suppl. **7**, 51–117 (1961)

ZÜLCH, K.J.: Allgemeine Prinzipien bei der Entstehung der Kollateralkreisläufe der Hirnarterien. Radiologe **9**, 396–406 (1969)

ZÜLCH, K.J., DREESBACH, H.A., ESCHBACH, O.: Occlusion of the middle cerebral artery with the formation of an abnormal arterial collateral system – Moyamoya type – 23 months later. Neuroradiology **7**, 19–24 (1974)

ZÜLCH, K.J., ESCHBACH, O.: The interhemispheric steal syndromes. Neuroradiology **4**, 179–184 (1972)

ZÜLCH, K.J., KLEIHUES, P., GABE, D.: Die aktuelle Problematik auf dem Gebiet der Pathogenese, Klinik und Therapie der Hirndurchblutungsstörungen. In: Der Hirnkreislauf in Forschung und Klinik, Kongreßband des II. Internat. Salzburger Symposiums 1964. Wien: Hallinek 1964

Ein Teil der Abbildungen ist mit Erlaubnis des Georg Thieme Verlages Stuttgart aus der „Zerebralen Angiographie für Klinik und Praxis“, KRAYENBÜHL/YASARGIL, 3. vollständig neubearbeitete Auflage von P. HUBER, Thieme Stuttgart 1979, übernommen worden. Die Übernahme der jeweils in der Legende bezeichneten Abbildungen ist dadurch bedingt, daß seit der Einführung der Computertomographie deutlich weniger Patienten mit zerebralen Infarkten angiographisch abgeklärt werden. Deshalb stehen innerhalb eines beschränkten Zeitraumes einer einzelnen neuroradiologischen Abteilung auch weniger für eine Wiedergabe geeignete seltenere Befunde zur Verfügung.

P. HUBER

Namenverzeichnis – Author Index

Die *kursiv* gesetzten Zahlen beziehen sich auf Literatur
Page numbers in *italics* refer to the references

Sachverzeichnis

(Deutsch – Englisch)

Bei gleicher Schreibweise in beiden Sprachen sind die Stichwörter nur einmal aufgeführt

Subject Index

(English – German)

Where English and German spelling of a word is identical, the German version is omitted